REPRODUCTIVE TECHNOLOGIES
AND THE LAW

REPRODUCTIVE TECHNOLOGIES AND THE LAW

Second Edition

Judith Daar
Associate Dean for Academic Affairs and Professor of Law
Whittier Law School

Clinical Professor of Medicine
University of California Irvine School of Medicine

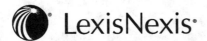 LexisNexis®

ISBN: 978-0-7698-4603-3
Looseleaf ISBN: 978-0-7698-4604-0
E-Book ISBN: 978-0-3271-7935-1

Library of Congress Cataloging-in-Publication Data

Daar, Judith.
Reproductive technologies and the law / Judith Daar. -- 2nd ed.
    p. cm.
Includes index.
ISBN: 978-0-7698-4603-3
1. Human reproductive technology--Law and legislation--United States. 2. Human reproductive technology--Law and legislation. I. Title.
KF3830.D33 2012
346.7301'7--dc23

2012035848

This publication is designed to provide authoritative information in regard to the subject matter covered. It is sold with the understanding that the publisher is not engaged in rendering legal, accounting, or other professional services. If legal advice or other expert assistance is required, the services of a competent professional should be sought.

LexisNexis and the Knowledge Burst logo are registered trademarks of Reed Elsevier Properties Inc., used under license. Moore's Federal Practice is a registered trademark of Matthew Bender & Company, Inc. Matthew Bender and the Matthew Bender Flame Design are registered trademarks of Matthew Bender Properties Inc.

> **NOTE TO USERS**
>
> To ensure that you are using the latest materials available in this area, please be sure to periodically check the LexisNexis Law School web site for downloadable updates and supplements at www.lexisnexis.com/lawschool.

Editorial Offices
121 Chanlon Rd., New Providence, NJ 07974 (908) 464-6800
201 Mission St., San Francisco, CA 94105-1831 (415) 908-3200
www.lexisnexis.com

MATTHEW◆BENDER

Dedication

For Eric and our beloved sons,

Evan, Jared, Adam and Ryan

Preface to the Second Edition

Tracking a field that is in constant motion poses unique challenges and opportunities. In the six years since the first edition of this book appeared, the field of assisted reproductive technologies (ART) has, at the same time, advanced, matured, stabilized and stalled. Each of these trajectories is explored alongside the particular area to which they attach. This new edition invites readers to plumb the origins of the world of assisted conception and then trace its development to the present day. Now that the world has welcomed more than 5 million children born via ART, and nearly 3 out of every 100 babies born in the United States are the product of assisted conception, the impact and import of the field cannot be overstated.

While the book contains an array of new cases, statutes, policies and commentaries, the fundamentals remain largely unchanged. ART continues to develop as an interdisciplinary field in which physicians and scientists work to create and improve techniques for family formation, and more recently medical therapy, while lawyers and lawmakers strive to understand and organize society's response to each new development. As more ART laws pepper the legal landscape, and demand for the technologies grow, so too will the need for informed practitioners who can represent the interests and needs of each stakeholder in the complicated equation. This book is designed to pique interest in ART as an academic discipline, as well as a robust and satisfying practice option.

This new edition is the work product of many generous students, colleagues, assistants and readers who have contributed their insights and efforts to help produce a book that is worthy of today's ART enthusiast. First, I want to thank the countless students who have pondered the book's material and reached out to share their thoughts and comments, many of which are incorporated throughout the pages that follow. Next, enormous credit and gratitude go to my tireless research assistants who have exhibited nothing but good cheer is responding to myriad requests over several years. My sincere thanks to Gerrick Warrington, Megan Emmer, Michael Ruttle and Nelly Ispiryan, all RAs extraordinaire. Finally, our institution is enormously benefitted by the services of an outstanding staff, including two members who worked with me throughout the writing process. Special thanks to Jennifer Maniscalco for her consistently superb administrative assistance and Rosalie Robles for her keen editing eye. Above all, any modicum of success this book or its author enjoys is made possible by the loving support of my husband Eric and our four sons. You are the light in my life.

Judith Daar

May 2012

Preface

The world of assisted reproductive technologies is a relative newcomer to the law school curriculum, making its perceptible entrance only within the past two decades or so. Yet the discipline mixing law and assisted conception seems to have established firm roots, sustained by a nearly daily dose of activity somewhere around the globe. The study of reproductive technologies has branched out from its founding in the late 1970s with the introduction of in vitro fertilization, to a field that includes such emerging topics as posthumous reproduction, embryonic stem cell research and human cloning. These topics often take center stage in our political and social world, making them ideal for dissection in the law school classroom.

This casebook is designed to introduce our students to the essentials in science, medicine, law and ethics that underpin and shape each of the topics that combine to form the law of reproductive technologies. As each new technology is introduced, an effort is made to fully inform the reader about the clinical application of the technique — that is, how the procedure is used to treat patients facing infertility or produce advances in medical research. Once comfortable with the science, students can then contemplate the legal parameters that do or should accompany the technology. Since so much of the law in this area is either nascent or wholly unformed, students are free, and indeed encouraged, to design legal systems that meet the needs of patients, parents, children and society at large — participants all in the world of assisted reproduction.

A cautionary note about the intensity of feelings that often attaches to discussions about the essential core of this book. At the heart of reproductive technologies beats the debate over the moral status of the early human embryo, and no book could do justice to the topic without fully exposing the depth and complexity of that debate. Early on, and continuing throughout the book, students are asked to contemplate, and even reveal, their views on the status of early human life so as to shape the various lenses through which the class will see the panoply of issues that implicate embryonic development. In my experience, this classroom discussion has been among the richest, often displaying a wide range of views yet always breeding respect for difference and the rights of expression that follow.

Writing this book has been nothing short of glorious. The mysterious world of a law professor is filled with many joys, from watching students blossom in the classroom to advancing one's own fund of knowledge through dialogue with gifted colleagues. For my already ideal academic world, the experience of preparing this casebook added an exquisite dimension that served to buoy my enthusiasm for this subject and for the art of writing in general. Though writing is a solitary sport, its very existence rests in the good graces of the many who patiently support the writer in her pursuit of the perfect turn of phrase. For me, those supporters were many and my gratitude is deep.

I want to first thank my dear friend Stacy Herman who assured me that she did indeed want to read the entire manuscript as each page slowly emerged from the printer. In her precious spare time, she diligently read every word, editing and making suggestions that undoubtedly added to the overall quality of the work. In life, such friends are rare and to be zealously cherished. Equal thanks are due Rosalie Robles, my law school assistant, who aided throughout the writing process, showing particular strength in helping secure

Preface

permission to include works from the many folks whose writing I have relied upon to present a comprehensive view of the field.

Finally, and most importantly, I am profoundly grateful to my husband Eric, whose unconditional love and abiding support has been the pillar of my existence for nearly a quarter century. Together we have been blessed with the privilege of reproduction four times over, and with the birth of each son I gained a further appreciation for the quest of parenthood that, when elusive, can shake one to the core. I hope this book helps and inspires our students to probe deeply into that quest, whether for academic or personal satisfaction.

Judith Daar

May 2005

Table of Contents

Preface

Acknowledgments

Chapter 1   **HUMAN REPRODUCTION: NATURAL AND ASSISTED METHODS OF CONCEPTION** **1**

SECTION I: THE WONDERS OF HUMAN REPRODUCTION 1
- A.   Natural Conception 2
  - Lawrence J. Kaplan & Carolyn M. Kaplan, *Natural Reproduction and Reproduction-Aiding Technologies* 2
  - Notes and Questions 6
- B.   Infertility: When Natural Conception Does Not Occur 9
  - 1.   Defining the Causes of Infertility 11
    - The New York State Task Force on Life and the Law, *Assisted Reproductive Technologies: Analysis and Recommendations for Public Policy* 11
  - 2.   Defining the Incidence of Infertility 12
    - Notes and Questions 13

SECTION II: JUDICIAL PERSPECTIVES ON THE MODERN ROLE OF REPRODUCTION 18
- A.   An Introductory Case 18
  - *Bragdon v. Abbott* 18
  - Notes and Questions 23

SECTION III: ASSISTED CONCEPTION 26
- A.   A Brief History of ART 26
  - 1.   The Earliest Years 26
  - 2.   Human Artificial Insemination 27
    - *Gursky v. Gursky* 29
    - Notes and Questions 33
- B.   Conception in the Laboratory — In Vitro Fertilization 35
  - 1.   Investigating the Possibility of Conception Outside the Body 35
  - 2.   Advances in IVF and the Future of ART 36
  - 3.   A Glossary of ART Terms 38
- C.   Successes and Failures in ART Medicine 40
  - 1.   Is ART Effective? 40
    - Notes and Questions 43
  - 2.   Is ART Safe for Children and Adults? 45
    - a.   Safety to Children 45

TABLE OF CONTENTS

Manon Ceelen, Mirjam M. Van Weissenbruch, Jan P.W. Vermeiden, Flora E. Van Leeuwen, and Henriette A. Delemarre-van de Wall, *Growth and Development of Children Born After In Vitro Fertilization* 45

George Kovalevsky, Paolo Rinaudo, and Christos Coutifaris, *Do Assisted Reproductive Technologies Cause Adverse Fetal Outcomes?* 48

Notes and Questions 49

b.   Safety to Adults 53

Edward G. Hughes and Mita Giacomini, *Funding In Vitro Fertilization Treatment for Persistent Subfertility: The Pain and the Politics* 53

Notes and Questions 54

SECTION IV: WHAT IS THE NATURE AND STATUS OF THE HUMAN EMBRYO? 56

A.   The Biological Status of the Human Embryo 56

Howard W. Jones, Jr. and Lucinda Veeck, *What Is An Embryo?* 56

Notes and Questions 59

B.   The Legal Status of the Human Embryo 60

1.   An Introductory Case 60

Davis v. Davis 60

Notes and Questions 69

2.   Legal Responses to the Status of the Human Embryo 70

Timothy Stoltzfus Jost, *Rights of Embryo and Foetus in Private Law* 70

Notes and Questions 73

C.   The Moral Status of the Human Embryo 74

Notes and Questions 76

Chapter 2   PROCREATIONAL LIBERTY: CONSTITUTIONAL JURISPRUDENCE AND THE RIGHT TO REPRODUCE **81**

SECTION I: TRADITIONAL REPRODUCTION AND THE CONSTITUTION . . 81

A.   Establishing Reproduction as a Fundamental Right 81

1.   The Early Cases 81

Meyer v. Nebraska 81

Notes and Questions 85

Skinner v. Oklahoma 87

Notes and Questions 90

2.   State Support for Mandatory Sterilization 92

Buck v. Bell 92

Notes and Questions 93

TABLE OF CONTENTS

Paul A. Lombardo, *Facing Carrie Buck* 95

B.   The Right to Avoid Procreation 100

   1.   Emerging Advances in Human Contraception 100

         Griswold v. Connecticut 100

         Notes and Questions 103

         Eisenstadt v. Baird 106

         Notes and Questions 108

   2.   Abortion 111

     a.   The Seminal Case 112

         Roe v. Wade 112

         Notes and Questions 119

     b.   The *Roe* Progeny 120

         Webster v. Reproductive Health Services 120

         Planned Parenthood of Southeastern Pennsylvania v. Casey . . 123

         Notes and Questions 128

     c.   The Latest Word on Abortion, For Now 130

SECTION II: ASSISTED REPRODUCTION AS A FUNDAMENTAL RIGHT . . 130

A.   Arguments for Recognizing ART as a Fundamental Right 130

         John A. Robertson, *Children of Choice: Freedom and the New*

         Reproductive Technologies 131

B.   Arguments Against Recognizing ART as a Fundamental Right 138

         Radhika Rao, *Constitutional Misconceptions* 138

         Ann MacLean Massie, *Regulating Choice: A Constitutional Law*

         Response to Professor John A. Robertson's Children of Choice . . . 143

         Notes and Questions 148

C.   Judicial Perspectives on ART as a Fundamental Right 150

   1.   Equating ART and Natural Conception 151

         Lifchez v. Hartigan 151

         Kass v. Kass 154

         Notes and Questions 157

   2.   Distinguishing ART from Natural Conception 158

         Davis v. Davis 158

         Notes and Questions 163

         Gerber v. Hickman 165

         Notes and Questions 171

Chapter 3   **THE BUSINESS OF ART: SELLING, DONATING AND INSURING ASSISTED REPRODUCTION** 173

SECTION I: UNDERSTANDING THE MARKET FOR REPRODUCTIVE TECHNOLOGIES 173

A.   Fertility Clinics as Providers of ART Services 173

TABLE OF CONTENTS

1.   A Patient's Perspective 173
            Notes and Questions 174
2.   The Physician's Perspective 179
            Ethics Committee of the American Society for Reproductive Medicine,
            Shared-Risk or Refund Programs in Assisted Reproduction 179
B.   Profiles of ART Clients 182
            Dorothy E. Roberts, *Race and the New Reproduction* 182

SECTION II: SPERM AND EGG "DONORS" 188

A.   Sperm Donations: Assessing Risks and Benefits 188
1.   Donor Disclosure: A Child's Perspective 191
            Notes and Problems 194
2.   The Pitfalls of Sperm Donation 196
            Johnson v. Superior Court 196
            Notes and Questions 204
B.   Egg Donations: Assessing Risks and Benefits 205
1.   The Business of Egg Donation 207
            Martha Frase-Blunt, *Ova-Compensating?; Women Who Donate Eggs
            To Infertile Couples Earn a Reward — But Pay a Price* 207
            Judith Daar, *Physical Beauty Is Only Egg Deep* 211
            Notes and Questions 213
2.   The Ethics of Egg Donation 215
            Ethics Committee of the American Society for Reproductive Medicine,
            Financial Compensation of Oocyte Donors 215
            Notes and Questions 219
3.   Informed Consent and Egg Donation 223
      a.   Informing Egg Donors of Risks and Benefits 223
            Gregory Stock, *Eggs for Sale: How Much Is Too Much?* 223
            Judith Daar, *Regulating the Fiction of Informed Consent in ART
            Medicine* 225
            Notes and Questions 227
      b.   Informing Donors About Gamete Placement 228
            Litowitz v. Litowitz 229
            Notes and Questions 232

SECTION III: THE BENEFITS AND BURDENS OF AN ART MARKET 233

A.   Should We Ban a Market for the Sale of Gametes? 233
1.   Arguments for Market Inalienability 233
            Mary Lyndon Shanley, *Collaboration and Commodification in Assisted
            Procreation: Reflections on an Open Market and Anonymous Donation
            in Human Sperm and Eggs* 234
            Notes and Questions 238
2.   Arguments In Support of a Gamete Market 239

TABLE OF CONTENTS

    Richard A. Posner, *The Ethics and Economics of Enforcing Contracts*
    of Surrogate Motherhood 239

B. Should the ART Market Be Open to All Willing Buyers and Sellers? . . 243

 1. Exclusions Based On Age 243
    Judith Daar, *Death of Aging Mother Raises More Questions About IVF*
    Rules 243
    Ethics Committee of the American Society for Reproductive Medicine,
    Oocyte Donation to Postmenopausal Women 245
    Notes and Questions 247

 2. Exclusions Based on Health Status 247
    Ethics Committee of the American Society for
    Reproductive Medicine, *Human Immunodeficiency Virus and Infertility*
    Treatment 248
    Notes and Problems 252

 3. Exclusions Based on Marital Status and Sexual Orientation 256
    North Coast Women's Care Medical Group, Inc. v. San Diego County
    Superior Court 256
    Notes and Questions 261

SECTION IV: INSURING ART SERVICES 262

A. The Market Landscape 262
 1. The Status of Infertility Insurance Coverage 262
  a. Statutory Law 262
  b. Case Law 266
    Lisa M. Kerr, *Can Money Buy Happiness? An Examination of the*
    Coverage of Infertility Services Under HMO Contracts 267
    Notes and Questions 270
    Saks v. Franklin Covey 271
    Notes and Questions 279

 2. The Politics of ART Insurance Coverage 280
    Edward G. Hughes & Mita Giacomini, *Funding In Vitro Fertilization*
    Treatment for Persistent Subfertility: The Pain and the Politics . . 280
    Questions 281

B. ART Insurance Coverage and the Effect on Clinical Outcomes 282
    Problem 283

Chapter 4   **CHOOSING OUR CHILDREN'S TRAITS: GENDER AND**
        GENETIC SELECTION IN ART **285**

SECTION I: THE CURRENT STATE OF TECHNOLOGY 288

A. Choosing a Child's Gender 289
 1. Preconception Gender Selection 292
    Ethics Committee of the American Society for Reproductive Medicine,

TABLE OF CONTENTS

        Preconception Gender Selection for Nonmedical Reasons 292

        Notes and Questions 296

2.   Postconception Gender Selection 299

        The Ethics Committee of the American Society for Reproductive
Medicine, *Sex Selection and Preimplantation Genetic Diagnosis* . 299

        Notes and Questions 305

        John A. Robertson, *Extending Preimplantation Genetic Diagnosis:
Medical and Non-medical Uses* 308

        The President's Council on Bioethics, *Beyond Therapy: Biotechnology
and the Pursuit of Happiness* 310

        Notes and Questions 311

B.   Choosing a Child's Genetic Make-Up 313

1.   Using Preimplantation Genetic Diagnosis to Cure Illness 314

        Notes and Questions 315

        Susan M. Wolf, Jeffrey P. Kahn, John E. Wagner, *Using
Preimplantation Genetic Diagnosis to Create a Stem Cell Donor:
Issues, Guidelines & Limits* 316

        *R (on The Application of Quintavalle) v. Human Fertilisation and
Embryology Authority* 323

        Notes and Questions 331

        Problem 333

2.   Using Preimplantation Genetic Diagnosis to Avoid Illness 334

  a.   PGD and the Meaning of Disability 334

        Notes and Questions 336

  b.   PGD and Adult-Onset Diseases 339

        Notes and Questions 341

3.   Using Preimplantation Genetic Diagnosis to Achieve Pregnancy ... 341

SECTION II: THE CURRENT STATE OF THE LAW 343

        Genetics & Public Policy Center, *Preimplantation Genetic Diagnosis: A
Discussion of Challenges, Concerns, and Preliminary Options Related to
the Genetic Testing of Human Embryos* 343

        Notes and Questions 347

SECTION III: ETHICAL AND LEGAL DEBATE SURROUNDING GENDER
        SELECTION 352

A.   Constitutional Analysis 353

        Carl H. Coleman, *Is There a Constitutional Right to Preconception Sex
Selection?* 353

        Notes and Questions 355

B.   Ethical Analysis 356

        Rebecca Dresser, *Cosmetic Reproductive Services and Professional
Integrity* 356

        Notes and Questions 357

TABLE OF CONTENTS

SECTION IV: ETHICAL AND LEGAL DEBATE SURROUNDING GENETIC
      SELECTION 358

A.   Ethical Dilemmas Surrounding Genetic Selection 358

        Maxwell J. Mehlman, *The Law of Above Averages: Leveling the New
        Genetic Enhancement Playing Field* 359

        Notes and Questions 362

B.   Legal Dilemmas Surrounding Genetic Selection 366

        Paretta v. Medical Offices for Human Reproduction 366

        Notes and Questions 369

        Problem 370

Chapter 5   **FAMILY LAW ISSUES IN ART: QUESTIONS OF
                            PARENTAGE AND PARENTAL RIGHTS** **371**

SECTION I: EARLY DILEMMAS IN FAMILY LAW 371

A.   Determining Paternity in AID Families 371

        Strnad v. Strnad 371

        Notes and Questions 372

        People v. Sorensen 373

        Notes and Questions 376

B.   Early Changes in the Law 377

        Jhordan C. v. Mary K. 379

        Notes and Questions 383

C.   The Problem of Known Donors 384

        Ferguson v. McKiernan 384

        Notes and Questions 392

SECTION II: BUILDING FAMILIES THROUGH SURROGATE PARENTING
      AGREEMENTS 394

A.   An Introductory Case 394

        In the Matter of Baby M 394

        Notes and Questions 404

B.   Distinguishing "Traditional" and "Gestational" Surrogacy 408

1.   Traditional Surrogacy 409

        R.R. v. M.H. 409

        Notes and Questions 413

2.   Gestational Surrogacy 415

        Johnson v. Calvert 415

        Notes and Questions 422

        A.H.W. v. G.H.B. 427

        Notes and Questions 429

3.   Profiles in Surrogate Parenting Arrangements 431

a.   Profile of a Traditional Surrogate Mother 432

TABLE OF CONTENTS

b.   Profile of a Gestational Surrogate Mother 433

c.   Profile of an Intended Mother 435

        Notes and Questions 435

C.   Statutory Responses to Surrogate Parenting Arrangements 439

   1.   Laws Regulating Surrogacy 439

    a.   Individual State Laws 439

        Notes and Questions 446

    b.   Uniform Laws on Surrogacy 447

        Notes and Questions 451

   2.   Constitutionality of Surrogacy Laws 453

        J.R., M.R. and W.K.J. v. Utah 453

        Notes and Questions 461

SECTION III: BUILDING FAMILIES THROUGH THE USE OF DONOR
        GAMETES 462

A.   The State of the Art in Donor Gametes 462

B.   The State of the Law in Donor Gametes 464

   1.   Judicial Perspectives 464

        In re Marriage of Buzzanca 464

        Notes and Questions 470

   2.   Statutory Perspectives on Donor Gametes 472

        Questions 474

SECTION IV: BUILDING FAMILIES IN SAME-SEX RELATIONSHIPS 474

A.   The Prevalence of Same-Sex Parents 474

B.   Family Law Dilemmas For Same-Sex Parents 478

   1.   Determining Paternity 478

        C.O. v. W.S. 478

        Lamaritata v. Lucas 479

        Notes and Questions 481

        Adoption of Tammy 483

        Notes and Questions 487

        K.M. v. E.G. 489

        Notes and Questions 496

SECTION V: MISHAPS IN THE LABORATORY: THE CHILDREN OF ART
        GAMETE MIX-UPS 498

A.   Defining the Problem 498

B.   Judicial Perspectives on Gamete Mix-Ups 500

   1.   The Case of Physician Malfeasance 500

        Prato-Morrison v. Doe 500

        Notes and Questions 504

   2.   Cases of Physician Negligence 506

        Robert B. v. Susan B. 506

        Notes and Questions 509

TABLE OF CONTENTS

    Perry-Rogers v. Fasano 510

    Leslie Bender, *Genes, Parents, and Assisted Reproductive*

    Technologies: ARTs, Mistakes, Sex, Race, & Law 514

    Notes and Questions 515

 C. Legislative Perspectives on Gamete Mix-Ups 517

Chapter 6   **LIFE AFTER DEATH: POSTMORTEM**
       REPRODUCTION **521**

SECTION I: THE POSSIBILITIES FOR POSTMORTEM REPRODUCTION . . 522

 A. Freezing Sperm 522

  1. Sperm Retrieval During Life 522

   a. Sperm Freezing — Past and Present 522

   b. Emerging Legal Disputes Over Frozen Sperm 524

     Hall v. Fertility Institute of New Orleans 525

     Notes and Questions 528

     Michael H. Shapiro, *Illicit Reasons and Means for Reproduction: On*

     Excessive Choice and Categorical and Technological Imperatives

     530

  2. Sperm Retrieval After Death 533

     Carson Strong, *Ethical and Legal Aspects of Sperm Retrieval After*

     Death or Persistent Vegetative State 535

     Notes and Questions 538

 B. Freezing Eggs: Retrieval During Life and After Death 540

     Problem 542

 C. Freezing Embryos 542

SECTION II: LEGAL DILEMMAS IN POSTMORTEM REPRODUCTION 545

 A. Family Law Questions: Who Is A Parent? 545

     In re Estate of Kolacy 546

     Notes and Questions 549

 B. Probate Law: Awarding Inheritance Rights and Death Benefits 551

     Woodward v. Commissioner of Social Security 551

     Notes and Questions 556

SECTION III: STATUTORY FRAMEWORKS FOR EVALUATING THE RIGHTS OF
POSTMORTEM CONCEPTION CHILDREN 560

 A. Uniform Laws Governing Postmortem Reproduction 561

  1. The Uniform Parentage Act 561

     Notes and Questions 562

  2. The Uniform Probate Code 563

     Notes and Questions 564

 B. Emerging Laws Governing the Rights of Posthumous Children 566

     Notes and Questions 567

TABLE OF CONTENTS

C.   Model Laws and Task Force Reports 569
  1.   The ABA Model Act 569
        Questions 570
  2.   The New York State Task Force on Life and the Law 570
        Questions 571

Chapter 7   ART AND DIVORCE: DISPUTES OVER FROZEN
                 EMBRYOS 573

SECTION I: THE POPULARITY AND FRAILTY OF EMBRYO
             CRYOPRESERVATION 574
             Frisina v. Woman and Infant Hospital of Rhode Island 575
             Miller v. American Infertility Group of Illinois, S.C. 580
             Notes and Questions 583
SECTION II: THE LEGAL LANDSCAPE SURROUNDING FROZEN EMBRYO
             DISPUTES 585
  A.   An Introductory Case 585
        Davis v. Davis 585
        Notes and Questions 589
  B.   The Contract Approach 591
        Kass v. Kass 591
        Notes and Questions 597
        Litowitz v. Litowitz 604
        Notes and Questions 611
  C.   The Public Policy Approach 612
        A.Z. v. B.Z. 612
        Judith F. Daar, Frozen Embryo Disputes Revisited: A Trilogy of
        Procreation-Avoidance Approaches 618
        Notes and Questions 621
        J.B. v. M.B. 625
        Notes and Questions 632
  D.   The Question of Parental Rights 634
        In re O.G.M. 634
        Notes and Questions 637
SECTION III: THE PROBLEM OF EXCESS AND ABANDONED EMBRYOS . 638
  A.   Excess Embryos and Patient Choice 639
  1.   Donate the Embryos for Research 639
    a.   Type of Research 639
    b.   State Law Prohibitions on Embryo Research 640
  2.   Discard the Embryos After a Designated Time Frame 641
  3.   Maintain the Embryos in Frozen Storage 642
  4.   Donate the Embryos to Another Couple 642

TABLE OF CONTENTS

B.   Excess Embryos and Lack of Patient Choice: The Problem of
Abandonment 645

        Notes and Questions 647

        York v. Jones 648

        Notes and Questions 652

        Problem 652

Chapter 8   **REGULATING REPRODUCTIVE TECHNOLOGIES** . . **655**

SECTION I: THE LEGAL LANDSCAPE FOR ART: AN INTRODUCTION . . . 656

A.   The Goals of Regulation 656

        Judith F. Daar, *Regulating Reproductive Technologies: Panacea or Paper
Tiger?* 656

        Notes and Questions 657

B.   The Current State of Regulation 659

   1.   Direct Regulation by the Federal Government 659

   2.   Indirect Regulation by the Federal Government 661

   3.   Direct Regulation by State Governments 662

   4.   Indirect Regulation by State Governments 663

   5.   Self-Regulation by the Fertility Industry 665

        Notes and Questions 666

SECTION II: IS (INCREASED) ART REGULATION NECESSARY? 668

A.   Protecting ART Patients 669

   1.   Luring Patients: False Advertising and Deceptive Statements 669

        Karlin v. IVF America, Inc. 669

        Notes and Questions 672

   2.   Lack of Informed Consent 673

        *Elements to Be Considered in Obtaining Informed Consent for
ART* 673

   3.   Treatment Errors: Negligence, Theft, and Fraud 675

   4.   Protecting Patient Health 677

B.   Protecting ART Offspring 680

        Doolan v. IVF America (MA), Inc. 680

        Notes and Questions 683

C.   Protecting ART Physicians 686

   1.   Enhancing Public Confidence 686

   2.   Authorizing Treatment Denials 687

        The Ethics Committee of the American Society for Reproductive
Medicine, *Child-Rearing Ability and the Provision of Fertility Services*
. . . . 687

        Notes and Questions 690

SECTION III: PROPOSED REGULATORY SCHEMES 691

TABLE OF CONTENTS

President's Council on Bioethics, *Reproduction & Responsibility: The Regulation of New Biotechnologies* 693

Notes and Questions 698

Chapter 9   HUMAN EMBRYONIC STEM CELL RESEARCH 703

SECTION I: THE SCIENCE OF EMBRYONIC STEM CELL RESEARCH 704

A.   Introduction to the Terms 704

Jennifer L. Enmon, *Stem Cell Research: Is the Law Preventing Progress?* 704

Notes and Questions 706

B.   Human and Animal Stem Cell Studies 712

Problem 716

C.   Framing the Debate Over Stem Cell Research 717

The President's Council on Bioethics, *Monitoring Stem Cell Research* 717

SECTION II: THE LEGAL FRAMEWORK SURROUNDING STEM CELL RESEARCH 718

A.   Laws Relating to Aborted Fetuses as Sources of Stem Cells 719

1.   Federal Law Relating to Aborted Fetuses as Sources of Stem Cells .. 719

National Bioethics Advisory Commission, *Ethical Issues in Human Stem Cell Research* 719

Notes and Questions 722

2.   State Laws Relating to Aborted Fetuses as Sources of Stem Cells ... 724

National Bioethics Advisory Commission, *Ethical Issues in Human Stem Cell Research* 724

Margaret S. v. Edwards 726

Notes and Questions 729

B.   Laws Relating to Embryos as Sources of Stem Cells 731

1.   Federal Law Relating to Embryos as Sources of Stem Cells 731

Kara L. Belew, *Stem Cell Division: Abortion Law and Its Influence on the Adoption of Radically Different Embryonic Stem Cell Legislation in the United States, the United Kingdom, and Germany* 731

Notes and Questions 734

Doe v. Shalala 735

Question 741

2.   State Laws Relating to Embryos as Sources of Stem Cells 741

National Bioethics Advisory Commission, *Ethical Issues in Human Stem Cell Research* 741

Notes and Questions 743

SECTION III: GOVERNMENT FUNDING OF STEM CELL RESEARCH 745

A.   Federal Funding of Stem Cell Research 746

TABLE OF CONTENTS

1. The First Presidential Proclamation: August 9, 2001 746
   Remarks by the President on Stem Cell Research 746
   Notes and Questions 749
2. Defending and Questioning the Bush Administration Policy 751
   O. Carter Snead, *The Pedagogical Significance of the Bush Stem Cell Policy: A Window into Bioethical Regulation in the United States*
   751
   James F. Childress, *An Ethical Defense of Federal Funding for Human Embryonic Stem Cell Research* 756
   Notes and Questions 758
   Problem 759
3. President Obama and a New Era of Stem Cell Research Policy 760
   The White House, *Removing Barriers to Responsible Scientific Research Involving Human Stem Cells* 760
   Notes and Questions 761
   Sherley v. Sebelius 764
B. State Funding of Stem Cell Research 768
   1. California 768
   2. New Jersey 770
   3. Other State Activities 772
   Problem 773

SECTION IV: INTERNATIONAL AND CROSS-CULTURAL PERSPECTIVES ON STEM CELL RESEARCH 774
A. International Perspectives 774
   Notes and Questions 785
B. Religious Perspectives on Embryonic Stem Cell Research 786
   National Bioethics Advisory Commission Summary of Presentations on Religious Perspectives Relating to Research Involving Human Stem Cells, May 7, 1999 787
   Notes and Questions 794

Chapter 10   HUMAN REPRODUCTIVE CLONING **797**

SECTION I: THE SCIENCE OF HUMAN REPRODUCTIVE CLONING 797
A. Three Types of Cloning 798
   1. Reproductive Cloning 798
   2. Therapeutic Cloning 799
   3. Embryo Cloning 800
B. Advances in Animal Cloning 801
   1. Safety and Efficacy Concerns 802
   2. Purposes of Animal Cloning 804
C. Inroads Into Human Cloning 805

TABLE OF CONTENTS

Judith F. Daar, *The Prospect of Human Cloning: Improving Nature or Dooming the Species?* 807

Lori B. Andrews, *Is There a Right to Clone? Constitutional Challenges to Bans on Human Cloning* 811

Notes and Questions 814

Problem 815

SECTION II: THE POLITICS OF HUMAN CLONING 816

A.   Initial Reaction from the Federal Government 816

National Bioethics Advisory Commission, *Cloning Human Beings* . 816

Notes and Questions 819

B.   Later Reactions from the Federal Government 822

The President's Council on Bioethics, *Human Cloning and Human Dignity* 823

Notes and Questions 825

C.   Reactions from the States 826

Notes and Questions 829

SECTION III: CONSTITUTIONAL ASPECTS OF HUMAN CLONING 831

A.   Cloning and Procreational Autonomy 831

Elizabeth Price Foley, *Human Cloning and the Right to Reproduce* 833

George J. Annas, Lori B. Andrews and Rosario M. Isasi, *Protecting the Endangered Human: Toward an International Treaty Prohibiting Cloning and Inheritable Alterations* 838

Notes and Questions 841

B.   Cloning and the Right to Scientific Inquiry 842

John Charles Kunich, *The Naked Clone* 842

Notes and Questions 846

GLOSSARY 849

TABLE OF CASES TC-1

INDEX I-1

ACKNOWLEDGMENTS

The author acknowledges the permissions kindly granted to reproduce excerpts from, or illustrations of, the materials indicated below.

Books and Articles

Andrews, Lori B., *Is There A Right To Clone? Constitutional Challenges to the Ban on Human Cloning*, 11 Harv. J. Law & Technology 643, 649-57 (1998). Copyright © 1998 by the President & Fellows of Harvard College and Lori B. Andrews. Reprinted by permission of the author.

_____, George J. Annas & Rosario M. Isasi, *Protecting the Endangered Human: Toward an International Treaty Prohibiting Cloning and Inheritable Alterations*, 28 Am. J. L & Med 151, 157-162 (2002). Copyright © 2005 by The American Society of Law, Medicine & Ethics. Reprinted by permission of the authors and the American Journal of Law & Medicine.

Belew, Kara L., *Stem Cell Division: Abortion Law and its Influence on the Adoption of Radically Different Embryonic Stem Cell Legislation in the United States, the United Kingdom, and Germany*, 39 Texas Int'l Law Journal 479, 499-506 (2004). Copyright © 2004 by the Texas International Law Journal. Reprinted by permission of the author and the Texas International Law Journal.

Bender, Leslie, *Genes, Parents, and Assisted Reproductive Technologies: ARTs, Mistakes, Sex, Race & Law*, 12 Colum. J. Gender & L. 1, 33-36 (2003). Copyright © 2003 by Leslie Bender. Reprinted by permission of the author.

California Cryobank Donor Essays. Copyright © 2012 by the California Cryobank, Inc. Reprinted by permission of the California Cryobank, Inc.

Ceelen, Manon, Mirjam M. Van Weissenbruch, Jan P.W. Vermeiden, Flora E. Van Ieeuwen & Henriette A. Delemarre-Vande Wall, *Growth and Development of Children Born After In Vitro Fertilization*, 90 Fertility & Sterility 1662 (2008). Copyright © 2008 by the American Society for Reproductive Medicine. Reprinted by permission of Elsevier, Inc.

Childress, James F., *An Ethical Defense of Federal Funding for Human Embryonic Stem Cell Research*, 2 Yale J. Health Policy, Law & Ethics 157 (2001). Copyright © 2001 by the Yale Journal of Health Policy, Law & Ethics. Reprinted by permission of the author.

Coleman, Carl H., *Is There A Constitutional Right To Preconception Sex Selection?*, 1 Am. J. Bioethics 27 (2001). Copyright © 2001 American Journal of Bioethics. Reprinted by permission of the author and Taylor & Francis, Inc., http://www.taylorandfrancis.com.

Daar, Judith, *Regulating Reproductive Technologies: Panacea or Paper Tiger?* 34 Hous. L. Rev. 609, 646-9 (1997). Copyright © 1997 by Judith F. Daar.

_____, *Physical Beauty Is Only Skin Deep*, Los Angeles Times, October 28, 1999 at B11. Copyright © 1999 by Judith F. Daar.

_____, *Regulating The Fiction of Informed Consent in ART Medicine*, 1 Am. J. Bioethics 19 (2001). Copyright © 2001 Taylor & Francis Inc. Reprinted by permission of the author and Taylor & Francis, Inc., http://www.taylorandfrancis.com.

ACKNOWLEDGEMENTS

_____, *Embryo Disputes Revisited: A Trilogy of Procreation-Avoidance Approaches*, 29 J Law Med & Ethics 197, 198-199 (2001). Copyright © 2001 by the Journal of Law Medicine & Ethics. Reprinted by permission of the author and the Journal of Law, Medicine & Ethics.

_____, *The Prospect of Human Cloning: Improving Nature or Dooming the Species?* 33 Seton Hall L. Rev. 511, 527-535 (2003). Copyright © 2003 by Judith F. Daar. Reprinted by permission of the author and the Seton Hall Law Review.

_____, *Death of Aging Mother Raises More Questions About IVF Rules*, Los Angeles Daily Journal, July 29, 2009. Copyright © 2009 by Judith F. Daar.

Dresser, Rebecca, *Cosmetic Reproductive Services and Professional Integrity*, 1 Am. J. Bioethics 11 (2001). Copyright ©2001 by the American Journal of Bioethics. Reprinted by permission of the author and Taylor & Francis, Inc., http://www.taylorandfrancis.com.

Enmon, Jennifer L., *Stem Cell Research: Is The Law Preventing Progress?* Utah Law Review 621, 622-628 (2002). Copyright © 2002 by the Utah Law Review. Reprinted by permission of the author and the Utah Law Review.

Ethics Committee of the American Society for Reproductive Medicine, *Shared-Risk or Refund Programs in Assisted Reproduction*, Vol. 70, no. 3 Fertility & Sterility 414-415 (1998). Copyright © 1998 by the American Society for Reproductive Medicine. Reprinted by permission of Elsevier, Inc.

_____, *Sex Selection and Preimplantation Genetic Diagnosis*, Vol. 72, no. 4 Fertility & Sterility 595-598 (1999). Copyright © 1999 by the American Society for Reproductive Medicine. Reprinted by permission of Elsevier, Inc.

_____, *Preconception Gender Selection for Nonmedical Reasons*, Vol. 75, no. 5 Fertility & Sterility 861-864 (2001). Copyright © 2001 by the American Society for Reproductive Medicine. Reprinted by permission of Elsevier, Inc.

_____, *Oocyte Donation to Postmenopausal Women*, Vol. 82, Fertility & Sterility, Supp. 1, pp. 254S -5S (2004). Copyright © 2004 by the American Society for Reproductive Medicine. Reprinted by permission of Elsevier, Inc.

_____, *Elements to Be Considered in Obtaining Informed Consent for ART*, Vol. 86 No. 4 Fertility & Sterility S272 (2006). Copyright © 2006 by the American Society for Reproductive Medicine. Reprinted by permission of Elsevier, Inc.

_____, *Financial Compensation of Oocyte Donors*, 88 Fertility & Sterility 305 (2007). Copyright © 2007 by the American Society for Reproductive Medicine. Reprinted by permission of Elsevier, Inc.

_____, *Child-Rearing Ability and the Provision of Fertility Services*, Vol. 92, no. 3 Fertility & Sterility 864-867 (2009). Copyright © 2009 by the American Society for Reproductive Medicine. Reprinted by permission of Elsevier, Inc.

_____, *Human Immunodeficiency Virus and Infertility Treatment*, Vol. 94, no. 1 Fertility & Sterility 11-15 (2010). Copyright © 2010 by the American Society for Reproductive Medicine. Reprinted by permission of Elsevier, Inc.

Frase-Blunt, Martha, *Ova-Compensating? Women Who Donate Eggs to Infertile Couples Earn a Reward — But Pay a Price*, Washington Post Dec. 4, 2001, at F1. Copyright © 2001 by Martha Frase-Blunt. Reprinted by permission of the author.

Genetic and Public Policy Center, *Preimplantation Genetic Diagnosis: A Discussion of Challenges, Concerns, and Preliminary Options Related to the Genetic Testing of*

ACKNOWLEDGEMENTS

Human Embryos, Jan. 2004, pp. 7-10. Copyright © 2004 by the Genetics & Public Policy Center/The Pew Charitable Trusts. Reprinted by permission of the Genetics and Public Policy Center.

Hughes, Edward G. & Mita Giacomini, *Funding In Vitro Fertilization Treatment For Persistent Subfertility: The Pain and the Politics*, Vol. 76, No. 3 Fertility & Sterility 434, 436 (2001). Copyright © 2001 by the American Society for Reproductive Medicine. Reprinted by permission of Elsevier, Inc.

_____, *Funding In Vitro Fertilization Treatment For Persistent Subfertility: The Pain and the Politics*, Vol. 76, no. 3 Fertility & Sterility 431-442 (2001). Copyright © 2001 by the American Society for Reproductive Medicine. Reprinted by permission of Elsevier, Inc.

Jones, Jr., Howard J. & Lucinda Veeck, *What Is An Embryo?*, Vol. 77, no. 4 Fertility & Sterility 658-659 (2002). Copyright © 2002 by the American Society for Reproductive Medicine. Reprinted by permission of Elsevier, Inc.

Jost, Timothy, *Rights of Embryo and Fetus in Private Law*, 50 Am. J. Comp Law 633 (2002). Copyright © 2002 by the American Journal of Comparative Law. Reprinted by permission of the author and the American Journal of Comparative Law.

Kahn, Jeffrey P, John E. Wagner & Susan M. Wolf, *Using Preimplantation Genetic Diagnosis to Create a Stem Cell Donor: Issues, Guidelines & Limits*, 31 Am. J. Law, Med. Ethics 327 (2003). Copyright © 2003 by The American Journal of Law, Medicine and Ethics. Reprinted by permission of the authors and The American Journal of Law, Medicine and Ethics.

Kaplan, Lawrence & Carolyn Kaplan, *The Ethics of Reproductive Technology* pp.15-19 (1992). Copyright © 1992 by Oxford University Press, Inc. Reprinted by permission of the author and Oxford University Press.

Kerr, Lisa M., *Can Money Buy Happiness? An Examination of the Coverage of Infertility Services Under HMO Contracts*, 49 Case W. Res. L. Rev. 599 (1999). Copyright © 1999 by Case Western Reserve University Law Review. Reprinted by permission of Case Western Reserve University.

Kovalevsky, George, Paolo Rinaudo, Christos Coutifaris, *Do Assisted Reproductive Technologies Cause Adverse Fetal Outcomes?* Vol. 79, no. 6 Fertility & Sterility 1270-1272 (2003). Copyright © 2003 by the American Society for Reproductive Medicine. Reprinted by permission of Elsevier, Inc.

Kunich, John Charles, *The Naked Clone*, 91 Kentucky L. J. 1, 48-55 (2002). Copyright © 2002 by the Kentucky Law Journal. Reprinted by permission of the author and the Kentucky Law Journal.

Lombardo, Paul, *Facing Carrie Buck*, 33 Hastings Center Report 14 (March-April 2003). Copyright © 2004 by The Hastings Center. Reprinted by permission of the author and The Hastings Center.

Massie, Ann M., *Regulating Choice: A Constitutional Law Response to Professor John A. Robertson's Children of Choice*, 52 Wash. & Lee Law Rev. 135 (1995). Copyright © 1995 by Washington and Lee Law Review. Reprinted by permission of the author and the Washington and Lee Law Review.

Mehlman, Maxwell, *The Law of Above Averages: Leveling the New Genetic Enhancement Playing Field*, 85 Iowa L. Rev. 517 (2000). Copyright © 2000 by Iowa Law

ACKNOWLEDGEMENTS

Review. Reprinted by permission of the author and the Iowa Law Review.

National Bioethics Advisory Commission, *Ethical Issues in Human Stem Cell Research*, pp. 29-33, 35-36, 99-104 (1999). Reprinted by permission of the National Bioethics Advisory Commission, http://bioethics.georgetown.edu/nbac.

_____, *Cloning Human Beings, Executive Summary I-V* (1997). Reprinted by permission of the National Bioethics Advisory Commission, http://bioethics.georgetown.edu/nbac.

New York State Task Force on Life and the Law, *Assisted Reproductive Technologies: Analysis and Recommendations for Public Policy*, pp. 8-10 (1998). NY State Dep't. of Health. Reprinted with permission from the New York State Department of Health.

Posner, Richard A., *The Ethics and Economics of Enforcing Contracts of Surrogate Motherhood*, 5 J. Cont. Health Law & Policy 21 (1989). Copyright © 1989 by Richard A. Posner. Reprinted by permission of the author.

President's Council on Bioethics, *Reproduction and Responsibility: The Regulation of the New Biotechnologies*, 151-153, 205-218 (2004). Copyright © 2004 by the President's Council on Bioethics. Reprinted by permission of the President's Council on Bioethics.

_____, *Monitoring Stem Cell Research*, 5-7 (2004). Copyright © 2004 by the President's Council on Bioethics. Reprinted by permission of the President's Council on Bioethics.

_____, *Human Cloning and Human Dignity, Executive Summary xxvii-xxix* (2002). Copyright © 2002 by the President's Council on Bioethics. Reprinted by permission of the President's Council on Bioethics.

Price Foley, Elizabeth, *Human Cloning and the Right to Reproduce*, 65 Albany L. Rev. 625, 638-46 (2002). Copyright © 2002 by the Albany Law Review Association. Reprinted by permission of the author and the Albany Law Review.

Rao, Radhika, *Constitutional Misconceptions*, 93 Michigan Law Review 1473 (1995). Copyright © 1995 by the Michigan Law Review Association. Reprinted by permission of the author and the Michigan Law Review.

Roberts, Dorothy E., *Race and the New Reproduction*, 47 Hast. L. Journal 935 (1996). Copyright © 1996 by University of California, Hastings College of Law. Reprinted by permission of the author and The Hastings Law Journal.

Robertson, John, *Children of Choice: Freedom and the New Reproductive Technologies*, pp. 22-42 (1994). Copyright © 1994 by Princeton University Press. Reprinted by permission of the author and Princeton University Press.

_____, *Extending Preimplantation Genetic Diagnosis: Medical and Nonmedical Uses*, 29 J. Med. Ethics 213 (2003). Copyright © 2003 BMJ Group. Reprinted by permission of the author and BMJ Group.

Shanley, Mary Lyndon. Collaborations and Commodification in Assisted Procreation: Reflections on an Open Market and Anonymous Donation in Human Sperm and Eggs. 37 Law & Society Rev. 257 (2002). Reprinted by permission of John Wiley & Sons, Ltd.

Shapiro, Michael H., *Illicit Reasons and Means for Reproduction: On Excessive Choice and Categorical and Technological Imperatives*, 47 Hast. L. J. 1081, 1127 (1996). Copyright ©1996 by University of California, Hastings College of the Law.

ACKNOWLEDGEMENTS

Reprinted by permission of the author and University of California, Hastings College of the Law.

Snead, O. Carter, *The Pedagogical Significance of the Bush Stem Cell Policy: A Window into Bioethical Regulation on the United States*, 5 Yale Journal of Health Policy, Law & Ethics 491 (2005). Copyright © 2005 by the Yale Journal of Health Policy, Law & Ethics. Reprinted by permission of the author.

Stock, Gregory, *Eggs For Sale: How Much Is Too Much?* 1 Am. J. Bioethics 26 (2001). Copyright © 2001 by Taylor & Francis, Inc. Reprinted by permission of Taylor & Francis, Inc., http://www.taylorandfrancis.com.

Strong, Carson, *Ethical and Legal Aspects of Sperm Retrieval After Death or Persistent Vegetative State*, 27 J. Law, Med., & Ethics 347 (1999). Copyright © 1999 by the American Society of Law, Medicine & Ethics. Reprinted by permission of the author and the American Society of Law, Medicine & Ethics.

Surrogacy.com, *One Surrogate's Experience*. Reprinted by permission of www.surrogacy.com.

_____, *Surrogate's Diary*. Reprinted by permission of www.surrogacy.com.

_____, *Thoughts On Becoming A Mommy*. Reprinted by permission of www.surrogacy.com.

Photographs and Illustrations

Blackmun, Harry. Photograph of Justice Harry A. Blackmun. Harris & Ewing Collection of the Supreme Court of the United States. Reproduced by permission.

Blood, Diane with Son Liam. Photograph. Copyright © by Reuters/CORBIS. Reproduced by permission

Brown, Louise, and her parents. Photograph by Adrian Arbib. Copyright © by Adrian Arbib/CORBIS. Reproduced by permission.

Brennan, William. Photograph of Justice William Brennan. Collection of the Supreme Court of the United States. Reproduced by permission.

Buck, Carrie, and her mother. Photograph. Arthur Estabrook Papers, M.E. Grenander Department of Special Collections and Archives, University at Albany, SUNY. Reproduced by permission.

Comstock, Anthony. Photograph. Copyright © by Bettmann/CORBIS. Reproduced by permission.

Dobbs, Alice, with Carrie baby Vivian. Photograph. Arthur Estabrook Papers, M.E. Grenander Department of Special Collections and Archives, University at Albany, SUNY. Reproduced by permission.

Douglas, William. Photograph of Justice William O. Douglas. Collection of the Supreme Court of the United States. Reproduced by permission.

Ginsburg, Ruth Bader. Official Photograph of Justice Ruth Bader Ginsburg. Courtesy of the Supreme Court of the United States. Reproduced by permission.

Glasbergen, Randy. Cartoon. Copyright © 1998 by Randy Glasbergen. Reproduced by permission of Randy Glasbergen.

Griswold, Estelle and Cornelia Jahncke. Photograph. Copyright © by Bettmann/CORBIS. Reproduced by permission.

Holmes, Oliver Wendell. Photograph of Justice Oliver Wendell Holmes. Collection of the Supreme Court of the United States. Reproduced by permission.

ACKNOWLEDGEMENTS

John, Elton, David Furnish and their son Zachary. Cover photo by Greg Gorman, from US Weekly, Jan. 18, 2011. Copyright © US Weekly LLC 2011. All Rights Reserved. Reprinted by Permission.

Kass, Leon. Photograph. Reproduced by permission of the President's Council on Bioethics.

Kennedy, Anthony M. Official Photograph of Justice Anthony M. Kennedy. Courtesy of the Supreme Court of the United States. Reproduced by permission.

Luckovich, Mike. Cartoon. Copyright © 1999 by Mike Luckovich. Reproduced by permission of Mike Luckovich.

McReynolds, James. Official Portrait of Justice James C. McReynolds. Vic Boswell, National Geographic Society, Courtesy of the Supreme Court of the United States. Reproduced by permission.

Mendel, Gregor. Portrait of Austrian Botanist. Photograph circa 1880. Copyright © by Bettmann/CORBIS. Reproduced by permission.

New Yorker, The. The New Yorker Magazine, Inc. Holds copyrights in the following cartoons: (1) cartoon by Dana Fradon Copyright © 1995; (2) cartoon by J.B. Handelsman Copyright © 1999; (3) cartoon by Donald Reilly Copyright © 1999; (4) cartoon by David Sipress Copyright © 2001. These cartoons are reprinted by permission of the Cartoon Bank, a division of The New Yorker Magazine (cartoonbank.com). All rights reserved.

O'Connor, Sandra Day. Photograph of Justice Sandra Day O'Connor. Dane Penland, Smithsonian Institute, Courtesy of the Supreme Court of the United States. Reproduced by permission.

Reeve, Christopher, Dr. John Gearhart and Dr. James Thomson. Photograph by Christy Bowe. Copyright © by Christy Bowe/CORBIS.Reproduced by permission.

Rehnquist, William. Official Photograph of Chief Justice William H. Rehnquist. Dane Penland, Smithsonian Institute, Courtesy of the Supreme Court of the United States. Reproduced by permission.

Steptoe, Patrick, and Robert Edwards. Photograph. Copyright © by Hulton-Deutsch Collection/CORBIS. Reproduced by permission.

Thibodeau, Gary, Anatomy and Physiology, Figure of female reproductive tract on p. 758, 11th Edition. Copyright © 1983 by C.V. Mosby Company. Reprinted by permission of Elsevier, Inc.

Van Leeuwenhoek, Antonie. Painting by Cornelis de Man. Copyright © by Bettmann/CORBIS. Reproduced by permission.

Werlin, Lawrence. Preimplantation Genetic Diagnosis. Photograph by Dr. Lawrence Werlin. Reproduced by permission of Dr. Lawrence Werlin.

_____, Zygote, Embryo, Blastocyst. Photographs by Dr. Lawrence Werlin. Reproduced by permission of Dr. Lawrence Werlin.

Wilmut, Ian with Dolly. Photograph by Najlah Feanny-Hicks. Copyright © by Najlah Feanny/CORBIS SABA. Reproduced by permission.

Chapter 1

HUMAN REPRODUCTION: NATURAL AND ASSISTED METHODS OF CONCEPTION

And when Rachel saw that she bare Jacob no children, Rachel envied her sister; and said unto Jacob, Give me children, or else I die. —

Genesis 30:1
King James Bible

One egg, one embryo, one adult — normality . . . Making ninety-six human beings grow where only one grew before. Progress. —

Aldous Huxley
Brave New World (1932)

SECTION I: THE WONDERS OF HUMAN REPRODUCTION

The mystery of human reproduction is a perennial source of intrigue and wonder, evoking both awe and curiosity from those who contemplate this method of species preservation. Throughout the ages mankind has striven to understand and master the process by which humans are conceived and brought into the world. Our journey will take us from the earliest accounts of scientific inquiry into human reproduction, to the current debates over developing technologies, such as cloning and stem cell research. Our focus throughout will be on *assisted reproductive technologies* (ART), which refers to the various medical techniques used to achieve a pregnancy by means other than sexual intercourse. ART is used when an individual is unable to have a child through the age-old process that combines egg and sperm inside a woman's body. We will learn that ART techniques are used to bypass or substitute for reproductive organs that are absent or do not function properly. Essential to any understanding of ART is a basic refresher on the wondrous workings of the human reproductive system. As you review the process of unassisted reproduction, consider how many opportunities there are for things to go awry.

A. Natural Conception

Lawrence J. Kaplan & Carolyn M. Kaplan
Natural Reproduction and Reproduction-Aiding Technologies
The Ethics of Reproductive Technology 15-19 (1992)

Sexual Reproduction

We begin our discussion with the biology and physiology of natural reproduction, that is, the conception of a child by a man and a woman through unaided and unsupplemented sexual intercourse and the subsequent biological processes.

Humans reproduce sexually, that is, through the union of two cells (gametes): the egg (ovum; plural, ova) from the female and the sperm from the male. These gametes carry the genetic code of the male and the female. In reproduction the egg and sperm combine to form a single cell from which a new individual develops. The genetic makeup of this new cell is a combination of the genes from the egg and the sperm.

The Male Reproductive System

The functions of the male reproductive system are to produce, store, and deliver sperm into the female's reproductive tract. The small sperm cell, about 0.06 mm in length, looks and moves like a tadpole, with a head and a long, wriggling tail. The head carries the vital genetic information in the nucleus of the cell, while the tail serves to propel the sperm in the reproductive tract of the female.

The primary structures of the male reproductive system are as follows:

Testes: two glandular organs in the scrotal sac that produce sperm and the male hormone testosterone

Penis: the external sex organ, with the urethral canal traversing its length

Tubes: the epididymis, vas deferens, and ejaculatory ducts that conduct sperm from the testes to the penis

Glands: several glands along the ejaculatory duct contributing secretions that constitute seminal fluid

Sperm is continuously produced in the mature male, and is stored in the epididymis and the first portion of the vas deferens. The stored sperm cells are haploid; that is, they contain only 23 chromosomes, half the original genetic information of the male. When a haploid sperm cell is combined with a haploid egg cell from the female, a diploid embryo results, each cell of which contains 46 chromosomes in 23 pairs. For the discussion of sex preselection below, it is important to note that the male sperm cell determines the sex of any offspring: whereas the sex chromosomes of females are always X chromosomes (female-determining), the sex chromosomes of males may be either X or Y chromosomes (male-determining). The sex of a child, then, is determined by whether the sperm that fertilizes the egg from which it develops happens to carry an X chromosome or a Y chromosome.

The production of sperm is controlled by a complex and delicate system of hormones: testosterone, follicle-stimulating hormone (FSH), and luteinizing hormone (LH). These hormones maintain a relatively constant number of sperm through negative feedback. When there is a dearth of sperm cells in the testes, hormones send a signal that increases production. Once sperm are replenished, production is shut down. Sperm cells take about 60-72 days to mature and are best produced at a temperature of around 95°F, slightly below normal body temperature — hence the location of the testes outside the body mass in the scrotal sac. Unejaculated sperm are reabsorbed into the body.

At ejaculation, muscular contractions propel sperm through the ejaculatory ducts, where fluids from the various glands are secreted to form semen. The seminal vesicles secrete a viscous alkaline fluid containing fructose (which supplies energy) and prostaglandins (which increase sperm motility and induce uterine contractions that help propel the sperm). The prostate gland contributes a milky fluid that protects the sperm from the acidic environment of the vagina, and a mucus-like lubricating substance is also added. The resulting semen (sperm and seminal fluids) is expelled through the urethra of the penis and into the woman's vagina. From there, the sperm move toward the egg, located higher in the female's reproductive tract, by whipping their tails and through involuntary muscular contractions of the uterus and fallopian tubes. During this period, the essential process of capacitation takes place, in which the sperm become capable of penetrating and fertilizing the egg. Only about 100 to 1000 sperm of the 50 to 250 million in a normal ejaculate reach the egg, taking about 15 minutes. Normally, only one sperm is able to unite with the egg and complete the process of fertilization.

The Female Reproductive System

The primary structures of the female reproductive system are as follows:

Ovaries: two walnut-sized organs located on either side of the lower abdomen in which eggs (ova) develop

Fallopian tubes or oviducts: thin tubes leading from each of the ovaries to the uterus, through which eggs travel and in which they are fertilized

Uterus: the womb, where the fertilized egg implants and develops in pregnancy

Cervix: passage from the uterus to the vagina

Vagina: a canal extending from the cervix to the outside of the body

The primary processes in the female reproductive system are as follows:

- Production of mature eggs

- Transportation of eggs from the ovaries to the uterus, during which time fertilization may occur

- Preparation of the uterus to receive the fertilized egg

- Development of the embryos in the uterus

- Parturition (giving birth)

The female reproductive system involves two distinct but intertwined systems under strict hormonal control. One system is the ovarian system, which is responsible for the production of eggs. The other is the uterine system, which prepares the lining of the uterus for implantation of a fertilized egg. These systems are regulated and synchronized by cyclical increases and decreases in the concentration of several hormones: estrogen, progesterone, gonadotropin-releasing hormone (GnRH), FSH, and LH.

Ovarian System

The ovaries contain cells (primordial sex cells) that, during a woman's reproductive life, mature into eggs. A woman's full complement of primordial sex cells (eggs in an incompletely developed form) is present from before birth, numbers about 7 million at the fifth month of fetal development, and declines to about 400,000 at birth. About 400-500 will mature during her active reproductive life.

In order to be capable of union with sperm, primordial sex cells must undergo further cell division and maturation. This ovarian process, along with the process of uterine development, takes place in a cycle of about 28 days throughout a woman's reproductive life (roughly from the early teens to the mid-forties).

Usually one egg will mature during each cycle, though more than one may develop, creating the possibility of fraternal twins, triplets, and so on. The cycle begins when FSH and LH secreted by the pituitary gland stimulate one or more primordial sex cells to resume development and the follicle surrounding the cells to enlarge. At about the middle of the 28-day cycle, ovulation takes place: FSH secretion decreases, the LH level rapidly rises (in what is often called the "LH surge"), and the enlarged follicle ruptures, releasing the maturing egg into the fallopian tube. Once in the fallopian tube, the egg is propelled down the tube toward the uterus.

Uterine System

After rupturing, the follicle in the ovary is transformed into a new structure called a corpus luteum. The corpus luteum secretes large amounts of estrogen and progesterone, which act on the wall of the uterus to prepare it for implantation and nourishment of the embryo. If fertilization does not occur, the enriched lining of the uterus will disintegrate and pass out of the body, along with the remains of the unfertilized egg, at menstruation.

Fertilization

Normally fertilization, if it is to occur, takes place in a fallopian tube and generally occurs within 10-15 hours of ovulation. In fertilization, a sperm penetrates the egg's jelly-like coat, the coat changes to prevent additional sperm from entering, and the egg undergoes one further cell division, allowing for the last stage of fertilization, the union of genetic materials of the egg and sperm. The result, if all goes well, is a single cell containing in its nucleus the full human complement of 23 pairs of chromosomes, half contributed by the sperm and half by the egg.

Implantation and Pregnancy

The fertilized egg is at first called a zygote. During the four or five days it takes to reach the uterus, the zygote undergoes several cell divisions. When it reaches the uterus, the mass of about 16 cells rearranges itself into a hollow ball of cells called a blastocyst. The cells in the blastocyst continue to divide until the outer layer of cells makes contact with the uterine lining and attaches to it in the process called implantation. Some of the cells of the blastocyst develop into the placenta and fetal membrane, and some develop into the fetus itself.

Following implantation, additional connections are made between the mother and the embryo to ensure that sufficient nutrients are available for development. As the embryo grows, membranous structures known as chorionic villi project into the uterine wall and provide firm attachment. The region of attachment is known as the placenta — the primary nutritive, respiratory, and excretory system for the embryo. A second membrane, the amnion, surrounds the embryo and provides the local environment in which the embryo grows. This extensive tissue system provides for the maintenance of the embryo during its continued division, differentiation, and development throughout pregnancy.

A number of important stages or events in the development of the embryo should be noted:

- At the two- and four-cell stage each cell is totipotential; that is, separated cells retain the potential to form separate embryos, which could result in the birth of identical twins.

- By about day 14 or 15 a heap of cells, called the "primitive streak," develops in the embryo. Two primitive streaks may develop; this is the last point at which identical twins can occur.

- Brain activity: primitive brain waves have been claimed to occur as early as the 40th day, though it is not clear how these electrical impulses relate to what we know as consciousness.

- Viability: the point at which the fetus can survive outside the womb. This point depends on the state of neonatal technology and presently occurs at around 24 weeks.

- Parturition: birth, usually around 40 weeks after conception.

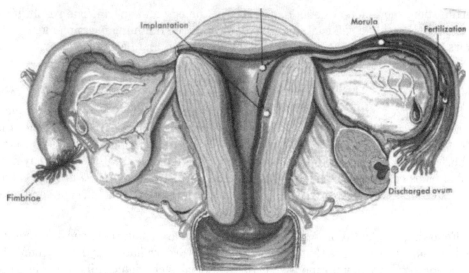

Figure 1. Appearance of the uterus and fallopian tubes from fertilization to implantation. Fertilization occurs in the outer third of the fallopian tube. Development reaches the blastocyst stage after the embryo has entered the uterus. The morula, the developing organism just after fertilization, is most commonly referred to as a preembryo.

Source: CATHERINE PARKER ANTHONY & GARY A. THIBODEAU, TEXTBOOK OF ANATOMY & PHYSIOLOGY 758 (1983).

NOTES AND QUESTIONS

1. The complex interworkings of the female reproductive system and the coalescing of male factors that are required for fertilization inspire awe that human reproduction works as well as it does. In fact, reproduction is not a model of efficiency; the majority of meetings between an egg and a sperm do not result in the birth of a child. It has been estimated that when sperm does reach the egg in natural reproduction via sexual intercourse, for every 100 eggs only 84 are fertilized, 69 implant, 42 survive the first week of pregnancy, and 31 survive to birth. Thus, even when both the male and the female are physiologically healthy and their relations are accurately timed, they face a 69% likelihood that they will fail to produce a child. Consistent with this figure are studies by embryologists, scientists who study the development of individuals before birth. These studies estimate that at least two-thirds of the products of egg and sperm fusion are in some way defective. If a fertilized egg is defective, generally it will not implant, or if it does implant, it will usually perish very early in development. For a detailed discussion of the processes of reproduction see Lawrence J. Kaplan and Carolyn M. Kaplan, *Natural Reproduction and Reproduction-Aiding Technologies*, in THE ETHICS OF REPRODUCTIVE TECHNOLOGY 15-31 (1992).

2. *A Glossary of Terms and Abbreviations.* The world of ART introduces many medical and scientific terms whose meanings are not generally intuitive and often

appear unaccompanied by further explanation. In addition, writings in the field of reproductive technologies rely on a veritable alphabet soup of abbreviations to shorthand the multi-worded medical techniques and procedures that are used to achieve a pregnancy. Whenever new terms or abbreviations are introduced, definitions and explanations will follow in the notes. For ease of reference, a glossary of terms and abbreviations appear at the end of the book. Do not despair at the number of times you find yourself turning to the glossary.

Thus far we have, or will soon, be introduced to the following terms:

ART Assisted reproductive technologies. A variety of medical procedures in which pregnancy is accomplished by means other than sexual intercourse. ART includes all fertility treatments in which the egg, the sperm, or both, are handled outside the body. The two most common ART procedures are: 1) artificial insemination, in which sperm is introduced into the female reproductive tract using an injection device, and 2) in vitro fertilization (IVF) which involves surgically removing eggs from a woman's ovaries, combining them with sperm in a laboratory, and returning the product of that union to the woman's uterus.

Blastocyst The developing embryo at approximately five days after fertilization. The blastocyst is composed of an inner cell mass and a trophectoderm, which is an outer layer of cells destined to become part of the placenta. The cells from the inner cell mass have the potential to form any cell type of the body and are commonly referred to as embryonic stem cells.

Egg The female sexual cell or gamete from inception until fertilization. Medical literature favors the term "oocyte."[1]

Embryo The developing human organism from approximately 14 days after fertilization of the egg by the sperm until the period when organs and organ systems begin to develop, at approximately the end of the second month.

Fertilization The union of male and female gametes leading to formation of a unique one-cell entity known as a zygote. Fertilization begins with the penetration of the oocyte by the sperm and is completed with the fusion of the male and female pronuclei (nuclear material containing chromosomes). When the pronuclei merge in human fertilization, the zygote contains the number of chromosomes characteristic of the species.

Fetus The developing human organism after the embryonic stage until birth. The fetus is described as the product of conception from approximately the end of the eighth week (or second month) until the moment of birth.

Gamete The oocyte (egg) or the spermatozoon (sperm); a mature reproductive cell which, upon union with another gametic cell, results in the development of a new individual.

Morula The developing human organism from the 16-cell preembryo stage until blastocyst formation; the stage commonly observed between 72-96 hours after

---

[1] One medical author, showing a clear preference for the medically accurate word "oocyte" to describe the female gamete, declared the term "egg" best reserved for the nutritive object often seen on the breakfast table! See Lucinda L. Veeck, AN ATLAS OF HUMAN GAMETES AND CONCEPTUSES 103 (1999).

fertilization.

Preembryo The developing human organism during early cleaving stages, which immediately follow fertilization, until development of the embryo. The preembryonic period immediately follows the zygote stage and ends at approximately 14 days after fertilization with the development of the primitive streak.

Sperm The male sexual cell or gamete, which serves to fertilize the female oocyte (egg). It consists of a head, neck, midpiece and tail. Medical literature uses the term "spermatozoon."

Zygote The one-cell stage of the developing human organism before the first cleavage, usually seen 18-24 hours after the sperm penetrates the egg.

3. Terminology and definitions themselves can be a source of controversy and debate. For example, STEDMAN'S MEDICAL DICTIONARY defines "conception" as "implantation of the blastocyst." This definition means that conception of a human being does not take place until approximately five days after the sperm has penetrated the egg. What are the implications of this medical definition for those who believe that life begins at conception, that is, when fertilization occurs? Would those who hold this view be persuaded that a one-celled zygote is not a life? Should laws that include reference to human conception be held to a medically accurate standard or should legislators be free to enact their own definitions of terms?

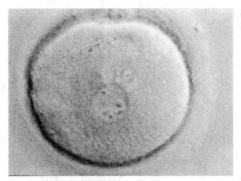

Photograph of a zygote

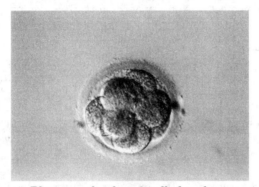

Photograph of an 8-celled embryo

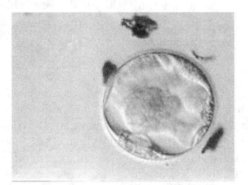

Photograph of a blastocyst

B.   Infertility: When Natural Conception Does Not Occur

Human history and literature is replete with stories of people who wish to have a child but are unable to reproduce naturally. The biblical mention of Rachel's desperate cry to Jacob, "Give me children or else I die" is only one of many tales involving the inability to have a child. Two other oft-told stories include Sarah, Abraham's wife, who is barren until the ripe-old age of 90 when she finally gives birth to Isaac, and Manoah's wife, who is likewise described as barren until she gives birth to Samson.² What these biblical women help us understand is that the inability to have children can be devastating to the individual or couple who suffer the perceived loss of family extension, but the condition need not be permanent.

The inability to conceive or carry a child to term is broadly known as *infertility*. The American Society for Reproductive Medicine (ASRM), a multidisciplinary organization of reproductive medicine professionals founded in 1944, defines infertility as:

> [A] disease of the reproductive system that impairs one of the body's most basic functions: the conception of children. Conception is a complicated process that depends upon many factors: on the production of healthy sperm by the man and healthy eggs by the woman; unblocked fallopian tubes that allow the sperm to reach the egg; the sperm's ability to fertilize the egg when they meet; the ability of the fertilized egg (embryo) to become implanted in the woman's uterus; and sufficient embryo quality.

> Finally, for the pregnancy to continue to full term, the embryo must be healthy and the woman's hormonal environment adequate for its development. When just one of these factors is impaired, infertility can result.

The ASRM defines infertility as the inability to conceive a child, but then expands upon this definition by including the inability to carry an embryo, and then later a fetus, to full term. The medical literature distinguishes between the inability to conceive and the inability to sustain a pregnancy as follows. *Infertility* is the inability to achieve conception. In most studies, infertility is defined as the failure of a couple to achieve pregnancy after one year of unprotected intercourse. More on this later. *Infecundity* is the inability to carry a pregnancy to term. Thus, a woman could suffer from infecundity but not infertility if she were able to become pregnant but suffered repeated miscarriages, or loss of pregnancy. *Sterility* is defined as permanent infertility, usually as a result of surgery which blocks or removes the body parts necessary for the gametes (egg or sperm) to travel and unite, or medical conditions which render essential reproductive body parts or processes incapacitated.

Taken together, the conditions of infertility, infecundity and sterility describe the inability of a woman to produce a child. A man cannot be described as suffering infecundity as men anatomically lack the ability to carry a child to term.³ A man can be diagnosed as infertile or sterile and thus be unable to effect the conception of a child. For the sake of simplicity, begging forgiveness for the slight inaccuracy in usage, hereafter the term infertility will be used to describe the inability of a man or woman to produce a child. That behind us, it is noteworthy that infertility affects men and women in equal proportions. In rough terms, one-third of infertility cases can be attributed to male factors, and one-third are attributable to female factors. For the remaining one-third of infertile couples, infertility is caused by a combina-

---

² These stories can be found respectively in *Genesis 17:17*, and *Judges 13:2, 24* in the King James version of the Bible.

³ Other than in contemporary cinema. Who can forget the image of a pregnant Arnold Schwarzenegger, finding himself in the family way after experimenting with a fertility potion in the 1994 hit comedy *Junior*, complaining to a sympathetic Emma Thompson about his nausea and sensitive nipples.

tion of problems in both partners or, in about 20 percent of cases, is unexplained. See www.asrm.org/awards/index.aspx?id=3012.

1. Defining the Causes of Infertility

Much research has been conducted and is ongoing into the causes of male, female and unexplained infertility. In April 1998, the New York State Task Force on Life and the Law, a state-created organization charged with recommending policy on a host of issues raised by medical advances, issued a report on ART. In its report, the Task Force summarized the available research into the causes of infertility. The following excerpts nicely describe where problems occur in both the female and male reproductive process.

The New York State Task Force on Life and the Law
Assisted Reproductive Technologies: Analysis and Recommendations for Public Policy 8-10
(April 1998)

The Female Reproductive Process — Where Problems Occur

For conception to occur, a woman must have at least one ovary capable of ovulation. Ovulation may not occur if ovaries are missing or damaged, if they never formed properly, if they have stopped responding adequately to hormones as menopause nears, or if hormonal signals are not sufficient, properly timed, or precisely coordinated. In addition, the ability of eggs to be fertilized and develop normally decreases with a woman's age.

At any point from the vagina to the ovaries, barriers may make it difficult or impossible for sperm, eggs, or embryos to pass. At the cervix, the opening from the vagina into the uterus, glands produce mucus that helps healthy sperm pass through. Hormonal or immunological problems may result in too little mucus or mucus with a texture or components that inhibit the passage of sperm. In addition, infection and scarring can block the fallopian tubes and keep the sperm from meeting the egg, or endometriosis[4] may prevent an egg from leaving the ovary or entering the fallopian tube. Blockages that keep the embryo from reaching the uterus can result in an ectopic pregnancy — one that lodges in the fallopian tube or another location outside the uterus.

Many fertilized eggs fail to implant in the uterus. Damage to the uterine lining may limit available sites. Hormones produced by the corpus luteum[5] may be

---

[4] Endometriosis is a condition in which tissue resembling the lining of the uterus occurs aberrantly in the pelvic and abdominal cavity, sometimes binding the reproductive organs and causing infertility. Endometriosis is thought to occur when the tissues that make up the lining of the uterus that are normally shed during a menstrual period, somehow flow back up through the ends of the fallopian tubes and implant in the abdominal and pelvic cavity. See SLOANE-DORLAND ANNOTATED MEDICAL-LEGAL DICTIONARY 217-218 (1992 Supp.) - Ed.

[5] Corpus luteum is the golden-colored body formed in the ovary immediately after ovulation when the ovum (egg) has been discharged from the ovary. The corpus luteum grows for 7 or 8 days, during which time it secretes hormones that are essential for a fertilized egg to develop and attach to the uterus. See

insufficient or improperly timed, leaving the lining unprepared to receive the fertilized egg and sustain the developing embryo. Chemical communications between the embryo and the woman's immune system, needed to allow the embryo to be recognized as a unique type of foreign tissue to be accepted and protected, may be faulty, resulting in a failure to implant or early miscarriage.

The Male Reproductive Process — Where Problems Occur

In a system in which 200 to 500 million sperm are ejaculated for one healthy sperm to fertilize an egg, anything that diminishes the production, delivery, movement, or capacitation of sperm can reduce the chance of pregnancy. In many infertile men, there is no detectable reason for a problem. The problems that are known break down into three broad areas. First, conditions that damage the testes or cells within the seminiferous tubules[6] can lead to the production of insufficient numbers of sperm (oligospermia) or no sperm at all (azoospermia). Second, inadequate or mistimed production of male hormones can result in problems in sperm production or sexual functioning. Third, missing or obstructed conduits at any point along the male genital tract can prevent sperm from being delivered.

---

2.   Defining the Incidence of Infertility

As we shall see, modern medical procedures make it possible for those affected by infertility, infecundity and sterility to have genetic offspring. Through a variety of drug therapies and surgical techniques, as well as the assistance of third parties, many who just a generation ago were diagnosed as unable to produce offspring, can today look to ART to assist in their quest for parenthood. Before journeying into the ways in which technology has aided in reproduction, let us investigate the prevalence of infertility in our country.

In 2005 the Centers for Disease Control and Prevention (CDC), an agency of the U.S. Department of Health and Human Services, issued a report on the status of women's health, including reproductive health. The report was based on a national survey conducted in 2002 by the National Center for Health Statistics. The results of this national survey are contained in the 2002 National Survey of Family Growth (NSFG) and reveal the following statistics.

- In 2002 about 7.4 percent of married women, or 2.1 million married women, were classified as infertile. In the survey, a married or cohabiting couple was defined as infertile if they had not used contraception and not become pregnant for 12 months or more. These figures show a decline from previous years, including 1988 with 2.3 million infertile women and 2.4 million, or 8.4%, in 1982.

- Approximately 61.6 million women of reproductive age (15-44 years) lived in

---

Catherine Parker Anthony & Gary A. Thibodeau, Textbook of Anatomy & Physiology 740-754 (11th ed. 1983) - Ed.

[6] Seminiferous tubules are coiled tubes located within the male testes which are responsible for the production of sperm. Id. At 717-720. - Ed.

the United States in 2002. Of this group, 12 percent (7.3 million) had used some kind of infertility service in their lifetime, compared with 16 percent (9.3 million) in 1995. Infertility services included medical advice, tests, drugs, surgery, or other treatments to get pregnant and to prevent miscarriage.

- Among childless women ages 35 to 39, 15 percent had received infertility services at some time in their lives, compared with 29 percent of childless women ages 40-44. Among all women of reproductive age, 2 percent (1.2 million) had an infertility-related medical appointment within the previous year and a total of 12 percent had received infertility treatment at some time in their lives.

- Infertility is higher among married couples where the wife is non-white. The incidence of infertility is highest, 27.7 percent, among childless married women categorized as "Black or African American, single race," compared with 24.3 percent of Hispanic or Latina women, and 15.9 percent of white, single race women.

- Infertility rates rise with age. The incidence of infertility is 6.3 percent among women 15-29 years, 8.1 percent among women 30-34 years and 9.4 percent among women 40-44 years. Interestingly, fertility improved in ages 35-39 with only 5.7 percent of married women experiencing infertility.

Table 1 contains the data on infertility collected by the 2002 National Survey of Family Growth. A draft of the full NSFG Report can be accessed at http://www.cdc.gov/nchs/data/series/sr_23/sr23_025.pdf.

NOTES AND QUESTIONS

1. *Defining Infertility.* Note that the NSFG adopts the common medical definition of infertility, placing the boundary between normal and abnormal fertility at one year of regular intercourse without contraceptives. This definition is not uniformly adopted by all health professionals. The World Health Organization, for example, expands the time frame to two years, suggesting that the criteria for determining infertility are not definitive. While we may jest that a woman cannot be "a little bit pregnant," apparently distinguishing between being fertile and infertile is far more difficult. One further study from the U.S. Office of Technology Assessment (OTA) supports the uncertainty in making a definitive infertility diagnosis. This OTA study found that only 16-21 percent of couples who are deemed infertile by the one-year definition will remain infertile throughout their lives.

Is it important to establish a definitive definition of infertility? If so, should such a definition focus on the lifelong inability to conceive and carry a pregnancy or should it be limited, as it currently seems to be, to discrete and measurable periods of time? What useful purpose does a uniform definition of infertility serve? Imagine, for comparison, the difficulties many individuals would have gaining access to health care if doctors were able to create their own definitions of illness.

Notice that the NSFG report looks only at infertility status among married women. For this reason alone, the report may underestimate the incidence of infertility in the U.S. because it excludes unmarried persons, including unmarried heterosexual couples, single women, single men, and same-sex couples[7] who are unable to naturally conceive and bear children. Reproduction among these latter groups of single individuals and same-sex couples is, of course, physiologically impossible without the aid of a gamete donor (egg donor for single and same-sex males, sperm donor for single and same-sex females), and in some cases a gestational carrier (woman who agrees to carry a child in her uterus to term), in the case of single and same-sex couple males.

Should data on infertility include the experience of individuals who have pursued pregnancy and childbirth in a non-traditional manner? If so, would the commonly accepted definition of infertility have to be modified since it is based on conception following regular sexual intercourse (presumably referring to intercourse between a man and a woman)? Perhaps a more inclusive definition of infertility would focus on individuals who have attempted and failed for one year to conceive by any means. While this modification may not drastically change the reported incidence of infertility in this country, information about the marital status and sexual orientation of those seeking infertility services may enlighten us as to changes and trends in the family structure.

At least one state lawmaker has considered broadening the definition of infertility to include "social" as well as "medical" infertility. In February 2011, Assembly Member Felipe Fuentes of California introduced a bill that would have expanded the definition of infertility for purposes of state health insurance coverage to include "[t]he desire to achieve pregnancy by means other than sexual intercourse." The bill, AB 1217, was amended shortly after it was introduced to exclude this expansive language.

2. *A Few Observations about the 2002 NSFG Report.* The NSFG data does provide some glimpse into the reproductive efforts of unmarried women. The report breaks down the percentage of childless women who have sought fertility services into to three marital status categories — married (23.8 percent), cohabitating (5.8 percent) and neither (2.5 percent). Recognizing and reporting that unmarried coupled and single women access assistance in reproduction reflect the growing percentage of U.S. infants who are born to unmarried women. According to the CDC, 41% of all births in 2008 were to unmarried women compared to 36% in 2002.

Finally, the NSFG report could be criticized for overestimating the incidence of infertility among married couples. The survey was based on in-home, in-person interviews with more than 12,000 respondents — 7,500 females and 5,000 males. The surveyor asked questions about contraception and pregnancy, but did not query interviewees about the regularity of their sexual relations. A woman was classified as infertile if she did not use contraception and did not become pregnant for 12 months or more. There is, of course, another key ingredient to this calculus, the romance. NSFG researchers, it seems, assume that married couples were having

---

[7] Today in the U.S. same-sex couples can no longer be automatically classified as "unmarried." According to the National Conference of State Legislatures, as of January 2013 a total of ten jurisdictions issue marriage licenses to same-sex couples (Connecticut, District of Columbia, Iowa, Maine, Maryland, Massachusetts, New Hampshire, New York, Vermont and Washington). The issue of ART and same-sex parenting is discussed in Chapter 5.

regular sex. This assumption is made explicitly in the previous NSFG study, published in 1997 in which surveyors measured infertility only for married couples because "the concept assumes continuous exposure to intercourse . . . which can be assumed only of currently married women."[8] Really? The problem with this assumption of "continuous exposure to intercourse" for married couples, is that if the interviewee fails to report months in which intercourse did not occur, or occurred very infrequently, a couple may be classified as infertile when they are not. A cover story appearing in Newsweek Magazine cites estimates by psychologists that 15 to 20 percent of married couples have sex no more than 10 times a year, which is how experts define sexless marriage. See Kathleen Deveny, *We're Not In The Mood*, Newsweek 41, 42 (June 30, 2003). Of course, most of the couples interviewed for the article already had children, raising interesting questions about the relationship between fertility and romance.

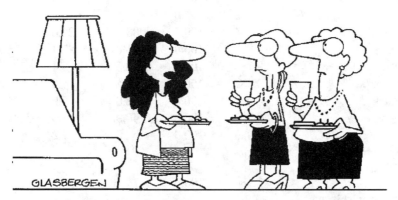

Copyright 1996 by Randy Glasbergen.
www.glasbergen.com

"My husband and I had to try 70 times before I got pregnant —that was one weekend I'll never forget!"

---

[8] For this proposition, the survey authors cite W.D. Mosher and W.F. Pratt, *Fecundity and Infertility in the United States, 1965-88*, Advance Data 192 (1990):1, 5. Do you agree that "continuous exposure to intercourse" can be assumed only of currently married women? Perhaps the authors would plumb a different source today, seeking the truth behind the glamorous portrayal of single life in HBO's wildly popular series, *Sex and the City* (1998-2004). Though Carrie, Miranda, Charlotte and especially Samantha seem to be the poster gals for "continuous exposure," in truth research consistently shows that married people engage in sexual activity more often than their non-married counterparts. In a report sponsored by the prestigious National Opinion Research Center at the University of Chicago, researchers reveal that sexual activity is 25-300% greater among married individuals compared to non-married individuals at various ages. See Tom W. Smith, American Sexual Behavior: Trends, Socio-Demographic Differences, and Risk Behavior 10 (April 2003).

Table 1. Number of married women 15-44 years of age and percent distribution by infertility status, according to selected characteristics: United States, 2002

Characteristic	Number in thousands	Total	Surgically sterile	Infertile	Fecund[*]
			Percent Distribution		
All women	28,327	100.0	34.8	7.4	57.8
Age					
15-29 years	7,246	100.0	12.2	6.3	81.5
30-34 years	6,351	100.0	26.0	8.1	65.9
35-39 years	6,989	100.0	45.6	5.7	48.7
40-44 years	7,740	100.0	53.4	9.4	37.3
Parity and Age[**]					
0 Births	5,142	100.0	9.1	16.6	74.3
15-29 years	2,364	100.0	1.6	11.0	87.4
30-34 years	1,279	100.0	2.4	16.9	80.7
35-39 years	684	100.0	33.1	22.6	44.3
40-44 years	815	100.0	21.0	27.4	51.5
1 or more births	23,185	100.0	40.5	5.4	54.2
15-29 years	4,882	100.0	17.4	4.0	78.6
30-34 years	5,072	100.0	32.0	5.9	62.1
35-39 years	6,305	100.0	46.9	3.9	49.2
40-44 years	6,925	100.0	57.2	7.2	35.6
Medical help to become pregnant					
Yes, at least once in last year	1,180	100.0	14.2	30.5	55.3
Yes, but not within last year	4,331	100.0	33.4	14.0	52.6
No	22,636	100.0	36.1	4.9	58.9
Education					
No high school diploma or GED	2,764	100.0	44.1	10.4	45.5
High school diploma or GED	6,092	100.0	44.0	6.5	49.5
Some college, no bachelor's degree . . .	8,189	100.0	37.9	6.6	55.5
Bachelor's degree or higher	8,521	100.0	23.0	8.4	68.6
Hispanic origin and race					
Hispanic or Latina . .	4,136	100.0	34.5	7.7	55.1
Non-Hispanic white, single race	20,061	100.0	35.1	7.0	57.9
Black or African American, single race	2,133	100.0	44.2	11.5	44.3

[*] Fecund refers to being fertile or capable of conceiving and bearing children - Ed.

[**] Parity refers to the state of having given birth - Ed.

NOTE: Percents may not add to 100 due to rounding.
Source: U.S. Department of Health and Human Services, Centers for Disease Control and
Prevention, National Center for Health Statistics: Fertility, Family Planning, and Women's Health:
New Data From the 2002 National Survey of Family Growth; Series 23, No. 25, p. 108.

2.   The term "infertility" can be seen as a medical diagnosis that follows from a
specific clinical observation — the failure to conceive after one year of unprotected
intercourse. Major health organizations that track women's health define infertility
as a disease, including the World Health Organization, the American Society for
Reproductive Medicine and the American College of Obstetrics and Gynecology.
But is the medicalization of the ability to bear a child a good thing for the infertile?
For the practice of medicine? For society? As you might imagine, there are several
views on the medicalization of infertility. Those in favor of defining infertility as a
medical condition are probably best represented by RESOLVE, a national support
and advocacy organization for the infertile founded in 1974. RESOLVE has argued
in a variety of forums, including state legislatures, that infertility is and therefore
should be addressed as a medical condition. Briefly stated, RESOLVE's goals are
twofold. First, defining infertility as a medical condition is fundamental to their goal
of mandatory insurance coverage. If state legislators can be convinced that
infertility is a medical problem with medical solutions then they may be more likely
to compel insurers to cover non-experimental treatments for the condition. Insurance coverage for infertility treatment is discussed in Chapter 3.

Second, advocates in RESOLVE hope that by deeming infertility a medical
condition, some of the blame (usually directed toward women) and stigma associated with infertility would be reduced. If we begin to view infertility as a strictly
medical condition solvable only by serious professional attention, we may ultimately
be willing to direct more resources toward its cure.

A counterbalancing view on the medicalization of infertility can be found in a
thoughtful book by Elizabeth Britt titled CONCEIVING NORMALCY. Professor Britt
argues that societal views of "involuntary childlessness," a term she prefers to the
medicalized "infertility," have become too focused on the physiological aspects of the
inability to have biological children. This focus, she urges, results in the categorization of women into groupings of *fertile* and *infertile*, which themselves create
perceptions of normalcy and abnormalcy. She continues:

> While the condition of being unable to have a biological child is often
> discussed as having social or cultural implications, it is nonetheless
> understood primarily as a medical condition with medical solutions. This
> medicalization of involuntary childlessness glosses over the complex cul-
> tural contexts within which the condition occurs and assumes its signifi-
> cance. In this sense, "infertility" may be understood as a metonym for the
> experience of involuntary childlessness. Kenneth Burke understands me-
> tonymy as a figure that reduces complexity by conveying "some incorporeal
> or intangible state in terms of the corporeal or tangible". The metonymic
> reduction of "involuntary childlessness" to "infertility" gives the condition
> a physical location in the body, where it can be investigated and treated.
> The reduction also temporalizes the experience so that social, economic,
> psychological, and cultural "factors" are understood as *implications* that

result from or *come after* the physical condition, not as conditions that are complicit in its construction. (*Italics* in the original).

ELIZABETH C. BRITT, CONCEIVING NORMALCY 6 (2001). Professor Britt discusses the broad implications of involuntary childlessness in today's society. What about the condition of voluntary childlessness? Should an individual or couple who chooses, for whatever reason, to remain childless be considered from a sociological or cultural perspective to be "abnormal"? How about from a legal perspective? Consider the following.

SECTION II: JUDICIAL PERSPECTIVES ON THE MODERN ROLE OF REPRODUCTION

A. An Introductory Case

BRAGDON v. ABBOTT
Supreme Court of the United States
524 U.S. 624 (1998)

JUSTICE KENNEDY delivered the opinion of the Court.

We address in this case the application of the Americans with Disabilities Act of 1990 (ADA), 104 Stat. 327, 42 U.S.C. § 12101 et seq., to persons infected with the human immunodeficiency virus (HIV). We granted certiorari to review, first, whether HIV infection is a disability under the ADA when the infection has not yet progressed to the so-called symptomatic phase . . .

I

Respondent Sidney Abbott (hereinafter respondent) has been infected with HIV since 1986. When the incidents we recite occurred, her infection had not manifested its most serious symptoms. On September 16, 1994, she went to the office of petitioner Randon Bragdon in Bangor, Maine, for a dental appointment. She disclosed her HIV infection on the patient registration form. Petitioner completed a dental examination, discovered a cavity, and informed respondent of his policy against filling cavities of HIV-infected patients. He offered to perform the work at a hospital with no added fee for his services, though respondent would be responsible for the cost of using the hospital's facilities. Respondent declined.

Respondent sued petitioner under state law and § 302 of the ADA, 104 Stat. 355, 42 U.S.C. § 12182, alleging discrimination on the basis of her disability. The state-law claims are not before us. Section 302 of the ADA provides:

> No individual shall be discriminated against on the basis of disability in the full and equal enjoyment of the goods, services, facilities, privileges, advantages, or accommodations of any place of public accommodation by any person who . . . operates a place of public accommodation. § 12182(a).

The term "public accommodation" is defined to include the "professional office of a health care provider." § 12181(7)(F) . . .

The District Court ruled in favor of the plaintiffs, holding that respondent's HIV infection satisfied the ADA's definition of disability. 912 F.Supp. 580, 585-587 (D.Me.1995) . . . The Court of Appeals affirmed. It held respondent's HIV infection was a disability under the ADA, even though her infection had not yet progressed to the symptomatic stage. 107 F.3d 934, 939-943 (C.A.1 1997). . . .

II

We first review the ruling that respondent's HIV infection constituted a disability under the ADA. The statute defines disability as:

(A) a physical or mental impairment that substantially limits one or more of the major life activities of such individual;

(B) a record of such an impairment; or

(C) being regarded as having such an impairment. § 12102(2).

We hold respondent's HIV infection was a disability under subsection (A) of the definitional section of the statute. In light of this conclusion, we need not consider the applicability of subsections (B) or (C).

Our consideration of subsection (A) of the definition proceeds in three steps. First, we consider whether respondent's HIV infection was a physical impairment. Second, we identify the life activity upon which respondent relies (reproduction and childbearing) and determine whether it constitutes a major life activity under the ADA. Third, tying the two statutory phrases together, we ask whether the impairment substantially limited the major life activity. In construing the statute, we are informed by interpretations of parallel definitions in previous statutes and the views of various administrative agencies which have faced this interpretive question.

A

1

. . . The first step in the inquiry under subsection (A) requires us to determine whether respondent's condition constituted a physical impairment. [The Court reviewed the natural history of HIV from acute, or initial, infection to the end stages of disease.] . . . In light of the immediacy with which the virus begins to damage the infected person's white blood cells and the severity of the disease, we hold it is an impairment from the moment of infection. As noted earlier, infection with HIV causes immediate abnormalities in a person's blood, and the infected person's white cell count continues to drop throughout the course of the disease, even when the attack is concentrated in the lymph nodes. In light of these facts, HIV infection must be regarded as a physiological disorder with a constant and detrimental effect on the infected person's hemic and lymphatic systems from the moment of infection. HIV infection satisfies the statutory and regulatory definition of a physical impairment during every stage of the disease.

2

The statute is not operative, and the definition not satisfied, unless the impairment affects a major life activity. Respondent's claim throughout this case has been that the HIV infection placed a substantial limitation on her ability to reproduce and to bear children. App. 14; 912 F. Supp., at 586, 107 F.3d, at 939. Given the pervasive, and invariably fatal, course of the disease, its effect on major life activities of many sorts might have been relevant to our inquiry. Respondent and a number of amici make arguments about HIV's profound impact on almost every phase of the infected person's life. See Brief for Respondent Abbott 24-27; Brief for American Medical Association as Amicus Curiae 20; Brief for Infectious Diseases Society of America et al. as Amici Curiae 7-11. In light of these submissions, it may seem legalistic to circumscribe our discussion to the activity of reproduction. We have little doubt that had different parties brought the suit they would have maintained that an HIV infection imposes substantial limitations on other major life activities.

From the outset, however, the case has been treated as one in which reproduction was the major life activity limited by the impairment. It is our practice to decide cases on the grounds raised and considered in the Court of Appeals and included in the question on which we granted certiorari. See, e.g., *Blessing v. Freestone*, 520 U.S. 329, 340, n. 3, 117 S.Ct. 1353, 1359, n. 3, 137 L.Ed.2d 569 (1997) (citing this Court's Rule 14.1(a)); *Capitol Square Review and Advisory Bd. v. Pinette*, 515 U.S. 753, 760, 115 S.Ct. 2440, 2445-2446, 132 L.Ed.2d 650 (1995). We ask, then, whether reproduction is a major life activity.

We have little difficulty concluding that it is. As the Court of Appeals held, "[t]he plain meaning of the word 'major' denotes comparative importance" and "suggest[s] that the touchstone for determining an activity's inclusion under the statutory rubric is its significance." 107 F.3d, at 939, 940. Reproduction falls well within the phrase "major life activity." Reproduction and the sexual dynamics surrounding it are central to the life process itself.

While petitioner concedes the importance of reproduction, he claims that Congress intended the ADA only to cover those aspects of a person's life which have a public, economic, or daily character. Brief for Petitioner 14, 28, 30, 31; see also id., at 36-37 (citing *Krauel v. Iowa Methodist Medical Center*, 95 F.3d 674, 677 (C.A.8 1996)). The argument founders on the statutory language. Nothing in the definition suggests that activities without a public, economic, or daily dimension may somehow be regarded as so unimportant or insignificant as to fall outside the meaning of the word "major." The breadth of the term confounds the attempt to limit its construction in this manner.

As we have noted, the ADA must be construed to be consistent with regulations issued to implement the Rehabilitation Act. See 42 U.S.C. § 12201(a). Rather than enunciating a general principle for determining what is and is not a major life activity, the Rehabilitation Act regulations instead provide a representative list, defining the term to include "functions such as caring for one's self, performing manual tasks, walking, seeing, hearing, speaking, breathing, learning, and working." 45 CFR § 84.3(j)(2)(ii) (1997); 28 CFR § 41.31(b)(2) (1997). As the use of the term "such as" confirms, the list is illustrative, not exhaustive.

These regulations are contrary to petitioner's attempt to limit the meaning of the term "major" to public activities. The inclusion of activities such as caring for one's self and performing manual tasks belies the suggestion that a task must have a public or economic character in order to be a major life activity for purposes of the ADA. On the contrary, the Rehabilitation Act regulations support the inclusion of reproduction as a major life activity, since reproduction could not be regarded as any less important than working and learning. Petitioner advances no credible basis for confining major life activities to those with a public, economic, or daily aspect. In the absence of any reason to reach a contrary conclusion, we agree with the Court of Appeals' determination that reproduction is a major life activity for the purposes of the ADA.

The determination of the Court of Appeals that respondent's HIV infection was a disability under the ADA is affirmed.

[The concurring opinion by Justice Stevens, joined by Justice Breyer, and the concurring opinion by Justice Ginsburg, are omitted.]

CHIEF JUSTICE REHNQUIST, joined by JUSTICE SCALIA and JUSTICE THOMAS, dissenting . . .

. . . [T]he Court is simply wrong in concluding as a general matter that reproduction is a "major life activity." Unfortunately, the ADA does not define the phrase "major life activities." But the Act does incorporate by reference a list of such activities contained in regulations issued under the Rehabilitation Act. 42 U.S.C. § 12201(a); 45 CFR § 84.3(j)(2)(ii) (1997). The Court correctly recognizes that this list of major life activities "is illustrative, not exhaustive," . . . but then makes no attempt to demonstrate that reproduction is a major life activity in the same sense that "caring for one's self, performing manual tasks, walking, seeing, hearing, speaking, breathing, learning, and working" are . . .

Instead, the Court argues that reproduction is a "major" life activity in that it is "central to the life process itself." . . . In support of this reading, the Court focuses on the fact that " 'major' " indicates " 'comparative importance,' " . . . ; see also Webster's Collegiate Dictionary 702 (10th ed. 1994) ("greater in dignity, rank, importance, or interest"), ignoring the alternative definition of "major" as "greater in quantity, number, or extent," . . . It is the latter definition that is most consistent with the ADA's illustrative list of major life activities.

No one can deny that reproductive decisions are important in a person's life. But so are decisions as to who to marry, where to live, and how to earn one's living. Fundamental importance of this sort is not the common thread linking the statute's listed activities. The common thread is rather that the activities are repetitively performed and essential in the day-to-day existence of a normally functioning individual. They are thus quite different from the series of activities leading to the birth of a child. Both respondent, Brief for Respondent Abbott 20, n. 24, and the Government Brief for United States as Amicus Curiae 13, argue that reproduction must be a major life activity because regulations issued under the ADA define the term "physical impairment" to include physiological disorders affecting the reproductive system. 28 CFR § 36.104 (1997). If reproduction were not a major life activity, they argue, then it would have made little sense to include the reproductive disorders in the roster of physical impairments. This argument is simply wrong. There are numerous disorders of the reproductive system, such as dysmenorrhea and endometriosis, which are so painful that they limit a woman's ability to engage in major life activities such as walking and working. And, obviously, cancer of the various reproductive organs limits one's ability to engage in numerous activities other than reproduction.

But even if I were to assume that reproduction is a major life activity of respondent, I do not agree that an asymptomatic HIV infection "substantially limits" that activity. The record before us leaves no doubt that those so infected are still entirely able to engage in sexual intercourse, give birth to a child if they become pregnant, and perform the manual tasks necessary to rear a child to maturity. See App. 53-54. While individuals infected with HIV may choose not to engage in these activities, there is no support in language, logic, or our case law for the proposition that such voluntary choices constitute a "limit" on one's own life activities.

The Court responds that the ADA "addresses substantial limitations on major life activities, not utter inabilities." . . . I agree, but fail to see how this assists the Court's cause. Apart from being unable to demonstrate that she is utterly unable to engage in the various activities that comprise the reproductive process, respondent has not even explained how she is less able to engage in those activities. Respondent contends that her ability to reproduce is limited because "the fatal nature of HIV infection means that a parent is unlikely to live long enough to raise and nurture the child to adulthood." Brief for Respondent Abbott 22. But the ADA's definition of a disability is met only if the alleged impairment substantially "limits" (present tense) a major life activity. 42 U.S.C. § 12102(2)(A). Asymptomatic HIV does not presently limit respondent's ability to perform any of the tasks necessary to bear or raise a child. Respondent's argument, taken to its logical extreme, would render every individual with a genetic marker for some debilitating disease "disabled" here and now because of some possible future effects.

In my view, therefore, respondent has failed to demonstrate that any of her major life activities were substantially limited by her HIV infection.

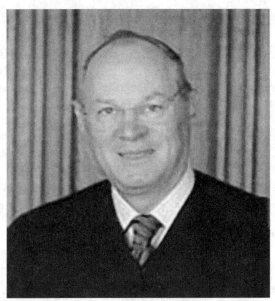

JUSTICE ANTHONY M. KENNEDY

NOTES AND QUESTIONS

1. The decision in *Bragdon v. Abbott* inspired numerous commentaries from legal scholars focusing on various aspects of the high court's decision, including the determination that reproduction is a major life activity for purposes of the Americans With Disabilities Act. A sampling of the commentaries that focus on whether the inability to reproduce naturally, i.e. infertility, should be considered a disability under the ADA include Shorge Sato, Note, *A Little Bit Disabled: Infertility and the Americans With Disabilities Act,* 5 N.Y.U. J. LEGIS. & PUB. POL'Y 189 (2001); Thomas D. Flanigan, *Assisted Reproductive Technologies and Insurance Under the Americans With Disabilities Act of 1990,* 38 BRANDEIS L.J. 777 (2000); Samuel R. Bagenstos, *Subordination, Stigma, and "Disability,"* 86 Va. L. Rev. 397 (2000); Peter K. Rydel, Comment, *Redefining the Right to Reproduce: Asserting Infertility as a Disability Under the Americans With Disabilities Act,* 63 ALB. L. REV. 593 (1999).

In 2008, Congress amended the ADA, effectively ending the debate over whether federal law regards infertility as a disability. The updated law defines "disability" as "a physical or mental impairment that substantially limits one or more major life activities," further specifying that a "major life activity also includes the operation of a major bodily function, including but not limited to . . . reproductive functions." 42 U.S.C. § 12102 (2008).

2. *Infertility and Stigma.* Professor Bagenstos, in his article cited in Note 1, suggests that the Court in *Bragdon v. Abbott* was correct in its result, but somewhat amiss in its reasoning. He proposes a method of assessing "disability" on the basis of social stigma and deprivation of opportunity, rather than strictly on a finding of "a physical or mental impairment that substantially limits one or more of the major

life activities of such individual" that the ADA employs. In the case of infertility, he observes:

> People who cannot have children suffer some degree of social stigma: Consider the shame historically attached to being labeled a "barren woman" or a man who could not pass on his name. And although a woman with HIV can reproduce, she can only do so by exposing her sexual partner and potential child to a deadly, progressively debilitating disease. Exposing others to a dread disease is itself widely stigmatized, and exposing one's unborn child to such a disease particularly so. Thus, while the Chief Justice was correct that no physical obstacles prevented Sydney Abbott from having a child or made it more difficult for her to do so, and a "truly disabled" approach would find no disabling limitation in reproduction, Abbott was "substantially limited" in the ability to reproduce. She could have a child, but only under a condition that itself would have subjected her to stigma. 86 Va. L. Rev. 486-491 (Citations omitted).

Under Professor Bagenstos' analysis, an HIV-positive individual would always be considered disabled because any attempt to reproduce would expose a partner or potential child to grave danger, thus engendering enormous stigma. In the years since *Bradgon* was decided, treatment for HIV has improved dramatically, so much so that Justice Kennedy may not have linked asymptomatic infection with reproductive impairment. Today, if an HIV-infected pregnant woman is treated with a drug regimen, she poses almost no risk of vertically transmitting the virus to her newborn. In 2005, the CDC reported that current therapies reduce the risk of mother to child transmission to less than two percent. Does this updated medical information call into question the Court's holding in *Bragdon*?

Professor Bagenstos also argues that an infertile HIV-negative individual could be considered disabled under a stigma approach, depending on the measures that are necessary to overcome the inability to reproduce. If a person's inability to conceive could be remedied quickly, for example by a single medical intervention involving little time and expense, then that individual would suffer little stigma and may not be considered disabled. If, on the other hand, a person expended significant sources of time and money in order to overcome infertility, such individual might be socially disadvantaged or stigmatized (by lost wages or loss of a job, for example) and thus be considered disabled.

Professor David Orentlicher voices a different take on the matter of infertility and stigma. He posits that, while as a historical matter, infertility has been considered a disability that confers disfavored status in society, recent changes in socioeconomic conditions have made procreation less desirable, thus reducing the stigma surrounding involuntary childlessness. "Infertility," he writes, "has become less stigmatized, and even seen by some as conferring protection from the disabling consequences of parenthood." David Orentlicher, *Discrimination Out of Dismissiveness: The Example of Infertility*, 85 IND. L. J. 143, 153 (2010).

3. Should the inability to conceive and bear a child through unprotected intercourse be considered a disability? That is, if the natural state of being infertile could be corrected through medical intervention, should the condition of being infertile still be regarded as a disability? The Supreme Court did not answer that

question in *Bragdon,* but it gave guidance as to how it might resolve that issue in a case decided the following court term. In *Sutton v. United Air Lines,* 527 U.S. 471 (1999), two sisters with severe myopia (nearsightedness), were denied positions as airline pilots based on their failure to meet minimum uncorrected vision requirements. With corrective lenses, each sister had vision that was 20/20 or better, but in their uncorrected state they were visually impaired. The sisters sued under the ADA, claiming discrimination on the basis of their "disability." Justice O'Connor, writing for the Court, said that the determination of whether an individual is disabled should be made with reference to measures, such as corrective lenses in the case of the sisters, that mitigate the individual's impairment. Since the sisters' vision impairment is mitigated by corrective measures, they are not regarded as disabled under the ADA.

In the context of infertility, the decision in *Sutton* could be interpreted to mean that a person who meets the clinical definition of infertile (i.e., failure to conceive after one year of unprotected intercourse) could only be regarded as disabled if corrective measures failed to reverse the impairment. In the case of vision impairment, the concept of "corrective measures" is fairly simple. Most people with vision impairment can achieve improved vision with corrective lenses (eyeglasses or contact lenses) and increasingly via laser surgery. But mitigation in the case of infertility is far more complicated. Instead of two or three, there are dozens of potential treatments to help a person have a biological child. These treatments often involve invasive surgical procedures costing tens of thousands of dollars. Moreover, as we shall see, many of these techniques are successful in only about one-third of cases. Should someone seeking the protections of the ADA be required to pursue all possible corrective measures before being considered disabled? Ironically, a person undergoing infertility treatment may face a job loss due to time away from work and at the same time fail to qualify as disabled because a court considers her impairment to be correctable.

4.   The designation of infertility as a medical condition or physical impairment has implications beyond federal disability law. For example, the question of whether infertility is an illness often arises in the context of health insurance contracts and reimbursement. We consider the issue of infertility and insurance in Chapter 3, but by way of introduction it may come as no surprise that courts differ on the question of whether a person who is unable to conceive naturally is considered to have an illness for purposes of insurance contract benefits.[9] The answer often rests on specific contract language. Compare *Egert v. Connecticut General Life Insurance Company,* 900 F.2d 1032 (7th Cir. 1990) (court rejects insurance company's claim that it does not consider infertility to be an illness or sickness where internal company memoranda refer expressly to the "illness of infertility"; company ordered to reimburse insured for infertility treatments) with *Kinzie v. Physician's Liability*

---

[9]   Distinguished members of the legislature likewise differ on the topic. In January 2005, Representative Casey Crane, a female member of the New Hampshire legislature, introduced a bill that would require health insurers to cover fertility treatments. Her colleague, Rep. Joseph Miller, a retired physician, chided Rep. Crane for believing that "every woman has a God-given right to get pregnant. These are assumptions you have made by coming here, which I don't think are accurate." *New Hampshire Bill Would Bar Arbitrary Denial of Fertility Treatments,* Health & Medicine Week, Jan. 31, 2005, at 1408. What God not giveth, the legislature not taketh away?

Insurance Company, 750 P.2d 1140 (Ok. Civ. App. 1987) (while plaintiff's infertility was considered a medical condition, she was still denied insurance coverage for treatment because conceiving a child was not considered medically necessary to the physical health of the insured).

SECTION III: ASSISTED CONCEPTION

Armed with a basic background in natural conception and the incidence of infertility, we can proceed to study the ways in which physicians and scientists have sought to assist infertile individuals in their quest to have children. From our early twenty-first century perspective, it appears that much of the progress in the field of ART has occurred in the past quarter-century, but in fact human curiosity and exploration surrounding reproduction dates back to the earliest periods of recorded history.

A.   A Brief History of ART

1.   The Earliest Years

The awareness of infertility as a treatable condition can be traced back to the fifth century B.C. writings of Hippocrates, a Greek physician regarded as the Father of Medicine. Hippocrates, who lived from 460 to 377 B.C., was very familiar with the problem of infertility and had a number of recipes inspired by the Egyptians to diagnose and treat it. One such recipe combined red nitre, cumin, resin and honey, used to open a woman's cervix that was thought to be "closed too tightly." Eight hundred years later, third century A.D. records show that Jewish thinkers discussed the possibility of human insemination by artificial means. Such references appear in the Talmud, a collection of Jewish law, which discusses the legal position of women who achieve pregnancy without physical contact. For the next millennium physicians postulated about the causes and cures for infertility, instituting treatments that may strike the modern mind as downright hilarious. During the Middle Ages, infertile men were prescribed a steady diet of testicles and livers from young stags, while women were diagnosed as infertile if their breath failed to display a garlicky odor after cloves of garlic were placed in their vagina.

A major breakthrough in medicine generally came in the mid-1600s with the invention of the microscope by Dutch scientist Antonie van Leeuwenhoek (1632-1723). In 1677, Leeuwenhoek observed his own sperm under the microscope, an experiment he "performed without defiling" himself, according to a letter he wrote reporting his findings to the Royal Society of England. In the letter, Leeuwenhoek described the microscopic sperm as a multitude of "animalcules," less than a millionth the size of a coarse grain of sand and with thin, undulating transparent tails. His colleague, Dutch mathematics and physics professor Nicolas Hartsoeker likewise observed the tiny, fast-moving structures, declaring that each sperm contained an already formed human. A 1692 drawing by Hartsoeker showing a perfectly formed little person contained in the head of a single sperm earned him the designation as a "preformationist," or those who believed that sperm contained "preformed" miniature people. *See* Robert Winston, *Playing God?*, 426 NATURE 603 (2003). Though the concept of preformation dates back to Aristotle, it withered as an explanation for reproduction as the eighteenth century dawned.

Armed with the ability to visualize sperm, scientists began to understand its role in the fertilization of the egg inside the body. In 1780, Italian priest and scientist, Lazzaro Spallanzani (1729-1799) developed the technique of artificial insemination in dogs. Spallanzani understood that the male ejaculate contained semen which carried the sperm; he further realized that the process of reproduction required that the sperm-carrying semen unite with the egg inside the body. He used this knowledge to inject sperm-carrying semen into the female canine reproductive tract, producing the earliest mammalian births by artificial insemination. Only a few years passed before this technique was used successfully in humans.

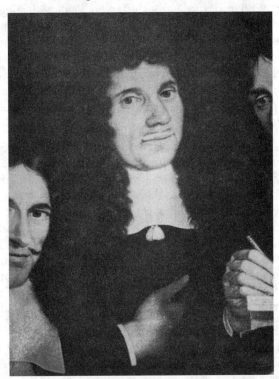

**Portrait of Antonie van Leeuwenhoek
by Cornelis de Man**

2. Human Artificial Insemination

In 1785 the first attempts at human artificial insemination were made by Scottish surgeon John Hunter (1728-1793).[10] In the late 1770s Dr. Hunter was approached by a London cloth merchant who suffered from hypospadia, a developmental

---

[10] John Hunter was a surgeon and founder of the field of pathological anatomy in England. He trained at Chelsea Hospital, became master of anatomy at Surgeon's Hall in 1753, and was elected surgeon at St. George's in 1758. Dr. Hunter was commissioned as an army surgeon in 1760 and became physician extraordinary to King George III in 1776 (one wonders what remedy he prescribed for King George's enormous headache brought on by those revolutionaries across the pond). Dr. Hunter's work relied heavily on investigation and experimentation. Rumor has it he even went so far as to infect himself

anomaly in which the opening of the penis is too low, thus inhibiting the projection of semen into the vagina. Dr. Hunter suggested that he collect the patient's sperm and inject it into his wife's vagina using a warm syringe. In 1785 Dr. Hunter's efforts to separate sexual intercourse and reproduction proved successful as the first child conceived through artificial insemination was born. Technically speaking, this eighteenth-century child's birth marks the beginning of the field of assisted reproductive technologies (ART), known modernly as the science of achieving a pregnancy by means other than sexual intercourse.

Despite Dr. Hunter's advancement in infertility treatment, medical journals were bereft of information about advances in artificial insemination for the next 100 years. In 1884 Dr. William Pancoast of Jefferson Medical College in Philadelphia published the first report of artificial insemination in a modern medical journal. What differentiated Dr. Pancoast's accomplishment from that of his predecessor Dr. Hunter was the source of the donor. Instead of using the woman's husband's sperm, Dr. Pancoast relied on a "donor," a man unrelated to the woman patient who produced his sperm to help her achieve pregnancy. The circumstances surrounding Dr. Pancoast's experiment are worthy of inclusion, leaving much for the modern medical ethicist to ponder.

Apparently the story begins with a wealthy merchant who complained to Dr. Pancoast of his inability to procreate. The good doctor took this as a golden opportunity to try out a new procedure. The couple was summoned to the doctor's medical facility. At some point during the visit, the patient's wife was anaesthetized. Before an audience of medical students, the doctor inseminated the woman using semen obtained from the "best looking member of the class." Nine months later, a child was born. The mother is reputed to have gone to her grave none the wiser as to the manner of her son's provenance. The husband was informed and was reputedly delighted. The son discovered his novel history at the age of 25 when enlightened by a former medical student who had been present at his conception. *See* A.D. Hard, *Artificial Impregnation*, 27 MEDICAL WORLD 163 (1909).

The technique of artificial insemination by donor (AID) grew in use and success over the next 50 years, with multipatient studies reporting promising results appearing in medical journals in the mid-1950s. AID gained popularity and practicality following reports of pregnancies using stored frozen semen in 1953. *See* R. Bunge & J. Sherman, *Fertilizing Capacity of Frozen Human Spermatazoa*, 172 NATURE 767 (1953). With freezing, or cryopreservation, of sperm, a woman could select a donor who could, over a relatively short period, produce enough semen to be stored for current and future use. If a woman became pregnant using the donor's sperm, she could later thaw the reserve sperm to attempt to conceive the child's genetic sibling, without having to request that the donor continue to make concurrent deposits.

The new technology created a family law scenario that was at the time, and remains today in some circles, controversial. AID enabled a married woman to give birth to a child who was not the biological child of her husband. This raised the

---

with syphilis so he could plot its course under treatment. *See* MACHELLE M. SEIBEL (ED.), INFERTILITY: A COMPREHENSIVE TEXT, 310 (1997).

possibility that the child would be, in the language used at the time, illegitimate. An illegitimate child was one "not recognized by law as lawful offspring; . . . born of parents not married to each other; conceived in fornication or adultery." WEBSTER'S NEW INTERNATIONAL DICTIONARY 1126 (3d ed. 1961). Illegitimacy was both a source of social stigma and the basis for denial of legal rights such as inheritance.

If a husband and wife agree that they will conceive and raise a child using AID, should that child be considered illegitimate? Consider one of the early cases in this area.

GURSKY v. GURSKY
Supreme Court of New York, Kings County
39 Misc.2d 1083, 242 N.Y.S.2d 406 (1963)

COSTANTINO, J.

The plaintiff alleged three causes of action in an amended pleading, the first of which was for annulment, and the others for separation on the ground of abandonment and cruel and inhuman treatment. Plaintiff also alleged that there was no issue of the marriage. The court dismissed plaintiff's action for annulment for failure of proof. Defendant wife had interposed an answer and counterclaimed for separation. On the trial and after plaintiff's dismissal defendant moved for leave to amend her answer to allege a counterclaim for annulment. The motion to amend was granted without objection thereto by plaintiff husband.

The believable testimony, the medical proof and other evidence in the case, including the formal admissions made on the part of the plaintiff husband, sustained defendant's position that there had been a failure of the consummation of the marriage between the parties.

After trial defendant was granted judgment of annulment.

The evidence indicated that the parties, upon discovery of the infirmities of plaintiff, sought medical advice. As a result of such advice and plaintiff's condition they then further consulted medically the possibility of artificially inseminating defendant wife.

Further testimony adduced at the trial revealed that the parties agreed that defendant wife would be artificially inseminated with the semen of a third party donor. The plaintiff and defendant both signed the consent to have her artificially inseminated. Plaintiff, in addition, promised to pay all expenses involved to effect such procedure. A contract was signed by the plaintiff for waiver of liability and for medical and/or surgical treatments . . .

As a result of said artificial insemination a child was born on September 14, 1961 — Minday Frances Gursky. It was conceded on the trial that the birth certificate listed Annette Gursky as the mother and Stanley Gursky as the father. In view of the issue of the legitimacy of the child raised in this litigation the statements in said certificate are neither controlling nor determinative of the parental status of the parties nor of the status of the infant.

We are now confronted with the problem of determining whether or not a child conceived by means of artificial insemination of a married woman through the use, with the husband's consent, of semen contributed by a donor other than the husband is legitimate. For the sake of convenience this practice will also be referred to in this opinion as heterologous artificial insemination or A.I.D.

The court wishes to emphasize at the outset that however much it is concerned with arriving at a solution that is least harmful to the child, it must in the final analysis be guided by the settled concepts of the common law as modified by statutory enactment. The court is, however, aware that any literal application of the law should be grounded in reason and logic if it is to lead to a proper and just adjudication.

The concept which historically is deeply imbedded in the law is that a child who is begotten through a father who is not the mother's husband is deemed to be illegitimate. This view is adverted to in *Com'r. of Public Welfare of City of New York, etc., v. Koehler*, 284 N.Y. 260 at page 264, 30 N.E.2d 587 at page 589, as follows:

> In judicial opinions, judges, according to their individual tastes or whims, had used indiscriminately the terms "natural child" or "child born out of wedlock" or "bastard" to describe a child whose father was not the mother's husband; and difference in the descriptive terms was not intended to carry any juridical consequences.

The foregoing concept has been judicially deemed to have been carried over into statutory law. Thus Judge Lehman, speaking for the Court of Appeals in the *Koehler*, supra, case, at page 264, 30 N.E.2d at page 589, points out that:

> The Legislature in different statutes enacted at different times has also used those terms indiscriminately to describe a child whose father is not the husband of the child's mother and the Legislature has conferred upon the Court of Special Sessions in the City of New York, and upon other courts elsewhere, jurisdiction in proceedings to establish the paternity of such a child for the purpose of compelling the father to pay for the child's support and education.

Unless there can be read into the statutory enactments of this State, dealing with persons born out of wedlock, an intention to modify the settled concept as to the status of a child whose father was not married to its mother, it must be presumed that the historical concept of illegitimacy with respect to such a child remains in force and effect. Turning to the statutes of this State involving the instant question, we find that the term "a child born out of wedlock" is deemed to be synonymous with and must be construed as meaning an "illegitimate child." (General Construction Law, § 59). A child born out of wedlock was defined in the Domestic Relations Laws, § 119 (which was in effect at the time of the child's birth) as "a child begotten and born: (a) Out of lawful matrimony; (b) while the husband of its mother was separate from her a whole year previous to its birth; or (c) during the separation of its mother from her husband pursuant to a judgment of a competent court." Reason and logic impel the conclusion that the phrase "out of lawful matrimony" refers not solely to the child of an unmarried woman, but also to the child of a married woman. In other words, subdivision (a) is to be deemed to refer to any child whose natural father was not married to its mother irrespective of the marital status of the mother (see *State of North Dakota v. Coliton*, 73 N.D. 582, 17 N.W.2d 546, 156 A.L.R. 1403). (*See also* SCHATKIN, DISPUTED PATERNITY PROCEEDINGS, 2nd Edition, Section 2).

That this construction accords with the intent of the legislature in passing the statute hereinabove referred to (Domestic Relations Law, § 119), the repeal of which went into effect on September 1, 1962, is manifest from the definition provided in Section 512 of the Family Court Act, which went into effect on September 1, 1962. That section of the Family Court Act defines a child born out of wedlock as being a child begotten and born out of lawful matrimony. The comment provided by way of annotation in McKinney's Consolidated Laws points out that the provision found in the definition contained in the Domestic Relations Law relating to the separation of the husband from the mother of the child for a period of a year previous to the birth of the child constituted proof of the fact that the child was born "out of lawful matrimony."

While Section 112 of the New York City Sanitary Code appears to constitute a recognition of the existence of the practice of artificial insemination by setting forth measures required to be adopted by physicians engaged in the practice, such provision of law must be read within the framework of the established concept of illegitimacy as hereinabove discussed and can in no wise be deemed to sanction the practice of artificial insemination or to render legitimate any issue thereof.

The State legislature has exercised its power to modify the concept of illegitimacy in certain respects when it has deemed it fitting to do so. Thus it has provided that the subsequent marriage of parents of an illegitimate child legitimatizes such child. (Domestic Relations Law, Sec. 24). The fact that it has not chosen to deal with the question of legitimacy as it relates to children begotten and born through heterologous artificial insemination must be deemed to manifest a disinclination to modify, by legislative fiat, a concept which must logically result only in a determination adverse to the legitimacy of a child begotten by a father other than the husband of the mother. Certainly, there has been increasing discussion and controversy generated on this subject sufficient to indicate that the ramifications and the myriad problems arising in this field of artificial insemination require legislative action if the historical concept of illegitimacy is to be modified so as to admit of the legitimacy of a child born through heterologous artificial insemination. Attempts have hereto been made to introduce legislation seeking in part the legitimization of A.I.D. children and such legislation has been defeated. This is another indication of a disinclination on the part of the legislature to disturb the application of the historical concept of illegitimacy to children begotten through heterologous artificial insemination.

The question with which we are here dealing has been the subject of somewhat conflicting judicial attitudes. It appears that the only case dealing with this subject in New York State is the case of *Strnad v. Strnad* (1948), 190 Misc. 786, 78 N.Y.S.2d 390. That case appears, on surface analysis, to hold that a child which is the offspring of heterologous artificial insemination, performed with the consent of the mother's husband, is legitimate. It must be borne in mind, however, that the precise question involved in that case was the husband's right of visitation as respects such child. The court concluded that the husband was entitled to rights of visitation as theretofore allowed as the evidence did not show him to be an unfit guardian, but did indicate that the best interests of the child called for reasonable visitations. The view expressed by the court in that case, that such child was not an illegitimate child, is supported by no legal precedent. Indeed, the further view expressed by the court, namely, that the child is deemed to have been "potentially adopted" or "semi-adopted" by the husband of its mother, constitutes an implicit recognition of the fact that the birth would otherwise be illegitimate. Since legal adoption can be accomplished only in accordance with the provisions of the Domestic Relations Law (Section 110), which specifically declares that no person shall be adopted except in pursuance thereof, and since in the *Strnad* case no legal adoption was alleged or provided, it would appear that the court's conclusion that the child was legitimate cannot logically be sustained.

Where the precise issue of legitimacy has been squarely presented for determination, it has been held that heterologous artificial insemination by a third party donor, with or without the consent of the husband, constitutes adultery on the part of the mother, and that a child so conceived is not a child born in wedlock and is therefore illegitimate (*Doornbos v. Doornbos*, No. 54 S. 14981 [Superior Court, Cook Co., December 13, 1954]).

It is my opinion, in light of all of the foregoing considerations, that the child in the instant case, which was indisputably the offspring of artificial insemination by a third-party donor with the consent of the mother's husband, is not the legitimate issue of the husband.

However, while the court is constrained to hold that the child of the defendant wife is not the legitimate issue of the plaintiff husband, it does not follow that the husband is thereby free of obligation to furnish support for the child in the opinion of the court. The husband's declarations and conduct respecting the artificial insemination of his wife by means of a third-party donor, including the husband's written "consent" to the procedure, implied a promise on his part to furnish support for any offspring resulting from the insemination. This, in the light of the wife's concurrence and submission to artificial insemination, was sufficient to constitute an implied contract . . .

The court concludes in the instant case that the husband is liable for the support of the child here involved, whether on the basis for an implied contract to support or by reason of application of the doctrine of equitable estoppel.

The court does not pass upon any personal rights, including property rights, that the child may have vis-a-vis the plaintiff husband. (See e. g. *Miller v. Elliott*, 266 App.Div. 428, 42 N.Y.S.2d 569).

There was testimony that plaintiff gave to defendant, for household expenses and incidentals, the sum of $80.00 per week prior to the birth of the child and the sum of $90.00 per week subsequent thereto.

Taking into consideration the financial requirements for the support of defendant and child and the ability of the plaintiff to meet this responsibility and upon all of the evidence adduced at the trial bearing thereon, the defendant wife is awarded the sum of $25.00 per week for her support and the sum of $20.00 per week for the maintenance and support of the infant . . .

The other causes of action alleged by plaintiff and defendant as hereinbefore set forth are dismissed.

NOTES AND QUESTIONS

1. *Clarification of Terms.* The *Gursky* court used the acronym "A.I.D." to refer to "heterologous artificial insemination." A bit confusing for those wondering what the "D" stands for in the term. There are two basic types of artificial insemination: homologous insemination, when the semen is obtained from the husband (AIH), and heterologous insemination, when the semen is obtained from a donor (AID). AIH is used when the man experiences physiological difficulties that make insemination through intercourse problematic, such as erectile dysfunction or low sperm production (where several ejaculates can be pooled for a single insemination).

2. *Early AID Cases. Gursky* is one of several early cases to tackle the family law aspect of AID. Justice Costantino refers to the first published opinion in this area, the 1948 decision in *Strnad v. Strnad*, 190 Misc. 786, 78 N.Y.S.2d 390 in which the court found that a child born using AID was not illegitimate. Justice Costantino criticizes his fellow New York brethren for creating out of whole cloth the rationale that the child had been "potentially adopted" or "semi-adopted" by the husband of the mother, and thus a legitimate child of the marriage. Since no legal adoption had taken place, the *Gursky* court rejected treating the parties as if that legal proceeding had taken place.

But perhaps the earliest ART jurists were on to something. The law is not immune to transforming actions and events into legal constructs that they are not, in order to serve public policy. The word *constructive* is a modifier familiar to all lawyers. It has been said that the word is a way of pretending that whatever word it modifies depicts a state of affairs that actually exists when actually it does not. The pretense is made whenever judges wish, usually for good but often undisclosed public policy reasons, a different reality from the one confronting them. Concepts such as "constructive possession" (ascribing the rights of a possessor to an absent landowner to prevent trespass) and "constructive eviction" (relieving an occupying tenant of the obligation to pay rent when the landlord substantially interferes with the beneficial enjoyment of the premises but does not actually evict the tenant) are a long-standing and essential part of our jurisprudence. *See* JESSE DUKEMINIER, JAMES KRIER, GREGORY ALEXANDER, MICHAEL SCHILL, PROPERTY 32, fn. 17 (7th ed. 2010).

Maybe what the 1948 New York court meant to suggest was that a child born into a marriage using AID is constructively adopted by the mother's husband who consents to the medical procedure. Is this a sensible approach or do you think a husband in this situation should be required to adopt the child born through AID? As the concepts of conception and intercourse move further apart in time and distance, questions of parentage become increasingly complex.

3. *AID and Adultery.* In the days before AID, if a married woman gave birth to a child who was not the biological child of her husband there could be only one explanation. Trouble in paradise. The woman could only have conceived by engaging in sexual intercourse with a man other than the woman's husband, i.e., by adultery.

Can AID be considered adultery in a technical sense? The argument seems strained because there is no intercourse involved in AID. Moreover, at the time of insemination the donor may be miles away or even dead, debunking the case that any interaction between the parties has occurred. But what about the case for a legal finding of adultery? After all, if we can agree to the concept of constructive adoption, why not constructive adultery? If you think this is far-fetched, take a look at *Doornbos v. Doornbos*, No. 54 S. 14981 (Superior Court, Cook Co., December 13, 1954), *aff'd*, 12 Ill. App. 2d 473, 139 N.E.2d 844 (1956) (artificial insemination by third-party donor, with or without consent of husband, constitutes adultery by mother; child is not a legitimate child of the marriage).

4. *Religious Objections to AID.* In addition to questions about paternity, AID raises concerns about the sanctity of the connection between conception and intercourse. An AID child is conceived without the benefit of sexual intercourse, and thus the practice departs from some religious tenets which hold sacred the unity between sex and procreation. These features caused some religious and policy leaders to condemn AID as "nothing more than mechanical adultery, equivalent to rape and clearly contrary to the law of God." *See* Albert R. Jonsen, *Reproduction and Rationality*, 4 CAMBRIDGE Q. HEALTHCARE ETHICS 263 (1995).

Roman Catholic theologians, in the main, have rejected AID. The official position of the Roman Catholic Church was stated in 1949 by Pope Pius XII. After condemning artificial insemination outside of marriage, the Pope went on to reject the practice within marriage as well:

> Artificial insemination in marriage with the use of an active element from a third person is equally immoral and as such is to be rejected summarily. Only the marriage partners have mutual rights over their bodies for the procreation of a new life, and these are exclusive, nontransferable, and inalienable rights. So it must be, out of consideration for the child.
>
> By virtue of this same bond, nature imposes on whoever gives life to a small creature the task of its preservation and education. Between the marriage partners, however, and a child which is the fruit of the active element of a third person — even though the husband consents — there is no bond of origin, no moral or juridical bond of conjugal procreation.

Pope Pius XII, *To Catholic Doctors*, THE CATHOLIC MIND (Vol. 48, No. 1048), 252, April 1950. In 2008, Pope Benedict XVI reiterated the Catholic Church's opposition to artificial insemination, stating that all forms of artificial fertilization that substitute for the conjugal act "are to be excluded." Congregation for the Doctrine of the Faith, Instruction *Dignitas Personae* on Certain Bioethical Questions (20 June 2008), available at: http://www.vatican.va/roman_curia/congregations/cfaith/documents/rc_con_cfaith_doc_20081208_dignitas-personae_en.html. For a broader analysis of religious perspectives on AID, see Daniel B. Sinclair, *Assisted Reproduction in Jewish Law*, 30 FORDHAM URBAN L. J. 71 (2002); Helen M. Alvare, *Catholic Teaching and the Law Concerning the New Reproductive Technologies*, 30 FORDHAM URBAN L. J. 107 (2002); Cynthia B. Cohen, *Protestant Perspectives on the Uses of the New Reproductive Technologies*, 30 FORDHAM URBAN L. J. 135 (2002); Hossam E. Fadel, *The Islamic Viewpoint on New Assisted Reproductive Technologies*, 30 FORDHAM URBAN L. J. 147 (2002).

While concerns may linger, AID is widely used today and accounts for nearly 60,000 births annually, far exceeding the number of families created through neonatal adoption. *See* Inst. for Sci., Law & Tech. Working Group, *ART Into Science: Regulation of Fertility Techniques*, 281 SCIENCE 651 (1998).

B.   Conception in the Laboratory — In Vitro Fertilization

1.   Investigating the Possibility of Conception Outside the Body

At the same time physicians were using and improving the technology of AID, scientists around the world began to wonder whether an embryo could be created outside the body by flushing eggs out of the woman's body and uniting them with sperm in a laboratory test tube. After all, AID proved that one-half of the reproductive formula, the sperm, could be captured and handled outside the body — why not investigate that same possibility for the female gametes? Experiments on this method of *in vitro* (literally, in glass) method of fertilization initially focused on animals. The earliest results began to be reported in the mid-1950s. In 1954, French scientists succeeded in fertilizing rabbit eggs in vitro and thereafter observed the embryos divide several times. Five years later, Chinese-American embryologist Min Chang successfully achieved a live rabbit birth using in vitro fertilization, mixing rabbit eggs and sperm in the laboratory and transferring the developing embryo back to a female rabbit's uterus. M. Chang, *Fertilization of Rabbit Ova In Vitro*, 184 NATURE 406 (1959).

The transfer of in vitro fertilization (IVF) technology from animals to humans seemed an inevitable and beneficial leap to many scientists, but as in the case of AID, opposition mounted. When scientists began to report success in the field of human IVF in the late 1960s, Paul Ramsey, a professor of religion at Princeton University, wrote a series of articles in 1972 urging against any further advancement in the field of reproductive technologies. At the outset of one piece he wrote, "I must judge that in vitro fertilization constitutes unethical medical experimentation on possible future human beings, and therefore is subject to absolute moral prohibition." Paul Ramsey, *Shall We "Reproduce?"* 220 JAMA 1346 (1972).[11]

Despite this and other dissenting voices, the wheels of science turned and, due largely to the efforts of two British scientists, the world's first "test tube baby" was born in 1978. British gynecologist Patrick Steptoe and Cambridge University scientist Robert Edwards met at a meeting of the Royal Society of Medicine in 1968 and for the next 10 years worked to perfect the process in which a woman's eggs are removed from her body just prior to ovulation, mixed with viable sperm in a hospitable test tube (or petri dish) environment, within hours fertilization occurs and within days embryos develop to the eight-cell stage and are transferred back to

---

[11] Some commentators believe that aspects of the early opposition to AID and IVF were replicated in the late twentieth century debate over human cloning. See Judith F. Daar, *The Future of Human Cloning: Prescient Lessons From Medical Ethics Past*, 8 So. Cal. Interdisciplinary L. J. 167 (1998). The reactions to the prospect of human cloning are discussed in Chapter 10.

the woman's uterus, implantation occurs, and a child is born nine months later.[12]

Louise Joy Brown was born on July 25, 1978 at a hospital outside London. She was the first child born following conception through IVF, in which Drs. Steptoe and Edwards removed one egg from her mother's ovary, placed it in a petri dish, fertilized it with her father's sperm and two days later transferred the resulting embryo back into her mother's uterus. In July 2003 Louise celebrated her 25th birthday at Bourn Hall, the British fertility clinic established by her pioneering British doctors, a facility that continues to offer IVF services today. Louise was joined at her birthday celebration by a thousand other children who share the manner in which she was conceived, including her younger sister Natalie who was the world's 40th IVF baby.[13] Dr. Steptoe died in 1988, long before he could appreciate the impact IVF would have on reproduction worldwide. His partner survives to this day, having recently added another entry in his biography — Nobel Laureate. Dr. Edwards was awarded the Nobel Prize in Medicine in 2010 for his work in developing IVF.

To date, it is estimated that more than five million children have been born worldwide using IVF and by all indications that number will continue to grow. In 2008, the U.S. Centers for Disease Control (CDC) reported that more than 61,000 babies were born as a result of IVF, more than two times higher than the nearly 31,000 infants born via IVF in 1999.[14] The combination of rising success rates using IVF, and delayed childbearing by many women can only add to the demand for this technology.

2.   Advances in IVF and the Future of ART

IVF remains the mainstay of ART medicine, with the past 35 years bringing refinements and improvements to the process. Like its predecessor technology AID, IVF turned to freezing methods in order to maximize a couple's chances of achieving a pregnancy while minimizing the amount of surgical treatment a woman had to undergo. As explained below, IVF requires that a woman be treated with hormone therapy, administered through a series of injections, so that she will produce multiple eggs rather than the single egg that is produced during a normal monthly cycle. Thereafter, the eggs are retrieved using a surgical procedure often requiring general anesthesia. Once the eggs and sperm are mixed in the laboratory, there may be more resulting embryos than can be safely transferred back to the woman's uterus. In that case, the embryos can be frozen for later use. This process

---

[12] The collaboration between Steptoe and Edwards may have produced a monumental accomplishment in the field of reproductive medicine, but it did seem to have its humble beginnings. Steptoe's clinic was located in the northern English town of Oldham, while Edwards laboratory was located in Cambridge, a distance of about 200 miles. In later years, Edwards recalled driving between the two towns for over a decade, clocking 250,000 miles on his car. Sometimes, as he drove home he had fresh eggs strapped to his side to keep them warm until he reached his lab. See Rosie Mestel, *Birth by Test Tube Turns 25*, Los Angeles Times, A1, July 24, 2003.

[13] Natalie Brown herself made history in 1999 when she became a mother, making her the first test tube baby to give birth to a child. But history did not repeat itself — Natalie conceived the old-fashioned way.

[14] These figures represent results from the nearly 440 ART clinics located in the United States. No similar collection and reporting of worldwide ART use is available at this time.

of cryopreservation allows a woman to avoid additional injections and surgeries if the initial IVF fails or she chooses to gestate the embryos at a later time. The first birth from a previously frozen embryo occurred on July 31, 1984 with the birth of Zoe Leyland in Australia. Today, frozen embryos are used in about 21% of all ART procedures.

Another improvement to the IVF technique was introduced in 1992 with a technique known as intracytoplasmic sperm injection (ICSI). ICSI involves the injection a single sperm into the center of an egg, making it possible for men with low sperm counts to become fathers. If the sperm is introduced directly into the egg, researchers have found a higher rate of success for fertilization and ultimately, pregnancy. The use of ICSI has risen dramatically since its introduction. In 2008, nearly two-thirds of all ART procedures (64%) relied on ICSI to accomplish fertilization. For a complete review of success rates and other statistics associated with ART *see 2008 Assisted Reproductive Technology Success Rates, National Summary and Fertility Clinic Reports* (December 2010), also available at: http://www.cdc.gov/art/ART2008/index.htm.

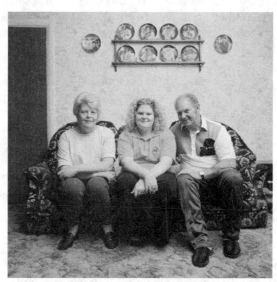

Louise Brown and Her Parents, Circa 2003

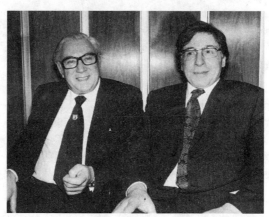

Doctors Patrick Steptoe and Robert Edwards (right), January 1979

A final refinement to the world of ART began to appear in the early 1990s and allowed scientists to view the health of an embryo before it was implanted back into a woman's uterus. Preimplantation genetic diagnosis (PGD) is a technique in which one cell of an early eight-celled embryo is removed and studied for its genetic composition. Researchers are now able to detect many genetically linked diseases and traits from a single embryonic cell, allowing couples an opportunity to select only healthy embryos for transport back into the woman's body. The embryo remains intact after the single cell is removed and continues to grow normally while the genetic review is being conducted. PGD is being used to detect inherited condition such as Down Syndrome, cystic fibrosis, and a variety of blood disorders. Early studies on children born following PGD show no deleterious effects from the procedure. See Yury Verlinsky et al., *Over a Decade of Experience with Preimplantation Genetic Diagnosis: A Multicenter Report*, 82 FERTILITY & STERILITY 292 (2004). The ethics and practice of PGD are discussed in more detail in Chapter 4.

The final episode of our current understanding of ART remains a futuristic concept, at least as of the writing of this text, but many predict it will take its place on the continuum of advances in human reproduction. Human cloning has stirred the imagination and ire of many contemporary researchers and policymakers, much in the same way AID and IVF were ushered into our contemporary mindset. But unlike previous technologies, which merely aided a man and a woman in their quest to combine gametes to form a healthy embryo, cloning uses the tissue from only one individual to produce an embryo with the exact genetic make-up of the tissue donor. To date, all human beings born in this world have a unique genome or genetic make-up. Cloning threatens to alter that reality and some argue threatens to alter the very core of human nature. The technology and controversy surrounding human cloning are left for later in our studies, beginning in Chapter 10.

3. A Glossary of ART Terms

The history of ART reveals that the condition of infertility has been studied from a variety of perspectives (i.e., male factor, female factor and unknown sources of infertility) and that advances have produced a variety of medical interventions. Though the treatments that make up the world of ART may be very familiar to those who dedicate their lives to helping others, or themselves, overcome infertility, to the rest of us the jargon can seem mammoth and confusing. What follows is a glossary of terms which spells out in more detail some of the terms and technologies associated with ART. The world of ART is a veritable alphabet soup of abbreviations and acronyms. Feel free to sample the provisions below as often as you like.

Assisted Reproductive Technologies Glossary of Terms

Artificial Insemination See Assisted Insemination

Assisted Insemination A medical procedure used to treat male factor infertility (for example, low sperm count or poor motility) or to assist women with no male partner achieve pregnancy. Assisted insemination requires that semen be obtained from the male, and then placed in the woman's reproductive tract using an injection device. There are three methods for performing assisted insemination: 1) intravaginal insemination involves placing semen in the vagina near the cervical opening and inserting a cap or other device on the cervix to hold the semen in place; 2) intracervical assisted insemination inserts a tube into the cervical opening and places a small amount of semen in the cervix, and 3) intrauterine insemination (IUI) requires the sperm be washed to remove bacteria and other components harmful to the uterus. Sperm is injected into the back of the uterus using a narrow tube threaded through the vagina, cervix and uterus.

ICSI Intracytoplasmic sperm injection. A medical procedure in which a single sperm is injected directly into the egg in order to achieve fertilization. ICSI involves placing sperm in a solution to slow their movement; a single sperm is selected from the solution and immobilized. Using a slim injection pipette, the sperm is inserted into the cytoplasm of the egg (the material surrounding the egg cell nucleus). ICSI is performed in the laboratory using eggs that have been retrieved from a woman's ovaries. Once the injection has taken place, the eggs are later studied to see if fertilization has occurred. The resulting embryos are then placed into the woman's uterus.

IVF In vitro fertilization. A medical procedure in which a woman's eggs are extracted from her ovaries, mixed with sperm in the laboratory, the resulting embryos are grown for three to five days, then transferred back to the woman's uterus through the cervix. IVF was originally designed to circumvent blockage of the fallopian tubes; today the indications for IVF have broadened enormously because the technique allows physicians to study the health of the embryos (we have recently learned that unhealthy embryos can be the cause of infertility).

An IVF cycle has four phases:

Phase 1: Ovarian Stimulation and Monitoring. A woman is treated with a sequence of drugs, generally administered through injection, to induce multiple follicles to mature so that several eggs can be retrieved. Drug treatment usually begins midway through a woman's menstrual cycle and continues until the eggs are retrieved.

Phase 2: Egg Collection. Egg retrieval is done in a surgical procedure in which either general anesthesia, or a combination of sedation and pain medications are administered to the woman. Physicians insert an ultrasound-guided needle through the vaginal wall and into a developed ovarian follicle. Using suction, the fluid inside the follicle is withdrawn, along with the egg it contains. This removal technique is repeated for each follicle that has developed.

Phase 3: Fertilization and Embryo Culture. Each normal appearing egg is placed in a separate petri dish containing culture medium. Semen is obtained from the male partner and is processed to obtain a high concentration of motile sperm. The sperm is then introduced into the dish. The contents of the dish are examined under a microscope after one day to determine if the egg is fertilized.

Phase 4: Embryo Transfer. Embryos are generally transferred to the woman's uterus two or three days after egg retrieval, when they are comprised of four to eight cells. Under certain circumstances the embryo will be transferred after five days when it has become a blastocyst. The transfer is accomplished using a sterile tube with a syringe on one end. Droplets of fluid containing one embryo are drawn into the tube which is inserted through the cervix and then injected into the uterus. Embryo transfer generally requires no anesthesia or sedation.

Following embryo transfer, a woman will wait approximately 10 to 14 days before undergoing a blood test to determine if she is pregnant.

GIFT Gamete intrafallopian transfer. A medical procedure in which a woman's eggs are retrieved following ovarian stimulation, mixed in the laboratory with sperm, and reintroduced into the fallopian tube using a fiber-optic instrument called a laparoscope which is inserted through small incisions in the woman's abdomen. GIFT assists the gametes (eggs and sperm) in reaching the fallopian tube, the location where natural fertilization takes place. In order to use GIFT, a woman must have at least one healthy fallopian tube.

ZIFT Zygote intrafallopian transfer. A medical procedure in which a woman's eggs are retrieved following ovarian stimulation, mixed in the laboratory with sperm, and allowed to develop into early embryos (also called zygotes, usually seen approximately one day after fertilization). The zygotes are transferred into a woman's fallopian tubes using a laparoscope, placed through the woman's abdomen, to guide placement of the early embryos. ZIFT combines some of the laboratory elements of IVF and the tubal transfer of GIFT.

C. Successes and Failures in ART Medicine

1. Is ART Effective?

In reproductive medicine, the measure of success is often referred to as the "take-home baby rate." Despite its somewhat crude name, the rate at which an individual or couple gives birth to a healthy baby is the only measure by which patients measure the success of any ART procedure. Patient and public access to success rates surrounding ART was greatly enhanced by a 1992 federal law requiring all clinics performing ART in the United States to annually report their success data to the CDC. Fertility Clinic Success Rate and Certification Act of 1992, 42 U.S.C. 263a-1. The CDC uses the data to publish an annual report detailing the ART success rates for each of the clinics reporting. In December 2010 the CDC issued its annual report for the calendar year 2008 (explaining the lag time between

ART procedure, a nine-month pregnancy, delivery and reporting of complete data for each procedure). In the year 2008, a total of 436 fertility clinics provided information about the ART cycles started in their clinics during the calendar year.[15]

The overall success rate for ART procedures for the year 2008 was 32%. This means that when a woman begins an ART cycle,[16] she has about a one in three chance of delivering a live baby. Interestingly, the average birth rate using natural conception is about 20% per menstrual cycle. This means that the likelihood of birth using ART outpaces the average rate of birth in natural conception by nearly 70%. Does this statistic suggest that couples should abandon the low-tech method of reproduction and jump right into an ART program? Certainly not. The physical burden of surgery and injection therapy alone should be enough to dissuade any fertile person from engaging the process. In addition, later chapters detail the expense and emotional burden that accompany ART therapy. No data suggests that anyone other than those diagnosed as infertile avail themselves of the services of an ART professional.

As the statistics reported in Table 2 reveal, the success of any ART procedure is impacted by two main factors: the age of the woman and the source of the eggs. Age plays a significant role in fertility; as a woman ages, her chances of achieving pregnancy and carrying a child to term diminish beginning at about age 35. Women younger than 35 had a 41% rate of live birth delivery, compared with 22% for women aged 38-40, and 5% for those aged 43-44. One way to increase the odds for success is to use eggs from another, preferably younger, woman. Today, women undergoing fertility treatment have the option of using their own eggs or eggs from another woman who agrees to act as a donor. Egg donors are typically in their 20s or early 30s. The egg donor undergoes the same ovarian stimulation and egg retrieval discussed in connection with IVF, but once her eggs are retrieved she turns over control of those eggs to a woman who is unable to produce viable eggs on her own. The success rate using donor eggs is impressive, averaging 58% per cycle. What is most hopeful to older women is that the rate of success does not drop dramatically once a woman reaches 40. We discuss the practice and ethics surrounding egg donation in Chapter 3.

---

[15] The CDC report defines ART as "all fertility treatments in which both egg and sperm are handled. In general ART procedures involve surgically removing eggs from a woman's ovaries, combining them with sperm in the laboratory, and returning them to the woman's body or donating them to another woman. They do NOT include treatments in which only the sperm are handled (i.e., intrauterine, or artificial, insemination) or procedures in which a woman takes drugs only to stimulate egg production without the intention of having eggs retrieved." 20028 Assisted Reproductive Technology Success Rates: National Summary and Fertility Clinic Reports (December 2010), at 3. Notice the CDC's definition of ART, derived from the 1992 Fertility Clinic Success Rate Act, is more narrow than the one we have adopted which includes all medical procedures in which pregnancy is accomplished by means other than sexual intercourse. Our definition includes techniques such as artificial insemination and intrauterine insemination, which do not involve the mixing of both male and female gametes. While the federal and CDC definitions of ART have been adopted for purposes of mandatory clinic reporting, the broader definition enjoys support among law and policymakers. See Assisted Reproductive Technologies: Analysis and Recommendations for Public Policy, The New York State Task Force on Life and the Law 1 (1998). As the new field of ART continues to evolve, a settled definition of its mainstay term may emerge. Until then, what remains important is clarifying the term ART to any relevant audience.

[16] According to the CDC Report, an ART cycles commences when a woman begins taking drugs to stimulate egg production or starts ovarian monitoring with the intent of having embryos transferred.

The dramatic increase in the number of babies born through ART corresponds directly with the increased use of infertility services. Table 2 shows a 69% increase in the number of ART cycles initiated from 1999 to 2008. One wonders whether this rise in demand is based on a rise in infertility among American women. According to the New York State Task Force on Life and the Law, surveys detect no overall rise in the prevalence of infertility, yet the demand for infertility treatment is increasing. The Task Force offers several reasons for this rise in demand:

First, medical services for infertile couples are more widely available, offer increasing options for treatment, and are well publicized. As the technologies expand, increasing the number of indications deemed appropriate for intervention, the number of infertile couples considered potentially treatable also rises. Recent examples include developments in the micromanipulation of sperm, which makes IVF possible for couples in which the man produces very few sperm; and the use of donor eggs, which makes it possible to treat postmenopausal women and others without functioning ovaries. As a greater number of services or more complicated or time-intensive services are offered to each couple, the number of patient visits will also increase.

Second, there are more women of reproductive age than in the past, so that even if the rate of infertility continues to decline or remains stable, the number of women with fertility problems may increase. The last of the baby boom generation will not reach the end of their reproductive years (approximately 44) until 2010.

Third, there is an ongoing trend toward delayed childbearing, particularly among professional and highly educated women. Between 1976 and 1986, the rate of first birth among women 40 years of age or older doubled. One in five women who reached 35 years of age by 1989 had not had children; in contrast, only 9 percent of women who turned 35 in 1970 were childless. According to a national survey, half of the women who are married and childless at 30 to 34 years of age expect to have at least one child. With increasing rates of divorce and remarriage, women who have already borne children, are also increasingly likely to attempt future childbearing in their later reproductive years. Since infertility increases with a woman's age, a higher proportion of these women will seek infertility services.

Fourth, important risk factors for infertility are increasing among younger women. In particular, increasing rates of chlamydia in the young may result in an increased prevalence of tubal infertility.

Finally, adoption is no longer an easy method of family building, which may increase the demand for medical intervention. Although the public impression may overstate the shortage of adoptable infants, adoption can be a slow and complicated process. According to one estimate, in a given year there are approximately 3.3 couples seeking adoption for every one who succeeds.

The New York State Task Force on Life and the Law, *Assisted Reproductive Technologies: Analysis and Recommendations for Public Policy* 15-16 (1998) (footnotes omitted).

Table 2. ART Success Rates Over a Ten-Year Period (1999-2008)

ART Event	1999	2008	Percentage Change
Number of ART Cycles Performed	87,636	148,055	+69%
Number of Live Babies Born	30,629	61,426	+100%
Live Births Per Transfer Using Fresh Non-Donor Eggs	32%	38%	+19%
Live Births Per Transfer Using Fresh Donor Eggs	43%	58%	+35%
Live Births Using Non-Donor Eggs By Age			
Under 35	38%	47%	+25%
35-37	32%	37%	+15%
38-40	24%	28%	+16%
41-42	14%	16%	+21%

Source: 2008 Assisted Reproductive Technology Success Rates, National Summary and Fertility Clinic Reports (Center for Disease Control and Prevention, December 2010).

NOTES AND QUESTIONS

1. Tracking the growing use of ART services in the United States is accomplished primarily through a reporting system administered by the Centers for Disease Control and Prevention (CDC). Since 1995, the CDC has issued an annual report detailing the overall success rates for U.S. fertility clinics as a whole, as well as publishing ART success rates for each individual fertility clinic that reported its results to the CDC. The impetus for this standardized reporting system came in part from patient complaints about false and exaggerated pregnancy success rates claimed by a number of fertility clinics. For example, in 1994, the New York City Department of Consumer Affairs investigated charges that Mount Sinai Medical Center had exaggerated success rates in promotional brochures and flyers, claiming a "take-home baby rate" of 20%, when in fact the delivery rate was between 10.9 and 13.7%. The hospital ultimately paid $4 million to hundreds of childless former patients in order to settle a lawsuit over false success rate claims. At the federal level, the Federal Trade Commission has won several cease-and-desist agreements over deceptive advertising claims with fertility clinics across the country. See Trip Gabriel, *High-Tech Pregnancies Test Hope's Limits*, N.Y. TIMES, Jan. 7, 1996, at 1.

2. In recent years, the CDC's methods of data collection and reporting have come under some criticism. The CDC does not collect data from fertility clinics on its own, but rather contracts with Westat, a statistical survey research organization, to gather information for the annual report. In December 2002, the CDC came under fire from clinics who claimed that data collectors failed to conduct on-site visits during that year, thus jeopardizing the accuracy of statistics collected for the 2002 report. According to a *Wall Street Journal* report, clinics are in fierce competition with one another to attract patients, thus without in-person oversight, data manipulation and misreporting is of significant concern. Manipulation of data

may come in the form of offering services only to those patients most likely to achieve a successful pregnancy, such as younger women or patients who agree to use donor eggs at the outset of treatment. In the most plain terms, one clinic director summarized the tactic as follows, "I can change the success rate of our clinic any time I want, not by lying but by choosing which patients I allow to do [IVF]." Amy Dockser Marcus, *Key Report on Fertility Clinics Is Under Fire*, WALL ST. J., Dec. 11, 2002, at D1.

Perhaps in response to these criticisms, Westat began to regularly conduct random site visits to verify the annual data submitted by fertility clinics. In 2008, Westat visited 35 of 436 reporting clinics. According to the 2008 CDC Report, "[i]n almost all cases, data available in the medical records on pregnancies and births were consistent with reported data." *2008 Assisted Reproductive Technology Success Rates, National Summary and Fertility Clinic Reports* (Center for Disease Control and Prevention, December 2010), at 7.

3. If you were a patient seeking ART services, what factors would be the most important to you? The clinic's success rate? We now see how clinic success rates can be manipulated simply by adjusting the pool of patients who are treated at a particular site. Moreover, a patient must carefully study the different measures of success, which can range from an initial positive blood test (which may later prove to be a false-positive), to a confirmed in utero pregnancy (which may later result in a miscarriage), to the delivery of a live infant (clearly what matters most to patients). How about looking at an individual doctor's success rate? As it turns out, skill levels can vary among ART doctors just as they vary among professionals in all fields. A patient is probably better off learning the individual success rate for her chosen doctor rather than looking to the clinics' rate overall. Whether a clinic is willing to share such data varies, probably according to the level of disparity in skills among the medical personnel.

Size also matters. It turns out that the more ART cycles a clinic performs, the higher their overall success rates. In 2008, clinics that performed more than 400 cycles per year boasted a 51% success rate for cycles using fresh (nonfrozen) donor eggs, compared to 43% for clinics performing less than 100 cycles. It stands to reason that experience improves outcomes, but there may be other, more subjective factors that go into the choice of a clinic.

Patients may also rely on a referral from a trusted friend. Patients themselves are probably the best judge of a clinic's merit. One patient tells a "Goldie Locks and the Three Bears" story of choosing a fertility clinic. She selected the first clinic because it was run by a doctor who had written numerous books in the field. Turns out, the doctor was so busy that the patient got little personal attention. She next tried a clinic with high CDC success rates, but didn't feel comfortable with the doctor. Finally, she found a third clinic that was just right for her, remarking "success rates don't mean a whole lot." Dockser Marcus, *supra* note 2.

Should a patient consider the convenience of the clinic location to home or work? Certainly the frequent in-clinic ultrasounds and blood work that accompany ART treatment should place location as a high priority. In the end, it seems there are many factors for every patient to consider in choosing a clinic. Typically not on that list, but of the utmost concern, is the health of any child born from the ART treatment. Having seen evidence of increases in demand and success surrounding ART, we now turn to the critical question of whether these technologies are safe for the adults they treat and the children they produce.

2.   Is ART Safe For Children and Adults?

The success of reproductive medicine has traditionally been measured by the pregnancy and delivery rates surrounding a particular intervention, but increasingly questions are raised about the health and well-being of children born following assisted conception, and adults who undergo repeated treatments with powerful hormones. In the early years of IVF, health concerns were rarely discussed because both the children and adults appeared to fit within normal parameters in terms of their health status. Moreover, the small number of children and patients made clinical trials difficult to conduct and accordingly of questionable validity. Today, more than three decades into the IVF world, the growing use and success of ART has caused medical researchers to turn their attention to the five million children born through ART and ask, "Is ART safe?" With this now large number of potential human research subjects, the data is starting to make its way into the pages of scientific journals and, for better or worse, into the popular press. As you read the study results and the spin on the study results, ask yourself whether any of the data would dissuade a patient bent on reproduction from availing herself of any reliable form of treatment.

a.   Safety to Children

Manon Ceelen, Mirjam M. Van Weissenbruch, Jan P.W. Vermeiden, Flora E. Van Leeuwen, and Henriette A. Delemarre-van de Wall
Growth and Development of Children Born After In Vitro Fertilization
90 Fertility & Sterility 1662 (2008)

In vitro fertilization used to overcome reproductive problems in humans is considered to be one of the most spectacular medical discoveries of the 20th century . . . Worldwide increasing delayed childbearing and the availability of new technologies, such as preimplantation genetic diagnosis to prevent transmission of severe or lethal diseases to offspring, will contribute to the increasing demand for IVF. Therefore, the need to evaluate the potential effects of fertility treatments is steadily growing.

Fortunately, for several years attempts to closely monitor the short- and long-term consequences of ART for both the mother and the child are increasing. This review will summarize current knowledge regarding the health of children born after IVF, including perinatal outcome after IVF, the incidence of congenital malformations, postnatal growth, and the occurrence of malignancies and imprinting disorders in children born after IVF.

Perinatal outcome IVF pregnancies

During the past two decades considerable interest has been focused on the perinatal health outcome of IVF pregnancies. Pregnancies after IVF have been reported to be at increased risk for adverse perinatal outcome, including preterm birth, low birth weight, and perinatal death. This has often been attributed to the increased incidence of multiple pregnancies after IVF and to confounding by maternal characteristics . . . Recently, several thorough systematic reviews of the existing literature on perinatal outcome after IVF have been published . . . All meta-analyses demonstrated that singletons conceived after IVF are at increased risk for preterm birth, low birth weight, being small for gestational age, perinatal mortality, and other adverse perinatal health outcomes, after correction for maternal age or parity . . . [Studies on the health of IVF twins varied in result, with some showing increased risks of preterm delivery and other perinatal problems compared to naturally conceived twins, while other studies showed no differences.]

Congenital anomalies

The term congenital anomaly refers to a broad spectrum of structural defects, which are apparent at birth or detected shortly after birth. In addition to genetic factors, various environmental conditions contribute to the etiology of congenital anomalies. . . . [T]he association between IVF and congenital anomalies has been extensively investigated and debated. Although various studies reported an increased risk of birth defects after IVF, others found that congenital abnormality rates among children born after IVF were not increased . . .

Although larger data sets are needed to detect specific risk increases for special malformations, certain organs systems have been suggested to be affected more often among children born after IVF including neural tube defects, gastrointestinal defects, orofacial defects, hypospadias and other genitourinary defects, cardiovascular defects, musculoskeletal defects, and chromosomal defects . . . It is still unclear whether the slightly increased risk of congenital malformations observed among infants born after IVF is inherent to factors associated with the underlying causes of infertility or factors associated with the IVF procedure . . .

Growth and physical development

During the past years, numerous studies on short-term outcome after IVF have reported increased rates of preterm birth, perinatal deaths, intrauterine growth retardation, and congenital malformations. Although preterm birth and low birth weight are known to be associated with childhood and adult morbidity and mortality, few well-designed studies have addressed postnatal growth and physical development of children born after IVF . . . [One] . . . study . . . showed that 5-year-old IVF singletons were more likely to have had a significant childhood illness, to have had a surgical operation, to require medical therapy, and to be admitted to hospital than naturally conceived children. Likewise, among IVF singletons as compared with spontaneously conceived infants, an increased cumulative incidence of different diseases diagnosed in outpatient or inpatient care was found during the 3-year follow-up period, especially regarding respiratory diseases and diarrhea . . . A possible explanation is that children born after IVF treatment might be more susceptible to morbidity, given the increased risk of perinatal complications among IVF infants. On the other hand, due to excessive parental concern IVF parents may seek medical help more often, or IVF children could be more easily referred to specialized pediatric care . . .

Epigenetic defects

. . . Recently published studies revealed a possible increased incidence of genomic imprinting disorders [genetic diseases] such as Beckwith-Wiedemann syndrome and Angelman syndrome among children conceived after ART . . . Angelman syndrome, which is associated with severe mental retardation, motor defects, lack of speech, and happy disposition . . . Beckwith-Wiedemann syndrome is characterized by a wide spectrum of symptoms including somatic overgrowth, congenital malformations, and a predisposition to embryonic neoplasia [early childhood cancers] . . .

Current implications

An accumulating body of evidence indicates that children born after IVF are at increased risk for several types of health problems. Although the influence of underlying fertility problems of the parents is not clear yet, health problems observed after IVF might (partially) originate from adaptations of the developing conceptus to the IVF procedure. The exposure of a gamete or an embryo to the different phases of an IVF treatment (e.g., fertility drugs, in vitro culture) during a critical period of development could have long-lasting developmental consequences. It is of great importance that during the following decades postnatal developmental and health aspects of children born after IVF will continue to be monitored worldwide . . .

In the above article, Dr. Ceelen and his colleagues collect and analyze some of the numerous studies published on the health and well-being of IVF-conceived children worldwide. While the authors conclude that IVF does increase the risk of infant and child health problems, the authors readily confess uncertainty as to the underlying cause. Below, a group of doctors at the University of Pennsylvania Center for Reproductive Medicine and Surgery react to the growing body of data linking IVF with health problems, calling into question some of the study results. Briefly stated, the Penn physicians question the methodology used in each study, raising doubts as to the cause and effect relationship between the use of ART and specific outcomes. Consider their views.

George Kovalevsky, Paolo Rinaudo, and Christos Coutifaris
Do Assisted Reproductive Technologies Cause Adverse Fetal Outcomes?
79 Fertility & Sterility 1270 (2003)

Treatment for infertility using assisted reproductive technologies (ART) is highly successful and has been used to help a steadily growing number of couples worldwide. In 1999, in the United States, more than 86,000 treatment cycles were performed resulting in the birth of more than 30,000 babies. Despite this widespread application, few follow-up studies of children conceived through ART have been performed, and more rigorous investigation of this important issue has clearly been needed. In recent months, three studies linking ART with several complications have been published in high profile and widely read general medical journals: Schieve et al. (1) reported that singletons conceived using ART were at an increased risk for low birth weight, whereas Hansen et al. (2) suggested an increased risk of major birth defects. Finally, Stromberg et al. (3) concluded that children conceived through IVF have an increased risk of neurological problems, especially cerebral palsy.

The importance of these studies is obvious as they provide clues of possible risks associated with ART. However, they are all retrospective analyses of data collected through registries and therefore are vulnerable to biases inherent to such study design. We must be careful not to overinterpret the data by concluding that the use of ART, whether from gamete or embryo manipulation or use of medications, is the direct cause of the complications — the observed associations may simply be explained by one or more confounders, such as an underlying infertility-related condition in the treated women. This short communication is an attempt to place these three articles in proper perspective for the clinician and to provide the impetus for conducting further studies to determine the true nature of the described associations.

At the outset, it should be stated that a major weakness of all three studies is the lack of proper controls. If the aim of a study is to determine whether a cause and effect relationship exists between the process of IVF and a specific outcome (i.e., low birth weight, major birth defects, neurological problems), the appropriate control population is that of babies born to infertile women achieving pregnancies by methods other than IVF. None of the three studies specifically included such a control population.

[The authors proceed to evaluate each of the three cited studies, calling into question the conclusions that the use of ART was the direct cause of the children's medical problems. The main critique of each study focus on the researchers' failure to consider the underlying infertility of the birth parent (or parents in the case of joint infertility) as a contributing factor or even the direct cause for the child's health status.]

The three articles we reviewed have suggested an association between use of ART and increased risk of problems in the resulting children. However, the validity of these associations and certainly the implication of a cause and effect relationship are weakened by potential limitations in the quality of the data inherent to registries. Furthermore, as highlighted, a major flaw of all three studies is the lack of appropriate controls, which ideally should have been babies born to infertile couples achieving pregnancy without the use of ART.

These studies should be applauded, as they have provided the groundwork and direction for future research. Carefully constructed, prospective, multicenter studies using the appropriate control patient population are clearly needed. It is imperative to determine whether use of ART results in increased risk to the children born after these procedures, as the answer may have profound clinical implications. For now we should make our patients aware of the possible associations (not risks) as part of obtaining informed consent for the treatment. However, we do not believe that altering patient selection for ART and reducing the treatment's utilization is justified at this time. Finally, it should not be forgotten that even if the described associations are accurate, infertile couples may still choose to accept the risk, as the chances of having a normal infant remain greatly in their favor, and lack of progeny may represent a greater personal tragedy than a potentially small risk of giving birth to an affected child.

Do the clinical and laboratory protocols used in ART cause adverse outcomes in infants conceived through these procedures? The present data suggest associations, but do not prove cause and effect relationships. We recommend that, until better evidence is available, our consent procedures should be modified, but our clinical practice should not.

NOTES AND QUESTIONS

1. The risk to children conceived using ART is generally evaluated in three distinct categories: 1) risks of congenital and genetic abnormalities (congenital referring to defects at birth that are not thought to be inherited, and genetic referring to birth defects inherited from one or both parents), 2) risks related to multiple pregnancy, and 3) psychological and psychosocial impacts on ART children. As to the first category of generalized health risks directly attributable to assisted conception, the Ceelen and Kovalevsky articles above reveal that studies are currently underway to investigate the cause and effect relationship between ART and health outcomes, but no definitive conclusions have yet emerged. At present, the studies show a higher association between problems such as low birth weight, major birth defects and neurological problems at birth following assisted conception (mostly IVF and ICSI) than is present in non-ART populations. But critics point out that "higher association" may mean a minor increase in the overall incidence of the problem because the risks remain very small.

In addition, questions have been raised as to whether ART is the cause for the offspring's health outcome, or whether other factors such as underlying parental infertility are more directly linked to children's health. A study published in 2012 in the *New England Journal of Medicine* attempts to address whether ART or infertility accounts for the greater percentage of birth defects experienced by ART-conceived children. The authors surveyed more than 300,000 births, about 2% of which were ART induced. The children's health records indicated a greater degree of birth defects in the ART group (8.3%) than in the non-ART group (5.8%). However, the authors also discovered that a history of infertility, with or without ART treatment, was associated with birth defects in offspring, thus concluding "[t]he increased risk of birth defects associated with IVF was no longer significant after adjustment for parental factors." Michael J. Davies et al., *Reproductive Technologies and the Risk of Birth Defects*, 366 NEW ENG. J. MED. 1803 (2012).

2. *Multiple Pregnancy.* The use of ART is often associated with multiple pregnancy, a pregnancy in which a woman carries two or more fetuses. The medical literature uses a number of different terms to refer to the gestation of more than one fetus, including multiple gestation pregnancy, multifetal pregnancy, multiple-fetus pregnancy, and high order multiple pregnancy to describe a pregnancy of three or more fetuses. In 2008, 31.6% of all babies born from fresh nondonor IVF cycles were the result of a multiple pregnancy (29.8% were twins, 1.8% were triplets or more). This rate is down from 37% in 1999. To compare, the rate of naturally occurring multiple pregnancy is 1-2% for twins, one in 8,100 births for triplets and 1 in 729,000 births for quadruplets. Mark I. Evans et al., *Selective Termination: Clinical Experience and Residual Risks*, 162 AM. J. OBSTETRICS & GYNECOLOGY 1668 (1990).

Why is there such a high risk of multiple pregnancy following treatment with ART? The answer is quite straightforward. Assisted reproductive treatment works by using powerful drugs to coax a woman's body to produce multiple eggs, which are then removed from her body and fertilized in the laboratory. Logic and research reveals that the more embryos that are transferred back to the uterus, the greater likelihood the woman will become pregnant. Thus, while there is a great deal of controversy over the appropriate number of embryos to transfer, nearly all treatments involve transferring at least two embryos, with nearly 40% all ART cycles involving transfer of three, four or more embryos back into the uterus. According to the CDC, in 2008 embryo transfers per cycles looked as follows: single embryo: 12%, two: 50%, three: 25%, four or more: 14%.

The risks to infants of multiple pregnancy arise primarily from premature birth. The rates of premature delivery increase from approximately 7% with a single gestation to 41% with twins and to 93% with triplets. See Edward G. Hughes & Mita Giacomini, *Funding In Vitro Fertilization Treatment for Persistent Subfertility: The Pain and the Politics*, 76 FERTILITY & STERILITY 431 (2001). Prematurity can result in low birth weight and respiratory distress syndrome, which can lead to severe physical and developmental impairments such as cerebral palsy and learning disabilities. Moreover, as the number of fetuses increases, the rate of neonatal (from birth to approximately the first 28 days of life) and infant death also rises. Advances in neonatal medicine have improved the medical outcomes for multiple pregnancy, but there is widespread consensus that reducing the multiple gestation rate should be a high priority for ART programs. See *Multiple Gestation Pregnancy: The ESHRE Capri Workshop Group*, 15(8) HUMAN REPRODUCTION 1856-64 (2000) (warning that the failure to reduce multiple pregnancy rates may invite overly restrictive legislation limiting ART practices).

We revisit the topic of ART multiple pregnancy in Chapter 8 when we discuss the potential regulatory responses that could be put in place to curb the number of twin and higher births now produced through IVF. Without peeking ahead, can you guess what those regulations might look like? Would you favor such a regulation?

3. *The Octomom Phenomenon.* Public attention to the issue of multiple pregnancy reached a fever pitch in January 2009 when Nadya Suleman gave birth to octuplets at a Los Angeles-area hospital. Dubbed "the Octomom," Ms. Suleman generated intrigue and scorn as a single, unemployed mother of six existing children, all conceived using IVF. The media frenzy that erupted in the wake of the octuplets birth continues to track the whereabouts of their infamous mother, from appearances on the interview-style *The View* to the must-see *Oprah Winfrey Show.* As the octo-experience reveals, our law does not limit the number of embryos a physician can transfer in any given IVF cycle. In some circles, "the Octomom" became a rallying cry for greater regulation of embryo transfer in the U.S. *See* David Orentlicher, *Multiple Embryo Transfers: Time for Policy,* HASTINGS CENTER RPT. 12 (May/June 2010); Naomi R. Cahn & Jennifer M. Collins, *Eight Is Enough,* 103 NORTHWESTERN U. L. REV. COLLOQUY 501 (2009).

The physician who treated Ms. Suleman, Michael Kamrava, was brought up on charges before the California Medical Board for gross negligence in his delivery of IVF services. At the hearing in October 2010, records showed that Ms. Suleman's 14 children were the result of 60 embryo transfers performed in seven IVF cycles, the last of which involved transfer of 12 embryos. Perhaps astonishingly but true, Ms. Suleman gave birth to four singletons and one set of twins from 48 embryos — an 8 to 1 ratio per child. In January 2011, the administrative law judge hearing the matter found Dr. Kamrava guilty of gross negligence, ordering probation rather than revocation of his medical license. The matter was referred to the Medical Board for final disposition. *See Witness Testifies "Octomom" Nadya Suleman's Fertility Doctor Improved Treatment, Recordkeeping,* L.A. TIMES, Oct. 20, 2010. On June 1, 2011, the Medical Board announced its decision to exact a harsher penalty, suspending Dr. Kamrava's license to practice medicine. *See* Rong-Gong Lin II & Jessica Garrison, *California Medical Board Revokes License of "Octomom" Doctor,* L.A. TIMES, June 2, 2011.

In his defense at the hearing, Dr. Kamrava claimed that he acted at his patient's insistence that multiple embryos be transferred at each cycle. Empiric data supports the doctor's claim. Research suggests patients often pressure physicians to pursue more aggressive treatment than they would otherwise recommend, preferring a riskier, multiple pregnancy to no pregnancy. Both financial and emotional pressures associated with overcoming infertility explain this dynamic. *See* Deborah L. Forman, *When "Bad" Mothers Make Worse Law: A Critique of Legislative Limits on Embryo Transfer,* 14 U. PA. J. CONST. L. 173 (2011). If a woman is fully informed about the risks of multiple pregnancy, should "patient-centered" physicians be held legally liable for following their patients' embryo transfer wishes?

4. *Self-Regulation of Embryo Transfer.* In November 2009, the American Society for Reproductive Medicine (ASRM) issued guidelines on the number of embryos to transfer in each IVF cycle. At the outset of the guidelines, ASRM propounds that the Society's goal is to "reduce the number of higher order multiple pregnancies [which are] an undesirable consequences of . . . ART." The guidelines set out recommended embryo transfer limits according to patient age, prognosis, embryo quality, and stage of development (three-day embryos vs. five-day blastocysts). Briefly, for patients with a good prognosis (defined as those with

good-quality embryos who have not failed prior IVF attempts), the following limits are recommended:

A. For patients under age 35, consideration should be given to transferring only a single embryo. No more than two embryos should be transferred.

B. For patients between 35 and 37, no more than two embryos should be transferred.

C. For patients between 38 and 40, no more than three embryos should be transferred.

D. For patients 41-42, no more than five embryos should be transferred.

See The Practice Committee of the American Society for Reproductive Medicine and the Practice Committee of the Society for Assisted Reproductive Technologies, *Guidelines on the Number of Embryos Transferred*, 92(5) FERTILITY & STERILITY 1518 (2009). The 2009 guidelines represent the fifth revision of these clinical standards since they were first issued in 1998. Each version of the guidelines has called for a progressive reduction in the number of embryos transferred.

5. *Psychological and Social Well-Being.* When Louise Brown, the world's first IVF baby, was born in 1978, critics worried that her life would become a "freak show," with media following her every developmental move from cutting her first tooth, to her first steps and beyond. Despite the understandable interest in Louise's development, by all accounts she managed to lead a relatively normal and private lifestyle. She made a rare public appearance in July 2003 while celebrating the 25th anniversary of IVF with hundreds of other similarly conceived children. When asked about her unique place in history, Louise remarked, "I used to think about how I was conceived quite a lot when I was about 10 or 11, but I don't think about it at all now that so many other babies have been born the same way." At the time of her 25th birthday, Louise was busy preparing for her wedding and keeping up her with job as a postal worker in England.

The psychological and social well-being of ART children and their parents is, of course, of enormous importance in assessing the overall success of reproductive medicine. To date, virtually every study focusing on the psychological well-being of parents and their children born after assisted reproduction has shown that ART families are no more likely than non-ART families to exhibit symptoms of psychological distress, and in fact may even be less likely to experience family-related stress. In a comprehensive look at empirical literature published from 1980 through June 2000 on the psychosocial well-being of parents and their children born after assisted reproduction, researchers found several common findings across the studies reviewed. First, with regard to quality of parenting and family functioning, mothers of children born using ARTs reported less parenting stress and more positive mother- and father-child relationships than mothers of naturally conceived children. Second, with regard to the children's well-being, researchers found no statistically significant differences in child functioning between ART and naturally conceived children in terms of emotions, behavior, self-esteem, or perceptions of family relationships. Chun-Shin Hahn, *Psychosocial Well-Being of Parents and*

Their Children Born After Assisted Reproduction, 26(8) J. PEDIATRIC PSYCHOLOGY 525-538 (2001).

For a comprehensive look at the moral and legal conundrums that arise when prospective parents use risky forms of reproductive technologies, *see* PHILIP G. PETERS, JR. HOW SAFE IS SAFE ENOUGH? (2004) (setting forth the contexts in which the state may reasonably assert an interest in the well-being of future persons).

6.   If you were a physician specializing in reproductive medicine, what information about risks to ART children would you provide to your patients? Would you disclose every study that has been conducted to date showing a possible link between infertility treatment and health risks? What about the risks of multiple pregnancy? Since one in every three IVF pregnancies results in a multiple birth, do you think this information would be material to a patient at the outset of treatment? What about discussing the technique of selective reduction in which a high order multifetal pregnancy is reduced, usually to a twin pregnancy, during the first trimester? Should patients be informed about the option of selective reduction before beginning treatment? Do you see any validity to the argument that telling patients about the option of selective reduction before treatment begins will lead those patients to demand more aggressive treatment, i.e. more embryos transferred, because they can then be assured of achieving pregnancy with the option to reduce to a safe number of fetuses during the first trimester?

b.   Safety to Adults

The health and safety risks to adults arising from infertility treatment fall into three basic categories: 1) risks from the drug and surgical treatments that comprise infertility therapy, 2) risks to women from multiple gestation, and 3) psychological and social harms from treatments and parenting following an ART birth. Though much of the research surrounding ART risks focuses on the children born following assisted conception, some research has emerged highlighting possible risks to the women who undergo the various ART treatments. The following excerpt briefly summarizes the medical and social risks infertility patients face when undergoing treatment that is, by its very nature, designed to bypass or enhance the natural process of conception.

Edward G. Hughes and Mita Giacomini
Funding In Vitro Fertilization Treatment for Persistent Subfertility: The Pain and the Politics
76 Fertility & Sterility 431 (2001)

Risks for Women

In addition to the perceived societal risks for women as a group, assisted reproductive technologies (ARTs) present some risks to the individual undergoing treatment. Ovulation induction agents must be used with caution to minimize the risk of severe ovarian hyperstimulation syndrome (OHSS). This may affect 2% to 5% of women undergoing treatment, some of whom require hospital admission and anticoagulant therapy to minimize the risk of thromboembolic disease. At least two deaths have been reported as a result of this phenomenon.

Concern has also been raised regarding ovarian cancer risk associated with fertility medications. Although clomiphene citrate [a drug used to induce the production of multiple eggs] use for >12 months has been cited as a potential source of increased risk, more recent data, including follow-up of approximately 30,000 Australian women, are reassuring. Maternal risks of multiple pregnancy are also significant: severe ovarian hyperstimulation syndrome, pre-eclampsia, antepartum and postpartum hemorrhage, gestational diabetes, and cesarian section are all more common than with single gestations.

A less visible risk to women might be summed up as the existential cost of going through IVF. Loss of personal control, objectification, and medicalization have all been linked with IVF. These may best be measured by women who have gone through treatment but have not conceived; they have an appreciation of the many costs of IVF that successful patients and society as a whole do not. Also, the cost to women of being denied access to treatment bears consideration.

The burden of illness from unresolved persistent subfertility is substantial. The individual women and men who experience this often bear tremendous personal and psychological pain. Some scholars argue that this suffering does not originate only from individuals' frustrated dreams but also from broader cultural, social or economic imperatives to procreate: this suffering is a product of a pronatal society, which values women largely for their ability to bear children. These imperatives in turn, contribute to the overvaluation of women as child bearers, which historically has perpetuated oppression and suffering that extends far beyond the realm of ART.

Some feminists argue that IVF and other technological opportunities, to bear children implicitly strengthens the imperative to have children, to the further detriment of women's status. This argument is perhaps best answered by individual women dealing with subfertility themselves. In industrialized Western societies, it seems paternalistic indeed to assume that women seeking infertility treatments act out of a sense of external obligation rather than out of authentic, self-interested desire. It is an empirical question whether the increased availability of assisted reproduction makes women in general more expected or obligated to bear children and whether this in turn undermines their power or status. There are many arguments — feminist as well as conventional — both in favor and against this possibility.

NOTES AND QUESTIONS

1. One major concern for women's health associated with infertility treatment is the possible link between the strong hormone-based drug therapies used to induce ovulation and later diagnoses of cancer. This risk became the subject of much concern in the early 1990s when the prestigious *New England Journal of Medicine* published a study showing an increased risk of cancerous ovarian tumors among women who had taken ovulation-inducing medications for a period of one year or longer. Mary Anne Rossing, Janet R. Daling, Noel S. Weiss, Donald E. Moore, and Steven G. Self, *Ovarian Tumors in a Cohort of Infertile Women*, 331 NEW ENG. J.

MED. 771-6 (1994). In the proceeding years, other studies were conducted that showed no such link. In the excerpt above, Drs. Hughes and Giacomini describe the current data as "reassuring," citing several large-scale studies. For example, in the year 2002 two major studies were published in which researchers concluded that data collected in the U.S. and Europe did not support any link between fertility treatment using ovarian stimulation and an increased incidence of breast, uterine or ovarian cancer. See Roberta B. Ness et al., *Infertility, Fertility Drugs, and Ovarian Cancer: A Pooled Analysis of Case-Control Studies*, 155 AM. J. EPIDEMIOLOGY 217-224 (2002); Pat Doyle et al., *Cancer Incidence Following Treatment for Infertility at a Clinic in the UK*, 17(8) HUMAN REPRODUCTION 2209-13 (2002).

2. *Multiple Pregnancy.* Carrying two or more fetuses poses greater risks to the woman than carrying a single fetus. Multiple gestation can adversely affect a woman's medical and psychological health both during pregnancy and after delivery. Pregnancy-related maternal complications include preterm labor, premature delivery, pregnancy-induced hypertension (high blood pressure), hemorrhage, severe anemia, preeclampsia, and postpartum blood transfusions. In addition to these serious complications, the mother of multiple fetuses must endure months of discomfort from uterine overdistention plus the boredom of long-term bed rest, often in a hospital, recommended beginning in the second trimester of pregnancy. As noted above, children born from a multiple pregnancy often suffer perinatal and even long-term health problems, adding to the physical, emotional and financial strains that typically befall new parents. Given these well-described risks associated with multiple pregnancy, one might guess that would-be parents would strive to avoid conceiving more than one child. In fact, studies show that a majority of patients undergoing ART treatment desire to conceive a twin pregnancy, an understandable reaction to years of infertility. *See* W.A. Grobman et al., *Patient Perceptions of Multiple Gestations: An Assessment of Knowledge and Risk Aversion*, 185(4) AM. J. OBSTETRICS & GYNECOLOGY 920-4 (2001); Mary D'Alton, *Infertility and the Desire to Multiple Births*, 81 FERTILITY & STERILITY 523 (2004) (noting 20% of women surveyed preferred multiple birth, 94% seeking twins).

3. *Blastocyst Transfer.* The current practice in most fertility clinics is to transfer embryos back to the woman's uterus on day 3, that is, three days after they are formed by the union of the egg and the sperm. Recent research shows promise in achieving pregnancy when the embryo transfer occurs on day five, two days after the traditional time for transfer. A five-day embryo is a blastocyst, a more highly developed entity containing approximately 120-200 cells, compared with the four- to eight-celled three-day embryo. In 2008, success rates for day 5 transfers were higher than for day three transfers across all age groups. Still, day 3 transfers remain the standard of care (56% of all cycles versus 35% for day 5 transfers). If blastocyst transfer proves successful for most ART patients, the elusive goal of reducing or eliminating multiple pregnancy may be within reach. See American Society for Reproductive Medicine and Society for Assisted Reproductive Technology, *Blastocyst Production and Transfer in Clinical Assisted Reproduction* (Practice Committee Report 2000).

4. Assume you are a physician specializing in reproductive medicine. A new patient and her husband, Mr. and Mrs. Baker, visit you in your office for an initial screening appointment. They tell you they have seen three other fertility doctors at

three different clinics where Mrs. Baker underwent a total of 12 IVF cycles, all unsuccessful. The Bakers say they are "desperate" to have a child and they want you to do "everything in your professional power" to help them achieve their dream of parenthood. What would you say to the Bakers? Would you agree to treat Mrs. Baker with additional fertility drugs and surgeries? At what point, if any, do you have a professional duty to decline to offer additional infertility therapies? *See* Ethics Committee of the American Society for Reproductive Medicine, *Fertility Treatment When the Prognosis is Very Poor or Futile*, 92 FERTILITY & STERILITY 1194 (2009).

SECTION IV: WHAT IS THE NATURE AND STATUS OF THE HUMAN EMBRYO?

Thus far our discussion has focused on the medical aspects of infertility and reproduction, with descriptions of the human embryo largely in technical and biological terms. But a deeper inquiry into the nature and status of the human embryo is essential to any analysis of the field of assisted reproductive technologies, as the embryo is at the very heart of all forms of reproduction. Your own view of the human embryo, whether you consider it to be a human life from the moment of conception or at some later time, has likely already been shaped by moral, religious, parental, or other influences that have helped make you the person you are today. The purpose of this section is not to challenge or change your views, but rather to present different perspectives on the nature and status of the human embryo in a variety of contexts. Specifically, we consider the human embryo by asking the following three-part question: What is the biological, the legal and the moral status of the human embryo? As you read the responsive materials, consider how each perspective would apply in a variety of situations, ranging from freezing spare embryos after an IVF cycle to harvesting cells from a blastocyst for stem cell research.

A.   The Biological Status of the Human Embryo

Howard W. Jones, Jr. and Lucinda Veeck
What Is An Embryo?
77 Fertility & Sterility 658 (2002)

What is an embryo? It depends who you ask. Merriam-Webster's Dictionary (Ninth Collegiate Edition) gives two definitions: "1) a vertebrate at any stage of development prior to birth or hatching, and 2) . . . the developing human individual from the time of implantation to the end of the eighth week after conception." Notice that the second definition excludes development before implantation. Stedman's Medical Dictionary (20th Edition) is quite vague, describing ". . . an individual from fertilization of the ovum to birth. In man, the stages beyond the third month of gestation are frequently designated as fetal." Notice that Stedman's appears to extend the embryonic period to 12 weeks.

In Developmental Stages in Human Embryos (Ronan O'Rahilly and Fabiola Muller, Carnegie Institution, Washington, DC, 1987, pp. 13–15), Carnegie stage 2 is defined as ". . . comprising specimens from 2 cells up to the appearance of the blastocystic (or segmentation) cavity . . .

In The Dictionary of Biology by Edwin B. Steen (Barnes and Noble Books/ Harper & Row, New York, 1971, p. 161), "embryo" is defined as, "In mammals, the stage between blastocyst and fetus, when organs and organ systems are coming into existence."

In the midst of this uncertainty, the concept of the preembryo was introduced in 1986 by the American Fertility Society, now the American Society for Reproductive Medicine, through its Ethics Committee with the issuance of the report of that committee (*Ethical Considerations of the New Reproductive Technologies*, Fertility and Sterility, 1986;46:1–93). At the same time, the Volunteer Licensing Authority, an arm of the Royal College of Obstetricians and Gynecologists, and the British Medical Research Council introduced the same term independently. The preembryo was identified as the interval up to the appearance of the primitive streak, which guarantees biologic individuation. This marker occurs at about 14 days. It was of some significance that quite independently the Ethics Advisory Board of the [U.S.] Department of Health, Education, and Welfare in its report in 1979 designated the period beyond 14 days as having attained special moral status.

The nonscientific, general public, next-door-neighbors are understandably quite unsure about the definition of an embryo, but remembering what they saw in a jar in biology class, generally think of an embryo as something shaped like a tadpole or perhaps even possessing arms and legs . . .

All this means that some precision is required in describing and defining accurately the various stages of development.

To be sure, the processes of spermatogenesis [development of sperm], oogenesis [development of eggs], fertilization and development are a continuum. Nevertheless, there are milestones, i.e., clear marker events, which conveniently segment various stages of development.

The events of the first few days of development are so biologically unique that they deserve to be described and segregated. This is the preembryonic period previously described (Jones and Schraeder, Fertility and Sterility 1989;52:189). This turbulent period has the following characteristics:

- Large numbers of abnormalities occur. Estimates vary as to the extent of these abnormalities which cause loss, but a conservative estimate is that at least two-thirds of the products of oocyte and sperm fusion are in some way defective, either chromosomally or perhaps more subtly at the molecular level. The carrier of these abnormalities is so abnormal that it never implants, or, if it does implant, usually perishes very early in development.

- During this early phase of development, most of the developing structures will be devoted to nourishing the subsequent embryo. The trophoblast predominates and is the predecessor of the placenta and extra-embryonic membranes that will be discarded at the time of birth. While the embryoblast segregates and is recognizable toward the end of this stage, it consists of only a few cells, rudiments of the subsequent actual embryo. It is from these cells that stem cells may be obtained.

- During the preembryonic time, twinning may occur. There is no guarantee that there will be a single individual until the end of the time of the preembryonic period, i.e., until only a single primitive streak differentiates.

- An individual may not develop at all. As a result of fertilization, the products of fertilization may end up as a tumor, a hydatidiform mole, or even worse, a chorioepithelioma that in the end may destroy the host.

- The lack of specificity of individual development is illustrated by the fact that during this interval, fusion of two preembryos can occur and result in the development of a single adult individual. This is well established in the human where fusion occasionally occurs with preembryos of different sexes. The presumption is that if it occurs under these circumstances there must be at least an equal number of instances where fusion occurs between two XX preembryos or between two XY preembryos. Thus, the primitive streak guarantees biological individuation and terminates the preembryonic period.

The subsequent embryonic period is far less turbulent. It is characterized by the appearance of fundamental tissues and with the formation of primitive organs and organ systems. Although the limb buds are identifiable, arms or legs are not yet present. As stated in Webster's, this period (embryonic) is generally considered to end at about 8 weeks, with transition into the fetal period. Thus, the terms "preembryo," "embryo," and "fetus" describe the products of very unique developmental intervals.

These developmental intervals are by no means acceptable to all members of the scientific community. This is especially true for those who came to study human material by way of the small animal laboratory where the 2- to 4-cell objects flushed from fallopian tubes were commonly referred to as "embryos." Although imprecise, this practice has been considered acceptable within the animal realm, but for the human where moral values may be assigned to development, we believe the animal terminology to be outdated and, more importantly, biologically inaccurate . . .

Wise men and women through the ages have used external signs, like quickening, audible heart sounds, and electrical brain activity, as evidence indicating change in moral status. The Supreme Court of the United States selected viability as its marker after which societal protection was considered required. The recent discussions about stem cells through print, visual, and audible media, and by both the general public and the scientific community, have indicated that there is considerable variation in the concepts of the stages of development and the significance thereof. We believe that the scientific community has a responsibility to be precise in these matters, both in communicating with ourselves and with the general public, in order to lend accuracy to the current debates.

NOTES AND QUESTIONS

1. Drs. Jones and Veeck strive to make the point that from a biologic standpoint, prenatal life can be divided into three distinguishable intervals, the preembryo, embryo and fetal stages. During the preembryo stage, they maintain, the developing entity consists of "only a few cells, rudiments of the subsequent actual embryo." This stage lasts until about 14 days after fertilization, at which point the full-fledged embryo emerges. The embryo becomes a fetus at the end of the eighth week of gestation. As we have discussed, all ARTs take place during the early stages of the preembryo period, often when the developing entity is three days old.

The division of prenatal life into three distinct stages is not universally accepted. For some, the notion of a preembryo is problematic because it suggests that the developing human at the earliest stages is less deserving of rights or moral status because it is "pre" or before the emergence of the embryo, often recognized as the beginning of human life. In response to the Jones and Veeck editorial set out above, two responders argue:

> . . . Jones infers that before implantation, an embryo does not exist and refers instead to the preembryo. In reality, it is the preembryo that does not exist. No human embryologist endorses the term preembryo. No textbook of human embryology endorses it. One text calls it "ill-defined, inaccurate, unjustified and equivocal." Furthermore, the Nomenclature Committee of the American Association of Anatomists has rejected the terms preembryo, preembryonic, and individuation for inclusion in the Terminologia Embryologica . . .

> The marvel of the continuum demonstrated in embryonic life should never be undermined by reducing the human essence to a function or some arbitrary pseudo-scientific stage. Human development does not end at birth. Just as in embryonic life, all of life is a continuum. To assign varying moral values at anytime during life is simply arbitrary and has nothing to do with science.

Richard Thorne & C. Ward Kischer, *Embryos, Preembryos, and Stem Cells*, Letter to the Editor, 78(6) FERTILITY & STERILITY 1355 (2002).

Note: Throughout this book we generally use the term "embryo" to refer to both the preembryo and embryo stages of development. We do so largely because most writers, be they scientists, judges or legislators, use the term *embryo* to refer to the developing human organism from the moment of conception. Our usage is not intended to favor one position over the other as to whether the preembryo exists, but rather to reflect the usage displayed in most excerpts contained in this book.

2. Does the Jones and Veeck three-stage description of the developing human remind you of other efforts to characterize prenatal life in three segments? In our next chapter we will review the United States Supreme Court's 1973 decision in *Roe v. Wade* in which Justice Harry Blackmun describes the pregnancy process in trimesters; three distinct stages of pregnancy from the first moments to the last, which take on legal significance in the context of abortion. Is a three-part description of the developing human organism also useful to help define the rights of patients, doctors, researchers and others toward prenatal life? Or should we favor

a description of the early life form that highlights its continual metamorphosis from a one-celled entity to a newborn infant? Clearly the law favors line-drawing to establish rights (i.e., a teenager becomes an adult on her 18th birthday, a worker becomes eligible for Social Security benefits on his 62nd birthday). What purpose is served by line-drawing at the earliest stages of life?

3. How do you answer the question, "When does life begin?" Do you believe that life begins at fertilization, when the sperm and egg fuse to form a genetically unique entity that has the capacity to grow into a fully formed human being? Or do you believe that life begins when the organism displays qualities that are associated with human life, such as brain activity or a beating heart? Or perhaps you associate life with more advanced human attributes such as consciousness and self-awareness. Have the explanations of the biologic development of the human being changed or influenced your answer to the question about the fundamental nature of life? If not, why not?

B. The Legal Status of the Human Embryo

1. An Introductory Case

DAVIS v. DAVIS
Supreme Court of Tennessee
842 S.W.2d 588 (1992)

DAUGHTREY, J.

This appeal presents a question of first impression, involving the disposition of the cryogenically-preserved product of in vitro fertilization (IVF), commonly referred to in the popular press and the legal journals as "frozen embryos." The case began as a divorce action, filed by the appellee, Junior Lewis Davis, against his then wife, appellant Mary Sue Davis. The parties were able to agree upon all terms of dissolution, except one: who was to have "custody" of the seven "frozen embryos" stored in a Knoxville fertility clinic that had attempted to assist the Davises in achieving a much-wanted pregnancy during a happier period in their relationship.

I. Introduction

Mary Sue Davis originally asked for control of the "frozen embryos" with the intent to have them transferred to her own uterus, in a post-divorce effort to become pregnant. Junior Davis objected, saying that he preferred to leave the embryos in their frozen state until he decided whether or not he wanted to become a parent outside the bounds of marriage.

Based on its determination that the embryos were "human beings" from the moment of fertilization, the trial court awarded "custody" to Mary Sue Davis and directed that she "be permitted the opportunity to bring these children to term through implantation." The Court of Appeals reversed, finding that Junior Davis has a "constitutionally protected right not to beget a child where no pregnancy has taken place" and holding that "there is no compelling state interest to justify [ ] ordering implantation against the will of either party." The Court of Appeals further held that "the parties share an interest in the seven fertilized ova" and remanded the case to the trial court for entry of an order vesting them with "joint control . . . and equal voice over their disposition."

Mary Sue Davis then sought review in this Court, contesting the validity of the constitutional basis for the Court of Appeals decision. We granted review, not because we disagree with the basic legal analysis utilized by the intermediate court, but because of the obvious importance of the case in terms of the development of law regarding the new reproductive technologies, and because the decision of the Court of Appeals does not give adequate guidance to the trial court in the event the parties cannot agree.

We note, in this latter regard, that their positions have already shifted: both have remarried and Mary Sue Davis (now Mary Sue Stowe) has moved out of state. She no longer wishes to utilize the "frozen embryos" herself, but wants authority to donate them to a childless couple. Junior Davis is adamantly opposed to such donation and would prefer to see the "frozen embryos" discarded. The result is, once again, an impasse, but the parties' current legal position does have an effect on the probable outcome of the case, as discussed below.

At the outset, it is important to note the absence of two critical factors that might otherwise influence or control the result of this litigation: When the Davises signed up for the IVF program at the Knoxville clinic, they did not execute a written agreement specifying what disposition should be made of any unused embryos that might result from the cryopreservation process. Moreover, there was at that time no Tennessee statute governing such disposition, nor has one been enacted in the meantime.[17]

In addition, because of the uniqueness of the question before us, we have no case law to guide us to a decision in this case. Despite the fact that over 5,000 IVF babies have been born in this country and the fact that some 20,000 or more "frozen embryos" remain in storage, there are apparently very few other litigated cases involving the disputed disposition of untransferred "frozen embryos," and none is on point with the facts in this case . . .

II. The Facts

Mary Sue Davis and Junior Lewis Davis met while they were both in the Army and stationed in Germany in the spring of 1979. After a period of courtship, they came home to the United States and were married on April 26, 1980. When their leave was up, they then returned to their posts in Germany as a married couple.

Within six months of returning to Germany, Mary Sue became pregnant but

---

[17] [n.1] At the time of trial, only one state had enacted pertinent legislation. A Louisiana statute entitled "Human Embryos," among other things, forbids the intentional destruction of a cryopreserved IVF embryo and declares that disputes between parties should be resolved in the "best interest" of the embryo. 1986 La. Acts R.S. 9:121 *et seq.* Under the Louisiana statute, unwanted embryos must be made available for "adoptive implantation."

unfortunately suffered an extremely painful tubal pregnancy, as a result of which she had surgery to remove her right fallopian tube. This tubal pregnancy was followed by four others during the course of the marriage. After her fifth tubal pregnancy, Mary Sue chose to have her left fallopian tube ligated, thus leaving her without functional fallopian tubes by which to conceive naturally. The Davises attempted to adopt a child but, at the last minute, the child's birth-mother changed her mind about putting the child up for adoption. Other paths to adoption turned out to be prohibitively expensive. In vitro fertilization became essentially the only option for the Davises to pursue in their attempt to become parents.

As explained at trial, IVF involves the aspiration of ova from the follicles of a woman's ovaries, fertilization of these ova in a petri dish using the sperm provided by a man, and the transfer of the product of this procedure into the uterus of the woman from whom the ova were taken.[18] Implantation may then occur, resulting in a pregnancy and, it is hoped, the birth of a child.

Beginning in 1985, the Davises went through six attempts at IVF, at a total cost of $35,000, but the hoped-for pregnancy never occurred. Despite her fear of needles, at each IVF attempt Mary Sue underwent the month of subcutaneous injections necessary to shut down her pituitary gland and the eight days of intermuscular injections necessary to stimulate her ovaries to produce ova. She was anesthetized five times for the aspiration procedure to be performed. Forty-eight to 72 hours after each aspiration, she returned for transfer back to her uterus, only to receive a negative pregnancy test result each time.

The Davises then opted to postpone another round of IVF until after the clinic with which they were working was prepared to offer them cryogenic preservation, scheduled for November 1988. Using this process, if more ova are aspirated and fertilized than needed, the conceptive product may be cryogenically preserved (frozen in nitrogen and stored at sub-zero temperatures) for later transfer if the transfer performed immediately does not result in a pregnancy. The unavailability of this procedure had not been a hindrance to previous IVF attempts by the Davises because Mary Sue had produced at most only three or four ova, despite hormonal stimulation. However, on their last attempt, on December 8, 1988, the gynecologist who performed the procedure was able to retrieve nine ova for fertilization. The resulting one-celled entities, referred to before division as zygotes, were then allowed to develop in petri dishes in the laboratory until they reached the four- to eight-cell stage.

Needless to say, the Davises were pleased at the initial success of the procedure. At the time, they had no thoughts of divorce and the abundance of ova for fertilization offered them a better chance at parenthood, because Mary Sue Davis could attempt to achieve a pregnancy without additional rounds of hormonal stimulation and aspiration. They both testified that although the process of cryogenic preservation was described to them, no one explained the ways in which

---

[18] [n.8] Alternatively, the fertilized ova may also be transferred to the uterus of a "surrogate mother," who carries through with the pregnancy for the gamete-providers, or they may be donated to a genetically unrelated couple.

it would change the nature of IVF for them.[19] There is, for example, no indication that they ever considered the implications of storage beyond the few months it would take to transfer the remaining "frozen embryos," if necessary. There was no discussion, let alone an agreement, concerning disposition in the event of a contingency such as divorce.

After fertilization was completed, a transfer was performed as usual on December 10, 1988; the rest of the four- to eight-cell entities were cryogenically preserved. Unfortunately, a pregnancy did not result from the December 1988 transfer, and before another transfer could be attempted, Junior Davis filed for divorce — in February 1989. He testified that he had known that their marriage "was not very stable" for a year or more, but had hoped that the birth of a child would improve their relationship. Mary Sue Davis testified that she had no idea that there was a problem with their marriage.[20] As noted earlier, the divorce proceedings were complicated only by the issue of the disposition of the "frozen embryos."

III. The Scientific Testimony

In the record, and especially in the trial court's opinion, there is a great deal of discussion about the proper descriptive terminology to be used in this case. Although this discussion appears at first glance to be a matter simply of semantics, semantical distinctions are significant in this context, because language defines legal status and can limit legal rights.[21] Obviously, an "adult" has a different legal status than does a "child." Likewise, "child" means something other than "fetus."[22] A "fetus" differs from an "embryo." There was much dispute at trial about whether the four- to eight-cell entities in this case should properly be referred to as "embryos" or as "preembryos," with resulting differences in legal analysis.

One expert, a French geneticist named Dr. Jerome Lejeune, insisted that there was no recognized scientific distinction between the two terms. He referred to the four- to eight-cell entities at issue here as "early human beings," as "tiny persons," and as his "kin." Although he is an internationally recognized geneticist, Dr. Lejeune's background fails to reflect any degree of expertise in obstetrics or gynecology (specifically in the field of infertility) or in medical ethics. His testimony revealed a profound confusion between science and religion. For example, he was

---

[19] [n.9] They also were not asked to sign any consent forms. Apparently the clinic was in the process of moving its location when the Davises underwent this last round and, because timing of each step of IVF is crucial, it was impossible to postpone the procedure until the appropriate forms were located.

[20] [n.10] Mary Sue Davis's testimony is contradictory as to whether she would have gone ahead with IVF if she had been worried about her marriage. At one point she said if she had known they were getting divorced, she would not have gone ahead with it, but at another point she indicated that she was so committed to the idea of being a mother that she could not say that she would not have gone ahead with cryopreservation.

[21] [n.11] For a thorough consideration of the implications of status, see Clifford Grobstein, Science and the Unborn, pages 58-62, Basic Books, Inc., New York (1988).

[22] [n.12] As Justice Stevens noted in *Thornburgh v. American College of Obstetricians and Gynecologists*, 476 U.S. 747, 779 n. 8, 106 S.Ct. 2169, 2188 n. 8, 90 L.Ed.2d 779 (1986) (Stevens, J., concurring), "No member of this Court has ever suggested that a fetus of [sic] a 'person' within the meaning of the Fourteenth Amendment."

deeply moved that "Madame [Mary Sue], the mother, wants to rescue babies from this concentration can," and he concluded that Junior Davis has a moral duty to try to bring these "tiny human beings" to term.[23]

Dr. LeJeune's opinion was disputed by Dr. Irving Ray King, the gynecologist who performed the IVF procedures in this case. Dr. King is a medical doctor who had practiced as a sub-speciality in the areas of infertility and reproductive endocrinology for 12 years. He established the Fertility Center of East Tennessee in Knoxville in 1984 and had worked extensively with IVF and cryopreservation. He testified that the currently accepted term for the zygote immediately after division is "preembryo" and that this term applies up until 14 days after fertilization. He testified that this 14-day period defines the accepted period for preembryo research. At about 14 days, he testified, the group of cells begins to differentiate in a process that permits the eventual development of the different body parts which will become an individual. Dr. King's testimony was corroborated by the other experts who testified at trial, with the exception of Dr. Lejeune. It is further supported by the American Fertility Society, an organization of 10,000 physicians and scientists who specialize in problems of human infertility. The Society's June 1990 report on Ethical Considerations of the New Reproductive Technologies[24] indicates that from the point of fertilization, the resulting one-cell zygote contains "a new hereditary constitution (genome) contributed to by both parents through the union of sperm and egg." Id. at 31S. Continuing, the report notes:

> The stage subsequent to the zygote is cleavage, during which the single initial cell undergoes successive equal divisions with little or no intervening growth. As a result, the product cells (blastomeres) become successively smaller, while the size of the total aggregate of cells remains the same. After three such divisions, the aggregate contains eight cells in relatively loose association . . . [E]ach blastomere, if separated from the others, has the potential to develop into a complete adult . . . Stated another way, at the 8-cell stage, the developmental singleness of one person has not been established. Beyond the 8-cell stage, individual blastomeres begin to lose their zygote-like properties. Two divisions after the 8-cell stage, the 32 blastomeres are increasingly adherent, closely packed, and no longer of equal developmental potential. The impression now conveyed is of a multicellular entity, rather than of a loose packet of identical cells.

> As the number of cells continues to increase, some are formed into a surface layer, surrounding others within. The outer layers have changed in properties toward trophoblast . . . , which is destined [to become part of the placenta]. The less-altered inner cells will be the source of the later embryo. The developing entity is now referred to as a blastocyst, charac- terized by a continuous peripheral layer of cells and a small cellular

---

[23] [n.13] For further rather uncomplimentary characterization of Lejeune's testimony, see Annas, A French Homunculus in a Tennessee Court, 19 Hastings Center Report (Nov/Dec 1989).

[24] [n.14] Published in the official Journal of the American Fertility Society, Volume 53, number 6, June 1990.

population within a central cavity . . . It is at about this stage that the [normally] developing entity usually completes its transit through the oviduct to enter the uterus.

Cell division continues and the blastocyst enlarges through increase of both cell number and [volume]. The populations of inner and outer cells become increasingly different, not only in position and shape but in synthetic activities as well. The change is primarily in the outer population, which is altering rapidly as the blastocyst interacts with and implants into the uterine wall . . . Thus, the first cellular differentiation of the new generation relates to physiologic interaction with the mother, rather than to the establishment of the embryo itself. *It is for this reason that it is appropriate to refer to the developing entity up to this point as a preembryo, rather than an embryo.*

Id. at 31S-32S (emphasis added). For a similar description of the biologic difference between a preembryo and an embryo, see Robertson, *In the Beginning: The Legal Status of Early Embryos*, 76 Va. L. Rev. 437 (1990), in which the author summarizes the findings of Clifford Grobstein in *The Early Development of Human Embryos*, 10 J.Med. & Phil. 213 (1984).

Admittedly, this distinction is not dispositive in the case before us.[25] It deserves emphasis only because inaccuracy can lead to misanalysis such as occurred at the trial level in this case. The trial court reasoned that if there is no distinction between embryos and preembryos, as Dr. Lejeune theorized, then Dr. Lejeune must also have been correct when he asserted that "human life begins at the moment of conception." From this proposition, the trial judge concluded that the eight-cell entities at issue were not preembryos but were "children in vitro." He then invoked the doctrine of parens patriae and held that it was "in the best interest of the children" to be born rather than destroyed. Finding that Mary Sue Davis was willing to provide such an opportunity, but that Junior Davis was not, the trial judge awarded her "custody" of the "children in vitro."

The Court of Appeals explicitly rejected the trial judge's reasoning, as well as the result. Indeed, the argument that "human life begins at the moment of conception" and that these four- to eight-cell entities therefore have a legal right to be born has apparently been abandoned by the appellant, despite her success with it in the trial court.[26] We have nevertheless been asked by the American Fertility Society, joined by 19 other national organizations allied in this case as amici curiae, to respond to this issue because of its far-reaching implications in other cases of this kind. We find the request meritorious.

---

[25] [n.15] It would be relevant, however, to the question of whether embryonic research is permissible, under regulations that limit such research to "preembryonic" stages. Such research is carried out principally in order to perfect in vitro fertilization techniques and to increase the success rate of pregnancies achieved through IVF and, as of 1986, was regulated by statute in some 25 states. See L.B. Andrews, *The Legal Status of the Embryo*, 32 Loyola L.Rev. 357, 396-397 (1986).

[26] [n.16] In her brief, the appellant now characterizes the preembryos as "potential life" rather than as "human beings."

IV. The "Person" vs. "Property" Dichotomy

One of the fundamental issues the inquiry poses is whether the preembryos in this case should be considered "persons" or "property" in the contemplation of the law. The Court of Appeals held, correctly, that they cannot be considered "persons" under Tennessee law:

> The policy of the state on the subject matter before us may be gleaned from the state's treatment of fetuses in the womb. . . . The state's Wrongful Death Statute, Tenn.Code Ann. § 20-5-106 does not allow a wrongful death for a viable fetus that is not first born alive. Without live birth, the Supreme Court has said, a fetus is not a "person" within the meaning of the statute . . . Other enactments by the legislature demonstrate even more explicitly that viable fetuses in the womb are not entitled to the same protection as "persons". Tenn.Code Ann. § 39-15-201 incorporates the trimester approach to abortion outlined in *Roe v. Wade*, 410 U.S. 113 [93 S.Ct. 705, 35 L.Ed.2d 147] (1973). A woman and her doctor may decide on abortion within the first three months of pregnancy but after three months, and before viability, abortion may occur at a properly regulated facility. Moreover, after viability, abortion may be chosen to save the life of the mother. This statutory scheme indicates that as embryos develop, they are accorded more respect than mere human cells because of their burgeoning potential for life. But, even after viability, they are not given legal status equivalent to that of a person already born. This concept is echoed in Tennessee's murder and assault statutes, which provide that an attack or homicide of a viable fetus may be a crime but abortion is not. See Tenn.Code Ann. §§ 39-13-107 and 39-13-210.

Junior Lewis Davis v. Mary Sue Davis, Tennessee Court of Appeals at Knoxville, No. 190, slip op. at 5-6, 1990 WL 130807 (Sept. 13, 1990).

Nor do preembryos enjoy protection as "persons" under federal law. In *Roe v. Wade*, 410 U.S. 113, 93 S.Ct. 705, 35 L.Ed.2d 147 (1973), the United States Supreme Court explicitly refused to hold that the fetus possesses independent rights under law, based upon a thorough examination of the federal constitution,[27] relevant common law principles, and the lack of scientific consensus as to when life begins. The Supreme Court concluded that "the unborn have never been recognized in the law as persons *Webster v. Reproductive Health Services* in the whole sense." Id. at 162, 93 S.Ct. at 731. As a matter of constitutional law, this conclusion has never been seriously challenged.[28] Hence, even as the Supreme Court in, 492 U.S. 490, 109 S.Ct. 3040, 106 L.Ed.2d 410 (1989), permitted the states some additional leeway in regulating the right to abortion established in *Roe v. Wade*, the *Webster* decision did no more than recognize a compelling state interest in potential life at the point when

---

[27] [n.17] The Fourteenth Amendment, for example, limits the equal protection and due process of law to "persons born or naturalized in the United States."

[28] [n.18] As Justice Stevens noted in *Thornburgh v. American College of Obstetricians and Gynecologists*, 476 U.S. 747, 779 n. 8, 106 S.Ct. 2169, 2188 n. 8, 90 L.Ed.2d 779 (1986) (Stevens, J., concurring), "No member of this Court has ever suggested that a fetus is a 'person' within the meaning of the Fourteenth Amendment."

viability is possible. Thus, as Justice O'Connor noted, "[v]iability remains the 'critical point.'" Id. at 529, 109 S.Ct. at 3062 (O'Connor, J., concurring). That stage of fetal development is far removed, both qualitatively and quantitatively, from that of the four-to eight-cell preembryos in this case.[29]

Left undisturbed, the trial court's ruling would have afforded preembryos the legal status of "persons" and vested them with legally cognizable interests separate from those of their progenitors. Such a decision would doubtless have had the effect of outlawing IVF programs in the state of Tennessee. But in setting aside the trial court's judgment, the Court of Appeals, at least by implication, may have swung too far in the opposite direction. The intermediate court, without explicitly holding that the preembryos in this case were "property," nevertheless awarded "joint custody" of them to Mary Sue Davis and Junior Davis, citing T.C.A. §§ 68-30-101 and 39-15-208, and *York v. Jones*, 717 F.Supp. 421 (E.D.Va.1989), for the proposition that "the parties share an interest in the seven fertilized ova." The intermediate court did not otherwise define this interest.

The provisions of T.C.A. §§ 68-30-101 et seq., on which the intermediate appellate court relied, codify the Uniform Anatomical Gift Act. T.C.A. § 39-15-208 prohibits experimentation or research using an aborted fetus in the absence of the woman's consent. These statutes address the question of who controls disposition of human organs and tissue with no further potential for autonomous human life; they are not precisely controlling on the question before us, because the "tissue" involved here does have the potential for developing into independent human life, even if it is not yet legally recognizable as human life itself.

The intermediate court's reliance on *York v. Jones*, is even more troublesome. That case involved a dispute between a married couple undergoing IVF procedures at the Jones Institute for Reproductive Medicine in Virginia. When the Yorks decided to move to California, they asked the Institute to transfer the one remaining "frozen embryo" that they had produced to a fertility clinic in San Diego for later implantation. The Institute refused and the Yorks sued. The federal district court assumed without deciding that the subject matter of the dispute was "property." The York court held that the "cryopreservation agreement" between the Yorks and the Institute created a bailment relationship, obligating the Institute to return the subject of the bailment to the Yorks once the purpose of the bailment had terminated. 717 F.Supp. at 424-425.

In this case, by citing to *York v. Jones* but failing to define precisely the "interest" that Mary Sue Davis and Junior Davis have in the preembryos, the Court of Appeals has left the implication that it is in the nature of a property interest. For purposes of clarity in future cases, we conclude that this point must be further addressed.

To our way of thinking, the most helpful discussion on this point is found not in the minuscule number of legal opinions that have involved "frozen embryos," but in

---

[29] [n.19] Left undisturbed in the mother's uterus, a viable fetus has an excellent chance of being brought to term and born live. In contrast, a preembryo in a petri dish, if later transferred, has only a 13-21 percent chance of achieving actual implantation. Of these pregnancies, between 56 percent and 75 percent result in live births. Jones and Rogers, *Clinical In Vitro Fertilization*, 51-62, cited in Poole, *Allocation of Decision-Making Rights to Frozen Embryos*, 4 J.Amer. Family L. 67 (1990).

the ethical standards set by The American Fertility Society, as follows:

> Three major ethical positions have been articulated in the debate over preembryo status. At one extreme is the view of the preembryo as a human subject after fertilization, which requires that it be accorded the rights of a person. This position entails an obligation to provide an opportunity for implantation to occur and tends to ban any action before transfer that might harm the preembryo or that is not immediately therapeutic, such as freezing and some preembryo research.
>
> At the opposite extreme is the view that the preembryo has a status no different from any other human tissue. With the consent of those who have decision-making authority over the preembryo, no limits should be imposed on actions taken with preembryos.
>
> A third view — one that is most widely held — takes an intermediate position between the other two. It holds that the preembryo deserves respect greater than that accorded to human tissue but not the respect accorded to actual persons. The preembryo is due greater respect than other human tissue because of its potential to become a person and because of its symbolic meaning for many people. Yet, it should not be treated as a person, because it has not yet developed the features of personhood, is not yet established as developmentally individual, and may never realize its biologic potential.

Report of the Ethics Committee of The American Fertility Society, supra, at 34S-35S.

Although the report alludes to the role of "special respect" in the context of research on preembryos not intended for transfer, it is clear that the Ethics Committee's principal concern was with the treatment accorded the transferred embryo. Thus, the Ethics Committee concludes that "special respect is necessary to protect the welfare of potential offspring . . . [and] creates obligations not to hurt or injure the offspring who might be born after transfer [by research or intervention with a preembryo]." Id. at 35S.

In its report, the Ethics Committee then calls upon those in charge of IVF programs to establish policies in keeping with the "special respect" due preembryos and suggests:

> Within the limits set by institutional policies, decision-making authority regarding preembryos should reside with the persons who have provided the gametes . . . As a matter of law, it is reasonable to assume that the gamete providers have primary decision-making authority regarding preembryos in the absence of specific legislation on the subject. A person's liberty to procreate or to avoid procreation is directly involved in most decisions involving preembryos.

Id. at 36S.

We conclude that preembryos are not, strictly speaking, either "persons" or "property," but occupy an interim category that entitles them to special respect because of their potential for human life. It follows that any interest that Mary Sue

Davis and Junior Davis have in the preembryos in this case is not a true property interest. However, they do have an interest in the nature of ownership, to the extent that they have decision-making authority concerning disposition of the preembryos, within the scope of policy set by law.

[The court goes on to address the constitutional rights of the parties to engage in assisted reproduction, discussed later in Chapter 2, and the disposition of the frozen embryos, a matter we take up in Chapter 7.]

REID, C.J., and DROWOTA, O'BRIEN and ANDERSON, JJ., concur.

NOTES AND QUESTIONS

1.   The *Davis* court was the first high court to consider the legal status of the early embryo in the context of ART. The court's position that embryos are neither persons nor property, "but occupy an interim category that entitles them to special respect because of their potential for human life" has not yet been widely adopted by subsequent courts considering disputes over the disposition of frozen embryos. For example, in *Kass v. Kass*, 91 N.Y.2d 554 (1998), the New York Court of Appeals considered a divorce scenario similar to the *Davis* dispute, only in this case the parties had signed an agreement with the fertility clinic. While the court agreed that the "pre-zygotes [are not] recognized as "persons" for constitutional purposes," it went on to state "we have no cause to decide whether the pre-zygotes are entitled to "special respect" because the parties' agreement resolved the question of disposition. Id. at 564-565. Likewise, the court in a Washington frozen embryo dispute ducked the question of the legal status of the early embryo, explaining "it is not necessary for this court to engage in a legal, medical or philosophical discussion whether the preembryos in this case are "children" . . ." because the contract resolves the dispute. *Litowitz v. Litowitz*, 146 Wash.2d 514, 533 (2002).

2.   The concept that embryos are entitled to special respect under the law has gained some support in cases in which the fate of disputed frozen embryos is not at stake. In these cases, courts have used the *Davis* language to reason by analogy that other reproductive material occupies a position of symbolic import in the law. For example, in *Janicki v. Hospital of St. Raphael*, 46 Conn. Supp. 204, 744 A.2d 963 (1999) a patient sued her physicians and hospital in tort after they performed an unauthorized autopsy on her nineteen week stillborn, nonviable fetus. Citing from the Davis decision, the Connecticut court held that the fetus "while not a person, was not "property" or "tissue" either. Instead, it occupied an intermediate category in the law entitled to a special respect that would not be given ordinary tissue." *Id.* at 220, 971. In *Janicki*, that special respect translated into a finding that plaintiff did state a claim for negligent infliction of emotional distress because "the hospital and its physicians were not entitled to dissect [the fetus] in the teeth of the mother's express instructions to the contrary." *Id. See also Hecht v. Superior Court*, 16 Cal. App. 4th 836 (1993) (frozen sperm willed to a decedent's girlfriend entitled to special respect because of its potential for human life). We will take up the matter of frozen sperm in the *Hecht* case in Chapter 6.

3.   The *Davis* court makes mention of United States Supreme Court precedent holding that a fetus is not considered a person within the meaning of the Fourteenth Amendment to the United States Constitution. At least one state explicitly rejects the finding that early human life is not entitled to the same rights as all persons under law. La. Rev. Stat. § 9:123 provides, "An in vitro fertilized human ovum exists as a juridical person until such time as the in vitro fertilized ovum is implanted in the womb; or at any other time when rights attach to an unborn child in accordance with law."

If the IVF human embryo exists as a "juridical person" (translation — a person in the eyes of the law), does this mean that infertile Louisiana couples cannot freeze any unused embryos during a fresh IVF cycle because to do so would potentially cause harm to the embryo in the freezing and thawing process? Does the Louisiana law require that all unwanted embryos be made available for adoption, as would be the case with children whose parents are unable or unwilling to care for them? If a Louisiana couple elects to freeze and then abandon their embryos, does this make the physicians "foster parents" to the embryos until an appropriate adoption can be arranged?

2.   Legal Responses to the Status of the Human Embryo

The legal status of the human embryo becomes important in a variety of legal contexts, many of which you have likely studied in your Torts and Criminal Law courses. For example, if a woman is murdered and, unbeknownst to her and the murderer, she was in the early stages of a pregnancy, should the act be considered a double homicide? Or is a physician liable for malpractice to an infant who is stillborn if the parents can prove that negligence caused the death of their fetus? The question of legal personhood and its accompanying rights, remedies and liabilities has been the source of debate at the judicial, legislative, and executive branches of government. Importantly, resolution of the debate over the legal status of the embryo has filled our law libraries, with solutions and suggestions finding their voice in constitutional law, statutory law and common law. What follows is a U.S. National Report to the Sixteenth International Congress of Comparative Law on the topic of American legal treatment of the embryo and fetus. The Report, authored by Professor Timothy Jost, provides an excellent summary of the many contexts in which the legal status of early human life is in question.

Timothy Stoltzfus Jost
Rights of Embryo and Foetus in Private Law
50 American. Journal of Comparative Law 633 (2002)

A. Embryo and Fetus: Concepts, In General

Neither the federal government of the United States nor any of its states have a specific law providing comprehensively for the protection of embryos and fetuses in all contexts. Rather the various states extend protection to embryos and fetuses to varying degrees and in various contexts. There is also no single legal definition of the terms embryo and fetus used throughout the United States, though the

Supreme Court has recognized the embryo and fetus as sequential stages in the development of an unborn human.

B. The Fetus as a 'Person' and Beginning of 'Personality'

In *Roe v. Wade* the Supreme Court expressly determined that: 'the word 'person,' as used in the Fourteenth Amendment of the United States Constitution does not include the unborn.' The Court also, however, recognized — and has reaffirmed even more strongly in subsequent cases — the ability of the states to protect the interests of the unborn. Perhaps because we are a common law jurisdiction, the states tend not to deal with the question of personhood or legal capacity of the unborn comprehensively, but rather address the issue on a case by case and issue by issue basis. One provision of the civil code of Louisiana proclaims that 'natural personality commences from the moment of live birth and terminates at death.' while another provision states: 'An in vitro fertilized human ovum exists as a juridical person until such time as the in vitro fertilized ovum is implanted in the womb.' But few states make such clear statements in their law. Rather the issue of legal status or capacity must be examined in a particular context. The only general statement one can make with some certainty with respect to all states is that legal personality exists from the point of birth, though full legal capacity may not attach until the date of majority (or even later if the person is incompetent). Every state, however, has common or statutory law protecting the interests of the unborn in some respects. Some states even protect the rights of fetuses born dead as against those who caused the death . . .

I. Remedies for the Protection of Embryo and Fetus

Historically, American common law courts did not permit wrongful death actions for injuries suffered in utero. This was true both because a fetus was considered a 'single entity' with his or her mother, and because of a fear of fraudulent claims. Beginning in the 1940s, American courts and state legislatures began to abandon this position. Currently, three major approaches can be found to this issue. First, it is clear in virtually all jurisdictions that have considered the issue that a personal injury action can be brought by a child born alive for fetal injuries, and wrongful death actions can be brought by the representatives of a child born alive for injuries suffered by the child before birth that resulted in death after birth, though in some jurisdictions it must be shown that the fetus was viable at the time of the injury. About half the states also allow wrongful death actions for fetuses that die from an injury suffered in utero if the fetus was viable when the injury occurred. Finally, a few jurisdictions allow wrongful death actions on the part of a fetus even if the fetus was not viable at the time of the injury. Where wrongful death damages are recoverable, the extent of damages recoverable depends on the damages permitted under the state's wrongful death statute. Courts generally permit recovery of medical care and funeral and burial expenses, with some going further to permit recovery based on the parents' loss of a potential child's society or of the child's future earning capacity. Finally, a few jurisdictions permit the mother to recover for her own sorrow, grieving and mental anguish for the loss of an unborn child.

Though courts have been increasingly open to permitting civil recoveries for the death of unborn fetuses, courts have been less willing to approve criminal prosecutions for murder or vehicular homicide involving the death of a fetus, except where a state's statutory law clearly authorizes such actions. When injury to a fetus caused the death of child born alive, however, homicide prosecutions are generally allowed. About half the states, moreover, currently have statutes criminalizing actions against a fetus either as homicide or feticide. These vary as to the point in fetal development after which causing death to a fetus becomes a crime, with some states criminalizing injuries causing the death of an unborn embryo or fetus from the date of conception, others only if the injury is caused after the point of 'quickening' or viability. Several states also penalize actions against pregnant women that result in miscarriage or injure the fetus. Legislation is currently pending in Congress that would make causing the death of, or causing bodily injury to, a child in utero a separate offense if the death or injury was caused while the perpetrator was in the course of committing one of a number of designated federal offenses . . .

The question of how to respond to women who expose their fetus to potential harm through drug abuse has proved particularly controversial in the United States. The problem has received a great deal of media coverage, and thirty-five states have adopted legislation addressing it. Though a few states have adopted statutes recognizing prenatal drug abuse as prima facie evidence of child abuse or neglect, most states have taken a more public health-oriented approach, emphasizing education and counseling. Despite the reluctance of state legislatures to adopt laws penalizing prenatal drug abuse, prosecutors in many states have brought criminal prosecutions against prenatal drug abusers under the general criminal laws. The United States Supreme Court has recently held that the practice of a state hospital which routinely tested the urine of pregnant patients for drugs and referred women who tested positive to the police for criminal prosecutions violated the constitutional prohibition against unreasonable searches.

American law distinguishes between wrongful birth cases (in which the parents of a child born with serious birth anomalies claim that they would not have chosen to conceive or would have aborted the child had they been given sufficient information about the child's probable condition); wrongful life cases (in which a child with serious anomalies presents the same claim); and wrongful conception cases (in which a healthy child's parents claim that the defendant's negligence resulted in the unwanted conception of the child.) Wrongful birth and conception cases have been widely accepted in the United States. Though seven states bar wrongful birth claims by statute, the courts of one of these states, North Carolina, have allowed a malpractice case based on defective genetic advising to proceed, noting that the parents could have chosen not to conceive had they been properly informed. Only three states permit 'wrongful life' cases, while nine states bar such claims by statute.

Courts in wrongful birth actions generally allow damages for the costs of the pregnancy and the extraordinary health care and educational costs associated with the child, but commonly do not permit recovery for the costs that would be incurred in raising a 'normal' child. States are divided as to whether emotional costs associated with the birth of a seriously ill child are recoverable. Where wrongful life actions are allowed, the damages allowed are similar to those permitted in wrongful birth cases. Courts in wrongful conception cases award medical expenses and lost earnings from the pregnancy, but most courts have not awarded the costs of raising the unwanted child, though this may be changing . . .

K. Summary and Conclusions

In summary, the law of the United States with respect to embryos and fetuses is far from consistent, representing the deep division in the United States over the issue of abortion. There are some recognizable tendencies in the law, however. Most states prohibit the abortion of viable fetuses except under very limited circumstances, while also allowing wrongful death actions and permitting criminal homicide or feticide prosecutions when a third party causes the death of the fetus. Most states, on the other hand do not permit wrongful death recoveries or criminal homicide prosecutions against one who causes the death of an embryo, and the states are forbidden by the Constitution, as currently interpreted, from penalizing abortion of an embryo. No state grants an embryo or fetus full recognition as a juridical person while in vivo, but neither does our law treat the embryo or fetus simply as property.

I do not foresee the possibility of the United States achieving a sufficient consensus as to the nature of the embryo and fetus to permit universal and consistent answers to the questions raised by this report. One recent opinion poll found that 52% of Americans agreed, and 37% disagreed, with the result of Roe v. Wade, while 50% identified themselves as pro-choice and 42% as pro-life. On the other hand, 50% believed that abortions were too easy to get in the United States (16% 'too hard'), while 42% supported new laws restricting abortion (38% opposed). With this level of division, and inconsistency, it is unlikely that we can hope for consistent laws the legitimacy of which will be widely accepted on these contentious topics in the near future.

NOTES AND QUESTIONS

1.   The growing recognition of the fetus as a legal person in the context of civil recovery for prenatal harm raises some interesting questions when applied to ART. For example, assume you practice law in a state that recognizes a claim for wrongful conception (typically for a botched vasectomy or tubal ligation) and awards damages equal to the cost of raising the unwanted child. Mr. and Mrs. Anderson visit your office with what they believe to be a legal dilemma. Nine months ago the couple welcomed quintuplets into their family, five babies born following infertility treatment using IVF. They explain that while they had hoped to have one or two children through assisted reproduction, they were clear to their physician, Dr. Benson, that they were not financially or emotionally prepared to handle a larger family. Dr. Benson assured the Andersons that "it was impossible" for them to have more than three babies because only three embryos were being transferred back into Mrs. Anderson's uterus. When the quintuplet pregnancy was discovered, Dr. Benson surmised that two of the embryos had split into twins following transfer, an extraordinarily rare, though possible, turn of events. The Andersons suspect a darker explanation, that Dr. Benson negligently transferred five embryos back, breaching a duty of care to the couple.

Is wrongful conception an appropriate cause of action in this case? Normally, such a claim flows from a couple who took action to avoid a pregnancy, but the Andersons sought out fertility services in order to achieve a pregnancy. Also, by admission the couple wanted at least two children. Does this mean that they must make a "Sophie's Choice" as to which of the quints are deemed "unwanted" for purposes of the lawsuit? Should too much of a good thing be actionable if the patient consents to ART treatment and is informed about the risks of multiple pregnancy? At least one couple thought so. An Australian patient sued her physician for excessive embryo transfer after giving birth to a healthy set of twins. According to the suit, the patient and her partner consented to single embryo transfer but the doctor transferred two embryos. The case was ultimately dismissed. *See Lesbian Couple Loses Bid to Sue IVF Doctor Over Birth of Twins When They Wanted 1 Child*, Welt Online July 25, 2008, available at http://www.welt.de/english-news/ article2248635/Lesbian-couple-loses-bid-to-sue-IVF-doctor-over-birth-of-twins-when-they-wanted-1-child.html.

2. Academic writing on the legal and moral status of the human embryo is abundant and elucidating. For a variety of views, see, e.g., Jessica Berg, *Owning Persons: The Application of Property Theory to Embryos and Fetuses*, 40 Wake Forest L. Rev. 159 (2005); Jean Reith Schroedel, *Is The Fetus a Person? A Comparison of Policies Across the Fifty States* (2000); Kayhan Parsi, *Metaphorical Imagination: The Moral and Legal Status of Fetuses and Embryos*, 4 DePaul J. Health Care L. 703 (1999); Carson Strong, *The Moral Standing of Embryos, Fetuses, and Infants*, in Ethics in Reproductive and Perinatal Medicine 41-62 (1997); Lori B. Andrews, *The Legal Status of the Embryo*, 32 Loy. L. Rev. 357 (1986).

C. The Moral Status of the Human Embryo

The moral status of the human embryo has been extensively and intensively debated within and across many disciplines. Thinkers in law, philosophy, science and religion have weighed in, producing a richly textured body of work reflecting myriad perspectives and arguments. To state the controversy at its most basic and dichotomous level, some assign full moral status to the human embryo from the moment of conception equal to that accorded a competent adult. This position is supported by the argument that fertilization produces a genetically unique, living human being capable of growing into an independent person. At the other end of the spectrum are those who believe the human embryo has no significant moral status because it lacks the usual attributes of rights-bearing persons, including consciousness, sentience and the ability to interact with others or its environment.

Professor John Robertson opines that "[w]ith such disparate views of the moral status of early embryos, a consensus to guide ethical and legal thinking may not be possible." Still, he presses to suggest a common ground that both sides can embrace. Addressing the perspective that human embryos have low (or no) moral status compared to higher evolved human beings, Professor Robertson suggests a shift in the moral calculus from status to respect. "Although not a person or a rights-bearing entity, the early embryo may still be accorded special respect because it is genetically unique, living human tissue that has the potential to develop into a fetus and newborn." Expounding on the concept of special respect,

Professor Robertson continues:

The abstract concept of respect must eventually confront the concrete situations in which the content of special respect is constituted. The notion of special respect will seem like empty rhetoric if it leads to no limits at all on what may be done with embryos. What substantive limits does respect then place on the many ends that persons seek through creation and disposition of early embryos? For example, does this reminder of our humanity permit the destruction of early embryos through abortion, contragestion, or failure to place an external embryo in the uterus? Does special respect allow embryos to be created externally, frozen, manipulated, donated to others, used in research, and genetically examined and altered? Are these activities consistent with the special respect due such a powerful symbol of the unique gift of human life?

Answers to such questions are not automatically given by an a priori appeal to the vague concept of special respect or even to the notion that the embryo is itself a person. Since technological change has only recently made early embryos independent objects of interest, there is no well established tradition defining special respect for the embryo. Thus, the content of respect must be forged across the various situations in which embryos and other human interests meet. In each case some important interest that requires a choice about embryos raises the possibility of conflict with the special respect that embryos are thought to deserve. In parsing these conflicts, views of the competing values at stake, as much as views of early embryo status, may determine evaluation of the activity in question.

...[C]onclusions about the embryo's legal status as defined by what trade offs are acceptable in defining special respect may depend very little on acceptance or rejection of theories that treat the early embryo as a subject of rights and duties. Only in a few areas such as contragestion, early abortion and research, and arguably not even there will legal status questions diverge because of the differing views held about the moral status of the early embryo. In most instances, the embryo's legal status will be determined by the importance of competing interests of bodily integrity, procreative choice, and family formation, and not by whether the early embryo is a prenatal subject of rights, or merely a living, human entity that deserves special respect...

In sum, except for the minority of persons who think that fertilization or implantation marks the emergence of a prenatal moral subject, most people hold that fertilized eggs and early embryos have no obligatory moral status. They are not owed anything in their own right, but may be assigned value or status because of the symbolic meaning that they carry for particular persons or communities. Whether this symbolic value must always be preserved will depend on the competing interests at stake in the various situations in which questions of disposition of the early embryo arise.

John A. Robertson, *In the Beginning: The Legal Status of Early Embryos*, 76 VA. L. REV. 437 (1990).

NOTES AND QUESTIONS

1.   Professor Robertson suggests that the degree and nature of the special respect due the early embryo may be entirely contextual. That is, our regard for the early embryo may not be based solely on how we view this biological entity (for example, as an existing person, as a potential person, as a nonperson), but rather how we treat the embryo relative to other life forms. As an example, consider a person who states, "I believe that life begins at conception and that all life forms are due equal respect." How would that person respond to a situation in which two life forms compete for survival? A common example offered to demonstrate this point is a pregnant woman whose fetus is growing in such a way as to threaten her life. Could an argument be made that aborting the fetus under these circumstances would be morally acceptable?

Public opinion polls show that some who oppose abortion make an exception for so-called tragic circumstances. These circumstances occur when the woman's life is endangered, when the pregnancy is the result of rape or incest, or when the child will be born with substantial handicaps. The justification for abortion under these circumstances is often based on the principle of indirect effect. The principle of indirect effect holds that although it is never morally right to "directly" perform a forbidden act (such as killing an embryo or fetus), it is morally permissible to undertake another act that may produce the forbidden action as an unintended consequence. For example, in the case of a pregnant woman with cancer of the uterus, although it would be wrong to surgically remove the fetus to treat the woman, it would be acceptable to treat the woman's uterus with radiation therapy, indirectly causing the death of the fetus. For a discussion of the moral and political debate surrounding abortion see KRISTIN LUKER, ABORTION AND THE POLITICS OF MOTHERHOOD (1984).

2.   The position that the early embryo possesses equal moral status to a fully formed human being is set forth by the Roman Catholic Church and is often a source of reference for those who subscribe to this view. The Catholic Church's position on the status of the embryo, as well as other teachings surrounding procreation, can be found in the Congregation For The Doctrine Of The Faith, *Instruction On Respect For Human Life In Its Origin And On The Dignity Of Procreation Replies To Certain Questions Of The Day*. In relevant part, the Church teaches:

> . . . Thus the fruit of human generation, from the first moment of its existence, that is to say from the moment the zygote has formed, demands the unconditional respect that is morally due to the human being in his bodily and spiritual totality. The human being is to be respected and treated as a person from the moment of conception; and therefore from that same moment his rights as a person must be recognized, among which in the first place is the inviolable right of every innocent human being to life. This doctrinal reminder provides the fundamental criterion for the solution of the various problems posed by the development of the biomedical sciences in this field: since the embryo must be treated as a person, it must also be defended in its integrity, tended and cared for, to the extent

possible, in the same way as any other human being as far as medical assistance is concerned.

The full Instruction can be found at: www.vatican.va/roman-curia/congregations/cfaith/documents.

3.   *The Identity Thesis.* The Church's position that embryos are distinct human beings from the moment of fertilization and thus have the same rights due every person already born influences its position on a host of reproductive and scientific technologies ranging from prenatal diagnosis to embryonic stem cell research. Professors Helga Kuhse and Peter Singer call this view the "identity thesis" and critique it from a biologic perspective:

> It is true that the life of the fertilized ovum is a genetically new life in the sense that it is neither genetically nor numerically continuous with the life of the egg or the sperm before fertilization. Before fertilization, there were two genetically distinct entities, the egg and the sperm; now there is only one entity, the fertilized egg or zygote, with a new and unique genetic code. It is also true that the zygote will — other things being equal — develop into an embryo, fetus and baby with the same genetic code . . . But, as we shall see, things are not always equal and some serious problems are raised for supporters of the identity thesis.
>
> Here are two scenarios of what might happen during early human development.
>
> In the first scenario, a man and a woman have intercourse, fertilization takes place, and a genetically new zygote, let's call it Tom, is formed. Tom has a specific genetic identity — a genetic blueprint — that will be repeated in every cell once the first cell begins to split, first into two, then into four cells, and so on. On day 8, however, the group of cells which is Tom divides into two separate identical cell groups. These two separate cell groups continue to develop and, some nine months later, identical twins are born. Now, which one, if either of them, is Tom? There are no obvious grounds for thinking of one of the twins as Tom and the other as Not-Tom; the twinning process is quite symmetrical and both twins have the same genetic blueprint as the original Tom. But to suggest that both of them are Tom does, of course, conflict with numerical continuity: there was one zygote and now there are two babies.
>
> People have thought in various ways about this: for example, that when the original cell split, Tom ceased to exist and that two new individuals, Dick and Harry, came into existence. But if that were conceded then it would, of course, no longer be true that the existence of the babies Dick and Harry began at fertilization: their existence did not begin until eight days *after* fertilization. Moreover (and we shall come back to this in a moment) if Tom died on day 8, how is it that he left no earthly remains?
>
> Now consider the second scenario. A man and a woman have intercourse and fertilization takes place. But this time, two eggs are fertilized and two zygotes come into existence — Mary and Jane. The zygotes begin to divide, first into two, then into four cells, and so on. But, then, on day 6, the two

embryos combine, forming what is known as a chimera, and continue to develop as a single organism, which will eventually become a baby. Now, who is the baby — Mary or Jane, both Mary and Jane, or somebody else — Nancy?

Helga Kuhse and Peter Singer, *Individuals, Humans and Persons: The Issue of Moral Status*, in EMBRYO EXPERIMENTATION 65-75 (1990). Professors Kuhse and Singer raise another challenge to the identity thesis — embryo totipotency. As explained in greater detail in Chapter 4, all the cells of the embryo remain totipotent, meaning "all potential," until about the fourth day of development. Totipotent embryonic cells are not yet differentiated, meaning that each cell by itself can grow into a whole and perfect enbryo, fetus and eventual infant. Kuhse and Singer observe:

> It is now believed that early embryonic cells are totipotent; that is, that, contrary to the "identity thesis", an early human embryo is not one particular individual, but rather has the potential to become one or more different individuals. Up to the 8-cell stage, each single embryonic cell is a distinct entity in the sense that there is no fusion between the individual cells; rather, the embryo is a loose collection of distinct cells, held together by the zona pellucida, the outer membrane of the egg. Animal studies on four-cell embryos indicate that each one of these cells has the potential to produce at least one fetus or baby.
>
> Take a human embryo consisting of four cells. On the assumption that this embryo is a particular human individual, we shall call it Adam. Because each of Adam's four cells is totipotent, any three cells could be removed from the zona pellucida and the remaining cell would still have the potential to develop into a perfect fetus or baby. Now, it might be thought that this baby is Adam, the same baby that would have resulted had all four cells continued to develop jointly. But this poses a problem because we could have left any one of the other three cells in the zona pellucida, each with the potential to develop into a baby. The same baby — Adam? Things are not made any easier by the recognition that the three 'surplus' cells, each placed into an empty zona pellucida, would also have the potential to develop into babies. We now have four distinct human individuals with the potential to develop into four babies. Because it does not make good sense to identify any one particular individual as Adam, let's call them Bill, Charles, David and Eddy . . .

The Kuhse and Singer argument that the early embryo is not a distinct human individual, and therefore is not due the same moral status of a more fully formed person, is based on scientific data which verifies the two developmental phenomena the authors speak of — twinning and fusing of embryos in the first week or so following fertilization. Twinning occurs when a single embryo divides to form two separate but genetically identical embryos. The twinning process can also yield conjoined twins, two genetically identical individuals who remain attached and often share vital organs, reflecting an incomplete separation of the embryos.

The idea that two embryos could fuse to form a single individual is less well studied. But in November 2003 scientists reported on the case of a 52-year-old woman who was discovered to be a chimera, a mixture of two individuals. When "Jane" needed a kidney transplant, her three adult sons were tested for tissue compatibility. Remarkably, doctors discovered that two of her sons were not genetically related to her, a shock to a woman who naturally conceived and gave birth to her children. After two years of searching, doctors concluded that Jane's mother had conceived two non-identical female embryos which had fused at the early stages of development to form a single embryo. Jane's body houses two full sets of genetic material, with certain body parts made up of one twin, and others comprised of the second twin. Jane's blood contains the genes from one twin, while her ovaries were found to contain eggs with the genetics of both twins. This explains why one son was found to be genetically related to her, while the other two, whose blood was not a genetic match, were found to be "genetically unrelated." To date, approximately 30 human chimeras have been identified and scientists expect that many more will emerge now that the phenomenon is better understood. See Claire Ainsworth, *The Stranger Within*, THE NEW SCIENTIST 34, Nov. 15, 2003.

4. *More on the Kuhse and Singer Argument.* The pair argue that the early embryo lacks a certain individualized identity because of its potential to twin or fuse, and therefore is not the appropriate marker for "when life begins." Instead, they look to the development of the primitive streak, at about 14 days post-fertilization, when the embryo can no longer become a chimera or two different individuals through twinning. In a later part of the chapter, not reproduced here, Kuhse and Singer argue that the early embryo has no moral standing as a human being because it lacks sentience, or the capacity to feel pleasure or pain. They conclude:

> Until that point [of sentience] is reached, the embryo does not have any interests and, like other non-sentient organisms (a human egg, for example), cannot be harmed — in a morally relevant sense — by anything we do. We can, of course, damage the embryo in such a way as to cause harm to the sentient being it will become, if it lives, but if it never becomes a sentient being, the embryo has not been harmed, because its total lack of awareness means that it never has had any interests at all.

Helga Kuhse & Peter Singer, *Individuals, Humans and Persons: The Issue of Moral Status*, in EMBRYO EXPERIMENTATION 73 (1990).

What do you think of the argument that an individual's moral status is based upon the ability to feel pain or pleasure? Is this a necessary quality to be considered a human being? Does this mean that people who suffer severe brain damage and languish in a coma are not human beings? Or is the argument really that the embryo has no history of ever experiencing or interacting with its environment? In your mind, what characteristics qualify an entity to be considered a human being? If you are unsure, don't worry. As we proceed with our exploration of reproductive technologies, we will revisit the moral status of the early embryo.

Chapter 2

PROCREATIONAL LIBERTY: CONSTITUTIONAL JURISPRUDENCE AND THE RIGHT TO REPRODUCE

In any human lifetime there are a handful of decisions that stand out as fundamental to the destiny and identity of the individual. Those decisions involve choices of utmost intimacy, shaping the basic parameters of one's life and even one's death. Decisions about whether or not to marry, whether or not to have children, whether or not to accept aggressive medical treatment in the face of a terminal illness, are generally made within the realm of personal morality, spirituality, religiosity and autonomy that are unique to the individual. The focus of our discussion, the decision whether or not to procreate, is prized in our society as a sacred and private choice. The mere thought that the government could either require or forbid us from having offspring is tantamount to contemplating the demise of our American constitutional system. Yet amid this aura of respect for the privacy of child-bearing decisions, questions remain about the source and strength of legal protections surrounding procreation. As you read the early Supreme Court cases that follow, ask yourself whether the language relating to reproduction can legitimately be extended to assisted reproduction, a science yet to be discovered at the time the justices enshrined procreation as a basic civil right.

SECTION I: TRADITIONAL REPRODUCTION AND THE CONSTITUTION

A.   Establishing Reproduction as a Fundamental Right

1.   The Early Cases

MEYER v. NEBRASKA
Supreme Court of the United States
262 U.S. 390 (1923)

JUSTICE MCREYNOLDS delivered the opinion of the Court.

Plaintiff in error was tried and convicted in the district court for Hamilton county, Nebraska, under an information which charged that on May 25, 1920, while an instructor in Zion Parochial School he unlawfully taught the subject of reading in the German language to Raymond Parpart, a child of 10 years, who had not attained and successfully passed the eighth grade. The information is based upon

"An act relating to the teaching of foreign languages in the state of Nebraska," approved April 9, 1919 (Laws 1919, c. 249), which follows:

> Section 1. No person, individually or as a teacher, shall, in any private, denominational, parochial or public school, teach any subject to any person in any language than the English language.

> Sec. 2. Languages, other than the English language, may be taught as languages only after a pupil shall have attained and successfully passed the eighth grade as evidenced by a certificate of graduation issued by the county superintendent of the county in which the child resides.

> Sec. 3. Any person who violates any of the provisions of this act shall be deemed guilty of a misdemeanor and upon conviction, shall be subject to a fine of not less than twenty-five dollars ($25), nor more than one hundred dollars ($100), or be confined in the county jail for any period not exceeding thirty days for each offense . . .

The Supreme Court of the state affirmed the judgment of conviction. 107 Neb. 657, 187 N. W. 100. [I]t held that the statute . . . did not conflict with the Fourteenth Amendment, but was a valid exercise of the police power. The following excerpts from the opinion sufficiently indicate the reasons advanced to support the conclusion:

> The salutary purpose of the statute is clear. The Legislature had seen the baneful effects of permitting foreigners, who had taken residence in this country, to rear and educate their children in the language of their native land. The result of that condition was found to be inimical to our own safety . . . The obvious purpose of this statute was that the English language should be and become the mother tongue of all children reared in this state. The enactment of such a statute comes reasonably within the police power of the state. *Pohl v. State*, 102 Ohio St. 474, 132 N. E. 20; *State v. Bartels*, 191 Iowa, 1060, 181 N. W. 508 . . . .

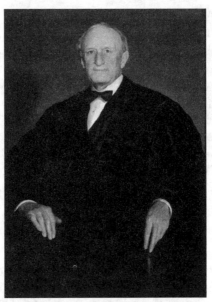

Justice James C. McReynolds

The problem for our determination is whether the statute as construed and applied unreasonably infringes the liberty guaranteed to the plaintiff in error by the Fourteenth Amendment:

No state * * * shall deprive any person of life, liberty or property without due process of law.

While this court has not attempted to define with exactness the liberty thus guaranteed, the term has received much consideration and some of the included things have been definitely stated. Without doubt, it denotes not merely freedom from bodily restraint but also the right of the individual to contract, to engage in any of the common occupations of life, to acquire useful knowledge, to marry, establish a home and bring up children, to worship God according to the dictates of his own conscience, and generally to enjoy those privileges long recognized at common law as essential to the orderly pursuit of happiness by free men. [citations omitted]. The established doctrine is that this liberty may not be interfered with, under the guise of protecting the public interest, by legislative action which is arbitrary or without reasonable relation to some purpose within the competency of the state to effect. Determination by the Legislature of what constitutes proper exercise of police power is not final or conclusive but is subject to supervision by the courts. *Lawton v. Steele*, 152 U. S. 133, 137, 14 Sup. Ct. 499, 38 L. Ed. 385.

The American people have always regarded education and acquisition of knowledge as matters of supreme importance which should be diligently promoted . . .

The challenged statute forbids the teaching in school of any subject except in English; . . . The Supreme Court of the state has held that "the so-called ancient or dead languages" are not "within the spirit or the purpose of the act." *Nebraska District of Evangelical Lutheran Synod, etc., v. McKelvie et al.* (Neb.) 187 N. W. 927 (April 19, 1922). Latin, Greek, Hebrew are not proscribed; but German, French,

Spanish, Italian, and every other alien speech are within the ban. Evidently the Legislature has attempted materially to interfere with the calling of modern language teachers, with the opportunities of pupils to acquire knowledge, and with the power of parents to control the education of their own . . .

That the state may do much, go very far, indeed, in order to improve the quality of its citizens, physically, mentally and morally, is clear; but the individual has certain fundamental rights which must be respected. The protection of the Constitution extends to all, to those who speak other languages as well as to those born with English on the tongue. Perhaps it would be highly advantageous if all had ready understanding of our ordinary speech, but this cannot be coerced by methods which conflict with the Constitution — a desirable end cannot be promoted by prohibited means.

For the welfare of his Ideal Commonwealth, Plato suggested a law which should provide:

> "That the wives of our guardians are to be common, and their children are to be common, and no parent is to know his own child, nor any child his parent. *** The proper officers will take the offspring of the good parents to the pen or fold, and there they will deposit them with certain nurses who dwell in a separate quarter; but the offspring of the inferior, or of the better when they chance to be deformed, will be put away in some mysterious, unknown place, as they should be."

In order to submerge the individual and develop ideal citizens, Sparta assembled the males at seven into barracks and intrusted their subsequent education and training to official guardians. Although such measures have been deliberately approved by men of great genius their ideas touching the relation between individual and state were wholly different from those upon which our institutions rest; and it hardly will be affirmed that any Legislature could impose such restrictions upon the people of a state without doing violence to both letter and spirit of the Constitution . . .

We are constrained to conclude that the statute as applied is arbitrary and without reasonable relation to any end within the competency of the state.

As the statute undertakes to interfere only with teaching which involves a modern language, leaving complete freedom as to other matters, there seems no adequate foundation for the suggestion that the purpose was to protect the child's health by limiting his mental activities. It is well known that proficiency in a foreign language seldom comes to one not instructed at an early age, and experience shows that this is not injurious to the health, morals or understanding of the ordinary child.

The judgment of the court below must be reversed and the cause remanded for further proceedings not inconsistent with this opinion.

Reversed.

Mr. Justice Holmes and Mr. Justice Sutherland, dissent.

NOTES AND QUESTIONS

1.   Undoubtedly it did not escape your notice that *Meyer v. Nebraska* is not a case involving reproduction. But *Meyer* is a foundational case in the road toward procreative liberty — the freedom to decide whether or not to have offspring and to control use of one's reproductive capacity. Professor John Robertson describes procreative liberty as follows:

> As a matter of constitutional law, procreative liberty is a negative right against state interference with choices to procreate or to avoid procreation. It is not a right against private interference, though other laws might provide that protection. Nor is it a positive right to have the state or particular persons provide the means or resources necessary to have or avoid having children.

John A. Robertson, Children of Choice: Freedom and the New Reproductive Technologies 23 (1994). If procreative liberty exists as a negative right protected by the U.S. Constitution, do you see how the *Meyer* case paves the way for establishment of that right?

2.   One noteworthy aspect of *Meyer* is the discussion of the Nebraska Supreme Court's selective enforcement of the foreign language law. Justice McReynolds mentions that the state high court has held that "the so-called ancient or dead languages are not within the spirit or purpose of the act" thus allowing Latin, Greek, and Hebrew to be taught while proscribing German, French, Spanish, Italian and other "modern" languages. Can you see how the practice of selective enforcement might apply to laws on reproduction?

Suppose a state legislature concludes that the best way to show special respect to the early embryo is to assure that it does not develop for more than five days post-fertilization in the laboratory setting. The legislature believes that all IVF-based embryos should be either cryopreserved (frozen for later use) or placed back in the uterus once they reach the blastocyst (5 day) stage because current research reveals that the longer the embryos remain in the laboratory, the greater the risk that they will develop abnormally or cease to further develop at all. To ensure the safe development of early embryos the legislature enacts the following law:

> (1) It shall be unlawful for any person to keep, place, manipulate or in any way contain a human embryo that has reached the age of six days post-fertilization or greater, in any location other than a woman's uterus. Violation of this Section shall constitute a felony, punishable by a fine of $25,000 per incident and imprisonment for up to ten years.

> (2) Section 1 herein shall not be violated if a six day or greater human embryo is cryopreserved for later use in compliance with established laboratory standards.

Suppose further that after this statute is enacted, doctors learn more about therapies that can be conducted on the early embryo. One such hypothetical therapy prevents the embryo from developing spina bifida, a birth defect of the spine in which part of the spinal cord is exposed through a gap in the backbone. The therapy involves injection of certain enzymes directly into the embryo, and the key to success is that it must be performed on a 10 day-old embryo; moreover, the embryo must be taken outside the uterus and placed in a special laboratory setting for the therapy to be effective. Granted, this scenario is wildly unrealistic but it is designed to illustrate the possibility of selective enforcement of laws affecting reproduction.

Under our hypothetical law, would a physician who performs this hypothetical therapy on a 10-day-old embryo that was naturally conceived be guilty of a felony? After all, the physician would be manipulating an embryo greater than six-days post fertilization, outside the woman's body. Clearly the physician would defend herself on the grounds that she is aiding the embryo, an act not within the "spirit or purpose of the act." Would a physician's reliance on this dicta from *Meyer v. Nebraska* be an effective defense? Should it be? If a court finds that the law was not intended to apply to embryos formed via natural conception, would this be an example of selective enforcement of laws pertaining to reproduction?

3.   The Supreme Court in *Meyer* moves away from a literal definition of Fourteenth Amendment "liberty" as the freedom from bodily restraint to a broader concept that recognizes certain aspects of family autonomy as fundamental rights. Included in this bundle of fundamental rights are the right "to marry, establish a home and bring up children." These rights do not appear in the text of the Constitution, but are nevertheless considered worthy of the highest degree of protection by the courts. Why? Should fundamental rights be limited to those liberties explicitly stated in the text of the Constitution or clearly intended by the framers, or should the Supreme Court be permitted to find fundamental rights according to contemporary societal values? For a discussion of the competing theories of constitutional interpretation *see* ERWIN CHEMERINSKY, CONSTITUTIONAL LAW: PRINCIPLES AND POLICIES 15-26 (4th ed. 2011). In 1923 the Supreme Court appeared willing to consider nontextual rights as fundamental and thus protected against certain forms of governmental interference. Given the broad language in *Meyer*, how do you think the Court is likely to respond to governmental interference in the area of procreation? Consider the next case.

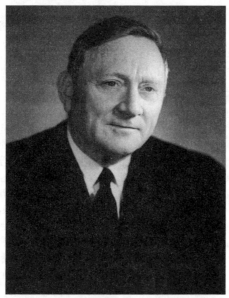

Justice William O. Douglas

SKINNER v. OKLAHOMA
Supreme Court of the United States
316 U.S. 535 (1942)

JUSTICE DOUGLAS delivered the opinion of the Court.

This case touches a sensitive and important area of human rights. Oklahoma deprives certain individuals of a right which is basic to the perpetuation of a race — the right to have offspring. Oklahoma has decreed the enforcement of its law against petitioner, overruling his claim that it violated the Fourteenth Amendment. Because that decision raised grave and substantial constitutional questions, we granted the petition for certiorari.

The statute involved is Oklahoma's Habitual Criminal Sterilization Act. Okl-.St.Ann. Tit. 57, § 171, et seq.; L.1935, p. 94 et seq. That Act defines an "habitual criminal" as a person who, having been convicted two or more times for crimes "amounting to felonies involving moral turpitude" either in an Oklahoma court or in a court of any other State, is thereafter convicted of such a felony in Oklahoma and is sentenced to a term of imprisonment in an Oklahoma penal institution. § 173. Machinery is provided for the institution by the Attorney General of a proceeding against such a person in the Oklahoma courts for a judgment that such person shall be rendered sexually sterile. §§ 176, 177. Notice, an opportunity to be heard, and the right to a jury trial are provided. §§ 177-181. The issues triable in such a proceeding are narrow and confined. If the court or jury finds that the defendant is an "habitual criminal" and that he "may be rendered sexually sterile without detriment to his or her general health", then the court "shall render judgment to the effect that said defendant be rendered sexually sterile" § 182, by the operation of vasectomy[1] in case of a male and of salpingectomy[2] in case of a female. § 174. Only one other provision of the Act is material here and that is § 195 which provides that "offenses arising out of the violation of the prohibitory laws, revenue acts, embezzlement, or political offenses, shall not come or be considered within the terms of this Act."

Petitioner was convicted in 1926 of the crime of stealing chickens and was sentenced to the Oklahoma State Reformatory. In 1929 he was convicted of the crime of robbery with fire arms and was sentenced to the reformatory. In 1934 he was convicted again of robbery with firearms and was sentenced to the penitentiary. He was confined there in 1935 when the Act was passed. In 1936 the Attorney General instituted proceedings against him. Petitioner in his answer challenged the Act as unconstitutional by reason of the Fourteenth Amendment. A jury trial was had. The court instructed the jury that the crimes of which petitioner had been convicted were felonies involving moral turpitude and that the only question for the jury was whether the operation of vasectomy could be performed on petitioner without detriment to his general health. The jury found that it could be. A judgment directing that the operation of vasectomy be performed on petitioner was affirmed by the Supreme Court of Oklahoma by a five to four decision. 189 Okl. 235, 115 P.2d 123.

Several objections to the constitutionality of the Act have been pressed upon us. It is urged that the Act cannot be sustained as an exercise of the police power in view of the state of scientific authorities respecting inheritability of criminal traits . . . It is argued that due process is lacking because under this Act, unlike the act . . . upheld in *Buck v. Bell*, 274 U.S. 200, 47 S.Ct. 584, 71 L.Ed. 1000, the defendant is given no opportunity to be heard on the issue as to whether he is the probable potential parent of socially undesirable offspring. See *Davis v. Berry*, D.C., 216 F. 413; *Williams v. Smith*, 190 Ind. 526, 131 N.E. 2. It is also suggested that the Act is penal in character and that the sterilization provided for is cruel and unusual punishment and violative of the Fourteenth Amendment. See *Davis v. Berry, supra.* Cf. *State v. Feilen*, 70 Wash. 65, 126 P. 75, 41 L.R.A., N.S., 418, Ann.Cas.1914B, 512; *Mickle v. Henrichs*, D.C., 262 F. 687. We pass those points without intimating an opinion on them, for there is a feature of the Act which clearly condemns it. That is its failure to meet the requirements of the equal protection clause of the Fourteenth Amendment.

We do not stop to point out all of the inequalities in this Act. A few examples will suffice. In Oklahoma grand larceny is a felony. Okl.St.Ann. Tit. 21, § 1705 (§ 5). Larceny is grand larceny when the property taken exceeds $20 in value. Id. § 1704. Embezzlement is punishable "in the manner prescribed for feloniously stealing property of the value of that embezzled." Id. § 1462. Hence he who embezzles property worth more than $20 is guilty of a felony. A clerk who appropriates over $20 from his employer's till (id. § 1456) and a stranger who steals the same amount are thus both guilty of felonies. If the latter repeats his act and is convicted three

---

[1] A vasectomy is the surgical excision of all or part of the sperm-carrying ducts of the testis, to induce sterility. Merriam-Webster Dictionary 808 (1997) - Ed.

[2] A salpingectomy is the removal of the fallopian tubes. Stedman's Medical Dictionary 1249 (1976) - Ed.

times, he may be sterilized. But the clerk is not subject to the pains and penalties of the Act no matter how large his embezzlements nor how frequent his convictions. A person who enters a chicken coop and steals chickens commits a felony (id. § 1719); and he may be sterilized if he is thrice convicted. If, however, he is a bailee of the property and fraudulently appropriates it, he is an embezzler. Id. § 1455. Hence no matter how habitual his proclivities for embezzlement are and no matter how often his conviction, he may not be sterilized. Thus the nature of the two crimes is intrinsically the same and they are punishable in the same manner . . .

It was stated in *Buck v. Bell, supra,* that the claim that state legislation violates the equal protection clause of the Fourteenth Amendment is "the usual last resort of constitutional arguments." 274 U.S. page 208, 47 S.Ct. page 585, 71 L.Ed. 1000. Under our constitutional system the States in determining the reach and scope of particular legislation need not provide "abstract symmetry". *Patsone v. Pennsylvania,* 232 U.S. 138, 144, 34 S.Ct. 281, 282, 58 L.Ed. 539. They may mark and set apart the classes and types of problems according to the needs and as dictated or suggested by experience . . . As stated in *Buck v. Bell, supra,* 274 U.S. page 208, 47 S.Ct. page 585, 71 L.Ed. 1000, "the law does all that is needed when it does all that it can, indicates a policy, applies it to all within the lines, and seeks to bring within the lines all similarly situated so far and so fast as its means allow."

But the instant legislation runs afoul of the equal protection clause, though we give Oklahoma that large deference which the rule of the foregoing cases requires. We are dealing here with legislation which involves one of the basic civil rights of man. Marriage and procreation are fundamental to the very existence and survival of the race. The power to sterilize, if exercised, may have subtle, far-reaching and devastating effects. In evil or reckless hands it can cause races or types which are inimical to the dominant group to wither and disappear. There is no redemption for the individual whom the law touches. Any experiment which the State conducts is to his irreparable injury. He is forever deprived of a basic liberty. We mention these matters not to reexamine the scope of the police power of the States. We advert to them merely in emphasis of our view that strict scrutiny of the classification which a State makes in a sterilization law is essential, lest unwittingly or otherwise invidious discriminations are made against groups or types of individuals in violation of the constitutional guaranty of just and equal laws. The guaranty of "equal protection of the laws is a pledge of the protection of equal laws." *Yick Wo v. Hopkins,* 118 U.S. 356, 369, 6 S.Ct. 1064, 1070, 30 L.Ed. 220. When the law lays an unequal hand on those who have committed intrinsically the same quality of offense and sterilizes one and not the other, it has made as an invidious a discrimination as if it had selected a particular race or nationality for oppressive treatment. *Yick Wo v. Hopkins, supra; Gaines v. Canada,* 305 U.S. 337, 59 S.Ct. 232, 83 L.Ed. 208. Sterilization of those who have thrice committed grand larceny with immunity for those who are embezzlers is a clear, pointed, unmistakable discrimination. Oklahoma makes no attempt to say that he who commits larceny by trespass or trick or fraud has biologically inheritable traits which he who commits embezzlement lacks. . . .

Reversed.

CHIEF JUSTICE STONE and JUSTICE JACKSON wrote separate concurring opinions.

[In his concurring opinion, Chief Justice Stone rejected the majority's recourse to the equal protection clause. Instead, he reasoned "I think the real question we have to consider is not one of equal protection, but whether the wholesale condemnation of a class to such an invasion of personal liberty, without opportunity to any individual to show that his is not the type of case which would justify resort to it, satisfies the demands of due process."]

NOTES AND QUESTIONS

1. *The Right to Procreate.* It may surprise you to learn that *Skinner v. Oklahoma* remains the only Supreme Court precedent to consider the positive right to procreate. As we shall see, every other high court analysis of procreative liberty involves the right to avoid procreation — either through the use of contraceptives or abortion. But the fundamental right to procreate established in *Skinner* has been reaffirmed by the Court on numerous occasions. The cases that look to *Skinner* for the proposition that our constitution protects "the basic liberty" of procreation, themselves involve conduct of the most personal nature. See, e.g., *Washington v. Glucksberg*, 521 U.S. 702 (1997) (challenge to state assisted suicide laws which deprive terminally ill patients the right to physician aid in dying); *Planned Parenthood of Southeastern Pennsylvania v. Casey*, 505 U.S. 833 (1992) (challenge to state abortion law, discussed beginning at page 120); *Cruzan v. Director*, Missouri Department of Health, 497 U.S. 261 (1990) (upholding right of competent adults to refuse life-sustaining medical treatment); *Michael H. v. Gerald D.*, 491 U.S. 110 (1989) (discussing right of biological father to establish paternity and right to visitation of child born to married woman living with her husband); *Bowers v. Hardwick*, 478 U.S. 186 (1986) (upholding constitutionality of Georgia sodomy statute as applied to homosexual conduct, later overturned in *Lawrence v. Texas*, 123 S. Ct. 2472 (2003)).

2. *Equal Protection v. Due Process.* Justice Douglas declared the Oklahoma Habitual Criminal Sterilization Act unconstitutional as violating equal protection because it discriminated among people in their ability to exercise a fundamental liberty — the right to procreate. As Professor Chemerinsky explains, "Usually equal protection is used to analyze government actions that draw a distinction among people based on specific characteristics, such as race, gender, age, disability, or other traits. Sometimes, though, equal protection is used if the government discriminates among people as to the exercise of a fundamental right." ERWIN CHEMERINSKY, CONSTITUTIONAL LAW: PRINCIPLES AND POLICIES 691 (4th ed. 2011). *Skinner* is unique in its reliance on equal protection to protect a fundamental right related to personal autonomy, as all future cases look to the liberty interest enumerated in the due process clause. Whether the right to procreate arising under the equal protection clause or the due process clause of the Fourteenth Amendment seems of little constitutional moment. Again, Professor Chemerinsky, ". . . the effect is the same whether a right is deemed fundamental under the equal protection clause or under the due process clause: Government infringements are subjected to strict scrutiny." Id. Thus, the *Skinner* legacy is the establishment of procreation as a fundamental right, requiring the government to present a

compelling interest to justify any infringement.

Do you think the right to procreate is more appropriately derived from the equal protection or due process clauses of the constitution? Though the remedy for state infringement may be the same under either framework, do you see a reason to favor one principle over the other as the basis for the fundamental right to procreate? Consider this question in the context of assisted reproduction. If a state enacted restrictions on the use of ARTs, such as limiting the number of embryos that a woman could implant, or prohibiting payment to gamete donors and surrogates, would an infertile couple who challenged the constitutionality of these laws be more likely to succeed using an equal protection or due process analysis? For an argument that current case law governing disposition of frozen embryos upon divorce violates equal protection by infringing on the rights of infertile women to exercise their fundamental right to control their early embryos, see Judith F. Daar, *Assisted Reproductive Technologies and the Pregnancy Process: Developing An Equality Model to Protect Reproductive Liberties*, 25 AMER. J. LAW & MED. 455 (1999).

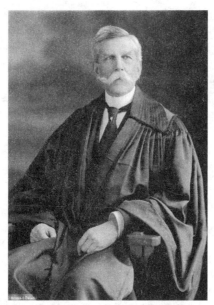

Justice Oliver Wendell Holmes

2. State Support for Mandatory Sterilization

BUCK v. BELL
Supreme Court of the United States
274 U.S. 200 (1927)

JUSTICE HOLMES delivered the opinion of the Court.

This is a writ of error to review a judgment of the Supreme Court of Appeals of the State of Virginia, affirming a judgment of the Circuit Court of Amherst County, by which the defendant in error, the superintendent of the State Colony for Epileptics and Feeble Minded, was ordered to perform the operation of salpingectomy upon Carrie Buck, the plaintiff in error, for the purpose of making her sterile. 143 Va. 310, 130 S. E. 516. The case comes here upon the contention that the statute authorizing the judgment is void under the Fourteenth Amendment as denying to the plaintiff in error due process of law and the equal protection of the laws.

Carrie Buck is a feeble-minded white woman who was committed to the State Colony above mentioned in due form. She is the daughter of a feeble-minded mother in the same institution, and the mother of an illegitimate feeble-minded child. She was eighteen years old at the time of the trial of her case in the Circuit Court in the latter part of 1924. An Act of Virginia approved March 20, 1924 (Laws 1924, c. 394) recites that the health of the patient and the welfare of society may be promoted in certain cases by the sterilization of mental defectives, under careful safeguard, etc.; that the sterilization may be effected in males by vasectomy and in females by salpingectomy, without serious pain or substantial danger to life; that the Commonwealth is supporting in various institutions many defective persons who if now discharged would become a menace but if incapable of procreating might be discharged with safety and become self-supporting with benefit to themselves and to society; and that experience has shown that heredity plays an important part in the transmission of insanity, imbecility, etc. The statute then enacts that whenever the superintendent of certain institutions including the above named State Colony shall be of opinion that it is for the best interest of the patients and of society that an inmate under his care should be sexually sterilized, he may have the operation performed upon any patient afflicted with hereditary forms of insanity, imbecility, etc., on complying with the very careful provisions by which the act protects the patients from possible abuse. The superintendent first presents a petition to the special board of directors of his hospital or colony, stating the facts and the grounds for his opinion, verified by affidavit. Notice of the petition and of the time and place of the hearing in the institution is to be served upon the inmate, and also upon his guardian, and if there is no guardian the superintendent is to apply to the Circuit Court of the County to appoint one. If the inmate is a minor notice also is to be given to his parents, if any, with a copy of the petition. The board is to see to it that the inmate may attend the hearings if desired by him or his guardian. The evidence is all to be reduced to writing, and after the board has made its order for or against the operation, the superintendent, or the inmate, or his guardian, may appeal to the Circuit Court of the County. The Circuit Court may consider the record of the board and the evidence before it and such other admissible evidence as may be offered, and may affirm, revise, or reverse the order of the board and enter such order as it deems just. Finally any party may apply to the Supreme Court of Appeals, which, if it grants the appeal, is to hear the case upon the record of the trial in the Circuit Court and may enter such order as it thinks the Circuit Court should have entered. There can be no doubt that so far as procedure is concerned the rights of the patient are most carefully considered, and as every step in this case was taken in scrupulous compliance with the statute and after months of observation, there is no doubt that in that respect the plaintiff in error has had due process at law.

The attack is not upon the procedure but upon the substantive law. It seems to be contended that in no circumstances could such an order be justified. It certainly is contended that the order cannot be justified upon the existing grounds. The judgment finds the facts that have been recited and that Carrie Buck 'is the probable potential parent of socially inadequate offspring, likewise afflicted, that she may be sexually sterilized without detriment to her general health and that her welfare and that of society will be promoted by her sterilization,' and thereupon makes the order. In view of the general declarations of the Legislature and the specific findings of the Court obviously we cannot say as matter of law that the grounds do not exist, and if they exist they justify the result. We have seen more than once that the public welfare may call upon the best citizens for their lives. It would be strange if it could not call upon those who already sap the strength of the State for these lesser sacrifices, often not felt to be such by those concerned, in order to prevent our being swamped with incompetence. It is better for all the world, if instead of waiting to execute degenerate offspring for crime, or to let them starve for their imbecility, society can prevent those who are manifestly unfit from continuing their kind. The principle that sustains compulsory vaccination is broad enough to cover cutting the Fallopian tubes. *Jacobson v. Massachusetts*, 197 U. S. 11, 25 S. Ct. 358, 49 L. Ed. 643, 3 Ann. Cas. 765. Three generations of imbeciles are enough.

But, it is said, however it might be if this reasoning were applied generally, it fails when it is confined to the small number who are in the institutions named and is not applied to the multitudes outside. It is the usual last resort of constitutional arguments to point out shortcomings of this sort. But the answer is that the law does all that is needed when it does all that it can, indicates a policy, applies it to all within the lines, and seeks to bring within the lines all similarly situated so far and so fast as its means allow. Of course so far as the operations enable those who otherwise must be kept confined to be returned to the world, and thus open the asylum to others, the equality aimed at will be more nearly reached.

Judgment affirmed.

Mr. Justice Butler dissents.

NOTES AND QUESTIONS

1. *A History of Eugenics in the U.S.* The word "eugenics" originates from the Greek word "eugenes," meaning "good in birth." The term eugenics was coined in the 1880s by Francis Galton, a Victorian aristocrat and nephew of Charles Darwin.

Galton and his colleagues harnessed the growing enthusiasm over the infant, yet burgeoning field of genetics to advance the concept of controlled human breeding. Eugenicists believed that most social problems were caused by hereditary faults of those afflicted by the problem, and they sought to eventually eliminate these problems from society through selective breeding. By the turn of the twentieth century, the eugenics movement had gained support in the United States, Germany and Britain, spawning well-funded movements. The movements won governmental support in the form of compulsory sterilization laws, such as the Virginia law at issue in *Buck v. Bell.* By the 1930s, more than 30 U.S. states had passed involuntary eugenic sterilization laws, typically applied to those deemed feeble-minded, insane, criminals, drug addicts, those with chronic, infectious diseases, the blind, the deaf, the deformed, and the dependent, including orphans, ne'er do wells, the homeless, tramps, and paupers. See Lisa Powell, *Eugenics and Equality: Does the Constitution Allow Policies Designed to Discourage Reproduction Among Disfavored Groups?*, 20 YALE LAW & POLICY REV. 481, 483 (2002), citing Harry Laughlin, *Model Eugenical Sterilization Law,* in EUGENICAL STERILIZATION IN THE UNITED STATES, A REPORT OF THE PSYCHOPATHIC LABORATORY OF THE MUNICIPAL COURT OF CHICAGO 445, 447 (1922). Between 1900 and 1963, at least 60,000 Americans were sterilized pursuant to eugenic sterilization laws. In response to a lawsuit, in 1974 the federal government adopted regulations banning sterilization without consent in hospitals that receive federal funds, but reports of violations surface periodically. For a thorough discussion of the eugenics movement and its impact on current ART dialogue, see Michael J. Malinowski, *Choosing the Genetic Makeup of Children: Our Eugenics Past — Present, and Future?*, 36 CONN. L. REV. 125 (2003).

2. *The Buck Legacy?* The decision in *Buck v. Bell* has never been explicitly overturned by the U.S. Supreme Court, and in fact has been cited more than a dozen times by the Court since Justice Holmes penned the words upholding compulsory sterilization of "mental defectives." For example, in *Roe v. Wade,* 410 U.S. 113 (1973), the first high court decision recognizing a woman's constitutional right to terminate her pregnancy, *Buck v. Bell* is favorably cited for the proposition that the Court has refused to recognize an unlimited right to do with one's body as one pleases. Id. at 154. Other cases cite *Buck* to showcase Justice Holmes' remark that a constitutional equal protection claim is "the usual last resort of constitutional arguments." See, e.g., *Regents of the University of California v. Bakke,* 438 U.S. 265, 326 (1978); *Zablocki v. Redhail,* 434 U.S. 374, 395 (1978). One of the most recent Supreme Court references to *Buck v. Bell* came in a 2001 decision in which state employees challenged their employer's claim of sovereign immunity from application of the Americans With Disabilities Act. Justice Rehnquist, writing for the majority, sided with the state, citing *Buck* in a footnote for the proposition that the Court has upheld the constitutionality of state laws which involve "extreme measures." *Board of Trustees of University of Alabama v. Garrett,* 531 U.S. 356, 365 (2001).

In the current world of ART, does *Buck v. Bell's* survival give any insight into how a court might rule on the constitutionality of laws restricting or even banning the use of reproductive technologies? Even if an argument could be made that limiting access to ARTs is the modern-day equivalent of state-sponsored sterilization by forcing genetic childlessness on infertile individuals, would a court necessarily have to overturn *Buck* in order to find such laws invalid?

3. *Does Skinner implicitly overrule Buck?* Fifteen years separate the Court's decisions in *Buck* (1927) and *Skinner* (1942). History reveals that this is a sufficient passage of time for the Court to overrule a precedent, though the *Skinner* court makes no mention of overruling Buck. Do you read *Skinner* (voiding a state law authorizing sterilization of repeat felons) as implicitly overruling *Buck* (upholding a state law authorizing sterilization of those in state custody "afflicted with hereditary forms of insanity, imbecility, etc.")? Professor Paul Lombardo, an acclaimed legal historian who has written extensively on the eugenics period, offers this analysis on the question:

> There is a common misconception that the Supreme Court decision in *Skinner* all but overruled *Buck* and that the postwar revelation of Nazi practices led to a general rejection of eugenics. But eugenically based assumptions about heredity as a basis for law survived well beyond *Skinner*, just as they outlived the Third Reich. Years after the case, Justice Douglas himself reiterated that there was no desire by the *Skinner* court to overrule *Buck*. Douglas was "very clear" on the case's constitutional validity. The eugenic foundations of *Buck* were safe because of the procedural protections that the Virginia law included.

PAUL A. LOMBARDO, THREE GENERATIONS NO IMBECILES 232 (2008).

4. The Virginia statute authorizing surgical sterilization is based on the empirical assumption that "mental defectives," once discharged from state confinement, will become a menace to society, but if rendered incapable of reproducing will become self-supporting "with benefit to themselves and to society." Do you agree with the Court's logic? Viewing this statement with an early twentieth-century eye which had little advantage of social science research, is the Court right to link involuntary infertility with social stability? Would a person who is involuntarily sterilized by the state be more likely to adhere to state-sponsored rules than a parent who is responsible for supporting a dependent child? Even if you see logic in the argument that people with children are more likely to be law-abiding and productive than those who have no dependents, that does little to address the Court's principal point that states have an interest in ridding society of "socially inadequate offspring." With these words the Court is referencing Carrie Buck and her child. Again, we can ask, where is the proof in this case? Consider the following essay.

Paul A. Lombardo
Facing Carrie Buck
33 Hastings Center Report 14 (March-April 2003)

Three generations of imbeciles are enough. Few phrases are as well known among scholars of bioethics as this remark by Oliver Wendell Holmes Jr. in his opinion in *Buck v. Bell.* The *Buck* case arose as a challenge to a 1924 Virginia law authorizing the sexual sterilization of people designated as "socially inadequate." The law explicitly adopted eugenic theory, affirming the proposition that tendencies to crime, poverty, mental illness, and moral failings are inherited in predictable patterns. The social costs of those conditions could be erased, the eugenicists thought, and Carrie Buck's case went to court to establish a constitutional precedent and ratify the practice of eugenic sterilization.

The sterilization law received a thundering endorsement from the U. S. Supreme Court in 1927. Holmes, by then perhaps the most revered judge in America, wrote an opinion that proclaimed: "It is better for all the world, if instead of waiting to execute degenerate off-spring for crime, or to let them starve for their imbecility, society can prevent those who are manifestly unfit from continuing their kind . . . ." His comment about generations of imbeciles was intended to summarize the evidence introduced in court about Carrie, her mother, and her daughter. Holmes' opinion became the rallying cry for American eugenicists. Within a decade of the decision, eugenic sterilization was enshrined in the laws of a majority of American states; the practice of state-mandated surgery remained intact for nearly three-quarters of the twentieth century, generating at least 60,000 victims.

When I met Carrie Buck in December 1982, it was clear that her frailty reflected the trials of a long, hard life. Her death only three weeks later was a surprise to no one. Weak from the infirmities of old age, she spoke sparingly, saving the little energy she had. In our brief conversation, little was said of the Supreme Court case that had settled her fate years earlier. In the decades since that meeting, I have searched for evidence that would shed light on the "three generations" condemned in Holmes's chilling phrase, particularly the young woman whose infamy it insured.

Slowly, the search yielded startling results. Virginia mental health agency records revealed that the sterilization law was originally written to protect a doctor who feared malpractice lawsuits from patients who had endured his freelance, coerced sterilization. Those records also confirmed that the lawyer paid to defend Carrie Buck actually betrayed her, by neglecting to challenge the claims of eugenicists who testified at her trial and colluding with the state's lawyer to guarantee that the sterilization law would remain in force. School report cards demonstrated the intelligence of Vivian, Carrie's daughter. The grade book I found showed her to be an "honor roll" student, contradicting the impression of trial witnesses that as an infant she was "peculiar," "not quite normal," and probably "feebleminded." Carrie's case turned out to be less about mental illness than about moralism, and the comments about her illegitimate baby served to hide the fact — confirmed by Carrie herself — that rape by a relative of her foster parents had left her pregnant.

But the records of lawyers and bureaucrats could never provide a complete perspective on Carrie Buck's story. As for my talk with Carrie: an aging woman's final recollections of the most painful memories of her adolescence were understandably brief, and some details continued to elude me. How did seventeen-year-old Carrie Buck feel as she faced a trial that would determine her future as a mother? What did this girl, described in court records as having "a rather badly formed face," really look like in 1924? Similar questions remained about the other two generations of the Buck family: Carrie's mother, Emma, and the baby Vivian.

Picturing Three Generations

Years after Carrie's sterilization, Dr. John Bell, the physician who eventually sterilized Carrie Buck, attempted to find pictures of Carrie and her baby that could be included in an article written by California eugenics enthusiast Paul Popenoe. Bell was successful in locating a photo of Carrie, but was frustrated in his search for a picture of Vivian, Carrie's baby, and wrote that the absence of documentation "has deprived the child of an opportunity to become a permanent figure in eugenic history." Bell submitted a portrait of himself to be paired with Carrie's image in the article celebrating the notorious case. He was unaware that any other photos of the Buck family existed and could not have known that, far from being a high point in American history, the eugenic sterilization movement would later be listed among the country's most shameful memories.

In my searches through university archives, I discovered two pictures that escaped Bell's attention. Both were taken at the time of the 1924 trial. The photographer was an expert witness who visited Virginia in preparation for his testimony in favor of Carrie Buck's sterilization. Our only perspective on the Bucks has been shaped by Holmes's callous proclamation. These photos show us the Buck family and provide the faces that we have thus far only imagined: three generations of the most famous but previously faceless victims of the eugenics movement in America.

Carrie Buck was committed to the Virginia Colony for Epileptics and Feeble-minded as a prelude to her sterilization. Her mother Emma preceded her at the Colony, arriving four years earlier . . .

The snapshots . . . of the Buck family have remained hidden among [the expert's] records since 1924. They are apparently the only surviving photos of the Bucks. One photo shows Carrie and her mother Emma . . . On one level, the photo is unremarkable. The women appear to have been posed. They are sitting together on a bench late on a cold November day. Emma wears a gingham house-dress . . . Her face shows no emotion. Carrie is wearing a long smock over a black, long-sleeved shirt. Her hands are formally cupped in her lap; her eyes seem slightly pained, and her mouth betrays hints of a frown. One cannot help but speculate about her state of mind. She had arrived at the Colony in June of 1924, separated from her baby soon after giving birth in late March. She was locked in an institution with strangers and interrogated repeatedly; within a month of her arrival she learned she would be the focus of a legal proceeding. At the time of the photograph she was seated next to the mother from whom she had been taken at least a dozen years earlier. In the photograph, the heads of the two women are tilted slightly away from each other.

[The] second picture includes . . . a mature woman . . . and an . . . infant . . . The woman is Alice Dobbs, Carrie's foster mother for more than a dozen years and now foster mother to Carrie's baby, Vivian. Dobbs appears to hold a coin in front of Vivian's face, perhaps in an attempt to catch her attention. The baby looks past her, staring into the distance.

Although copies of intelligence tests given to Carrie and Emma remain among Colony records, no evidence of formal mental testing of Vivian appears in the Colony files . . . It is clear that . . . plans had been made to get a "mental test" of the baby . . . At that time, testing for an infant would have included attempts to gauge neurological development through simple exercises. Exercises for children as young as three and six months included turning the head toward a source of sound, following a moving light, and balancing the head while sitting. At the age of one year, children were expected to show visual coordination of the head and eyes while following a moving object. If [an observer] is holding a coin in this picture, it is plausible that the photo is a reenactment of some portion of an I.Q. test . . . [The Colony's expert's] testimony about Vivian came the day after the photos were taken. He described his short encounter, saying: "I gave the child the regular mental test for a child of the age of six months, and judging from her reaction to the tests I gave her, I decided she was below the average." This comment, coupled with a nurse's recollection that Vivian was "not quite normal," sealed the conclusion that the Buck family defects spanned three generations.

The Apology

The seventy-fifth anniversary of the Supreme Court decision in *Buck v. Bell* was 2 May 2002. In Carrie Buck's hometown of Charlottesville on that day, a historic marker was erected to commemorate the case. Virginia Governor Mark Warner sent an official apology that was read at the marker's dedication, denouncing his state's involvement in the eugenics movement as a "shameful effort." The state's flagship newspaper, which applauded the eugenics movement during its heyday, condemned sterilization as "state sanctioned butchery." The story drew national press attention, reminding readers that the sterilization of Carrie Buck was the first of more than 8,000 state-mandated operations performed under Virginia's 1924 eugenic sterilization law. The Virginia law paved the way for more than 60,000 operations in more than thirty American states with similar laws and provided a precedent for 400,000 sterilizations that would occur in Nazi Germany.

Oregon, North and South Carolina recently followed Virginia in repudiating their history of eugenics.

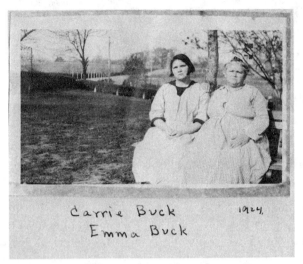

Carrie Buck (left) and mother Emma, Circa 1924

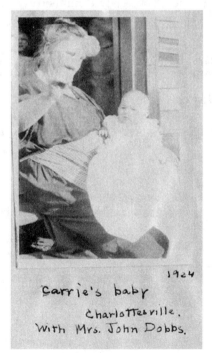

Alice Dobbs with Carrie's baby Vivian, Circa 1924

B. The Right to Avoid Procreation

1. Emerging Advances in Human Contraception

GRISWOLD v. CONNECTICUT
Supreme Court of the United States
381 U.S. 485 (1965)

JUSTICE DOUGLAS delivered the opinion of the Court.

Appellant Griswold is Executive Director of the Planned Parenthood League of Connecticut. Appellant Buxton is a licensed physician and a professor at the Yale Medical School who served as Medical Director for the League at its Center in New Haven — a center open and operating from November 1 to November 10, 1961, when appellants were arrested.

They gave information, instruction, and medical advice to married persons as to the means of preventing conception. They examined the wife and prescribed the best contraceptive device or material for her use. Fees were usually charged, although some couples were serviced free.

The statutes whose constitutionality is involved in this appeal are §§ 53 — 32 and 54 — 196 of the General Statutes of Connecticut (1958 rev.). The former provides:

Any person who uses any drug, medicinal article or instrument for the purpose of preventing conception shall be fined not less than fifty dollars or imprisoned not less than sixty days nor more than one year or be both fined and imprisoned.

Section 54 — 196 provides:

Any person who assists, abets, counsels, causes, hires or commands another to commit any offense may be prosecuted and punished as if he were the principal offender.

The appellants were found guilty as accessories and fined $100 each, against the claim that the accessory statute as so applied violated the Fourteenth Amendment. The Appellate Division of the Circuit Court affirmed. The Supreme Court of Errors affirmed that judgment. 151 Conn. 544, 200 A.2d 479. We noted probable jurisdiction . . .

We think that appellants have standing to raise the constitutional rights of the married people with whom they had a professional relationship . . .

Coming to the merits, we are met with a wide range of questions that implicate the Due Process Clause of the Fourteenth Amendment . . . This law . . . operates directly on an intimate relation of husband and wife and their physician's role in one aspect of that relation.

The association of people is not mentioned in the Constitution nor in the Bill of Rights. The right to educate a child in a school of the parents' choice — whether public or private or parochial — is also not mentioned. Nor is the right to study any particular subject or any foreign language. Yet the First Amendment has been construed to include certain of those rights.

By *Pierce v. Society of Sisters*, [268 U.S. 510], the right to educate one's children as one chooses is made applicable to the States by the force of the First and Fourteenth Amendments. By *Meyer v. State of Nebraska*, [262 U.S. 390], the same dignity is given the right to study the German language in a private school. In other words, the State may not, consistently with the spirit of the First Amendment, contract the spectrum of available knowledge. The right of freedom of speech and press includes not only the right to utter or to print, but the right to distribute, the right to receive, the right to read . . . Without those peripheral rights the specific rights would be less secure. And so we reaffirm the principle of the Pierce and the Meyer cases . . .

The foregoing cases suggest that specific guarantees in the Bill of Rights have penumbras, formed by emanations from those guarantees that help give them life and substance. See *Poe v. Ullman*, 367 U.S. 497, 516-522, 81 S.Ct. 1752, 6 L.Ed.2d 989 (dissenting opinion). Various guarantees create zones of privacy. The right of association contained in the penumbra of the First Amendment is one, as we have seen. The Third Amendment in its prohibition against the quartering of soldiers 'in any house' in time of peace without the consent of the owner is another facet of that privacy. The Fourth Amendment explicitly affirms the 'right of the people to be secure in their persons, houses, papers, and effects, against unreasonable searches and seizures.' The Fifth Amendment in its Self-Incrimination Clause enables the citizen to create a zone of privacy which government may not force him to surrender to his detriment. The Ninth Amendment provides: 'The enumeration in the Constitution, of certain rights, shall not be construed to deny or disparage others retained by the people.' . . .

We have had many controversies over these penumbral rights of 'privacy and repose.' [citations omitted] These cases bear witness that the right of privacy which presses for recognition here is a legitimate one.

The present case, then, concerns a relationship lying within the zone of privacy created by several fundamental constitutional guarantees. And it concerns a law which, in forbidding the use of contraceptives rather than regulating their manufacture or sale, seeks to achieve its goals by means having a maximum destructive impact upon that relationship. Such a law cannot stand in light of the familiar principle, so often applied by this Court, that a 'governmental purpose to control or prevent activities constitutionally subject to state regulation may not be achieved by means which sweep unnecessarily broadly and thereby invade the area of protected freedoms.' *NAACP v. Alabama*, 377 U.S. 288, 307, 84 S.Ct. 1302, 1314, 12 L.Ed.2d 325. Would we allow the police to search the sacred precincts of marital bedrooms for telltale signs of the use of contraceptives? The very idea is repulsive to the notions of privacy surrounding the marriage relationship.

We deal with a right of privacy older than the Bill of Rights — older than our political parties, older than our school system. Marriage is a coming together for better or for worse, hopefully enduring, and intimate to the degree of being sacred. It is an association that promotes a way of life, not causes; a harmony in living, not political faiths; a bilateral loyalty, not commercial or social projects. Yet it is an association for as noble a purpose as any involved in our prior decisions.

Reversed.

MR. JUSTICE GOLDBERG, whom THE CHIEF JUSTICE and MR. JUSTICE BRENNAN join, concurring.

I agree with the Court that Connecticut's birth-control law unconstitutionally intrudes upon the right of marital privacy, and I join in its opinion and judgment. Although I have not accepted the view that 'due process' as used in the Fourteenth Amendment includes all of the first eight Amendments . . . , I do agree that the concept of liberty protects those personal rights that are fundamental, and is not confined to the specific terms of the Bill of Rights. My conclusion that the concept of liberty is not so restricted and that it embraces the right of marital privacy though that right is not mentioned explicitly in the Constitution . . . is supported both by numerous decisions of this Court, referred to in the Court's opinion, and by the language and history of the Ninth Amendment . . .

The Ninth Amendment reads, 'The enumeration in the Constitution, of certain rights, shall not be construed to deny or disparage others retained by the people.' . . .

The Ninth Amendment simply shows the intent of the Constitution's authors that other fundamental personal rights should not be denied such protection or disparaged in any other way simply because they are not specifically listed in the first eight constitutional amendments . . .

The entire fabric of the Constitution and the purposes that clearly underlie its specific guarantees demonstrate that the rights to marital privacy and to marry and raise a family are of similar order and magnitude as the fundamental rights specifically protected.

Although the Constitution does not speak in so many words of the right of privacy in marriage, I cannot believe that it offers these fundamental rights no protection. The fact that no particular provision of the Constitution explicitly forbids the State from disrupting the traditional relation of the family — a relation as old and as fundamental as our entire civilization — surely does not show that the Government was meant to have the power to do so. Rather, as the Ninth Amendment expressly recognizes, there are fundamental personal rights such as this one, which are protected from abridgment by the Government though not specifically mentioned in the Constitution . . .

MR. JUSTICE HARLAN, concurring in the judgment.

I fully agree with the judgment of reversal, but find myself unable to join the Court's opinion . . .

In my view, the proper constitutional inquiry in this case is whether this Connecticut statute infringes the Due Process Clause of the Fourteenth Amendment because the enactment violates basic values 'implicit in the concept of ordered liberty'. . . . I believe that it does. While the relevant inquiry may be aided by resort to one or more of the provisions of the Bill of Rights, it is not dependent on them or any of their radiations. The Due Process Clause of the Fourteenth Amendment stands, in my opinion, on its own bottom.

[Justice White filed a separate concurring opinion.].

MR. JUSTICE BLACK, with whom MR. JUSTICE STEWART joins, dissenting.

. . . I do not to any extent whatever base my view that this Connecticut law is constitutional on a belief that the law is wise or that its policy is a good one. In order that there may be no room at all to doubt why I vote as I do, I feel constrained to add that the law is every bit as offensive to me as it is my Brethren . . . who, reciting reasons why it is offensive to them, hold it unconstitutional . . .

The Court talks about a constitutional 'right of privacy' as though there is some constitutional provision or provisions forbidding any law ever to be passed which might abridge the 'privacy' of individuals. But there is not . . .

I get nowhere in this case by talk about a constitutional 'right or privacy' as an emanation from one or more constitutional provisions. I like my privacy as well as the next one, but I am nevertheless compelled to admit that government has a right to invade it unless prohibited by some specific constitutional provision. For these reasons I cannot agree with the Court's judgment and the reasons it gives for holding this Connecticut law unconstitutional.

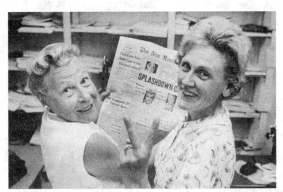

Planned Parenthood League of Connecticut Executive Director Estelle Griswold (left), with the League's president, Cornelia Jahncke, celebrates the landmark U.S. Supreme Court decision that bears her name.

NOTES AND QUESTIONS

1. *A Brief History of Contraception.* The events that led to the *Griswold* case transpired in 1961, corresponding almost exactly with the introduction of the first human birth control pill in 1960. While the pill may have revolutionized female contraception (and perhaps inspired a sexual revolution in the latter part of the decade), the daily ingestible was not a stand-alone choice, but rather joined a long list of established and evolving methods of preventing pregnancy. Like the methods

of treating infertility described in Chapter 1 beginning at page 25, the practice of contraception dates back to ancient times. A brief perusal of these methodologies serves to remind today's lovers that they enjoy freedom from such niceties as crocodile dung and tobacco juice, preferring as we do a whiff of Chanel.

As far back as 1850 B.C., ancient Egyptians searched for a formula that could be inserted in a woman's vagina to inhibit conception. A mixture of crocodile dung, honey and sodium bicarbonate proved popular. Other concoctions included olive oil, pomegranate pulp, ginger, and tobacco juice, smeared in or around the vagina to kill or slow the sperm before reaching the egg. The Egyptians further advanced the field by developing a tampon-like object that contained lactic acid anhydride, a chief ingredient in modern contraceptive jellies. Two millennia later, in the second century A.D., Greek gynecologists understood that women were fertile during ovulation, but wrongly believed that ovulation occurred during menstruation. In fact, it would take until the 1930s for physicians to understand precisely when ovulation occurs.

Barrier methods of birth control, including the modern day condom and diaphragm also have their place in contraception history. A well-worn condom myth attributes the first sperm-catching device to Dr. Condom, who invented the penis sheath for King Charles II in the seventeenth century to prevent him from fathering illegitimate children. But in fact ancient Egyptians wore condoms made out of fabric, not as a contraceptive but as protection from insect bites. The condom as we know it today was developed in the 1840s by Charles Goodyear, alas of tire fame. Goodyear used the recently developed vulcanized rubber to create a strong elastic material that gradually fell out of favor in the 1930s when latex was substituted as a preferable material. Female barrier devices evolved from near barbaric beginnings to the current choice of a diaphragm (a dome shaped rubber device placed over the cervix to prevent sperm from passing through to the uterus) or a female condom (fitting inside the vagina to catch and contain semen). Early barriers for women included half a lemon stuck in the vagina, and the ever comfortable large wooden block inserted in the vagina. Hard to understand why the latter method was later deemed a device of torture.

Historians attribute the intrauterine device (IUDs) to the Arabs. Reportedly they would stick pebbles into the uteruses of their camels to prevent pregnancy on long trips across the desert. Today's IUD is a T-shaped device measuring approximately 2 inches, made of either steel, plastic or copper. The device is inserted in the uterus, causing the environment within the uterus to be unsuitable for the embryo to implant.

Oral contraceptives began life as eclectic mixtures of various substances made into a drink, including urine, animal parts, mercury, arsenic and strychnine. Greek scientists suggested drinking the water used by blacksmiths to cool hot metals. The modern history of oral contraception is often associated with nurse Margaret Sanger (1879-1966), a lifelong advocate for affordable and effective birth control. In the 1950s, while in her 80s, Sanger underwrote the research necessary to create the first human birth control pill, raising $150,000 to support the project. The "pill" was introduced into the U.S. market in May 1960, known as Enovid-10. Birth control pills are made of synthetic hormones that mimic the way real estrogen and progestin work in a women's body. The pill prevents ovulation by "tricking" the body into believing the woman is already pregnant.

The popularity of the pill grew from 1.2 million users in 1962, to 10 million women in 1973, to over 80 million users worldwide in the mid-1980s. For a thorough history of the pill, set out in timeline fashion, visit the PBS website, featuring "American Experience: The Pill" at: http://www.pbs.org/wgbh/amex/pill/timeline/index.html.

Research into new forms of contraception continues, with recent efforts focused on a contraceptive patch worn on the abdomen or back, contraceptive injections, nasal sprays and implants for men. Today's legal battles over contraception seem not to focus on its availability to married couples, as in *Griswold*, but on its availability to minors, low- and no-income individuals, and individuals whose health insurance denies contraceptive benefits. For a discussion of the health insurance industry's policies on birth control benefits, see Lisa A. Hayden, *Gender Discrimination Within the Reproductive Health Care System: Viagra v. Birth Control*, 13 J. L. & HEALTH 171 (1999).

To learn more about the history of contraception, consider visiting The History of Contraception Museum, located just outside Toronto, Canada. Where else could you see a display of over 600 different IUDs, sponges, condoms and other contraceptive devices? For a comprehensive read about the history of birth control see ANGUS MCLAREN, A HISTORY OF CONTRACEPTION: FROM ANTIQUITY TO THE PRESENT DAY (1991).

2.   The decision in *Griswold v. Connecticut* is an interesting case study because of the wide-ranging views presented by individual and groupings of justices. Justice Douglas found the state law prohibiting the use and distribution of contraceptives unconstitutional because he believed such governmental activity violated a right of privacy, a fundamental right he saw emanating from the penumbras (defined: shadows) of the Bill of Rights. Justices Goldberg, Chief Justice Warren and Justice Brennan found the Ninth Amendment proper authority for the Court to protect nontextual rights such as privacy. Justice Harlan found the right of privacy in the liberty of the due process clause of the Fourteenth Amendment. In dissent, Justices Black and Stewart saw no such right of privacy, because the constitution lacks any explicit reference to privacy or any right thereto. From your contemporary vantage point, which of these views best describes your view of marital privacy?

3.   The Connecticut statute at issue in *Griswold* was originally enacted in 1879 under the sponsorship of P.T. Barnum, the circus promoter, who was then serving in the Connecticut legislature. Notice that, on its face, the law was not limited to married individuals ("any person who uses . . ."). But Estelle Griswold was charged under the statute for giving contraceptive information to married persons. And importantly, the decision focuses on the marital relationship as deserving constitutional protection. What of the rights of unmarried individuals to engage in sexual activity, with or without the use of birth control? Perhaps no single individuals found their way to the Planned Parenthood League of Connecticut, but as the decade wore on, that became increasingly unlikely. This next case tests the limits of restricting contraceptives on the basis of marital status.

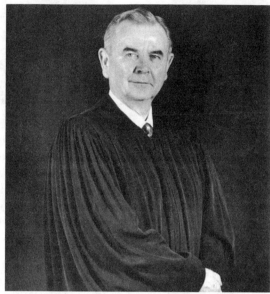

Justice William J. Brennan, Jr.

EISENSTADT v. BAIRD
Supreme Court of the United States
405 U.S. 438 (1972)

JUSTICE BRENNAN delivered the opinion of the Court.

Appellee William Baird was convicted at a bench trial in the Massachusetts Superior Court under Massachusetts General Laws Ann., c. 272, § 21, first, for exhibiting contraceptive articles in the course of delivering a lecture on contraception to a group of students at Boston University and, second, for giving a young woman a package of Emko vaginal foam at the close of his address.[3] The Massachusetts Supreme Judicial Court unanimously set aside the conviction for exhibiting contraceptives on the ground that it violated Baird's First Amendment rights, but by a four-to-three vote sustained the conviction for giving away the foam. Commonwealth v. Baird, 355 Mass. 746, 247 N.E.2d 574 (1969). Baird subsequently filed a petition for a federal writ of habeas corpus, which the District Court dismissed. 310 F.Supp. 951 (1970). On appeal, however, the Court of Appeals for the First Circuit vacated the dismissal and remanded the action with directions to grant the writ discharging Baird. 429 F.2d 1398 (1970). This appeal by the Sheriff of Suffolk County, Massachusetts, followed, and we noted probable jurisdiction. 401 U.S. 934, 91 S.Ct. 921, 28 L.Ed.2d 213 (1971). We affirm.

Massachusetts General Laws Ann., c. 272, § 21, under which Baird was convicted, provides a maximum five-year term of imprisonment for 'whoever . . . gives away

---

[3] [n.4] The Court of Appeals below described the recipient of the foam as 'an unmarried adult woman.' 429 F.2d 1398, 1399 (1970). However, there is no evidence in the record about her marital status.

. . . any drug, medicine, instrument or article whatever for the prevention of conception,' except as authorized in § 21A. Under § 21A, '(a) registered physician may administer to or prescribe for any married person drugs or articles intended for the prevention of pregnancy or conception. (And a) registered pharmacist actually engaged in the business of pharmacy may furnish such drugs or articles to any married person presenting a prescription from a registered physician.' . . . As interpreted by the State Supreme Judicial Court, these provisions make it a felony for anyone, other than a registered physician or pharmacist acting in accordance with the terms of § 21A, to dispense any article with the intention that it be used for the prevention of conception. The statutory scheme distinguishes among three distinct classes of distributees — first, married persons may obtain contraceptives to prevent pregnancy, but only from doctors or druggists on prescription; second, single persons may not obtain contraceptives from anyone to prevent pregnancy; and, third, married or single persons may obtain contraceptives from anyone to prevent, not pregnancy, but the spread of disease . . .

[W]e hold that the statute, viewed as a prohibition on contraception per se, violates the rights of single persons under the Equal Protection Clause of the Fourteenth Amendment . . .

II

The basic principles governing application of the Equal Protection Clause of the Fourteenth Amendment are familiar. As The Chief Justice only recently explained in *Reed v. Reed*, 404 U.S. 71, 75 — 76, 92 S.Ct. 251, 253, 30 L.Ed.2d 225 (1971): 'In applying that clause, this Court has consistently recognized that the Fourteenth Amendment does not deny to State the power to treat different classes of persons in different ways . . . The Equal Protection Clause of that amendment does, however, deny to State the power to legislate that different treatment be accorded to persons placed by a statute into different classes on the basis of criteria wholly unrelated to the objective of that statute. A classification 'must be reasonable, not arbitrary, and must rest upon some ground of difference having a fair and substantial relation to the object of the legislation, so that all persons similarly circumstanced shall be treated alike.' *Royster Guano Co. v. Virginia*, 253 U.S. 412, 415, 40 S.Ct. 560, 64 L.Ed. 989 (1920).'

The question for our determination in this case is whether there is some ground of difference that rationally explains the different treatment accorded married and unmarried persons under Massachusetts General Laws Ann., c. 272, §§ 21 and 21A [4] For the reasons that follow, we conclude that no such ground exists . . .

[W]hatever the rights of the individual to access to contraceptives may be, the rights must be the same for the unmarried and the married alike.

If under *Griswold* the distribution of contraceptives to married persons cannot

---

[4] [n.7] Of course, if we were to conclude that the Massachusetts statute impinges upon fundamental freedoms under *Griswold*, the statutory classification would have to be not merely rationally related to a valid public purpose but necessary to the achievement of a compelling state interest . . . But just as in *Reed v. Reed*, 404 U.S. 71, 92 S.Ct. 251, 30 L.Ed.2d 225 (1971), we do not have to address the statute's validity under that test because the law fails to satisfy even the more lenient equal protection standard.

be prohibited, a ban on distribution to unmarried persons would be equally impermissible. It is true that in *Griswold* the right of privacy in question inhered in the marital relationship. Yet the marital couple is not an independent entity with a mind and heart of its own, but an association of two individuals each with a separate intellectual and emotional makeup. If the right of privacy means anything, it is the right of the individual, married or single, to be free from unwarranted governmental intrusion into matters so fundamentally affecting a person as the decision whether to bear or beget a child . . .

We hold that by providing dissimilar treatment for married and unmarried persons who are similarly situated, Massachusetts General Laws Ann., c. 272, §§ 21 and 21A, violate the Equal Protection Clause. The judgment of the Court of Appeals is affirmed.

[Justice Douglas wrote a concurring opinion advocating for analysis under the First Amendment because the basis for Baird's conviction was giving a female member of the audience a contraceptive foam following his hour lecture, an activity the justice deemed "a permissible adjunct of free speech." 405 U.S. at 460.]

JUSTICE WHITE and JUSTICE BLACKMUN issued a separate concurring opinion.

CHIEF JUSTICE BURGER issued a dissenting opinion.

JUSTICE POWELL and JUSTICE REHNQUIST took no part in the consideration or decision of this case.

NOTES AND QUESTIONS

1. *The Advent of Comstock Laws.* The criminal contraception statutes at issue in both *Griswold v. Connecticut* and *Eisenstadt v. Baird* derive from the nineteenth century advocacy of Anthony Comstock, a self-appointed anti-vice crusader from New York. By all accounts, Mr. Comstock managed to shepherd through Congress the Comstock Act of 1873, a federal law which banned the importation or transportation in interstate commerce of matter pertaining to abortion or contraception. A criminal statute, the Comstock Act was designed "for the suppression of trade in and circulation of obscene literature and articles of immoral use." Act of March 3, 1873, ch. 258, § 2, 17 Stat. 599 (1873). In the same era, Comstock-type statutes gained favor in state legislatures, with many state lawmakers enacting laws that forbade the dissemination or, in some cases as we have seen, even the use of contraceptives. Comstock was so zealous and effective in the enforcement of these laws that by the late nineteenth century, the subject of contraception had become unmentionable, even in major medical textbooks. During his reign, Comstock orchestrated the arrest of more than 3,000 individuals in the name of public morals, believing as he did that "anything remotely touching upon sex was . . . obscene." *See* HEYWOOD CAMPBELL BROUN & MARGARET LEECH, ANTHONY COMSTOCK 265 (1927). For a behind-the-scenes look at the events surrounding the arrest and opinion in *Eisenstadt v. Baird, see* Roy Lucas, *New Historical Insights on the Curious Case of Baird v. Eisenstadt,* 9 ROGER WILLIAMS U.L. REV. 9 (2003).

2.   The Comstock laws were handed an unrecoverable defeat in 1972, but it would still be another decade before all remnants of Comstockery would be laid to rest. In *Carey v. Population Services International*, 431 U.S. 678 (1977), the Supreme Court declared unconstitutional a New York criminal statute banning the sale or distribution of contraceptives to minors under age 16. The law also limited distribution of contraceptives to licensed pharmacists and criminalized the advertisement or display of contraceptives by any person. Justice Brennan, writing for the Court, again took up the mantle of family and procreational autonomy, stating that "[t]he decision whether or not to beget or bear a child is at the very heart of this cluster of constitutionally protected choices." 431 U.S. at 685. Importantly, Justice Brennan also set the constitutional standard that must be met for the government to justify a law restricting access to contraceptives. " 'Compelling' " he wrote, "is of course the key word; where a decision as fundamental as that whether to bear or beget a child is involved, regulations imposing a burden on it may be justified only by compelling state interests, and must be narrowly drawn to express only those interests." Id. At 686.

A final challenge to the original Comstock law came in *Bolger v. Youngs Drug Products Corp.*, 463 U.S. 60 (1983) in which a manufacturer and distributor of contraceptives brought action contesting the constitutionality of a federal statute prohibiting unsolicited mailing of contraceptive advertisements. The Court found in favor of the company, holding that the statutory ban was an unconstitutional restriction on commercial speech. Thus, while the court in *Bolger* did not focus on the same privacy rights discussed in previous contraception cases, the case is noteworthy for its rejection of the last vestige of Victorian era morals law.

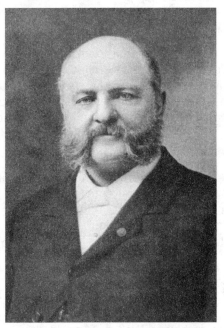

Anthony Comstock (1844-1915)

3.   Let us revisit Justice Brennan's oft-quoted language in *Eisenstadt v. Baird*. "If the right of privacy means anything, it is the right of the individual, married or single, to be free from unwarranted governmental intrusion into matters so fundamentally affecting a person as the decision whether to bear or beget a child . . ." 405 U.S. at 453. From the perspective of reproductive technologies, the decision in *Eisenstadt v. Baird* could prove essential in determining whether federal or state laws that regulate the use of ARTs are constitutional. Do you see why?

4.   Notice that the decision in *Eisenstadt v. Baird* is based on the equal protection clause of the Fourteenth Amendment to the constitution, which the Court held prohibited the state of Massachusetts from providing dissimilar treatment for married and unmarried persons who are similarly situated. The similar situation that affected both groups was their desire for access to contraceptives. As to equal protection at the federal level, interestingly there is no provision in the constitution that prohibits the federal government from denying equal protection of the laws. However, in a mid-twentieth-century case the Court held that the guarantee of equal protection applies to the federal government through the due process clause of the Fifth Amendment. See *Bolling v. Sharpe*, 347 U.S. 497 (1954). For a discussion of the Court's interpretation of the Fifth Amendment as including an implicit requirement for equal protection, see Kenneth Karst, *The Fifth Amendment's Guarantee of Equal Protection*, 55 N.C.L.REV. 540 (1977).

What if a federal law required that doctors practicing reproductive medicine treat their patients unequally in some manner. Could the concept of federal equal protection be used to prohibit unequal treatment of, say, women who are treated with low-tech medical therapies versus women who undergo high-tech treatments such as in vitro fertilization?

A child born as a result of IVF may look and act the same as a naturally conceived child, but the origin of the IVF child's conception raises questions and concerns that are unique to ART. For example, while we as a society may recoil at the thought of delving into the circumstances surrounding a spontaneous pregnancy, we may find it totally acceptable to monitor the activities that give rise to an assisted conception. By way of example, imagine the following conversations taking place in adjacent rooms in a physician's office:

Patient A: Hello Doctor. I am here because I would like to have a baby but I haven't become pregnant after three months of trying.

Doctor: I see. Are you interested in learning about fertility treatments such as in vitro fertilization?

Patient A: Absolutely not. I am only interested in conception that occurs inside the body.

Doctor: Fine. Then I will treat you with a hormone regimen that may enable you to become pregnant by increasing the number of eggs that your ovaries release. The prescribed treatment and your response to the treatment will be kept completely confidential.

Patient A: Thank you, Doctor.

In the next room, Patient B awaits her turn. When asked if she is interested in IVF, she says she would be willing to consider any treatment that could help her have a child.

Doctor:	If you choose to undergo IVF, you will be treated with hormone injections for about one month. Then you will undergo a surgical retrieval of any eggs produced. The surgery will be performed under general anesthesia.
Patient B:	That sounds invasive.
Doctor:	If you think the treatment is invasive, wait until you hear about the reporting requirements. If I treat you with IVF, I am required to report to the federal government the fact that you began a treatment cycle, whether you had any embryos transferred to your uterus, whether you became pregnant and whether and how many babies you gave birth to.
Patient B:	Who has access to that information?
Doctor:	Anyone with interest. The data is available on the website for the Centers for Disease Control. But don't worry, your name is not reported.
Patient B:	Doctor, I need to think about all you have said.

Do you think a federal law that treated patients differently depending on whether their pregnancies were conceived in vivo (inside the body) or ex vivo (outside the body) could withstand a constitutional challenge? What possible important governmental objectives could be offered to justify this differential treatment?

2. Abortion

The topic of abortion, the voluntary termination of a pregnancy, could itself occupy the pages of an entire law school casebook. Mindful of the breadth of analysis and intensity of feeling that is characteristic of the debate over abortion, the goal herein is admittedly limited. The section that follows is intended to provide you the basic parameters of the Supreme Court's abortion decisions. Since our focus is on the constitutional right to reproduce using reproductive technologies, try to read the abortion cases with an eye toward their applicability to the use of ART. How is it that cases which explain the rights and limitations of a woman's right to terminate her pregnancy could control the rights of infertile individuals to access reproductive technologies? As we shall see, the jury is still out on that question.

a.   The Seminal Case

ROE v. WADE
Supreme Court of the United States
410 U.S. 113 (1973)

JUSTICE BLACKMUN delivered the opinion of the Court.

This Texas federal appeal and its Georgia companion, *Doe v. Bolton*, 410 U.S. 179, 93 S.Ct. 739, 35 L.Ed.2d 201, present constitutional challenges to state criminal abortion legislation. The Texas statutes under attack here are typical of those that have been in effect in many States for approximately a century. The Georgia statutes, in contrast, have a modern cast and are a legislative product that, to an extent at least, obviously reflects the influences of recent attitudinal change, of advancing medical knowledge and techniques, and of new thinking about an old issue.

We forthwith acknowledge our awareness of the sensitive and emotional nature of the abortion controversy, of the vigorous opposing views, even among physicians, and of the deep and seemingly absolute convictions that the subject inspires. One's philosophy, one's experiences, one's exposure to the raw edges of human existence, one's religious training, one's attitudes toward life and family and their values, and the moral standards one establishes and seeks to observe, are all likely to influence and to color one's thinking and conclusions about abortion . . .

I

The Texas statutes that concern us here are Arts. 1191-1194 and 1196 of the State's Penal Code, Vernon's Ann.P.C. These make it a crime to 'procure an abortion,' as therein defined, or to attempt one, except with respect to 'an abortion procured or attempted by medical advice for the purpose of saving the life of the mother.' Similar statutes are in existence in a majority of the States.

Texas first enacted a criminal abortion statute in 1854. Texas Laws 1854, c. 49, § 1, set forth in 3 H. Gammel, Laws of Texas 1502 (1898) . . .

II

Jane Roe,[5] a single woman who was residing in Dallas County, Texas, instituted this federal action in March 1970 against the District Attorney of the county. She sought a declaratory judgment that the Texas criminal abortion statutes were unconstitutional on their face, and an injunction restraining the defendant from enforcing the statutes.

Roe alleged that she was unmarried and pregnant; that she wished to terminate her pregnancy by an abortion 'performed by a competent, licensed physician, under safe, clinical conditions'; that she was unable to get a 'legal' abortion in Texas

---

[5] [n.4] The name is a pseudonym.

because her life did not appear to be threatened by the continuation of her pregnancy; and that she could not afford to travel to another jurisdiction in order to secure a legal abortion under safe conditions. She claimed that the Texas statutes were unconstitutionally vague and that they abridged her right of personal privacy, protected by the First, Fourth, Fifth, Ninth, and Fourteenth Amendments.

V

The principal thrust of appellant's attack on the Texas statutes is that they improperly invade a right, said to be possessed by the pregnant woman, to choose to terminate her pregnancy. Appellant would discover this right in the concept of personal 'liberty' embodied in the Fourteenth Amendment's Due Process Clause; or in personal marital, familial, and sexual privacy said to be protected by the Bill of Rights or its penumbras, see *Griswold v. Connecticut*, 381 U.S. 479, 85 S.Ct. 1678, 14 L.Ed.2d 510 (1965); *Eisenstadt v. Baird*, 405 U.S. 438 (1972); id., at 460, 92 S.Ct. 1029, at 1042, 31 L.Ed.2d 349 (White, J., concurring in result); or among those rights reserved to the people by the Ninth Amendment, *Griswold v. Connecticut*, 381 U.S., at 486, 85 S.Ct., at 1682 (Goldberg, J., concurring) . . .

VII

Three reasons have been advanced to explain historically the enactment of criminal abortion laws in the 19th century and to justify their continued existence. It has been argued occasionally that these laws were the product of a Victorian social concern to discourage illicit sexual conduct. Texas, however, does not advance this justification in the present case, and it appears that no court or commentator has taken the argument seriously. The appellants and amici contend, moreover, that this is not a proper state purpose at all and suggest that, if it were, the Texas statutes are overbroad in protecting it since the law fails to distinguish between married and unwed mothers.

A second reason is concerned with abortion as a medical procedure. When most criminal abortion laws were first enacted, the procedure was a hazardous one for the woman. This was particularly true prior to the development of antisepsis. Antiseptic techniques, of course, were based on discoveries by Lister, Pasteur, and others first announced in 1867, but were not generally accepted and employed until about the turn of the century. Abortion mortality was high. Even after 1900, and perhaps until as late as the development of antibiotics in the 1940's, standard modern techniques such as dilation and curettage were not nearly so safe as they are today. Thus, it has been argued that a State's real concern in enacting a criminal abortion law was to protect the pregnant woman, that is, to restrain her from submitting to a procedure that placed her life in serious jeopardy.

Modern medical techniques have altered this situation. Appellants and various amici refer to medical data indicating that abortion in early pregnancy, that is, prior to the end of the first trimester, although not without its risk, is now relatively safe. Mortality rates for women undergoing early abortions, where the procedure is legal, appear to be as low as or lower than the rates for normal childbirth. Consequently, any interest of the State in protecting the woman from an inherently hazardous procedure, except when it would be equally dangerous for her to forgo it, has largely disappeared. Of course, important state interests in the areas of health and medical standards do remain. The State has a legitimate interest in seeing to it that abortion, like any other medical procedure, is performed under circumstances that insure maximum safety for the patient. This interest obviously extends at least to the performing physician and his staff, to the facilities involved, to the availability of after-care, and to adequate provision for any complication or emergency that might arise. The prevalence of high mortality rates at illegal 'abortion mills' strengthens, rather than weakens, the State's interest in regulating the conditions under which abortions are performed. Moreover, the risk to the woman increases as her pregnancy continues. Thus, the State retains a definite interest in protecting the woman's own health and safety when an abortion is proposed at a late stage of pregnancy.

The third reason is the State's interest-some phrase it in terms of duty-in protecting prenatal life. Some of the argument for this justification rests on the theory that a new human life is present from the moment of conception. The State's interest and general obligation to protect life then extends, it is argued, to prenatal life. Only when the life of the pregnant mother herself is at stake, balanced against the life she carries within her, should the interest of the embryo or fetus not prevail. Logically, of course, a legitimate state interest in this area need not stand or fall on acceptance of the belief that life begins at conception or at some other point prior to birth. In assessing the State's interest, recognition may be given to the less rigid claim that as long as at least potential life is involved, the State may assert interests beyond the protection of the pregnant woman alone . . .

It is with these interests, and the weight to be attached to them, that this case is concerned . . .

VIII

— The Constitution does not explicitly mention any right of privacy. In a line of decisions, however, going back perhaps as far as *Union Pacific R. Co. v. Botsford*, 141 U.S. 250, 251, 11 S.Ct. 1000, 1001, 35 L.Ed. 734 (1891), the Court has recognized that a right of personal privacy, or a guarantee of certain areas or zones of privacy, does exist under the Constitution. In varying contexts, the Court or individual Justices have, indeed, found at least the roots of that right in the First Amendment, in the Fourth and Fifth Amendments, in the penumbras of the Bill of Rights, in the Ninth Amendment, or in the concept of liberty guaranteed by the first section of the Fourteenth Amendment [citations omitted]. These decisions make it clear that only personal rights that can be deemed 'fundamental' or 'implicit in the concept of ordered liberty,' . . . are included in this guarantee of personal privacy. They also make it clear that the right has some extension to activities relating to marriage, *Loving v. Virginia*, 388 U.S. 1, 12, 87 S.Ct. 1817, 1823, 18 L.Ed.2d 1010 (1967); procreation, *Skinner v. Oklahoma*, 316 U.S. 535, 541-542, 62 S.Ct. 1110, 1113-1114, 86 L.Ed. 1655 (1942); contraception, *Eisenstadt v. Baird*, 405 U.S., at 453-454, 92 S.Ct., at 1038-1039, id., at 460, 463-465, 92 S.Ct. at 1042, 1043-1044 (White, J., concurring in result); family relationships, *Prince v. Massachusetts*, 321 U.S. 158, 166, 64 S.Ct. 438, 442, 88 L.Ed. 645 (1944); and child rearing and education, *Pierce v. Society of Sisters*, 268 U.S. 510, 535, 45 S.Ct. 571, 573, 69 L.Ed. 1070 (1925), *Meyer v. Nebraska, supra.*

~ This right of privacy, whether it be founded in the Fourteenth Amendment's concept of personal liberty and restrictions upon state action, as we feel it is, or, as the District Court determined, in the Ninth Amendment's reservation of rights to the people, is broad enough to encompass a woman's decision whether or not to terminate her pregnancy. The detriment that the State would impose upon the pregnant woman by denying this choice altogether is apparent. Specific and direct harm medically diagnosable even in early pregnancy may be involved. Maternity, or additional offspring, may force upon the woman a distressful life and future. Psychological harm may be imminent. Mental and physical health may be taxed by child care. There is also the distress, for all concerned, associated with the unwanted child, and there is the problem of bringing a child into a family already unable, psychologically and otherwise, to care for it. In other cases, as in this one, the additional difficulties and continuing stigma of unwed motherhood may be involved. All these are factors the woman and her responsible physician necessarily will consider in consultation.

On the basis of elements such as these, appellant and some amici argue that the woman's right is absolute and that she is entitled to terminate her pregnancy at whatever time, in whatever way, and for whatever reason she alone chooses. With this we do not agree. Appellant's arguments that Texas either has no valid interest at all in regulating the abortion decision, or no interest strong enough to support any limitation upon the woman's sole determination, are unpersuasive. The Court's decisions recognizing a right of privacy also acknowledge that some state regulation in areas protected by that right is appropriate. As noted above, a State may properly assert important interests in safeguarding health, in maintaining medical standards, and in protecting potential life. At some point in pregnancy, these respective interests become sufficiently compelling to sustain regulation of the factors that govern the abortion decision. The privacy right involved, therefore, cannot be said to be absolute . . .

Where certain 'fundamental rights' are involved, the Court has held that regulation limiting these rights may be justified only by a 'compelling state interest . . . and that legislative enactments must be narrowly drawn to express only the legitimate state interests at stake.

IX

The District Court held that the appellee failed to meet his burden of demonstrating that the Texas statute's infringement upon Roe's rights was necessary to support a compelling state interest, and that, although the appellee presented 'several compelling justifications for state presence in the area of abortions,' the statutes outstripped these justifications and swept 'far beyond any areas of compelling state interest.' 314 F.Supp., at 1222-1223. Appellant and appellee both contest that holding. Appellant, as has been indicated, claims an absolute right that bars any state imposition of criminal penalties in the area. Appellee argues that the State's determination to recognize and protect prenatal life from and after conception constitutes a compelling state interest. As noted above, we do not agree fully with either formulation.

A. The appellee and certain amici argue that the fetus is a 'person' within the language and meaning of the Fourteenth Amendment. In support of this, they outline at length and in detail the well-known facts of fetal development. If this suggestion of personhood is established, the appellant's case, of course, collapses, for the fetus' right to life would then be guaranteed specifically by the Amendment. The appellant conceded as much on reargument. On the other hand, the appellee conceded on reargument that no case could be cited that holds that a fetus is a person within the meaning of the Fourteenth Amendment.

The Constitution does not define 'person' in so many words. Section 1 of the Fourteenth Amendment contains three references to 'person.' The first, in defining 'citizens,' speaks of 'persons born or naturalized in the United States.' The word also appears both in the Due Process Clause and in the Equal Protection Clause. 'Person' is used in other places in the Constitution. . . . But in nearly all these instances, the use of the word is such that it has application only postnatally. None indicates, with any assurance, that it has any possible prenatal application.

All this, together with our observation, supra, that throughout the major portion of the 19th century prevailing legal abortion practices were far freer than they are today, persuades us that the word 'person,' as used in the Fourteenth Amendment, does not include the unborn . . .

This conclusion, however, does not of itself fully answer the contentions raised by Texas, and we pass on to other considerations.

B. The pregnant woman cannot be isolated in her privacy. She carries an embryo and, later, a fetus, if one accepts the medical definitions of the developing young in the human uterus. See Dorland's Illustrated Medical Dictionary 478-479, 547 (24th ed. 1965). The situation therefore is inherently different from marital intimacy, or bedroom possession of obscene material, or marriage, or procreation, or education, with which Eisenstadt and Griswold, Stanley, Loving, Skinner and Pierce and Meyer were respectively concerned. As we have intimated above, it is reasonable and appropriate for a State to decide that at some point in time another interest, that of health of the mother or that of potential human life, becomes significantly involved. The woman's privacy is no longer sole and any right of privacy she possesses must be measured accordingly.

Texas urges that, apart from the Fourteenth Amendment, life begins at conception and is present throughout pregnancy, and that, therefore, the State has a compelling interest in protecting that life from and after conception. We need not resolve the difficult question of when life begins. When those trained in the respective disciplines of medicine, philosophy, and theology are unable to arrive at any consensus, the judiciary, at this point in the development of man's knowledge, is not in a position to speculate as to the answer . . .

X

In view of all this, we do not agree that, by adopting one theory of life, Texas may override the rights of the pregnant woman that are at stake. We repeat, however, that the State does have an important and legitimate interest in preserving and protecting the health of the pregnant woman, whether she be a resident of the State or a non-resident who seeks medical consultation and treatment there, and that it has still another important and legitimate interest in protecting the potentiality of human life. These interests are separate and distinct. Each grows in substantiality as the woman approaches term and, at a point during pregnancy, each becomes 'compelling.'

With respect to the State's important and legitimate interest in the health of the mother, the 'compelling' point, in the light of present medical knowledge, is at approximately the end of the first trimester. This is so because of the now-established medical fact . . . that until the end of the first trimester mortality in abortion may be less than mortality in normal childbirth. It follows that, from and after this point, a State may regulate the abortion procedure to the extent that the regulation reasonably relates to the preservation and protection of maternal health. Examples of permissible state regulation in this area are requirements as to the qualifications of the person who is to perform the abortion; as to the licensure of that person; as to the facility in which the procedure is to be performed, that is, whether it must be a hospital or may be a clinic or some other place of less-than-hospital status; as to the licensing of the facility; and the like.

This means, on the other hand, that, for the period of pregnancy prior to this 'compelling' point, the attending physician, in consultation with his patient, is free to determine, without regulation by the State, that, in his medical judgment, the patient's pregnancy should be terminated. If that decision is reached, the judgment may be effectuated by an abortion free of interference by the State. With respect to the State's important and legitimate interest in potential life, the 'compelling' point is at viability. This is so because the fetus then presumably has the capability of meaningful life outside the mother's womb. State regulation protective of fetal life after viability thus has both logical and biological justifications. If the State is interested in protecting fetal life after viability, it may go so far as to proscribe abortion during that period, except when it is necessary to preserve the life or health of the mother.

Measured against these standards, Art. 1196 of the Texas Penal Code, in restricting legal abortions to those 'procured or attempted by medical advice for the purpose of saving the life of the mother,' sweeps too broadly. The statute makes no distinction between abortions performed early in pregnancy and those performed later, and it limits to a single reason, 'saving' the mother's life, the legal justification for the procedure. The statute, therefore, cannot survive the constitutional attack made upon it here . . .

XI

To summarize and to repeat:

1. A state criminal abortion statute of the current Texas type, that excepts from

criminality only a life-saving procedure on behalf of the mother, without regard to pregnancy stage and without recognition of the other interests involved, is violative of the Due Process Clause of the Fourteenth Amendment.

(a) For the stage prior to approximately the end of the first trimester, the abortion decision and its effectuation must be left to the medical judgment of the pregnant woman's attending physician.

(b) For the stage subsequent to approximately the end of the first trimester, the State, in promoting its interest in the health of the mother, may, if it chooses, regulate the abortion procedure in ways that are reasonably related to maternal health.

(c) For the stage subsequent to viability, the State in promoting its interest in the potentiality of human life may, if it chooses, regulate, and even proscribe, abortion except where it is necessary, in appropriate medical judgment, for the preservation of the life or health of the mother.

It is so ordered.

Affirmed in part and reversed in part.

JUSTICE STEWART, CHIEF JUSTICE BURGER, and JUSTICE DOUGLAS issued separate concurring opinions.

JUSTICE REHNQUIST and JUSTICE WHITE issued dissenting opinions.

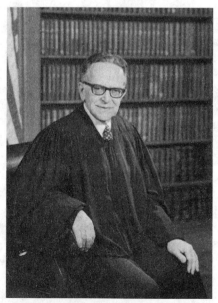

Justice Harry A. Blackmun

NOTES AND QUESTIONS

1.   How does the decision in *Roe v. Wade* affect the law of assisted reproductive technologies? As we learned in Chapter 1, the technology that enabled physicians to create embryos outside the human body, in vitro fertilization, was not developed until the mid-1970s, after the Court's landmark abortion decision. Clearly the justices did not analyze the constitutionality of state abortion laws with an eye toward analogous reasoning being applied to state regulation of ARTs. But we also learned from reading the decisions in *Griswold v. Connecticut* and *Eisenstadt v. Baird* that some justices view the constitution as a flexible instrument, capable of protecting rights not explicitly enumerated in the text of the great document. Justices of this same constitutional persuasion could also find that the protections surrounding a woman's rights vis-a-vis the early fetus likewise apply to protect an ART patient from state interference with her right to pursue fertility treatment. Other justices advocate a strict construction of the words of the constitution, which lack any mention of abortion, procreative liberty, or contraception. These justices may be disinclined to advance by analogy the abortion jurisprudence to the debate over regulation of ART. Of the hundreds and hundreds of commentaries that flowed from the decision in *Roe v. Wade*, two are noteworthy for their critique of this tension between the application of a flexible versus a strict construction of constitutional language. Compare John Hart Ely, *The Wages of Crying Wolf: A Comment on Roe v. Wade*, 82 YALE L. J. 920, 935 (1973) . . . ("What is frightening about *Roe* is that this super-protected right is not inferable from the language of the Constitution, the framers' thinking respecting the specific problem in issue, any general value derivable from the provisions they included, or the nation's governmental structure . . .") with Philip B. Heymann & Douglas E. Barzelay, *The Forest and the Trees: Roe v. Wade and Its Critics*, 53 B.U.L.REV. 765, 772 (1973) . . . ("*Roe* is amply justified by precedent and by those principles that have long guided the Court in making the ever-delicate determination of when it must tell a state that it may not pursue certain measures, because to do so would impinge on those rights of individuals that the Constitution explicitly or implicitly protects."). For a discussion of the ongoing debate over how the Court should interpret the Constitution and when, if at all, it is permissible for the judiciary to protect unenumerated rights, *see* ERWIN CHEMERINSKY, CONSTITUTIONAL LAW: PRINCIPLES AND POLICIES 15-26 (4th ed. 2011).

2.   No doubt you are struck by the yin-yang relationship between *Roe v. Wade* and the use of ART. Under the right of privacy articulated in *Roe*, a woman seeks to end her pregnancy without state interference; in an ART scenario, a woman seeks to initiate a pregnancy without limitations imposed by the state. Given these obviously divergent goals, is Roe even a relevant, let alone a useful, precedent in determining the rights that ART users might seek in their quest for parenthood? Would you expect courts to be more willing to expand rights so as to expand opportunities for parenthood? Or do you see courts favoring only certain types of families, for example those formed through traditional reproduction, such that rights to create families outside established norms might incur stringent regulation?

3.   *The Roe Progeny.* In the nearly 40 years since the landmark decision in *Roe*, the Court has twice reevaluated the wisdom of its 1973 decision, both times leaving

the precedent in place (read, not overruled), but creating ample opportunity for law professors and others to wax eloquent about the dooming of women's autonomy or the decay in respect for early life, depending upon the author's perspective. In 1989, the Court reviewed a comprehensive Missouri abortion law in *Webster v. Reproductive Health Services*, 492 U.S. 490 (1989). Three years later, following the resignation of Justices Brennan and Marshall who voted with the majority in *Roe*, the Court agreed to hear a challenge to the constitutionality of amendments to the Pennsylvania abortion statute in *Planned Parenthood of Southeastern Pennsylvania v. Casey*, 505 U.S. 833 (1992). The decision in *Webster v. Reproductive Health Services* is discussed below, followed by the (highly edited) opinion in *Planned Parenthood v. Casey.*

b. The *Roe* Progeny

WEBSTER v. REPRODUCTIVE HEALTH SERVICES
Supreme Court of the United States
492 U.S. 490 (1989)

CHIEF JUSTICE REHNQUIST delivered the plurality opinion of the Court, joined by JUSTICE WHITE and JUSTICE KENNEDY.

This appeal concerns the constitutionality of a Missouri statute regulating the performance of abortions. The United States Court of Appeals for the Eighth Circuit struck down several provisions of the statute on the ground that they violated this Court's decision in Roe v. Wade, 410 U.S. 113, 93 S.Ct. 705, 35 L.Ed.2d 147 (1973), and cases following it. We noted probable jurisdiction, 488 U.S. 1003, 109 S.Ct. 780, 102 L.Ed.2d 772 (1989), and now reverse . . .

II

Decision of this case requires us to address four sections of the Missouri Act: (a) the preamble; (b) the prohibition on the use of public facilities or employees to perform abortions; (c) the prohibition on public funding of abortion counseling; and (d) the requirement that physicians conduct viability tests prior to performing abortions. We address these seriatim.

A

The Act's preamble, as noted, sets forth "findings" by the Missouri Legislature that "[t]he life of each human being begins at conception," and that "[u]nborn children have protectable interests in life, health, and well-being." . . .

Certainly the preamble does not by its terms regulate abortion or any other aspect of appellees' medical practice. The Court has emphasized that *Roe v. Wade* "implies no limitation on the authority of a State to make a value judgment favoring childbirth over abortion." *Maher v. Roe*, 432 U.S., at 474, 97 S.Ct., at 2382-83. The preamble can be read simply to express that sort of value judgment . . .

B

Section 188.210 provides that "[i]t shall be unlawful for any public employee within the scope of his employment to perform or assist an abortion, not necessary to save the life of the mother," while § 188.215 makes it "unlawful for any public facility to be used for the purpose of performing or assisting an abortion not necessary to save the life of the mother." The Court of Appeals held that these provisions contravened this Court's abortion decisions. 851 F.2d, at 1082-1083. We take the contrary view.

. . . the State's decision here to use public facilities and staff to encourage childbirth over abortion "places no governmental obstacle in the path of a woman who chooses to terminate her pregnancy." *[Harris v.] McRae*, 448 U.S., at 315, 100 S.Ct., at 2687 . . . Having held that the State's refusal to fund abortions does not violate *Roe v. Wade*, it strains logic to reach a contrary result for the use of public facilities and employees. If the State may "make a value judgment favoring childbirth over abortion and . . . implement that judgment by the allocation of public funds," *Maher [v. Roe], supra*, [432 U.S.] at 474, 97 S.Ct., at 2382, surely it may do so through the allocation of other public resources, such as hospitals and medical staff . . .

[In part D, the Court examines the viability-testing provision of the Act, which creates a presumption of viability at 20 weeks, which the physician must rebut with tests indicating that the fetus is not viable prior to performing an abortion. Under the trimester framework in *Roe v. Wade*, presumably a statute which proscribed abortion of a viable fetus would meet constitutional muster, thus the Missouri statute seems designed to expand the realm of state restriction of abortion while complying with existing law. The Court plurality addresses the *Roe* trimester analysis, making no secret of its dislike for the controversial precedent.]

. . . Stare decisis is a cornerstone of our legal system, but it has less power in constitutional cases, where, save for constitutional amendments, this Court is the only body able to make needed changes . . . We have not refrained from reconsideration of a prior construction of the Constitution that has proved "unsound in principle and unworkable in practice. . . . We think the *Roe* trimester framework falls into that category.

In the first place, the rigid *Roe* framework is hardly consistent with the notion of a Constitution cast in general terms, as ours is, and usually speaking in general principles, as ours does. The key elements of the *Roe* framework — trimesters and viability — are not found in the text of the Constitution or in any place else one would expect to find a constitutional principle. Since the bounds of the inquiry are essentially indeterminate, the result has been a web of legal rules that have become increasingly intricate, resembling a code of regulations rather than a body of constitutional doctrine . . . [T]he trimester framework has left this Court to serve as the country's "*ex officio* medical board with powers to approve or disapprove medical and operative practices and standards throughout the United States." . . .

In the second place, we do not see why the State's interest in protecting potential human life should come into existence only at the point of viability, and that there should therefore be a rigid line allowing state regulation after viability but prohibiting it before viability . . . "[T]he State's interest, if compelling after viability, is equally compelling before viability." *Thornburgh [v. American College of Obstetricians and Gynecologists]* 476 U.S., at 795, 106 S.Ct., at 2197 (White, J., dissenting); see id., at 828, 106 S.Ct., at 2214 (O'Connor, J., dissenting) ("State has compelling interests in ensuring maternal health and in protecting potential human life, and these interests exist 'throughout pregnancy' ") (citation omitted) . . .

[W]e are satisfied that the requirement of these tests permissibly furthers the State's interest in protecting potential human life, and we therefore believe § 188.029 to be constitutional . . .

Because none of the challenged provisions of the Missouri Act properly before us conflict with the Constitution, the judgment of the Court of Appeals is reversed.

[Justice O'Connor issued a separate opinion, concurring in part and concurring in the judgment. She evaluated each of the challenged provisions of the Missouri law and found each constitutionally permissive. But as to the viability of *Roe v. Wade*, she simply stated, "[t]here is no necessity to accept the State's invitation to reexamine the constitutional validity of *Roe v. Wade.*" 492 U.S. at 525. Justice Scalia, in a separate concurring opinion, wrote that the plurality opinion "effectively would overrule *Roe*" adding, "I think that should be done, but would do it more explicitly." Id. at 532. Justice Blackmun filed a dissenting opinion, in which Justice Brennan and Justice Marshall joined, lamenting what he perceives to be *Roe's* low prospects for ultimate survival. "For today, at least" he writes, "the law of abortion stands undisturbed. For today, the women of this Nation still retain the liberty to control their destinies. But the signs are evident and very ominous, and a chill wind blows." Id. at 561.]

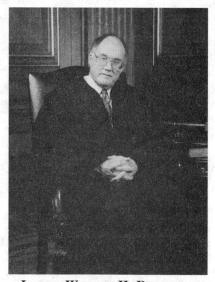

JUSTICE WILLIAM H. REHNQUIST

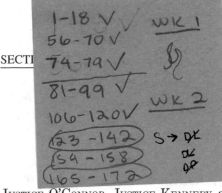

_____OOD OF SOUTHEASTERN _____ ANIA v. CASEY

the United States, 1992

_____ U.S. 833

JUSTICE O'CONNOR, JUSTICE KENNEDY, and JUSTICE SOUTER announced the judgment of the Court.

[The Court evaluates five provisions of the Pennsylvania Abortion Control Act of 1982. The law does not prohibit abortions, but rather regulates them by creating a 24-hour waiting period before an abortion is performed, requiring physicians to inform women of the availability of information about the fetus, requiring parental consent for unmarried minors' abortions, creating requirements for reporting and recordkeeping, and requiring married women notify their husbands of their intended abortions. The Court upheld all but the last provision requiring spousal notification, but in so doing changed the framework for evaluating state regulation of abortion.]

Liberty finds no refuge in a jurisprudence of doubt. Yet 19 years after our holding that the Constitution protects a woman's right to terminate her pregnancy in its early stages, _Roe v. Wade_, 410 U.S. 113, 93 S.Ct. 705, 35 L.Ed.2d 147 (1973), that definition of liberty is still questioned. Joining the respondents as amicus curiae, the United States, as it has done in five other cases in the last decade, again asks us to overrule _Roe_ . . .

After considering the fundamental constitutional questions resolved by _Roe_, principles of institutional integrity, and the rule of stare decisis, we are led to conclude this: the essential holding of _Roe v. Wade_ should be retained and once again reaffirmed.

It must be stated at the outset and with clarity that _Roe's_ essential holding, the holding we reaffirm, has three parts. First is a recognition of the right of the woman to choose to have an abortion before viability and to obtain it without undue interference from the State. Before viability, the State's interests are not strong enough to support a prohibition of abortion or the imposition of a substantial obstacle to the woman's effective right to elect the procedure. Second is a confirmation of the State's power to restrict abortions after fetal viability, if the law contains exceptions for pregnancies which endanger the woman's life or health. And third is the principle that the State has legitimate interests from the outset of the pregnancy in protecting the health of the woman and the life of the fetus that may become a child. These principles do not contradict one another; and we adhere to each.

II

Constitutional protection of the woman's decision to terminate her pregnancy derives from the Due Process Clause of the Fourteenth Amendment. It declares that no State shall "deprive any person of life, liberty, or property, without due process of law." The controlling word in the cases before us is "liberty." Although a literal reading of the Clause might suggest that it governs only the procedures by which a State may deprive persons of liberty, for at least 105 years, since *Mugler v. Kansas*, 123 U.S. 623, 660-661, 8 S.Ct. 273, 291, 31 L.Ed. 205 (1887), the Clause has been understood to contain a substantive component as well, one "barring certain government actions regardless of the fairness of the procedures used to implement them." *Daniels v. Williams*, 474 U.S. 327, 331, 106 S.Ct. 662, 665, 88 L.Ed.2d 662 (1986) . . .

Men and women of good conscience can disagree, and we suppose some always shall disagree, about the profound moral and spiritual implications of terminating a pregnancy, even in its earliest stage. Some of us as individuals find abortion offensive to our most basic principles of morality, but that cannot control our decision. Our obligation is to define the liberty of all, not to mandate our own moral code. The underlying constitutional issue is whether the State can resolve these philosophic questions in such a definitive way that a woman lacks all choice in the matter, except perhaps in those rare circumstances in which the pregnancy is itself a danger to her own life or health, or is the result of rape or incest . . .

Our law affords constitutional protection to personal decisions relating to marriage, procreation, contraception, family relationships, child rearing, and education. *Carey v. Population Services International*, 431 U.S., at 685, 97 S.Ct., at 2016 . . . These matters, involving the most intimate and personal choices a person may make in a lifetime, choices central to personal dignity and autonomy, are central to the liberty protected by the Fourteenth Amendment. At the heart of liberty is the right to define one's own concept of existence, of meaning, of the universe, and of the mystery of human life. Beliefs about these matters could not define the attributes of personhood were they formed under compulsion of the State.

These considerations begin our analysis of the woman's interest in terminating her pregnancy but cannot end it, for this reason: though the abortion decision may originate within the zone of conscience and belief, it is more than a philosophic exercise. Abortion is a unique act. It is an act fraught with consequences for others: for the woman who must live with the implications of her decision; for the persons who perform and assist in the procedure; for the spouse, family, and society which must confront the knowledge that these procedures exist, procedures some deem nothing short of an act of violence against innocent human life; and, depending on one's beliefs, for the life or potential life that is aborted. Though abortion is conduct, it does not follow that the State is entitled to proscribe it in all instances. That is because the liberty of the woman is at stake in a sense unique to the human condition and so unique to the law. The mother who carries a child to full term is subject to anxieties, to physical constraints, to pain that only she must bear. That these sacrifices have from the beginning of the human race been endured by woman with a pride that ennobles her in the eyes of others and gives to the infant a bond of love cannot alone be grounds for the State to insist she make the sacrifice. Her suffering is too intimate and personal for the State to insist, without more, upon its own vision of the woman's role, however dominant that vision has been in the course of our history and our culture. The destiny of the woman must be shaped to a large extent on her own conception of her spiritual imperatives and her place in society.

It should be recognized, moreover, that in some critical respects the abortion decision is of the same character as the decision to use contraception, to which *Griswold v. Connecticut, Eisenstadt v. Baird,* and *Carey v. Population Services International* afford constitutional protection. We have no doubt as to the correctness of those decisions. They support the reasoning in Roe relating to the woman's liberty because they involve personal decisions concerning not only the meaning of procreation but also human responsibility and respect for it . . .

[The Court next discusses the role of *stare decisis,* the obligation to follow precedents. It concludes that the rationales that justify overruling a prior case do not exist with respect to *Roe v. Wade.* Specifically, the Court writes, "[t]he sum of the precedential inquiry to this point shows *Roe's* underpinnings unweakened in any way affecting its central holding. While it has engendered disapproval, it has not been unworkable. An entire generation has come of age free to assume *Roe's* concept of liberty in defining the capacity of women to act in society, and to make reproductive decisions; no erosion of principle going to liberty or personal autonomy has left *Roe's* central holding a doctrinal remnant; *Roe* portends no developments at odds with other precedent for the analysis of personal liberty; and no changes of fact have rendered viability more or less appropriate as the point at which the balance of interests tips. Within the bounds of normal stare decisis analysis, then, and subject to the considerations on which it customarily turns, the stronger argument is for affirming *Roe's* central holding, with whatever degree of personal reluctance any of us may have, not for overruling it.]

From what we have said so far it follows that it is a constitutional liberty of the woman to have some freedom to terminate her pregnancy. We conclude that the basic decision in *Roe* was based on a constitutional analysis which we cannot now repudiate. The woman's liberty is not so unlimited, however, that from the outset the State cannot show its concern for the life of the unborn, and at a later point in fetal development the State's interest in life has sufficient force so that the right of the woman to terminate the pregnancy can be restricted . . .

We conclude the line should be drawn at viability, so that before that time the woman has a right to choose to terminate her pregnancy. We adhere to this principle for two reasons. First, as we have said, is the doctrine of stare decisis . . . The second reason is that the concept of viability, as we noted in *Roe,* is the time at which there is a realistic possibility of maintaining and nourishing a life outside the womb, so that the independent existence of the second life can in reason and all fairness be the object of state protection that now overrides the rights of the woman. See *Roe v. Wade,* 410 U.S., at 163, 93 S.Ct., at 731 . . .

Roe established a trimester framework to govern abortion regulations. Under this elaborate but rigid construct, almost no regulation at all is permitted during the first trimester of pregnancy; regulations designed to protect the woman's health, but not to further the State's interest in potential life, are permitted during the second trimester; and during the third trimester, when the fetus is viable, prohibitions are permitted provided the life or health of the mother is not at stake. *Roe, supra,* 410 U.S., at 163-166, 93 S.Ct., at 731-733 . . .

The trimester framework no doubt was erected to ensure that the woman's right to choose not become so subordinate to the State's interest in promoting fetal life that her choice exists in theory but not in fact. We do not agree, however, that the trimester approach is necessary to accomplish this objective. A framework of this rigidity was unnecessary and in its later interpretation sometimes contradicted the State's permissible exercise of its powers.

Though the woman has a right to choose to terminate or continue her pregnancy before viability, it does not at all follow that the State is prohibited from taking steps to ensure that this choice is thoughtful and informed. Even in the earliest stages of pregnancy, the State may enact rules and regulations designed to encourage her to know that there are philosophic and social arguments of great weight that can be brought to bear in favor of continuing the pregnancy to full term and that there are procedures and institutions to allow adoption of unwanted children as well as a certain degree of state assistance if the mother chooses to raise the child herself. " '[T]he Constitution does not forbid a State or city, pursuant to democratic processes, from expressing a preference for normal childbirth.' " *Webster v. Reproductive Health Services*, 492 U.S., at 511, 109 S.Ct., at 3053 (opinion of the Court) (quoting *Poelker v. Doe*, 432 U.S. 519, 521, 97 S.Ct. 2391, 2392, 53 L.Ed.2d 528 (1977)). It follows that States are free to enact laws to provide a reasonable framework for a woman to make a decision that has such profound and lasting meaning. This, too, we find consistent with *Roe's* central premises, and indeed the inevitable consequence of our holding that the State has an interest in protecting the life of the unborn.

We reject the trimester framework, which we do not consider to be part of the essential holding of *Roe* . . . A logical reading of the central holding in *Roe* itself, and a necessary reconciliation of the liberty of the woman and the interest of the State in promoting prenatal life, require, in our view, that we abandon the trimester framework as a rigid prohibition on all previability regulation aimed at the protection of fetal life. The trimester framework suffers from these basic flaws: in its formulation it misconceives the nature of the pregnant woman's interest; and in practice it undervalues the State's interest in potential life, as recognized in *Roe* . . .

The very notion that the State has a substantial interest in potential life leads to the conclusion that not all regulations must be deemed unwarranted. Not all burdens on the right to decide whether to terminate a pregnancy will be undue. In our view, the undue burden standard is the appropriate means of reconciling the State's interest with the woman's constitutionally protected liberty . . .

A finding of an undue burden is a shorthand for the conclusion that a state regulation has the purpose or effect of placing a substantial obstacle in the path of a woman seeking an abortion of a nonviable fetus. A statute with this purpose is invalid because the means chosen by the State to further the interest in potential life must be calculated to inform the woman's free choice, not hinder it. And a statute which, while furthering the interest in potential life or some other valid state interest, has the effect of placing a substantial obstacle in the path of a woman's choice cannot be considered a permissible means of serving its legitimate ends . . .

Some guiding principles should emerge. What is at stake is the woman's right to make the ultimate decision, not a right to be insulated from all others in doing so. Regulations which do no more than create a structural mechanism by which the State, or the parent or guardian of a minor, may express profound respect for the life of the unborn are permitted, if they are not a substantial obstacle to the woman's exercise of the right to choose . . . Unless it has that effect on her right of choice, a state measure designed to persuade her to choose childbirth over abortion will be upheld if reasonably related to that goal. Regulations designed to foster the health of a woman seeking an abortion are valid if they do not constitute an undue burden . . .

We give this summary:

(a) To protect the central right recognized by *Roe v. Wade* while at the same time accommodating the State's profound interest in potential life, we will employ the undue burden analysis as explained in this opinion. An undue burden exists, and therefore a provision of law is invalid, if its purpose or effect is to place a substantial obstacle in the path of a woman seeking an abortion before the fetus attains viability.

(b) We reject the rigid trimester framework of *Roe v. Wade*. To promote the State's profound interest in potential life, throughout pregnancy the State may take measures to ensure that the woman's choice is informed, and measures designed to advance this interest will not be invalidated as long as their purpose is to persuade the woman to choose childbirth over abortion. These measures must not be an undue burden on the right.

(c) As with any medical procedure, the State may enact regulations to further the health or safety of a woman seeking an abortion. Unnecessary health regulations that have the purpose or effect of presenting a substantial obstacle to a woman seeking an abortion impose an undue burden on the right.

(d) Our adoption of the undue burden analysis does not disturb the central holding of *Roe v. Wade*, and we reaffirm that holding. Regardless of whether exceptions are made for particular circumstances, a State may not prohibit any woman from making the ultimate decision to terminate her pregnancy before viability.

(e) We also reaffirm *Roe's* holding that "subsequent to viability, the State in promoting its interest in the potentiality of human life may, if it chooses, regulate, and even proscribe, abortion except where it is necessary, in appropriate medical judgment, for the preservation of the life or health of the mother." *Roe v. Wade*, 410 U.S., at 164-165, 93 S.Ct., at 732 . . .

It is so ordered.

[JUSTICE BLACKMUN and JUSTICE STEVENS concurred in the judgment in part, and dissented in part. These justices agreed that *Roe v. Wade* should be reaffirmed, but would have upheld the trimester framework and the use of strict scrutiny to evaluate state interference with a woman's right to control her early pregnancy. CHIEF JUSTICE REHNQUIST and JUSTICE SCALIA each wrote opinions concurring in the judgment in part and dissenting in part. These justices joined each other's opinions and JUSTICE WHITE and JUSTICE THOMAS joined each. These four justices agreed that "*Roe* was wrongly decided, and that it can and should be overruled consistently with our traditional approach to *stare decisis* in constitutional cases." 505 U.S. at 944.]

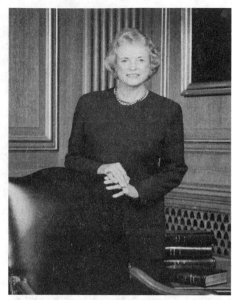

JUSTICE SANDRA DAY O'CONNOR

NOTES AND QUESTIONS

1. *The Right to Avoid Procreation.* The decisions in *Roe, Webster,* and *Casey* speak of a woman's right to avoid procreation by terminating her pregnancy via the medical procedure of abortion. The cases focus on the government's authority to regulate that private decision. Earlier in this chapter we looked at case law surrounding state restrictions on the use and sale of contraceptives, an area that likewise implicates the right to avoid procreation. The contraception and abortion cases could be distinguished on gender grounds; the right to avoid procreation via abortion is unique to women[6], while the right to avoid procreation through the use of contraceptives applies equally to women and men. Suppose we looked at the right to avoid procreation as a time line, which charted various events along the reproductive path. Such events might include the purchase and later use of contraceptives such as condoms, or the act of sexual intercourse, or the ingestion of an abortifacient drug following sex to inhibit the formation and attachment of an embryo. The Supreme Court cases suggest that the woman's right to avoid procreation begin with the opportunity to use contraceptives and continue until the fetus reaches viability at which point the state can proscribe abortion altogether. But what about the man's right? Does he lose his right to avoid procreation once his sperm enters the woman's body? If so, why?

---

[6] Recall that the joint opinion in *Planned Parenthood v. Casey* held invalid the Pennsylvania statute requiring that a woman notify her husband that she is about to undergo an abortion. Relying on its previous decision in *Planned Parenthood of Central Missouri v. Danforth,* 428 U.S. 52 (1976), the Court reiterated that the Constitution does not permit a state to require a married women to obtain her husband's consent before undergoing an abortion, largely because "it is the woman who physically bears the child and who is the more directly and immediately affected by the pregnancy, as between the two, the balance weighs in her favor." Id. at 71.

Do you think the right to avoid procreation looks any different in an ART scenario? Does the fact that an embryo forms outside the woman's body change the constitutional rights traditionally accorded procreation? Should a woman get fewer rights to control the early embryo because it is not physically implanted in her uterus? Should a man get more rights to control the early embryo because it is not implanted in a woman's uterus? Since an ART pregnancy does not involve intercourse, we may have to rethink the traditional parameters that govern reproductive rights. Professor Glenn Cohen does just that, envisioning the right not to procreate as a bundle of rights rather than a monolithic right to avoid procreation in general. For a discussion on the right not to be a legal, genetic or gestational parent, *see* I. Glenn Cohen, *The Constitution and the Rights Not to Procreate*, 60 STAN. L. REV. 1135 (2008).

2. *The Casey Legacy.* In the years since *Planned Parenthood v. Casey*, the Supreme Court has cited the 1992 case in a handful of decisions discussing the constitutionally protected liberty interest. In *Washington v. Glucksberg*, 521 U.S. 702 (1997), the Court heard a challenge from terminally ill patients and their physicians to the constitutionality of a state criminal ban on assisted suicide. Relying on *Casey*, the plaintiffs argue that the ban places an undue burden of the exercise of their constitutionally protected liberty interest in the right to die by committing physician-assisted suicide. The Court reviews our nation's long history of outlawing assisted suicide, and rejects the plaintiffs' claim, explaining, "the asserted 'right' to assistance in committing suicide is not a fundamental liberty interest protected by the Due Process Clause." 521 U.S. at 728. The Court reaches this conclusion via *Casey*, which figures prominently in this portion of the opinion. "The opinion [in *Casey*] moved from the recognition that liberty necessarily includes freedom of conscience to the observation that 'though the abortion decision may originate within the zone of conscience and belief, it is *more than a philosophic exercise.*'" *Glucksberg*, 521 U.S. at 727 citing *Casey* at 505 U.S. at 852 [emphasis added by Court in Glucksberg]. From this recognition of liberty, the Court moves on to its limitation: "That many of the rights and liberties protected by the Due Process Clause sound in personal autonomy does not warrant the sweeping conclusion that any and all important, intimate, and personal decisions are so protected . . . and *Casey* did not suggest otherwise." 521 U.S. at 727-728.

While the decision in *Washington v. Glucksberg* may lead one to conclude that the liberty interest in *Casey* is limited to the traditionally protected intimacies of marriage, child-rearing and procreation, a more recent case defies such character-ization and livens up the legal landscape. In *Lawrence v. Texas*, 539 U.S. 558 (2003), the Court declared unconstitutional a Texas statute making it a crime for two persons of the same sex to engage in certain intimate sexual conduct, as applied to adult males engaging in consensual sodomy. The question of sexual practices common to a homosexual lifestyle, the Court said, are private matters protected by the right to liberty under the Due Process Clause. "The State cannot demean their existence or control their destiny by making their private sexual conduct a crime . . . 'It is a promise of the Constitution that there is a realm of personal liberty which the government may not enter.'" Id. at 578, citing *Casey*, 505 U.S. at 847. If the right of intimate association can be interpreted to include the free sexual expression of all consenting adults, can the right to procreate likewise be interpreted to include freedom to choose one's method of reproduction?

c. The Latest Word on Abortion, For Now

In 2000 and again in 2007, the Court heard cases involving a particular form of abortion, late term or so-called partial-birth abortion, performed in the later stages of pregnancy. In *Stenberg v. Carhart*, 530 U.S. 914 (2000), the Court invalidated a Nebraska law criminalizing partial-birth abortion, defined as an abortion procedure in which the person performing the technique "partially delivers vaginally a living unborn child before killing the unborn child and completing the delivery." Neb. Rev. Stat. Ann. § 28-326(9). The Court found that the statute's broad language would ban the most commonly used method of second trimester previability abortion and thus placed an undue burden on a woman's right to make an abortion decision.

Three years after *Stenberg*, Congress enacted the Partial-Brith Abortion Ban Act of 2003, a federal law banning a specific type of procedure used in late term abortion, an intact dilation and evacuation. The Court upheld the federal law in a 5-4 decision. In *Gonzales v. Carhart*. 550 U.S. 124 (2007), the Court distinguished the invalidated Nebraska law from the federal law at issue, finding the latter acceptably narrow in its scope and effect. As to the question of whether the law posed a "substantial obstacle in the path of a woman seeking an abortion before the fetus attains viability," the standard set out in *Casey*, Justice Kennedy, writing for the majority, found no such constitutional infraction. He reasoned that because the law banned only one type of procedure, thus leaving other methods of late term abortion available, the law could not be deemed an undue burden on women seeking late term abortion. "[T]he State may use its regulatory power to bar certain procedures and substitute others, all in furtherance of its legitimate interests in regulating the medical profession in order to promote respect for life, including life of the unborn." *Id.* at 158. Does the Court's language open the door to greater regulation of reproductive technologies which intimately tie the medical profession with the life of the unborn? More broadly, does the constitutional jurisprudence surrounding the right to avoid procreation through the use of contraception and abortion support or inform a right to access procreation through the use of ART? The materials that follow explore this question in detail.

SECTION II: ASSISTED REPRODUCTION AS A FUNDAMENTAL RIGHT

A. Arguments for Recognizing ART as a Fundamental Right

The previous materials make clear that the Supreme Court has never directly addressed the question of whether procreation via assisted reproductive technologies is a fundamental right protected under the Constitution. We know that if a right is deemed to be a fundamental right, any governmental restrictions on exercise of that right will be evaluated by a court using strict scrutiny, and can only be justified as achieving a compelling state purpose. The materials that follow address the question, "Is the right to procreate a fundamental right, and if so, does it include the right to assisted conception?" We begin with an answer in the affirmative and then hear rebuttal.

John A. Robertson
Children of Choice: Freedom and the New Reproductive Technologies
22-42 (1994)

The Presumptive Primacy of Procreative Liberty

Procreative liberty has wide appeal but its scope has never been fully elaborated and often is contested. The concept has several meanings that must be clarified if it is to serve as a reliable guide for moral debate and public policy regarding new reproductive technologies.

WHAT IS PROCREATIVE LIBERTY?

At the most general level, procreative liberty is the freedom either to have children or to avoid having them. Although often expressed or realized in the context of a couple, it is first and foremost an individual interest. It is to be distinguished from freedom in the ancillary aspects of reproduction, such as liberty in the conduct of pregnancy or choice of place or mode of childbirth . . .

In this book the terms "procreative liberty" and "reproductive freedom" will mean the freedom to reproduce or not to reproduce in the genetic sense, which may also include rearing or not, as intended by the parties. Those terms will also include female gestation whether or not there is a genetic connection to the resulting child . . .

As a matter of constitutional law, procreative liberty is a negative right against state interference with choices to procreate or to avoid procreation. It is not a right against private interference, though other laws might provide that protection. Nor is it a positive right to have the state or particular persons provide the means or resources necessary to have or avoid having children. The exercise of procreative liberty may be severely constrained by social and economic circumstances. Access to medical care, child care, employment, housing, and other services may significantly affect whether one is able to exercise procreative liberty. However, the state presently has no constitutional obligation to provide those services. Whether the state should alleviate those conditions is a separate issue of social justice . . .

THE IMPORTANCE OF PROCREATIVE LIBERTY

Procreative liberty should enjoy presumptive primacy when conflicts about its exercise arise because control over whether one reproduces or not is central to personal identity, to dignity, and to the meaning of one's life. For example, deprivation of the ability to avoid reproduction determines one's self-definition in the most basic sense. It affects women's bodies in a direct and substantial way. It also centrally affects one's psychological and social identity and one's social and moral responsibilities. The resulting burdens are especially onerous for women, but they affect men in significant ways as well.

On the other hand, being deprived of the ability to reproduce prevents one from an experience that is central to individual identity and meaning in life . . .

Decisions to have or to avoid having children are thus personal decisions of great import that determine the shape and meaning of one's life. The person directly involved is best situated to determine whether that meaning should or should not occur. An ethic of personal autonomy as well as ethics of community or family should then recognize a presumption in favor of most personal reproductive choices. Such a presumption does not mean that reproductive choices are without consequence to others, nor that they should never be limited. Rather, it means that those who would limit procreative choice have the burden of showing that the reproductive actions at issue would create such substantial harm that they could justifiably be limited. Of course, what counts as the "substantial harm" that justifies interference with procreative choice may often be contested . . .

A closely related reason for protecting reproductive choice is to avoid the highly intrusive measures that governmental control of reproduction usually entails. State interference with reproductive choice may extend beyond exhortation and penalties to Gestapo and police state tactics.

In China, forcible abortion and sterilization have occurred in the service of a one-child-per-family population policy. Village cadres have seized pregnant women in their homes and forced them to have abortions. A campaign of forcible sterilization in India in 1977 was seen as an "attack on women and children" and brought Indira Ghandi's government down. In the United States, state-imposed sterilization of "mental defectives," sanctioned in 1927 by the United States Supreme Court in *Buck v. Bell*, resulted in 60,000 sterilizations over a forty-year period. Many mentally normal people were sterilized by mistake, and mentally retarded persons who posed little risk of harm to others were subjected to surgery . . .

TWO TYPES OF PROCREATIVE LIBERTY

To see how values of procreative liberty affect the ethical and public policy evaluation of new reproductive technologies, we must determine whether the interests that underlie the high value accorded procreative liberty are implicated in their use . . .

An essential distinction is between the freedom to avoid reproduction and the freedom to reproduce . . .

AVOIDING REPRODUCTION: THE LIBERTY NOT TO REPRODUCE

One sense in which people commonly understand procreative liberty is as the freedom to avoid reproduction — to avoid begetting or bearing off-spring and the rearing demands they make . . . A decision not to procreate could occur prior to conception through sexual abstinence, contraceptive use, or refusal to seek treatment for infertility . . . Countervailing interests concern societal interests in increasing population, a partner's interest in sexual intimacy and progeny, and moral views about the unity of sex and reproduction.

Once pregnancy has occurred, reproduction can be avoided only by termination of pregnancy. Procreative freedom here would involve the freedom to abort the pregnancy. Competing interests are protection of embryos and fetuses and respect for human life generally, the most heated issue of reproductive rights. They may also include moral or social beliefs about the connectedness of sex and reproduction, or views about a woman's reproductive and work roles . . .

Legal Status of Avoiding Reproduction

Legally, the negative freedom to avoid reproduction is widely recognized, though great controversy over abortion persists, and there is no positive constitutional right to contraception and abortion. The freedom to avoid reproduction is clearest for men and women prior to conception . . .

Constitutional recognition of the right to use contraceptives — to have sex and not reproduce — occurred in the 1965 landmark case of *Griswold v. Connecticut.* A doctor and a married couple challenged a Connecticut law that made it a crime to use or distribute contraceptives. The United States Supreme Court found that the law violated a fundamental liberty right of married couples, which it later extended to unmarried persons, to use contraceptives as a matter of personal liberty or privacy . . .

Once conception has occurred, the right to avoid reproduction differs for the woman and man involved. In the United States and most of Western Europe, abortion in early stages of the pregnancy is widely permitted. Under *Roe v. Wade*, whose central holding was reaffirmed in 1992 in *Planned Parenthood v. Casey*, women, whether single or married, adult or minor, have a right to terminate pregnancy up to viability . . .

The father, once conception through sexual intercourse has occurred, has no right to require or prevent abortion, and cannot avoid rearing duties of financial support once birth occurs. This is true even if the woman has lied to him about her fertility or her use of contraceptives. However, he is free to relinquish custody and give up for adoption. He is also free to determine whether IVF embryos formed from his sperm should be implanted in the uterus . . .

THE FREEDOM TO PROCREATE

In addition to freedom to avoid procreation, procreative liberty also includes the freedom to procreate — the freedom to beget and bear children if one chooses. As with avoiding reproduction, the right to reproduce is a negative right against public or private interference, not a positive right to the services or the resources needed to reproduce. It is an important freedom that is widely accepted as a basic, human right. But its various components and dimensions have never been fully analyzed, as technologies of conception and selection now force us to do.

As with avoiding reproduction, the freedom to procreate involves the freedom to engage in a series of actions that eventuate in reproduction and usually in child rearing. One must be free to marry or find a willing partner, engage in sexual intercourse, achieve conception and pregnancy, carry a pregnancy to term, and rear offspring. Social and natural barriers to reproduction would involve the unavailability of willing or suitable partners, impotence or infertility, and lack of medical and child-care resources. State barriers to marriage, to sexual intercourse, to conception, to infertility treatment, to carrying pregnancies to term, and to certain child-rearing arrangements would also limit the freedom to procreate. The most commonly asserted reasons for limiting coital reproduction are overpopulation, unfitness of parents, harm to offspring, and costs to the state or others . . .

An entirely different set of concerns arises with noncoital reproductive techniques. Charges that noncoital reproduction is unethical or irresponsible arise because of its expense, its highly technological character, its decomposition of parenthood into genetic, gestational, and social components, and its potential effects on women and offspring. To assess whether these effects justify moral condemnation or public limitation, we must first determine whether noncoital reproduction implicates important aspects of procreative liberty.

The Right to Reproduce and Noncoital Technology

If the moral right to reproduce presumptively protects coital reproduction, then it should protect noncoital reproduction as well. The moral right of the coitally infertile to reproduce is based on the same desire for offspring that the coitally fertile have. They too wish to replicate themselves, transmit genes, gestate, and rear children biologically related to them. Their infertility should no more disqualify them from reproductive experiences than physical disability should disqualify persons from walking with mechanical assistance. The unique risks posed by noncoital reproduction may provide independent justifications for limiting its use, but neither the noncoital nature of the means used nor the infertility of their beneficiaries mean that the presumptively protected moral interest in reproduction is not present . . .

Are Noncoital Technologies Unethical?

. . . Judgment about the reproductive importance of noncoital technologies is crucial because many people have serious ethical reservations about them, and are more than willing to restrict their use. The concerns here are not the fears of overpopulation, parental unfitness, and societal costs that arise with allegedly irresponsible coital reproduction. Instead, they include reduction of demand for hard-to-adopt children, the coercive or exploitive bargains that will be offered to poor women, the commodification of both children and reproductive collaborators, the objectification of women as reproductive vessels, and the undermining of the nuclear family . . .

These criticisms are powerful ones that explain much of the ambivalence that surrounds the use of certain reproductive technologies. They call into question the wisdom of individual decisions to use them, and the willingness of society to promote or facilitate their use. Unless one is operating out of a specific religious or deontological ethic, however, they do not show that all individual uses of these techniques are immoral, much less that public policy should restrict or discourage their use . . .

Legal Status of the Right to Reproduce

Because there have been few attempts by government to limit reproduction, there is little explicit law concerning the right to reproduce. However, judges in dicta often refer to such a right, and there seems little doubt that the right to procreate would be protected in most circumstances. Such statements generally assume a married couple that seeks to reproduce coitally . . .

In the United States laws restricting coital reproduction by a married couple would have to withstand the strict scrutiny applied to interference with fundamental constitutional rights. Although no right to reproduce is explicitly mentioned in the Constitution, dicta in many cases suggest that such a right exists.

The strongest precedent here is the case of *Skinner v. Oklahoma*, a 1942 case in which the Court struck down a state law that authorized thieves but not embezzlers to be sterilized without consent after a third conviction. Although relying on an equal protection rationale, the Court stressed the importance of marriage and procreation as among "the basic civil rights of man" and noted that "marriage and procreation are fundamental to the very existence and survival of the race." Under this principle, persons cannot be selectively deprived of their right of procreation, and the state must justify any deprivation by showing a compelling state interest that could not be satisfied in alternative ways.

Many other Supreme Court cases contain statements that support the protected status of decisions to reproduce. In *Meyer v. Nebraska,* . . . the Court stated that constitutional liberty includes "the right of an individual to marry, establish a home and bring up children." In *Stanley v. Illinois*, the Court, . . . stated that "rights to conceive and raise one's children have been deemed 'essential,' 'basic civil rights of man,' and 'rights far more precious than property rights.'" *Cleveland Bd. of Education v. LaFleur* recognized . . . "freedom of personal choice in matters of marriage and family life is one of the liberties protected by the Due Process clause of the Fourteenth Amendment." The most ringing endorsement of this right occurred in *Eisenstadt v. Baird* when . . . Justice Brennan, in an opinion for the Court, stated: "If the right of privacy means anything, it is the right of the individual, married or single, to be free of unwarranted governmental intrusion into matters so fundamentally affecting a person as the decision whether to bear or beget a child." Most recently, in the 1992 decision in *Casey v. Planned Parenthood*, Justices O'Connor, Kennedy, and Souter stated that "our law affords constitutional protection to personal decisions relating to marriage, procreation, contraception, family relationships, childrearing and education. [These] matters, involving the most intimate and personal choices a person may make in a lifetime, choices central to personal dignity and autonomy, are central to the liberty protected by the Fourteenth Amendment."

Such statements suggest that a married couple's right to reproduce would be recognized even by conservative justices if a case restricting coital reproduction ever reached the Supreme Court . . .

Unmarried persons may have strong interests in reproducing outside of marriage, and in many cases may be excellent child rearers. It is unclear, however, whether unmarried persons have the same constitutional rights to reproduce coitally that married persons do . . .

As a practical matter, however, the state's possible constitutional power to ban nonmarital forms of sexual intercourse gives it only a limited tool to restrict nonmarital reproduction. With over 28 percent of births in 1990 occurring out of wedlock, it is unrealistic to think that laws prohibiting nonmarital sex or penalizing unmarried reproduction would accomplish much . . .

The Legal Status of Noncoital Reproduction

The law has not yet dealt with legal claims of infertile persons to procreate, yet the principles that underlie a constitutional right to reproduce would seem to apply to the infertile as well. If so, they would have a negative constitutional right to use a wide variety of reproductive technologies to have offspring.

If married (and possibly even single) persons have a presumptive right to reproduce coitally, what then about persons who cannot reproduce coitally? Coital infertility is no indication of a couple's adequacy as child rearers. Their desire to have a family — to beget, bear, and rear offspring — is as strong as in fertile couples. Because the values and interests that undergird the right of coital reproduction clearly exist with the coitally infertile, their actions to form a family also deserve respect. If so, the same standard of scrutiny applied to state action that restricts coital re-production should apply to state restrictions on noncoital means of treating infertility.

Yet some people have challenged this notion, arguing that there is no legal right to reproduce if one lacks the physical ability to do so. But consider the analogous effect of blindness on the First Amendment right to read books. Surely a blind person has the same right to acquire information from books that a sighted person has. The inability to read visually would not bar the person from using braille, recordings, or a sighted reader to acquire the information contained in the book. Because receipt of the book's information is protected by the First Amendment, the means by which the information is received does not itself determine the presence or absence of First Amendment rights.

Similarly, if bearing, begetting, or parenting children is protected as part of personal privacy or liberty, those experiences should be protected whether they are achieved coitally or noncoitally. In either case they satisfy the basic biologic, social, and psychological drive to have a biologically related family. Although full genetic reproduction might not exist in each case, the interest of the couple in rearing children who are biologically related to one or both rearing partners is so close to the coital model that it should be treated equivalently. Noncoital reproduction should thus be constitutionally protected to the same extent as is coital reproduction, with the state having the burden of showing severe harm if the practice is unrestricted.

This conclusion is clearest with noncoital techniques that employ the couple's egg and sperm, as occurs with IVF or artificial insemination with husband sperm. Religious or moral objections to the separation of sex and reproduction should not override the use of these techniques for forming a family . . .

Similar protection should extend to the use of gamete donation to overcome gametic infertility in one member of the couple, as occurs in sperm and egg donation. Gamete donation permits the married couple to raise offspring biologically related to one or both parents (as in the case of egg donation). Again, moral objections to the noncoital nature per se of the conception or to the involvement of a third party without further indication of harm should not suffice to ban such procedures . . .

Use of a surrogate should also be presumptively protected, since it enables an infertile couple to have and rear the genetic offspring of both husband and wife in the case of gestational surrogacy, and of the husband in the case of full surrogacy. Indeed, recognizing the couple's right to use a surrogate is necessary to avoid discrimination against infertile wives. If an infertile male can parent his wife's child through the use of donor sperm, an infertile woman should be free to parent her husband's child through use of a surrogate. This is all the clearer if the surrogate is carrying the embryo of the couple.

Of course, finding that the interests that underlie coital reproduction are present in noncoital and collaborative reproduction does not eliminate the harms or ill effects that some persons fear. Presumptive protection of these techniques, however, shifts the burden to those who would restrict them to establish the compelling harm that would outweigh the couple's reproductive liberty. As later chapters will show, it is difficult to show that the alleged harms of noncoital reproduction are sufficient to justify overriding procreative liberty . . .

RESOLVING DISPUTES OVER PROCREATIVE LIBERTY

. . . If procreative liberty is taken seriously, a strong presumption in favor of using technologies that centrally implicate reproductive interests should be recognized. Although procreative rights are not absolute, those who would limit procreative choice should have the burden of establishing substantial harm. This is the standard used in ethical and legal analyses of restrictions on traditional reproductive decisions. Because the same procreative goals are involved, the same standard of scrutiny should be used for assessing moral or governmental restrictions on novel reproductive techniques . . .

To take procreative liberty seriously, then, is to allow it to have presumptive priority in an individual's life. This will give persons directly involved the final say about use of a particular technology, unless tangible harm to the interests of others can be shown . . .

THE LIMITS OF PROCREATIVE LIBERTY

. . . Recognition of procreative liberty will protect the right of persons to use technology in pursuing their reproductive goals, but it will not eliminate the ambivalence that such technologies engender. Societal ambivalence about reproductive technology is recapitulated at the individual level, as individuals and couples struggle with whether to use the technologies in question. Thus recognition of procreative liberty will not eliminate the dilemmas of personal choice and responsibility that reproductive choice entails. The freedom to act does not mean that we will act wisely, yet denying that freedom may be even more unwise, for it denies individuals' respect in the most fundamental choices of their lives.

B. Arguments Against Recognizing ART as a Fundamental Right

Radhika Rao
Constitutional Misconceptions
93 Michigan Law Review 1473 (1995)

"59-Year-Old Woman Becomes a Mother"; "Black mother, white baby: artificial conception stirs Europe[an] debate"; "South Africa Woman Gives Birth to 3 Grandchildren, and History"; "Healthy Baby Is Born After Test to Screen Out Deadly Gene"; "The Hot Debate About Cloning Human Embryos"; "Infertility doctors plan to use eggs from aborted foetuses." This bewildering barrage of headlines reveals a reproductive revolution in the making. *Children of Choice: Freedom and the New Reproductive Technologies* ambitiously endeavors to shed light upon and bring order to the chaotic brave new world spawned by advances in reproductive technology. Professor John A. Robertson proposes a unifying principle — the presumptive primacy of procreative liberty — that is elegant in its simplicity. Applying this principle, he methodically canvasses each technology and concludes that almost every practice necessary to procreate should receive constitutional protection. He finds a constitutional right to reproduce technologically, to purchase sperm, eggs, and gestational services, and even to enforce preconception agreements to rear offspring.

Robertson's principle of procreative liberty possesses merit as an ethical precept, but it falters as an axiom of constitutional law because it lacks a solid foundation in Supreme Court jurisprudence. In his effort to distill a single principle that encompasses myriad contexts, moreover, Robertson forgoes a more nuanced constitutional analysis, one that takes into account the many ways in which individuals experience liberty in various categories and clauses of the Constitution. He focuses almost exclusively upon the right to procreate, overlooking other constitutional privacy interests, such as the right of body integrity and the right of parental autonomy.

More fundamentally, Robertson's effort to constitutionalize conception is unavailing because global constitutional principles are ill-suited to resolve the problems posed by the new reproductive technologies. Perhaps for this reason, Robertson's approach, though cast in constitutional terms, traces its roots more closely to contractual principles. He conceives reproductive freedom in terms of an individual's right to participate in a free market — a market whose commodity is the means of producing children. In so doing, Robertson actually constitutionalizes freedom of contract in the name of protecting procreative rights.

I. A Constitutional Right to Procreate by any Means Necessary

Robertson begins with a brief description of "the scope of the reproductive revolution that technological change has now wrought." The reproductive revolution originated in the 1960s when the development of the pill made possible sex without procreation. This revolution has culminated in the 1990s with the development of technology that allows procreation without sex . . .

Armed with his principle of procreative liberty — which protects "the freedom to decide whether or not to have offspring and to control the use of one's reproductive capacity" — Robertson enters the fray, mapping out a framework for resolving the controversies engendered by the new reproductive technologies. He defines procreative liberty as "the freedom to reproduce or not to reproduce in the genetic sense", and extends the term to include gestation as well because "gestation is a central experience for women and should enjoy the special respect or protected status accorded reproductive activities". Procreative liberty, according to this view, consists of a negative right to be free from state interference, rather than a positive right to call upon the state to provide the means or resources necessary to exercise procreative choice . . .

Attempting to ground his principle of procreative liberty in the constitutional right to privacy, Robertson parses it into its component parts — the right not to procreate and the right to procreate. The former aspect of procreative liberty finds a firm footing in Supreme Court precedents that clearly delineate a constitutional right to avoid reproduction by means of contraception and abortion. Constitutional jurisprudence provides sketchy support, however, for the latter aspect of procreative liberty. Robertson points primarily to *Skinner v. Oklahoma* . . .

Building upon his reading of the case law, Robertson makes the following argument: if fertile persons possess a constitutional right to reproduce under *Skinner*, then infertile persons must possess such a right as well because "the values and interests that undergird the right of coital reproduction clearly exist with the coitally infertile" . . .

After analyzing technologies that prevent reproduction, Robertson turns his attention to those that facilitate procreation. He focuses his discussion upon in vitro fertilization (IVF), a procedure that involves collecting eggs surgically after ovarian stimulation, fertilizing them in the laboratory, and then implanting them in the uterus. In order to maximize the probability of a pregnancy, Robertson explains, most IVF practitioners hyperstimulate the ovaries to retrieve multiple eggs. If too many fertilized eggs are placed in the uterus at one time, however, there is an increased risk of multiple pregnancy, which may, in turn, require selective abortion. Therefore, such practitioners usually implant only three or four embryos in the uterus; the extra embryos generated by the process may be cryogenically frozen and later thawed for use in subsequent IVF cycles . . .

Robertson predicts that a law banning IVF altogether "would no doubt be found unconstitutional because it [would] directly impede[ ] the efforts of infertile married couples to have offspring, thus interfering with their fundamental right to procreate" . . .

Indeed, Robertson's principle of procreative liberty appears to possess no logical stopping point, expanding to the outer limits of technological possibility and human ingenuity. It protects not only the right to conceive by means of reproductive technologies such as IVF, but also the right to engage the services of reproductive collaborators, such as gamete donors and surrogates. If a couple lacks the physical capacity to conceive through coitus, Robertson contends, the right to procreate "should include the right to use noncoital means of conception to form families". Likewise, "[i]f the couple lacks the gametes or gestational capacity to produce offspring, a commitment to procreative liberty should also permit them the freedom to enlist the assistance of willing donors and surrogates" . . .

After sketching out the ramifications of his constitutional principle of procreative liberty, Robertson finally recounts and rebuts three major critiques of this approach. First, the "class critique" capitalizes upon the fear that collaborative reproduction could result in "a breeder class of poor, minority women whose reproductive capacity is exploited" by the rich and powerful. Robertson responds by saying that "denying poorer women [such] opportunity . . . denies them a reproductive role which they find meaningful. Given that poorer women serve as nannies, babysitters, housekeepers, and factory workers, gestational services might also be sold, even though it will offend the respect that some persons have for maternal gestation". Second, the "feminist critique" suggests that such practices may "further patriarchal domination of women by reinforcing the traditional identification of women with childbearing and childrearing". According to Robertson, this criticism falters because it fails to recognize that precisely the opposite result is likely: collaborative reproductive arrangements actually upset and overturn gender-role stereotypes by "undercut[ting] traditional notions of reproductive orthodoxy that identify women with gestation and childrearing". This argument also "overlooks the many ways in which technology offers options that expand the freedom of women . . . [and] assures women a large measure of control over their reproductive lives". Collaborative reproduction, for example, affords infertile women the chance to experience the joys of gestating or rearing biologically related children, and it offers fertile women an opportunity to earn money by serving as surrogates. "On balance," Robertson concludes, "there is no reason to think that women do not end up with more rather than less reproductive freedom as a result of technological innovation". Third, the "communitarian critique" contends that "[d]isaggregation and recombination of reproductive components [may] undermine the traditional importance of genetic and gestational bonds", thereby contributing to the destruction of the traditional family. Robertson rejects this argument as well, avowing that "[r]ather than undermin[ing] family, these practices present new variations of family and community that could help fill the void left by flux in the shape of the American family".

II. A CONSTITUTIONAL LAW CRITIQUE

. . . Robertson's constitutional framework views the landscape of reproductive conflict through the lens of procreative liberty, inquiring whether the constitutional right to procreate or avoid procreation encompasses each one of these new technologies. From the Supreme Court's decision to strike down a compulsory sterilization law in *Skinner* and from broad dicta in several other cases, Robertson derives "a negative constitutional right to use a wide variety of reproductive technologies to have offspring". Based upon this freshly minted constitutional right, he extrapolates not only a constitutional right to employ gamete donors and surrogates to assist in the reproductive venture, but also a constitutional right to obtain court enforcement of preconception contracts that purport to bargain away rearing rights to the resulting child.

Robertson erects this elaborate edifice upon *Skinner*, but *Skinner* is too weak a reed to carry so much constitutional weight. As the sole precedent supporting the constitutional right to procreate, *Skinner* is indeterminate: the case may be read in several different ways, all of which are equally consistent with current constitutional doctrine. Just as the constitutional right to an abortion established in *Roe* and reaffirmed in *Casey* does not preclude states from prohibiting the destruction of extracorporeal embryos, so the constitutional right not to be sterilized announced in *Skinner* may not prevent states from regulating extracorporeal reproduction. The result in *Skinner* may simply rest upon the constitutional right to privacy of person, which prohibits state intrusions upon bodily integrity. If this is its rationale, then *Skinner* protects only the right to refuse abortion and carry a coital pregnancy to term, as well as the right to resist compulsory contraception or sterilization. Thus it is not at all clear that *Skinner* extends constitutional protection to noncoital methods of reproduction, such as artificial insemination and in vitro fertilization.

Moreover, recognition of a negative right to procreate does not imply a positive right to call upon the apparatus of the state for assistance in procreation. Therefore, even if *Skinner* does create a constitutional right to be free from state interference with the use of reproductive technology, it does not follow that the state possesses an affirmative obligation to assure the exercise of procreative choice by placing its prestige and power behind the enforcement of preconception contracts. If government need not supply the financial resources necessary to exercise the right to procreate, it is not clear why government must supply the judicial resources necessary to exercise the right either . . .

Yet the real problem with interpreting the constitutional right to procreate to require court enforcement of preconception contracts is not a question of semantics — of whether the right is labelled positive or negative. Rather, it is that recognition of such an expansive version of the right to procreate may diminish other constitutional rights and disregard the constitutional rights of others. Robertson's reading of this right conflates procreation and parenting, but the two are distinct. Even if *Skinner* supports a constitutional right to procreate, therefore, parental prerogatives need not follow. The right to reproduce does not necessarily entail the right to rear one's biological child. Should one right accompany the other, moreover, how do we determine which procreator — the gamete contributors, the gestator, or the intending parents — possesses these related rights? . . . These questions are often more illuminating and instructive than any available answers.

Robertson's difficulties stem from the fact that constitutional rights "have a way of bumping into each other in cases involving husbands, wives, and unmarried individuals when all are claiming parental rights." Protecting the parental rights of one procreator risks denying the rights of other procreators . . . By requiring a court to enforce a preconception agreement that would wrest a child from the arms of one biological parent and transfer her to the home of another, Robertson's right to procreate has become so broad as to impinge upon parental rights. Such a sweeping right of reproduction threatens to swallow up other constitutional privacy rights.

All these weaknesses evidence a deeper flaw in Robertson's all-encompassing constitutional framework. Robertson strives to reduce the manifold issues raised by the new reproductive technologies to one constitutional right. In his search for simplicity, however, he forgoes a more nuanced constitutional analysis. He relies almost exclusively upon one constitutional principle — the primacy of procreative liberty. Yet a comprehensive constitutional analysis cannot apply procreational privacy rights in isolation; rather, it must take into account all of the ways in which an individual experiences liberty in various categories and clauses of the Constitution. At a minimum, it must reconcile the right to privacy of procreation with two other elements of the constitutional right to privacy, which I shall term privacy of person and privacy of parenting. Robertson's framework falls short because it focuses upon procreational privacy, seldom considering personal privacy and almost entirely ignoring parental privacy.

III. Toward a New Taxonomy

. . . Robertson's constitutional framework defines the right to procreate as the right to create genetically or gestationally connected progeny. In so doing, it specifies that the initial entitlement belongs to those who are biologically reproducing. But by assuming without justifying why it is that this entitlement can be bargained away, Robertson seems to be operating in the Coasian[7] world of contract and not in the realm of constitutional rights. Though it employs the rhetoric of rights, Robertson's constitutional model reveals itself to be a version of the contract law model. It concentrates upon policy questions central to contract law, ignoring or overlooking the question of the alienability of constitutional rights that lies at the core of constitutional law. Robertson has simply constitutionalized freedom of contract in the name of advancing reproductive rights.

Perhaps Robertson reverts to contract law because of the awkwardness of constitutional law in adjudicating family conflicts. Constitutional law's strength lies in addressing disputes that pit the individual against the state. Cases that present a multiplicity of conflicting rights and a plethora of adverse parties, however, are less readily resolved by resort to global constitutional principles. The new reproductive technologies, moreover, raise issues too complex to be decided according to constitutional principles that permanently balance basic values, setting them in constitutional stone. Robertson's quest to constitutionalize conception is misguided because it would freeze the law in an area of rapidly developing technology with as yet unknown and potentially far-reaching implications for society . . .

---

[7] Professor Rao is referring to the Coase Theorem, first articulated in a classic essay by Ronald Coase, *The Problem of Social Cost*, 3 J. L. & Econ. 1 (1960). Briefly stated, the Coase Theorem holds that, in the absence of transaction costs, the initial allocation of entitlements to various parties is not binding because the parties are free to bargain around them. The Theorem posits that parties will bargain to achieve an efficient allocation of resources. In the world of ART, this can mean that the decisive factor in determining the right to parent a child born with the aid of third parties (gamete donors, gestational surrogates, for example) is intent. The parties who intend to parent should prevail even if their "entitlement" to do so is not based on a genetic or gestational tie to the child. Such a case is made by Carmel Shalev, Birth Power: The Case For Surrogacy (1989). -Ed.

Ann MacLean Massie
Regulating Choice: A Constitutional Law Response to Professor John A. Robertson's Children of Choice
52 Washington & Lee Law Review 135 (1995)

I. Introduction

. . . Professor Robertson's central thesis is the primacy of "procreative liberty — the freedom to decide whether or not to have offspring and to control the use of one's reproductive capacity." Noting that "this value is widely acknowledged when reproduction occurs *au naturel*," the author states that "it should be equally honored when reproduction requires technological assistance." In Robertson's view, "procreative liberty deserves presumptive respect because of its central importance to individual meaning, dignity, and identity"; hence, his succinctly stated proposition: "I propose that procreative liberty be given presumptive priority in all conflicts, with the burden on opponents of any particular technique to show that harmful effects from its use justify limiting procreative choice."

Given this hypothesis, "[a] central question in this enterprise is to determine whether effects on embryos, families, women, and other participants rise to the level of severity necessary to justify infringing a basic right." Professor Robertson . . . devotes substantial portions of the book to arguments that almost no conceivable counterinterest actually sustains the burden of proving the sufficiency of its importance. In Robertson's words, "it is difficult to show that the alleged harms of noncoital reproduction are sufficient to justify overriding procreative liberty."

. . . One might think, as do a number of commentators, that the well-being of the children resulting from assisted conception would constitute precisely the sort of weighty counterinterest that could justify restrictions on the procreative liberty of adult would-be parents whenever there were grounds to think that the use of reproductive technologies might threaten or jeopardize the welfare of resulting offspring. Professor Robertson readily admits that impact on offspring is an important consideration, but he invariably trumps its potential to restrict adult procreative interests by noting that, with respect to any given child born with the use of assisted conception, its only choice would be either existence under the limitations imposed by the parental behavior or total nonexistence . . .

[I]nstances of persons desiring access to reproductive technologies — HIV-positive women, single persons, gay or lesbian couples, individuals or couples who do not need the service for reasons of infertility, and women well above natural childbearing age — present situations in which reasonable persons might well differ on issues of whether such access ought to be permitted and in which many might consider society's stake in the outcomes to be high. Specifically, it might well be argued that a due regard for the welfare of the resulting children would militate in favor of particular kinds of regulations, or at least in favor of proceeding cautiously during the next few years as we make our way through the thorny social considerations raised by advancing reproductive technologies.

Yet Professor Robertson's analysis would, as a matter of constitutional law, decide for us that in each of the situations posed the would-be parent's procreative liberty overrides competing considerations and prevents any regulations other than those designed purely to ensure safe medical practices. The effect of his constitutional interpretation is to foreclose debate and remove the issues from the public forum, for, in this view, the "rights" of adults preclude the possibility of regulation that public consensus might deem desirable. The conversation is over before it has had a chance to begin . . .

I submit . . . that Professor Robertson's definition of "procreative liberty" paints with too broad a brush insofar as constitutional interpretation is concerned. By foreclosing discussion and the possibility of social control over issues important to the future of us all, he reaches results that are unnecessary for the protection of constitutional values and undesirable from the standpoint of public policy. His glib recitation of the rubric that, from the perspective of any individual, it is invariably better to have been born than not to have been born makes too short a shrift of a concern central to the reproductive technologies debate — namely, what we should do to ensure the physical, mental, and psychological well-being of the children whom we are deliberately bringing into existence . . .

II. The Constitutional Argument

A. Robertson's Thesis

Much of the discussion in *Children of Choice* of the primacy of procreative liberty as an overriding value is couched in terms of social policy arguments, not necessarily constitutional ones. From a purely social policy perspective, I do not disagree with Professor Robertson that the procreative interests of would-be parents is a primary value, worthy of a great deal of respect and accommodation as we consider the increasing sophistication and usage of reproductive technologies . . . As a matter of social policy, my disagreement with Professor Robertson is more one of emphasis than of kind. I would endow the procreative interests of would-be parents with a less thoroughgoing primacy and would place more weight on the interests of the children resulting from the use of these technologies.

Where I differ from Professor Robertson is with his insistence that procreative liberty as a constitutionally protected fundamental right should be broadly construed in a manner that protects from all but minimal regulation virtually any means of achieving biological parenthood for virtually any would be parent. . . . [H]is basic phraseology throughout the book mirrors the constitutional parlance of fundamental rights language . . .

B. The Current Constitutional Status of Procreative Liberty

1. Supreme Court Decisions

To assess Professor Robertson's arguments, it is first necessary to determine as precisely as possible what interests the Supreme Court has held to be subject to heightened protection under the Constitution. Identifying the core values at stake in defined liberty interests should then lead to logical conclusions about the potential scope of procreative liberty as an element of the right of privacy.

Professor Robertson and other commentators have accurately noted that the Supreme Court's clearest jurisprudence in this area concerns the right not to procreate — i.e., not to bear unwanted children. [Professor Massie next reviews the decisions in *Griswold v. Connecticut* (1965), *Eisenstadt v. Baird* (1972), *Carey v. Population Services International* (1977), *Roe v. Wade* (1973), and *Planned Parenthood v. Casey* (1992), agreeing with Professor Robertson that the government must respect an individual's right to prevent procreation by the use of contraception or by previability abortion.]

[B]ut what is the picture when we look to the positive side of procreative liberty — the right to procreate? . . . [I]n *Skinner v. Oklahoma* [1942], the Court in dictum referred to procreation as "one of the basic civil rights of man" and noted that "marriage and procreation are fundamental to the very existence and survival of the race." *Skinner*, however, was an equal protection case concerning the state's power to render someone permanently sterile, and its reference was to natural procreative *capacity*, not to procreative acts.

Since *Skinner*, in construing the liberty interest protected by the Due Process Clause of the Fourteenth Amendment, the Court has delineated, in Justice Powell's words, "[a] host of cases . . . [that] have consistently acknowledged a 'private realm of family life which the state cannot enter.' " This realm includes personal decisions "relating to marriage, procreation, contraception, family relationships, and child rearing and education." Accordingly, the Court has struck down policies restricting an individual's choice of whom and when to marry, zoning regulations burdening rights of blood relatives to live together in a single household, and laws deemed to interfere with parental rights to raise and educate children as one sees fit . . .

Yet we must also keep in mind some sharp cutoff points that the Court has earmarked in its delineation of the constitutionally protected right of privacy. In *Bowers v. Hardwick* [1986], the Court refused to characterize homosexual behavior as an aspect of the freedom of intimate association. Instead, the Court upheld a state prohibition against homosexual sodomy on the grounds that the practice had long constituted a criminal offense and hence did not fit within the "fundamental liberties . . . 'deeply rooted in this Nation's history and tradition.' " . . .

2. Values Underlying the Decisions

Professor Robertson's reading of the privacy cases leads him to conclude that coital reproduction within marriage is a fundamental right subject to the highest degree of constitutional protection. Because the underlying motivations and desires are the same, he argues that noncoital reproduction should receive the same degree of constitutional deference. Are these conclusions justified? I submit that the first one is, but the second one is not. The distinction becomes apparent upon an examination of the values underlying the cases involving procreative choice.

Professor Robertson argues that the primary value at stake here is the "central importance [of procreative liberty] to individual meaning, dignity, and identity" for both fertile and infertile couples. In other words, what matters is the shared wish of both fertile and infertile couples "to replicate themselves, transmit genes, gestate, and rear children biologically related to them." The desire is the same, the motivations are the same, and the goal is the same. Therefore, he reasons, infertile couples should have the same protected right to noncoital reproduction that fertile couples have to coital reproduction. This syllogism has an appealing ring to it and, as a social policy proposition, deserves respect if not wholesale accommodation. In the realm of constitutional law, however, there are many instances in which there is a sharp distinction between the degree of protection specifically provided to a belief or motivation and the degree of protection provided to the conduct arising from that belief or motivation.

3. The Belief/Conduct Distinction

. . . [I]t is also true that our system of constitutional government, for all its emphasis upon individual liberties as particularly recognized in the Bill of Rights, has always insisted upon the importance of the distinction between beliefs, on the one hand, and conduct stemming from those beliefs, on the other. Beliefs often possess, for the believer, the quality of the absolute; certainly, from the standpoint of government, they possess the quality of the unregulable. The government may attempt to influence beliefs, but it ultimately lacks the power either to instill or to expunge them from the minds of those who hold them. Conduct, on the other hand, is the stuff with which regulation is concerned. Given that beliefs are both central to self-definition and essentially ungovernable, while conduct is both the natural outgrowth of beliefs and the arena of regulation, the important question becomes: To what extent must government accommodate conduct in order to respect belief and to preserve the right of self-definition, as it simultaneously acts in the best interests of all by promulgating regulations that seem desirable to a majority? . . .

The privacy cases themselves also leave broad scope for the regulation of conduct. Although the cases most directly related to procreative liberty speak in terms of the "right to decide whether to bear or beget a child" (a mental process), the holdings fall far short of protecting all possible behaviors related to that choice. Instead, the cases defining constitutionally protected conduct invariably implicate not only the value of self-fulfillment or self-definition, but one or more other values as well. Generally, these values are characterizable either as respect for an individual's bodily integrity or as social concerns related to the privacy of marital intimacy and the integrity of the family unit . . .

The marriage relationship, with its concomitant intimacy, thus lies at the heart of the constitutionally protected right of privacy. Within the context of marriage, consensual behavior that might normally be expected to result in procreation — in other words, coital reproduction — certainly comes within the ambit of this protection.

Notice, however, that with respect to other so-called "procreative liberty" decisions, this syllogism does not apply. The Court has made very clear, for example, that outside the context of the marriage relationship, protection of the right of access to contraception does not mean protection of the right to engage in the behavior that makes contraception necessary or desirable, particularly in the case of minors. Thus, laws against fornication and adultery and those prohibiting sexual activities with or on the part of minors are perfectly valid. Similarly, the abortion cases, although protecting the rights of a woman to bodily integrity against the burden of an unwanted pregnancy, have specifically refused to hold that "one has an unlimited right to do with one's body as one pleases."

The clear message is that not all procreative behavior is subject to the heightened protection of the constitutional right of privacy. The next question is whether the special privacy right that inheres in the marriage relationship nonetheless encompasses all consensual procreative behavior, including use of the means of assisted reproduction.

I submit that the answer is no. Unlike coital reproduction, assisted reproduction does not directly implicate the values — bodily integrity, marital intimacy, or integrity of the family unit — that are central to the privacy cases. Heightened protection is not triggered simply by the fact that any particular conduct represents a search for meaning in life or because the persons involved are seeking self-fulfillment central to their self-definition. When invoked, those values have proven to be an insufficient basis for a claim to constitutional protection of the resulting behavior. In *Bowers v. Hardwick*, Justice Blackmun's dissent vehemently called upon these values to protect, as part of the right of intimate association, the conduct prohibited by Georgia's antisodomy statute. The majority, however, disagreed and noted that "the law . . . is constantly based on notions of morality."

4. Conclusions

. . . Professor Robertson himself concedes that sufficient harm to a third party's interests is an appropriate limit on procreative liberty; however, he repeatedly discounts the notion of harm to the third parties most directly affected by an individual's or a couple's use of reproductive technologies — namely, the resulting children. I believe that Robertson underplays the interests of the children deliberately created by assisted reproduction and in so doing neglects a primary value that must be given due weight in any responsible social policy concerning these "children of choice." . . . .

III. The Welfare of Third Parties: The Interests of "Children of Choice"

Throughout *Children of Choice*, whenever Professor Robertson contemplates any potentially negative effects of adults' reproductive choices on the resulting children, he favors the adults' procreative liberty on the ground that, from the standpoint of the children, the only alternative is nonexistence, and it is always "better to have been born than not to have been born." This rubric decides the issue for him: The adults have a fundamental right "to decide whether to bear or beget a child"; the children have no fundamental right to nonexistence and undoubtedly would not choose it if they could.

It seems to me that this approach is conceptually flawed and morally inadequate . . .

Current social policy, which respects autonomous patient choice for end-of-life decision-making, reflects a humane awareness that there are conditions under which life may be intolerable to the individual living it. Surely that can be just as true for infants as for those who have lived much longer.

Even if one concedes that children who owe their existence to assisted reproduction are virtually certain to find their lives to be net benefits rather than net burdens, a social policy choice that is content to rest upon this minimum threshold as the appropriate criterion for acceptability strikes me as highly questionable . . .

Robertson's contentions are highly controversial . . . What I wish to suggest here is that the same consideration — the optimal (not minimal) well-being of the future children — is the appropriate basis upon which to shape social policy with regard to the use of assisted reproduction. This assertion is not novel. In the area of family law, generally, issues involving the welfare of children are invariably decided on the ground of serving the children's best interests, even when doing so means infringing upon the rights or interests of adults.

The resolution of issues raised by assisted reproduction need not, in fact, go so far. Determining the "best interests" of children whose existence we are planning is a speculative enterprise. We do not even know the nature or extent of potential harms that might uniquely affect children born of assisted reproduction. Commentators raise such considerations as the effect upon self-identity when one does not know who one or both genetic parents are, the confusion of "too many parents" or the psychological harm perhaps engendered by custody battles when surrogate mothers wish to maintain contact with the babies that they have delivered, and the need for full and accurate family medical profiles. A child born to a postmenopausal woman or a child born as a clone of someone else, especially when that child is named after a deceased sibling, may suffer from a heavy burden of preconceived expectations. Deliberate planning for nontraditional families, such as single-parent situations or households in which both parents are of the same gender, poses other issues. The possibilities raised by increasing sophistication in genetic engineering may present the most far-reaching and unpredictable problems likely to arise.

IV. Conclusion

Certainly, society as a whole, as well as the individuals involved in the use of assisted reproduction, has a stake in the welfare of the future citizens that we are deliberately creating — not only their physical health, but their psychological and emotional well-being. We already have some parallels upon which to base our judgments, such as the experiences of adopted children or children from divorced or "blended" families. Careful deliberation and due regard for potential pitfalls should enable us to anticipate and to plan carefully to provide resolutions of social policy that will accommodate not only the procreative desires of would-be parents, but also the optimum conditions of health and nurturance for their "children of choice."

NOTES AND QUESTIONS

1. Professor Rao and Professor Massie are two of many commentators who reviewed and critiqued John Robertson's book, CHILDREN OF CHOICE: FREEDOM AND THE NEW REPRODUCTIVE TECHNOLOGIES (1994). As would be expected with a topic of this import, the commentators varied in their level of (dis)agreement with Professor

Robertson's theories, yet all agreed that the book made a valuable contribution to the dialogue surrounding reproductive technologies. *See, e.g.*, Gilbert Meilaender, *Products of the Will: Robertson's Children of Choice*, 52 WASH. & LEE L. REV. 173 (1995); Laura M. Purdy, *Children of Choice: Whose Children? At What Cost?*, 52 WASH. & LEE L. REV. 197 (1995); Jon F. Merz, *The Search for Coherence in Reproductive Policy*, 17 J. LEGAL MED. 169 (1995); Dan W. Brock, *Procreative Liberty*, 74 TEX. L. REV. 187 (1995): Duane R. Vlaz, *Book Review: Children of Choice: Freedom and the New Reproductive Technologies*, 10 HIGH TECH. L. J. 201 (1995); *Book Review*, Gregory P. Smith, 36 JURIMETRICS 115 (1995). For a more recent and summative assessment of the law and legal literature surrounding the constitutional right to access ART, *see* Sonia M. Suter, *The "Repugnance" Lens of Gonzales v. Carhart and Other Theories of Reproductive Rights: Evaluating Advanced Reproductive Technologies*, 76 GEO.WASH. L. REV. 1514 (2008).

Professor Robertson makes the case that constitutional law protects the right to procreate, either naturally or with assisting technologies, with the state having the burden of demonstrating a compelling interest if it restricts the practice in any way. The primacy of procreative liberty, in Robertson's view, derives largely from *Skinner v. Oklahoma* (1942), a case declaring procreation "a basic civil right of man." Professor Rao is skeptical that a case decided well before the advent of any type of reproductive technology (recall artificial insemination wasn't introduced to the general public until the 1950s) can be the foundation for such a comprehensive right. "*Skinner,*" she argues, "is too weak a reed to carry so much constitutional weight." Do you agree? Certainly the basic principle articulated by Justice Douglas has never been repudiated, and in fact has been reaffirmed in numerous cases (See Note 1 following *Skinner v. Oklahoma*, at page 90). But Rao argues that the right to be free from state interference with reproduction does not necessarily translate into a right to use ART unfettered by any regulation. What seems to emerge from this critique is a sense that reproductive rights can be classified as either negative (right to be free from government interference) or positive (right to enlist state's assistance to access means of procreation). Do you think reproductive rights are positive or negative rights? Does your answer help shape your view of the constitutional right to procreate using ART?

2.   One of Professor Massie's major concerns is that a constitutional primacy of procreative liberty accords insufficient weight to the well-being of ART children when the interests of would-be parents are weighed against state interests in restricting assisted reproduction. As we learned in Chapter 1, the subject of harm of ART offspring is of growing and significant concern to physicians and families worldwide. A formal expression of concern for the welfare of children born via assisted conception was voiced by the President's Council on Bioethics, an executive-level advisory panel created by President George W. Bush on November 28, 2001, by means of Executive Order 13237. The Council issued a report in March 2004 titled, "Reproduction and Responsibility: The Regulation of New Biotechnolo-gies." In its discussion of assisted reproduction, the Council summarizes the clinical studies to date that suggest a link between the use of ART and birth defects and developmental difficulties in children. The Council observes that "[n]one of these studies provide a causal link between ART and the dysfunctions observed . . . [n]evertheless, these findings have raised some concerns." Report at 40. In the end,

the Council recommends that the federal government undertake a "federally funded longitudinal study of the impact of assisted reproductive technologies on the health and development of children born with their aid." *Id.* at xlvi.

In the years since the Council report, a number of studies have been conducted looking at the impact of ART on the resulting offspring. These studies are discussed in greater detail in Chapter 1. Some studies suggest no difference in the health status of ART-conceived children and spontaneously conceived children, while others find ART increases the likelihood of a major birth defect by up to 1.5 times. *Compare* Tracy Skevell et al., *Assisted Reproductive Technology and Pregnancy Outcomes*, 106 OBSTETRICS & GYNECOLOGY 1039 (2005) (finding no increased rate of chromosomal or structural abnormalities in ART offspring) *with* Michéle Hanson et al., *Assisted Reproductive Technology and the Risk of Birth Defects — A Systematic Review*, 20 HUMAN REPROD. 328 (2005) (reporting 1.3 to 1.35 times more likely rate of birth defects). Should the results of medical studies be relevant to the regulation of ART? If so, should individuals who pose a substantial risk of transmitting a genetic or infectious disease to their offspring through natural conception likewise be subject to procreative restrictions?

C.　Judicial Perspectives on ART as a Fundamental Right

The academic commentaries in the previous section engage in classic analogical reasoning, a cornerstone of legal analysis. That is, the authors look to existing law and try to predict how a case with different but related facts might be decided using the principles and policies from the known precedents. Analogical reasoning is particularly apt in discussing the constitutionality of ART because scant case law exists to shed light on judicial attitudes toward ART and its regulation. Professor Robertson argues that assisted reproduction should be treated the same as natural conception as far as legal constraints are concerned, because both processes share a common value of individual expression. Professors Massie and Rao find the direct analogy between coital and noncoital reproduction more troubling, calling into question the primacy of procreative liberty over the rights of children and others who assist in the reproductive process.

Ultimately, the strength of procreative liberty in the use of ART will be decided by the courts in the same case-by-case approach that has brought us our rich history in the field of avoiding procreation through sterilization, contraception, and abortion. What follows are the few cases that involve the use of some form of ART, cases that may someday form the foundation of the right to assisted conception.

1. Equating ART and Natural Conception

LIFCHEZ v. HARTIGAN
United States District Court, Northern District of Illinois
735 F. Supp. 1361 (1990)

WILLIAMS, J. Dr. Lifchez represents a class of plaintiff physicians who specialize in reproductive endocrinology and fertility counselling. Physicians with these medical specialities treat infertile couples who wish to conceive a child. Dr. Lifchez is suing the Illinois Attorney General and the Cook County State's Attorney, seeking a declaratory judgment that a provision of the Illinois Abortion Law is unconstitutional. He also seeks a permanent injunction against the defendants from enforcing the statute. The provision at issue concerns fetal experimentation. Ill.Rev.Stat., Ch. 38 ¶ 81-26, § 6(7) (1989). Both sides move for summary judgment, alleging that there are no disputed facts and that each side is entitled to judgment as a matter of law. The court finds that § 6(7) of the Illinois Abortion Law violates the Constitution in two ways: (1) it offends Fourteenth Amendment principles of due process by being so vague that persons such as Dr. Lifchez cannot know whether or not their medical practice may run afoul of the statute's criminal sanctions, and (2) the statute impinges upon a woman's right of privacy and reproductive freedom as established in *Roe v. Wade*, 410 U.S. 113, 93 S.Ct. 705, 35 L.Ed.2d 147 (1973), *Carey v. Population Services International*, 431 U.S. 678, 97 S.Ct. 2010, 52 L.Ed.2d 675 (1977), and their progeny. The court therefore declares § 6(7) of the Illinois Abortion Law to be unconstitutional and permanently enjoins the defendants from enforcing it.

Vagueness

[1] Section 6(7) of the Illinois Abortion Law provides as follows:

(7) No person shall sell or experiment upon a fetus produced by the fertilization of a human ovum by a human sperm unless such experimentation is therapeutic to the fetus thereby produced. Intentional violation of this section is a Class A misdemeanor. Nothing in this subsection (7) is intended to prohibit the performance of in vitro fertilization.

Ill.Rev.Stat., Ch. 38 ¶ 81-26, § 6(7) (1989). Dr. Lifchez claims that the Illinois legislature's failure to define the terms "experimentation" and "therapeutic" renders the statute vague, thus violating his due process rights under the Fourteenth Amendment. The court agrees.

[Dr. Lifchez, argued that the absence of clear guidance from the legislature as to the meaning of these significant terms left him uncertain about the lawfulness of his work using IVF. Even though the statute exempts "the performance of in vitro fertilization," there are several related techniques, such as embryo transfer and genetic screening of IVF-derived embryos, that are not explicitly exempt under the statute and might have subjected Dr. Lifchez and others to liability. Moreover, Dr. Lifchez worried that if he tried to improve upon current IVF techniques, even these subtle changes would be undertaken "at his peril." Any variation of the IVF technique may be therapeutic to the woman trying to conceive, but it is decidedly non-therapeutic to embryos that might be lost in the initial stages of experimentation. Thus, even though the statute exempted IVF from prosecution, it left uncertainty as to how the technique could be undertaken. The court agreed that the failure to define key terms rendered the statute impermissibly vague because it subjected physicians to uncertainty and possible criminal liability for engaging in seemingly protected conduct.]

Reproductive Privacy[8]

Section 6(7) of the Illinois Abortion Law is also unconstitutional because it impermissibly restricts a woman's fundamental right of privacy, in particular, her right to make reproductive choices free of governmental interference with those choices. Various aspects of this reproductive privacy right have been articulated in a number of landmark Supreme Court cases, including *Griswold v. Connecticut*, 381 U.S. 479, 85 S.Ct. 1678, 14 L.Ed.2d 510 (1965) (striking down statute which forbid use of contraceptives on grounds that statute invaded zone of privacy surrounding marriage relationship); *Eisenstadt v. Baird*, 405 U.S. 438, 92 S.Ct. 1029, 31 L.Ed.2d 349 (1972) (striking down statute forbidding distribution of contraceptives to unmarried persons on equal protection grounds, but observing in dicta that: "If the right of privacy means anything, it is the right of the individual, married or single, to be free from unwarranted governmental intrusion into matters so fundamentally affecting a person as the decision whether to bear or beget a child." Id. at 453, 92 S.Ct. at 1038); *Roe v. Wade*, 410 U.S. 113, 93 S.Ct. 705, 35 L.Ed.2d 147 (1973) (establishing unrestricted right to an abortion in first trimester); and *Planned Parenthood of Missouri v. Danforth*, 428 U.S. 52, 96 S.Ct. 2831, 49 L.Ed.2d 788 (1976) (striking down provisions of abortion statute requiring spousal consent and parental consent). In *Carey v. Population Services International*, 431 U.S. 678, 97 S.Ct. 2010, 52 L.Ed.2d 675 (1977), the Court struck down a statute which forbid the sale of contraceptives to minors, forbid anyone other than pharmacists from distributing contraceptives to anyone, and forbid all advertising of contraceptives. The Court reviewed its prior privacy cases and declared that

> The decision whether or not to beget or bear a child is at the very heart of this cluster of constitutionally protected choices. That decision holds a particularly important place in the history of the right of privacy, a right first explicitly recognized in an opinion holding unconstitutional a statute prohibiting the use of contraceptives . . . and most prominently vindicated in recent years in the contexts of contraception . . . and abortion.

Id. at 685, 97 S.Ct. at 2016 (citations omitted).

Section 6(7) intrudes upon this "cluster of constitutionally protected choices." Embryo transfer and chorionic villi sampling[9] are illustrative. Both procedures are

---

[8] [n.8] Although neither party has raised the issue, the court notes that Dr. Lifchez has standing to assert the reproductive privacy rights of his patients. See *Singleton v. Wulff*, 428 U.S. 106, 117-18, 96 S.Ct. 2868, 2875-76, 49 L.Ed.2d 826 (1976) and *Doe v. Bolton*, 410 U.S. 179, 188-89, 93 S.Ct. 739, 745-46, 35 L.Ed.2d 201 (1973).

[9] In an earlier part of the decision, the court describes chorionic villi sampling (CVS) as a diagnostic procedure used in pregnancy, designed to give genetic information about the developing fetus. CVS

"experimental" by most definitions of that term. Both are performed directly, and intentionally, on the fetus. Neither procedure is necessarily therapeutic to the fetus. In embryo transfer, it is not therapeutic to remove the embryo from a woman's uterus after it has been fertilized and expose it to the high risk associated with trying to implant it in the infertile woman. In chorionic villi sampling, it is not therapeutic to the fetus to invade and snip off some of its surrounding tissue. Both embryo transfer and chorionic villi sampling violate any reasonable interpretation of § 6(7).

Both procedures, however, fall within a woman's zone of privacy as recognized in *Roe v. Wade, Carey v. Population Services International*, and their progeny. See also John A. Robertson, *"The Right To Procreate and In Utero Fetal Therapy,"* 3 J. Leg. Med. 333, 339 (1982). Embryo transfer is a procedure designed to enable an infertile woman to bear her own child. It takes no great leap of logic to see that within the cluster of constitutionally protected choices that includes the right to have access to contraceptives, there must be included within that cluster the right to submit to a medical procedure that may bring about, rather than prevent, pregnancy. Chorionic villi sampling is similarly protected. The cluster of constitutional choices that includes the right to abort a fetus within the first trimester must also include the right to submit to a procedure designed to give information about that fetus which can then lead to a decision to abort. Since there is no compelling state interest sufficient to prevent a woman from terminating her pregnancy during the first trimester, *Roe v. Wade*, 410 U.S. at 163, 93 S.Ct. at 731; *Akron v. Akron Center for Reproductive Health*, 462 U.S. 416, 450, 103 S.Ct. 2481, 2503, 76 L.Ed.2d 687 (1983), there can be no such interest sufficient to intrude upon these other protected activities during the first trimester. By encroaching upon this protected zone of privacy, § 6(7) is unconstitutional.

CONCLUSION

The court grants Dr. Lifchez' motion for summary judgment and denies the defendants' motion for summary judgment. Section 6(7) of the Illinois Abortion Law is unconstitutional and the defendants are permanently enjoined from enforcing it.

The decision in *Lifchez v. Hartigan* weighs the possible constitutional infringements *should* the Illinois Abortion Law be used to prevent physicians from offering a range of reproductive services, including assisted conception. In anticipation of such application, the federal district court declares the law unconstitutional. The next case presents an actual controversy in which the parties make arguments about the applicability of traditional reproductive jurisprudence to the use of ARTs. The court takes a definitive stand on whether noncoital reproduction should be treated the same as natural reproduction.

------

involves inserting a catheter through the cervix in order to take a biopsy of the chorionic tissue, which is tissue surrounding the fetus. The tissue is then analyzed to determine the genetic health of the fetus. 735 F. Supp. At 1367. - Ed.

KASS v. KASS
Supreme Court of Nassau County, New York, 1995
1995 WL 110368 (Not reported in N.Y.S.2d)

RONCALLO, J. The parties to this matrimonial action have settled all outstanding issues but one — possession of five (5) frozen fertilized pre-embryos presently in the possession of the *In Vitro* Fertilization program operated by John T. Mather Memorial Hospital. The parties have agreed that the remaining issue shall be submitted for determination on the affidavits and memoranda of law previously filed. The relevant facts are these.

The parties were married in July of 1988. Childless, they attempted *in vitro* fertilization on six (6) occasions prior to May of 1993. Each attempt ended in failure. At that time they enrolled in the *In Vitro* program conducted by physicians at John T. Mather Memorial Hospital with the hope that ova of the wife fertilized by her husband's sperm could be successfully implanted in an oocyte donee — the wife's sister. A pregnancy did not result. Of the original ova taken and fertilized, five (5) remain. When the parties enrolled in the program they executed informed consent forms.

All frozen ova are at a stage of development of less than fourteen (14) days after fertilization. The term zygote refers to the cell formed by the union of two (2) reproductive cells or gametes. The term most commonly used to describe the zygote during the first two (2) weeks following creation is pre-embryo. Here I will use both terms interchangeably.

On July 21st, 1993 the wife instituted the within action for divorce. As noted, the only remaining issue is possession of the zygotes. The wife seeks to recover the zygotes for purposes of implantation in herself. Her husband seeks a direction that the zygotes be turned over to John T. Mather Hospital for use in connection with embryo research.

The issues raised do not appear to have been considered by the Courts of this State nor the vast majority of our sister states. One Court, the highest appellate court of the State of Tennessee — the Tennessee Supreme Court — has confronted the issue head on in *Davis v. Davis* (842 S.W.2d 588) decided in the spring of 1992. The conclusions reached there will be discussed subsequently . . .

Of necessity the starting point of any discussion of the parties' rights must be a categorization of the nature of the zygotes. The only available choices would appear to be the legal dichotomy of person or property. While one jurisdiction has attempted to grant "judicial person" status to "in vitro human ovum" (see Louisiana Revised Statutes 9:129) and one Court has determined they are not property (see *Del Zio v. Columbia Presbyterian Hosp.*, S.D.N.Y., Index # 74-358, slip op 11/14/78) it appears clear, that a gamete provider's interest in a zygote/pre-embryo should be considered in the nature of a property interest (see, *York v. Jones*, 717 F.Supp. 421 [E.D.VA1989], *Davis v. Davis*, 842 S.W.2 588 . . .)

The fact that zygotes are not persons from a legal standpoint does not establish they are property within the ordinary sense of that term. They most assuredly are not. As life inchoate they represent the ultimate in nascency and potentiality.

Equating zygotes with washing machines and jewelry for purposes of a marital distribution borders on the absurd. The issues involved transcend such a context. To paraphrase Shakespeare, they are the "stuff" of procreation. As such the rights involved are "far more precious than property rights" (see, *Stanley v. Illinois*, 405 U.S. 645, 651 (1972)). Unlike ordinary property, possession of the zygotes is secondary to the right to control their destiny. If the wife is awarded possession the pre-embryos will be afforded an opportunity to realize their potential; if the husband is successful such potential will be extinguished as part of a scientific inquiry.

The unique nature of the subject matter precludes a solution which divides the pre-embryos between the parties. To adopt such a course would be simplistic and accomplish nothing more than a sidestepping of the real issues, i.e., a determination as to which party has the right to determine the embryos' fate.

As might be expected, the rights involved in the relationship between husband, wife, zygote and state reach constitutional proportions. Justice Doughtrey's scholarly decision in *Davis v. Davis (supra)* relieves me of the obligation of setting forth an in depth analysis of such rights. It is sufficient here to note the existence of a constitutionally protected right of privacy involving "procreational autonomy", a right which includes both a "right to procreate" and a "right to avoid procreation" (see *Meyer v. Nebraska*, 262 U.S. 390 (1923); *Roe v. Wade*, 410 U.S. 113 (1973); *Griswold v. Connecticut*, 381 U.S. 479 (1965), *Davis v. Davis, supra*, pg. 598, 599).

A resolution here requires that I discuss the issue of rights from two standpoints. The rights that all gamete providers have with respect to the product of their donation and the rights that these providers have under the circumstances present here. Or put another way, what rights do the parties have in the abstract and the concrete.

As I perceive it, the key to an intelligent discussion is the question of whether there is a conceptual or propositional difference between the product of an *in vitro* fertilization and the product of an *in vivo* fertilization.

It cannot seriously be argued that a husband has a right to procreate or avoid procreation following an *in vivo* fertilization. He cannot force conception. He cannot compel or prevent an abortion (*Roe v. Wade, supra, Planned Parenthood of Missouri v. Danforth*, 428 U.S. 52 (1976)). The simple fact of the matter is that an *in vivo* husband's rights and control over the procreative process ends with ejaculation. From that moment until such time as the fetus reaches a stage of development sufficient to trigger the State's interest in its life the fetus' fate rests with the mother to the exclusion of all others.

> The obvious fact is that when the wife and the husband disagree on this decision [abortion], the view of only one of the two marriage partners can prevail. Inasmuch as it is the woman who physically bears the child and who is the more directly and immediately affected by the pregnancy, as between the two, the balance weighs in her favor. (cf. *Roe v. Wade*, 410 U.S. at 153), *Planned Parenthood of Missouri v. Danforth, supra*, pg. 52, 71.

It is clear then if there is no difference between *in vivo* and *in vitro* fertilizations the rights of the wife must be considered paramount and her wishes with respect to disposition must prevail.

In my opinion there is no legal, ethical or logical reason why an *in vitro* fertilization should give rise to additional rights on the part of the husband. From a propositional standpoint it matters little whether the ovum/sperm union takes place in the private darkness of a fallopian tube or the public glare of a petri dish. Fertilization is fertilization and fertilization of the ovum is the inception of the reproductive process. Biological life exists from that moment forward. The fact that an *in vitro* zygote does not seek to fulfill its biological destiny immediately upon such fertilization does not alter that fact. The rights of the parties are dependent upon the nature of the zygote not the stage of its development or its location. To deny a husband rights while an embryo develops in the womb and grant a right to destroy while it is in a hospital freezer is to favor situs over substance.

Just as an *in vivo* husband's "right to avoid procreation" is waived and ceases to exist after intercourse in a coital reproduction, such right should be deemed waived and non-existent after his participation in an *in vitro* program. Upon entering he knows, or should have known, that technology is such that the possibility and probability of a delayed implantation are very real. Absent some indication of a contrary intent, the agreement to participate, if it does not expressly provide for such an eventuality, must be deemed an agreement to permit a delayed implantation. Such consent should not be abolished *nunc pro tunc* merely because of a change in circumstances which could and should have been anticipated. As will be seen from the Informed Consent Forms quoted subsequently, the parties here acknowledge that frozen pre-embryos will be distributed in accordance with the directives of a Divorce Court. Under such circumstances it cannot be said that a divorce was an unforeseen eventuality which would negate the husband's prior intent.

Before leaving the subject I would make one further observation. If I were to overlook what to me is the obvious conclusion that a "right to avoid procreation" cannot logically survive the initial act of procreation, and posit such a right, the right has been transformed from one founded in restraint into a right to take positive steps to terminate a potential human life. The Supreme Court of the United States has expressly refused to recognize such a right (see, *Planned Parenthood of Missouri v. Danforth, supra*) . . .

I conclude therefore between the parties, plaintiff Maureen Kass has the exclusive right to determine the fate of the subject zygotes. That being so, the question becomes whether that right has been expressly or impliedly waived by her conduct or agreement either before or after entering the *in vitro* program.

[The court reviews the consent forms signed by the parties prior to receiving treatment at the IVF Program and concludes that Mrs. Kass did not waive her right to determine the future of the subject zygotes. We will take up this part of the case, as well as other cases dealing with the disposition of frozen embryos upon divorce, in Chapter 7.]

In reaching my determination in this matter I am not unmindful of the difficult situation confronting defendant. While I have determined that he does not have the right to prevent his wife from attempting conception,[10] I do not believe his potential for parenthood should remain open ended. At the very least he is entitled to a directive that plaintiff exercise her right to implant the zygotes within a medically reasonable time after the entry of judgment. I have not considered the defendant's obligation to support or his possible claims against plaintiff, if any, if he is forced to contribute. Such matters are more properly considered, if and when, a pregnancy results.

Accordingly it is my determination that plaintiff, if she so elects, is entitled to take possession to the five (5) zygotes presently in the possession of the John T. Mather Hospital In Vitro Fertilization Program for purposes of attempting conception, any such attempt to be made within a medically reasonable time after entry of the judgment to be submitted hereon . . .

NOTES AND QUESTIONS

1.   The courts in *Lifchez v. Hartigan* and *Kass v. Kass* both seem supportive of the application of existing constitutional principles to reproductive technologies. Do the courts rely on the same constitutional principles? If you believe the courts rely on different principles, which principles do you believe are features in each opinion? What do you see as the similarities and differences between these two trial court decisions? Do you agree with either case?

2.   As we shall see in Chapter 7, the trial court decision in *Kass v. Kass* was reversed by the Court of Appeals of New York Court in 1998. Thus, Judge Roncallo's dicta that "it matters little whether the ovum/sperm union takes place in the private darkness of a fallopian tube or the public glare of a petri dish" is not necessarily the case in New York. The situs of fertilization, it would seem, does affect the status of the resulting embryo and the rights of those who brought about conception in the first place. Certainly the law is no stranger to the concept that the situs, or location, of a particular event is relevant to the rights that arise out of that event. In your Civil Procedure course you likely studied issues surrounding personal jurisdiction, specifically the ability of a plaintiff to "haul" a defendant into an out-of-state court when there was little if any activity linking the defendant to the forum state. Recall the concept of minimum contacts, which investigates the nexus between the forum contacts and the cause of action; if the nexus is too attenuated, it violates fundamental fairness to force a defendant with non-continuous or non-systematic contacts to defend a lawsuit in that forum. See *International Shoe Co. v. Washington*, 326 U.S. 310 (1945).

Does the trial court in *Kass* make a "minimum contacts" argument? Do you read Judge Roncallo to say that once the husband's sperm had contact with the egg, no matter the location of the union, any resulting embryo could be subject to the fundamental rights of the wife to control the early embryo, as delineated in *Roe v. Wade*? Thus, the essential nexus for assertion of the primacy of a woman's right to continue or terminate a pregnancy would rest in the man's consensual surrender of his sperm. Do you think this nexus between the voluntary provision of sperm and

---

[10] Does the court mean pregnancy? Technically, hasn't conception already occurred by the fusing of the egg and sperm in the laboratory petri dish? -Ed.

the preemption of the man's right to avoid procreation is the same in cases of natural and assisted conception? Asked another way, does the situs of fertilization matter when it comes to assigning fundamental rights?

2.   Distinguishing ART from Natural Conception

Today virtually every ART dispute that reaches an appellate court will be a case of first impression, giving the panel of judges an opportunity to analyze and explain their view on the question of fundamental rights and assisted conception. Where the courts in *Lifchez v. Hartigan* and *Kass v. Kass* saw important similarities between natural and assisted conception, the following two cases point out essential differences.

DAVIS v. DAVIS
Supreme Court of Tennessee
842 S.W.2d 588 (1992)

[Recall our previous look at this case in Chapter 1 in connection the legal status of the human embryo. Briefly, Mary Sue and Junior Davis filed for divorce and were unable to resolve the "custody" of seven frozen embryos stored in a Knoxville fertility clinic. The embryos were the result of a seventh attempt at in vitro fertilization, all previous attempts having failed. At the time the embryos were frozen, the couple did not indicate their intentions concerning the disposition in the event of divorce, either formally in writing or informally by way of oral expression. The Tennessee Supreme Court evaluated the biologic, legal and moral status of the 3-day old embryos, concluding that they "are not, strictly speaking, either "persons" or "property," but occupy an interim category that entitles them to special respect because of their potential for human life." What follows is the court's discussion of the parties' constitutional rights with respect to the disputed embryos.]

DAUGHTREY, JUSTICE.

VI. *The Right of Procreational Autonomy*

Although an understanding of the legal status of preembryos is necessary in order to determine the enforceability of agreements about their disposition, asking whether or not they constitute "property" is not an altogether helpful question. As the appellee points out in his brief, "[as] two or eight cell tiny lumps of complex protein, the embryos have no [intrinsic] value to either party." Their value lies in the "potential to become, after implantation, growth and birth, *children*." Thus, the essential dispute here is not where or how or how long to store the preembryos, but whether the parties will become parents. The Court of Appeals held in effect that they will become parents if they both agree to become parents. The Court did not say what will happen if they fail to agree. We conclude that the answer to this dilemma turns on the parties' exercise of their constitutional right to privacy.

The right to privacy is not specifically mentioned in either the federal or the Tennessee state constitution, and yet there can be little doubt about its grounding in the concept of liberty reflected in those two documents. In particular, the Fourteenth Amendment to the United States Constitution provides that "[n]o state shall . . . deprive any person of life, liberty, or property, without due process of law." Referring to the Fourteenth Amendment, the United States Supreme Court in *Meyer v. Nebraska* observed:

> While this court has not attempted to define with exactness the liberty thus guaranteed, the term has received much consideration and some of the included things have been definitely stated. Without doubt, it denotes not merely freedom from bodily restraint but also the right of the individual to contract, to engage in any of the common occupations of life, to acquire useful knowledge, to marry, establish a home and bring up children, to worship God according to the dictates of his own conscience, and generally to enjoy those privileges long recognized at common law as essential to the orderly pursuit of happiness by free men. 262 U.S. 390, 399, 43 S.Ct. 625, 626, 67 L.Ed. 1042 (1923).

The right of privacy inherent in the constitutional concept of liberty has been further identified "as against the [power of] government, the right to be let alone — the most comprehensive of rights and the right most valued by civilized men." *Olmstead v. United States*, 277 U.S. 438, 478, 48 S.Ct. 564, 572, 72 L.Ed. 944 (1928) (Brandeis, J., dissenting). As to scope, "the concept of liberty protects those personal rights that are fundamental, and it is not confined to the specific terms of the Bill of Rights." *Griswold v. Connecticut*, 381 U.S. 479, 486, 85 S.Ct. 1678, 1683, 14 L.Ed.2d 510 (1965) (Goldberg, J., concurring) . . .

Here, the specific individual freedom in dispute is the right to procreate. In terms of the Tennessee state constitution, we hold that the right of procreation is a vital part of an individual's right to privacy. Federal law is to the same effect.

In construing the reach of the federal constitution, the United States Supreme Court has addressed the affirmative right to procreate in only two cases. In *Buck v. Bell*, 274 U.S. 200, 207, 47 S.Ct. 584, 584, 71 L.Ed. 1000 (1927), the Court upheld the sterilization of a "feebleminded white woman." However, in *Skinner v. Oklahoma*, 316 U.S. 535, 62 S.Ct. 1110, 86 L.Ed. 1655 (1942), the Supreme Court struck down a statute that authorized the sterilization of certain categories of criminals. The Court described the right to procreate as "one of the basic civil rights of man [sic]," 316 U.S. at 541, 62 S.Ct. at 1113, and stated that "[m]arriage and procreation are fundamental to the very existence and survival of the race." *Id.*

In the same vein, the United States Supreme Court has said:

> If the right of privacy means anything, it is the right of the *individual*, married or single, to be free from unwarranted governmental intrusion into matters so fundamentally affecting a person as the decision whether to bear or beget a child. *Eisenstadt v. Baird*, 405 U.S. 438, 453, 92 S.Ct. 1029, 1038, 31 L.Ed.2d 349 (1972) (emphasis in original). *See also Carey v. Population Services International*, 431 U.S. 678, 685, 97 S.Ct. 2010, 2016, 52 L.Ed.2d 675 (1977) (decision whether or not to beget or bear a child fundamental to individual autonomy).

That a right to procreational autonomy is inherent in our most basic concepts of liberty is also indicated by the reproductive freedom cases, *see, e.g., Griswold v. Connecticut*, 381 U.S. 479, 85 S.Ct. 1678, 14 L.Ed.2d 510 (1965); and *Roe v. Wade*, 410 U.S. 113, 93 S.Ct. 705, 35 L.Ed.2d 147 (1973), and by cases concerning parental rights and responsibilities with respect to children. *See, e.g., Wisconsin v. Yoder*, 406 U.S. 205, 92 S.Ct. 1526, 32 L.Ed.2d 15 (1972); *Prince v. Massachusetts*, 321 U.S. 158, 64 S.Ct. 438, 88 L.Ed. 645 (1944); *Cleveland Board of Education v. LaFleur*, 414 U.S. 632, 94 S.Ct. 791, 39 L.Ed.2d 52 (1974); *Pierce v. Society of the Sisters of the Holy Names of Jesus and Mary*, 268 U.S. 510, 45 S.Ct. 571, 69 L.Ed. 1070 (1925); and *Bellotti v. Baird*, 443 U.S. 622, 99 S.Ct. 3035, 61 L.Ed.2d 797 (1979). In fact, in *Bellotti v. Baird*, the Supreme Court noted that parental autonomy is basic to the structure of our society because the family is "the institution by which we inculcate and pass down many of our most cherished values, morals and cultures." *Bellotti*, 443 U.S. at 634, 99 S.Ct. at 3043.

The United States Supreme Court has never addressed the issue of procreation in the context of *in vitro* fertilization. Moreover, the extent to which procreational autonomy is protected by the United States Constitution is no longer entirely clear. Justice Blackmun noted, in his dissent, that the plurality opinion in *Webster v. Reproductive Health Services*, 492 U.S. 490, 109 S.Ct. 3040, 106 L.Ed.2d 410 (1989), "turns a stone face to anyone in search of what the plurality conceives as the scope of a woman's right under the Due Process Clause to terminate a pregnancy free from the coercive and brooding influence of the State." *Id.* at 538, 109 S.Ct. at 3067. The *Webster* opinion lends even less guidance to those seeking the bounds of constitutional protection of other aspects of procreational autonomy.[11]

For the purposes of this litigation it is sufficient to note that, whatever its ultimate constitutional boundaries, the right of procreational autonomy is composed of two rights of equal significance — the right to procreate and the right to avoid procreation. Undoubtedly, both are subject to protections and limitations. *See e.g., Prince v. Massachusetts*, 321 U.S. 158, 64 S.Ct. 438, 88 L.Ed. 645 (1944) (parental control over the education or health care of their children subject to some limits); *Roe v. Wade*, 410 U.S. 113, 93 S.Ct. 705, 35 L.Ed.2d 147 (1973) (states' interests in potential life overcomes right to avoid procreation by abortion in later states of pregnancy).

The equivalence of and inherent tension between these two interests are nowhere more evident than in the context of *in vitro* fertilization. None of the concerns about a woman's bodily integrity that have previously precluded men from controlling abortion decisions is applicable here.[12] We are not unmindful of the fact that the trauma (including both emotional stress and physical discomfort) to which women

---

[11] [n.23] Justice O'Connor did note in her concurring opinion in *Webster* that the plurality's position might threaten the development of IVF programs. Despite her concern, she voted to uphold the Missouri statute at issue, because she found the possibility "too hypothetical to support the use of declaratory judgment procedures and injunctive remedies" since there was no indication that Missouri might seek to prohibit IVF programs. *Webster*, 492 U.S. at 523, 109 S.Ct. at 3054 (O'Connor, J., concurring).

[12] [n.24] See *Planned Parenthood v. Danforth*, 428 U.S. 52, 71, 96 S.Ct. 2831, 2842, 49 L.Ed. 788 (1976) ("Inasmuch as it is the woman who physically bears the child and who is the more directly and immediately affected by the pregnancy, as between the two, the balance weighs in her favor."). *See* discussion in *Developments in the Law — Medical Technology and the Law*, 103 Harv. L. Rev. 1519, 1544-45 (1990).

are subjected in the IVF process is more severe than is the impact of the procedure on men. In this sense, it is fair to say that women contribute more to the IVF process than men. Their experience, however, must be viewed in light of the joys of parenthood that is desired or the relative anguish of a lifetime of unwanted parenthood. As they stand on the brink of potential parenthood, Mary Sue Davis and Junior Lewis Davis must be seen as entirely equivalent gamete-providers.

It is further evident that, however far the protection of procreational autonomy extends, the existence of the right itself dictates that decisional authority rests in the gamete-providers alone, at least to the extent that their decisions have an impact upon their individual reproductive status . . . [N]o other person or entity has an interest sufficient to permit interference with the gamete-providers' decision to continue or terminate the IVF process, because no one else bears the consequences of these decisions in the way that the gamete-providers do.

Further, at least with respect to Tennessee's public policy and its constitutional right of privacy, the state's interest in potential human life is insufficient to justify an infringement on the gamete-providers' procreational autonomy. The United States Supreme Court has indicated in *Webster*, and even in *Roe*, that the state's interest in potential human life may justify statutes or regulations that have an impact upon a person's exercise of procreational autonomy. This potential for sufficiently weighty state's interests is not, however, at issue here, because Tennessee's statutes contain no statement of public policy which reveals an interest that could justify infringing on gamete-providers' decisional authority over the preembryos to which they have contributed . . .

Certainly, if the state's interests do not become sufficiently compelling in the abortion context until the end of the first trimester, after very significant developmental stages have passed, then surely there is no state interest in these preembryos which could suffice to overcome the interests of the gamete-providers. The abortion statute reveals that the increase in the state's interest is marked by each successive developmental stage such that, toward the end of a pregnancy, this interest is so compelling that abortion is almost strictly forbidden. This scheme supports the conclusion that the state's interest in the potential life embodied by these four- to eight-cell preembryos (which may or may not be able to achieve implantation in a uterine wall and which, if implanted, may or may not begin to develop into fetuses, subject to possible miscarriage) is at best slight. When weighed against the interests of the individuals and the burdens inherent in parenthood, the state's interest in the potential life of these preembryos is not sufficient to justify any infringement upon the freedom of these individuals to make their own decisions as to whether to allow a process to continue that may result in such a dramatic change in their lives as becoming parents.

The unique nature of this case requires us to note that the interests of these parties in parenthood are different in scope than the parental interest considered in other cases. Previously, courts have dealt with the child-bearing and child-rearing aspects of parenthood. Abortion cases have dealt with gestational parenthood. In this case, the Court must deal with the question of genetic parenthood. We conclude, moreover, that an interest in avoiding genetic parenthood can be significant enough to trigger the protections afforded to all other aspects of parenthood. The technological fact that someone unknown to these parties could gestate these preembryos does not alter the fact that these parties, the gamete-providers, would become parents in that event, at least in the genetic sense. The profound impact this would have on them supports their right to sole decisional authority as to whether the process of attempting to gestate these preembryos should continue. This brings us directly to the question of how to resolve the dispute that arises when one party wishes to continue the IVF process and the other does not.

VII. *Balancing the Parties' Interests*

Resolving disputes over conflicting interests of constitutional import is a task familiar to the courts. One way of resolving these disputes is to consider the positions of the parties, the significance of their interests, and the relative burdens that will be imposed by differing resolutions. In this case, the issue centers on the two aspects of procreational autonomy — the right to procreate and the right to avoid procreation. We start by considering the burdens imposed on the parties by solutions that would have the effect of disallowing the exercise of individual procreational autonomy with respect to these particular preembryos.

Beginning with the burden imposed on Junior Davis, we note that the consequences are obvious. Any disposition which results in the gestation of the preembryos would impose unwanted parenthood on him, with all of its possible financial and psychological consequences. The impact that this unwanted parenthood would have on Junior Davis can only be understood by considering his particular circumstances, as revealed in the record.

Junior Davis testified that he was the fifth youngest of six children. When he was five years old, his parents divorced, his mother had a nervous break-down, and he and three of his brothers went to live at a home for boys run by the Lutheran Church. Another brother was taken in by an aunt, and his sister stayed with their mother. From that day forward, he had monthly visits with his mother but saw his father only three more times before he died in 1976. Junior Davis testified that, as a boy, he had severe problems caused by separation from his parents. He said that it was especially hard to leave his mother after each monthly visit. He clearly feels that he has suffered because of his lack of opportunity to establish a relationship with his parents and particularly because of the absence of his father.

In light of his boyhood experiences, Junior Davis is vehemently opposed to fathering a child that would not live with both parents. Regardless of whether he or Mary Sue had custody, he feels that the child's bond with the non-custodial parent would not be satisfactory. He testified very clearly that his concern was for the psychological obstacles a child in such a situation would face, as well as the burdens it would impose on him. Likewise, he is opposed to donation because the recipient couple might divorce, leaving the child (which he definitely would consider his own) in a single-parent setting.

Balanced against Junior Davis's interest in avoiding parenthood is Mary Sue Davis's interest in donating the preembryos to another couple for implantation. Refusal to permit donation of the preembryos would impose on her the burden of knowing that the lengthy IVF procedures she underwent were futile, and that the preembryos to which she contributed genetic material would never become children. While this is not an insubstantial emotional burden, we can only conclude that Mary Sue Davis's interest in donation is not as significant as the interest Junior Davis has in avoiding parenthood. If she were allowed to donate these preembryos, he would face a lifetime of either wondering about his parental status or knowing about his parental status but having no control over it. He testified quite clearly that if these preembryos were brought to term he would fight for custody of his child or children. Donation, if a child came of it, would rob him twice — his procreational autonomy would be defeated and his relationship with his offspring would be prohibited.

The case would be closer if Mary Sue Davis were seeking to use the preembryos herself, but only if she could not achieve parenthood by any other reasonable means. We recognize the trauma that Mary Sue has already experienced and the additional discomfort to which she would be subjected if she opts to attempt IVF again. Still, she would have a reasonable opportunity, through IVF, to try once again to achieve parenthood in all its aspects — genetic, gestational, bearing, and rearing.

Further, we note that if Mary Sue Davis were unable to undergo another round of IVF, or opted not to try, she could still achieve the child-rearing aspects of parenthood through adoption. The fact that she and Junior Davis pursued adoption indicates that, at least at one time, she was willing to forego genetic parenthood and would have been satisfied by the child-rearing aspects of parenthood alone . . .

REID, C.J., and DROWOTA, O'BRIEN and ANDERSON, JJ., concur.

NOTES AND QUESTIONS

1. The court in *Davis v. Davis* acknowledges that reproductive autonomy is composed of two equally important rights — the right to engage in reproduction and the right to avoid reproduction. Under the case facts, the court concludes that Junior Davis' right to avoid procreation outweighs Mary Sue's interest in donating the frozen embryos to another couple for gestation. But what if Mary Sue were in the early stages of pregnancy when the couple split. Would Junior be able to exercise his right to avoid procreation and demand that Mary Sue abort the pregnancy? Would Junior's right become stronger if Mary Sue planned to place the child out for adoption? After all, the husband could argue that his ex-wife's "interest in donation is not as significant as the interest Junior Davis has in avoiding parenthood." What distinguishes the frozen embryo from the adoption scenario?

Clearly the distinguishing feature is the pregnancy. When a woman is pregnant her rights to unilaterally decide whether to continue or terminate the pregnancy are solidly protected, but when she is merely in the process of becoming pregnant through assisted conception, she shares equally any rights to determine the status of the prospective pregnancy with her male counterpart. Should pregnancy be the gatekeeper for reproductive rights? If so, then does the requirement of pregnancy create roadblocks for infertile women in the exercise of their procreational liberty? Consider one perspective:

An infertile woman's fundamental right to procreate is essentially suspended, rather than wholly deprived. It can be asserted that both a fertility patient and a nonfertility patient stand equally on the brink of the reproductive process with their fundamental right to procreate intact. But once the physiological process begins, their fundamental rights are viewed differently. A woman who experiences an in vivo pregnancy is fully protected by *Roe* and its progeny, while a fertility patient essentially loses her fundamental right to procreate once the egg is harvested from her ovary. The fertility patient's rights are not restored until the embryo is returned to her body and attaches itself to her uterine wall.

Judith F. Daar, *Assisted Reproductive Technologies and the Pregnancy Process: Developing an Equality Model to Protect Reproductive Liberties*, 25 AM. J. LAW 7 Med. 455, 465 (1999).

2. In traditional (coital) reproduction, the exercise of procreational rights is always genetically based. That is, the rights at stake involve the act of passing (or refusing to pass) one's genetic heritage to a child through one's gametes. What if the reproduction does not involve passing one's genetic heritage, such as when donor gametes are used? Does a person's reproductive liberty lessen when his or her actions toward conception, gestation and child rearing are unaccompanied by a genetic link to the resulting child? For example, under the *Davis* facts, would the outcome be the same if the embryos were procured with the aid of a sperm donor? If Junior consented to the use of a sperm donor and assisted Mary Sue in the IVF process, would his right to avoid procreation still outweigh his wife's interest in assuring that the embryos are donated to another couple?

3. Suppose that Husband and Wife wish to have a child but need assistance from third parties because the wife is unable to produce eggs or gestate a child due to a previous hysterectomy in which her ovaries and uterus were removed. Using H's sperm and a donor's eggs, five embryos are created. Three are implanted in a woman who agrees to gestate the couple's embryos for a fee. The remaining two embryos are frozen for later use. If the gestational carrier becomes pregnant, does she have the right to terminate the pregnancy even if the couple strongly opposes such action? What if a prenatal test reveals that the child will suffer from a severe and painful handicap? Can the couple force the pregnant woman to abort "their" fetus? Whose reproductive rights are at stake in this scenario?

What about W's rights with regard to the two frozen embryos? What if the couple divorces and battles over the disposition of the remaining embryos? If H wants to enlist the same woman to gestate the embryos but W wants them destroyed, is W's right to avoid procreation at stake? See *Litowitz v. Litowitz*, 10 P.3d 1086 (Wash. App. 2000), *rev'd*, 48 P.3d 261 (Wash. 2002) (spouse who does not contribute gametes to embryo does not have a constitutional right to procreate). What if W wants to hire a surrogate to gestate the embryos and H objects? Are her rights to control the early embryo reduced or even abrogated because she lacks a genetic tie to the embryo? See Lainie M.C. Dillon, *Conundrums With Penumbras: The Right to Privacy Encompasses Non-Providers Who Create Preembryos With the Intent to Become Parents*, 78 WASH. L. REV. 625 (2003) (arguing gamete and non-gamete providers who create preembryos with the intent to become a parent have made an intimate decision involving procreation, marriage, and family life that falls squarely within the right to privacy and should be afforded equal constitutional protection).

The exercise of the right to procreate grows complicated as third parties enter the reproductive relationship. But the right can be equally complicated when only two parties are involved, if one of those parties is an inmate in a state prison serving a 100 years to life sentence. Consider the next case.

GERBER v. HICKMAN
United States Court of Appeals, Ninth Circuit
291 F.3d 617 (2002)

SILVERMAN, C.J.

William Gerber, an inmate in the California State prison system, filed an amended complaint in federal court in which he alleged: "Petitioner asserts that Mule Creek State Prison is violating his Constitutional Rights by not allowing him to provide his wife with a sperm specimen that she may use to be artificially inseminated." Gerber sought an order of the court directing the institution to permit him to provide "a sample of sperm to artificially inseminate his wife."

The district court dismissed Gerber's suit for failure to state a claim, ruling that a prisoner does not have a constitutional right to procreate while incarcerated. *Gerber v. Hickman*, 103 F.Supp.2d 1214, 1216-18 (E.D.Cal.2000). Because we agree with the district court that the right to procreate is fundamentally inconsistent with incarceration, we affirm.

I. BACKGROUND

We adopt the statement of facts from the district court's thoughtful opinion: Plaintiff, a forty-one year old man, is an inmate at Mule Creek State Prison serving a sentence of 100 years to life plus eleven years. Plaintiff's wife, Evelyn Gerber, is forty-four years old. Plaintiff and his wife want to have a baby. The California Department of Corrections ("CDC") prohibits family visits for inmates "sentenced to life without the possibility of parole [or] sentenced to life, without a parole date established by the Board of Prison Terms." Cal.Code Regs. tit. 15 § 3174(e)(2). No parole date has been set for plaintiff, and according to plaintiff, due to the length of his sentence, no parole date seems likely. Accordingly, he wishes to artificially inseminate his wife. To accomplish this, plaintiff requests that (1) a laboratory be permitted to mail him a plastic collection container at the prison along with a prepaid return mailer, (2) he be permitted to ejaculate into the container, and (3) the filled container be returned to the laboratory in the prepaid mailer by overnight mail. Alternatively, plaintiff requests that his counsel be permitted to personally pick up the container for transfer to the laboratory or health care provider. Plaintiff represents that he and his wife will bear all of the costs associated therewith, including any costs incurred by the CDC. Defendant [Hickman] refuses to accommodate plaintiff's request.

Gerber, 103 F.Supp.2d at 1216 (first alteration in original).

II. JURISDICTION AND STANDARD OF REVIEW

We have jurisdiction over this appeal pursuant to 28 U.S.C. § 1291, and we review de novo a district court's dismissal for failure to state a claim. *Monterey Plaza Hotel, Ltd. v. Local 483*, 215 F.3d 923, 926 (9th Cir. 2000).

III. ANALYSIS

A. Fundamental Rights in the Prison Setting

It is well-settled that "[p]rison walls do not form a barrier separating prison inmates from the protections of the Constitution." *Turner v. Safley*, 482 U.S. 78, 84, 107 S.Ct. 2254, 96 L.Ed.2d 64 (1987). A state could not, for example, decide to ban inmate access to mail or prohibit access to the courts. However, "while persons imprisoned . . . enjoy many protections of the Constitution, it is also clear that imprisonment carries with it the . . . loss of many significant rights." *Hudson v. Palmer*, 468 U.S. 517, 524, 104 S.Ct. 3194, 82 L.Ed.2d 393 (1984). The very fact of incarceration thus "withdraw[s] or limit[s] . . . many privileges and rights," and this "retraction [is] justified by the considerations underlying our penal system." *Pell v. Procunier*, 417 U.S. 817, 822, 94 S.Ct. 2800, 41 L.Ed.2d 495 (1974) (internal quotation marks omitted). Prisoners retain only those rights "not inconsistent with [their] status as . . . prisoner[s] or with the legitimate penological objectives of the corrections system." *Hudson*, 468 U.S. at 523, 104 S.Ct. 3194 (quoting *Pell*, 417 U.S. at 822, 94 S.Ct. 2800) (alterations in original).

Gerber challenges the prison's refusal to allow him to artificially inseminate his wife from prison. In order to determine whether this amounts to an impermissible deprivation of Gerber's constitutional rights, our inquiry is two-fold. First, we must determine whether the right to procreate while in prison is fundamentally inconsistent with incarceration. *Turner*, 482 U.S. at 94-96, 107 S.Ct. 2254. If so, this ends our inquiry. Prisoners cannot claim the protection of those rights fundamentally inconsistent with their status as prisoners.

Only if we determine that the asserted right is not inconsistent with incarceration do we proceed to the second question: Is the prison regulation abridging that right reasonably related to legitimate penological interests? *Turner*, 482 U.S. at 96-99, 107 S.Ct. 2254. If it is, the regulation is valid; if not, it is unconstitutional.

B. Whether the Right to Procreate is Fundamentally Inconsistent with Incarceration

1.

We begin our analysis by inquiring whether the right to procreate is fundamentally inconsistent with incarceration. Incarceration, by its very nature, removes an inmate from society. *Pell*, 417 U.S. at 822-23, 94 S.Ct. 2800. A necessary corollary to this removal is the separation of the prisoner from his spouse, his loved ones, his friends, family, and children . . . Once released from confinement, an inmate "can be gainfully employed and is free to be with family and friends and to form the other enduring attachments of normal life." *Morrissey v. Brewer*, 408 U.S. 471, 482, 92 S.Ct. 2593, 33 L.Ed.2d 484 (1972). But not until then.

During the period of confinement in prison, the right of intimate association, "a fundamental element of personal liberty," *Roberts v. United States Jaycees*, 468 U.S. 609, 618, 104 S.Ct. 3244, 82 L.Ed.2d 462 (1984), is necessarily abridged. Intimate association protects the kinds of relationships "that attend the creation and sustenance of a family — marriage, childbirth, the raising and education of children, and cohabitation with one's relatives . . ." *Id.* at 619, 104 S.Ct. 3244 (citations omitted). The loss of the right to intimate association is simply part and parcel of being imprisoned for conviction of a crime.

"[M]any aspects of marriage that make it a basic civil right, such as cohabitation, sexual intercourse, and the bearing and rearing of children, are superseded by the fact of confinement." *Goodwin v. Turner*, 702 F.Supp. 1452, 1454 (W.D.Mo.1988). Thus, while the basic right to marry survives imprisonment, *Turner*, 482 U.S. at 96, 107 S.Ct. 2254, most of the attributes of marriage — cohabitation, physical intimacy, and bearing and raising children — do not. "Rights of marital privacy, like the right to marry and procreate, are necessarily and substantially abridged in a prison setting." *Hernandez v. Coughlin*, 18 F.3d 133, 137 (2d Cir.1994) (citing *Turner*, 482 U.S. at 95-96, 107 S.Ct. 2254). Incarceration is simply inconsistent with the vast majority of concomitants to marriage, privacy, and personal intimacy . . .

[I]t is well-settled that prisoners have no constitutional right while incarcerated to contact visits or conjugal visits. See *Kentucky Dep't of Corrs. v. Thompson*, 490 U.S. 454, 460, 109 S.Ct. 1904, 104 L.Ed.2d 506 (1989) (no due process right to unfettered visitation); *Block v. Rutherford*, 468 U.S. 576, 585-88, 104 S.Ct. 3227, 82 L.Ed.2d 438 (1984) (pretrial detainees have no constitutional due process right to contact visits); *Hernandez*, 18 F.3d at 137 (no constitutional right to conjugal visits); *Davis v. Carlson*, 837 F.2d 1318, 1319 (5th Cir.1988) (same); *Toussaint v. McCarthy*, 801 F.2d 1080, 1113-1114 (9th Cir.1986) (denial of contact visits does not violate Eighth Amendment). The fact that California prison officials may choose to permit some inmates the privilege of conjugal visits is simply irrelevant to whether there is a constitutional right to conjugal visits or a right to procreate while in prison.

It is difficult, if not impossible, to reconcile the holdings of cases like *Turner, Hudson,* and *Pell* and an understanding of the nature and goals of a prison system, with a wholly unprecedented reading of the constitution that would command the warden to accommodate Gerber's request to artificially inseminate his wife as a matter of right.

2.

One issue that arose during oral argument was the effect of technological advancement on the issue before us. If, for example, science progressed to the point where Gerber could artificially inseminate his wife as easily as write her a letter, would this change our analysis? It would not. Our conclusion that the right to procreate is inconsistent with incarceration is not dependent on the science of artificial insemination, or on how easy or difficult it is to accomplish. Rather, it is a conclusion that stems from consideration of the nature and goals of the correctional system, including isolating prisoners, deterring crime, punishing offenders, and providing rehabilitation. See generally Jack B. Weinstein & Catherine Wimberly, *Secrecy in Law and Science*, 23 Cardozo L.Rev. 1, 9-11 (2001) (discussing the interaction between law and science).

3.

Gerber argues that the right to be free from forced surgical sterilization, *Skinner v. Oklahoma*, 316 U.S. 535, 62 S.Ct. 1110, 86 L.Ed. 1655 (1942), combined with the right to marry while in prison, *Turner*, 482 U.S. at 96, 107 S.Ct. 2254, inevitably leads to the conclusion that inmates have a constitutional right to procreate while in prison. This argument fails for two reasons. First, *Skinner* stands only for the proposition that forced surgical sterilization of prisoners violates the Equal Protection Clause. The Court in *Skinner* recognized that procreation is fundamental to the existence of the race, and thus the state's "power to sterilize, if exercised, may have subtle, far-reaching and devastating effects." *Skinner*, 316 U.S. at 541, 62 S.Ct. 1110. Sterilization is intrusive, permanent, and irreparable. By no stretch of the imagination, however, did *Skinner* hold that inmates have the right to exercise their ability to procreate while still in prison. The right to procreate while incarcerated and the right to be free from surgical sterilization by prison officials are two very different things. "There is simply no comparison between sterilization . . . and denial of the facilitation of artificial insemination." *Goodwin*, 702 F.Supp. at 1454 (citation omitted). The Second Circuit in *Hernandez*, 18 F.3d at 136, has recognized this crucial distinction, noting in its discussion of *Skinner* that "inmates possess the right to maintain their procreative abilities for later use once released from custody. . . ." Later use, not current use.

Second, the Supreme Court in Turner recognized that an inmate's right to marry while in prison did not include the inmate's right to consummate the marriage while in prison or to enjoy the other tangible aspects of marital intimacy . . .

A holding that the State of California must accommodate Gerber's request to artificially inseminate his wife as a matter of constitutional right would be a radical and unprecedented interpretation of the Constitution. We hold that the right to procreate while in prison is fundamentally inconsistent with incarceration. Accordingly, we do not reach the second part of the analysis to inquire whether the prison's regulation is related to a valid penological interest . . .

Gerber also argues that denial of his artificial insemination request violates the Eighth Amendment's prohibition against cruel and unusual punishment. Because the state's denial of his request to artificially inseminate his wife can by no means be considered a deprivation of "the minimal civilized measure of life's necessities," *Hudson v. McMillian*, 503 U.S. 1, 9, 112 S.Ct. 995, 117 L.Ed.2d 156 (1992), granting leave for Gerber to allege an Eight Amendment claim would have been futile . . . The district court therefore acted within its discretion in dismissing Gerber's complaint without permitting leave to amend.

AFFIRMED.

[This en banc decision was joined by Chief Judge Schroeder and Judges O'Scannlain, Rymer, Gould, and Rawlinson. Judge Tashima filed a dissenting opinion in which Judges Kozinski, Hawkins, Paez, and Berzon joined. A second dissenting opinion follows.]

KOZINSKI, CIRCUIT JUDGE, with whom JUDGES PAEZ and BERZON join, dissenting:

The majority hinges its opinion on the proposition that "the right to procreate is fundamentally inconsistent with incarceration," Maj. Op. at 620, but does not explain how. Let's consider the possibilities. Gerber asks for permission to:

1. Ejaculate

2. into a plastic cup, which is then to be

3. mailed or given to his lawyer

4. for delivery to a laboratory

5. that will try to use its contents to artificially inseminate Mrs. Gerber.

I gather that the first step of this process is not fundamentally inconsistent with incarceration and prison guards don't patrol cell blocks at night looking for inmates committing Onan's transgression. Similarly, the prison has no penological interest in what prisoners do with their seed once it's spilt; a specimen cup would seem to be no worse a receptacle, from the prison's point of view, than any other.

Nor is there anything remotely inconsistent with incarceration in mailing a package, or handing it to your lawyer. Sure, the prison is entitled to make sure it doesn't contain prison escape plans, but Gerber is not claiming an exemption from routine security checks. That a package contains semen, rather than a book or an ashtray or some other such object, would seem to make no rational difference from the prison's point of view.

Once the package is outside prison walls, the prison's legitimate interest in it is greatly diminished. That it is to be delivered to a laboratory, rather than to any other willing recipient, seems to make no difference to prison authorities; certainly they have offered no proof that it does. Nor, I would think, does the prison have a legitimate interest in what the recipient does with the package. Whether it is used to inseminate Mrs. Gerber, to clone Gerber or as a paperweight has no conceivable effect on the safe and efficient operation of the California prison system. Thus, what Gerber seeks to do is not inconsistent with incarceration the way it would be if he wanted to carry a Glock or conduct nuclear fission experiments in his cell. Production of the semen and delivery to a laboratory neither compromises security, nor places a strain on prison resources beyond that required to mail any other package.

Perhaps the majority is talking about a different kind of inconsistency altogether. Prison is meant to deny inmates certain rights enjoyed by free people; loss of those rights is the punishment. It would be inconsistent with Gerber's status as an inmate for him to vacation in Paris or spend the weekend at home, because the very point of incarceration is to deny prisoners freedom of movement and the comforts of home. When the legislature imposes imprisonment as punishment for a crime, it necessarily curtails all those other rights that require freedom of physical movement for their exercise.

Is procreation one of those rights the exercise of which is inconsistent with the prisoner's loss of his freedom of locomotion? Apparently not, at least as Gerber proposes to exercise it. Gerber is not asking to go home for a conjugal visit, nor to enjoy such a visit within the prison; he does not seek to loosen the strictures of his confinement in the least. Gerber asks only to engage in activities that prisoners are already free to engage in (see steps 1-3 above). That these activities might result in the creation of a life outside prison walls is no more inconsistent with Gerber's status as a prisoner than is any other consequence of mailing materials from prison to the outside world. Thus, a prisoner might become a best-selling author by sending out a manuscript for a novel or biography. *See, e.g.*, O.J. Simpson, *I Want to Tell You* (1995); . . . These activities may give the prisoner great wealth and satisfaction . . . but they are not inconsistent with his status as a prisoner because the physical acts required to accomplish them are entirely consistent with incarceration . . .

[T]here is . . . nothing inherently inconsistent about the mechanics of procreation — at least as Gerber proposes to practice them — that would compromise prison security, unduly burden prison resources or otherwise interfere with the safe and efficient operation of the California prison system.

What then is left? It is nothing more than the ad hoc decision of prison authorities that Gerber may not procreate. But, as the majority seems to admit, and as *Griswold v. Connecticut*, 381 U.S. 479, 85 S.Ct. 1678, 14 L.Ed.2d 510 (1965), clearly holds, procreation (at least within the marital relationship) is a fundamental right. Such a right may be abrogated only pursuant to lawful authority and for compelling reasons. The reasons here must be particularly strong because the burden of this prohibition falls not only on Gerber but also on Mrs. Gerber, who is precluded from bearing a child fathered by her husband. As the Supreme Court noted in *Turner*, when a prison regulation creates a "consequential restriction on the [constitutional] rights of those who are *not* prisoners," it will be subjected to more searching scrutiny than when the burden falls only on inmates. *Turner*, 482 U.S. at 85, 107 S.Ct. 2254 . . .

The majority suggests that abrogating the right to procreate serves the goals of "isolating prisoners, deterring crime, punishing offenders, and providing rehabilitation . . . But such judgments must be made by the legislature in setting the nature and degree of punishment for particular crimes. Prison administrators may not supplement the punishment imposed by the legislature because they believe doing so would enhance "deterrence and retribution." By cutting off Gerber's fundamental right to procreate, prison authorities have enhanced Gerber's punishment beyond that authorized by statute, and consigned Mrs. Gerber to a childless marriage. These are rights far too important to be abrogated based on nothing more than the personal opinion of prison bureaucrats that we would be better off as a society if the Gerbers were prevented from parenting an offspring. For these reasons . . . I respectfully dissent.

NOTES AND QUESTIONS

1.   The Ninth Circuit decision in *Gerber v. Hickman* is an *en banc* decision by the appellate court. *En banc*, meaning "full bench," refers to a session where the entire membership of the court participates in the decision rather than the regular quorum of three judges. According to the rules of the Ninth Circuit, an *en banc* panel consists of the Chief Judge of the circuit and 10 additional judges drawn by lot from the active judges of the court. United States Court of Appeals for the Ninth Circuit Rule 35-3. The Ninth Circuit's Rules provide the ground for granting a petition for *en banc* review as follows:

> When the opinion of a panel directly conflicts with an existing opinion by another court of appeals and substantially affects a rule of national application in which there is an overriding need for national uniformity, the existence of such conflict is an appropriate ground for suggesting a rehearing *en banc*.

United States Court of Appeals for the Ninth Circuit Rule 35-1. The *en banc* decision reverses an earlier decision by the Ninth Circuit, which held that Gerber's fundamental right to procreate was not inconsistent with his status as a prisoner and thus survived his incarceration. Further, the court held that the prison regulation abridging his right to procreate was not reasonably related to legitimate penological interests. *Gerber v. Hickman*, 264 F.3d 882 (9th Cir. 2001). With this 2001 decision, the Ninth Circuit became the first court in the nation to hold that the right to procreate does survive incarceration. With all other appellate decisions to the contrary, the first Ninth Circuit decision became an "option of a panel [that] directly conflicts with an existing opinion by another court of appeals," opening the opportunity for *en banc* review. For a discussion of the other cases addressing prisoners' rights to procreate, see Richard Guidice Jr., *Procreation and the Prisoner: Does the Right to Procreate Survive Incarceration and Do Legitimate Penological Interests Justify Restrictions on the Exercise of the Right*, 29 FORDHAM URBAN L. J. 2277 (2002).

2.   *An International Perspective.* Prisoners in other countries have also petitioned to preserve their right to reproduce. In a few cases, courts have granted these requests, paving the way for the delivery of sperm outside the prison walls. In Israel, the assassin who gunned down Prime Minister Yitzhak Rabin in 1995 was allowed to father a child using insemination according to a High Court of Justice decision in 2006. Unlike the court in *Gerber*, the Israeli court held that the prisoner "has basic human rights that were not appropriated from him when he went to prison." *See* Yuval Yoaz, *High Court Rules Amir May Inseminate Partner*, Haaretz.com, June 14, 2006, available at: http://www.haaretz.com/print-edition/news/high-court-rules-amir-may-inseminate-partner-he-has-basic-human-rights-1.190228. In 2007, the Grand Chamber of the European Court of Human Rights granted a British prisoner's request for access to artificial insemination. *See* Steve Doughty, *Killer in Prison Wins Right to Father a Child by Artificial Insemination*, MailOnline, Dec. 4, 2007, available at: http://www.dailymail.co.uk/news/article-499744/Killer-prison-wins-right-father-child-artificial-insemination.html.   What's more, the convicted murderer was awarded approximately $25,000 in damages, to be paid by the British government, for trampling his right to reproduce.

3. *Does Gender Matter?* If a U.S. court found that a prisoner's right to procreate survived incarceration, presumably it would have to apply that ruling in a gender-neutral fashion. If male prisoners are permitted to provide their semen for use in artificial insemination, then female prisoners should likewise be able to harvest their eggs for use in IVF. Eggs could be combined with a husband or partner's sperm and the resulting embryos could either be transferred to a gestational carrier or frozen for later use by the prisoner. Do you think the court had this female scenario in mind when it ruled that the right to procreate while in prison is fundamentally inconsistent with incarceration? The fact is there are fundamental differences when it comes to assisted conception by males and females. As the dissent points out, a male prisoner's provision of gametes requires conduct that causes minimal, if any, deviation from his normal, permissive routine. While a female prisoner who wishes to produce, retrieve and send off eggs would require a significant deviation from routine prison practices. Moreover, if a female prisoner could exercise her right to procreate by sending her eggs outside the prison walls, why couldn't she exercise the same right by importing her husband's sperm into her prison cell? With a simple plastic tube, procreation could be achieved in a relatively unobtrusive manner. See Sarah L. Dunn, *The "ART" of Procreation: Why Assisted Reproduction Technology Allows For The Preservation of Female Prisoner's Right to Procreate*, 70 FORDHAM L. REV. 2561 (2002) (arguing the right to procreate while in prison should be recognized for both men and women). For an argument that males are afforded less protection of their procreative liberty than females, *see* Daniel Sperling, *'Male and Female He Created Them': Procreative Liberty, Its Conceptual Deficiencies and the Legal Right to Access Fertility Care of Males*, 7(3) INT'L J. L. IN CONTEXT 375 (2011).

4. *The Cost Factor.* The decisions in *Davis v. Davis* and *Gerber v. Hickman* suggest that the right to procreate is not absolute and, like other fundamental rights, must be weighed against competing interests such as the right to avoid procreation (*Davis*) and the right to an orderly administration of prison life (*Gerber*). Whether the right to procreate via assisted conception is on equal footing with the right to coital reproduction remains unclear, but what will come into sharp focus in the next chapter are the striking differences in costs. Mr. and Mrs. Gerber offered to pay for the cost of procuring and sending the specimen. But had the genders been reversed and Mrs. Gerber behind bars, how many couples (relying in a single income) could afford the expense associated with egg retrieval and IVF? Even when both spouses are liberated and employed, the costs of ART are staggering, leading to questions about market regulation and insurance reimbursement, to which we now turn.

Chapter 3

THE BUSINESS OF ART: SELLING, DONATING AND INSURING ASSISTED REPRODUCTION

The miracles of modern science always come at a cost, and the techniques of assisted reproduction are no exception. It is estimated that patients in this country spend approximately $4 billion annually on infertility-related goods and services. The bulk of those dollars are spent on IVF, which costs an average of $12,000 per attempt. In the vast majority of cases, patients must pay out-of-pocket for their infertility treatment, as ART is rarely covered by medical insurance. In addition to expenses for medical services, those needing assistance with childbearing may also incur costs associated with egg and sperm donors (an obvious misnomer since all non-relative gamete providers are paid), or women willing to serve, for a fee, as gestational carriers. The business of assisted reproductive technologies is undeniable and growing, despite a commonly held sentiment that the association between money and offspring is disquieting, if not downright unseemly. Let us now explore this association, delving into the question of who pays and who profits in the provision of ART services.

SECTION I: UNDERSTANDING THE MARKET FOR REPRODUCTIVE TECHNOLOGIES

A. Fertility Clinics as Providers of ART Services

1. A Patient's Perspective

Today there are no shortage of articles, interviews, autobiographies and blogs documenting a patient's journey through ART. Watching assisted conception become just another form of family formation means hearing from the thousands of individuals who journey to the nation's fertility clinics each year. While every patient's experience is unique to his or her circumstances, certain themes do emerge from the collected works of ART storytellers. First, fertility treatment is expensive. For most people, the expense is an unaffordable burden on the household budget. As one newspaper story recounts, prospective patients will spend more than they have on the chance for biologic parenthood. Documenting the case of one woman who spent four years and $300,000 to have a baby, the reporter writes:

> Most couples cannot afford what she spent: she charged the bills for her treatment on her husband's credit card. But more and more women are entering the fertility vortex and finding that despite themselves, they will go as far as needed, spend whatever they can scrape up, take out second and third mortgages on their homes, and travel across the country and even

overseas for tests and treatments, all in the hope of becoming pregnant.

Gina Kolata, *The Heart's Desire*, NY Times, May 11, 2004, at F1. A second theme that emerges from first hand accounts of ART is that the diagnosis and treatment of infertility is emotionally difficult, even devastating. Such is the case even when the patient has ample funds to afford multiple cycles of IVF. World famous singer Celine Dion spoke publically about her attempt to conceive a second child using in vitro. She told People magazine that her five failed IVF cycles were physically and emotionally exhausting. In a cover story titled "My Private Heartbreak," the then 41-year old artist confessed "I'm going to try until it works." She detailed the strain of giving herself daily hormone injections and enduring the "roller-coaster ride of emotions they bring." Marisa Laudadio, Celine Dion's Struggle for a Second Baby, People, Feb. 10, 2010. For Celine and her manager-husband Rene Angélil, the sixth time was the charm. In November 2010, the couple welcomed twin sons Nelson and Eddy.

NOTES AND QUESTIONS

1. *The Costs of IVF.* The above brief vignettes are intended to demonstrate that a diagnosis of infertility can be both emotionally and financially devastating. For every women like Celine Dion who decides to jump aboard the ART train, there are hundreds of infertile individuals who simply lack the economic resources to access the costly treatments. The cost for a single IVF cycle will typically fall somewhere between $10,000 to $14,000, this figure representing the "no-frills" treatment option, that is, IVF excluding ICSI, freezing costs for extra embryos and any fees paid to gamete donors.

For anyone facing the prospect of IVF treatment, a legitimate question arises: How much can I expect to pay to give birth to a live baby? That question looks beyond the cost of a single IVF cycle to take into account the probability of achieving a delivery as a result of that cycle. In a study published in the New England Journal of Medicine, researchers investigated the average cost of a successful delivery with IVF. The study examined the costs associated with IVF, including the fees for initial consultation, laboratory tests, medications, ultrasonography, egg retrieval, gamete culturing, embryo transfer, and physician and nursing services. The cost assumptions also included calculations for time away from work, maternal complications associated with the procedure, and neonatal complications due to multiple births. On average, researchers concluded that the cost incurred per successful delivery with IVF increases from $66,667 for the first cycle to $114,286 by the sixth cycle. For couples in which the woman is older and there is a diagnosis of male-factor infertility, the cost rises from $160,000 for the first cycle to $800,000 for the sixth. *See* Peter J. Neumann, Soheyla D. Gharib, & Milton C. Weinstein, *The Cost of a Successful Delivery With In Vitro Fertilization*, 331 New Eng. J. Med. 239 (1994).

2. *Fertility Tourism.* If you already have concerns about the impact outsourcing of jobs has on the U.S. economy, consider the emerging phenomenon of fertility tourism. A January 2005 news report reveals that a small but growing number of U.S. couples are seeking treatment for their infertility in countries like South Africa, Israel, Italy, Germany and Canada, where the costs for IVF are generally

much lower than those in the U.S. Though costs may be lower, it is often difficult to measure other factors such as safety records, pregnancy success rates, and quality of donor gametes in other countries. Still, according to a South African fertility specialist, "For the price of one I.V.F. cycle in the U.S.A. the patient can come to South Africa, have the treatment done here in Cape Town and have a lovely holiday at the same time and still take some cash home." Felicia R. Lee, *Fertility Clinics Overseas Draw More From U.S.*, N.Y. TIMES, Jan. 25, 2005, at A1.

Fertility tourism, also called cross-border reproductive care, is a global reality. Three main factors motivate citizens to travel outside their country of domicile in search of fertility services abroad: cost, access and law. Let's look briefly at each of these factors.

The Cost of ART Worldwide. The cost of ART varies widely worldwide, incentivizing cross-border travel from departure countries with higher average IVF costs to more bargain-friendly destination jurisdictions. Compare the approximate cost of a single cycle of IVF in five different countries, measured in U.S. dollars:

United States	$12,000
United Kingdom	$6,000
Hungary	$3,000
South Africa	$3,000
Russia	$2,000

Clearly a woman in London could travel to Budapest for treatment and still spend less money than she would walking down the street to her local fertility clinic (assuming she opted out of the UK National Health Service system that does cover certain ART services). Fertility tourism is so common it has garnered its own phraseology. Google the term "IVF holiday" and you can slog through over 2,670,000 hits, including numerous specialty travel services including "IVF Travel Solutions" and "IVF Vacation.com." While traveling for treatment may save money for the intended parents, fertility tourism can add costs for the departure countries in the form of added health care expenses. In England, for example, a quarter of all ART-related multiple pregnancies originate outside the UK. British couples and individuals who travel abroad for IVF escape not just high prices, but restrictions that limit embryo transfers to one or two per cycle. These fertility tourists return home with twins or greater and seek medical care through the National Health Service for a high-risk pregnancy that their home country's laws are designed to avoid. *See* A. McKelvey, A.L. David, F. Shenhield, E.R. Jauniaux, *The Impact of Cross-Border Reproductive Care or "Fertility Tourism" on NHS Services*, BRIT. J. OBSTETRICS & GYNECOLOGY 1520 (2009).

Access to ART. Limited availability of ART services, including donor gametes, is often cited as a reason would-be parents travel abroad for treatment. Even if the home country does not prohibit the service or treatment, legal structures can limit access to the point where citizens calculate they are better off seeking ART outside the jurisdiction. For example, Canada and the UK ban compensation to gamete donors, relying instead on altruism. As a result, supplies of eggs and sperm are low and waiting times are long. Travel across borders to the U.S. (from Canada) and Spain (from countries in the European Union), where gamete supplies are buoyed by a system of compensation, is well-documented. *See* Louise Frances, *Passports, Tickets, Suncream, Sperm*, OBSERVER, Jan. 15, 2006. Traveling to access services not readily available in one's country of origin can produce unexpected consequences. At least one report warns that patients traveling to access donor eggs are surprised to discover their growing offspring display physical characteristics that are unlike those of either genetic parent — including the egg donor whose profile was carefully screened. The suspected culprit? A high stakes bait-and-switch by local agents. *See* Eric Blyth, *Tackling Issues in Cross-Border Reproductive Care*, BioNews.org.uk (May 18, 2009), available at: www.bionews.org.uk/commentary.lasso?storyid=4348%20.

Should it be unlawful in the departure country to travel abroad to access a product or service that is either banned or limited for reasons of national policy? Should fertility tourists be arrested when they re-enter their jurisdictional border for violating the law of their country? At least one country purports to punish women who travel abroad for donor insemination, banned in the homeland. *See* Jonathan Head, *Turkey Bans Trips Abroad for Artificial Insemination*, BBC News, Mar. 15, 2010, available at: http://news.bbc.co.uk/2/hi/8568733.stm.

Law as a Motivation for Fertility Travel. The patchwork of laws governing ART worldwide reflects legal schemes ranging from heavily restrictive to highly permissive. Some countries restrict *who* can access treatment (banning access to women over a certain age, to unmarried individuals, to same-sex couples), while others ban *what* can be accessed (prohibiting the use of donor gametes, embryo cryopreservation, genetic screening of preimplantation embryos, sex selection). Patients who want a banned service or fit a banned category have no other choice for biologic parenthood than to travel abroad for treatment. In December 2003, Italy passed what may be considered the most restrictive ART law in the world, prohibiting the use of donor gametes, genetic embryo screening, embryo freezing (making IVF more expensive because an egg retrieval surgery is required for each cycle), posthumous use of gametes, and treatment for unmarried women. A 2006 study revealed that Italian citizens are on the move in search of ART. In the years since the new law went into effect, Italian fertility tourism quadrupled, with several Spanish clinics reporting that Italians comprise 50% of their patient population. *See* Fabio Turone, *Italians are Forced to Go Abroad for Assisted Reproduction*, 333 BRITISH MED. J. 1192 (2006).

Scholars and policymakers have raised concerns about the impact fertility tourism has or might have on those in the destination countries. As with many goods and services heavily purchased by tourists, the costs of those items rise, often pricing local populations out of the market. More troubling, some see the marketing of women egg donors to foreigners as akin to sex tourism. Do you agree? *See* Richard F. Storrow, *Quests for Conception: Fertility Tourists, Globalization and Feminist Legal Theory*, 57 HAST. L.J. 295 (2005).

3. *Competition Among Doctors.* The high cost of infertility treatment certainly prices many out of the market, at the same time creating a competitive environment among fertility clinics to attract paying clients. In the U.S. there are approximately 1,700 reproductive endocrinologists (physicians specializing in reproductive medicine) staffing some 480 fertility clinics. By all accounts, these clinics vie for

patients using aggressive marketing and novel payment arrangements designed to land the highly sought-after patient of means. The hoopla surrounding the opening of one clinic in New Jersey in late 2001 seems telling of the fiercely competitive market for patients. When Reproductive Medicine Associates opened its doors in Morristown, they hired a marketing consultant, started weekly support group meetings for infertile couples and invited doctors to dinners, including a wine-tasting dinner with a sommelier flown in from France. See Gina Kolata, *Fertility Inc.: Clinics Race to Lure Clients*, N.Y. TIMES, January 1, 2002, at D1.

What impact do you think the competition for patients has on the area of reproductive medicine? You might guess, on the one hand, that competition lowers prices and enhances quality as doctors seek to attract patients with their technical skills and reasonable costs. But do you see another side to competition in this area? If a patient is attracted to a particular clinic, it is likely because of the patient's belief that the physician will succeed in helping her become pregnant and deliver a healthy child. With this in mind, what sort of behaviors might the clinic engage in to meet the patient's expectations?

4. *Novel Payment Arrangements.* Later in this chapter we will take a look at the availability of health insurance for infertility treatments. Suffice it to say that a majority of patients receive little or no coverage for the expensive treatments that comprise ART. Realizing that out-of-pocket payment of tens of thousands of dollars is not a possibility for most patients, physicians began to think about ways to make ART more accessible while still maintaining a reasonable profit margin. One novel payment arrangement involves the concept of a money back guarantee. The program is described in an issue of *Kiplinger's Personal Finance* magazine:

> . . . To make [IVF] more affordable and attract new patients, many clinics are offering a package deal, or "shared risk" approach. Such deals have become almost as controversial as the infertility technique used to be.

> Think of shared risk as a three-cycle special. You may be asked to pay $25,000 up front — much more than the $10,000 you would for a single standard IVF cycle — and in exchange you're promised three tries. If you become pregnant on the first attempt, you've spent more than you would have otherwise. If the second attempt is successful, you roughly break even. If you become pregnant on the third attempt — at this point, your odds have risen to a decent 75% or better — then you've saved money.

> Depending on the type of shared-risk plan you purchase, you may be guaranteed a refund of a portion of your original outlay if you do not deliver a live baby. For a couple who may want to adopt if they're not successful, the refund option assures them that they won't exhaust all of their resources on futile IVF attempts . . .

A STACKED DECK

. . . [C]ouples . . . see shared risk as a win-win proposition: You maximize your chances of success while placing an upper limit on what you spend. Either you get a baby or you get some of your money back.

But critics say clinics are the big winners because shared risk results in higher profit margins. For starters, shared-risk programs accept only those patients with the best chances of IVF success — those who, based on their age and diagnosis, have a 50% to 60% probability of getting pregnant on the first try. Women are probably not eligible if they're 39 or older, or if they have poor egg quality, unless they agree to use donor eggs.

In other words, the clinic stacks the deck in its favor. "I am convinced that with a shared-risk program, a clinic will at least break even, and will probably make money, even if the patient doesn't get pregnant at all and the refund kicks in," says Dr. David Grainger, a reproductive endocrinologist in Wichita, Kan.

Nevertheless, the lure of a money-back guarantee is so irresistible for many patients that they're willing to put up with a certain amount of price gouging as long as their story has a happy ending. "We as an industry are making a product that has an inestimable value — a baby — and patients are being exploited in the process," says Thatcher, whose own clinic charges a relatively low $6,500 per IVF cycle and does not use the shared-risk approach.

CONFLICTS OF INTEREST

Medical ethicists have also expressed concern about potential conflicts of interest inherent in shared-risk programs. Do doctors, for example, have an incentive to take inappropriate risks in order to get patients pregnant faster and improve the clinic's bottom line?

That's of particular concern with clinics that have initiated stand-alone shared-risk programs: Doctors themselves bear the risk of producing too few babies, and packaged-plan payments may be commingled with general clinic funds. To protect yourself, choose a clinic that belongs to a shared-risk network, the largest of which are Advanced Reproductive Care (ARC) and Integramed. Both sidestep the conflict-of-interest issue by having patients purchase the packaged plan through the network rather than through the individual clinic. The network then reimburses the clinic for each round of IVF, just as an insurance company would do.

"Our physicians get paid for the care they give regardless of whether the patient gets pregnant, so they aren't biased to change the care inappropriately," says Dr. David Adamson, a reproductive endocrinologist and surgeon who founded ARC five years ago. "Doctors are trained to do the best that they can and should be paid for their effort, not the outcome," adds Jay Higham of Integramed.

ARC and Integramed customers are also insulated from the risk that a clinic will go out of business and be unable to pay a refund. ARC's refund guarantee is backed by the network, which in turn is reinsured through Lloyd's of London. Integramed is a publicly held company that pays refunds out of its own reserve fund.

Melynda Dovel Wilcox, *What Price A Miracle?*, Kiplinger's Personal Finance (September 2002).

In a recent survey of U.S. fertility clinic refund programs, Professor Jim Hawkins concludes that a majority of programs engage in deceptive practices that exploit patients in the fertility industry. For example, Professor Hawkins' research revealed that 60% of programs do not disclose that the fee paid does not include a host of other expenses such as office visits, pregnancy testing and medications. In some instances, the non-covered costs can be more than the services included in the one-time fee. Jim Hawkins, *Financing Fertility*, 47 HARV. J. LEGIS. 115 (2010). See also Lisa Barrett Mann, *A Baby, or Cash Back: Some IVF Centers Offer Risk-Sharing Deals*, WASH. POST (May 18, 2004), at F1 (describing a warranty program in which patients pay some $28,000 up front but receive back $20,000 if the treatment fails).

Does the practice of a money-back guarantee for IVF strike you as a good idea? Would this same practice be transferable to other medical treatments such as cosmetic surgery or laser eye correction? These examples are provided because they generally require a patient to pay for treatment without the aid of health insurance reimbursement. If so, who should decide whether the facelift, for example, was successful? The patient? The doctor? A neutral third party? You can see the problem with a "guarantee" in other areas of medicine (e.g., cancer treatment, heart bypass surgery). Either the outcome is too subjective or the patient's condition is not susceptible to cure through no fault of the physician. Backers of the shared-risk plan for ART argue that the desired outcome is objective and easily measured, with little opportunity for the patient's conduct to shape the treatment outcome. Yet a potential conflict of interest, pitting the physician's desire to succeed (i.e., keep the funds) against standard treatment that will likely not produce a pregnancy, looms large in the field. Let us hear from the American Society for Reproductive Medicine (ASRM), the largest professional organization of reproductive medicine specialists.

2. The Physician's Perspective

Ethics Committee of the American Society for Reproductive Medicine
Shared-Risk or Refund Programs in Assisted Reproduction
70 Fertility & Sterility 414 (1998)

Some assisted reproduction programs now offer in vitro fertilization (IVF) on a "shared-risk," "warranty," "refund," or "outcome" basis, in addition to traditional fee-for-service pricing. Initially, shared-risk patients pay a higher fee. If a shared-risk patient achieves an ongoing pregnancy or delivery, the provider keeps the entire fee. If treatment fails, however, 90-100% of the fee is returned. Pretreatment screening costs, which can be considerable, and the costs of drugs are ordinarily not covered in these plans.

Such programs have been criticized as being exploitative, misleading, and contrary to long-standing professional norms against charging contingent fees for medical services. Proponents, on the other hand, argue that this form of payment is a legitimate response to the lack of health insurance coverage for IVF and to patient concerns about the high cost and substantial risk of IVF failure. If IVF fails in these programs, the patient is still left with resources to pursue other options such as adoption.

In assessing such programs, the Committee focused on the impact of such plans on patients, and not on the profit motive or entrepreneurial impulse that may also have motivated their emergence. It concluded that such plans are in principle ethically acceptable, but that great care is needed in their implementation to ensure that patients are fully aware of the advantages and disadvantages of shared risk programs, including the likelihood of success, the costs that are not covered, and the incentives that providers offering this plan have to take risks to assure success.

The Committee found that shared risk programs may be viewed as a form of insurance against the risk of failure of IVF that might appeal to some couples seeking IVF. The appeal arises from the absence generally of health insurance coverage for IVF, and the loss which treatment failure causes couples who purchase IVF with their own funds. Although both insured and uninsured patients experience disappointment when a treatment cycle fails, those patients who have paid for IVF out of their own pocket have also paid a substantial financial cost . . .

One set of ethical concerns raised about shared risk programs is that they are misleading or exploitive in that they induce patients who are desperate to have a child into purchasing a more expensive form of IVF service than is necessary. The Committee found, however, that the plans it examined provided sufficient information to enable patients to make an informed choice about whether to choose this option. For example, patients who meet program qualifications for these plans should know that they are otherwise good candidates for successful IVF, and thus might not need to purchase this form of insurance. Also, while there are difficulties with patients comparing clinics in terms of efficacy, those problems exist independently of financial arrangements such as shared risk.

A second set of ethical concerns has arisen because shared-risk programs appear to violate long-standing ethical prohibitions against paying contingency fees in medicine. This concern is based on Opinion 6.01 of the AMA Code of Medical Ethics, which states that "a physician's fee should not be made contingent on the successful outcome of medical treatment." However, . . . the . . . reason . . . given in support of Opinion 6.01 [does not] appl[y] to IVF shared-risk plans . . .

The . . . reason cited in support of Opinion 6.01 is that hinging fees on the success of medical treatment implies that "successful outcomes from treatment are guaranteed, thus creating unrealistic expectations of medicine and false promises to consumers." While it is unethical to create unrealistic expectations or make false promises, shared-risk plans do not appear to have that intent or effect. Providers charge a substantial premium to those who enter the plan, compared to their conventional fee-for-service charge. While the provider's willingness to assume some of the risk of failure may convey a message of confidence in its services, no patient is likely to interpret the arrangement as a guarantee of success. On the contrary, the substantial "premium" built into shared-risk fees signals to the patient that the provider needs to be compensated for assuming some of the risk of failure precisely because there is a significant risk that treatment will fail. What is guaranteed is obviously not success, but a refund if treatment fails.

Another rationale, not mentioned in Opinion 6.01, that might justify an ethical objection to contingent fees in medicine is that it is often hard to define medical success and determine whether it has occurred in a given case. Where the measure of success is not clearly specifiable, contingent fees will inevitably spawn doctor-patient disputes over whether a fee has been earned. But this rationale also is inapplicable to IVF shared-risk plans, where measures of success are clearly stated, either delivery of a child or a pregnancy of specified duration.

A third set of concerns is that such programs have a built-in conflict of interest which is likely to skew clinical decision-making toward achieving pregnancy regardless of the impact on the patient in order to avoid paying a refund. Two such dangers may be cited. One is that the provider will be biased in favor of stimulation protocols that tend to produce more oocytes but pose relatively large risks to the woman's health. The other is that the provider will be biased in favor of transferring a relatively large number of embryos, thereby increasing the likelihood not only of pregnancy but of multiple gestation, which can harm women, fetuses, and potential offspring.

The Committee recognizes this potential danger, but has not seen any evidence that either danger has materialized. It also noted that non-shared risk fee-for-service programs also have incentives to overstimulate the ovaries or transfer multiple embryos in order to have high enough success rates to attract future patients. The Committee did not find that the incentives are so much greater in shared-risk plans that they deserve condemnation independently of comparable risks in fee-for-service plans. In both cases the ethical solution is to assure that patients are provided with reliable information about their chances of success, and the costs and benefits of different financing arrangements.

Conclusion

The Committee finds that the shared-risk form of payment for IVF is an option that might be ethically offered to patients without health insurance coverage for IVF if certain conditions that protect patient interests are met. These conditions are that the criterion of success is clearly specified, that patients are fully informed of the financial costs and advantages and disadvantages of such programs, that informed consent materials clearly inform patients of their chances of success if found eligible for the shared risk program, and that the program is not guaranteeing pregnancy and delivery. It should also be clear to patients that they will be paying a higher cost for IVF if they in fact succeed on the first or second cycle than if they had not chosen the shared-risk program, and that, in any event, the costs of screening and drugs are not included.

The Committee was especially concerned about the incentives that shared-risk programs create for providers to take actions that might harm patients in order to achieve success and avoid a refund. For shared-risk programs to be ethical, it is imperative that patients be aware of this potential conflict of interest, and that shared-risk programs not over-stimulate patients to obtain a large supply of eggs or transfer more embryos than is safe for the patient, fetus, and prospective offspring.

Patients should be fully informed of the risks of multifetal gestation for mother and fetus, and have had ample time to discuss and consider them prior to egg retrieval.

B.   Profiles of ART Clients

The cost of ART is obviously linked to the demographics of the clients who can and do avail themselves of such treatments. We learned in Chapter 1 that infertility does not affect racial groups equally. According to the 2002 National Survey of Family Growth (NSFG), infertility is higher among married couples where the wife is non-white, compared to couples in which the wife is white. The incidence of infertility is highest, 27.7 percent, among childless married women categorized as "Black or African American, single race," compared with 24.3 percent of Hispanic or Latina women, and 15.9 percent of white, single-race women.

These differentials in the incidence of infertility may lead us to question whether the delivery of fertility services mirrors the disparity of infertility among racial groups. The Centers for Disease Control and Prevention (CDC) collects data about the use of ART in the U.S., but does not include information about the race or ethnicity of the patients utilizing the services. The only identifying information published by the CDC is the age of women undergoing ART cycles. In 2008, nearly 40% of all ART users were under age 35, and 20% were over age 40. *See 2008 Assisted Reproductive Technology Success Rates: National Summary and Fertility Clinic Reports* (December 2010), at 17. Current data on other demographic features of ART users is not available through the CDC collection process but less formal sources indicate that the majority of fertility clinic patients are Caucasian. For example, websites that advertise the availability of egg donors generally have only a handful of black donors, compared to about 5-15% Asian donors, 5-15% Hispanic donors, with the rest Caucasian. This mix is likely proportional to the race of individuals and couples seeking an egg donor, assuming that prospective parents are seeking same-race donors.

The lack of representation by black women and couples may be attributable to a number of factors. Professor Dorothy Roberts, a well-known scholar in the area of race and reproduction, presents her perspective on the role of race in assisted conception in the excerpt that follows.

Dorothy E. Roberts
Race and the New Reproduction
47 Hastings Law Journal 935 (1996)

. . . In this essay I will explore how [reproductive] technologies reflect and reinforce the racial hierarchy in America. I will focus primarily on in vitro fertilization because it is the technology least accessible to Black people and most advantageous to those concerned about genetic linkages. The salient feature of in vitro fertilization that distinguishes it from other means of assisted reproduction is that it enables an infertile couple to have a child who is genetically-related to the husband.

I. The Role of Race in the New Reproduction

A. Racial Disparity in the Use of Reproductive Technologies

One of the most striking features of the new reproduction is that it is used almost exclusively by white people. Of course, the busiest fertility clinics can point to some Black patients; but they stand out as rare exceptions. Only about one-third of all couples experiencing infertility seek medical treatment at all; and only 10 to 15 percent of infertile couples use advanced techniques like IVF. Blacks make up a disproportionate number of infertile people avoiding reproductive technologies.

When I was recently transfixed by media coverage of battles over adopted children, "surrogacy" contracts, and frozen embryos, a friend questioned my interest in the new methods of reproduction. "Why are you always so fascinated by those stories?," he asked. "They have nothing to do with Black people." Think about the images connected with reproduction-assisting technologies: They are almost always of white people. And the baby in these stories often has blond hair and blue eyes — as if to emphasize her racial purity . . .

In January, 1996, the New York Times launched a prominent four-article series entitled *The Fertility Market*, and the front page photograph displayed the director of a fertility clinic surrounded by seven white children conceived there while the continuing page featured a set of beaming IVF triplets, also white.

When we do read news accounts involving Black children created by these technologies they are always sensational stories intended to evoke revulsion at the technologies' potential for harm. In 1990, a white woman brought a lawsuit against a fertility clinic which she claimed had mistakenly inseminated her with a Black man's sperm, rather than her husband's, resulting in the birth of a Black child. Two reporters covering the story speculated that "if the suit goes to trial, a jury could be faced with the difficult task of deciding the damages involved in raising an interracial child." Although receiving the wrong gametes was an injury in itself, the fact that the gametes were of the wrong race added a unique dimension of harm to the error . . .

It is easy to conclude that the stories displaying blond-haired blue-eyed babies born to white parents are designed to portray the positive potential of the new reproduction, while the stories involving the mixed-race children reveal its potential horror.

These images and the predominant use of IVF by white couples indisputably reveal that race in some way helps to shape both the use and popularity of IVF in America. What are the reasons underlying this connection between race and the new reproduction?

First, the racial disparity in new reproduction has nothing to do with rates of infertility. Married Black women have an infertility rate one and one-half times higher than that of married white women. In fact, the profile of people most likely to use IVF is precisely the opposite of those most likely to be infertile. The people in the United States most likely to be infertile are older, poorer, Black and poorly educated. Most couples who use IVF services are white, highly educated, and affluent . . .

[T]he reason for the racial disparity in fertility treatment appears to be a complex interplay of financial barriers, cultural preferences, and more deliberate professional manipulation. The high cost of the IVF procedure places it out of reach of most Black people whose average median income falls far below that of whites. The median cost of one procedure is about $8,000; and, due to low success rates, many patients try several times before having a baby or giving up. Most medical insurance plans do not cover IVF, nor is it included in Medicaid benefits. IVF requires not only huge sums of money, but also a privileged lifestyle that permits devotion to the arduous process of daily drug injections, ultrasound examinations and blood tests, egg extraction, travel to an IVF clinic, and often multiple attempts — a luxury that few Black people enjoy. As Dr. O'Delle Owens, a Black fertility specialist in Cincinnati explained, ' "For White couples, infertility is often the first roadblock they've faced — while Blacks are distracted by such primary roadblocks as food, shelter and clothing.' " Black people's lack of access to fertility services is also an extension of their more general marginalization from the health care system.

There is evidence that some physicians and fertility clinics may deliberately steer Black patients away from reproductive technologies. For example, doctors are more likely to diagnose white professional women with infertility problems such as endometriosis that can be treated with in vitro fertilization. In 1976, one doctor found that over 20 percent of his Black patients who had been diagnosed as having pelvic inflammatory disease, often treated with sterilization, actually suffered from endometriosis.

Screening criteria not based specifically on race tend to exclude Black women, as well. Most Black children in America today are born to single mothers, so a rule requiring clients to be married would work disproportionately against Black women desiring to become mothers. One IVF clinic addresses the high cost of treatment by offering a donor oocyte program that waives the IVF fee for patients willing to share half of their eggs with another woman. The egg recipient in the program also pays less by forgoing the $2000 to $3000 cost for an oocyte donor. I cannot imagine that this program would help many Black patients, since it is unlikely that the predominantly white clientele would be interested in donations of *their* eggs.

The racial disparity in the use of reproductive technologies may be partially self-imposed. The myth that Black people are overly fertile may make infertility especially embarrassing for Black couples. One Black woman who eventually sought IVF treatment explained, "Being African-American, I felt that we're a fruitful people and it was shameful to have this problem. That made it even harder." Blacks may find it more emotionally difficult to discuss their problem with a physician, especially considering the paucity of Black specialists in this field. Blacks may also harbor a well-founded distrust of technological interference with their bodies and genetic material at the hands of white physicians.

Finally, Blacks may have an aversion to the genetic marketing aspect of the new reproduction. Black folks are skeptical about any obsession with genes. They know that their genes are considered undesirable and that this alleged genetic inferiority has been used for centuries to justify their exclusion from the economic, political and social mainstream . . .

Blacks have understandably resisted defining personal identity in biological terms. Blacks by and large are more interested in escaping the constraints of racist ideology by defining themselves apart from inherited traits. They tend to see group membership as a political and cultural affiliation. Their family ties have traditionally reached beyond the bounds of the nuclear family to include extended kin and non-kin relationships.

My experience has been that fertility services simply are not a subject of conversation in Black circles, even among middle-class professionals. While I have recently noticed stories about infertility appearing in magazines with a Black middle-class readership such as Ebony and Essence, these articles conclude by suggesting that childless Black couples seriously consider adoption. Black professional women I know are far more concerned about the assault that recent welfare reform efforts are inflicting on our poorer sisters' right to bear children — an assault that devalues all Black women and children in America.

Moreover, Black women are also more concerned about the higher rates of sterilization in our community, a disparity that cuts across economic and educational lines. One study found that 9.7 percent of college-educated Black women had been sterilized, compared to 5.6 percent of college-educated white women. The frequency of sterilization increased among poor and uneducated Black women. Among women without a high school diploma, 31.6 percent of Black women and 14.5 percent of white women had been sterilized . . .

II. Implications for Policy Regarding the New Reproduction

What does it mean that we live in a country in which white women disproportionately use expensive technologies to enable them to bear children, while Black women disproportionately undergo surgery that prevents them from being able to bear any? Surely this contradiction must play a critical part in our deliberations about the morality of these technologies. What exactly does race mean for our own understanding of the new reproduction?

Let us consider three possible responses. First, we might acknowledge that race influences the use of reproductive technologies, but decide this does not justify interfering with individuals' liberty to use them. Second, we could work to ensure greater access to these technologies by lowering costs or including IVF in insurance plans. Finally, we might determine that these technologies are harmful and that their use should therefore be discouraged.

A. The Liberal Response: Setting Aside Social Justice

The liberal response to this racial disparity is that it stems from the economic and social structure, not from individuals' use of reproductive technologies. Protection of individuals' procreative liberty should prohibit government intervention in the choice to use IVF, as long as that choice itself does not harm anyone. Currently, there is little government supervision of reproduction-assisting technologies, and many proponents fear legal regulation of these new means of reproduction. In their view, financial and social barriers to IVF are unfortunate but inappropriate reasons to interfere with the choices of those fortunate enough to have access to this technology. Nor, according to the liberal response, does the right to use these technologies entail any government obligation to provide access to them. And if for cultural reasons Blacks choose not to use these technologies, this is no reason to deny them to people who have different cultural values.

Perhaps we should not question infertile couples' motives for wanting genetically-related children. After all, people who have children the old-fashioned way may also practice a form of genetic selection when they choose a mate. The desire to share genetic traits with our children may not reflect the eugenic notion that these particular traits are superior to others; rather, as Barbara Berg notes, "these characteristics may simply symbolize to the parents the child's connection to past generations and the ability to extend that lineage forward into the future." Several people have responded to my concerns about race by explaining to me, "White couples want white children not because of any belief in racial superiority, but because they want children who are like them." . . .

B. The Distributive Solution

. . . Obviously the unequal distribution of wealth in our society prevents the less well off from buying countless goods and services that wealthy people can afford. But there may be a reason why we should be especially concerned about this disparity when it applies to reproduction.

Reproduction is special. Government policy concerning reproduction has tremendous power to affect the status of entire groups of people. This is why the Supreme Court in *Skinner v. Oklahoma* declared the right to bear children to be "one of the basic civil rights of man." "In evil or reckless hands," Justice Douglas wrote, the government's power to sterilize "can cause races or types which are inimical to the dominant group to wither and disappear." This explains why in the *Casey* opinion Justices O'Connor, Kennedy, and Souter stressed the importance the right to an abortion had for women's equal social status. It is precisely the connection between reproduction and human dignity that makes a system of procreative liberty that privileges the wealthy and powerful particularly disturbing.

Procreative liberty's importance to human dignity is a compelling reason to guarantee the equal distribution of procreative resources in society. Moreover, the power of unequal access to these resources to entrench unjust social hierarchies is just as pernicious as government interference in wealthy individuals' expensive procreative choices. We might therefore address the racial disparity in the use of reproductive technologies by ensuring through public spending that their use is not concentrated among affluent white people. Government subsidies, such as Medicaid coverage of IVF, and legislation mandating private insurance coverage of IVF would allow more diverse and widespread enjoyment of the new reproduction.

C. Should We Discourage the New Reproduction?

If these technologies are in some ways positively harmful, will expanding their distribution in society solve the problem? The racial critique of the new reproduction is more unsettling than just its exposure of the maldistribution of fertility services. It also challenges the importance that we place on genetics and genetic ties.

But can we limit individuals' access to these technologies without critically trampling our protection of individual freedom from unwarranted government intrusion? After all, governments have perpetrated as much injustice on the theory that individual interests must be sacrificed for the public good as they have on the theory that equality must be sacrificed for individual liberty. This was the rationale justifying eugenic sterilization laws enacted earlier in this century.

Even for liberals, individuals' freedom to use reproductive technologies is not absolute. Most liberals would place some limit on their use, perhaps by defining the legitimate reasons for procreation. If a core view of reproduction can limit individuals' personal procreative decisions, then why not consider a view that takes into account reproduction's role in social arrangements of wealth and power? If the harm to an individual child or even to a core notion of procreation can justify barring her parents from using the technique of their choice, then why not the new reproduction's potential for worsening group inequality? . . .

Black women in particular would be better served by a focus on the basic improvement of conditions that lead to infertility, such as occupational and environmental hazards, diseases, and complications following childbirth and abortion.

Taking these social justice concerns more seriously, then, might justify government efforts to reallocate resources away from expensive reproductive technologies.

Conclusion

These are thorny questions. It is extremely difficult to untangle white couples' reasons for using reproduction-assisting technologies and Black couples' reasons for avoiding them. Evidence is hard to come by: what doctor or fertility clinic will admit (at least publicly) to steering Black women away from their services? Few people seem to want to confront the obvious complexion of this field. Moreover, the problems raised by the racial disparity in the use of these technologies will not be solved merely by attempting to expand their distribution. Indeed, the concerns I have raised in this essay may be best addressed by placing restrictions on the use and development of the technologies, restrictions imposed by the government or encouraged by moral persuasion. This possibility is met by a legitimate concern about protection of our private decisions from government scrutiny. Indeed, Black women are most vulnerable to government efforts to control their reproductive lives.

Nonetheless, we cannot ignore the negative impact that the racial disparity and imagery of the new reproduction can have on racial inequality in America. Our vision of procreative liberty must include the eradication of group oppression, and not just a concern for protecting the reproductive choices of the most privileged. It must also include alternative conceptions of the family and the significance of genetic relatedness that truly challenge the dominant meaning of family.

———————

Professor Roberts has written extensively on the topic of race and reproduction. For a fuller look at her keen analysis, see DOROTHY ROBERTS, KILLING THE BLACK BODY: RACE, REPRODUCTION, AND THE MEANING OF LIBERTY (1997), reviewed by Timothy Zick, *Re-Defining Reproductive Freedom: Killing the Black Body: Race, Reproduction, and the Meaning of Liberty*, 21 HARVARD WOMEN'S L. J. 327 (1998).

SECTION II: SPERM AND EGG "DONORS"

The financial costs of assisted conception, already considered exorbitant by many prospective patients, can grow even higher if a successful outcome depends upon the use of a third party's gametes. In that case, individuals and couples often turn to egg and sperm "donors," a clear misnomer given that men and women who supply their gametes to the infertile are typically paid for said contribution. Of course, gratuitous transfers are made between family members and even between friends, but the vast majority of gamete donations involve payment from the intended parent(s) to the egg or sperm donor. Gamete donors play a role in the birth of tens of thousands of children annually. Recent data suggests that approximately 60,000 children are born each year to women using sperm donors, while the CDC reports that in the year 2008 there were nearly 7,200 babies born to women who used donor eggs. See 2008 Assisted Reproductive Technology Success Rates, National Summary and Fertility Clinic Reports 63 (Center for Disease Control and Prevention, December 2010).

The structures in place for soliciting and paying gamete donors have similarities and differences for egg and sperm donors, as well as for the intended parents who look to purchasing eggs or sperm to complete their families. Below we explore the world of gamete donation, with an eye toward hearing from all parties involved in this adventure of collaborative reproduction.

A.   Sperm Donations: Assessing Risks and Benefits

In Chapter 1 we learned a bit about the history of ART, including the development of the technique of artificial insemination by donor (AID) in the late nineteenth century wherein the sperm of a donor is injected into a woman's reproductive tract using a narrow tube or catheter. AID was made popular and practical by the ability to freeze sperm, a technique that was first developed in the 1950s. By freezing and then intermittently thawing the sperm of a single donor, doctors can assist a woman in creating a family in which all of the siblings are of the same genetic origin. If a single woman or couple selects a donor to provide the sperm for a pregnancy, that same donor's sperm can be cryopreserved (frozen, from the Greek word "kryos," meaning cold or frost) until such time as the parents wish to have another child. The donor need not return to provide a specimen for the later born child, and the parents need not seek out a sperm donor with like characteristics to those of the first donor. Sperm freezing has become so sophisticated that it is now possible to preserve sperm in frozen storage for a full generation. *See Baby Born from 21-year old Defrosted Sperm, Chicago Sun-Times,* May 26, 2004, at 32 (reporting birth of healthy child to married couple who used thawed sperm 21 years after husband stored specimens before undergoing treatment for testicular cancer).

The development of new technologies often spawns new industries, and the technique of sperm freezing was no exception. In the early 1970s the first commercial sperm bank opened, collecting, storing and providing sperm on a fee-for-service basis. The world's largest sperm bank, California Cryobank, opened its doors in Los Angeles (where else?) in 1977. Today California Cryobank can be found in several locations, including three sites near the campuses of UCLA, Stanford and Harvard, presumably based near these prestigious institutes of higher learning to recruit donors of ample intellectual endowment. But lest you think that selling sperm is the light-hearted chap's answer to an easy dollar, here are some cold hard facts:

- Donors are paid around $100 per specimen, up to a maximum of $1200 per month[1]

- Donors are asked to provide an average of 2 to 3 specimens per week for a period of 12 to 18 months

- Donors must abstain from sex for 48 hours prior to the time of donation

- Donors must undergo quarterly blood draws to be tested for various infectious diseases

- Money earned via sperm donation is reported to the IRS

California Cryobank reports that only about 1% of the men who apply to become sperm donors are ultimately accepted into the program. The screening process includes laboratory analysis of the applicant's sperm and blood, an extensive review of family and medical history, genetic and infectious disease screening, physical examination, and the completion of a donor profile for prospective recipients to review. Applicants are rejected for a host of reasons, including a family history of diabetes, current use of certain anti-depression medications, and height (generally donors must be at least 5'9" to qualify).

Once an applicant is accepted into the program, he is asked to provide an audio interview for prospective recipients to listen to and a baby photo to view. His profile will be placed in the Donor Registry which will identify him by a random "Donor ID" number. Prospective recipients can browse the Donor Registry, manually or online, to learn a donor's race, religion, educational background, and the results of a personality test. The website's newest feature — a "donor look-alike" section, lists the famous celebrities and athletes the donor is thought to resemble. In addition to this descriptive information, each donor is asked to handwrite (for purposes of later handwriting analysis) a short essay. The donor essay is a one-

---

[1] On the other end of the retail chain, sperm banks charge recipients about $400 per vial (and recommend 2-3 vials per insemination for maximum effectiveness), plus miscellaneous costs for donor handwriting analysis ($20), donor baby photos ($25), facial features reports ($20), and shipping. The cost for donor insemination, including physician services, can run as high as $2000.

page form containing four standard questions. The following are a few sample donor essays that give a glimpse into the motivations and aspirations of the men who participate in the sperm donation process.

DONOR 3735

Race: Two or More

Religion: Catholic

Ethnic Origin: Irish, Czech, Pacific Islands, English

Why do you want to be a donor?

I need help financially to put myself through college. I am donating to make money.

Describe your relationship with your family. How has your family shaped your values and who you are today?

I am very close with my family. I was brought up to treat others with respect and to treat myself with respect. My parents were stern and commanded respect. This turned me into a disciplined man who follows through with that I say I am going to do. I respect myself and others.

What makes you unique?

I had and still have the opportunity to compete at an extremely high level athletically and academically. I don't think there are too many people who are successful at both these levels.

What are you most proud of and why?

I am most proud of the way I've lived my life. I have been able to enjoy my life and accomplish goals I've set. I've been able to live my life without regrets.

If we could pass on a message to the recipients or their children, what would that message be?

Enjoy everyday you are alive because it goes so fast. Make good friends, love your family, love the person you marry, and be excited to start a family of your own. It's the best gift you can give back to the world.

DONOR 3743

Race: Caucasian

Religion: None

Ethnic Origin: Irish, Scottish, English, Italian

Why do you want to be a donor?

I have a very close friend who had a baby through a similar program. I have seen how much happiness it has brought them and I would like to help others.

Describe your relationship with your family. How has your family shaped your values and who you are today?

My parents were very hard workers. They always put the kids first. I believe that has helped me develop a strong work ethic and to think of others first.

What makes you unique?

I have the ability to fit in with all types of people and be comfortable. My career has helped with this as well, but I know from experience not everyone can do that.

What are you most proud of and why?

I paid for my own college tuition. I worked all 4 years and paid for all expenses.

If we could pass on a message to the recipients or their children, what would that message be?

Good luck and don't be afraid to take risks.

DONOR 5609

Race: Caucasian

Religion: None

Ethnic Origin: English, Welsh

Why do you want to be a donor?

I feel lucky, very blessed. Life has generally been very easy for me, and if I can help someone else's life become a little easier I'd like to.

Describe your personality and character.

Honest, driven, compassionate, curious, independent, witty, loving (I'm not making this up). I set very high standards for myself and work hard to exceed them — you never know who might view you as a role model.

What are your hobbies, interests, and talents?

Sports, travel, adventure, history, music, filmmaking (and watching, of course), animals, camping . . . I'm interested in nearly everything!

If you could pass on a message to the recipient(s) of your semen, what would that message be?

Good luck to you! Hope it helps!

1.   Donor Disclosure: A Child's Perspective

A parent's decision to enlist the aid of a sperm donor is a difficult one, and the birth of a child following AID raises the question of whether and when a child should be told of his or her genetic heritage. For single women or lesbian couples who conceive with donor sperm, the decision to disclose the circumstances surrounding the child's conception may be easier than for a married couple who are less likely to face questions from a curious child.[2] Armed with the knowledge that one's rearing parent or parents used a sperm donor to conceive, a child will no doubt wonder about the characteristics, and perhaps even the whereabouts, of the donor. Sperm banks are generally free to develop and enforce their own donor identity policies, that is, whether the bank is willing to reveal identifying information about the donor to the child upon reaching the age of majority. Increasingly, sperm banks are becoming more open to providing adult children information about their biological heritage. For example, the California Cryobank has adopted the following "Openness Policy":

> California Cryobank recognizes the concerns regarding the rights to privacy and confidentiality on the part of the sperm donor, all parents, and the child. To best balance these concerns with a donor conceived child's real and legitimate needs to know about his or her biological heritage, CCB has developed our Anonymous Donor Contact Policy:
>
> - We will never destroy patient or donor files. They will remain securely stored by CCB indefinitely.
>
> - Upon reaching the age of eighteen, any CCB child has the right to request additional information about his/her genetic father. Cryobank will make all reasonable efforts to supply that information either from our records or by attempting to contact the donor on the child's behalf.
>
> - Upon reaching the age of eighteen, any CCB child has the right to request contact with his/her genetic father. Cryobank will make all reasonable efforts to contact the donor on the child's behalf. If the donor is willing, CCB will help facilitate the initial contact.
>
> - A parent may not, either for themselves or on behalf of their underage child, receive any additional information on their donor beyond the available profile. Any medical concerns or genetic questions should be directed to the CCB Genetic Counselors . . .
>
> - While we are NOT opposed in principal to breaking anonymity between the donor and the adult child, it must be by mutual consent of both parties. We are obligated by mutual agreements to maintain the anonymity and privacy of the donor, child, and parent. **The only exceptions to this rule are in instances of mutual consent by both the adult child and donor.**

Reprinted from http://www.cryobank.com.

---

[2] A growing percentage of sperm bank clientele are single women and lesbian couples. According to one medical director, single women (presumably including lesbian couples - Ed.) make up 40 percent of the sperm bank clientele. The other 60 percent are married couples with fertility problems who "seek a donor similar to the husband." Once a child is born to the married couple, 80 percent keep the process a secret from family and friends. See Gail Schmoller Philbin, *Web of Conception: Couples Turning to Internet Sites to Secure Donated Sperm*, CHICAGO TRIBUNE, Aug. 20, 2003, at 1.

No doubt each child who learns of their conception via sperm donation will form an individualized opinion about merits of seeking out information or contact with the donor. For some, knowing their biological father is an essential piece of their own life story. According to one report, "Internet chat rooms dedicated to issues surrounding donor insemination teem with messages from offspring desperate to find their biological fathers. The kids are not seeking to be raised or supported by the donor fathers. Rather, they pine for knowledge of and connection to the missing halves of their very selves. One adult offspring at a sperm-donors group recently wrote: 'We don't want money . . . We have the fundamental questions that everyone has growing up. Where did I come from? Who am I? Do I have their eyes, their nose, their hair?' " Jennifer Wolff, *Sperm Donor Ruling Could Open Door For Offspring*, USA TODAY, June 15, 2004, at A13.

Not surprisingly, the Internet has played a vital role in connecting donor-conceived children with their half-siblings and even their genetic fathers. In 2000, Wendy Kramer, the mother of a donor-conceived son, founded The Donor Sibling Registry, an online site that facilitates match-ups between children who share the same sperm donor. Available at www.thedoorsiblingregistry.com, the website also dispenses advice to children, parents and donors about how to incorporate the news and the presence of a genetic relative into their lives. The website urges full disclosure about the use of gamete donors. "It is never too early to begin telling your child the circumstances of her conception and birth." Study data supports this admonition. Research into the well-being of parents and their donor-conceived children tend to show that early disclosure reduces the stress and anxiety associated with secrecy, producing a healthier familiar environment. *See* Emma Lycett, Ken Daniels, Ruth Curson, Susan Golombok, *Offspring Created as a Result of Donor Insemination: A Study of Family Relationships, Child Adjustment, and Disclosure*, 82 FERTILITY & STERILITY 172 (2004).

In its first decade, the Donor Sibling Registry has attracted 30,000 members and made 8,000 matches. In some cases, donors were willing to come forward to meet their genetic progeny. Jeffrey Harrison, previously known as Donor 150, was one such donor. Popular in the late 1980s, Donor 150 was described in his profile as "6 foot and blue-eyed with interest in philosophy, music and drama." After reading a newspaper article profiling two teenage girls looking for their donor father — Donor 150 — Mr. Harrison agreed to connect with his genetic daughters. The donor, now 50, lives with his four dogs in a recreational vehicle near Venice, California. Mr. Harrison hesitated at first, concerned the girls would be disappointed by his humble circumstances. But after meeting her biological father, Harrison's "daughter" exclaimed, "He's sort of a free spirit, and I don't care what career he has. I got to talk to his dogs." *See* Amy Harmon, *Sperm Donor Father Ends His Anonymity*, N.Y. TIMES, Feb. 14, 2007, at A15. It turns out Donor 150 produced more than a dozen children. Other popular donors are reputed to have dozens of offspring. With no formal system in place to alert donor-conceived children to their genetic heritage, should we worry they might unwittingly meet as adults and fall in love? Would this be considered incest?

NOTES AND PROBLEMS

1.   The United States, unlike the United Kingdom, does not have a nationwide policy regarding sperm, egg or embryo donor anonymity. Under a British law enacted in 2004, children born as a result of sperm, egg or embryo donated after April 2005 will be able to access the identity of their donor when they reach age 18. What about the many children who are the product of donor gametes provided prior this date? According to the British Human Fertilisation and Embryology Authority, the governmental body that regulates and inspects all UK fertility clinics, more than 25,000 children have been born in the UK as a result of donated sperm, eggs or embryos since 1991, the year the HFEA established a registry of information about donors. To address these children's desire for identification of their genetic parents, the government instituted a voluntary contact registry called UK Donor-Link. Using DonorLink, donors and children are invited to exchange information and, where desired, contact each other. The registry is limited to children over the age of 18 who were conceived using gametes donated in the UK before 1991, thus leaving 25,000 children born from gametes donated from 1991-2005 under the anonymity policy that governed during that period.

The idea of a gamete registry has been suggested in the U.S., but to date the idea has gained little operational traction. While the idea of a national registry has gained support among patient and physician groups, no organization has been willing to provide the funds necessary to create and maintain such a repository. *See* Naomi Cahn, *Necessary Subjects: The Need for a Mandatory National Donor Gamete Databank*, 12 DePaul J. Health Care L. 203 (2009). For a critique of Professor Cahn's position that the U.S. should adopt prohibitions on donor gamete anonymity, *see* Gaia Bernstein, *Regulating Reproductive Technologies: Timing, Uncertainty, and Donor Anonymity*, 90 Boston U. L. Rev. 1189 (2010).

One not-so-unexpected result of the British law mandating access to donor identity is the impact on supply of donor gametes in the UK. Immediately after the new policy took effect, reports of sperm shortages began to surface. One report was particularly dire — revealing there was only one active sperm donor in all of Scotland. These shortages have caused long waits for British patients, and you know by now that time is not the friend of the infertile. As shortages persisted and waiting times increased, British prospective parents began to travel abroad for their fertility treatment, including assisted conception using donor sperm. Lack of donor anonymity and its consequential gamete shortage is but one of many reasons spurring fertility tourism, as discussed earlier in this Chapter. A recent study shows that lack of access to donor gametes is a real and measured motivator for cross-border reproductive care. *See* F. Shenfield et al., The ESHRE Taskforce on Cross Border Reproductive Care, *Cross Border Reproductive Care in Six European Countries*, 25 Human Reprod. 1361 (2010).

In the UK and other countries where open donor mandates have caused sperm shortages, law and policy makers have tried to generate supply in a variety of ways, including public awareness campaigns, financial incentives in which a cycle of IVF is discounted if the male partner also agrees to donate sperm, and one particularly patriotic approach. In Australia, an IVF clinic asked members of Parliament under age 45 to donate sperm to boost the country's dwindling supply, blamed on a 1998 law allowing children to trace the identity of donors. *See Victorian MPs Asked To Donate Sperm*, Australian Broadcast Corp., Jan. 13, 2005. No word emerged on whether the plea for legislative sperm boosted Aussie supply.

2. The State of Washington was the first, and so far the only, U.S. jurisdiction to statutorily address the issue of gamete donor identity disclosure. Effective July 2011,

> (1) A person who donates gametes to a fertility clinic in Washington to be used in assisted reproduction shall provide, at a minimum, his or her identifying information and medical history to the fertility clinic. The fertility clinic shall keep the identifying information and medical history of its donors and shall disclose the information as provided under subsection (2) of this section.

> (2) (a) A child conceived through assisted reproduction who is at least eighteen years old shall be provided, upon his or her request, access to identifying information of the donor who provided gametes for the assisted reproduction that resulted in the birth of the child, unless the donor has signed an affidavit of nondisclosure with the fertility clinic that provided the gamete for assisted reproduction.

Revised Code of Washington, as amended by House bill 1267 (effective July 22, 2011). The law defines "identifying information" as "the first and last name of the person; and the age of the person at the time of the donation." Note that the law allows donors to avoid being identified to their adult offspring by filing an "affidavit of nondisclosure" at the time that gametes are provided. Given what some might call a soft approach to disclosure, what impact do you think the new law will have on gamete donation in Washington? On donor-conceived offspring? Can you think of any other constituency that might be affected by the new law? Hint: Think about our neighbors to the north.

3. The American Society for Reproductive Medicine has considered the issues associated with gamete donor identification, looking at the effects of disclosure on parents, donors, and, most significantly, children. The ASRM addresses the questions of whether to disclose and how much to tell children about their genetic origins, by suggesting five essential guideposts:

> 1. While ultimately the choice of recipient parents, disclosure to offspring of the use of donor gametes is encouraged.

> 2. Parties should agree in advance on how and when ART programs and sperm banks will release donor information to the recipients.

> 3. Programs and sperm banks should gather and store medical and genetic information concerning donors.

> 4. Counseling and informed consent about disclosure are essential for the donor and recipients.

> 5. Programs and sperm banks should expect inquiries from donor offspring and consider developing a written policy to respond to these inquiries.

Ethics Committee of the American Society for Reproductive Medicine, *Informing Offspring of their Conception by Gamete Donation*, 81 FERTILITY & STERILITY 527 (2004).

4. Suppose that your brother, William, came to you for advice. He is a 21-year-old college student, attending a prestigious university in the northeastern part of the U.S. He has been intrigued by a daily advertisement that runs in his college newspaper that reads, "Help Build a Family. Wanted: College-age males who wish to make the ultimate gift of kindness. Help others overcome nature's barriers to have the family they have dreamt about. Compensation up to $300 per week, for less than 3 hours commitment." William explains that he is in need of money to pay his tuition and living expenses. The compensation sounds excellent, especially in light of the limited time commitment. After you explain that the ad is soliciting sperm donors, he remains interested in responding to the ad. What advice would you give to your brother? Would you give the same advice to a friend? Why?

5. The sperm bank in your local community, let's call it The Family Bank (TFB), has come to you for advice. TFB is considering revising its donor anonymity policy and seeks your input. The policy has always been one of strict anonymity, meaning that TFB has refused to provide any identifying information to donors or children without a court order. But TFB believes that the atmosphere surrounding gamete donation is increasingly one of openness, and thus the bank is interested in rethinking its anonymity policy. What advice would you offer TFB? Would you advise TFB to adopt a policy similar to the UK law that allows donor-conceived children to access their donor's identity when they reach 18? What do you see as the upsides and downsides to openness in gamete donation?

2. The Pitfalls of Sperm Donation

JOHNSON v. SUPERIOR COURT
California Court of Appeal, Second District
80 Cal. App. 4th 1050, 95 Cal. Rptr. 2d 864 (2000)

MALLANO, J.

INTRODUCTION

Petitioners Diane L. Johnson and Ronald G. Johnson, along with their minor daughter Brittany L. Johnson, filed an action against real parties in interest, California Cryobank, Inc., Cappy M. Rothman, M.D., and Charles A. Sims, M.D., claiming that real parties failed to disclose that the sperm they sold came from a donor with a family history of kidney disease called Autosomal Dominant Polycystic Kidney Disease (ADPKD). That sperm was used to conceive Brittany who has been diagnosed with this serious kidney disease. When petitioners sought to take the deposition and obtain documents of John Doe, the person believed to be the anonymous sperm donor, real parties (including John Doe) filed motions to quash the deposition subpoena. At the same time, petitioners filed a motion to compel compliance with the deposition subpoena. The trial court denied petitioners' motion and granted the motions to quash the deposition subpoena. By their petition, petitioners seek a writ of mandate directing the superior court to vacate its order and issue a different order compelling John Doe's deposition and the production of records.

The novel issue presented here is whether parents and their child, conceived by the sperm of an anonymous sperm donor, may compel the donor's deposition and production of documents in order to discover information relevant to their action against the sperm bank for selling sperm that they alleged transmitted ADPKD to the child. As fully discussed below, we conclude that the alleged sperm donor in this case must submit to a deposition and answer questions, as well as produce documents, which are relevant to the issues in the pending action, but that his identity should remain undisclosed to the fullest extent possible.

FACTUAL AND PROCEDURAL HISTORY

The Second Amended Complaint

Petitioners sued Cryobank, as well as its employees, officers, and directors, Doctors Sims and Rothman, for professional negligence, fraud, and breach of contract. In their second amended complaint, petitioners allege as follows. Diane and Ronald Johnson decided to conceive a child through the use of a sperm donor upon the recommendation of their infertility doctors. The Johnsons contacted Cryobank's sperm bank facility in Los Angeles. Ultimately, Cryobank sold the Johnsons frozen sperm specimens donated by donor No. 276. At or near the time of sale, the Johnsons signed Cryobank's form agreement that provided, in relevant part, that "Cryobank shall destroy all information and records which they may have as to the identity of said donor, it being the intention of all parties that the identity of said donor shall be and forever remain anonymous."

At the time of their purchase, Cryobank assured the Johnsons that the anonymous sperm donor had been fully tested and genetically screened. The Johnsons' doctors then implanted the purchased sperm in one of Diane Johnson's fallopian tubes. The procedure was successful and Brittany was born on April 18, 1989. In May 1995, the Johnsons were informed that Brittany was positively diagnosed with ADPKD.

As neither Ronald nor Diane Johnson has ADPKD or a family history of the disease, it was donor No. 276 who genetically transmitted ADPKD to Brittany. At the time donor No. 276 sold his sperm to Cryobank in December 1986, Doctors Sims and Rothman at Cryobank interviewed him and learned that the donor's mother and his mother's sister both suffered from kidney disease and hypertension, and the donor's mother suffered a 30 percent hearing loss before the age of 60. The presence of multiple instances of kidney disease coupled with hypertension and neurological disorders, such as deafness, are red flag indicators of the presence of ADPKD in donor No. 276's family, and thus, Cryobank and Doctors Sims and Rothman knew that donor No. 276's sperm could be at risk of genetically transferring kidney disease.

Even though Cryobank knew of donor No. 276's family history of kidney disease, none of this information was provided to the Johnsons at or prior to the time they purchased the sperm specimens. Despite this knowledge, Cryobank's staff falsely represented to the Johnsons that the sperm they were purchasing was tested and screened for infectious and genetically transferable diseases and safe to effectuate their pregnancy. Cryobank failed properly to test and screen donor No. 276 and conduct further investigation or testing of the donor once they learned that he had a family history of kidney disease.

The Answer

Cryobank answered, asserting several affirmative defenses to petitioners' action, including comparative fault. Cryobank alleges that "persons or parties not named [in] this action . . . may have contributed to a certain degree to the injuries alleged to have been sustained by plaintiffs."

The Discovery Dispute

During the course of the action, petitioners propounded discovery to Cryobank seeking information regarding donor No. 276, including his name, address, and medical history. Cryobank objected to providing any information regarding donor No. 276, claiming the donor's right to privacy and his physician-patient privilege. Cryobank did, however, produce two donor consent agreements that were in use at the time donor No. 276 sold his sperm. Both of these agreements state that the donor will be compensated for each sperm specimen, that he will not attempt to discover the identity of the persons to whom he is donating his sperm, and that his identity "will be kept in the strictest confidence unless a court orders disclosure for good cause. . . ." Cryobank also produced a document showing that on September 6, 1991, Cryobank informed Diane Johnson that donor No. 276 had been withdrawn from the donor program because "new information on his family members . . . indicates that he is at risk for kidney disease" and that a "few small cysts were found" after performing a "renal ultrasound." Cryobank's responses to interrogatories indicated that donor No. 276 had sold 320 deposits of his semen to Cryobank. Donor No. 276's agreement with Cryobank indicated that he received approximately $35 per semen specimen. Donor No. 276 thus received a total of $11,200 for his sperm . . .

Petitioners moved to compel further responses to their discovery requests regarding the identity and medical history of donor No. 276. They also moved to compel answers to questions asked of Cryobank's genetic counselor regarding donor No. 276's identity and medical history. Petitioners argued that they were entitled to have all of donor No. 276's medical information in Cryobank's possession and disclosure of donor No. 276's identity so that they could question him directly because the information (1) was relevant to the issues in the litigation, and (2) was necessary "as a predictor of the medical fate of Brittany" and is "one of the most reliable indicators of Brittany's future." . . .

[P]etitioners' counsel located real party in interest John Doe, who they believe is donor No. 276. John Doe does not admit that he is in fact donor No. 276. Petitioners served him with deposition and trial subpoenas in September 1998.

Petitioners and John Doe, through his counsel, then negotiated and signed a detailed and comprehensive stipulation in June 1999 concerning his testimony in the case. The stipulation would have maintained the confidentiality of John Doe's identity and limited his testimony at deposition and trial to (a) his involvement with Cryobank and (b) his, as well as his family's, medical history as it relates to ADPKD.

Prior to a September 1999 hearing at which petitioners asked the trial court to approve the stipulation and enter a protective order, John Doe submitted a declaration stating that he did not want his deposition taken. In addition, Cryobank objected to the stipulation and protective order and opposed any deposition of John Doe. The trial court denied petitioners' request to approve the stipulation . . .

DISCUSSION

. . . Here, we review whether petitioners may subject John Doe to a nonparty deposition and force him to produce documents concerning his and his family's medical history with ADPKD notwithstanding his right to privacy. Because of the novel issue presented by this case — whether parents and their child, conceived by the sperm of an anonymous donor, may compel the donor's deposition and production of documents in order to discover information relevant to their action against the sperm bank for selling sperm which allegedly transmitted a serious kidney disease — we granted an alternative writ of mandate . . .

The Physician-Patient Privilege

Cryobank and Doctor Rothman contend that petitioners are not entitled to John Doe's deposition, even if he is donor No. 276, because all the communications between him and the physicians at Cryobank are protected by the physician-patient privilege. We disagree.

Evidence Code section 994 provides that "the patient, whether or not a party, has a privilege to refuse to disclose, and to prevent another from disclosing, a confidential communication between patient and physician." . . .

In order for a party to invoke the physician-patient privilege under Evidence Code section 994, there must be a patient. A "patient" is defined under section 991 as "a person who consults a physician or submits to an examination by a physician for the purpose of securing a diagnosis or preventative, palliative, or curative treatment of his physical or mental or emotional condition." Therefore, if a person does not consult a physician for diagnosis or treatment of a physical or mental ailment, the privilege does not exist . . .

Real parties in interest have failed to demonstrate that the physician-patient privilege is applicable in this case. The evidence presented to the trial court revealed that donor No. 276 visited Cryobank for the sole purpose of selling his sperm. That he consulted with Cryobank's physicians and medical personnel as part of the process of donating his sperm does not change the dominant purpose for his visit. There was no evidence presented to the trial court that donor No. 276 visited Cryobank "for the purpose of securing a diagnosis or preventative, palliative, or curative treatment of his physical or mental or emotional condition." Thus, we conclude that the physician-patient privilege has no application here.

John Doe's Status as Third Party Beneficiary

John Doe next claims that petitioners are not entitled to discover his identity because their contract with Cryobank prohibits it. John Doe argues that petitioners' agreement with Cryobank providing that the sperm donor's identity would never be disclosed was made for his benefit and thus, as a third party beneficiary, he is entitled to keep his identity confidential as the agreement requires. While we agree that John Doe is a third party beneficiary, we disagree that the agreement precludes disclosure of his identity or related information under any circumstance.

1. John Doe Is a Third Party Beneficiary

"Under California law third party beneficiaries of contracts have the right to enforce the terms of the contract under Civil Code section 1559 which provides: 'A contract, made expressly for the benefit of a third person, may be enforced by him at any time before the parties thereto rescind it.'" (*Harper v. Wausau Ins. Co.* (1997) 56 Cal.App.4th 1079, 1086 [66 Cal.Rptr.2d 64].) . . .

In this case, the Johnsons promised in their contract with Cryobank that they would, among other things, "not now, nor at any time, require nor expect [Cryobank] to obtain or divulge . . . the name of said donor, nor any other information concerning characteristics, qualities, or any other information whatso-ever concerning said donor." The Johnsons further agreed "that, following the said insemination, [Cryobank] shall destroy all information and records which they may have as to the identity of said donor, it being the intention of all parties that the identity of said donor shall be and forever remain anonymous." The agreement bound the Johnsons as well as their heirs and assigns.

We conclude that the Cryobank agreement with the Johnsons expresses the clear intent of both the Johnsons and Cryobank that the donor's identity and related information would be kept confidential and that such intent was for the benefit of all parties, including the donor. Our conclusion is further supported by Diane Johnson's testimony at her deposition in this case where she stated it was her intent by executing the Cryobank agreement that the donor's identity would not be disclosed to her and that her identity would not be disclosed to the donor. While John Doe or Donor No. 276 are not specifically named in the agreement, it is clear that he belongs to the class of persons — Cryobank sperm donors — who are to benefit from the agreement's confidentiality provisions.

But, our analysis does not end here. We must determine whether the Cryobank agreement with the Johnsons is contrary to an express provision of law, the policy of express law, or public policy and, hence, unenforceable. (Civ. Code, § 1667; *Metropolitan Creditors Service v. Sadri* (1993) 15 Cal.App.4th 1821, 1825-1826 [19 Cal.Rptr.2d 646] [contracts contrary to public policy are unlawful and unenforceable].) We conclude for the reasons stated below, that the Cryobank agreement goes too far in precluding disclosure of the donor's identity and related information under all circumstances and thus conflicts with public policy.

2. Cryobank's Agreement Conflicts with Public Policy

Family Code section 7613 provides: "(a) If, under the supervision of a licensed physician and surgeon and with the consent of her husband, a wife is inseminated artificially with semen donated by a man not her husband, the husband is treated in law as if he were the natural father of a child thereby conceived. The husband's consent must be in writing and signed by him and his wife. The physician and surgeon shall certify their signatures and the date of the insemination, and retain the husband's consent as part of the medical record, where it shall be kept confidential and in a sealed file. However, the physician and surgeon's failure to do so does not affect the father and child relationship. *All papers and records pertaining to the insemination, whether part of the permanent record of a court or of a file held by the supervising physician and surgeon or elsewhere, are subject to inspection only upon an order of the court for good cause shown.* [¶] (b)." (Italics added.) . . .

[W]e conclude that based on the policy expressed in Family Code section 7613, inspection of insemination records, including a sperm donor's identity and related information contained in those records, may be disclosed under certain circumstances. Thus, to prohibit disclosure of the donor's identity and related information in every situation and under all circumstances, as Cryobank and John Doe attempt to do here by the Johnsons' agreement with Cryobank, would be contrary to the policy expressed in the statute. We note that Cryobank has apparently recognized that disclosure of a donor's identity could be allowed under certain circumstances as its agreement with all of its donors provides that the donor's identity "will be kept in the strictest confidence unless a court orders disclosure for good cause."

And enforcement under all circumstances of a confidentiality provision such as the one in Cryobank's contract with the Johnsons conflicts with California's compelling interest in the health and welfare of children, including those conceived by artificial insemination. (See, e.g., *Mansfield v. Hyde* (1952) 112 Cal.App.2d 133, 139 [245 P.2d 577] [the state, as parens patriae, is charged with continuing interest in minor children's welfare and has surrounded the matter with many protective laws].) There may be instances under which a child conceived by artificial insemination may need his or her family's genetic and medical history for important medical decisions. For example, such genetic and medical history can lead to an early detection of certain diseases and an increased chance of curing them. In some situations, a person's ability to locate his or her biological relative may be important in considering lifesaving transplant procedures . . . While in most situations the donor's genetic and medical information may be furnished without the need of disclosing the donor's identity, there may be other situations that require disclosure of the donor's identity in order to obtain the needed information. In either event, a contract that completely forecloses the opportunity of a child conceived by artificial insemination to discover the relevant and needed medical history of his or her genetic father is inconsistent with the best interests of the child.

We conclude that Cryobank's agreement with the Johnsons precluding disclosure of the donor's identity and other information pertaining to the donor under all circumstances is contrary to public policy and therefore unenforceable. Because a third party beneficiary such as John Doe can only enforce a contract where there is a " 'valid and subsisting obligation between the promisor and the promisee' " (*Principal Mutual Life Ins. Co. v. Vars, Pave, McCord & Freedman*,65 Cal.App.4th at pp. 1485-1486; 1 Witkin, Summary of Cal. Law, § 662, p. 601), we hold that the Cryobank agreement with the Johnsons does not preclude disclosure of the donor's identity and related information about the donor.

THE CONSTITUTIONAL RIGHT OF PRIVACY

Finally, real parties in interest contend that petitioners are precluded from deposing John Doe because to do so would violate his constitutional right of privacy under the federal and California Constitutions. We agree with real parties that donor No. 276 has a right of privacy in his medical history and his identity. We disagree, however, that such a right precludes his deposition and the production of the records requested in the deposition subpoena.

The California Constitution expressly provides that all people have the inalienable right to privacy. (Cal. Const., art. I, § 1; see also *American Academy of Pediatrics v. Lungren* (1997) 16 Cal.4th 307, 325-326 [66 Cal.Rptr.2d 210, 940 P.2d 797] [the California Constitution expressly recognizes a right of privacy and is considered broader than the implied federal right to privacy].) "In *Hill v. National Collegiate Athletic Assn.* (1994) 7 Cal.4th 1, 52-57 [26 Cal.Rptr.2d 834, 865 P.2d 633] our high court . . . advanced an analytical framework for deciding questions arising under this constitutional right of privacy, and found that a violation of the constitutional right of privacy is only established where three conditions are shown: '(1) a legally protected privacy interest; (2) a reasonable expectation of privacy in the circumstances; and (3) conduct by defendant constituting a serious invasion of privacy.' (*Id.* at pp. 39-40.)" (*Rains v. Belsh* (1995) 32 Cal.App.4th 157, 167 [38 Cal.Rptr.2d 185].) . . .

1. Legally Recognized Privacy Interest

A person's medical history undoubtedly falls within the recognized zones of privacy . . . Because donor No. 276's identity is necessarily linked with his medical history, he likewise has a privacy interest in the disclosure of his identity.

2. Reasonable Expectation of Privacy in the Circumstances

" 'Even when a legally cognizable privacy interest is present, other factors may affect a person's reasonable expectation of privacy.' . . . 'In addition, customs, practices, and physical settings surrounding particular activities may create or inhibit reasonable expectations of privacy. [Citations.]' " . . .

The record before us reveals that Cryobank routinely told its sperm donors that nonidentifying medical history and related information could be disclosed to the purchasers of the sperm. Such warnings naturally lessen the donor's expectation that nonidentifying medical information will not be revealed to purchasers of the sperm. Indeed, some of donor No. 276's nonidentifying medical history has already been disclosed to petitioners. We thus conclude that donor No. 276's reasonable expectation as to the disclosure of nonidentifying medical information was substantially diminished.

And donor No. 276's reasonable expectation of privacy in his identity was substantially diminished by his own conduct. This is not a case of a donor making isolated donations of his sperm in order to help one woman conceive a child. Rather, the record before us reveals that donor No. 276 deposited over 320 specimens of his semen with Cryobank. Donor No. 276's 320 semen deposits earned him over $11,000. Thus, donor No. 276's connection with Cryobank involved a substantial commercial transaction likely to affect the lives of many people.

We conclude that although donor No. 276 does indeed have a limited privacy interest in his identity as a sperm donor and in his medical history, under the circumstances of this case, it would be unreasonable for donor No. 276 to expect that his genetic and medical history, and possibly even his identity, would never be disclosed . . .

While donor No. 276 has an interest in maintaining the confidentiality of his identity and medical history, we hold that in the context of the particular facts of this case the state's interests, as well as those of petitioners, outweigh donor No. 276's interests. Accordingly, John Doe must appear at his deposition and answer all questions and produce documents that are relevant to the issues raised in the litigation. But this does not mean that John Doe's identity must automatically be disclosed if he indeed is donor No. 276 . . .

For example, an order could be fashioned which would allow John Doe's deposition to proceed and documents produced on matters relevant to the issues in the litigation but in a manner which maintains the confidentiality of John Doe's identity and that of his family. Attendance at the deposition could be limited to the parties' counsel and the deposition transcript might refer simply to "John Doe" as the deponent. But we leave it to the trial court to craft the appropriate order . . .

CONCLUSION

We conclude that the trial court abused its discretion in denying petitioners' motion to compel John Doe's deposition and production of documents and in granting real parties' motion to quash. The trial court failed to consider the state and petitioners' countervailing interests that favor disclosure and failed to consider an order with " ' "partial limitations rather than [an] outright denial of discovery." [citation omitted] Petitioners are entitled to take John Doe's deposition and inquire whether he is donor No. 276, and if he is, delve into his and his family's health and medical history, and his communications with Cryobank, but only as to those issues which are relevant to the pending litigation. Similarly, we conclude that petitioners are entitled to the production of documents identified in their renotice of John Doe's deposition which are relevant and in the possession, custody, or control of John Doe. But John Doe's identity is to be protected to the fullest extent possible and the identities of his family members are not to be disclosed . . .

BOREN, P. J., and NOTT, J., concurred.

(The petitions of real parties in interest for review by the California Supreme Court were denied August 23, 2000.)

NOTES AND QUESTIONS

1.   Diane and Ronald Johnson won the right to depose Donor No. 276 and they did so on May 29, 2001. At the deposition, the Johnsons received a copy of the Donor Profile contained in Donor No. 276's file. The Donor Profile revealed that Donor No. 276 had answered affirmatively when asked about the presence of kidney disease in his mother and his aunts and uncles. On the same form, in different colored ink than that used by the donor, appeared question marks and the notation "at risk for kidney disease" next to the kidney-related questions. Armed with this apparent knowledge by Cryobank of Donor No. 276's family history of kidney disease, the Johnsons pursued their lawsuit against the sperm bank for damages relating to their daughter's health. In August 2002, the California Court of Appeal (a three-judge panel with two of the same justices from the 2000 case), ruled against the Johnsons, concluding that "[r]egardless of what petitioners allege with respect to causation, it cannot be said that Cryobank, Sims and Rothman *caused* Brittany's inherited abnormalities by improperly approving Donor No. 276 as a sperm donor. Brittany's kidney condition was *caused* by the gene contained within the sperm provided by Donor No. 276." *Johnson v. Superior Court*, 101 Cal. App. 4th 869, 124 Cal. Rptr. 2d 650 (2002). The court denied the Johnsons' claim for general damages and damages for Brittany's lost earnings.

2.   The incidence of disease transmission through artificial insemination by donor (AID) is rare, but as the facts in *Johnson* reveal, not nonexistent. AID poses potential harm to offspring through the transmission of a deleterious gene from the sperm donor. Sporadic but heartbreaking reports do appear in which researcher identify a cluster of donor-conceived children with rare and often live-threatening genetic disorders. The donors' genetic anomalies are typically not detected by commercial sperm banks because they are quite rare and therefore not included in routine tests, or genetic tests for the disorder did not exist at the time the donor's sperm was procured. *See, e.g.*, B. Maron, J. Lesser, J. Schiller, K. Harris, C. Brown, H. Rehm, *Implications of Hypertrophic Cardiomyopathy Transmitted by Sperm Donor*, 302 JAMA 1681 (2009).

In addition to passing on a genetic disorder, a sperm donor could pose harm to both the woman who is inseminated and her resulting child if the donor is infected with a sexually transmitted disease such as HIV or AIDS. See M. R. Araneta et al., *HIV Transmission Through Donor Artificial Insemination*, 273 JAMA 854 (1995) (describing incidence of HIV transmission to inseminated women via AID prior to 1986, when testing for the virus became available). Today, the incidence of HIV transmission via AID is exceedingly low because of intensive screening methods that are routinely used to evaluate donor and sperm health. In addition to HIV testing of all donors and all semen specimens, sperm banks often quarantine frozen sperm for at least six months in order to retest the donor for the presence of HIV. That said, cases of HIV transmission through donor insemination are intermittently reported. See, e.g., Shaikh Azizur Rahman, *Sperm Donor Transmits HIV To Woman*, COURIER MAIL, May 22, 2003, at 18 (reporting transmission of HIV to 35-year-old woman from Calcutta, as first such case in Asia).

3.   Mishaps in artificial insemination can also take the form of human error on the part of the physician. In 2004 a Connecticut woman sued a fertility clinic to turn over information on a man whose sperm she accidentally received and thereafter became pregnant. The woman and her fiancé, a black couple, visited the clinic with a vial of the fiance's sperm. After the insemination when the woman was leaving the clinic, the doctor chased after her and admitted he actually gave her the sperm of another man. The possible sources, she surmised, were one of the two white males sitting in the waiting area. The woman decided to go ahead with the pregnancy despite her knowledge that the child she was carrying was not the biological offspring of her fiancé. She brought suit after the doctor and clinic refused to provide her nonidentifying information about the biological father's medical history. See Mary Vallis, *Patient Sues Fertility Clinic for Receiving Wrong Sperm*, NAT'L POST, July 16, 2004, at A10.

B.   Egg Donations: Assessing Risks and Benefits

The practice of egg donation is of more recent origin than the decades-old practice of sperm donation. In 1984 scientists from Australia reported the world's first birth resulting from a donor egg. The delay between the advent of sperm and egg donation is understandable, given the differences in technological know-how needed to retrieve each type of gamete. For a man to provide sperm, he requires little more than a plastic cup and a vivid imagination. But a woman cannot provide eggs on her own. She must commit to a month-long medical regimen involving hormone injections and surgery. Physicians continue to fine-tune and improve the technology used for egg retrieval, as the current process can pose risks to the young women who comprise the donor pool. In one reported case, a 22-year-old graduate student suffered a massive stroke after beginning the daily hormone injections required to stimulate egg production. See Joan O'C. Hamilton, *What Are the Costs*, Standford Magazine, Nov./Dec., 2000.

Each fertility clinic likely has its own system for recruiting and treating egg donors. One author summarizes the egg donation procedure as follows:

> The harvesting of donor eggs is a complicated and intricate process. The first step in the egg donation process is the recruitment of a donor, preferably under age 30. Recruitment practices range from private "egg brokers" to medical centers with affiliated fertility clinics to freestanding, independent fertility centers. Enticing monetary offers of "generous compensation for time and inconvenience" usually prompt the prospective donor to contact the fertility center.

> As part of the screening and recruitment process, the prospective donor is asked to complete a detailed profile and questionnaire, requesting information ranging from physical characteristics, personality traits, and estimated exposure to radiation, to photographs of the donor and her offspring, if any. The process includes psychological screening, consulta-

tions, and evaluation, as well as completion of a detailed medical exam, history, physical, and possibly genetic testing. The egg donation agency will match the donor to a number coded recipient, and frequently, the potential parents request knowledge of the donor's first name. In time, the donor is matched with the recipient and scheduled to begin the process of priming the ovaries, coordinating the donor's and recipient's cycles, and retrieving the eggs.

Some agencies include legal consultation for the recipient couple as part of the overall process to facilitate and review the contracts and financial commitments, however, the donor is only provided with a list of available attorneys and legal consultation is not a prerequisite. The informed consent process is not standardized, and again varies depending on the type of fertility center and medical center/hospital affiliation. Since most fertility clinics are privately run enterprises, the requisite informed consent documents vary from a general reference to the "legal aspects of donating" to generalized legal aspects of egg donation. Note, however, neither of these selected FAQ's or Contract Considerations specifically include a framework for how to define the key legal terms, such as informed consent, confidentiality, liability, or future child custody/support expectations. One egg donation group provides a sample "Consent for Egg Donation" and other egg donation centers include general legal information, but it is unknown how a Court would treat this egg donation contract in terms of enforcement since to date no cases have been filed on this exact issue.

Presuming the hurdle of informed consent is overcome, and the donor chooses to move forward, the donor then picks up a dozen pinkie size vials full of powdered hormones and dilutents, along with the first cash payment. Thus begins ten days of daily injections of a high dose hormone, such as Lupron, which suppresses her own ovarian function and synchronizes her menstrual cycle with the recipient's. These injections are crucial, and must be administered on a strict schedule and regimen; dauntingly enough, an injection delayed by a few hours can ruin the entire process. Later, the donor is given another hormone injection to stimulate the egg production and harvesting, which results in the production of ten or more eggs during one cycle.

The donor's eggs are extracted using a large needle inserted into the vagina while the patient is under anesthesia. The eggs are then inseminated immediately with sperm from the recipient's husband (or possibly with donor sperm) and the resulting embryos are implanted into the recipient. Recent statistics estimate that ART procedures result in a live birth rate of 39 percent. However, the donor's set compensation is guaranteed as soon as egg retrieval is complete. Some women on fertility drugs harvest an excess of 40 eggs per cycle - other women harvest 8-10. No matter the number of eggs, however, the compensation remains the same . . . an envelope with numerous $100 bills; cash payment for services, or rather - time and inconvenience rendered.

Kari L. Karsjens, *Boutique Egg Donations: A New Form of Racism and Patriarchy*, 5 DePaul J. Health Care L. 57, 61-64 (2002).

1. The Business of Egg Donation

The practice of egg donation is both emerging and largely unregulated. Thus, we learn about the potential legal parameters of the field through the stories of those who have ventured into an egg donation agreement and through a handful of judicial decisions in which the practice has played a role in the litigation. As you read the stories and the inevitable lawsuits, think about whether and how the growing practice of egg donation should be addressed by the law.

Martha Frase-Blunt
Ova-Compensating?; Women Who Donate Eggs To Infertile Couples Earn a Reward — But Pay a Price
Washington Post, December 4, 2001, at F1

"Pay Your Tuition With Eggs," reads one ad in an Ivy League campus newspaper. Another promises $50,000 to an "intelligent, athletic egg donor" who "must be at least 5-10 and have a 1400 SAT score."

Shantel Balentine just shakes her head in wonder when she sees such ads. The 32-year-old North Texas woman has never completed college, but in the opinion of many fertility specialists, she has ideal donor characteristics: maturity, demonstrable fertility — she is a mother of three — and an altruistic motivation. Her academic record, they believe, is far less important than these attributes.

"Your heart has to be fully involved," says Balentine, who is undergoing her fourth egg donation process. "It can be painful. There are delays — cycles can stretch out for weeks. But I won't walk away. This couple is counting on me."

Egg donors can be stereotyped as college students eager to pay off their student loans with a sudden windfall, and it's true that some clinics target such women. For a student, the lure of easy money for what may seem to be no more than a minor surgical procedure can be compelling: Those Ivy League ads notwithstanding, a $50,000 payment can't be expected, but a donor typically pockets several thousand dollars for having artificially ripened eggs extracted from her youthful ovary.

But despite the preferences that many infertile couples have for the eggs of younger, better-educated donors, experts cite psychological, physiological and even logistical reasons to steer these couples away from college students and toward a less-elite group of candidates.

According to Patricia Mendell, a New York psychotherapist who assesses and counsels would-be egg donors, these women are as diverse as any societal group, except that virtually all are healthy and between the ages of 18 and 32; many are also organ donors and blood donors.

Mendell has also found that their demographics vary by geographic area: "Egg donors in Boston and New York are predominantly students, because of the large student population in these cities. In California, it's split evenly between childless women and mothers, and in the South, you'll tend to find the majority of donors to be young mothers. Besides that, there is a lot of diversity when it comes to personalities and backgrounds."

There's no doubt that biologically, very young egg donors are ideal. But do they make the best egg donors psychologically? "That's the question mark," says Pamela Madsen, executive director of the American Infertility Association, which is based in New York. "Are we . . . leading them to make a decision that later in life they may regret? The money will be spent and, in the end, she has given up her genetic child forever. We have to really care about these women, and the babies that will be born as a result." . . .

Competition for egg donors is heated. Clinics and brokers advertise in print and on the radio, place flyers in health clubs and even buy ads on movie screens, all in an effort to reach a broad swath of the young female population. The more egg donors an organization can secure, the more choices it can give the recipient couples — or, sometimes, the single women — who pay the donor's fee. A significant element of the transaction, after all, is the couple's ability to select a donor who seems ideal.

Some clinics, including the Genetics & IVF Institute in Fairfax, allow casual visitors to their Web sites to read profiles of prospective donors. At the Annapolis office of the Center for Surrogate Parenting and Egg Donation, recipients are invited to peruse the organization's database of some 350 donors, searching by variables such as state, ethnic background, hair color, eye color and physical build. Once they focus on a likely candidate, they can also view a picture of the donor, along with some details from her application . . .

After the client has selected several prospects, the donors' status is checked, and the recipient couple receives additional information and photos, medical data "and more subjective information, like personality details," said Smith. This openness is unique: Most fertility clinics and agencies provide recipients only the most basic information about donors.

On the other hand, the women who donate their eggs through the firm are given scant information about the recipients — a one-page statement about how the couple met, how long they've been married, their infertility history. The donor sees no photos of the prospective parents, whom she knows only by their first names.

A college student hoping to pay her tuition with eggs — or any prospective donor — may be surprised to learn how much is required of her.

Following an extensive application process, she could wait months, even years, to be selected by a couple. After that come tests for genetic and infectious diseases and a complete physical examination. Screenings are also conducted by psychotherapists who explore the donor's reasons for participating, the extent of her family's support and what she will tell her current or future children about the donation process. Approval may also hinge on attaining a particular score on the Minnesota Multiphasic Personality Inventory, which assesses psychological traits.

After clearing these hurdles, the donor can prepare to have her eggs harvested. Her associated medical expenses are paid by the recipient couple, who are also required to buy short-term life insurance for the donor. She in turn must commit to multiple doctor appointments and give herself daily or twice-daily hormone injections in the thigh or abdomen for three weeks or longer; these drugs mature or "ripen" the follicles in her ovaries, which produce several eggs ready for extraction.

The donor is monitored daily until the ripening is complete; then she receives an injection of a powerful hormone that prepares the ovaries to release the mature follicles. The eggs are removed in a vaginal procedure conducted under light anesthesia in a fertility clinic or the office of the recipient's doctor.

Side effects of the injections can be unpleasant, with PMS-like symptoms such as bloating, abdominal pain, nausea and moodiness. In 3 to 5 percent of cases, hyperstimulation of the ovaries occurs, causing severe abdominal pain; on rare occasions, surgery is required and the patient can be left infertile. Other risks of retrieval include lacerations, ovarian trauma, infection and anesthesia-related complications.

Once retrieved, the eggs are promptly fertilized in vitro, and in two or three days the resulting embryos — three of them, frequently — are transferred to the recipient, whose uterus has been primed with hormones to receive them.

The donor is generally not hospitalized, but needs two to three days of rest to recover. Only then is she paid.

"It's definitely not easy money," says Balentine. And to discourage those who think otherwise, most reputable clinics and agencies try to weed out donors who are motivated solely by money, preferring a woman with an altruistic urge to undergo the procedure.

Agency officials say it's often an infertile couple who presses them to solicit college students with large cash offers — like the pair who placed a half-page advertisement in the Stanford Daily last year offering $100,000 for the eggs of a donor "with proven college-level athletic ability."

In a statement, the couple's agent, Families 2000+, said the offer was intended to attract women who might not otherwise consider becoming donors. But such large sums amount to improper enticement, says Madsen of the infertility association. "We don't object to advertising for donors, and we agree that donors must be compensated for their time, effort and the pain and suffering involved in the procedure," she says. "But we have to be concerned and careful about the amounts of money being offered. We are dealing with young women who are smart and savvy and know their bodies and minds. But if she would say no to $2,500, and yes to $7,000, then maybe we're enticing her."

Although Families 2000+ says it cannot discuss the results of the $100,000 offer, the ad apparently added to its pool of college-age donors. According to the Los Angeles Times, the ad was answered by about 200 women. One of them told the paper she was not matched with the couple who initiated the ad but did give her eggs to another couple and received a fee of $18,000. At the time, Karen Synesiou, director of Egg Donation's main office in Beverly Hills, Calif., told the Times she believed that many big-money advertisements were "fake," designed "to attract media attention and a lot of donors."

Is it a bait-and-switch game? "I wouldn't go that far," says Madsen. "But we have to be wary as a community that offering women that kind of money for this service puts a tremendous burden on other infertile couples, on other donors, and ultimately on that child. When you put such high expectations on a potential baby, it becomes something different and, in my mind, a bit ugly. This should just be about women helping women. It should be about families."

Smith says that only rarely would her organization advertise in a college paper, and only if a couple insists. "We just don't get the return," she says. Egg Donation has a strict age limit of 21, she says, and "college students are often hard to reach, they have exams, their schedules are unpredictable. Donors have to be dependable, particularly with their medications." And because the Annapolis office deals with client couples throughout the United States and overseas, she says, "our donors have to be available to travel on short notice" to the home cities of the recipients.

Smith recruits on the Internet and through ads in "pennysaver" publications and parenting magazines, hoping to attract those she considers the best donors — young mothers like Balentine. "Not only is their fertility proven, but they tend to be more mature, and have a better understanding of what it means to donate their genetic material. And they really empathize with the infertile couple. They know what it means to want to be pregnant and give birth." In other words, money is less likely to be the main motivator.

Sharon Owens says she and her husband independently hit on the idea of donating her eggs after each heard news reports about the practice. So at the decidedly mature age of 32, the mother of three called Egg Donation. "I thought it would be a wonderful experience to help an infertile couple. I was finished having kids and didn't need my eggs anymore," says Owens, who lives in Towson, Md.

To her surprise, she was selected by two couples within a few months. She doesn't really know why. "There is no way of knowing when a donor will be selected," says Owens, who now coordinates the egg donor program at the Annapolis office. "Each couple has different wants and priorities. For some it's mandatory that the donor be under a certain age. Others are looking at physical similarities to themselves. For some it's a combination of a number of factors. It's an incredibly personal choice."

Owens shares Madsen's concerns about enticing young childless women with large sums of money and can imagine the regrets down the line if the donor later suffered infertility problems of her own. "A donor that is truly mature and ready won't look at it as giving someone their child, but as giving someone the possibility of having a child of their own," she says.

The American Society for Reproductive Medicine has recommended that donor fees not go above $5,000 — any higher can be seen as coercive, the group declared last year. In the Washington area they average about $3,000 for a first donation, slightly more for a donor who has proven herself.

But according to Madsen, fees in New York have risen to $7,000 in recent months, and in New Jersey average fees have topped $6,000. Jewish and African American donors can command even higher fees because of their scarcity.

Madsen doesn't blame the clinics for nudging prices up. "Practitioners are just trying to meet the growing demand and shorten waiting lists," she says, and fees are one of the few ways a clinic or agency can differentiate itself from its peers.

Nor does Madsen fault couples who scour donor databases for educated, accomplished women who meet certain height and coloring criteria. "I don't think they are looking for a 'Faberge egg.' That's not the goal. These couples just want to find someone like themselves. And the reality is, those who seek — and can afford — egg donation tend to be highly educated, professional women in the upper income brackets." In addition to the fee paid to the donor, the cost of this type of in vitro fertilization can range from $8,000 to $20,000.

Smith counsels many couples through the selection process, often downplaying the donors' educational qualifications and stressing instead the attributes of the young mothers in her database: They are compassionate, dedicated parents who are committed to the process and truly want to ease another couple's pain. Many started their families young, and didn't have time for advanced degrees or glamorous careers.

Smith also explains to clients that genetics is basically a crapshoot. "I tell couples, 'The perfect donor is not on any database — because it is you. We can't predict which genes your child will be born with. Choose the donor who would best fit into your family.' "

Judith Daar,
Physical Beauty Is Only Egg Deep
Los Angeles Times, October 28, 1999, at B11

I nearly choked over my coffee and eggs last weekend as I read about the exploits of sixtysomething Ron Harris, a sometime Playboy photographer and horse breeder who has launched a Web site auctioning human eggs from models and actresses. Just log on to http:www.ronsangels.com and you too can bid on the eggs of an "actress" whose finest moment was playing the part of a dead body on "Homicide, Life on the Street" and whose sole self-proclaimed defect is that she exercises too much.

The assisted reproductive technology community has responded with horror, sounding its usual battle cry that regulation is needed to stop profiteers like Harris from preying on vulnerable people whose only desire is to overcome infertility and become parents. Unethical and distasteful, decries the American Society for Reproductive Medicine, a private voluntary group of infertility specialists.

Maybe so. But moral and ethical revulsion do not always translate into unlawful conduct, and this eggs-for-sale Web site exemplifies the (fre)e-market influence that has invaded our social fabric. Advertising human eggs for sale is not illegal under federal law, although it may be prohibited under some states' surrogate parenting laws. The sale of eggs and sperm is likewise not illegal and in fact has been a flourishing industry for more than a decade, since the 1985 introduction of cryopreservation, or freezing, of human embryos. While federal law does prohibit the sale of nonreplenishable solid organs such as kidneys, lungs and hearts, regenerating tissues such as blood, sperm and eggs are not covered under the act.

But while federal law may not specifically prohibit the sale of human gametes, it is not totally silent on the booming infertility industry. The Fertility Clinic Success Rate and Certification Act of 1992 contains reporting and certification requirements for programs offering in vitro fertilization and other reproductive technologies. This act was designed in part to prevent infertility clinics from defrauding patients by overinflating their advertised success rates. The law's author, Sen. Ron Wyden (D-Ore.), said he would be looking into the activities of Harris.

Would a federal law banning the sale of human eggs and sperm be in the best interest of those individuals that such a law would be designed to protect? I think not. The "ronsangels" Web site is one of dozens advertising the services of women who, for a host of reasons, are seeking payment for the surrender of their eggs. What seems particularly repellent about Harris' approach is that he is flaunting two characteristics that we would like to think are dissociated with reproduction — greed and physical beauty.

But even in the noncyber world, these factors often have played a role in issuing of offspring, and we are seemingly none the worse off for it. In the quaint, old-fashioned world of coital reproduction, mates seek out their reproductive soul mate to give their children the best opportunity for a quality life. Infertility patients are no less concerned with maximizing the quality of life for their children and may even be in the market for an egg to avoid passing on a genetic disease.

I join with the masses who deplore the sale of "beautiful" eggs for its borderline eugenic assertion that society values physical beauty above all else. But any student of genetic logic understands that the egg is only half the equation and the spermatic influence could be overwhelming.

Moreover, infertility is not a condition of choice. Couples seeking egg donors would much prefer to procreate naturally and thus tend to seek out donors who best mirror their characteristics, physical and otherwise, so as to produce a child as genetically close to them as possible.

As for www.ronsangels.com, I suggest that Harris save any commissions he receives from these postings for his legal defense fund. Trouble is already brewing with the beauties. One was taken off the site because "she was unstable," to quote Harris; another aged two years overnight when her listed age was changed from 18 to 20.

Sloppiness like this portends lawsuits for fraud, negligence and the like. And unlike many of his competitors, Harris does not provide medical, psychological or genetic screening of his models, making his donors far less attractive to individuals who are earnest in their quest to become parents and must rely on technology to do so.

If women feel particularly offended by the idea of beauty eggs, suggesting our only worth is in our reflection, take heart. Harris says he will soon be posting male model sperm donors. And in an era of concerns about comparable worth, consider that beautiful sperm will go for about $5,000 a vial while beautiful eggs are expected to garner up to $150,000 each.

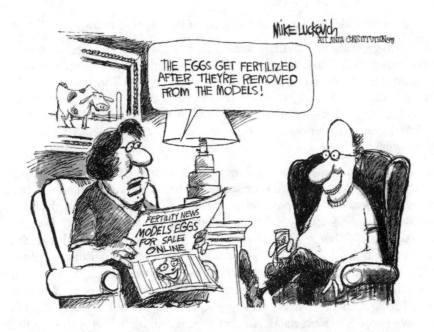

NOTES AND QUESTIONS

1.   A 2005 visit to www.ronsangels.com revealed an enterprise less about supplying model eggs to infertile couples and more about advertising Mr. Harris' ancillary businesses, including his work as an aerobic exercise guru and "fashion" photographer (for Playboy Magazine, where readers flock to view the haute couture). Despite these high-profile outlier offers to pay tens of thousands of dollars for Vogue and Ivy League eggs, the vast majority of egg donors are paid, on average, approximately $5,000 per donation cycle. This figure derives from a 2007 survey of several hundred fertility clinics that offer egg donation services. *See* Sharon Covington & William Gibbons, *What Is Happening to the Price of Eggs?*, 87 FERTILITY & STERILITY 1001 (2007) (finding national average for egg donor compensation is $4,200, with regional variations). As with sperm donation, the gamete purchaser can expect to pay far more than the donor's fee to procure the surrendered gametes. One Southern California egg donation agency tells prospective parents that they can expect to pay up to $20,000 for donated eggs, $5,000 to $10,000 for the donor's fee, up to $5,000 for the donor's medical expenses, and $6,000 for administrative costs, including psychological screening of the donor and legal fees. See www.thedonorsource.com.

2.   In 2008, more than one in every 10 ART cycles involved a donor egg (12.3% of all ART procedures involved either a fresh or frozen embryo created with a donor egg). See 2008 Assisted Reproductive Technology Success Rates, National Summary and Fertility Clinic Reports 16 (December 2010). The reason for the widespread use of donor eggs has little to do with a couple's desire to birth a lanky, intelligent, musical, and athletic child, but more to do with the pregnancy success rates using donor eggs. Overall, a woman has a 50% chance of delivering a live baby if she uses a fresh (nonfrozen) donor egg. Most importantly, these success rates

hold up even for older women who experience the highest rates of ART failure.

3.   Most egg donation agencies accept donors between the age of 20 and 30ish who are college educated, healthy and "height and weight" proportional. Many female law students would be well qualified applicants, and in fact would likely be highly desirable based on objective factors including SAT scores and college grades. In all probability, either you or someone very close to you would qualify as an egg donor. Would you consider donating eggs or encouraging those close to you to do so? What are your reasons?

On the other hand, would you encourage a friend or relative to use donated eggs? Would you use them in your own reproductive efforts? As was discussed with sperm donation, egg donation can pose serious harm to offspring if the donor has an undiagnosed genetic anomaly. In 2006, a California gay male couple learned their infant daughter — born with the help of an egg donor — had Tay-Sachs, a devastating neurological disease that usually leads to death within a few years of birth. The donor was unaware of her carrier status, as was the partner who supplied the sperm. *See* William Heisel, *Registry May Track Egg, Sperm Donors*, L.A. TIMES, Jan. 3, 2008, at B1. Some suggest that a gamete registry would alert prospective parents to material donor features, including health status, drug use or psychological problems. Critics warn collection of such data in a public place would be an invasion of donor privacy that would chill gamete donation.

4.   You have just been elected to the legislative body in your state. A constituent from your district calls your local office and reports that her 25-year old daughter is considering donating her eggs to an egg donation agency. Your constituent is worried that her daughter will be harmed by the process, either physically or psychologically, and that she will regret the decision to surrender her eggs once she decides to become a mother herself. She asks you to sponsor a law prohibiting egg donation in the state. Would you be willing to sponsor such a bill? If so, would your bill ban the practice entirely or just for commercial purposes? If you are not willing to legislate away the practice, would you be willing to regulate it in any way? What types of restrictions do you think would aid the citizens of your state?

There are a handful of state laws addressing the practice of egg donation, though none bans the practice entirely. For purposes of our discussion on the business of egg donation, consider the following Florida law: "Only reasonable compensation directly related to the donation of eggs, sperm, and preembryos shall be permitted." Fla. Stat. Ann. § 742.14 (West 2004). "Reasonable compensation" is not specifically defined in the bill. What compensation would you consider reasonable? Would that same amount be reasonable to your sister? Your best friend? A model with a six-figure income who wants to assist a childless couple? Do you see the problem with the term "reasonable?"

2. The Ethics of Egg Donation

Ethics Committee of the American Society for Reproductive Medicine
Financial Compensation of Oocyte Donors
88 Fertility & Sterility 305 (2007)

During the last 2 decades, oocyte donation increasingly has been accepted as a method of assisting women without healthy oocytes to have children. In addition to coordinating the voluntary and unpaid donation of oocytes from friends and relatives, a number of programs offer financial incentives to prospective oocyte donors. These remunerations take the form of monetary payment to donors or reduced IVF fees to women undergoing IVF who agree to provide oocytes to others. Programs also provide services to couples who have recruited their own offers of payment or through agencies that recruit oocyte donors . . .

The use of financial incentives raises two ethical questions: [1] do recruitment practices incorporating remuneration sufficiently protect the interests of oocyte donors, and [2] does financial compensation devalue human life by treating oocytes as property or commodities? . . .

ETHICAL CONCERNS RAISED BY REMUNERATION

[M]onetary compensation . . . create[s] the possibility of undue inducement and exploitation in the oocyte donation process. Women may agree to provide oocytes in response to financial need. High payments could lead some prospective donors to conceal medical information relevant to their own health or that of their biological offspring . . . With . . . compensation, there is a possibility that women will discount the physical and emotional risks of oocyte donation out of eagerness to address their financial situations . . . Financial compensation also could be challenged on grounds that it conflicts with the prevailing belief that gametes should not become products bought and sold in the marketplace.

Concerns Raised by Payment

Women undergoing retrieval purely to provide oocytes to others are exposed to physical and psychological burdens they would not otherwise face. There is some risk of unintentional pregnancy, because hormonal contraceptives must be discontinued for donation to occur. Donors also are exposed to risks of morbidity risks and a remote risk of mortality risk from [superovulation] and oocyte retrieval. Although the data are unclear at this time, it is possible that fertility drugs and procedures involved in oocyte donation could increase a woman's future health risks, including the risk of impaired fertility. Young women may be prone to dismiss the potential psychological consequences of donation, particularly those that could arise if they later experience infertility problems themselves. In addition, they may underestimate the psychological and legal consequences of their agreement to forgo parental rights and future contact with children born to oocyte recipients.

Another ethical concern is that payment for oocytes implies that they are property or commodities, and thus devalues human life. Many people believe that payment to individuals for reproductive and other tissues is inconsistent with maintaining important values related to respect for human life and dignity. This view is reflected in state and federal laws prohibiting direct payment to individuals providing organs and tissues for transplantation. Yet such laws generally permit organ and tissue donors to receive reimbursement for expenses and other costs associated with the donation procedure. In the analogous circumstances of biomedical research, human subjects exposed to physical and psychological risks are often reimbursed for expenses. Moreover, they may receive additional payments to compensate for the time and inconvenience associated with study participation.

Compensation based on a reasonable assessment of the time, inconvenience, and discomfort associated with oocyte retrieval can and should be distinguished from payment for the oocytes themselves. Payment based on such an assessment is also consistent with employment and other situations in which individuals are compensated for activities demanding time, stress, physical effort, and risk.

As payments to women providing oocytes increase in amount, the ethical concerns increase as well. The higher the payment, the greater the possibility that women will discount risks. High payments, particularly for women with specific characteristics, also convey the idea that oocytes are commercial property. Moreover, high payments are disturbing because they could be used to promote the birth of persons with traits deemed socially desirable, which is a form of positive eugenics. Such efforts to enhance offspring are morally troubling because they objectify children rather than assign them intrinsic dignity and worth. Finally, high payments could make donor oocytes available only to the very wealthy . . .

JUSTIFICATIONS FOR PERMITTING REMUNERATION

Although potential harm must be acknowledged and addressed, financial incentives may be defended on ethical grounds. First, providing financial incentives increases the number of oocyte donors, which in turn allows more infertile persons to have children. Second, the provision of financial or in-kind benefits does not necessarily discourage altruistic motivations; indeed, in surveys of women receiving such benefits, most reported that helping childless persons remained a significant factor in their decisions to donate. In a recent survey of donors who had been compensated up to $5,000, 88% of subjects reported that the best thing about the donation experience was "being able to help someone."

Third, financial compensation may be defended on grounds that it advances the ethical goal of fairness to donors . . .

The failure to provide financial or in-kind benefits to oocyte donors would arguably demean their significant contribution. Such an approach also would treat female gamete donors differently from sperm donors, who typically receive a financial benefit (albeit a modest one) for a much less risky and intrusive procedure. Fourth, the pressures created by financial incentives do not necessarily exceed and may be less than those experienced by women asked to make altruistic donations to relatives or friends.

Although the physical and psychological risks entailed in oocyte donation are real, they are not so severe as to justify intervention to limit the decision-making authority of adult women. Programs offering financial incentives should take steps to minimize the possibility of undue influence and exploitation by incorporating certain safeguards into the disclosure and counseling process. Programs can also structure the provision of incentives in ways that reduce the likelihood that women will be improperly influenced to donate. Such steps would reflect good ethical practice and reduce the likelihood of later legal action by dissatisfied donors.

DISCLOSURE AND COUNSELING

To discourage improper decisions to donate oocytes, programs should adopt an effective information disclosure and counseling process. Regardless of how prospective donors are recruited, programs should ensure that they receive accurate and meaningful information on the potential physical, psychological, and legal effects of oocyte retrieval and donation. The potential negative health and psychological consequences should be openly acknowledged . . . Prospective donors should understand the measures they must take to avoid unwanted pregnancy during a stimulation cycle. They also should understand that they could later develop desires to establish contact with genetically related children, desires that may be difficult or impossible to satisfy because of legal or other barriers.

Donor candidates should be encouraged to explore their possible emotional responses, particularly those that could develop if they have infertility problems themselves. To reduce the incidence of subsequent psychological problems, it would be prudent to limit donors to those who are 21 or older and have the emotional maturity to make such decisions.

To enhance the likelihood that information relevant to donation will be fully explored, programs are encouraged to designate an individual with psychological training and expertise to counsel prospective donors. This individual's primary responsibilities are to ensure that the prospective oocyte donor understands and appreciates the relevant information and feels free to decide against donation if doubts arise at any point before completion of the procedure. The prospective donor's motivation should be explored during the session, with the goal of ascertaining whether she fails to appreciate the full consequences of her donation or is improperly discounting the risks because of her economic status or infertility problems.

Some empirical data show that egg donors may want to know whether children are born as a result of their donations. Others may have preferences about how their donated eggs are used. For example, they may not want eggs to be provided to unmarried persons or unused embryos produced with their eggs to be destroyed. Program staff should discuss with prospective donors the amount of information they will be given about whether a birth occurs and any control they will have over oocyte disposition.

THE INCENTIVE STRUCTURE

Payment

Payments to women providing oocytes should be fair and not so substantial that they become undue inducements that will lead donors to discount risks. Monetary compensation should reflect the time, inconvenience, and physical and emotional demands associated with the oocyte donation process.

A 1993 analysis estimated that oocyte donors spend 56 hours in the medical setting, undergoing interviews, counseling, and medical procedures related to the process. According to this analysis, if men receive $25 for sperm donation, which this analysis estimated as taking 1 hour, oocyte donors should receive at least $1,400 for the hours they spend in the donation process. In 2000, the average payment to sperm donors was $60–$75, which this analysis suggests would justify a payment of $3,360–$4,200 to oocyte donors.

The above analysis fails to consider the time spent by sperm donors undergoing interviewing and screening. Even if this additional time is taken into account, however, the lengthier time commitment of women providing oocytes supports substantially higher payments to them than to sperm donors. Moreover, because oocyte donation entails more discomfort, risk, and physical intrusion than sperm donation, sperm donor reimbursement rates may not be a good model for determining payments to women providing oocytes.

It has been suggested that compensation for oocyte donors should be given for the hours spent on medication and on clinic visits, with the hourly rate based on the mean hourly wage of persons with demographic characteristics similar to those of the donor. This method of establishing payment rates presents practical difficulties and arguably would be unfair to women from lower income groups.

Although there is no consensus on the precise payment that oocyte donors should receive, at this time sums of $5,000 or more require justification and sums above $10,000 are not appropriate. Programs recruiting oocyte donors and those assisting couples who have recruited their own donors should establish a level of compensation that minimizes the possibility of undue inducement of donors and the suggestion that payment is for the oocytes themselves . . .

Payment also should reflect the amount of time expended and the burdens of the procedures performed. Thus, a woman who withdraws for medical or other reasons should be paid a portion of the fee appropriate to the time and effort she contributed. To protect the donor's right to withdraw, oocyte recipients must accept the risk that a donor will change her mind. In no circumstances should payment be conditioned on successful retrieval of oocytes or number of oocytes retrieved. Likewise, donors should never be required to cover the costs of the interrupted cycle. To avoid putting a price on human gametes or selectively valuing particular human traits, compensation should not vary according to . . . the number or quality of oocytes retrieved, the outcome of prior donation cycles, or the donor's ethnic or other personal characteristics . . .

ADDITIONAL ETHICAL CONSIDERATIONS

Once the donation process begins, oocyte donors become patients owed the same duties present in the ordinary physician-patient relationship. Programs should ensure that every donor has a physician whose primary responsibility is caring for the donor. Oocyte program staff should recognize that physicians providing services to both donors and recipients could encounter conflicts in promoting the best interests of both parties and should create mechanisms ensuring equitable and fair provision of services.

Programs offering . . . financial incentive[s] should adopt and disclose policies regarding coverage of an oocyte donor's medical costs should she experience health complications from the procedure. Ideally, programs should ensure that donors will be covered for any health care costs resulting from the procedure. Programs also should consider whether to make psychological services available to oocyte donors who experience subsequent distress related to the procedure.

Programs offering financial incentives should ensure that advertisements for donors are accurate and responsible. If financial or other benefits are noted in advertisements, the existence of risks and burdens also should be acknowledged . . .

To limit the health risks of donation and to avoid inadvertent consanguinity among offspring, programs should limit the number of times a woman may undergo retrieval procedures purely to provide oocytes to others. A good faith effort should be made to avoid accepting women who have already made a high number of donations elsewhere. Finally, all IVF programs offering oocyte donation should encourage further study of the medical and psychological effects on donors. Findings from such research could improve evaluation of risks and benefits and allow programs to provide more accurate information to prospective donors.

NOTES AND QUESTIONS

1. The ASRM guidelines on the ethics of commercial egg donation conclude that payment to women donors are, on balance, justified "on grounds that they advance the ethical goal of fairness to donors." The ASRM Ethics Committee suggests that financial incentives under $5,000 are justified in light of the time and effort that is required to complete an oocyte donation cycle. In contrast, they argue that payments of $10,000 or more cannot be justified on this same basis, as such large financial inducements shift focus from appropriate incentive to heavy-handed coercion. Do you agree? Does the amount that someone is paid for an activity determine whether that activity is ethical? If an activity is deemed ethical, can it become unethical because certain people who engage in the activity earn more than others? If so, can you think of other industries that might be affected by such an ethical yardstick? Been to the movies or a sporting event lately?

2. *Egg Donation and the SATs.* A survey of two months of advertisements for egg donors in 306 college newspapers found that nearly half of all ads exceeded the ASRM's $10,000 recommended limit on compensation. Notably, the higher the median SAT score of the college or university, the more likely the ads exceeded the

recommended limit, suggesting that "donor agencies and couples valued specific donor characteristics and based compensation on those preferences." *See* Aaron D. Levine, *Self-Regulation, Compensation, and the Ethical Recruitment of Oocyte Donors*, 40 HAST. CTR. RPT. 25 (2010). On paying for a smarter egg donor, one commentator remarked, "[W]e allow individuals to choose their mates and sperm donors on the basis of such characteristics. Why not choose egg donors similarly?" John Robertson, *Is There an Ethical Problem Here?*, 40 HAST. CTR. RPT. 3 (2010).

3.   *Egg Donation and Antitrust Law.* In April 2011, a former egg donor filed suit against the ASRM, its affiliate the Society for Assisted Reproductive Technology, and a Northern California fertility center alleging violations of Section 1 of the Sherman Act, a major federal antitrust law that dates back to 1890. The suit, a class action on behalf of all women who donated eggs during a certain period, claims the ASRM policy reprinted above is a conspiracy to fix the price of donor services purchased in the U.S. by requiring that clinics adhere to its policies in order to remain in good standing with the Society. ASRM policies include its compensation guidelines for egg donation. Thus, according to the suit, the organization has illegally suppressed and fixed the price of donor services since 2000. The complaint quotes, and was perhaps inspired by a law professor who labeled egg donor compensation practices in the U.S. "naked price-fixing . . . [by a] buyers' cartel." Kimberly Krawiec, *Sunny Samaritans and Egomaniacs: Price-Fixing in the Gamete Market*, 72 LAW & CONTEMP. PROBS. 59 (2009).

4.   The ethics of egg donation has been discussed by many policy-oriented organizations, but undoubtedly the most high-level group to issue a written report on the topic is the President's Council on Bioethics. Created by Executive Order on November 28, 2001, the Council was charged with advising President George W. Bush on bioethical issues that "may emerge as a consequence of advances in biomedical science and technology." See Exec. Order No. 13237, 66 Fed. Reg. 59,851 (Nov. 28, 2001). The Council first tackled the controversial issue of human cloning, which we take up in Chapter 10, and then moved on to explore other aspects of human reproduction. In March 2004 the Council issued a report on the regulation of biotechnologies that touch on human reproduction. The Council's report, titled *Reproduction and Responsibility: The Regulation of New Biotechnologies*, devotes Chapter 6 to the topic of "Commerce." It reads in relevant part:

> Payments for human gametes raise several ethical concerns. Some argue that the commercialization of reproductive tissues might diminish respect for the human body and human procreation. By putting human reproductive tissue — the seeds of the next generation — up for sale in the marketplace, it is argued that we stand to introduce a commercial character into human reproduction, and to introduce commercial concerns into the coming-to-be of the next generation. If the essential materials of human procreation are regularly bought, sold, and esteemed in accordance with market valuations (and indeed valued differently based on the desirability of certain traits, as in ads in college newspapers that offer premium prices for donors with particular characteristics), the human meaning of bringing forward the next generation may be obscured or undermined.

Others see such concerns as misleading and unjustified. They argue that commerce in human gametes is no different from commerce in other meaningful activities of life (like paying one's doctor) or commerce in other articles of special significance (like a religious text or a wedding ring). They point out that the clinics and laboratories are making money from assisting reproduction, and they suggest that it is unfair that only the donor is excluded from financial benefit. They further argue that the ability to buy and sell gametes helps otherwise infertile couples to participate in the activities of human procreation and child-rearing.

Ovum sales raise additional ethical concerns. The process of retrieving ova is onerous and risky for donors. The high fees paid to ovum donors — who are often from financially vulnerable populations, such as full-time students — might create pressure to undergo these invasive procedures . . . An additional concern is that a free market in ova could lead to discrimination and greater inequality. The 1994 National Institutes of Health (NIH) Human Embryo Research Panel speculated that an open market for ova would lead to a two-tiered system in which wealthy white ovum donors would receive high payments primarily from IVF patients, whereas poor minority women would receive substantially lower payments primarily from researchers.

Finally, financial incentives for donation encourage individuals to become the biological parents — sometimes many times over — of children they will never know. Alternatively, with the advent of laws providing children with the right to know their biological parentage, such donors may become involved in the lives of these children despite their wish to remain anonymous.

However, *not* compensating individuals for donating gametes raises still other ethical concerns. Financial incentives increase supply in other markets and are likely to do the same in the market for gametes for IVF. If there are no payments for gametes, some couples might remain childless because of an inadequate supply of eggs and sperm. Furthermore, given the sacrifice that is made by many gamete donors — especially ova donors — many argue that it would be unjust not to compensate them. Finally, some argue that a free market in gametes ultimately benefits all parties: those willing to provide their gametes get the compensation they desire, and those willing to pay for such gametes get the reproductive tissues they need to undergo assisted reproduction.

The President's Council on Bioethics, *Reproduction and Responsibility: The Regulation of the New Biotechnologies*, 151-53 (March 2004).

The Council's report, one could argue, is neutral in its view of the ethics of egg donation for financial remuneration, merely pointing out the arguments of both sides. In an earlier document issued by the Council, a more disfavored view of commercial egg donation emerged. In July 2003 the Council's staff issued a working paper to aid in the discussion of issues of human reproduction, suggesting restrictions on gamete donation could be in order:

(F) *Commodification of Nascent Human Life/Human Procreation:*

The commodification of human procreation is, for some, a further cause for concern, and an additional potential target for regulation. At present, the buying and selling of gametes is essentially unrestricted in most states, as is, in principle, the buying and selling of embryos . . .

Possible policies in this arena include:

(a) *Limits or restrictions on the buying and selling of gametes:* If trade in human gametes is a concern, the government could set certain limits, potentially including a ceiling on the price of eggs, limits on advertising for or by gamete donors, or perhaps even a restriction on the selling of gametes altogether . . .

President's Council on Bioethics, Staff Working Paper, U.S. Public Policy and the Biotechnologies That Touch the Beginnings of Human Life: Some Policy Options (July 2003) (according to the working paper, "the staff working paper was discussed at the Council's July 2003 meeting. It was prepared by staff solely to aid discussion, and does not represent the official views of the Council or of the United States Government."). It appears the Council's final report did not adopt the staff's possible policy in the area of egg donation, opting instead to enunciate the ethical parameters of the practice.

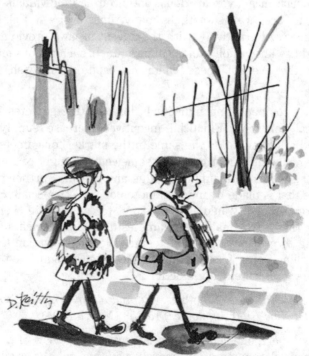

"I told my parents that if grades were so important they should have paid for a smarter egg donor."

3.   Informed Consent and Egg Donation

a.   Informing Egg Donors of Risks and Benefits

In part the discussion about the ethics of egg donation focuses on the vulnerability of women likely to offer their services as an egg donor. There is no dispute that potential donors should be informed about the risks and benefits of the process, just as any patient is entitled to similar information before undergoing any medical procedure. But the physician/patient relationship may be complicated in an egg donor scenario by the fact that the donor patient is undergoing treatment not for her medical benefit, but for the benefit of the sponsoring individual or couple. Moreover, typically patients are not paid to undergo medical treatment, an element that could influence the dynamic between the physician and the patient.

Even before the donor meets a physician to discuss medical risks, she is screened by an ART clinic or egg donation agency. It would seem natural that prospective donors would have questions and concerns about the potential risks involved in egg retrieval. In the late 1990s researchers at the University of Pennsylvania conducted a study to evaluate the risk information provided by egg donor programs to prospective donors who made a preliminary telephone call inquiry to the program. Interviewers posed as prospective egg donors who responded to ads placed in college newspapers. The study assessed the programs' responses when asked questions about the risks of egg donation. The majority of programs surveyed did not volunteer any risk information, and those that volunteered or responded to questions provided incomplete and/or inaccurate risk information. Andrea D. Gurmankin, *Risk Information Provided to Prospective Oocyte Donors in a Preliminary Phone Call*, 1 AM. J. BIOETHICS 3 (2001).

The University of Pennsylvania study evoked a number of commentaries, two of which are reprinted below.

Gregory Stock
Eggs for Sale: How Much Is Too Much?
1 Am. J. Bioethics 26 (2001)

. . . Egg donation brims with difficult issues of informed consent, conflicting physician responsibilities, appropriate recruitment procedures, and the impact of financial incentives upon donors. The author's concern about the impact of misinformation upon donors and how this might interact with large recruitment fees is commendable, and her pilot data provide useful pointers to further studies. Her policy recommendations, however, have little to do with the actual data she has collected, and the implication that her suggestions somehow flow from that data is misleading.

The author makes four basic policy proposals:

   1. That medically trained personnel be required to receive initial calls from egg donors;

   2. That a standard information packet be provided all donors;

   3. That third party screeners be used; and

4. That donor fees be reduced.

It is difficult to see, however, why the modest and unsurprising conclusion of her small pilot study, namely that "some oocyte donor programs are providing incomplete and inaccurate information to prospective oocyte donors in preliminary phone inquiries," warrant these actions.

It is important to look at the author's proposed policies within the framework of practices that are commonplace throughout medicine and other realms of society. The first suggestion — that medically trained personnel should answer preliminary phone calls — strikes me as the kind of regulatory micromanagement that creates significant overhead without accomplishing much. Ads are placed routinely for cosmetic surgery, hi-tech screening tests, weight-loss treatments, blood donation, and infertility treatment. All these procedures involve some risk, and rarely do medical personnel field initial phone inquiries for any of them. Nor should they. Not only would it be a highly inefficient use of trained medical professionals, it would convey the false impression that these are not essentially sales pitches. It is unreasonable to assume that someone responding to an ad offering tens of thousands of dollars for oocyte donation — especially an educated young woman at a premier academic institution — is entirely naive about the motivations of those placing that ad . . .

The author also suggests providing donors with standard information packets. This is a good idea, but it stands on its own merit. Such a packet would be useful to prospective donors no matter how much risk information most agencies were providing. The information would be cheap and easy to distribute and would insure access to up-to-date authoritative information about the procedure. The author's own failure to include potential psychosocial risks in her pilot study shows just how easy it is to neglect some risk factors. The author's proposal for third-party screeners, on the other hand, is dubious. It is cumbersome, it has operational pitfalls, and it would be unnecessary if donors got information packets.

The author's final suggestion — to reduce donor fees — is so weakly connected to her data that it seems like a preconceived point she has grafted to her discussion. Her pilot study does not attempt to look at whether organizations that pay more for eggs are more deceptive about discussing risks with their clients, nor does it look at whether high fees distort donor-risk perceptions. Agencies that pay the highest fees may be more, not less forthright about discussing risks with their potential donors. We just do not have the data. Moreover, if a woman is being misled about the risks she is subjecting herself to, why is it worse if she is motivated by financial gain rather than altruism?

The core issue about high fees for donors is not whether such compensation is a strong motivator, but whether there is anything wrong with monetary incentives. If we accept that a freely accepted payment is coercion, then are we not coerced when we sell our home at a hefty profit or take a high-paying job? Money is a meaningful part of modern life; and we do things for money that we would not do in its absence. The idea that monetary reward constitutes coercion cheapens the entire concept of coercion.

It is not clear why it should matter whether donors are motivated primarily by altruism or by money, but if it somehow did matter, then lowering donor fees might not shift the motivations of donors so much as shift their demographics. A specific fee that will appropriately balance the equation of personal benefit and altruism does not exist. People have different tendencies toward altruism and different needs for money. Many agencies use a maximum fee of $5,000 for donors. For some women that is a lot of money for egg donation; for others, five times as much would seem like very little for the procedure. The idea of compensating egg donors at the same hourly wage as sperm donors shows how absurd the rationales for setting price limits might become. If we think it is wrong to tempt donors with money, then we should not pay donors anything. If it is not wrong, then we do not need to regulate prices.

The only criticism the author hazards for her suggestion to reduce donor fees is that oocyte donation programs might be left with unmet demand for oocytes. But there is no shortage of donors in general, just a shortage of donors with certain profiles of intelligence, beauty, education, religion, and other factors. If $5,000 is a big incentive for some women and is an acceptable fee to regulators, it is hard to see why a higher amount, which will be a strong incentive to other women with other profiles, is wrong. These higher figures will not be a temptation to most potential donors, because most women cannot command these prices. Anecdotal evidence suggests that the high donor fees mentioned in college newspaper ads are primarily a come-on to get inquiries from potential donors.

The author has brought up an important issue: Full risk disclosure is critical for egg donors and should occur early in the recruitment process. Her suggestion of providing a standardized risk statement to potential oocyte donors would be a good way of ensuring that they get the information they need and seems to have very little downside. The author, however, has not made an adequate case for more aggressive policies such as regulating fees, using third-party screeners, or requiring medical professionals to do sales work.

Judith Daar
Regulating the Fiction of Informed Consent in ART Medicine
1 Am. J. Bioethics 19 (2001)

Andrea Gurmankin bravely ventures into the harrowing and dynamic world of reproductive medicine to investigate its most vulnerable feature, the practice of informed consent. Her empirical research explores the level of frank risk disclosure provided by assisted reproductive technology (ART) programs to young women who contemplate selling their eggs to infertile couples. Not surprisingly, Gurmankin's research reveals that most programs do not volunteer risk information and many provide inaccurate or incomplete risk information when queried by potential egg donors. The article's empirical foundation and dismaying conclusions prompt inquiry into whether informed consent can ever be a practical reality in a field of medicine grounded in the trilogy of rapidly advancing technologies, emotionally-charged expectations, and commercialism.

To begin, the fiction of informed consent in the broader doctor-patient relationship is well described. Studies indicate that as physicians feel increased pressure to see more patients, particularly in the managed care setting, full disclosure and an open discussion is less likely to occur. At the same time, patient comprehension is low and decision making about medical choices is often based on factors other than accurate information, such as fear, emotion and religious beliefs. To posit that egg donors receive less risk information and therefore have less opportunity for informed consent than patients in other medical specialty areas is truly a bleak prospect . . .

The role of informed consent in oocyte donation is further complicated by the way in which egg donors are perceived in the overall treatment plan for the infertile couple. Granted an egg donor is essential to successful treatment of the couple, but is she treated as a patient, quasi-patient, or even non-patient by the physician monitoring her progress in the donation process? If a single physician is retained to perform both egg retrieval from the donor and IVF for the intended mother, a clear conflict of interest arises. The physician must simultaneously maximize the opportunity for pregnancy by retrieving as many eggs as possible, while minimizing the risk of harm to the donor by limiting the number of eggs that are produced. Since it is the infertile couple who generally pays the physician's fees, it seems likely this conflict would more often be resolved in favor of the sponsoring couple. Perhaps physicians are not fully cognizant of this conflict because they don't view the egg donor as a patient. Because she gains no medical benefit from the physician's services, she may be perceived as a pure instrumentality to the doctor's therapeutic capabilities, directed solely at the infertile couple.

Even if the egg donor is cared for by an independent physician, one who is not involved in the treatment of the infertile couple, the doctor-patient relationship still defies traditional parameters. In the course of (euphemistically) donating her eggs, the donor derives and the physician provides no medical benefit. If informed consent is truly a doctrine in which risks and benefits are disclosed for the sake of rational balancing, it is logical that the absence of benefit in the egg donor scenario would confound the disclosure process. If a doctor can offer no medical benefits, she may be inclined to minimize the medical risks. Commercial gain is such a rare patient goal that at this juncture it simply can't be reconciled with the informed consent doctrine.

In California, lawmakers became aware of the potential vulnerability of egg donors and drafted legislation to address some of those concerns. In February 2000, State Senator Tom Hayden introduced Senate Bill 1630 into the California Senate. Initially, the ambitious bill contained a wide array of provisions, including language mandating insurance coverage for infertility treatment, a limitation on the number of times a woman could donate eggs during her lifetime (4), the establishment of a registry for all egg donors in the state, and an assortment of disclosure requirements directed at ART patients and oocyte donors. After numerous amendments, a bare bones bill was passed by the legislature and presented to Governor Davis. Even in its pared down form, the bill required ART physicians to provide oocyte donors with a standardized written summary of "health and consumer issues", including disclosures about:

> [t]he potential risks of oocyte donation, including the risk of decreased
> fertility and the risks associated with using the drugs, medications, and

hormones prescribed for ovarian stimulation during the oocyte donation process.

Regrettably, Governor Davis vetoed the bill, citing an ongoing effort by the state Department of Health Services to develop guidelines for informing ART patients of the potential risks of treatment. Despite this setback, there is hope that lawmakers in California, home to 51 of the 360 fertility clinics located in the United States, will revisit the issue of ART disclosure and consent. If such a standardized disclosure pamphlet is developed, perhaps it can serve as a model for state lawmakers and ART program directors across the country.

Of course, standardizing and mandating risk disclosure to oocyte donors does not resolve the myriad problems attendant to decision making in this area. Donors may continue to ignore or downplay known risks in the face of overwhelmingly attractive financial incentives. But at the very least, egg donors can join the ranks of other medical patients whose irrational decisions are made in the face of full and fair risk disclosure.

NOTES AND QUESTIONS

1.   In 2009, California law makers did enact and Governor Schwarzenegger did sign a new law mandating standardized disclosure to women who provide their eggs for another's fertility treatment. The law places the burden on clinics and egg donor agencies who advertise for prospective donors. California Health & Safety Code § 125325 provides in relevant part:

> The person or entity posting an advertisement seeking oocyte donation associated with the delivery of fertility treatment that includes assisted oocyte production and a financial payment or compensation of any kind, shall include the following notice in a clear and conspicuous manner:
>
>> "Egg donation involves a screening process. Not all potential egg donors are selected. Not all selected egg donors receive the monetary amounts or compensation advertised. As with any medical procedure, there may be risks associated with human egg donation. Before an egg donor agrees to begin the egg donation process, and signs a legally binding contract, she is required to receive specific information on the known risks of egg donation. Consultation with your doctor prior to entering into a donor contract is advised."

What, if any, impact do you think this new law will have on the practices and attitudes of women who contemplate becoming egg donors for cash? Does knowing "not all potential egg donors are selected" make women more or less likely to enter the marketplace?

2.   The new California law described in Note 1 became effective on January 1, 2010, at the height of the worst economic recession in many decades. If lawmakers intended to suppress or dampen the egg market, their efforts were overwhelmed by a flood of prospective egg (and sperm) donors who entered the market during the recession. In a recent *Wall Street Journal* article, egg donation agencies reported a substantial increase in the number of inquiries by prospective egg donors during

the economic downturn. "We're even getting men offering up their wives," one agency reported, adding, "It's pretty scary." *See* Melinda Beck, *Ova Time: Women Line Up to Donate Eggs — For Money*, WALL STREET JOURNAL, Dec. 9, 2008, at D1.

----

b.   Informing Donors About Gamete Placement

What control do sperm and egg donors retain over their gametes once they are removed from the body? Sperm donors traditionally retain no control over their surrendered sperm. Once the donation is made, the sperm bank directs the disposition of the sperm to an interested client. For egg donors, the procedure may be slightly different because often couples will solicit a particular donor rather than relying on a database available through an egg donor program. A prospective donor may be inclined to donate her eggs because she is interested in assisting a particular couple, rather than adding her profile to an existing pool of available donors.

A typical ad soliciting a particular egg donor may read as follows: **"Chinese/Asian Egg Donor Needed.** We are a loving, committed couple seeking a woman age 21-30. Reasonable compensation and expenses paid. Please contact our attorney at . . ." (This ad appeared in the *Tufts Daily* on May 3, 2004). A woman responding to this ad may have the opportunity to meet the couple before deciding to become a donor. This is known as an "open donation" and by all accounts, is not a widespread practice among commercial egg donation programs. Most egg donation agencies offer anonymous donations, much like their sperm donor counterparts. With an anonymous donation system, donors do not have the opportunity to either meet the recipient of their eggs or direct the disposition in anyway. This generalized practice may be the norm, but disputes do arise.

For example, a Texas egg donor sued two married couples for what she considered unlawful sharing of her donated eggs. The donor alleged she agreed to donate eggs to one couple via an Internet site. She later learned that some of her eggs had been given to another couple by their treating physician who proposed the egg-sharing between the two couples. According to the donor, no one sought her permission — or compensated her — for providing her eggs to anyone other than the couple with whom she originally contracted. The attorney for the treating physician defended his client's actions saying, "Once you donate those eggs, you have no rights to those eggs or to the child of those eggs." *See* Jo Ann Zuniga, *Fertile Ground for Dispute*, HOUS. CHRONICLE, June 1, 2002, at A33. If the attorney is correct that the donor lost dispositional control over her excised eggs, where did the control go? To the doctor, as the attorney suggests? To the original couple who contracted with the donor? To the agency that solicited the donor via the Internet?

The issue of dispositional authority over human eggs that have left the donor's body but not yet made their way into the body of an intended parent or gestational surrogate remains controversial. If a donated egg is fertilized by the sperm of an intended parent, does this act settle the issue of dispositional authority? Consider the next case.

LITOWITZ v. LITOWITZ
Supreme Court of Washington
48 P.3d 261 (2002)

SMITH, J. Petitioner Becky M. Litowitz seeks review of a decision of the Court of Appeals, Division Two, which affirmed an order of the Thurston County Superior Court in favor of Respondent David J. Litowitz in a dissolution action in which Respondent was awarded two cryopreserved [3] preembryos[4]. The Court of Appeals affirmed the trial court and awarded the preembryos to Respondent. This court granted review. We reverse . . .

STATEMENT OF FACTS

On February 27, 1982 Petitioner Becky M. Litowitz and Respondent David J. Litowitz were married. Respondent adopted Petitioner's two children from a previous marriage. On July 15, 1980, prior to their marriage, Petitioner and Respondent had a child together, Jacob Litowitz. Shortly after Jacob was born Petitioner Litowitz had a hysterectomy leaving her unable to produce eggs or to naturally give birth to a child.

Petitioner and Respondent decided to have another child through *in vitro* fertilization. They sought the services of the Center for Surrogate Parenting, Loma Linda University Gynecology and Obstetrics Medical Group, in Loma Linda, California. Five preembryos were created with eggs received from an egg donor. The eggs were fertilized by Respondent Litowitz' sperm. Three of the five preembryos were implanted in a surrogate mother, producing a female child, M., who was born January 25, 1997. The two remaining preembryos were cryopreserved and stored in the clinic in Loma Linda, California.

Petitioner and Respondent entered into a contract in Beverly Hills, California with the egg donor. The contract was signed by Petitioner Becky M. Litowitz on March 20, 1996, by Respondent David J. Litowitz on March 21, 1996 and by the egg donor, J.Y., and her husband, E.Y., on April 1, 1996. The contract defined Petitioner as the "Intended Mother" and Respondent as the "Natural Father." The "Intended Mother" and "Natural Father" are further defined as the "Intended Parents." The egg donor contract provided in part:

---

[3] [n.1] STEDMAN'S MEDICAL DICTIONARY 416 (26th ed.1995) ("cryopreservation" is defined as the "[m]aintenance of the viability of excised tissues or organs at extremely low temperatures.").

[4] [n.2] Clerk's Papers at 177-78. "The term 'preembryo' denotes that stage in human development immediately after fertilization occurs. The preembryo 'comes into existence with the first cell division and lasts until the appearance of a single primitive streak, which is the first sign of organ differentiation. This [primitive streak] occurs at about fourteen days of development.'" Donna A. Katz, Note, *My Egg, Your Sperm, Whose Preembryo? A Proposal for Deciding Which Party Receives Custody of Frozen Preembryos*, 5 Va. J. Soc. Pol'y & L. 623, 628-29 n. 42 (1998) (alteration in original) (quoting Clifford Grobstein, *Human Development from Fertilization to Birth, in Encyclopedia of Bioethics* 847 (Warren Thomas Reich ed., 1995)).

PARAGRAPH 13

All eggs produced by the Egg Donor pursuant to this Agreement shall be deemed the property of the Intended Parents and as such, the Intended Parents shall have the sole right to determine the disposition of said egg(s). In no event may the Intended Parents allow any other party the use of said eggs without express *written* permission of the Egg Donor.

Respondent and Petitioner entered into two contracts with the Loma Linda Center for Fertility and In Vitro Fertilization in Loma Linda, California. One, a consent and authorization for preembryo cryopreservation (freezing) following *in vitro* fertilization, dated March 25, 1996, provided for freezing the preembryos The other was an agreement and consent for cryogenic preservation (short term), dated March 25, 1996 . . .

Petitioner and Respondent separated before their daughter, M., was born. In the dissolution proceedings in the Pierce County Superior Court, Respondent on October 21, 1998 indicated his wish to put the remaining preembryos up for adoption. In those proceedings Petitioner on October 26, 1998 indicated her wish to implant the remaining preembryos in a surrogate mother and bring them to term. On December 11, 1998 the trial court, the Honorable Waldo F. Stone, awarded the preembryos to Respondent David J. Litowitz based upon the "best interest of the child." . . .

In affirming the trial court, the Court of Appeals concluded the contracts signed by Petitioner and Respondent in California did not require Respondent to continue with their family plan to have another child and that Respondent's right not to procreate compelled the court to award the preembryos to him . . .

CONTRACTUAL ISSUES

This is the first case in which this court has been asked to resolve a dispute over disposition of frozen preembryos in a dissolution action. There is limited case law in other jurisdictions involving disputes over disposition of frozen preembryos . . .

This case involves a dispute over frozen preembryos between Petitioner, who is not a progenitor,[5] and Respondent, who is a progenitor. In the four cases cited from Tennessee, Massachusetts, New York and New Jersey, one party to each dispute contributed the egg and the other party contributed the sperm. They were all progenitors. In this case Petitioner did not produce the eggs used to create the preembryos. She has no biological connection to the preembryos and is not a progenitor. Any right she may have to the preembryos must be based solely upon contract.

The egg donor contract provides:

All eggs produced by the Egg Donor pursuant to this Agreement shall be deemed *the property of the Intended Parents and as such, the Intended Parents shall have the sole right to determine the disposition of said egg(s).*

---

[5] [Footnote 41 in text] STEDMAN'S MEDICAL DICTIONARY 1434 (26th ed. 1995) (A "progenitor" is "[a] precursor, ancestor; one who begets.").

In no event may the Intended Parents allow any other party the use of said eggs without express *written* permission of the Egg Donor (Emphasis added).

Petitioner Becky M. Litowitz correctly asserts that the egg donor contract gives her and Respondent equal rights to the eggs even though she is not a progenitor. The contract defines Petitioner Litowitz as the "Intended Mother" and Respondent David J. Litowitz as the "Natural Father." It defines the "Intended Parents" as the Natural Father and the Intended Mother. The contract provides that the intended parents, Petitioner and Respondent, have a right to determine disposition of the eggs. Even though Respondent Litowitz, as the intended father, indeed has a biological connection to the preembryos, he has no greater contractual right to the eggs than Petitioner Litowitz has as the intended mother. Under that contract, Petitioner and Respondent would have equal rights to the eggs. But the egg donor contract does not relate to the preembryos which resulted from subsequent sperm fertilization of the eggs . . .

Petitioner claims the decision of the Court of Appeals is internally inconsistent because it held that the contract did not control the dispute between the intended parents while it could be used to extinguish the rights of the egg donor. She asserts the Court of Appeals extinguished the rights of the egg donor when it allowed Respondent the right to transfer the preembryos to a third party without the egg donor's consent as required by the egg donor contract.

Respondent asserts the Court of Appeals did not determine the rights of the egg donor. He maintains the court chose not to determine the egg donor's rights under the contract because he had not sought transfer of the preembryos under terms of that contract, but based his claim only upon the cryopreservation contract. Respondent points out that the egg donor has not been a party at any stage in this litigation and no issues relating to any rights the egg donor might have to the preembryos have been brought before the court.

The Court of Appeals correctly concluded the egg donor contract, at any rate, did not prevent Respondent from donating the preembryos to another couple. The court indicated Respondent would not need written permission from the egg donor to donate the preembryos because the egg donor contract only required written permission for transfer of the donated eggs. The court correctly observed that the eggs no longer existed as they were identified in the egg donor contract because they were later fertilized by Respondent's sperm and their character was then changed to preembryos. The Court of Appeals did not rule on the rights of the egg donor under the egg donor contract because that matter has not been before the court at any stage of these proceedings. Even if it were, it is doubtful that the egg donor would have a remaining contractual right once the eggs have been fertilized and become preembryos . . .

[The court goes on to decide the fate of the contested frozen embryos, a topic we take up in Chapter 7.]

NOTES AND QUESTIONS

1.   The reported litigation in Texas over the disposition of donor eggs and the *Litowitz* case focus on a contract signed by an egg donor prior to the retrieval process. If the egg donor contract in the Texas case had the identical language to Paragraph 13 of the Litowitzs' contract, would the plaintiff egg donor be likely to prevail at a trial on the merits?

2.   The Washington Supreme Court concludes that the egg donor contract (and the egg donor by extension) no longer controlled the disposition of the Litowitzs' embryos because "the eggs no longer existed" because they were fertilized and then changed to embryos. Whatever property interest the egg donor had, including the right to control the disposition of the surrendered tissue, was lost because the property itself no longer exists. In 1990, the California Supreme Court confronted a similar issue, although the tissue involved was not of reproductive potential. In *Moore v. Regents of the University of California*, 51 Cal. 3d 120, 271 Cal. Rptr. 146, 793 P.2d 479 (1990), *cert. denied*, 499 U.S. 936 (1991), the court evaluated the claim of John Moore, a patient whose spleen had been removed to cure his leukemia, but was later used by researchers to create a valuable cell line that was the subject of lucrative commercial agreements. The patient claimed a property interest in the cell line because his spleen cells had been used, without his consent, to develop the valuable product. The court rejected Mr. Moore's claim largely on the grounds that the valuable cell line "is both factually and legally distinct from the cells taken from Moore's body." Instead, the court determined the cell line was the product of the inventive effort put forth by the researchers, not the property of the one who provided the raw ingredients.

How does the decision in *Moore v. Regents of the University of California* affect disputes over the disposition of donated eggs? Is an egg donor, like Mr. Moore, a mere provider of raw ingredients who loses any claim to her eggs once they have changed in form into embryos? Do you see any distinctions between the *Moore* case and the case of an egg donor?

3.   Should gamete donors be informed about the placement of their donations? What are the benefits and possible drawbacks of informing donors about gamete placement? What about informing gamete donors about the birth of children from their donation? It might surprise you to learn that most sperm and egg agencies do not notify donors about the birth of children following a donation. In some cases, sperm banks and egg donation agencies will provide limited data to donors who follow up after a donation. In the case of sperm donors, some banks will tell inquiring donors that a live birth has occurred but will rarely reveal the exact number of children born. In egg donation scenarios, often recipient couples are asked whether they wish the egg donor to know about a live birth. If the couple declines, the donor is not privy to the fruits of her labor.

SECTION III: THE BENEFITS AND BURDENS OF AN ART MARKET

We have learned about the integral role that money plays in assisted conception, from the cost of IVF to the payments made to gamete donors. Now we turn to evaluate the merits and risks of intertwining commercialization and reproduction. As you read the commentaries, you may want to reflect on whether your expenditure of money on a cherished activity affects your attitude and actions toward that activity.

A.   Should We Ban a Market for the Sale of Gametes?

1.   Arguments for Market Inalienability

Some view the interaction of commercial enterprise and human reproduction as inherently problematic, even immoral. The scenario in which want-to-be parents pay money in order to produce a child, usually one that is genetically related to one parent, threatens to bring such unwanted byproducts as commodification of children (treating children as a product, with expectations such as value, performance and even exchangeability dominating the parents' view of the child), and the denigration of the dignity of human procreation. Arguments against teaming procreation and money began to surface before the advent of the sale of human eggs; such arguments were initially aimed at the practice of surrogate parenting in which the contracting woman is paid for her gestation (and sometimes egg/genetic) services.

An early critic of marketing reproductive services was Professor Margaret Radin, whose seminal article on the concept of market-inalienability has been the cornerstone for discussion about the sale of reproductive goods and services. In her article, *Market-Inalienability*, 100 HARV. L.R. 1849 (1987), Professor Radin begins by defining market-inalienability as the notion that some things may be given away but not sold. She argues that surrogacy services should be inalienable, which would allow women to gratuitously provide reproductive services but not to sell them on the open market. The worry she expresses is that commercial surrogacy will lead to the commodification of women and children. For women, her fear is that their attributes (height, eye color, measured intelligence) will be commodified and they will be valued not as individual persons but rather as goods that can be purchased on the open market. For children, her concern is that they may be perceived as products of a baby-selling scheme, a wholly illegal and very dangerous trade.

Ultimately, Professor Radin concludes that market-inalienability is the only way to assure and support the ideal of "human flourishing." She argues that the concept of personhood involves an ideal of individual uniqueness that is inconsistent with the idea that a person's attributes are fungible, that they have a monetary equivalent. An open market to human attributes reduces people to fungible units totally lacking in individuating characteristics. For these reasons, she concludes that commercial surrogacy should be disfavored, instead looking to altruism to meet the needs of infertile individuals. *See* 100 HARV. L. R. at 1885, 1932-36.

As can be expected, the concept of market-inalienability for reproductive services has its fans and detractors. Let's hear from both sides.

Mary Lyndon Shanley
Collaboration and Commodification in Assisted Procreation: Reflections on an Open Market and Anonymous Donation in Human Sperm and Eggs
36 Law & Society Rev. 257 (2002)

The practices through which we regulate the transfer of human gametes (eggs and sperm) reflects and shapes our understanding of our relationship to our genetic material, the extent to which family bonds are created by nature and by human will, and the role the market should play in forming families. The ways in which we think about and justify these practices engages important themes of liberal political theory: the understanding of individuals as autonomous or defined (at least in part) by relationships that entail dependence, interdependence, and care; the meaning of reproductive freedom; and the extent to which a free market may protect or undercut individual liberty. Here, I approach these theoretical issues by focusing on [the] ethical and policy question . . . that arise when people form families with gametes supplied by other persons. [S]hould the sale of eggs and sperm be prohibited, regulated, or left to the open market?

An Argument Against Marketing Human Gametes

In the United States, unlike many other countries, the mechanism by which gametes are transferred from one person to another has largely been the market. In market transactions . . . an anonymously produced object becomes part of a store on which others draw. Preserving the social anonymity of market goods is fundamental to the supposition that goods are available for all. Because gametes are separable from the provider they can appear to have certain characteristics of commodities, objects "produced" by the body that become part of a common store — as the term "sperm bank" suggests. Control over eggs or sperm can be transferred from provider to doctor or fertility clinic, and from these to the recipient. They can be treated as a generalized "resource" that can be traded in the market. . . . [T]he market analogy has already done its work: we think so freely of the providing and purchasing of goods and services that transactions in gametes is already a thought-of act of commerce . . . And once people conceptualize gametes as commodities, it becomes very difficult to argue against allowing a market in gametes.

The fact that it is appropriate for people to regard gametes as the possession of the provider in the sense that no one (including the government and medical research facilities) may commandeer them does not mean, however, that a gamete provider has a right to sell that material; the right to exclude others from use does not entail the right to sell. The liberal ideal of "self ownership" does not mean that we can do whatever we like with all our body parts, selling off what we don't need or want. The law allows people to sell hair, and sometimes blood, but prohibits the sale of body organs. Even someone willing and able to live with only one kidney or eye may not sell the other, nor may the kidney, eye, heart, or liver from a deceased person be sold. The distinction here is not simply that between renewable and nonrenewable material, or between material necessary and unnecessary to sustain life. It also involves a judgment that some parts of the body should not be for sale either because of the significance of reserving aspects of the human body from commodification, or because economic need might lead poor people to sell body parts. What kind of "body parts" are gametes, and how should we think about the ways in which they should be transferred from one person to another for purposes of procreation? To what extent should gametes be regarded as personal property, and providers as owners of those gametes?

Buying and selling gametes, whether by differential or uniform pricing, suggests that they are property and that the person in whose body they originate has rights of ownership until he or she transfers the gametes (and the rights of ownership) to someone else. Differential pricing of gametes based on characteristics like the provider's height, skin and hair color, athletic or academic achievement, and musical ability seems to validate the assumption that persons with such attributes — both providers and as-yet-unborn (indeed, as-yet-unconceived) children — are "worth more" than others. Certain characteristics people are born with are valued more than others: lighter-skinned people encounter less employment discrimination than darker-skinned individuals; men are paid more than women with comparable education. It is bad enough that these and other differences, which are accidents of birth, generate economic inequality in the labor market; it is far worse when these traits lead to differential compensation for the provider's gametes. When people know that the genetic material that made a particular child's existence possible was bought for a higher (or lower) price than that of some other child, such knowledge may undermine the proposition that all persons are of equal dignity regardless of their wealth or social status.

Some people believe that paying a flat rate to providers (higher for eggs than sperm donation because egg donation is much more difficult) avoids the affront to human dignity involved in an open market in eggs and sperm and is not improper. They point out that in gamete transfer, unlike adoption, there is no existing child and no social relationship between provider and gamete. Hence the prohibitions on baby-selling do not apply, and the gamete may be sold by the person from whom it is extracted. But treating gametes as property that can be sold, even for a uniform price, suggests that individuals "own" their gametes in the same way that they own other transferable property. This is the wrong way to conceptualize human beings' relationship to their genetic material . . . [T]he kind of ownership which we can be said to possess in relation to our gametes is conditional: we are not allowed to do anything we like with them, because they are not unequivocally ours. They are held in common with past and future generations . . . A person's relationship to his or her genetic material is better thought of as a kind of stewardship than as ownership. To shape social practices to avoid conveying the idea that gametes are properly thought of as individually owned property, we must move either to a system of paying for the activities involved in providing gametes (not for gametes themselves), or to pure donation (gift), options I discuss in the next section.

Transforming the Practice of Gamete Transfer

If [an] open market buying and selling of gametes is [un]desirable, what are possible policy alternatives and how would each of these shape the "tale told by law and public policy" with respect to gamete transfer? Ideally . . . gamete transfer would be a gift relationship with reimbursement only for medical, child-care, transportation, and other necessary expenses. "The gift of life" should be just that, a "gift," if it is to reflect the proper understanding of both provider's and recipient's relationship to this genetic material, and the significance of collaborative procreation to the person who comes into being. I believe it is possible and desirable to devise policies and practices that would recognize the relational as well as the individualistic aspects of human procreation, and would give proper place to the potential child and the adult he or she will become . . .

If buying and selling eggs and sperm were prohibited, gamete transfer might take place either by payment of an "inconvenience allowance" or by gift. The previous section argued that an unregulated market is an assault on the human dignity of both providers and persons who come into being, and it falsely conflates human freedom with the exercise of market choice. While uniform payment is less objectionable than differential pricing, it still entails the commodification of human gametes. Some people have suggested that payment of an "inconvenience allowance," which would compensate providers for the time and discomfort of transferring gametes, not for the gametes themselves, would avoid the morally unacceptable aspects of gamete transfer . . .

Payment of an inconvenience allowance that is linked to the actual procedures performed is preferable to payment for gametes themselves because it does not treat gametes as private property, and it directs attention to the provider and the activity or process of transfer rather than to the gamete as a commodity. But portraying gamete transfer as analogous to labor or participation in medical trials brings with it problems of its own. For one thing, an effort to increase the supply of gametes may push up inconvenience allowances to the point where payment becomes an inappropriate inducement to serve as a provider, and where money provides a sufficient reason for donating.

In addition, while an inconvenience allowance avoids treating gametes as property, it treats labor or the use of the body as something that can be bought and sold in a way analogous to remuneration for participating in a clinical trial. Because gamete transfer involves the creation of a new human being it is not analogous to forms of labor or use of the body that do not involve procreation. Bringing a human life into being is an act of tremendous import. If gamete transfer is analogized to other forms of labor or participation in clinical trials, the gamete is viewed as having no particular significance to the provider, it is simply matter that is detachable from the body, not materials that will have psychological and social significance both for the recipient and for the person who may be brought into being . . . I suggest that commodification not only of human gametes but also of certain kinds of labor and uses of the body, including selling the use of one's body for the purpose of procreation by someone else, should not be regarded as the societal norm. Participation in human procreation is not properly thought of as a market transaction, the essence of which is that the owner can alienate — definitively separate from the self — either procreative material or labor . . .

Providing eggs is so much more complicated than providing sperm that people who are concerned to maintain a supply of eggs balk at the suggestion that eggs be transferred only by unpaid gift. Gender equity suggests that since sperm providers are paid, egg providers should also be paid, especially since egg retrieval requires both hormone manipulation and a surgical procedure, both of which entail discomfort and some risk. In England, unlike the United States, egg providers were not traditionally paid, and some feminists denounced a practice that treated women as altruists and men as economic actors . . . To reflect a commitment to sexual equality, however, one would not have to pay egg providers; one could just as well stop paying sperm providers.

Some people oppose moving to a regime of unpaid gamete transfer because they believe that payment is necessary to get men and women to provide sperm and eggs in sufficient quantity to meet the demand of those wishing to purchase gametes. I am not convinced that this is so, or that if it is, that satisfying demand justifies a practice that is in itself improper. Some evidence suggests that unless egg providers receive some payment beyond reimbursement for expenses, the supply of gametes will fall well below the demand. England prohibited remuneration of more than £ 15 (about U.S. $24) for egg providers. This amount is inadequate at present to recruit a sufficient number of egg providers; the waiting period to receive eggs is about five years . . .

The United States has never tried a vigorous campaign to try to recruit unpaid sperm and egg providers. Little public discussion about the plight of the infertile and the ability of others to contribute to their effort to procreate has taken place. It is impossible to know how much donations might be increased by a vigorous public education and advertising campaign explaining the help that providers could provide to the infertile. It is known that . . . when a system incorporates both paying and nonpaying elements, the altruistic element will suffer . . . The United States was able to move from a system of payment for blood, combined with a small amount of unpaid donation, to a largely unpaid system through a vigorous public education campaign . . .

Reimagining gamete transfer as something other than a market activity will be an uphill struggle, but is not inevitably doomed to failure. It is possible to envision gamete transfer as either a market activity or as a way to collaborate in others' efforts to conceive a child. Altruistic transfer is preferable to paid transfer because it leads society at large, not only provider and recipient, to reflect on and discuss what participation in human procreation means. Subsuming collaborative procreation into other kinds of buying and selling commodifies either human gametes or the use of the body, or both. Payment suggests that the transfer is a complete and discrete event, that the action of the person providing gametes has no intrinsic relationship to that of the person receiving the gametes. It would be far preferable if the collaborative acts necessary to bring a new life into being were acknowledged rather than obscured in the practices surrounding gamete transfer . . .

Gamete transfer has not existed long enough for many children and adults created with third-party genetic material to share their perspectives, although these will be very important to future moral reasoning. In the present absence of such first-person testimony, I would suggest that respect for the equal worth of human beings precludes setting different monetary values on genetic material to be used in procreation. And respect for each individual's right to establish his or her own sense of identity requires that society not withhold from anyone information about his or her origins. The deep conceptual transformations necessitated by the creation of families from gamete transfer are not encompassed by a false dichotomy suggesting that family bonds are grounded either in "nature" or in "convention." Rather, these transformations require us to frame an ethic of interpersonal and intergenerational responsibility under conditions of unprecedented choice. They challenge us to alter our conceptual models of human gametes from one of ownership to one of stewardship, and of individual autonomy from bounded separation to self-direction in relationship with others. It is possible to change both our thinking about and the policies governing the transfer of human gametes to be used in procreation, and we should do so for the sake of all those involved.

NOTES AND QUESTIONS

1.   Numerous commentators have evaluated the wisdom of a market in repro-ductive goods and services. A brief list includes Thomas H. Murray, The Worth of a Child (1996); Margaret Jane Radin, Contested Commodities (1996), Kenneth Baum, *Golden Eggs: Towards the Rational Regulation of Oocyte Donation*, 2001 BYU L. Rev. 107; Marjorie M. Schultz, *Questioning Commodification*, 85 Cal. L. Rev. 1841 (1997); Joan Heifetz Hollinger, *From Coitus to Commerce: Legal and Social Consequences of Noncoital Reproduction*, 18 Mich. J. of Law Reform 865 (1985); Martin H. Johnson, *The Culture of Unpaid and Voluntary Egg Donation Should Be Strengthened*, 314 British Medical J. 1401 (1997).

Another commentator, Professor Martha M. Ertman, succinctly summarizes what she perceives to be the main arguments against an artificial insemination (AI) market:

> At least four aspects of the AI market could be described as negative. First, the donor selection process appears to be highly racialized, raising eugenic concerns. Second, poor women lack access to the market. Third, anonymity may deprive some children of the opportunity to know their biological fathers and also deprive them of potential financial support. Fourth and finally, a parenthood market might harm children by treating them like chattel.

Martha M. Ertman, *What's Wrong With A Parenthood Market?*, 82 N.C.L. Rev. 1, 26 (2003). Arguably each of these reasons could be likewise applied to an egg market. Do you agree with these conclusions? If so, do you think that a prohibition on all commercial exchanges is the best solution? Do you see any other way to address Professor Ertman's concerns while preserving a market in human gam-etes?

2. Arguments In Support of a Gamete Market

One of the most well-known and well-regarded legal scholars to write in the area of law and economics is Judge Richard A. Posner, currently a judge on the United States Court of Appeals for the Seventh Circuit and a Senior Lecturer at the University of Chicago Law School. Since the early 1970s, Judge Posner has written extensively about the economic analysis of legal rules and institutions. In the excerpt that follows, Judge Posner makes the case for enforceability of surrogate parenting contracts, agreements in which a woman contracts to gestate a child for another couple or individual in exchange for a money payment. Though our current topic focuses on the merits of a gamete market (rather than a surrogacy market), Judge Posner's reasoning and analysis are highly transferable to the objections raised over the sale of human eggs and sperm.

Richard A. Posner
The Ethics and Economics of Enforcing Contracts of Surrogate Motherhood
5 J. Contemporary Health Law and Policy 21 (1989)

My topic is surrogate motherhood, and specifically the issue — the central issue in the controversy over surrogacy — whether contracts of surrogate motherhood, that is contracts whereby a woman agrees, in exchange for money, to become impregnated through artificial insemination and to give up the newly born child to the father, should be legally enforceable, whether by damages or specific performance. I shall not consider whether such contracts are enforceable under existing law, nor the intricate legal questions that such contracts even when enforceable could be expected to raise, but whether they should be enforceable. To this question of policy, issues of economics and ethics are central, and are the focus of this paper . . .

The case for allowing people to make legally enforceable contracts of surrogate motherhood is straightforward. Such contracts would not be made unless the parties to them believed that surrogacy would be mutually beneficial. Suppose the contract requires the father and his wife to pay the surrogate mother $10,000 (apparently this is the most common price in contracts of surrogate motherhood. The father and wife must believe that they will derive a benefit from having the baby that is greater than $10,000, or else they would not sign the contract. The surrogate must believe that she will derive a benefit from the $10,000 (more precisely, from what she will use the money for) that is greater than the cost to her of being pregnant and giving birth and then surrendering the baby. So ex ante, as an economist would say (i.e., before the fact), all the parties to the contract are made better off . . .

There are various objections to this simple economic analysis. The one that fits the framework of economic theory most comfortably is that the analysis fails to consider that a contract of surrogate motherhood has effects on nonparties, in particular on the baby that the surrogate gives birth to. The presence of an affected but nonconsenting third party makes it difficult to say that the transaction is Pareto superior (i.e., that at least one person is made better off by the transaction and no one is made worse off) — the strongest normative concept of efficiency. In fact, however, it is very likely that the baby is made better off by the contract of surrogate motherhood, and certainly not worse off. For without the contract the baby probably wouldn't be born at all. With the contract, he (or she) becomes a member of a family consisting of the biological father and his wife. The baby's position is much like that of a baby whose mother dies during the baby's infancy and whose father then remarries. If there is any evidence that such babies, when they become adults, decide they'd rather not have been born, I am not aware of it . . .

The remaining possibility is that knowledge that surrogate mothers are paid will blight the child's life. The child will know that his natural mother gave him up for money. But this knowledge will surely be less wrenching than knowledge that one's mother had sold one (as in baby selling). For the mother had agreed from the outset to bear the child for the father and the father's wife. Are children conceived after artificial insemination with sperm obtained from a sperm donor devastated to learn that their parents had bought the sperm? Are children embarrassed or distressed to discover that they are the product of in vitro fertilization which may have cost their parents thousands of dollars? The world is changing, and practices that seem weird and unnatural to members of the current adult generation will seem much less so, I predict, to the next generation . . .

The most frequent argument one hears against contracts of surrogate mother-hood is that they are not truly voluntary, because the surrogate mother doesn't know what she is getting into and would not sign such a contract unless she was desperate. The first point has a more secure foundation in economics than the second. Information costs provide a traditional reason for doubting whether a particular contract is actually value-maximizing ex ante. If women who agree to make surrogate contracts don't know how distressed they will be when it comes time to surrender the baby, then the contracts may not result in a net increase in welfare. To put this differently, the tendency in economics to evaluate welfare on an ex ante rather than ex post basis depends on an assumption that expectations are not systematically biased. Contracts cannot be depended on to maximize welfare if parties signing them don't know what they're committing themselves to.

However, there is no persuasive evidence or convincing reason to believe that, on average, women who agree to become surrogate mothers underestimate the distress they will feel at having to give up the baby . . . Hundreds of babies have been born to surrogate mothers, and since very few of these arrangements have been drawn into litigation one's guess is that most surrogate mothers do not balk when it comes time to surrender the baby. Newspaper and magazine interviews with surrogate mothers confirm this impression. Oblique but important corrobora-tive evidence is that most surrogate mothers already have children and that few are under 20 years of age. A mature woman who has borne children should be able to estimate the psychic cost to her of giving up her next baby . . .

Are these desperate women — women who value $10,000 more than a baby only because society has failed to spread a safety net under them? Even if they were, this might not justify a ban on the enforcement of surrogate contracts. To someone who is desperately in need of $10,000, a court's refusal to allow her to obtain it will seem a hypocritical token of concern for her plight, especially since the court has no power to alleviate that plight in some other way. At all events, there is no evidence that surrogate mothers are drawn from the ranks of the desperately poor, and it seems unlikely they would be . . . A couple would be unlikely to want the baby of a desperately poor woman; they would be concerned about her health, and therefore the baby's. Interviews with surrogate mothers indicate not only that they are not poor, but that they have made a careful tradeoff between the use they can make of $10,000 (or whatever the contract price is) and the costs (including regret) of bearing a child for another couple. When asked what they plan to do with the $10,000, they give standard middle-class answers (home improvement, a new car, a better education for their children). For many surrogate mothers, moreover, regret at giving up the child is balanced by empathy for the father's infertile wife. This is particularly likely where the surrogate mother has already had children — but that is, as I have noted, usually the case with surrogate arrangements.

There is, in short, no persuasive evidence that contracts of surrogate motherhood are less likely to maximize value than the classes of contracts that the law routinely enforces. However, other arguments are also made against the enforcement of surrogacy contracts. One is that such enforcement is inequitable because only middle-class couples can afford the price of a surrogate contract and because invariably the surrogate mother comes from a lower income class than the father and his wife. But society does not forbid contracts for luxury goods or contracts that involve the purchase of services from persons lower on the income ladder. Only wealthy people employ butlers, and butlers are invariably less well off than their employers. Nevertheless employment contracts with butlers are enforceable. Moreover, while probably no truly poor person could afford the price of a surrogate contract, it is hardly the case that only wealthy people can pay $10,000 for a good or service. Most Americans can afford a new car, and most new cars cost more than $10,000. In any event, unless envy is very intense and widespread, it is very difficult to see how people who can't afford to pay for surrogate arrangements are helped by a law that forbids those who can afford to pay to enter into enforceable contracts of surrogacy.

Next it is argued — and not only by Marxists as one might have expected — that to enforce surrogacy contracts is to endorse the 'commodification' of motherhood. It is true that our society does not permit every good or service to be bought and sold, even where there are no palpable or demonstrable third-party effects. People are not permitted to make contracts of self-enslavement, to enter into suicide pacts, to agree to enter gladiatorial contests (or even to box without gloves), or to sign loan agreements enforceable by breaking the borrower's knees in the event of default. And some forms of 'commodification' that are permitted, such as the sale of blood to blood banks, are heavily criticized. Apart from objections, based on a variety of grounds unrelated to surrogate motherhood, to specific forms of 'commodification,' there is a widespread aversion, particularly but not only among intellectuals, to placing all relations and interactions in society on a strictly pecuniary basis. It is feared that pervasive reliance on the 'cash nexus' would extinguish altruism and foster anomie, anxious privatism, and other alleged ills of a capitalist system.

I am skeptical. People are what they are, and what they are is the result of millions of years of evolution rather than of such minor cultural details as the precise scope of the market principle in a particular society. I don't think we would be more selfish than we are if the market sector in this country were larger than it is, or less selfish if it were smaller. People in countries that have less 'commodifi-cation' than we — countries ranging from Sweden to Ethiopia — do not appear to be less selfish than Americans. Anyway, allowing the enforcement of contracts of surrogate motherhood isn't going to have any significant effect on underlying norms and attitudes in our society. Very few fertile couples will be interested in surrogate motherhood; most couples are fertile; and the fraction of infertile couples is bound to decline with continued advances in medical technology, even as women marry later (fertility problems increase with age).

The last ethical argument that I will consider against the enforcement of surrogacy contracts is mounted by feminists. They argue that surrogacy is akin to prostitution in that it also involves the sale of female sexuality; and just as prostitution is widely regarded as exploitive of women, so surrogacy is (these feminists argue) inevitably exploitive of the deluded women who agree to market their reproductive capacity. Moreover, there is a small but irreducible risk of death or serious illness to the surrogate mother.

The argument is unconvincing. It overlooks, to begin with, the fact that the surrogates are not the only women in the picture. There are also the infertile wives to be considered. Not only are they hurt if their ability to obtain a baby (necessarily not borne by them) is impeded by a ban on the enforcement of contracts of surrogate motherhood, but their already weak bargaining position in a marriage to a fertile husband is further weakened, for under modern permissive divorce law he is always free to 'walk,' and seek a fertile woman to marry. Beyond this, the idea that women who 'sell' (really, rent) their reproductive capacity, like women who sell sexual favors, are 'exploited' patronizes women. Few would argue that a gigolo or a sperm donor or a man who marries for money or a male prostitute is 'exploited.' These men might not be admirable, but they are not victims. The idea that women are particularly prone to be exploited in the marketplace hearkens back to the time (not so long ago) when married women were deemed legally incompetent to make enforceable contracts. I am surprised that feminists — not all of them, however — should want to resurrect the idea in the surrogacy context. It is only worse when the argument is bolstered by pointing out that hormonal changes incident to pregnancy may induce a regret at parting with the baby that the surrogate mother could not have foreseen when she signed the contract. The idea that women are peculiarly dominated by their hormones (and not men by their testosterone?) is a traditional rationalization for limiting women's access to responsible employment.

The feminist criticisms of surrogacy are inconsistent with mainstream feminist thought. They reinforce the anti-feminist stereotype summed up in the slogan, 'biology is destiny.' The unintended implication of the feminist position on surrogate motherhood (but I emphasize that this is the position of some, not all, feminists) is, if you're infertile, you shouldn't have a baby; and if you are fertile, and have a baby, you should keep it. A main thrust of modern feminism has been to deny that biology is destiny, that it is woman's predestined lot to be a bearer and raiser of children. Some women don't want to have children; some want to have children but not in the traditional setting of heterosexual marriage; some want to have but not bear children and some, finally, want to bear but not have children (or more children — they are the surrogate mothers). Feminism seeks to expand the opportunities of women beyond the traditional role, felt as stifling by many, of being a housewife and mother who makes a career of bearing and raising children. The opportunity to hire a surrogate mother and the opportunity to be a surrogate mother are two unconventional opportunities now open to women. It is curious that feminists, of all people, should want to close the door on these opportunities.

The last and least argument against surrogate motherhood is that it is just another form of 'baby selling.' This is argumentation by epithet. The surrogate mother no more 'owns' the baby than the father does. What she sells is not the baby but her parental rights, and in this respect she is no different from a woman who agrees in a divorce proceeding to surrender her claim to custody of the children of the marriage in exchange for some other concession from her husband — or from a sperm donor who receives cash, but no parental rights, in exchange for his donation . . .

B. Should the ART Market Be Open to All Willing Buyers and Sellers?

1. Exclusions Based On Age

Judith Daar
Death of Aging Mother Raises More Questions About IVF Rules
Los Angeles Daily Journal, July 29, 2009

The death of Guinness World Record holder Maria del Carmen Bousada at age 69 refocuses attention on the very feat that earned her distinction. In December 2006, the Spanish native gave birth to twin boys, conceived at a Los Angeles fertility clinic using in vitro fertilization with (much younger) donor eggs. The unmarried 66-year old became the world's oldest woman to give birth, though that record has since been surpassed by a 70-something matriarch in India. Motherhood for septuagenarians, like the birth of octuplets using IVF, raises legitimate questions about the math surrounding infertility treatment. How many is too many, how old is too old?

Orphaning minor children is always tragic, regardless of parental age . . . Arguably the case of the Spanish twins is deserving of special attention because their mother put them at risk of orphan-status by intentionally birthing them without a partner, at an age she was statistically unlikely to see them blossom into adulthood.

Three key factors coalesced around this and other post-menopausal births, each sharing equal responsibility for introducing the term "granny-mom" into our lexicon. The patient's desire, the physician's willingness, and the law's silence all play a role when a woman of advanced maternal age gives birth. Since the science of IVF with donor eggs is largely unaffected by the age of the gestator, it is the players and the rules they operate under that are fairly subject to scrutiny.

Patients whose age place them beyond the bounds of natural reproduction often have strong desires for biologic parenthood. Some are newly wed, others wait until their social and financial foundations are strong, still others feel the wrench of childlessness later than most. So fierce is their fervor that some, like Bousada, falsify their birth records to meet clinic age restrictions. Dr. Vicken Sahakian, the physician who provided treatment explained that his clinic does limit service to single women age 55 or younger, but confessed, "we don't ask for passports . . . we're not detectives here."

It's no surprise that patients will go to great lengths to obtain ill-advised medical therapies — IVF, prescription drugs, excessive cosmetic surgeries. So what responsibility do physicians have to police their own operations? In the case of reproductive technology services, most clinics do impose age restrictions on patients and often on spouses as well. A typical ceiling is 55 for women, with some practices imposing a combined age limit of 110 for both partners . . .

By all news accounts, Maria Bousada was a good candidate for treatment based on her medical, social and genetic background. Her mother died at age 101 (which if disclosed, should have provided a clue to her actual age) and the cancer that took her life did not present until a year after the babies were born. If she did live as long as her maternal ancestor, would we have the same reaction to the doctor's half-hearted age verification? . . .

The legal landscape governing reproductive medicine, like the law surrounding every other medical specialty, wisely does not impose practice guidelines as a substitute for physician judgment. No federal or state law in the U.S. restricts the age at which women can obtain infertility treatment. Accordingly, American women enjoy far greater reproductive autonomy than any of their counterparts worldwide.

The lack of formal law, however, does not equate to a lack of guidance and considered opinion on the subject. The American Society for Reproductive Medicine issued an ethics opinion on the use of egg donation by post-menopausal women in 1996. The ASRM opinion urges physicians to consider and counsel patients on the medical risks to both woman and child, as well as the long-term parenting plan should the family, as envisioned, change. "It is permissible" the ASRM concludes, "for programs to decline to provide these procedures to women over 50 based on these concerns." As noted, many clinics do impose such age limits, though the rules have been known to operate in the breach.

Our cultural and historic allegiance to medical and reproductive autonomy explains the nation's laissez faire approach to regulating IVF and other forms of assisted conception. While other countries do restrict access to fertility treatments, including the UK which limits IVF to women 40 and under, the U.S. entrusts doctors to provide treatment as they deem medically appropriate. While such discretion can be abused, at times begetting heartbreaking family scenarios, the absence of provider discretion threatens even more dire outcomes. State-sponsored restrictions on reproduction are certain to thwart far more happy families than they create. Leaving math to the mathematicians and medicine to the physicians makes sense, so long as the welfare of both mother and child are at the heart of any treatment decision.

———

Maria Bousada's story reveals much about the emotional and logistical journey an older woman might endure in order to give birth to a child. A successful outcome requires two key ingredients — donated oocytes (eggs) and a willing physician. As mentioned in the above editorial, the Ethics Committee of the American Society for Reproductive Medicine has considered the issues surrounding late-late motherhood. The following report contains arguments for and against assisting so-called "Granny Moms."

Ethics Committee of the American Society for Reproductive Medicine
Oocyte Donation to Postmenopausal Women
82 Fertility & Sterility, Supp. 1, 254S (2004)

The reported success of oocyte donation to older women makes pregnancy feasible in virtually any woman with a normal uterus, regardless of age or the absence of ovaries and ovarian function. A women's reproductive age, once a dictate of nature, now has been artificially extended. Both women with premature ovarian failure and women of postreproductive age may give birth by using donated oocytes fertilized in vitro and transferred to their uteri . . .

[C]ircumstances may lead some postmenopausal women to request the procedure. For example, a postmenopausal woman who loses her only child may seek to have another, or a postmenopausal woman with no prior children may desire to start a family. Is the use of a technology that extends a woman's reproductive life appropriate and sensible, and, if so, should limits be recommended for its application?

Arguments For and Against Oocyte Donation

Arguments in favor of oocyte donation to postmenopausal women are based on societal practices, gender equality, and reproductive freedom. In our society, it is not unusual for children to be raised by grandparents who take on most of the parenting role, and often bring economic stability, parental responsibility, and maturity to the family unit. There is therefore no reason to assume that society will be harmed by allowing older individuals to procreate or that older women and their partners lack the physical and psychological stamina for raising children. Also, because older men may father children, denying women a successful alternative for reproduction at ages equivalent to men is sexist and prejudicial, especially as women generally live longer than men. Finally, our society respects the rights of individuals to make reproductive choices regardless of age or life expectancy. For example, individuals with life-limiting illnesses are not prohibited from reproduction because of their shortened life expectancy. Given the possibility that postmenopausal reproduction may satisfy the strong desire of a couple for an offspring, it would be wrong to deny women the use of donated oocytes solely because of their age.

One major argument against oocyte donation to postmenopausal women is that there is a "natural" limit in reproductive capacity that is intrinsic to being human, and to transcend this limit is "unnatural." Just as oocyte donation to prepubertal girls is unacceptable, so should it be unacceptable for postmenopausal women to bear children. Because parenting is both an emotionally stressful and physically demanding experience, older women and their partners may be unable to meet the needs of a growing child and maintain a long parental relationship. Additionally, the fact that some grandparents can successfully raise children is not necessarily sufficient to justify using new technologies to establish pregnancies after menopause. Children also are being successfully raised by teenage mothers, which does not mean teenage pregnancy should be encouraged by physicians. Finally, because some older men can father children does not mean that it would be unfair to deny older women the opportunity to bear children. Nor would this redress gender inequality in reproduction. In postmenopausal pregnancy, the woman does not genetically reproduce, yet she alone faces increased medical risk of hypertension, diabetes, multiple gestation, preterm labor, pre-eclampsia and other complications of pregnancy and childbirth. These medical risks are significant enough to support the argument against oocyte donation to postmenopausal women. Thus, it is argued that pregnancy after menopause serves neither the interests of older women nor the interests of the children they bear.

Medical and Ethical Issues

There are no tests to detect the propensity of older women to develop hypertension during pregnancy. In addition, older women face increased risks of cardiovascular complications, gestational diabetes, and operative delivery. Because pregnancy rates with donor IVF do not seem adversely affected by age, there also is the possibility of multiple gestation, which poses significant maternal risks and the need for women to consider pregnancy reduction. Finally, women face the uncertain genetic risks associated with conception, especially when the male partner is 50 or more years of age. It is therefore vitally important for physicians to conduct a thorough medical and psychological evaluation of women and their partners and carefully counsel prospective parents about the medical and genetic risks of conception at an advanced age. Furthermore, because women may accept the genetic risks associated with using sperm from older men, and children cannot, physicians and prospective parents have a significant moral responsibility to ensure that reproductive choices are protective of both the well-being and welfare of resulting children.

The central ethical issue is whether the interests of women and children are served by this technology. These interests can be served when the desire for a child and the ultimate bearing and rearing of a child contribute to mutual well being. On the other hand, given the societal and cultural constraints of women to be mothers, it is possible women might be pressured to have a child. Moreover, children could resent having mothers old enough to be grandmothers and be adversely affected psychologically and socially by having older parents. Finally, the interests of mothers and their children are so inextricably intertwined that any serious discussion of the ethics of postmenopausal pregnancy must focus on considerations of maternal and child interests together. These considerations must include issues of parenting and child support, especially in couples where both partners are old.

Conclusion

Medical, psychological, and ethical factors weigh heavily in the decision to have a child at any age. However, when the sole concern is the age of the prospective mother, there seems to be no medical or ethical reason compelling enough to judge the practice as unethical in every case. Just as fertility is the norm during reproductive years and treating physicians are justified in their efforts to correct deficient reproductive functions, including premature ovarian failure, infertility should remain the natural characteristic of menopause. Because of this, and the physical and psychological risks involved, postmenopausal pregnancy should be discouraged. Prospective parents and their treating physicians must carefully consider the specifics of each case before using oocyte donation, including a woman's health, medical and genetic risks, and the provision for child-rearing.

NOTES AND QUESTIONS

1.   The ASRM Ethics Committee concludes that pregnancy should be discouraged for older women because of the physical and psychological risks involved, yet they acknowledge the existing double standard as older men face little or none of the social stigma associated with senior parenting. Perhaps one reason for the differing social reactions is that when older men become fathers they tend to mate with much younger women, who presumably will survive their geriatric spouse to care for the offspring. Famous examples of such pairings abound, including actor Michael Douglas and Catherine Zeta Jones, whose reported 35-year age gap did not prevent the couple from marrying in 2000 and having two children, despite Mr. Douglas' eligibility for social security. Fellow 60-something CNN interviewer Larry King twice became a father with fifth wife Shawn, 26 years his junior. And the obituary for *The Odd Couple*'s beloved Tony Randall noted his joy at becoming a first-time dad at age 77 with his 26-year-old wife, Heather. When Randall died at age 84 in May 2004, he was survived by his wife and two children, ages 7 and 6.

2.   Should age be a lawful barrier to reproductive services? If you believe so, how would you advise a lawmaker to draft regulations that would establish such limitations on access to ART services? Would your plan distinguish between men and women? Between singles and married persons? What age would you set as the upper limit for accessing ART services? Do you think a lobby group such as the American Association of Retired Persons (AARP) would favor your proposed law? How about the Children's Defense Fund?

2.   Exclusions Based on Health Status

The controversy over older women using donated eggs to become pregnant largely focuses on the social plight of children born to mothers who may not survive long enough to see their children graduate from high school, or otherwise rear their offspring during the critical years of childhood. The question of access to ART services becomes even more hotly contested when it comes to parents who could potentially harm their offspring just by the act of conception.[6] When a parent is afflicted by a genetic or infectious disease that can be passed to a child through the

---

[6]   In Chapter 8 we consider the broader question of whether ART providers should be able to refuse to treat individuals they believe will be unfit parents. Unfitness can be based on a prospective parent's health status, but psychological and social factors can also impact an individual's ability to act in the best interest of their child.

reproductive process, serious questions arise about the tension between the welfare of the child and the right to reproductive autonomy. One such scenario that has garnered public attention is the desire of individuals infected with the human immunodeficiency virus (HIV, the virus that causes acquired immunodeficiency syndrome or AIDS) to use ART services in order to reduce the chance of transmitting HIV to their offspring. While an HIV-infected person may view the enlistment of ART professionals as a positive, risk-reducing act, others may see only the potential risk to the child that should be avoided by denying services (and some may argue reproduction) altogether.

The dilemma posed by HIV-infected prospective parents for ART professionals can be briefly summarized as follows. On the one hand, typically an HIV-infected individual can reproduce naturally, without any medical assistance, but such conduct poses a risk of transmission of the virus to the infected individual's partner and child. On the other hand, reproduction using ART can significantly reduce the risk of transmission of HIV to a partner and the resulting child, but the ART professional can do nothing about the fact that a new parent is afflicted with a serious disease that may deprive the child of a rearing parent at a young age. Some ART professionals have seen this as a "no win" situation and have refused to aid HIV-infected individuals and couples in their quest to become parents in the safest manner possible.

Recent breakthroughs in treatment for HIV prompted the American Society for Reproductive Medicine to rethink the issue of infertility treatment for HIV-infected individuals. In 1994, the Ethics Committee of the ASRM cautioned practitioners to counsel patients about the consequences of reproducing when one partner is HIV-infected, suggesting that physicians discuss alternative options such as gamete donation, adoption, or not having children. Ethics Committee of the American Society for Reproductive Medicine, *Special Considerations Regarding Human Immunodeficiency Virus and Assisted Reproductive Technologies*, 62 FERTILITY & STERILITY 85S (1994). In 2002, the ASRM reconsidered its position in light of new and highly effective drug therapy for HIV and further developments in ART techniques that drastically reduce the risk of transmission to partner and offspring. The topic was again revisited in 2010, as new research continued to suggest that HIV and ART are not incompatible. The Committee's most recent reasoning is set forth in the following report.

Ethics Committee of the American Society for Reproductive Medicine
Human Immunodeficiency Virus and Infertility Treatment
94 Fertility & Sterility 11 (2010)

Human immunodeficiency virus (HIV) has infected people of all ages. The largest group affected (86%) are persons of active reproductive age (15-44 years), about one-third of whom report that desire to have children. This fact underscores the concern of viral transmission to sexual partners and offspring. Because women make up approximately 20% of cases, and because HIV has become more prevalent among heterosexual couples than in the past, some infected persons will probably ask their health care providers for advice about and assistance with having children who are free of the virus . . .

Several methods of limiting the risk for HIV transmission to partner and offspring have . . . been developed. For example, zidovudine [AZT] has reduced the vertical transmission of infection from 16%–24% to 5%–8% when given to HIV-infected pregnant women during the second and third trimesters and to their newborns for 6 weeks . . .

[S]tudies conducted in North America and Europe concluded that elective (planned) cesarean section added to antiviral treatment would decrease the vertical transmission rate to 2% compared with 7.6% in children of treated women who deliver vaginally. Subsequent studies have found that cesarean section is not needed to lower the risk of transmission if viral levels in the pregnant woman are undetectable.

Lack of apparent transmission of HIV to partner or child with intrauterine insemination (IUI), or with IVF with . . . ICSI has been reported for discordant (male-positive) couples. Highly active antiretroviral therapy can lessen the viral burden in a person's serum and semen. Testing of sperm by using a polymerase chain reaction assay has improved the ability to determine whether the virus is present in the washed sperm preparation . . .

This paper addresses ethical issues concerning [1] infertility treatment when one partner is HIV-infected, [2] infertility treatment when both partners are infected, [3] knowingly conceiving a child who may be born with HIV, [4] HIV testing for couples seeking fertility assistance, and [5] potential risks to the caregivers of patients who are HIV infected.

INFERTILITY TREATMENT WHEN ONE PARTNER IS HIV POSITIVE

The presence of HIV may not affect the reproductive potential of a seropositive person unless he or she is ill owing to an opportunistic infection. The HIV transmission rate to an uninfected partner is estimated to be approximately 1 in 500 to 1,000 episodes of unprotected intercourse. The risk of viral transmission increases dramatically if the HIV-infected partner's viral load is high or if the HIV-uninfected partner has a concomitant genital infection, inflammation, or abrasions.

If a woman is HIV-infected and her male partner is HIV-uninfected, transmission of infection to the male partner can be avoided by using homologous [artificial] insemination with the partner's sperm . . .

If an HIV-infected pregnant woman is not actively treated with antiviral drugs, the risk of HIV transmission to the infant is greater than 20% regardless of the viral load. Administration of zidovudine [AZT] to pregnant women and newborns during the first 6 weeks of life can substantially reduce the risk of HIV transmission to 5%–8%. Delivery by cesarean section and avoidance of breast-feeding may further reduce the chance of infection to approximately 2%.

Attempts at conception between HIV-infected men and their HIV-uninfected female partners that rely on using condoms except at the time of ovulation appear to reduce, but not eliminate the risk of seroconverstion compared with complete avoidance of condom use . . . Even though some HIV-discordant couples have established pregnancies through timed unprotected intercourse without infecting the uninfected partner or child, this practice is unsafe and is not recommended.

Several reports have described specific methods for sperm preparation and testing that can substantially reduce the chance of HIV transmission to the female partner and child. [Studies assessing these techniques report that all children and all mothers tested were HIV negative.] . . .

When male-positive discordant couples want to have their own genetically related children, they should be informed of available risk-reduction techniques and encouraged to seek assistance at institutions that can provide the most effective methods of sperm preparation as well as the rigorous testing and treatment necessary to minimize the chance of HIV transmission to partner and offspring. To determine the true efficacy of the chosen method of treatment, these centers should use strict study protocols with proper informed consent and thorough follow-up of patients, partners, and offspring.

INFERTILITY TREATMENT WHEN BOTH PARTNERS ARE HIV POSITIVE

As with any couple presenting for evaluation and treatment, both persons may have normal fertility potential or one or both may have impaired fertility. If an HIV-infected couple asks for medical advice regarding pregnancy, they must be encouraged to adopt protocols that have been demonstrated to be safe and effective in . . . research studies . . . If the viral load can be suppressed to undetectable levels in both partners, the couple may have a child who is free of HIV. Aggressive drug therapy with protease inhibitors and other antiretroviral therapy can extend life and improve health in HIV-infected persons; however, it is unknown whether they will ultimately have a normal or near-normal life expectancy. The child may lose one or both parents to AIDS before he or she reaches adulthood, although recent success with [drugs] has significantly reduced death rates of infected persons.

ETHICAL ISSUES RAISED BY KNOWINGLY RISKING THE BIRTH OF A CHILD WITH HIV

The risk of HIV transmission to offspring . . . can be greatly reduced but not eliminated. This risk raises ethical issues concerning the scope of freedom to reproduce, what is considered to be harm sufficient to justify restricting that freedom, and the responsibilities of health care professionals faced with a request to provide services to HIV-infected patients.

Does a couple's desire to have genetic offspring justify the risk of transmitting a serious disease to their child? Although the risk can be reduced in many ways, and recent data show no instances of vertical transmission using sperm-prepared IUI or IVF with ICSI, theoretically the risk cannot be completely eliminated. Those who assess the ethics of assisting such patients to have children must address the question of whether offspring born with HIV are harmed despite the preventive steps taken. They must consider that some risk remains that the child will be born with HIV. Until sperm preparation techniques prove completely effective, there may be no way, short of refraining from reproduction altogether, to completely prevent some cases of HIV transmission. In situations in which a child could be born with a serious disease, one can argue that individuals are not acting unethically in proceeding with reproduction if they have taken all reasonable precautions to prevent disease transmission and are prepared to love and support the child, regardless of the child's medical condition. Similarly, one can argue that health care providers are not acting unethically if they have taken all reasonable precautions to limit the risk of transmitting HIV to offspring or to an uninfected partner. It would not, however, be ethically acceptable for a physician, clinic, or institution to proceed with reproductive assistance if they lacked the clinical and laboratory resources needed to effectively care for HIV-infected couples who wish to have a child. In such instances, the medical care provider should refer couples to a center that has these resources.

The ethical issues raised here are similar in some respects to those in couples who know that they are carriers of an autosomal recessive disease, such as Tay-Sachs disease, sickle-cell anemia, or cystic fibrosis. Such couples may choose to take the risk of having an affected child rather than use IVF plus preimplantation genetic diagnosis, which enables prospective parents to deselect embryos found to express certain genetic anomalies, forgo biologic parenthood; adopt; use a gamete donor; or, if a test result is positive, terminate the pregnancy. The risk of transmitting an autosomal recessive genetic disease cannot be reduced below 25%, whereas the risk of HIV transmission can be reduced to a substantially lower number — in some cases, to less than 2% . . . . Health care workers who are willing to provide reproductive assistance to couples whose offspring are irreducibly at risk for a serious genetic disease should find it ethically acceptable to treat HIV-infected individuals or couples who are willing to take reasonable steps to minimize the risks of transmission.

TESTING INFERTILE COUPLES FOR HIV

. . . It is ethically appropriate for practitioners to encourage HIV testing for all couples who want to have children, not just those who request infertility treatment. To mandate that people be tested solely because they request medical assistance in having a child would infringe on their personal liberty and introduce an unjustifiable distinction between those who seek treatment for infertility and those who do not . . .

HIV AND THE HEALTH PROFESSIONAL

Health professionals care for patients with serious and potentially contagious diseases, knowing that they themselves could become infected. Knowledge of diseases, combined with careful hygienic practices, has allowed caregivers to lessen that risk . . .

If standard universal precautions to prevent infectious disease transmission are taken, the risk of virus transmission to medical caregivers is very small and, in itself, is not a sufficient reason to deny reproductive services to HIV-infected individuals and couples. Clinicians have the same obligation to care for those infected with HIV as to care for patients with other chronic diseases. Concern about the public's perception of a clinic or provider that cares for HIV-infected patients is insufficient cause to deny services.

Clinicians faced with requests for reproductive assistance from persons who are HIV positive should be aware of the 1998 United States Supreme Court decision in *Bragdon vs. Abbott*. The Court ruled that a person with HIV is considered "disabled" and therefore protected under the Americans with Disabilities Act. According to that decision, persons who are HIV-infected are entitled to medical services unless a physician can demonstrate "by objective scientific evidence" that treatment would pose "a significant risk" of infection. The Court determined that having HIV was a disability because it interfered with the "major life activity" of reproduction due to the risk of transmitting HIV to offspring. Unless health care workers can show that they lack the skill and facilities to treat HIV-positive patients safely or that the patient refused reasonable testing and treatment, they may be legally, as well as ethically, obligated to provide requested reproductive assistance.

IMPROVING ACCESS TO CARE FOR HIV-INFECTED INDIVIDUALS

Despite improved outcomes in the use of IUI and IVF with ICSI to virtually eliminate the risk of vertical and horizontal transmission of HIV, access to these reproductive technologies for seropositive individuals is extremely limited. Fewer than 3% of U.S. ART practices registered with the Society for Assisted Reproductive Technologies provide service to couples in whom one or both partners are HIV infected. This lack of access is attributable to concerns about transmission to clinic personnel, fear of cross-contamination by gametes and embryos being cultured and stored on clinic premises, lack of expertise by clinicians in handling infectious patients and their gametes, and the high cost to clinics for providing separate laboratory space and equipment to minimize the risk of cross contamination, as recommended by ASRM.

To date, there have been no reported cases of occupational transmission to ART personnel or contamination of gametes or embryos in the clinic setting that would support denial of service to HIV-infected individuals or couples. The few centers that do provide care report seeing happy and grateful families, many of whom travel a great distance for access to the safest method of reproduction currently available. To the extent it is economically and technically feasible, ART providers should widen access to HIV-infected patients who desire to procreate in a manner that minimizes the risk of viral transmission to their partners and offspring.

NOTES AND PROBLEMS

1.   The ASRM Ethics Committee cautions physicians that despite their personal predilections about providing ART services to HIV-infected individuals, federal law may prohibit denial of reproductive assistance on the basis of the patient's HIV status alone. Recall our discussion of *Bragdon v. Abbott*, 524 U.S. 624 (1998) in Chapter 1. In that case, the Supreme Court deemed HIV a disability under the

Americans With Disabilities Act because the virus interferes with the major life activity of reproduction by posing a risk of transmission to a partner or child. Does this mean that an ART provider would run afoul of the ADA if she denied reproductive services to an HIV-infected individual because she had concerns about the well-being of any resulting child? How about denials of service based on other medical conditions, such as carrier-status for a genetic disease? If a physician knows that a particular couple has a 50% chance of passing a deleterious gene to a child (for example, in a case where one parent is afflicted with the gene for Huntington's Disease, a life-threatening disease that causes degeneration of brain cells), would a physician violate federal law by refusing to aid the couple to reproduce? Is a desire to avoid harm to offspring a sufficient counterweight to the ADA's goal of preventing discrimination against people with disabilities?

Professor Carl Coleman has addressed these questions in a comprehensive and thoughtful article focusing on the history and meaning of the ADA in the context of ART services. At the outset of his article, Professor Coleman explains:

> Applying the ADA to denials of treatment by ART practitioners raises particularly challenging legal and ethical issues. On the one hand, the danger that physicians will inappropriately deny treatment to patients with disabilities — a serious concern in all areas of medicine — is especially worrisome in the context of ARTs. Our society has a long history of efforts to prevent people with disabilities from having children, a history in which the medical profession played an especially prominent role. While we no longer embrace the coercive eugenics policies of the early twentieth century, the perception that some individuals with disabilities are inherently incapable of being parents remains common in our society. Hence, there is a real danger that disability-related denials of ARTs will be based on ignorance or bias against people with disabilities, even more so than when physicians deny individuals with disabilities other types of medical care.
>
> On the other hand, ARTs are fundamentally different from other medical treatments because their goal is the conception and birth of a child. In some cases, patients' disabilities may have potentially devastating implications for any child born to the patient, including the possibility that the child will be born with life-threatening or seriously debilitating impairments. Some physicians may have strong ethical objections to helping patients become pregnant in the face of such risks. Physicians also may be concerned about indirect risks to the child from patients' disabilities, such as the possibility that patients with life-threatening disabilities will die while the child is still young. To the extent physicians' objections to providing ARTs to patients with disabilities are based on the disability's implications for the future child's welfare, they raise unique considerations that do not apply to the use of disability-related eligibility criteria for other types of medical care.

Professor Coleman carefully analyzes the history and language of the ADA as it relates to denial of medical services, pointing out that even if an ART practitioner's refusal constitutes disability discrimination, he could avoid liability by proving that such denial of treatment was necessary to avoid "a direct threat to the health and safety of others." Thus, the question of whether ART denials on the basis of HIV or some other disability are lawful under federal law depends upon whether the "direct threat defense" can be invoked by physicians who fear for the welfare of future children. Professor Coleman concedes that physician objections to providing ARTs based on concerns about a future child's welfare can be sufficiently compelling to justify a disability-related denial of care if it is "clear that there is a significant likelihood the child's health status will fall below a minimally decent threshold." When this is the case, Professor Coleman proposes a comparative approach, in which courts could evaluate the risks and benefits of ARTs in relation to the other reproductive parenting options available under the circumstances, including embryo screening techniques, use of donor gametes, gestational surrogacy, or adoption. This comparative approach, he urges, is optimal because:

> [e]nsuring equitable access to medical treatment for individuals with disabilities is a critically important societal value, but so too is avoiding unnecessary suffering in future generations and recognizing physicians' standing as moral agents. In some cases, it will be impossible to reconcile all of these values. When such cases arise, a court must reach a resolution, knowing that whichever values it favors will have both advantages and costs.
>
> The framework proposed in this Article seeks to balance the competing factors on a case-by-case basis, comparing the risks and benefits of the patient's requested treatment with the other available reproductive and parenting options. The advantage of this approach is that it recognizes each of the considerations as important values, and it prioritizes them based on an individualized assessment of a particular case. The drawback, however, is the difficulty of line-drawing. The line between appropriate and inappropriate denials of treatment is far from bright, and undoubtedly it will prove difficult to determine when that line has been crossed. There is a real danger that seemingly objective determinations about a future child's best interests will be influenced by pervasive, and often unconscious, biases and stereotypes about people with disabilities. To the extent that consistency and predictability are important legal values, an argument can be made for a bright-line solution — either treating ART practitioners like common carriers, with an obligation to accept any patient who is willing to pay, or giving them unbridled discretion to select patients as they please.
>
> But, while any system that requires drawing distinctions is prone to error, the tolerable margin of error depends on the purpose of the distinctions. It would be one thing if the law sought to specify circumstances in which physicians would be prohibited from providing ARTs to particular patients. In such a system, the tolerable margin of error would be extremely narrow, as the ability of individuals with disabilities to use ARTs would depend exclusively on how those circumstances were defined. The framework proposed in this Article, by contrast, seeks only to identify circumstances in which concerns about the future child should be accepted as a reasonable justification for withholding treatment — if a physician chooses to assert those concerns. Physicians would still be permitted to provide treatment in such situations if doing so were consistent with their own ethical views, and

it can be expected that many physicians will do so. Thus, the tolerable margin of error is greater, because the consequences of drawing the line in a particular place are far less severe.

Moreover, while consistency and predictability are important considerations, they are not the only values the law must consider. Attempting to accommodate competing considerations is unlikely to yield a simple solution, but in ethically charged contexts simplicity is rarely an attainable goal. Courts confronted with ADA challenges to decisions about ARTs should avoid the temptation to find an easy way out of the ethical thicket. The comparative framework proposed in this Article provides an approach to resolving these dilemmas that takes seriously the risk of disability discrimination in the context of reproduction, while acknowledging physicians' legitimate desire to avoid serious risks to the future child's well-being.

Carl H. Coleman, *Conceiving Harm: Disability Discrimination in Assisted Reproductive Technologies*, 50 UCLA L. REV. 17, 20-21, 65, 67-68 (2002). For another keen analysis of the ADA's protection of people with substantial disabilities from being denied access to ART, *see* Kimberly M. Mutcherson, *Disabling Dreams of Parenthood: The Fertility Industry, Anti-Discrimination, and Parents with Disabilities*, 27 LAW & INEQUALITY 311 (2009) (using HIV and quadriplegia as paradigm cases).

    2.   You are an ART practitioner at a university-based fertility clinic in a state that recognizes civil unions between same-sex partners. John and David, both age 30-something, make an appointment to consult with you about their desire to have a child. They explain that they have been together as a couple for 10 years, having registered with the state as civil partners since the civil union law first went into effect. The couple has always dreamed of raising a family together, a goal endorsed by John's sister Betsy, who has agreed to act as an egg donor and gestational carrier for her brother and his partner. John and David reveal to you that both are HIV-infected, having been diagnosed at the same time in 2001. They are both on drug therapy and according to their doctor, are "doing well, with undetectable viral loads, meaning they have very little virus in their systems." In all likelihood, the doctor reports, both John and David will live a normal life with a normal life span "if the drug therapy continues to perform as it has." Betsy is aware of the couple's HIV status, and has agreed to undergo retrieval of her eggs so they can be fertilized by David's sperm (to avoid consanguinity). Further, she is willing to gestate the resulting embryos and disclaim any parental rights to the child or children so that her brother and David can fulfill their dreams of parenthood.

    How would you respond to John and David's request for ART services? Which factor or factors most influenced your decision? Would you give the same response to Brian and Rochelle, a married couple who are both carriers of the recessive Tay-Sachs gene, meaning that neither individual is afflicted with the disease but their offspring face a 25% chance of inheriting both recessive genes and suffering an early and painful death? How are the dilemmas posed by the two couples similar? How are they different? In your mind, how weighty a factor is potential harm to offspring compared to an individual's right to procreate? Does it matter that one couple is married and the other is not? Marital status, it turns out, can be a factor in gaining access to ART services. Please read on.

3. Exclusions Based on Marital Status and Sexual Orientation

NORTH COAST WOMEN'S CARE MEDICAL GROUP, INC. v. SAN DIEGO COUNTY SUPERIOR COURT
Supreme Court of California
44 Cal. 4th 1145, 189 P.3d 959 (2008)

KENNARD, J.

Do the rights of religious freedom and free speech, as guaranteed in both the federal and the California Constitutions, exempt a medical clinic's physicians from complying with the Unruh Civil Rights Act's prohibition against discrimination based on a person's sexual orientation? Our answer is no.

I

This case comes to us after the trial court granted plaintiff's motion for summary adjudication of one affirmative defense, thereby determining that no triable issue of material fact existed as to the defense and that plaintiff was entitled to judgment on the defense as a matter of law . . . The Court of Appeal issued a writ of mandate setting aside that ruling on the ground that it failed to completely dispose of the affirmative defense and thus was contrary to the statutory requirements for summary adjudication . . . Because this case reached us pretrial, after the trial court granted plaintiff's motion for summary adjudication, our factual description comes primarily from the parties' statements of undisputed facts filed in connection with that motion.

Plaintiff Guadalupe T. Benitez is a lesbian who lives with her partner, Joanne Clark, in San Diego County. They wanted Benitez to become pregnant, and they decided on intravaginal self-insemination, a nonmedical process in which a woman inserts sperm into her own vagina. Benitez and Clark used sperm from a sperm bank. In 1999, after several unsuccessful efforts at pregnancy through this method, Benitez was diagnosed with polycystic ovarian syndrome, a disorder characterized by irregular ovulation, and she was referred to defendant North Coast Women's Care Medical Group, Inc. (North Coast) for fertility treatment.

In August 1999, Benitez and Clark first met with defendant Christine Brody, an obstetrician and gynecologist employed by defendant North Coast. Benitez mentioned that she was a lesbian. Dr. Brody explained that at some point intrauterine insemination (IUI) might have to be considered. In that medical procedure, a physician threads a catheter through the patient's cervix and inserts semen through the catheter into the patient's uterus. Dr. Brody said that if IUI became necessary, her religious beliefs would preclude her from performing the procedure for

Benitez.[7] According to Dr. Brody, she told Benitez and Clark at that initial meeting that her North Coast colleague, Dr. Douglas Fenton, shared her religious objection to performing IUI for an unmarried woman, but that either of two other North Coast physicians, Dr. Charles Stoopack and Dr. Ross Langley, could do the procedure for Benitez. According to Benitez, however, Dr. Brody said that she was the only North Coast physician with a religious objection to performing IUI for Benitez, and that "all other members of her practice — whom she believed lacked her bias — would be available" to do this medical procedure.

From August 1999 through June 2000, Dr. Brody treated Benitez for infertility. The treatment consisted chiefly of prescribing Clomid, an ovulation-inducing medication, followed by Benitez's use of intravaginal self-insemination with sperm obtained from a sperm bank. To determine whether Benitez's fallopian tubes were blocked, Dr. Brody had her take a medical test (hysterosalpingiogram), which was negative. After performing a surgical procedure (diagnostic laparoscopy), Dr. Brody determined that Benitez's infertility was not the result of endometriosis.[8]

According to Benitez, when in April 2000 she still had not become pregnant, she decided "with the advice and consent of Dr. Brody," to try IUI, which, as explained earlier, is a medical procedure in which a physician uses a catheter to insert sperm directly into the patient's uterus. Instead, in May 2000, Benitez resorted to the nonmedical procedure of intravaginal self-insemination that she had used before; but this time, rather than using sperm from a sperm bank as she had done earlier, she used fresh sperm donated by a male friend. When Benitez thereafter missed a menstrual period, she thought she was pregnant. But a home pregnancy test was negative, and a pregnancy test done at defendant North Coast's facilities on July 5, 2000, confirmed that she was not pregnant. Benitez then decided to try IUI, using her friend's fresh sperm.

The parties agree that when Benitez told Dr. Brody she wanted to use her friend's donated fresh sperm for the IUI, Brody replied that this would pose a problem for North Coast. Its physicians had performed IUI either with fresh sperm provided by a patient's husband or sperm from a sperm bank, but never with fresh sperm donated by a patient's friend. To do the latter, Dr. Brody said, might delay the procedure as North Coast would first have to confirm that its protocols

---

[7] [n.1] The parties dispute the factual basis for Dr. Brody's religious objection to performing IUI for plaintiff. Dr. Brody claims that her religious beliefs preclude her from active participation in medically causing the pregnancy of any unmarried woman, and therefore her refusal to perform IUI for Benitez was based on Benitez's marital status, not her sexual orientation. But Benitez, whose complaint does not allege marital status discrimination, asserts that Dr. Brody objected to performing IUI for a lesbian, and consequently the alleged denial of the medical treatment at issue constituted sexual orientation discrimination. The trial court ruled that the factual basis for Dr. Brody's objection presented a disputed issue of material fact to be resolved at trial.

In so ruling, the trial court apparently concluded that, at the times relevant here, California's Unruh Civil Rights Act did not prohibit discrimination based on marital status. The Court of Appeal in this case expressly so held. Because Benitez's claim for relief under the Unruh Civil Rights Act is not based on marital status discrimination, we do not address that issue.

[8] [n.2] "Endometriosis is a condition in which tissue similar to the lining of the uterus" occurs on the ovaries, the fallopian tubes, or elsewhere in the body. Between 30 and 40 percent of women with this condition may suffer from infertility. (See <http://www.endo metriosis.org/endometriosis.html> [as of Aug. 18, 2008].)

pertaining to donated fresh sperm would satisfy the requirements of North Coast's state tissue bank license and the federal Clinical Laboratory Improvement Amendment (42 U.S.C. § 263). After hearing this, Benitez opted to have the IUI with sperm from a sperm bank. Dr. Brody so noted in Benitez's medical records and then left for an out-of-state vacation.

During Dr. Brody's absence, her colleague, Dr. Douglas Fenton, took over Benitez's medical care. Dr. Fenton contends that he was unaware of Dr. Brody's record notation of Benitez's decision not to use her friend's fresh sperm for the IUI, because the secretary who had typed that notation in Benitez's file left it in Dr. Brody's in box awaiting her return from vacation. Therefore, according to Dr. Fenton, he mistakenly believed that Benitez intended to have IUI with fresh sperm donated by a friend. The parties agree that unlike sperm from a sperm bank, fresh sperm (even when provided by a patient's husband) requires "certain preparation" before it can be used for IUI, and that "[c]ertain licensure" is necessary to do the requisite sperm preparation. Of North Coast's physicians, only Dr. Fenton was licensed to perform these tasks. But he refused to prepare donated fresh sperm for Benitez because of his religious objection. Two of his colleagues, Drs. Charles Stoopack and Ross Langley, had no such religious objection, but unlike Dr. Fenton, they were not licensed to prepare fresh sperm. Dr. Fenton then referred Benitez to a physician outside North Coast's medical practice, Dr. Michael Kettle.

The IUI performed by Dr. Kettle did not result in a pregnancy. Benitez was unable to conceive until June 2001, when Dr. Kettle performed in vitro fertilization.

In August 2001, Benitez sued North Coast and its physicians, Brody and Fenton, seeking damages and injunctive relief on several theories, notably sexual orientation discrimination in violation of California's Unruh Civil Rights Act. Defendants' answer to the complaint asserted a variety of affirmative defenses. Pertinent here is affirmative defense No. 32 stating that defendants' "alleged misconduct, if any" was protected by the rights of free speech and freedom of religion set forth in the federal and state Constitutions.

Benitez moved for summary adjudication of that defense. The trial court granted the motion, ruling that neither the federal nor the state Constitution provides a religious defense to a claim of sexual orientation discrimination under California's Unruh Civil Rights Act. Defendants challenged that ruling through a petition for writ of mandate filed in the Court of Appeal. That court granted the petition with respect to the two physician defendants only, thereby allowing Drs. Brody and Fenton to later assert at trial that their constitutional rights of free speech and religious freedom exempt them from complying with the Unruh Civil Rights Act's prohibition against sexual orientation discrimination. We granted Benitez's petition for review.

II

Benitez's claim of sexual orientation discrimination is based on California's Unruh Civil Rights Act (hereafter sometimes Act). (Civ.Code, § 51, subd. (a).) At the times relevant here, it provided: "All persons within the jurisdiction of this state are free and equal, and no matter what their sex, race, color, religion, ancestry, national origin, disability, or medical condition are entitled to the full and equal accommodations, advantages, facilities, privileges, or services in all business establishments of every kind whatsoever." (Civ.Code, § 51, former subd. (b), as amended by Stats.2000, ch. 1049.)

The Unruh Civil Rights Act's antidiscrimination provisions apply to business establishments that offer to the public "accommodations, advantages, facilities, privileges, or services." . . . A medical group providing medical services to the public has been held to be a business establishment for purposes of the Act . . .

In 1999 and 2000, the period relevant here, the Unruh Civil Rights Act did not list sexual orientation as a prohibited basis for discrimination. But before 1999, California's reviewing courts had, in a variety of contexts, described the Act as prohibiting sexual orientation discrimination. [citations omitted] Through an amendment to the Act in 2005, the Legislature expressly prohibited sexual orientation discrimination. (Stats.2005, ch. 420, § 2.)

The Unruh Civil Rights Act subjects to liability "[w]hoever denies, aids or incites a denial, or makes any discrimination or distinction contrary to [the Act]." (Civ.Code, § 52, subd. (a).) Thus, liability under the Act for denying a person the "full and equal accommodations, advantages, facilities, privileges, or services" of a business establishment (Civ.Code, § 51, subd. (b)) extends beyond the business establishment itself to the business establishment's employees responsible for the discriminatory conduct.

Below, we discuss defendant physicians' claims, first under the federal Constitution, and then under the California Constitution.

III

The First Amendment to the federal Constitution states that "Congress shall make no law respecting an establishment of religion, or prohibiting the free exercise thereof; or abridging the freedom of speech. . . ." (U.S. Const., 1st Amend.) This provision applies not only to Congress but also to the states because of its incorporation into the Fourteenth Amendment . . .

[The court next reviews several key U.S. Supreme Court cases in which individual challenged state laws as infringing on their First Amendment right to free exercise of religion.]

[I]n 1990 . . . the high court . . . announced that the First Amendment's right to the free exercise of religion "does not relieve an individual of the obligation to comply with a 'valid and neutral law of general applicability on the ground that the law proscribes (or prescribes) conduct that his religion prescribes (or proscribes).'" [citations omitted]

Thus, under the United States Supreme Court's most recent holdings, a religious objector has no federal constitutional right to an exemption from a neutral and valid law of general applicability on the ground that compliance with that law is contrary to the objector's religious beliefs . . .

In this case . . . with respect to defendants' reliance on the First Amendment, we apply the high court's . . . test. California's Unruh Civil Rights Act, from which defendant physicians seek religious exemption, is "a valid and neutral law of general applicability". As relevant in this case, it requires business establishments to provide "full and equal accommodations, advantages, facilities, privileges, or services" to all persons notwithstanding their sexual orientation. (Civ.Code, § 51, subds. (a) & (b).) Accordingly, the First Amendment's right to the free exercise of religion does not exempt defendant physicians here from conforming their conduct to the Act's antidiscrimination requirements even if compliance poses an incidental conflict with defendants' religious beliefs . . .

To avoid any conflict between their religious beliefs and the state Unruh Civil Rights Act's antidiscrimination provisions, defendant physicians can simply refuse to perform the IUI medical procedure at issue here for any patient of North Coast, the physicians' employer. Or, because they incur liability under the Act if they infringe upon the right to the "full and equal" services of North Coast's medical practice . . . defendant physicians can avoid such a conflict by ensuring that every patient requiring IUI receives "full and equal" access to that medical procedure though a North Coast physician lacking defendants' religious objections . . .

DISPOSITION

The judgment of the Court of Appeal is reversed.

WE CONCUR: GEORGE, C.J., and BAXTER, WERDEGAR, CHIN, MORENO, and CORRIGAN, JJ.

Concurring Opinion by BAXTER, J.

I join the majority's narrow conclusion that, on the facts of this case, defendants have no affirmative defense, based on the free exercise of religion clauses of the federal and state Constitutions, against plaintiffs' Unruh Civil Rights Act claims of discrimination on the basis of sexual orientation . . .

As the majority indicates, defendants in this case, who are members of a group medical practice, can avoid any conflict between their religious beliefs and the Unruh Civil Rights Act's requirements "by ensuring that every patient requiring [intrauterine insemination] receives 'full and equal' access to that medical procedure through a North Coast physician lacking defendants' religious objections."

I am not so certain this balance of competing interests would produce the same result in the case of a sole practitioner, who arguably is a "business establishment[ ]" for purposes of the Unruh Civil Rights Act . . . but who lacks the opportunity to ensure the patient's treatment by another member of the same establishment. At least where the patient could be referred with relative ease and convenience to another practice, I question whether the state's interest in full and equal medical treatment would compel a physician in solo practice to provide a treatment to which he or she has sincere religious objections . . .

NOTES AND QUESTIONS

1. *State Antidiscrimination Laws.* The California law at issue in *North Coast* today offers protection against discrimination across a broad range of categories, including sex, race, color, religion, ancestry, national origin, disability, medical condition, marital status and sexual orientation. Unruh Civil Rights Act, Cal. Civ. Code § 51(b). At the time Guadalupe Benitez sought treatment, the law did not explicitly include marital status or sexual orientation as protected categories, but both were subsequently added by the legislature. Antidiscrimination protection varies from state to state. In the U.S., about half of all states protect against discrimination on the basis of marital status in public accommodations (which includes medical offices), while less than a third cover sexual orientation discrimination. *See* Judith F. Daar, *Accessing Reproductive Technologies: Invisible Barriers, Indelible Harms*, 23 BERK. J. GENDER, LAW & JUSTICE 18 (2008). If the North Coast physicians practiced in a state that did not protect against discrimination on the basis of marital status or sexual orientation, could they have refused to provide ART services to Ms. Benitez because of her personal characteristics? Should they be permitted to exercise such discretion?

2. *Physician Autonomy.* A physician is free to determine whether or not to enter into a doctor/patient relationship with a prospective patient. The only exceptions to this principle of physician autonomy are the antidiscrimination provisions embedded in federal and state civil rights laws. How do ART practitioners exercise this discretion to refuse to provide services to some patients? A survey released in 2005 polled physicians on their attitudes and practices in treating patients with different social backgrounds. When asked about hypothetical patients, the following percentage of respondents said they would be "very or extremely likely to turn away" the following:

A single man	53%
A gay male couple in search of a surrogate	48%
A couple on welfare	38%
A single woman	20%
A gay female couple in search of a sperm donor	17%

See A. Gurmankin, A. Caplan, & A. Braveman, *Screening Practices and Beliefs of Assisted Reproductive Technology Programs*, 83 FERTILITY & STERILITY 61 (2005).

3. *ART and the Single Woman.* Lawmakers in several states have attempted to limit ART to married individuals. In late 2005 and early 2006, legislators in Indiana and Virginia, respectively, introduced legislation that would prohibit health care providers from offering or performing any medical procedure on an unmarried woman for the purpose of conception or procreation. The Indiana bill, introduced by State Senator Patricia Miller (R-Indianapolis) in October 2005, would have required that couples who seek assistance to become pregnant, such as through IUI, donor eggs, sperm and embryos, IVF or "other medical means" would have to be married to each other. While the Senator ultimately dropped the bill, its mere introduction caused alarm among those who favor equal access to ART regardless of marital status. *See* Mary Beth Schneider, *Assisted Reproduction Bill Dropped*, INDIANAPO-

LIS STAR, Oct. 6, 2005 (Sen. Miller is quoted upon dropping the bill, "The issue has become more complex than anticipated.").

A similar bill was introduced into the Virginia Legislature in January 2006. Virginia House Bill 187 provides in relevant part:

> No individual licensed by a health regulatory board shall assist with or perform any intervening medical technology, whether in vivo or in vitro, for or on an unmarried woman that completely or partially replaces sexual intercourse as the means of conception, including, but not limited to, artificial insemination by donor, cryopreservation of gametes and embryos, in vitro fertilization, embryo transfer, gamete intrafallopian tube transfer, and low tubal ovum transfer.

The bill was not enacted, but if it were would it mean that a single woman who develops cancer and wants to have her eggs cryopreserved (frozen for later use), could not enlist the assistance of a Virginia doctor because he or she would risk loss of a medical license?

SECTION IV: INSURING ART SERVICES

A.   The Market Landscape

1.   The Status of Infertility Insurance Coverage

a.   Statutory Law

At the beginning of this Chapter we learned of the high cost of infertility treatment, leading many couples to surrender their life's savings in an effort to become parents. This voluntary impoverishment follows from the fact that, for the most part, the American health insurance system does not provide coverage for infertility-related medical expenses. Health insurance coverage in the U.S. is a complex web of public programs (primarily Medicare, covering those 65 and older, and Medicaid, covering mostly the indigent) and private insurers who are largely accessed by individuals through their workplaces. Even under major health reform enacted by the Patient Protection and Affordable Care Act in 2010, responsibility for health insurance remains primarily with individuals, rather than the government. The government provides little or no coverage for infertility services,[9] so any reimbursement for services will necessarily be accessed through private health insurance policies.

Whether an individual's health insurance policy covers infertility services may depend upon whether the state in which the policy is issued requires insurers to provide such coverage. According to the National Conference of State Legislatures, currently 14 states have passed laws that require insurers to either cover (known as a "mandate to provide" or "hard mandate") or offer coverage ("mandate to

---

[9] Surprisingly, infertility services are covered under Medicaid and Title X, although there is little information available on the amount of public funds actually spent on infertility treatment. See 42 C.F. R. § 59.5(a)(1).

offer" or "soft mandate") for fertility diagnosis and treatment. Twelve of the states have laws that require insurance companies to cover infertility treatment (hard mandate states), while two states have laws that require insurance companies to offer coverage for treatment (soft mandate states). That said, the level of coverage in each state is highly variable. For example, Massachusetts and Rhode Island have the most comprehensive statutes, mandating health insurance companies to provide coverage for diagnosis and treatment of infertility. But the Massachusetts law actually provides wider coverage because the Rhode Island statute is limited to married couples. In 2007, the governor of Rhode Island vetoed a bill that would have extended infertility insurance coverage to unmarried women. Texas and California are both "soft mandate" states, and require insurers to offer coverage to employers, which they may accept or decline. Even if employers in both of these states elect to offer coverage, Californians will see fewer benefits because the state law specifically excludes coverage for IVF. Relevant portions of the Massachusetts and Texas statutes are set forth below. In addition, Table 1 shows each state law related to infertility insurance coverage, including the date of original enactment plus significant amendments.

A further limitation to access to infertility care is a 1974 federal law designed to standardize pension benefits for American workers. While it remains the case in the U.S. that the regulation of health insurance is largely left to the states, an astute student of the law of insurance will be quick to point out that federal law does significantly impact the insurance industry through the Employee Retirement Income Security Act of 1974 (ERISA), 29 U.S.C. § 1001 et seq. Briefly stated, ERISA is a federal statute regulating employee benefit plans, including health benefit plans. The importance of ERISA to infertility insurance coverage is that in some cases, particularly when employers self-insure their health insurance coverage, the federal law preempts (or makes void) state laws that relate to employee benefit plans. Thus, even if a state requires insurers to cover infertility treatments, ERISA may preempt such a state law and allow health insurance providers to decline to offer infertility coverage. For a comprehensive analysis of ERISA, *see* BARRY R. FURROW, THOMAS L. GREANEY, SANDRA H. JOHNSON, TIMOTHY STOLTZFUS JOST & ROBERT L. SCHWARTZ, HEALTH LAW 418-60 (2d ed. 2000).

Mandate to Offer

Texas Insurance Code § 1366.003-005

Offer of Coverage Required

(a) [A]n issuer of a group health benefit plan that provides pregnancy-related benefits for individuals covered under the plan shall offer and make available to each holder or sponsor of the plan coverage for services and benefits on an expense incurred, service, or prepaid basis for outpatient expenses that arise from in vitro fertilization procedures.

(b) Benefits for in vitro fertilization procedures required under this section must be provided to the same extent as benefits provided for other pregnancy-related procedures under the plan.

Conditions Applicable to Coverage

The coverage offered under Section 1366.003 is required only if . . .

(2) the fertilization or attempted fertilization of the patient's oocytes is made only with the sperm of the patient's spouse;

(3) the patient and the patient's spouse have a history of infertility of at least five continuous years' duration.

Mandate to Provide

Mass. Gen. Laws Ann. ch. 176A, § 8K

Infertility diagnosis and treatment benefits

Any contract . . . between a subscriber and the corporation under an individual or group hospital service plan which is delivered, issued for delivery or renewed in the commonwealth while this provision is effective and which provides pregnancy-related benefits shall provide as a benefit for all individual subscribers or members within the commonwealth . . . , to the same extent that benefits are provided for other pregnancy-related procedures, coverage for medically necessary expenses of diagnosis and treatment of infertility . . . For purposes of this section, "infertility" shall mean the condition of an individual who is unable to conceive or produce conception during a period of 1 year if the female is age 35 or younger or during a period of 6 months if the female is over the age of 35.

Do you agree as a matter of public policy that infertility benefits should be provided on par with pregnancy-related benefits? Notice that Texas limits coverage to married couples who use their own gametes. Notice also that Texans must experience infertility for five years before becoming eligible for coverage. From what you know about the relationship between infertility and age, how useful is the Texas law in assisting those in need of ART?

Table 1. 50 States Summary of Legislation Related To Infertility Insurance Coverage

State	Coverage
Arkansas	**Ark. Stat. Ann. §§ 23-85-137 and 23-86-118 (1987, 2011)** requires health insurance companies to cover the expenses of IVF procedures at licensed facilities.
California	**Cal. Insurance Code § 10119.6 (1989)** requires insurers to offer coverage of infertility treatments, except for IVF. Infertility may be a result of a medical condition or may refer to the inability to carry a pregnancy during a one-year or more period of time. Infertility treatment refers to diagnosis, diagnostic tests, medication, surgery, and gamete intrafallopian transfer.

State	Coverage
Connecticut	**Conn. Gen. Stat. § 38a-536 and 38a-509 (1989, 2005)** requires health insurance organizations provide coverage for medically necessary expenses of the diagnosis and treatment of infertility, including IVF. Infertility refers to an otherwise healthy individual's inability to retain a pregnancy during a one-year period.
Hawaii	**Hawaii Rev. Stat. §§ 431:10A-116.5 and 432.1-604 (1989, 2003)** requires health insurance policies that provide pregnancy-related benefits to include a one-time-only benefit for outpatient expenses arising from IVF. In order to qualify for IVF, the couple must have a history of infertility for at least 5 years or prove that the infertility is a result of specified medical conditions.
Illinois	**Ill. Rev. Stat. ch. 215, § ILCS 5/356m (1991, 1996)** requires certain insurance policies that provide pregnancy-related benefits to provide coverage for the diagnosis and treatment of infertility. Coverage includes IVF, uterine embryo lavage, embryo transfer, artificial insemination, GIFT, zygote intrafallopian tube transfer, and low tubal ovum transfer.
Maryland	**Md. Insurance Code Ann. § 15-810, Md. Health General Code Ann. § 19-701 (2000)** prohibits health insurers that provide pregnancy-related benefits from excluding benefits for outpatient expenses arising from IVF. Law requires a history of infertility of at least 2 years duration and infertility associated with one of several listed medical conditions. An insurer may limit coverage to 3 IVF attempts per live birth, not to exceed a maximum lifetime benefit of $100,000. An insurer or employer may exclude coverage if it conflicts with the religious beliefs and practices of a religious organization. Infertility care included in definition of health care services.
Massachusetts	**Mass. Gen. Laws Ann. ch. 175, § 47H, ch. 176A, § 8K, ch. 176B, § 4J, ch. 176G, § 4, and 211 CMR 37.00 (1987, 2010)** requires health insurance policies that provide pregnancy-related benefits to also provide coverage for diagnosis and treatment of infertility, including IVF. "Infertility" is defined as the condition of a presumably healthy individual who is unable to conceive or produce conception during a period of one year if female is 35 or younger or 6 months if the female is over 35.
Montana	**Mont. Code Ann. § 33-22-1521 (1987)** revises Comprehensive Health Association, the state's high-risk pool, and clarifies that covered expenses do not include charges for artificial insemination or treatment for infertility. **Mont. Code Ann. § 33-31-102(2)(v), et seq. (1987)** requires HMOs to provide basic health services on a prepaid basis, including infertility care.

State	Coverage
New Jersey	**N.J. Laws, Chap. 236 (2001)** requires health insurers to provide coverage for medically necessary expenses incurred in diagnosis and treatment of infertility, including medications, surgery, IVF, embryo transfer, artificial insemination, GIFT, ZIFT, ICSI and four completed egg retrievals per lifetime of the covered person. The law has a religious exemption for employers that provide health coverage to less than 50 employees.
New York	**N.Y. Insurance Law §§ 3216 (13), 3221 (6) and 4303 (1990, 2002)** prohibits individual and group health insurance policies from excluding coverage for hospital, surgical and medical care for diagnosis and treatment of correctable medical conditions otherwise covered by the policy solely because the condition results in infertility. The law does not require coverage for IVF.
Ohio	**Ohio Rev. Code Ann. § 1751.01(A)(7)(1991)** requires insurers offer basic health care services, including infertility services when medically necessary.
Rhode Island	**R.I. Gen. Laws §§ 27-18-30, 27-19-23, 27-20-20 and 27-41-33 (1989, 2007)** requires any contract, plan or policy of health insurance, nonprofit hospital service, nonprofit medical service and HMO to provide coverage for medically necessary expenses of diagnosis and treatment of infertility. Co-payments for infertility services may not exceed 20 percent. Infertility is defined as the condition of an otherwise healthy married individual who is unable to conceive or produce conception during a period of one year.
Texas	**Tex. Insurance Code Ann. § 3.51-6, Sec. 3A (1987, 2003)** health insurers must offer and make available coverage for services and benefits on an expense incurred or prepaid basis for outpatient expenses that may arise from IVF procedures. In order to qualify for IVF services, the couple must have a history of infertility for at least five years or have specified medical conditions resulting in infertility.
West Virginia	**W. Va. Code § 33-25A-2 (1995)** requires health insurers to offer "basic health care services," which include infertility services. Applies to HMOs only.

Source: National Conference of State Legislatures, available at:
http://www.ncsl.org/default.aspx?tabid=14391

b.   Case Law

In addition to specific and explicit statutory language governing infertility insurance coverage, the law has taken up the question of insurance reimbursement through a number of appellate court decisions. When, for example, a woman seeks treatment for infertility through IVF and her insurance policy does not specifically address coverage for this medical procedure, she may submit the expense to her insurance carrier. If the carrier refuses to reimburse her for these expenses, she may sue on the ground that the IVF is a covered service under the general terms of the policy. In the article that follows, the author has nicely summarized the case law surrounding the battle between health insurance carriers and their policyholders over the coverage of infertility services.

Lisa M. Kerr
Can Money Buy Happiness? An Examination of the Coverage of Infertility Services Under HMO Contracts
49 Case W. Res. L. Rev. 599 (1999)

Courts have dealt with the question of whether insurance companies will be required to cover infertility services in four main contexts: 1) as reversal of sterilization, 2) as an illness, 3) as "medically necessary," and 4) as experimental . . . The case law is conclusive on some issues — e.g., that insurance companies do not have to pay for the reversal of voluntary sterilization and that most infertility procedures are no longer experimental. Frustratingly, however, decisions dealing with infertility as an illness and infertility services as medically necessary do not offer any definite answers.

1. Reversal of Voluntary Sterilization

Insurers consistently refuse to cover expenses related to reversal of voluntary sterilization and the courts have supported this position. In *Reuss v. Time Insurance Co.*, [340 S.E.2d 625 (Ga. Ct. App. 1986)] the court held that expenses for a procedure designed to reverse a vasectomy were not covered under the policy language. Similarly, in *Marsh v. Reserve Life Insurance Co.*, [516 So.2d 1311 (La. Ct. App. 1987)] the court held that the insurer was not obligated to pay for surgery to reverse tubal ligation that the Plaintiff had elected to have some years earlier. The reasoning behind these exclusions is that voluntary sterilization procedures, which have infertility as their purpose, do not constitute a "sickness" under the policy for which the insurer is obliged to pay. Viewed in this light, the exclusion makes sense: If a person purposefully undergoes a procedure designed to produce sterility, it seems illogical that the person's infertility is a result of an illness. Rather, the infertility is a result of a conscious decision not to have children.

2. Infertility as a Disease

Insurance companies also deny coverage for infertility treatments under the rationale that infertility is not a "disease." This argument has had less success in the courts. A number of definitions of disease have been advanced by courts, such as "(a) deviation from the healthy or normal condition of any of the functions . . . of the body" or "(a) disturbance in function or structure of any . . . part of the body." Infertility fits into both these definitions. When an otherwise healthy couple can not reproduce because of a physical or genetic impairment, there is obviously a deviation from the normal reproductive function of the body.

Two decisions which have adopted this type of reasoning are *Witcraft v. Sundstrand Health and Disability Group Benefit Plan* [420 N.W.2d 785 (Iowa 1988)] and *Egert v. Connecticut General Life Insurance Co.* [900 F.2d 1032 (7th Cir.

1990)]. In *Witcraft*, the court considered whether infertility was an "illness" within the meaning of the Plaintiffs' insurance policy. Physical examinations of the Plaintiffs revealed that the husband had a low sperm count and the wife experienced irregular ovulation. The couple received infertility treatments and eventually conceived a child. They then underwent a second set of treatments in order to have another child, but this course of AI [artificial insemination] was unsuccessful. This second AI procedure, as well as all prior treatments had been paid for by the insurance company, but when the Plaintiffs submitted a claim for an additional treatment to the husband's sperm, their third overall, it was denied.

Their health care insurance policy stated that all "expenses relating to injury or illness" would be covered, and provided no exclusion for infertility. The plan defined "illness" as "any sickness occurring to a covered individual which does not arise out of or in the course of employment . . . ." The trial court found that "the dysfunctioning of the reproductive organs of both Mr. and Mrs. Witcraft came within the plan's definition of an 'illness.' " On appeal, the Supreme Court of Iowa affirmed the trial court's decision, stating that "the natural function of the reproductive organs is to procreate" and that the stated procedures did "help to reverse the dysfunction of the reproductive organs of both parties."

The insurance company was also required to pay for infertility services in *Egert v. Connecticut General Life Insurance Co.* The health insurance policy at issue stated therein that participants would be reimbursed for services "essential for the necessary care and treatment of an (i)njury or a (s)ickness." The *Egert* court ordered the insurance company to pay for the procedures because the Defendant's own internal memorandum referred to infertility as an illness.

3. Medical Necessity of Infertility Services

Medical necessity is another consideration traditionally affecting whether insurance companies will pay for infertility treatment. In *Kinzie v. Physician's Liability Insurance Co.*, [750 P.2d 1140 (Okla. Ct. App. 1987)] the court held that "in vitro fertilization (is) not a medically necessary service because it (is) elective and (is) not required to cure or preserve Mrs. Kinzie's health." The court reasoned that "(t)he infertile condition of Mrs. Kinzie's body was not corrected by in vitro fertilization. Although Mrs. Kinzie and her husband did indeed become parents, Mrs. Kinzie's infertile medical condition was in no way reversed or cured." Finally, the court stated that "(t)he conception of a child, although certainly important to married couples who have a problem conceiving, was not 'medically necessary' to the physical health of the insured." This decision is inconsistent with the *Witcraft* analysis, which held that infertility procedures did help cure the dysfunction of the Plaintiff's reproductive organs.

The insurer in *Egert* employed the same line of reasoning to argue that IVF was not medically necessary. It asserted that the IVF treatment at issue would not cure the infertility. The insurer argued that IVF was "not essential because it cannot make (the Plaintiff) fertile again unlike microsurgery (which was covered by the policy) which might repair her fallopian tubes." This argument is frequently used to deny coverage for assisted reproduction procedures, such as IVF, GIFT or ZIFT, because these procedures do not permanently correct an underlying physical problem, but rather circumvent the problem area. Insurance companies continue to embrace the notion that if a treatment does not cure a condition it should not be covered. One insurance representative stated that IVF should not be covered because "(i)t doesn't treat a disease, it bypasses the condition." The *Egert* court did not, unfortunately, come to a conclusion on this issue.

4. Assisted Reproductive Technologies Excluded as Experimental

A final method employed by insurance companies to deny coverage for infertility services is to label such services as "experimental." Insurers regularly seek to exclude such experimental services in order to keep their costs down. There are, however, other more socially responsible reasons for denying coverage of experimental treatments. Exclusion of experimental treatments promotes elimination of worthless procedures from the medical field. Before insurers agree to pay for a treatment they want to make sure that it is safe and efficacious, thereby protecting the public from quackery.

A number of factors must be considered in deciding whether a treatment is experimental. These include cost, expert testimony, the patient's condition, the possibility of alternative treatments, professional consensus regarding the treatment's effectiveness and the extent to which the treatment is prescribed. In *Reilly v. Blue Cross & Blue Shield United*, [846 F.2d 416 (7th Cir. 1988)] the insurance company claimed that IVF was excluded under the policy's general exclusion of experimental treatments because it had a success rate of less than fifty percent. The court suggested that the insurance company's success ratio of fifty percent was arbitrary and unrealistic, pointing out that the insurance company did not use a success ratio in determining whether other diseases should be covered by the policy.

Despite the decision in *Reilly*, many insurers are still excluding coverage for IVF by continuing to consider it experimental, with one insurer recently announcing a lifetime limit on payments for infertility services of $5000. In reality, most advanced technologies carry high price tags, and thus, this limit is barely adequate to cover one attempt. On the other hand, $5000 is adequate to pay for a number of more traditional services, such as drug therapy and artificial insemination. In short, this amount reinforces the belief that the assisted reproductive technologies are still experimental and therefore undeserving of coverage from insurance companies. Once a procedure has gained widespread acceptance in the medical community, it should no longer be considered experimental. Insurance policies should recognize as acceptable and useful treatments, and in turn should provide coverage for, those procedures that have been deemed safe and effective by either the American Society for Reproductive Medicine or the American College of Obstetricians and Gynecologists . . .

5. Traditional Contract Principles

Courts have also applied traditional principles of contract and insurance law to decide if an insurance policy covers infertility treatments. Courts examine what both parties intended the contract to mean and the contract is construed against the insurer as the drafter of the document. All ambiguities must be resolved in favor of the insured and the insurance company bears the burden of proving that the disputed treatment is not covered by the policy. One important reason behind this jurisprudence is it takes into account the reasonable expectations of the insured. This is an important factor because when the insured signs a contract he or she has a present expectation about what will and will not be covered. If the contract is misleading it will prevent the insured from seeking out another contract which may cover the desired type of treatment. By the time the insured gets sick and needs the insurance, it is too late to look for another policy, and therefore the insured's reasonable expectations must be taken into account in any judicial determination of the meaning of a contract. After courts began interpreting insurance contracts to include coverage for infertility treatments, insurers began to specifically exclude infertility services from the plans.

NOTES AND QUESTIONS

1.   The issues surrounding insurance coverage for infertility can be viewed strictly in the context of private health insurance, where we learned that most providers do not provide or even offer coverage for their insureds. One study estimates that only 14% of large health plans and 16% of preferred plans offer IVF coverage. *See* P.J. Neumann, *Should Health Insurance Cover IVF? Issues and Options*, 22 J. HEALTH POLIT. POLICY LAW 1215 (1997). Alternatively, coverage for ARTs can be viewed in the larger picture of health care access in general. In the U.S., it is estimated that 50 million Americans lack access to any type of health insurance and thus lack access to even the most basic health care services. While it may seem obvious and even necessary to discount the plight of the under or uninsured infertile individual compared to the basic health needs of millions, consider the economics involved. To provide health coverage for the nearly 20% of Americans who lack access would require an expenditure of resources that all sides of the political spectrum agree would be enormous and perceptible by the ranks of all taxpayers. On the other hand, providing infertility coverage for all privately insured employee-based health plans would raise annual premiums about $3.00. See Edward G. Hughes & Mita Giacomini, *Funding In Vitro Fertilization Treatment for Persistent Subfertility: The Pain and the Politics*, 76 FERTILITY & STERILITY 431 (2001). Would you be willing to add $3.00 to your insurance bill to fund infertility? Would your answer depend upon whether you perceived yourself at risk of experiencing infertility at some point in your life?

2.   The article by Lisa Kerr sets forth the strategy that insured individuals have employed to overturn decisions by their health insurers that coverage is not required by the terms of the policy. In the described cases, insured and carriers focus on the language of insurance policies to tease out whether infertility is a covered illness, or whether certain treatments are medically necessary. What avenues does a patient have if her policy explicitly and unequivocally excludes coverage for infertility treatment?

Mary Jo Krauel was such a patient. After several years of trying to become pregnant naturally, Ms. Krauel sought treatment at a fertility clinic and gave birth to a daughter following GIFT (gamete intrafallopian transfer, in which the egg and sperm are retrieved and placed into the fallopian tube). Her employer, Iowa

Methodist Medical Center (IMMC), self-insured its employees' health insurance with a plan that explicitly excluded treatment of infertility problems. Instead of looking for leeway in the policy language, Ms. Krauel sued IMMC on the ground that denial of insurance coverage for her fertility treatments violated the Americans With Disabilities Act because her infertility limited her ability to reproduce naturally and therefore constituted a disability under the ADA. The United States Court of Appeals for the Eighth Circuit rejected Ms. Krauel's claim, reasoning that infertility does not substantially affect a major life activity, as required as a qualifying condition under the ADA. The court defines the term "major life activity" as "functions such as caring for oneself, performing manual tasks, walking, seeing, hearing, speaking, breathing, learning, and working." The court found that Ms. Krauel's infertility in no way prevented her from performing her full job duties at the hospital or engaging in any of the enumerated activities that comprise major life activities. Thus, the court granted summary judgment to the Medical Center on the ADA Claim. *Krauel v. Iowa Methodist Medical Center*, 95 F.3d 674 (8th Cir. 1996).

Do you think the decision in *Bragdon v. Abbott*, 524 U.S. 624 (1998), which we read in Chapter 1, affects the decision in *Krauel v. Iowa Methodist Medical Center*? Did the Supreme Court intend to elevate infertility to a federally recognized disability under federal law when it found that HIV is a disability because it impairs the major life activity of reproduction? It seemed inevitable that this question would be litigated, as the next case reveals.

SAKS v. FRANKLIN COVEY
United States District Court, Southern District New York
117 F. Supp. 2d 318 (2000)

McMahon, District Judge. Infertility blights the lives of thousands of American families. Fortunately, modern medicine has devised ways that enable some of those who suffer from infertility to conceive biological children and carry them to term. Like so many of the extraordinary advances in medicine, these treatments are quite expensive. It is a testament to the basic nature of the reproductive drive that people who are desperate to have children will go to great lengths to conceive — often enduring extreme physical discomfort and incurring expenses that bring them close to bankruptcy. The physical discomforts are, of course, unavoidable. Whether the financial discomfort can be avoided by one family, at least, is the central issue in this case.

From March 1995 through October 1999, plaintiff Rochelle Saks was employed by defendant Franklin Covey, a seller of products and services related to time management, organization and business communication training. During that period, plaintiff and her husband were endeavoring to have a child. Saks and her husband had numerous treatments, prescribed by two different doctors, to enable her to conceive and carry a child, including a regimen of clomiphine ("Clomid") and progesterone and intrauterine insemination ("IUI"), which were unsuccessful. She also completed two cycles of in vitro fertilization ("IVF"), in April 1999 and August 1999. She became pregnant three times between September 1997 and August 1999. All three pregnancies ended in miscarriages.

Saks made claims for insurance reimbursement for her treatments. For purposes of this motion, defendants concede that plaintiff suffered from the condition known as infertility and that all of the treatments prescribed to help her become pregnant, including in vitro fertilization and intra-uterine implantation, were "medically necessary" as that term is defined in Franklin Coveys' self-insured health benefits plan. Ms. Saks' surgical fertilization procedures, which were rendered by American medical professionals, qualify as "a service required for the treatment of an active illness" (that illness being the inability to conceive a child in the usual way).

Nonetheless, Franklin Covey has declined to cover the cost of those procedures. Its insurance Plan specifically excludes coverage for "surgical impregnation procedures," including artificial insemination and in vitro fertilization. Saks contends in this lawsuit that this exclusion violates three separate Federal statutes: The Americans with Disabilities Act ("ADA"), 42 U.S.C. § 12101 *et seq.;* Title VII of the Civil Rights Act of 1964, as amended ("Title VII"), 42 U.S.C. § 2000e *et seq.;* and the Pregnancy Discrimination Act ("PDA"), 42 U.S.C. § 2000e(k) . . . After discovery, both parties have moved for summary judgment — defendants for dismissal of the complaint, plaintiff for partial summary judgment on the issue of liability.

For the reasons stated below, I am dismissing plaintiff's claim that Franklin Covey's refusal to cover surgical procedures that create pregnancy violates the law.

Standards for Summary Judgment

The usual standards for an award of summary judgment apply: a party is entitled to judgment if there is no dispute of material fact and that party is entitled to judgment as a matter of law. *See Anderson v. Liberty Lobby, Inc.*, 477 U.S. 242, 250, 106 S.Ct. 2505, 91 L.Ed.2d 202 (1986). I view the facts most favorably to plaintiff for purposes of considering defendants' motion, which I elect to consider first since, if granted, it would dispose of the entire case.

Statement of Facts

The following facts are undisputed for purposes of this motion. Plaintiff was employed by defendant Franklin Covey Co. as a store manager at the company's retail store from March 1995 until she resigned in October 1999. As part of its benefits package, Franklin Covey offers a self-insured health benefits plan ("the Plan") that provides coverage to all full-time employees and their dependents. The company has a contractual arrangement with The TPA, Inc. ("The TPA"), an administrator for self-insured health benefit plans, to act as the third-party processing agent for claims made under the Company's Plan.

The Plan provides coverage for all "medically necessary" treatments, which are defined under the Plan as "any service or supply required for the diagnosis or treatment of an active illness or injury that is rendered by or under the supervision of the attending physician, generally accepted by medical professionals in the United States and non-experimental."

An "illness" is defined as "any bodily sickness, disease, mental/nervous disorder or pregnancy." Jane Clark, a Claim Support Manager for the TPA, testified that infertility is a "disease" or "illness" within the meaning of the Plan. Ms. Clark also testified that fertility drugs and assisted reproductive techniques such as intrauterine insemination ("IUI") and in vitro fertilization ("IVF") are not considered experimental treatments for the disease of infertility. However, the Plan excludes coverage for "surgical impregnation procedures," including IVF and IUI. "[C]omplications arising from any non-covered surgery" are also excluded from coverage.

Plaintiff has unsuccessfully attempted to conceive since May 1994. In July 1995, she consulted with Dr. Ralph Berardi, an OB/GYN, who suspected that plaintiff suffered from polycystic ovarian syndrome. Plaintiff underwent a test that ruled out that possibility, and Dr. Berardi recommended that plaintiff and her husband, Joel Saks, continue to attempt a pregnancy through sexual relations. In February 1996, Plaintiff began seeing another OB/GYN, Dr. Deborah Cerar, who recommended that plaintiff undergo several diagnostic tests to determine the cause of her infertility. None of these tests revealed the source of plaintiff's infertility. Upon Dr. Cerar's recommendation, plaintiff began using ovulation kits to determine when she was ovulating so that intercourse with her husband could be timed to maximize the likelihood of conception. This approach, however, proved unsuccessful.

In November 1996, Plaintiff consulted with Dr. John Stangel, a specialist in the area of reproductive endocrinology. Dr. Stangel prescribed for plaintiff the drug Clomid in order to induce and regulate ovulation, and recommended that this treatment be accompanied by intrauterine inseminations ("IUI") and regular intercourse to increase the chances for a successful conception. Because patients who take Clomid must be monitored for potential side effects, plaintiff underwent ultrasounds and blood tests while on that medication. Plaintiff also continued to use ovulation kits in conjunction with her other treatments. She completed two IUI's with Dr. Stangel, neither of which resulted in pregnancy.

By May or June 1997, plaintiff had become dissatisfied with Dr. Stangel's insemination procedures, and decided to switch to a new reproductive endocrinologist, Dr. Gad Lavy. In or about May or June 1997, plaintiff called defendants' third-party administrator ("TPA") to determine the benefits to which plaintiff was entitled under the Plan for her initial visit with Dr. Lavy. The TPA informed plaintiff that, except for the $15 co-payment required for all doctor visits, the initial consultation would be covered under the Plan.

Plaintiff consulted with Dr. Lavy in or about July or August 1997. Lavy diagnosed plaintiff as having a hormonal imbalance and, consequently, ovulation disorder. Dr. Lavy recommended (1) treatment with Clomid, estrogen and progesterone to regulate plaintiff's ovulation, and (2) continued IUI and regular intercourse to increase the likelihood of successful conception. Plaintiff underwent the first cycle of IUI in August 1997. The administration of Clomid to plaintiff had to be monitored with blood work and ultrasound tests, as did her course of estrogen and progesterone treatment.

Plaintiff submitted claims to the TPA for all the expenses incurred in connection with Dr. Lavy's treatment. However, the TPA authorized reimbursement only for venipuncture that Lavy had performed on plaintiff, as well for the cost of the drugs estradiol and progesterone administered on August 29, 1997. Payment for the remainder of Lavy's treatment was denied.

On September 8, 1997, plaintiff learned that she was pregnant. During the following two weeks, her pregnancy was closely monitored with ultrasound and blood tests, which defendants refused to cover. Her first ultrasound revealed a heartbeat, as well as a possible second gestational sac. Her second ultrasound, however, on or about September 27, revealed no heartbeat in the first gestational sac, and a follow-up blood test showed a decrease in HCG, the pregnancy hormone. A subsequent test on October 6 confirmed that plaintiff had miscarried, and she underwent a dilation and curettage ("D & C") the next day to remove the miscarried fetus. Further tests on the fetus to determine the cause of the miscarriage were inconclusive.

The TPA refused to reimburse plaintiff for the cost of the D & C, hysterosalpingogram, and the pathology tests performed after plaintiff's miscarriage. Plaintiff successfully appealed that denial, however, and in October 1998, the TPA provided coverage for her pregnancy-related expenses.

Plaintiff continued her treatments with Dr. Lavy through December 1998, or thereabouts, during which time she underwent ten more IUIs. From November 1997 until April 1998, she continued the course of Clomid, progesterone and estrogen accompanied by IUIs. Beginning in May 1998, Dr. Lavy prescribed Humagon, an injectable drug (plaintiff does not recall whether the Humagon was administered in place of, or in conjunction with, the Clomid). Plaintiff continued the course of progesterone, estrogen and IUIs and the monitoring with ultrasounds and blood work that her treatment entailed. Dr. Lavy also advised plaintiff to undergo another hysterosalpingogram, the results of which came back negative. Dr. Lavy then told plaintiff that the next appropriate treatment step was in vitro fertilization ("IVF"). Plaintiff claims that she was unable to pursue that course of action because of defendants' refusal to cover the cost of her treatment with Dr. Lavy. The TPA refused coverage for all of the IUIs and related drug and monitoring expenses that plaintiff incurred while in Dr. Lavy's care. Consequently, plaintiff and her husband were forced to pay for this treatment personally.

In December 1998, Dr. Lavy informed plaintiff that he would not continue to provide her with further treatment until she paid in full the outstanding balance of Lavy's fee, which totaled approximately $6,000. Plaintiff was unable to pay this amount, and ended her relationship with Lavy.

Plaintiff found another reproductive endocrinologist, Dr. Zev Rosenwaks, at the Center for Reproductive Medicine and Infertility in Manhattan. Rosenwaks determined that plaintiff was a good candidate for IVF, and in or about March and early April 1999, prescribed a course of Lupron, Humagon, HCG and Follostim to stimulate superovulation. This treatment, too, required that plaintiff be monitored through blood and ultrasound tests. Plaintiff began the IVF procedure on April 16, 1999, including progesterone therapy to support a potential pregnancy. On April 30, a blood test reflected HCG levels indicating a positive pregnancy, but by the following day, the levels had dropped. Plaintiff was informed that she had a chemical pregnancy, but that it was not sustained.

In July 1999, plaintiff began a second cycle of IVF, including the same course of drugs that she had taken in March and April. Three embryos were implanted on August 7, 1999, and plaintiff again began progesterone therapy. On August 25, 1999, plaintiff's HGC levels indicated another pregnancy, though they were lower than the normally expected level. Testing over the following few days revealed low estrogen levels, and plaintiff experienced some blood spotting. In late August, plaintiff miscarried again. She was told that her pregnancy had been ectopic.

The TPA denied coverage for nearly all of plaintiff's treatment under Dr. Rosenwaks' care, including her consultation and other office visits, diagnostic tests, the injectable drugs, the IVF's, and blood work and ultrasound monitoring costs. It is not disputed that Plaintiff complied with the Plan's procedural requirements for submission of claims.

On an unidentified date, plaintiff filed a charge with the EEOC against Franklin Covey alleging the same ADA, Title VII and Pregnancy Discrimination Act violations as in the instant action. In a determination dated April 27, 1999, the New York District Director found reasonable cause that Franklin Covey had violated those statutes by denying coverage to plaintiff in connection with her infertility treatments.

Plaintiff filed this suit on September 9, 1999. On March 21, 2000, defendants moved for summary judgment as to all of plaintiff's claims. On that same date, plaintiff cross-moved for partial summary judgment as to her ADA, PDA, Title VII and breach of contract claims. For the reasons that follow, defendant's motion is granted, and the case is dismissed.

Conclusions of Law

1. *Franklin Covey's Exclusion of Surgical Impregnation Procedures Does Not Violate the Americans with Disabilities Act*

Congress passed the Americans with Disabilities Act in order to, *inter alia*, "provide a clear and comprehensive national mandate for the elimination of discrimination against individuals with disabilities" and "provide clear, strong, consistent, enforceable standards addressing discrimination against individuals with disabilities." 42 U.S.C. § 12101(b)(1),(2). To those ends, the statute prohibits discrimination by any "covered entity" against "a qualified individual with a disability because of the disability of such individual in regard to job application procedures, the hiring, advancement, or discharge of employees, employee compensation, job training, and other terms conditions, and privileges of employment." 42 U.S.C. § 12112(a). The "terms and conditions" of employment, within the meaning of the Act, include the provision of fringe benefits. *See Castellano v. City of New York*, 142 F.3d 58, 66 (2d Cir.), *cert. denied*, 525 U.S. 820, 119 S.Ct. 60, 142 L.Ed.2d 47 (1998).

Before I can reach the merits of plaintiff's claim, I must dispose of a challenge to her ability to maintain this action. The parties do not dispute that Rochelle Saks is infertile, or that infertility is a physical impairment. Defendant does, however, contend that plaintiff is not a "person with a disability," and thus lacks standing to sue under the ADA, because her impairment does not substantially limit her in any major life activity.

This is an unsupportable contention. Plaintiff is substantially limited in her ability to reproduce — i.e., to conceive and bear children. In *Bragdon v. Abbott*, 524 U.S. 624, 118 S.Ct. 2196, 141 L.Ed.2d 540 (1998), the United States Supreme Court declared "reproduction" to be a major life activity. *See Bragdon*, 524 U.S. at 638, 118 S.Ct. 2196. Defendant has not articulated any principled basis upon which this Court could refuse to apply that rather clear-cut rule to the facts at bar.

Defendants recognize that *Bragdon* is on the books and binding on this Court. So they urge that, when ruling that "reproduction" constituted a major life activity, the Supreme Court actually meant to say that the plaintiff in *Bragdon* was limited in her ability to engage in "sexual activity."

Defendants make this argument on a rather strained reading of *Bragdon*. In that case, the plaintiff suffered from AIDS. She alleged that she was a "person with a disability" because she was substantially limited in her ability to reproduce — that is, to conceive and bear a child. In *Bragdon*, there was no indication that the plaintiff was physically unable to have sexual intercourse. Nor was there any suggestion that she *could not* conceive if she had "unprotected" sexual intercourse. Instead, plaintiff argued that she was reproductively limited because she could not conceive while having "safe sex" — i.e., while using a condom. Thus, any limitation on reproduction, while a by-product of her AIDS, was the result of a conscious, voluntary — and, I hasten to add, socially responsible — choice on the part of the plaintiff. Nonetheless, the Supreme Court ruled that she was substantially limited in the major life activity of reproduction by virtue of her disease.

Viewing *Bragdon* in this (the only fair) light, the fallacy in defendants' argument is immediately apparent. On the record before me, it appears that plaintiff Saks *cannot* become pregnant without some sort of chemical or surgical assistance. That is, her condition (infertility) physically impairs her in such a way that her reproductive organs do not work like those of a fertile woman of her age. There can be no question that Saks' infertility "substantially limits" her ability to reproduce — indeed, it appears to prevent it altogether, absent outside intervention of a very drastic nature. Thus, she is a "person with a disability" within the meaning of the ADA.

Defendants' contention that *Bragdon* does not answer "the central question in this case" — which it identifies as "whether infertility is a limitation on the *activity* of reproduction" — is simply silly. Notwithstanding *Bragdon*, Defendants assert that an individual cannot be reproductively limited unless she is unable to engage in sexual activity. (*See* Def. Br. at 8-9.) Indeed, defendants fairly imply that "reproduction" is not an activity in and of itself, and that the only "activity" connected with reproduction is sex. That is a ridiculous argument. As anyone who has given birth can attest, sex is the least of it . . .

Defendants urge that *Murphy* [*v. United Parcel Service*, 527 U.S. 471 (1999)] and *Sutton* [*v. United Airlines*, 527 U.S. 471 (1999)] compel a finding that infertility is not a disability, precisely because it can be overcome in certain people by various treatments, including some that are covered under its insurance plan. The short answer to this argument is that there is a critical distinction between *Murphy* and *Sutton*, on the one hand, and plaintiff Saks: the treatment prescribed for Murphy (who suffered from high blood pressure that could be alleviated by medication) and the plaintiffs in *Sutton* (who had myopic vision that could be corrected by wearing glasses) worked, whereas Ms. Saks' infertility has yet to be either cured or "bypassed." Defendants note that Saks has managed to become pregnant three times while receiving various fertility treatments. However, she has miscarried each time. She has never achieved a successful pregnancy — one that resulted in the birth of a child. Therefore, her condition has not been successfully overcome, as were the conditions of the plaintiffs in *Murphy* and *Sutton*.

Nonetheless, defendants raise an interesting and difficult point. The full scope of *Murphy* and *Sutton* has yet to be fleshed out, of course, but in the opinion of this Court, the Supreme Court did not intend to rule that no disease or organic defect can qualify as an ADA disability as long as some treatment can ameliorate its impact in some percentage of persons afflicted, however small that percentage may be. Indeed, I think it highly likely that courts will, over time, develop a spectrum of "disability" along which various diseases will fall, depending on some case-by-case analysis of their seriousness, their susceptibility to treatment, the rate at which treatment succeeds in curing them altogether or lessening their impact, and the impact of available treatments on the plaintiff at bar. For example, I find it inconceivable that persons who suffer from chronic conditions involving organ failure, like Type I diabetes or kidney failure, are not "substantially limited" in certain major life activities, simply because they can lead relatively normal lives by taking multiple injections of insulin everyday or by hooking themselves up to dialysis machines (I use the phrase "relatively normal" advisedly). And I view it as highly unlikely that courts will decide that "cancer" as a class of diseases does not substantially limit certain major life activities, just because *some* cancers in *some* people (though not *all* cancers in *all* people) can be successfully treated.

Infertility is the chronic failure of an organ system. It can be treated, but the success rate (with success defined as becoming pregnant and carrying to term) is far from compelling — closer to that of certain cancers than to the all-but-universally correctable conditions discussed in *Murphy* and *Sutton*. Indeed, treatment has not succeeded in this very case. Whether the availability of draconian regimens that avoid the consequences of infertility in a small percentage of individuals places this particular impairment closer to the *Murphy/Sutton* end of the spectrum or the diabetes/cancer/kidney failure end could not possibly be determined on the present record. But the position espoused by defendants is not so self-evident (as demonstrated by the fact that they relegate this argument to a footnote) that I would dismiss on *Murphy/Sutton* grounds at this juncture.

Finally, Defendants argue that infertility *cannot* be a disability, because people become infertile for many reasons, including reasons that have nothing whatever to do with a disease or defect — age being the obvious one. For this unremarkable proposition, defendants cite *McGraw v. Sears Roebuck & Co.*, 21 F. Supp.2d 1017 (D. Minn.1998), in which Judge Rosenbaum concluded that menopause was not a disability — a proposition that enlightened women have been espousing for centuries.

This Court harbors no doubt that infertility that results from the natural aging process, rather than from some disease or defect, is not a "disability" within the meaning of the ADA — just as age-induced inability to focus optically, which crops up in all of us at about the age of 50, is not a "disability," even though it limits (in some cases substantially) an older person's ability to see. The American College of Obstetricians and Gynecologists defines "infertility" as the *abnormal* functioning of the reproductive system. *See* American College of Obstetricians and Gynecologists, *Infertility: Causes and Treatment* 1 (1992). A post-menopausal woman cannot conceive, but she is not "disabled" because her reproductive system — or, rather, her non-reproductive system — is in fact functioning normally. When passing the ADA, Congress was not trying to undo the inevitable effects of aging, like some legislative King Canute commanding in vain that the tide not come in. But this does not mean that a pre-menopausal women in her child-bearing years is not "disabled" if she is unable to become pregnant when, absent some physical abnormality, she would ordinarily be able to do so.

Thus, plaintiff has standing to pursue an ADA claim. That said, however, plaintiff's claim under the ADA must be dismissed, for two reasons.

First, it is undisputed that Franklin Covey's plan offers the same insurance coverage to all its employees. It does not offer infertile people less pregnancy and fertility-related coverage than it offers to fertile people. Therefore, as a matter of law, the Plan does not violate the ADA. In *EEOC v. Staten Island Savings Bank*, 207 F.3d 144 (2d Cir.2000), the Court of Appeals, joining the Third, Seventh and Eighth Circuits, held that insurance distinctions that apply equally to all insured employees do not discriminate on the basis of disability. In that case (brought by the EEOC on behalf of the defendant bank's employees, pursuant to the Commission's Interim Guidance on the Applicability of the ADA to Health Insurance that forms the linchpin of plaintiff's argument here), the employer's policy significantly limited coverage for mental health care while providing much greater coverage for physical illnesses. The Commission argued that defendant's failure to offer employees equivalent benefits for mental and physical illness discriminated on the basis of disability. The Court disagreed, stating:

> We . . . agree with our sister circuits that "so long as every employee is offered the same plan regardless of that employee's contemporary or future disability status, then no discrimination has occurred even if the plan offers different coverage for various disabilities."

Staten Island Savings Bank, 207 F.3d at 150 (quoting *Ford v. Schering-Plough Corp.*, 145 F.3d 601, 608 (3d Cir.1998)). The Court went on to observe:

> It is fully consistent with an understanding that the ADA protects the individual from discrimination based on his or her disability to read the Act to require no more than that access to an employer's fringe benefit program not be denied or limited on the basis of his or her particular disability.

Id. at 151. The panel also noted that requiring equivalent coverage for every type of disability "would destabilize the insurance industry in a manner definitely not intended by Congress." *Id.* at 152 (quoting *Ford*, 145 F.3d at 608). Finally, the Court expressly declined to defer to the Commission's Interim Guidance on this question. *See id.*

Plaintiff suggests that *Staten Island Savings Bank* does not compel dismissal of her claim because there the challenge was to non-equivalent levels of coverage for two gross categories of impairment, physical and mental, while here the issue is failure to provide coverage for certain types of procedures that overcome infertility. With respect, I fail to see any difference. Insurance policies have historically contained exclusions for particular types of procedures. Indeed, surgical impregnation procedures are not the only treatments expressly excluded from coverage under Franklin Covey's Plan. The policy also excludes artificial heart implantation, penile prosthetic implants, Kerato-refractive eye surgery and non-human organ transplants. It is beyond dispute that, under this Plan, people with cancer have access to a greater range of treatment for their problem than do people with infertility. But all employees face exactly the same limitation. That the limitation hits infertile employees like Ms. Saks harder than it hits other employees is of course true, but the limitation on mental health coverage in *Staten Island Savings Bank* was more disruptive to bank employees whose family members needed therapy than to those who did not. Nonetheless, the Circuit held that there was no ADA discrimination.

Second, and even more fundamental, Franklin Covey's Plan is not covered by the ADA. It is undisputed that Franklin Covey's Plan is a bona fide benefit plan under the Employment Retirement Insurance Security Act of 1974, ("ERISA"), 29 U.S.C. § 1001 *et seq.* It is also a self-insured plan. Thus, it falls within the so-called "safe harbor" provision found at § 501(c)(3) of the ADA, 42 U.S.C. § 12201 (c)(3), which provides that nothing in the ADA shall be construed to prohibit or restrict an employer from "establishing, sponsoring, observing or administering the terms of a bona fide benefit plan that is not subject to State laws that regulate insurance." *See also* 29 C.F.R. § 1630.16(f). The only self-insured plans that fall outside the ADA Safe Harbor are those that are used as a subterfuge to evade the purposes of the statute. However, the Second Circuit recently held, in *Leonard F. v. Israel Discount Bank of New York*, 199 F.3d 99, 104 (2d Cir.1999), that a benefit exclusion adopted by a self-insured Plan prior to the passage of the ADA by definition cannot have been adopted as a subterfuge to avoid the statute. Franklin Covey's insurance plans have excluded surgical impregnation procedures since 1989, if not earlier. The ADA became law in 1991. That ends the discussion.

For the above reasons, plaintiff's claim for relief under the ADA is dismissed . . .

Conclusion

The Clerk is directed to enter judgment in favor of defendants, dismissing the complaint, with costs on the motion to defendants.

NOTES AND QUESTIONS

1.   The decision in *Saks v. Franklin Covey* was affirmed by the United States Court of Appeals for the Second Circuit, at 316 F.3d 337 (2d Cir. 2003). In the appeal, the plaintiff's position was supported by the American Society for Reproductive Medicine, which filed an amicus brief in favor of Ms. Saks. ASRM argued that the Franklin Covey health insurance plan violated Title VII of the Civil Rights Act of 1964, which prohibits discrimination on a number of bases, including sex. The prohibition extends to discrimination in providing health insurance and other fringe

benefits. Essentially, ASRM argued that the defendant's plan discriminates on the basis of sex under Title VII because it excludes coverage for procedures that are performed exclusively on women (namely, IVF), and therefore the exclusion affects only female employees. In response, the three-judge panel explained:

> In a different context the exclusion of surgeries that are performed solely on women from an otherwise comprehensive plan might arguably constitute a violation of Title VII, but here we are faced with the unique circumstance of surgical impregnation procedures performed for the treatment of infertility. Although the surgical procedures are performed only on women, the need for the procedures may be traced to male, female, or couple infertility with equal frequency. Thus, surgical impregnation procedures may be recommended regardless of the gender of the ill patient. For example, where a male suffers from poor sperm motility or low sperm count, resulting in his infertility, his healthy female partner must undergo the surgical procedure. In addition, treatment by surgical impregnation procedures requires the participation of both the male and the female partners. Because male and female employees afflicted by infertility are equally disadvantaged by the exclusion of surgical impregnation procedures, we conclude that the Plan does not discriminate on the basis of sex.

316 F.3d at 347. True enough that the causes of infertility are shared equally by men and women, but is there merit in the argument that women are disproportionately the patient when surgical treatment for infertility is performed and therefore are disproportionately harmed when coverage is denied? For an argument that exclusion of infertility treatment in private health insurance does amount to discrimination in violation of Title VII and the ADA, see Elizabeth A. Pendo, *The Politics of Infertility: Recognizing Coverage Exclusions as Discrimination*, 11 CONN. INS. L. J. 293 (2005).

2.   In your view, do the opinions in *Bragdon* and *Saks* bode well or ominously for the future of ART? Does the recognition of infertility as a disability under federal law have any meaning when the recognition seems to be unaccompanied by any tangible benefit? Are there intangible benefits to such a recognition? *See, e.g.,* *Laporta v. Wal-Mart Stores, Inc.*, 103 F. Supp. 2d 758 (W.D. Mich. 2001) (viable ADA claim when employer refuses to reasonably accommodate disability of infertility by denying a day off for IVF treatment).

2.   The Politics of ART Insurance Coverage

Edward G. Hughes & Mita Giacomini
Funding In Vitro Fertilization Treatment for Persistent Subfertility: The Pain and the Politics
76 Fertility & Sterility 431 (2001)

. . . The question of whether failure to conceive a wanted pregnancy is a medical or social problem is central to the debate over who should pay for treatment. Public debate currently tends to follow two separate themes. The first concerns whether *subfertility in general* [the authors use this term to mean infertility] is a legitimate problem for social subsidy via medical insurance . . . [U]sing Canada as an example, the answer to this question has been relatively uncontentious: Both the Royal Commission on New Reproductive Technologies and provincial ministries of health have explicitly affirmed subfertility as a legitimate medical concern for public funding. Indeed, "lower tech" subfertility treatments such as ovulation induction and tubal surgery have been covered without contest by health insurance in many jurisdictions. Clearly, IVF has raised new concerns.

The second theme concerns whether *IVF in particular* is more than just a treatment for subfertility. Are the diverse applications of IVF, such as surrogacy, medically insurable and socially acceptable, and does IVF unduly medicalize social and personal problems? Indeed, IVF techniques have introduced a number of reproductive options and practices besides the simple opportunity to bear a child. These include sex selection of embryos, the identification of certain genetic abnormalities before implantation, the ability to contract out one's biological child bearing to a surrogate, the creation of a market for human ova and the advent of childbearing after menopause. These raise serious ethical questions, including who should be obliged to pay for such choices if they are to be allowed at all. Crucial policy questions include whether such ethical challenges are integral or incidental to IVF technology and whether IVF coverage can be limited to address more conventional understandings of subfertility without supporting a plethora of socially questionable uses of the technology.

QUESTIONS

1.   Authors Hughes and Giacomini argue that the question of insurance funding for IVF engenders a larger debate over the ethics of all forms of assisted reproductive technologies, including egg donation, surrogacy and genetic screening of embryos (a topic we take up next in Chapter 4). Do you agree? Do you believe there are other medical treatments that likewise raise questions about behaviors that may be a consequence of the requested therapy? Consider, for example, the ancillary consequences of the drug Viagra, a compound that treats erectile dysfunction. What analogies, if any, do you see between Viagra and ART as they affect third persons?

2.   Are there other stakeholders who might oppose subsidizing IVF for reasons unrelated to the costs of the procedure and its impact on insurance rates? If couples or individuals could not afford IVF, would they be likely to turn to adoption to meet their desires for parenthood? Professors Glenn Cohen and Daniel Chen investigated this "substitution theory," looking at data to determine if state mandates for IVF coverage diminish adoption in those jurisdictions. Their findings? "We do not find strong evidence that increased access to IVF through state-level insurance mandates decreases domestic or international adoptions." I. Glenn Cohen & Daniel L. Chen, *Trading-Off Reproductive Technology and Adoption: Does Subsidizing IVF Decrease Adoption Rates and Should it Matter?*, 95 MINN. L. REV. 485 (2010).

B. ART Insurance Coverage and the Effect on Clinical Outcomes

The availability of infertility insurance coverage certainly affects access to ART therapy and the debt burden that patients incur to pay for desired treatment. But researchers also became interested in another aspect of infertility insurance coverage — the impact that coverage has on clinical outcomes. Working under the hypothesis that greater access to treatment improves overall treatment success, researchers at Harvard Medical School conducted a study to determine whether coverage for IVF services is associated with increased use of services and improved outcomes for patients and offspring. The study was conducted using data collected and published by the Centers for Disease Control and Prevention (CDC) on success rates at 360 fertility clinics in the U.S. The Harvard team divided the clinics into three groups, according to the state in which the clinic was located: 1) states that mandate complete insurance coverage for IVF (31 clinics), 2) states that mandate partial coverage for IVF (27 clinics), and 3) states that did not require any coverage (302 clinics). The results were as follows:

- States that require complete insurance coverage for IVF services have the highest rates of utilization of such services

- States that do not require insurance coverage for IVF services have the lowest rates of utilization of such services

- States that do not require insurance coverage have the highest number of embryos transferred per cycle, the highest rates of pregnancy and live birth from IVF, and the highest rates of births of multiple infants (especially three or more)

The researchers explain the relationship between higher rates of pregnancy and lack of insurance coverage is attributable to the pressure that patients (and correspondingly physicians) feel to succeed during the first IVF cycle, since many patients will surrender all their resources for a single chance at a pregnancy. Specifically, the researchers surmise:

Although the rates of pregnancy and live births from in vitro fertilization are higher in states that do not require insurance coverage, so are the rates of pregnancies with three or more fetuses, probably because more embryos are transferred per cycle in these states than in states that require complete insurance coverage. It is also possible that because patients must pay out of pocket in states without mandated coverage, physicians are under pressure to obtain a "successful" outcome the first time and therefore transfer more embryos per cycle.

Tarun Jain, Bernard L. Harlow & Mark D. Hornstein, *Insurance Coverage and Outcomes of In Vitro Fertilization*, 347 N. ENG. J. MED. 661, 665 (2002). From an economic standpoint, the researchers argue, the net result of saving health insurance dollars by not covering IVF may be a greater expenditure of dollars to care for multiple birth newborns. For example, "[i]n 1991, hospital charges for the delivery of twins were 4 times as high and charges for triplets were 11 times as high as charges for a singleton delivery." *Id.* at 665. Moreover, the lifetime health care costs to care for multiple birth infants can be staggering due to the higher risk of respiratory distress syndrome, cerebral palsy, blindness and other physical and developmental disabilities that are associated with higher order multiple birth.

The Harvard study results prompted ART professionals to ponder whether as a matter of public policy IVF insurance coverage should be mandated by all states. One such physician reflected as follows:

> Does the association between required insurance coverage and lower rates of multifetal pregnancy (as a fraction of total pregnancies) suggest that all states should require coverage for in vitro fertilization? In my opinion, the answer is no. Even in states that require complete coverage for in vitro fertilization, the rate of multifetal pregnancy is still much too high; according to the data reported by Jain et al., in these states, 36 percent of live births from in vitro fertilization involve multiple infants, and 10 percent of pregnancies from in vitro fertilization involve three or more fetuses. The estimated direct medical expenses of a gestation involving three or more fetuses are about $340,000, and this figure does not include the costs of long-term care and special education for disabilities resulting from prematurity.

> As a matter of clinical practice and public health, rates of multifetal pregnancy from in vitro fertilization must be lowered. Improved clinical and laboratory methods should help reduce these rates . . . [A]nother approach is to impose restrictions on the number of embryos transferred, as had been done through government regulation in several European countries. Although it may not be politically realistic to suggest that the European approach can be extended to the United States, reasonable national limits on the number of embryos transferred to the uterus would go a long way toward reducing multifetal pregnancies.

David S. Guzick, *Should Insurance Coverage For In Vitro Fertilization Be Mandated?* 347 New Eng. J. Med. 686, 687-88 (2002). As noted in Chapter 1, high order multiple pregnancy rates have dropped from 3% of all ART births in 1999 to 1.8% in 2008. Still, a more recent study of insurance coverage and IVF outcomes confirmed what the Harvard study found. Clinics in states without insurance mandates have higher pregnancy, live-birth and multiple pregnancy rates because they transfer more embryos than clinics in states with coverage. *See* J. Ryan Martin, Jason C. Bromer, Denny Sakkas, Pasquale Patrizio, *Insurance Coverage and In Vitro Fertilization Outcomes: A U.S. Perspective*, 95 Fertility & Sterility 964 (2011). Would you rather live in a mandated state with lower pregnancy rates or a nonmandated state with higher multiple pregnancy rates?

PROBLEM

Imagine you are an ART provider in a state that does not mandate insurance coverage for IVF. In your practice experience, virtually all of your patients pay for IVF services out of pocket because private and employer-based health insurance plans specifically exclude ART services. Anabel and Joshua Germaine are a married couple who have tried unsuccessful to conceive naturally for two years. The couple visits your ART practice in search of assistance. Test results show that

Anabel has blocked fallopian tubes, a condition you believe can be successfully treated using IVF (which bypasses the fallopian tubes by placing the embryos directly into the uterus). Anabel agrees to undergo hormone therapy and egg retrieval in preparation for IVF. Three days after her eggs are retrieved and mixed with her Joshua's sperm, yielding eight viable embryos from the laboratory process. You meet with the couple to report the happy news that they have three opportunities for embryo transfer, using two embryos now, freezing the remaining six and then transferring two or three at a later cycle and the remainder at yet another time. The Germaines explain that they have mortgaged their house and borrowed money from their credit cards in order to pay for the IVF treatment. As a result, they can only afford this single cycle and ask that you transfer back all eight embryos. You explain the risks associated with high order multiple pregnancy, the high likelihood of success if two, or perhaps three embryos are transferred. You explain the relatively low cost of freezing the remaining embryos and transferring them back at a later point. The couple seems to fully comprehend the ramifications of their request, and yet they continue to insist that you "give them their best shot" at a successful outcome, stressing that they had always dreamed of having a large family.

What action would you take at this point? Whose interests are at stake if you proceed to transfer all eight embryos? Whose interests are at stake if you refuse to transfer all eight embryos? In your view, would the availability of insurance coverage change the Germaines' requested transfer of all the viable embryos?

Chapter 4

CHOOSING OUR CHILDREN'S TRAITS: GENDER AND GENETIC SELECTION IN ART

Each human being possesses a combination of qualities that makes that individual a unique member of the human species. The qualities of gender, height, weight, intelligence, hair color, skin tone, eye shade and a host of other characteristics converge in each person to create a one-of-a-kind individual whose lifetime accomplishments and challenges may be shaped in part by those defining characteristics. The age-old debate over "nature versus nurture," that is, whether we are guided more by our inherent biological make-up or by external and environmental forces, remains a source of intrigue and investigation, but most experts agree that both "nature" and "nurture" play a critical role in human development. Until very recently, parents understood that they had no control over the "nature" of their children; once a couple made a decision to procreate, the resulting child's inherent qualities would be a random mixing of the gamete providers' genes, the material that determines the structure and function of the human body. But interest and advancements in assisted conception, in which the early embryo develops outside the body, placed focus on the ability to screen or even alter the genetic make-up of our offspring.

The mechanics that might enable a parent to select for a girl, or a redhead, or a child free of cystic fibrosis (a gene-linked disease) require an in-depth explanation best left for a graduate seminar in Molecular Biology. For our purposes, a brief overview of genetics and its role in human development should suffice. The story begins with an Austrian monk named Gregor Mendel, whose mid-nineteenth-century experiments with pea plants demonstrated that hereditary traits could be explained by certain factors in the parent plants. By mating plants with different traits (round v. wrinkled seeds, tall v. dwarf size, white v. purple flowers) Mendel noted that offspring plants often resembled one parent, leading him to theorize that each plant inherits one factor from each parent; he further theorized that one factor was dominant, the other recessive, thus explaining the outward appearance of each offspring.

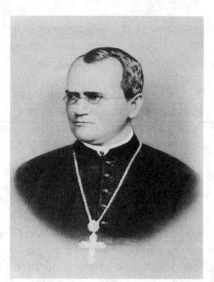

Portrait of Austrian Botanist Gregor Mendel (1822-1884)
Photograph circa 1880

Mendel's "factors" theorem lay dormant for nearly 40 years until it gained the attention of early twentieth-century scientists who verified his results, coined the term "gene" and founded the branch of biology known as genetics. The factors that Mendel observed are today known as genes, which form the basis of human heredity. During this same early 1900s era, cell biologists discovered structures in cells that lined up in pairs as each cell undergoes division, with one copy of each structure transmitted to the new cell. These structures were dubbed "chromosomes," a Latin term meaning colored things, because scientists stained the structures with colored dyes in order to observe their movement.

Chromosomes, we now know, are contained in the nucleus, or center, of each human cell. Humans have two types of chromosomes, sex chromosomes (which determine our gender) and autosomes (which largely determine our other human traits such as height, eye color, predisposition toward certain genetic diseases). Each human cell (except egg and sperm cells, more on this in a moment) contains 23 pairs of chromosomes — 22 pairs of autosomes and one pair of sex chromosomes. The two sex chromosomes (Pair 23) determine the sex of an individual, and they are called the X chromosome and the Y chromosome. If you are female, you have two Xs, and if you are male, you have one X and one Y. A picture of the 23 pairs of human chromosomes in found in Figure 1, depicting a male individual. Notice that the pairs are numbered 1 through 22, plus an additional XY pair, in order from the largest pair (Pair 1) to the smallest pair (Pair 22).

During conception the egg and sperm fuse to create a new entity known as the zygote. The zygote contains a unique complement of chromosomes because it combines one set from each of its parents. Egg and sperm cells contain only 23 individual chromosomes (as opposed to the 23 pairs, or 46 individual chromosomes contained in other cells), the egg contributing an X and the sperm containing either an X or a Y. Thus, it is the male sperm that determines if the offspring will be a boy or a girl. Thinking ahead to our discussion of selecting for the gender of offspring, you can begin to see the role that chromosomes play in the selection process. If the X- and Y-bearing sperm can be separated and isolated, selecting for a preferred gender can be accomplished by mixing the egg with only the X or Y sperm.

One final yet essential point in our brief review focuses on genes. A gene is the fundamental physical and functional unit of heredity. It is comprised of an ordered sequence of DNA, short for deoxyribonucleic acid, a molecule shaped like a twisted ladder that encodes trait information.[1] Each gene is located on a particular position on the chromosome and encodes for a specific trait. Over the past decade we have learned much about the identity and role of genes in human development, thanks in large measure to the Human Genome Project (HGP), an international, collaborative research program whose goal was the complete mapping and understanding of all the genes in a human being. Launched in 1990, the HGP gained worldwide attention in 2001 when researchers from both public and private consortia announced that a rough map of the entire human genome had been completed. In the intervening 11 years, researchers funded by the HGP were able to identify and locate numerous genes associated with diseases such as cystic fibrosis, Huntington's Disease and an inherited form of breast cancer.[2]

Again, in terms of assisted conception, you can begin to understand how the discovery of disease-linked genes could play a vital role for families whose children have been affected by genetic diseases. If physicians could somehow detect the presence or absence of the specific gene *before* the embryo is transferred back to the uterus, then parents could select only healthy embryos for transfer and thereby avoid transmission of the deleterious gene into their family line.

The selection of a child's genetic traits such as gender and disease predisposition raise a number of legal, ethical and social issues that, because of the fresh nature of the technology, we are only beginning to grapple with. In the pages that follow, we explore the current state of genetic selection technology, the developing legal landscape surrounding the nascent technology, and the anticipated future uses and potential misuses of genetic manipulation.

---

[1] Great discoveries in the field of human genetics are often attributed to the Nobel Prize winning work of Francis Crick and James Watson who, in the 1950s, revealed the structure of DNA and its ability to pass on information to later generation cells.

[2] For a detailed discussion of the history and current advances in the field of genetics, see LORI B. ANDREWS, MAXWELL J. MEHLMAN, MARK A. ROTHSTEIN, GENETICS: ETHICS, LAW AND POLICY (2d ed. West 20062).

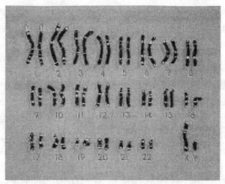

Figure 1. Human Chromosomes

This is a male genome, as indicated by the "XY" pair in chromosome 23

SECTION I: THE CURRENT STATE OF TECHNOLOGY

Generations from now our grandchildren will likely look back on today's genetic technology and marvel at how we managed to get by during these "olden days." Acknowledging our state of infancy, we can proceed to review the technologies that have been developed, primarily over the past 20 years. We will briefly describe the technologies below, and fill in with more details as the ethical and legal implications of each are discussed.

There are three areas in which the manipulation of human genes — genetic selection — is most often discussed: 1) gender selection, 2) medical selection, and 3) trait selection.

In terms of gender genetics, scientists have developed two methods to assist in gender selection. First, using microscopes and laser beam technology, researchers can now separate X- and Y-bearing sperm to create single gender-rich specimens for artificial insemination. Second, scientists can study the chromosomes in a three-day old embryo that is maturing in the laboratory following IVF, thus enabling parents to "sex select" by choosing to transfer back into the uterus either the XX (girl) or XY (boy) embryo.

In terms of selection for medical reasons, scientists can use this same method of studying the chromosomes of the early embryo to detect whether a given embryo has the correct number of chromosomes. For example, an embryo that has an additional chromosome in Pair 21 will be affected with Down Syndrome, sometimes referred to as Trisomy 21 (meaning a third, or extra chromosome in Pair 21). Extra or missing chromosomes are associated with life-threatening and life-altering diseases and thus parents who learn that their early embryos have more or less than 46 chromosomes can select to discard those affected embryos. In addition, scientists have discovered the location and workings of certain genes (located at exact points on particular chromosomes) that are directly responsible for serious diseases. These "single gene disorders" include cystic fibrosis and hemophilia, to name two of the more than 1,000 diseases that are caused by defects in single genes.[3] If an embryo is found to have the deleterious gene, parents can decide whether to gestate the affected embryo or avoid the risk of producing a seriously ill child.

In addition to genetic selection for gender and medical purposes, there is discussion about selection for certain benign traits such as hair color, height, and intelligence. This type of selection is often referred to as "genetic enhancement" and is not currently an existing technology. In fact, many theorize that genetic enhancement may never emerge as an available technology for two reasons. First, most human traits are polygenic, meaning they are controlled by many genes scattered throughout the genome, rather than a single gene. Second, it is well-established that many traits, such as height, are also controlled by environmental factors (such as diet) and thus are not amenable to genetic manipulation. But the futuristic nature of genetic enhancement has not prevented researchers, policymakers and others from commenting on the prospect of such technology.

As we proceed through the thorny debates over sex selection, selection of embryos for medical reasons, and genetic enhancement, consider whether any of these technologies would be attractive to you as a prospective parent, a prospective child, or a member of a society in which such technologies were employed.

A. Choosing a Child's Gender

The selection of gender has been a quest of couples for as far back as recorded history allows. Early drawings from prehistoric times suggest that sex selection efforts were being investigated by our earliest ancestors. Later history shows intense interest in sex selection by early Chinese, Egyptian and Greek cultures. This history is followed by documented scientific efforts beginning in the 1600s to sway the chances of achieving a gender-specific pregnancy by a variety of methods including the consumption of particular foods, the use of various vaginal douches and the timing of intercourse in relation to ovulation. By and large these methods proved unreliable, with gender seemingly determined on a random, even basis. Under normal circumstances, the chances of any child being a particular sex is around 50%; typically 102-106 boys are born for every 100 girls.

Recently, research and work carried out in the 1980s and 1990s have yielded methods of sex selection that are fairly reliable, offering couples a high likelihood of producing a child of their gender choice. There are two basic methods of sex selection — sperm sorting and preimplantation genetic diagnosis (PGD). There are currently two methods used for sperm sorting and one method for PGD. The methods are described herein:

---

[3] See Michael J. Smith, *Population-Based Genetic Studies: Informed Consent and Confidentiality*, 18 COMPUTER & HIGH TECH. L.J. 57, 62 (2001) (reporting that "over 5,000 human disorders are known to have a genetic basis and over 1,000 of those disorders have been mapped to specific regions of the genome").

Sperm Sorting

The Ericsson Technique

The Ericsson Technique was developed in the 1970s and is considered "low-tech" by today's standards. Sperm are poured into a glass jar containing a top layer of albumin, a viscous fluid. The sperm naturally swim down, due to their head-heavy structure. Sperm carrying Y chromosomes swim faster than sperm carrying X chromosomes, reaching the bottom of the jar sooner. Depending on whether a girl or a boy is desired, a different fraction of sperm is recovered and used to artificially inseminate the woman. Supporters of this low-cost method claim a 78-85% chance of having a boy, while critics say it does not improve the chances of having a particular gender at all.

MicroSort

Developed in the mid-1990s, the MicroSort technology is based on the fact that the X chromosome is substantially larger than the Y chromosome. Since chromosomes are made of DNA, human sperm cells having an X chromosome will contain approximately 2.8% more total DNA than sperm cells having a Y chromosome. With this weight difference in mind, sperm are stained with a fluorescent dye that binds to chromosomes. Since X chromosomes are bigger they soak up more dye than Y chromosomes. The sperm are passed through a laser that illuminates the dye; X chromosomes glow brighter because they contain more dye. Next, the sperm pass by an electrode that gives Xs a positive charge and Ys a negative one. Charged plates then attract and separate Xs and Ys, channeling them into different receptacles. The sorted sperm sample can then be used with either intrauterine insemination (IUI) or with IVF and intracytoplasmic sperm injection (ICSI) in which a single sperm is injected directly into the cytoplasm of the egg. Currently, MicroSort sperm separation for female gender selection (X-Sort) results in an average 93% success rate for selecting girls. Separation for male selection (Y-Sort) results in an average 82% success rate for selecting boys. The benefits of MicroSort seem to be that it significantly improves the chances of having a child of a particular gender (from 50% to 82 or 93%) and it is a preconception method of sex selection, meaning that no embryos or fetuses are purposefully destroyed in the selection process.

Preimplantation Genetic Diagnosis (PGD)

PGD was developed in late 1980s in England to detect the presence of genes associated with inheritable diseases, including cystic fibrosis, muscular dystrophy and Huntington's disease. Because PGD allows scientists to visualize the chromosomes of an early embryo, it can also be used to select for gender because the sex chromosomes (Pair 23) are visible along with the other 22 pairs.

PGD is a technique that is performed on a three-day-old embryo, which typically is comprised of 8 cells. The goal of PGD is to remove and analyze a single embryonic cell, known as a blastomere. To extract the blastomere, an opening is made in the covering of the embryo and a single cell is removed via aspiration using a pipette. Figure 2 shows a single blastomere being aspirated from an 8-

celled embryo. After the blastomere is removed, the embryo is placed in an incubator while the extracted cell is analyzed. The extracted cell is analyzed using a technique called fluorescence in-situ hybridization or FISH. This technique uses probes — small pieces of DNA — that are a match for the chromosomes present in the cell. Each probe is labeled with a different fluorescent dye. These fluorescent probes are applied to the extracted cell and they attach to the chromosomes. Under a fluorescent microscope, scientists can visualize the dye-colored chromosomes that are in that cell. This visualization allows scientists to count if the cell has the correct number of chromosomes and also to determine the gender of the embryo because the sex chromosomes can be dyed and seen under the microscope.

Testing of the cell destroys that particular cell because it must be glued to a glass slide and repeatedly heated and cooled. Importantly, removing the cell causes no damage to the developing embryo. No part of the future fetus will be lacking because one or even two cells are removed from the embryo three days after fertilization. All the cells of the embryo remain totipotent, meaning "all potential," until about the fourth day of development. Totipotent embryonic cells are not yet differentiated, meaning that each cell by itself can grow into a whole and perfect fetus. Thus, removing a single totipotent cell to perform PGD does not interfere with the remaining seven cells' ability to develop into a fully formed human being. The procedure merely delays continued cell division for a few hours, after which the embryo reaches the same number of cells as before and continues its normal development. *See Embryo Biopsy Safe for Singleton Pregnancies, Largest Study of PGD Children Suggests*, SCIENCE DAILY (Dec. 23, 2009), available at: http://www. sciencedaily.com/releases/2009/12/091222105103.htm.

The PGD results tell parents the health status and gender of their developing embryos. Armed with this information, parents can decide which embryos to transfer back to the woman's uterus for gestation. Since 1990, physicians have performed more than 6,000 clinical cycles of PGD, with more than 1,000 children born as a result. See Yury Verlinsky et al., *Over A Decade of Experience With Preimplantation Genetic Diagnosis: A Multicenter Report*, 82 FERTILITY & STERIL-ITY 292 (2004).

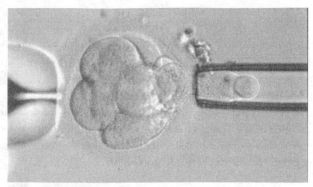

Figure 2: Preimplantation Genetic Diagnosis

One cell (known as a blastomere) is removed from an 8-celled embryo using an injection pipette.

The increasing availability and reliability of sex selection technology may encourage us to pause and think deeply about the benefits and harms of choosing a child's gender. One way to approach the analysis is by distinguishing between the technologies in terms of their impact on early life. Sperm sorting techniques are used *before* conception and thus selecting to use X or Y sperm will have no impact on a developing embryo. In contrast, PGD is performed *after* conception and thus selecting to implant only male or female embryos can have an impact on the remaining embryos of the disfavored gender. With these technological truths in mind, let's explore the current analysis surrounding pre- and post-conception gender selection.

1.   Preconception Gender Selection

Ethics Committee of the American Society for Reproductive Medicine
Preconception Gender Selection for Nonmedical Reasons
75 Fertility & Sterility 861 (2001)

. . . The use of preconception techniques for nonmedical gender selection raises important ethical and social concerns that need thorough attention before these techniques become available for nonmedical purposes.

. . . [T]his report will discuss the ethical arguments for and against the use of such techniques. Drawing on the Ethics Committee's previous analysis of preimplantation genetic diagnosis for sex selection, it recognizes the serious ethical concerns that such a practice raises and counsels against its widespread use. It concludes, however, that sex selection aimed at increasing gender variety in families may not so greatly increase the risk of harm to children, women, or society that its use should be prohibited or condemned as unethical in all cases . . .

THE ETHICAL DILEMMA RAISED BY PRECONCEPTION GENDER SELECTION

The Ethics Committee's report on sex selection and preimplantation genetic diagnosis identified several general ethical concerns with sex selection.[4] These include "the potential for inherent gender discrimination, inappropriate control over nonessential characteristics of children, unnecessary medical burdens and costs for parents, and inappropriate and potentially unfair use of limited medical resources." The report also identified concerns over possible sex ratio imbalances and "psychological harm to sex-selected offspring (i.e., by placing on them too high expectations), increased marital conflict over sex selective decisions, and reinforcement of gender bias in society as a whole."

At the same time, the Ethics Committee recognized that parents have traditionally had great discretion in their procreative decisions and that sex selection might provide "perceived individual and social goods such as gender balance or distribution in a family with more than one child, parental companionship with a child of one's own gender, and a preferred gender order among one's children."

This report discusses how these competing concerns should be balanced if safe and effective preconception techniques to select the gender of offspring become available.

ARGUMENTS FOR PRECONCEPTION GENDER SELECTION

The argument for permitting preconception gender selection is that it serves the desires of couples who have strong preferences about the gender of their offspring, some of whom might use abortion or embryo selection to realize their goal or be unhappy with children of the undesired gender. In some cases, couples with one or more children of a particular sex might strongly prefer to have a child of the opposite sex and might choose not to have another child unless they can use preconception gender selection to provide gender variety in their offspring. In other cases, they might have such strong preferences for a first-born child's gender that they might resort to postconception selection methods or not reproduce at all unless preconception methods are available.

Because the strength of their desire for a child of a particular gender is largely self-imposed, one can question whether their desire alone justifies acceptance of their preference. Proponents of the choice, however, would argue that ethics, law, and social practice, while not regarding procreative liberty as absolute or unlimited, ordinarily accord couples and individuals wide choice in reproductive matters. They argue that unless substantial harm to others resulted from a reproductive practice, couples should in many circumstances be permitted to act on preferences for children of a particular gender. However, these proponents of choice also recognize that just because a practice falls within the scope of one's personal liberty does not mean that that practice is good in itself or that it should be positively encouraged, but disagreement with a choice is not by itself a sufficient basis to prohibit it.

---

[4] The Ethics Committee 1999 report on sex selection and PGD referred to herein is reprinted *infra* in the next section, focusing on postconception gender selection. -Ed.

ARGUMENTS AGAINST PRECONCEPTION GENDER SELECTION

Although preconception selection methods do not destroy embryos and fetuses or intrude on a woman's body as prenatal or preimplantation sex selection does, these procedures do raise other important issues. One concern is the potential of such techniques to increase or reinforce gender discrimination, either by allowing more males to be produced as first children or by encouraging parents to pay greater attention to gender itself. A second concern is the welfare of children born as a result of gender selection, who may be expected to act in certain gender-specific ways when the technique succeeds and who may disappoint parents when it fails. A third concern is societal. Widely practiced, preconception gender selection could lead to sex ratio imbalances, as have occurred in some parts of India and China because of female infanticide, gender-driven abortions, and a one-child family policy.

Another societal concern is the emphasis that gender selection places on a child's genetic characteristics, rather than his or her inherent worth. This emphasis contributes to the commodification of offspring that many critics of assisted reproduction decry. Such practices also lead physicians to use their skills for nonmedically indicated purposes, thereby possibly diverting medical resources from more important uses.

EVALUATION OF ETHICAL AND SOCIAL ISSUES

Concerns about sex ratio imbalances, the welfare of offspring, and instrumentalizing reproduction may be less central to debates over nonmedical uses of sex selection than whether such practices would contribute to gender discrimination. If few persons choose to use preconception gender selection, sex ratio imbalances may never be a problem. If imbalances did occur, gender preferences would likely alter to bring the two genders into a better balance. If the threat of sex ratio imbalances were severe, laws or guidelines that required providers to select for males and females in equal numbers could be enacted, without unjustifiably violating procreative liberty.

It may also be difficult to show that individual children born after preconception sex selection were harmed by the technique. If the child is born with the desired gender, the child presumably will be wanted and loved. Parents who choose preconception sex selection should be informed of the risks that the technique will not succeed and counseled about what steps they will take if a child of the undesired gender is born. If counseling of couples indicates that they are committed to the well-being of the child, whatever its gender, the risk to children may be slight. However, even with counseling and a couple's claim that they will accept the resulting child, whatever its gender, there is still the risk that some couples will abort a fetus or reject a child of the undesired sex. Also, parental desires to select a child's gender, particularly if motivated by a wish for gender variety in the family, do not mean that the parents have such rigid expectations of gender stereotypical behavior that the child is likely to be harmed.

The question of diverting medical resources to nonmedical purposes must be evaluated in the context of a medical system in which physicians often provide services that have no direct medical benefit but that do have great personal value for the individual. Given the acceptance of these practices, one could not, without calling that system into question, condemn a practice merely because it uses medicine for lifestyle or child-rearing choices. Nor is preconception gender selection likely to consume a substantial amount of resources, particularly if used only to conceive children of the gender opposite to that of an existing child or children. As a relatively low-cost procedure (intrauterine insemination after mechanical separation of sperm), preconception gender selection is unlikely to drain substantial resources from the medical system.

The question of whether any nonmedical use of sex selection is inherently discriminatory is more complicated. Because women in many societies have been subject to disadvantage and discrimination solely because of their gender, some investigators have argued that any concern with gender, male or female, is per se wrong and should be discouraged regardless of whether one can show an intention to harm women or that adverse consequences for them will likely result. Proponents of this view believe that even if one's intention in using preconception gender selection is not to denigrate or harm women, acting on the basis of any gender preference for offspring lends credence to existing gender stereotypes. Indeed, those stereotypes are likely to have created or influenced individual and social preferences for rearing children of different genders. Under this view, a couple with three boys who now would like to have a girl may be acting on the basis of deeply engrained sexual stereotypes that harm women. Similarly, a couple who wanted to have only a girl might be contributing to unjustified gender discrimination against both men and women, even if they especially valued females and would insist that their daughter receive every benefit and opportunity accorded males.

The opposing view in favor of preconception gender selection asserts that gender "similarity and complementarity are morally acceptable reasons for wanting a child of a certain sex." This view is based on the claim that there are actual physical and psychological differences between male and female children that affect parental child-rearing experiences. These well-established differences provide legitimate reasons for some couples to prefer to rear a girl rather than a boy, or vice versa, without reflecting discriminatory attitudes or inherently disadvantaging women, particularly if they already have one or more children of the opposite gender.

Under this view, a couple who sought to have a child of a particular gender because they recognize that the experience of rearing a child of one gender is different from the experience of rearing a child of a different gender might do so without thinking that one gender is superior to another. If preconception selection occurred in a social and legal context where equal rights and status of women are respected, its use would not be likely to deny women the equal rights, opportunities, or value as persons, the disallowance of which constitutes unacceptable gender discrimination.

The Committee believes that reasonable persons might legitimately disagree over which view of gender discrimination best agrees with values of equal respect and concern for both genders. Until a more clearly persuasive ethical argument emerges, or there is stronger empirical evidence that most choices to select the gender of offspring would be harmful, policies to prohibit or condemn as unethical all uses of nonmedically indicated preconception gender selection are not justified.

Nor would it be unethical for parents to use or for physicians to provide safe and effective means of preconception gender selection to have a child of the gender opposite to that of an existing child or children. Similarly, it would not be unethical for parents to prefer that their first-born or only child be of a particular gender because of the different meaning and companionship experiences that they expect to have.

COMMITTEE RECOMMENDATIONS

Until a method of separating X- and Y-bearing producing sperm is established as safe and effective in statistically valid, properly executed clinical trials, preconception gender selection should be labeled as experimental and treated accordingly. If such trials show that preconception gender selection based on sperm separation or other techniques is safe and effective, the most prudent approach at present for the nonmedical use of these techniques would be to use them only for gender variety in a family, i.e., only to have a child of the gender opposite of an existing child or children. If the social, psychological, and demographic effects of those uses of preconception gender selection have been found acceptable, then other nonmedical uses of preconception selection might be considered.

If flow cytometry [such as MicroSort] or other methods of preconception gender selection are found to be safe and effective, physicians should be free to offer preconception gender selection in clinical settings to couples who are seeking gender variety in their offspring if the couples [1] are fully informed of the risks of failure, [2] affirm that they will fully accept children of the opposite sex if the preconception gender selection fails, [3] are counseled about having unrealistic expectations about the behavior of children of the preferred gender, and [4] are offered the opportunity to participate in research to track and assess the safety, efficacy, and demographics of preconception selection. Practitioners offering assisted reproductive services are under no legal or ethical obligation to provide nonmedically indicated preconception methods of gender selection.

NOTES AND QUESTIONS

1. *Opposing Views within the Medical Community.* The American College of Obstetricians and Gynecologists, which defines itself as "the nation's leading group of professionals providing health care to women" issued an opinion on sex selection in February 2007. The ACOG Committee on Ethics accepted, "as ethically permissible, the practice of sex selection to prevent sex-linked genetic disorders." However, the Committee opposed "meeting other requests for sex selection . . . for personal and family reasons, including family balancing, because of the concern that such requests may ultimately support sexist practices." *Sex Selection*, AGOC Committee Opinion No. 360, 109 OBSTETRICS & GYNECOLOGY 475 (2007). It would not be uncommon for a reproductive endocrinologist (a physician who delivers ART treatment) to belong to both ACOG and ASRM. If such a physician were approached by a patient seeking sex selection for family balancing, how should the doctor respond given the conflicting opinions issued by these professional groups?

2. *Safety and Efficacy.* The ASRM Ethics Committee gives tentative approval to preconception gender selection for "gender variety" in a family, with the caveat that the technique proves safe and effective in properly executed clinical trials. A clinical trial is a study in which patients agree to participate as human subjects to test a new drug, medical device, or medical technique. To date, clinical trials investigating the safety and efficacy of MicroSort (the technique that separates X- and Y-bearing sperm using fluorescent dyes) have been ongoing at the Genetics & IVF Institute (GIVF) in Fairfax, Virginia. GIVF helped develop the sperm sorting technology in the mid-1990s, reporting the first human birth following MicroSort in 1996. Since that time, GIVF has enrolled more than 1,500 patients in its clinical trial. The preliminary results show promise for both safety and efficacy. As to safety, no adverse outcomes have been reported related to the technique. Measuring efficacy by comparing results to naturally occurring gender ratios of 50/50, MicroSort researchers report a 93% success rate for girls (879/945) and a 82% rate for boys (239/291). *See* www.microsort.com. One cautionary note: these results are self-reported and have yet to be published as full articles in a peer-reviewed medical journal.

3. *Medical Reasons for Gender Selection.* The majority of ethical and legal debate surrounding preconception sex selection focuses on *nonmedical* reasons that parents have for choosing one gender over another (e.g., having a child of a different gender than an existing child or children, anticipating a particular rearing experience, believing a boy or girl can best "carry on" a family trait, name or enterprise). In contrast, most commentators generally favor gender selection for *medical* reasons — to avoid transmitting a sex chromosome-linked disease to a child. Sex-linked diseases are recessive genetic disorders which are inherited through a genetic defect on the X or Y chromosome. Examples of the hundreds of known X-linked disorders include hemophilia and muscular dystrophy, diseases that most often affect males. The reason that males are primarily affected has to do with the concept of dominant and recessive genes. A recessive genetic disorder will only express itself (by manifesting the disease) in a female if she inherits the deleterious recessive gene from both parents. For a girl (XX), this means that both the mother and father's X chromosome will contain the recessive gene. For a boy (XY), if either the mother or father passes the recessive gene on the X chromosome, the boy will be affected since he only has one X chromosome. Inheritance of a defect attached to that one copy of the X chromosome will cause the disorder.

The ongoing MicroSort clinical trials referenced in Note 1 initially limited enrollment to two categories of participants: 1) married couples with a known history of an X-linked disease and 2) married couples with at least one child who are selecting for a child of the opposite gender (this is often referred to as "family balancing"). If the clinical trials confirm that MicroSort is a safe and effective method of sex selection, should the technology be limited to use for medical reasons and family balancing? What if a couple is delighted with their two daughters and wants to ensure a female triumvirate in their family? Should this couple be prevented from accessing the technology? If restrictions are put in place, who are the appropriate regulators of the technology? The fertility clinics? The states? The federal government? Who would you trust most/least to make these decisions about access to ART?

While the ASRM Ethics Committee offered its approval of preconception gender selection for family balancing, the U.S. government is another matter. In 2010, the U.S. Food and Drug Administration notified GIVF that it could no longer offer MicroSort for family balancing, but was limited to using the technique for genetic disease prevention. The rationale? The federal agency reasoned there is no public health benefit in offering nonmedical gender selection. Do you agree? Is the public better off if individual parents have greater control over the sex of their offspring, and perhaps greater happiness with their children, or does such power corrupt the family dynamic and thus negatively impact the public at large?

4. *Opposition to Selection for Medical Reasons.* Not everybody agrees that sex selection to avoid transmission of a genetic disorder is ethically permissible. In the United Kingdom, the Parliamentary Office of Science and Technology (POST), an office of both Houses of Parliament charged with providing independent and balanced analysis of public policy issues, issued a report on sex selection in July 2003. In this report, POST summarized the opposition to sex selection for medical reasons as follows:

> Where sex selection is used for medical reasons there is a clear intention to benefit the health of a prospective child. However, there is concern from disability and religious groups that sex selection technology will be used to select against progressively milder conditions (an extreme example of this would be colour blindness). The definition of "serious" disease is not an issue specific to sex selection but applies to any medical intervention that aims to avoid the birth of people with disabilities.

Parliamentary Office of Science and Technology, Postnote: Sex Selection 4 (July 2003), located at www.parliament.uk/post. The concern about sex selection for medical reasons expressed by POST is that the concept of "medical" or "disease" is ill-defined, at best. What may be considered a serious disease worthy of selecting against by some, may be an acceptable health status for others. While this argument is rarely, if ever, made in connection with the two most common X-linked diseases, hemophilia and muscular dystrophy, arguments about selecting against disabilities in general raise cautionary warnings about eugenics. Author Margaret Talbot, writing in response to the ASRM Ethics Report, above, sanctioning sex selection for family balancing, warns, "The era of consumer-driven eugenics has begun." She concludes:

> [I]f we allow people to select a child's sex, then there is really no barrier to picking embryos — or, ultimately, genetically programming children — based on any whim, any faddish notion of what constitutes superior stock . . . A world in which people (wealthy people, anyway) can custom-design human beings unhampered by law or social sanction is not a dystopian sci-fi fantasy any longer but a realistic scenario. It is not a world most of us would want to live in.

Margaret Talbot, *Jack or Jill? The Era of Consumer-Driven Eugenics Has Begun*, 289 Atlantic Monthly 25 (March 2002). Do you agree that selecting the sex of one's child is the same as selecting for other genetically linked traits such as height, hair color, and perhaps intelligence?

From a developmental standpoint, these types of selections can be distinguished on the basis of when the decision to favor one trait over another is made. Using sperm sorting, sex selection can be accomplished before conception (by selecting to introduce the egg to only X or Y sperm), and thus does not involve the intentional destruction of embryos for reasons of gender. In contrast, trait selection (provided it should ever become a scientific reality) can only be accomplished after conception because only then does an embryo possess the traits a parent might choose to select for or against. The state of knowledge today tells us that human traits such as height, eye color or even perfect pitch, are determined only after the male and female chromosomes combine to form a unique genome. Thus, trait selection would necessarily involve selecting among existing embryos, and possibly discarding those lacking a desired trait. The distinction between gender and trait selection blurs, however, when the concept of postconception gender selection is introduced. Using preimplantation genetic diagnosis (PGD), parents can select for gender after their embryos are formed, raising additional concerns about the prospect of sex selection.

2. Postconception Gender Selection

The Ethics Committee of the American Society of Reproductive Medicine
Sex Selection and Preimplantation Genetic Diagnosis
72 Fertility & Sterility 595 (1999)

. . . Interest in sex selection has a long history dating to ancient cultures. Methods have varied from special modes and timing of coitus to the practice of infanticide. Only recently have medical technologies made it possible to attempt sex selection of children before their conception or birth. For example, screening for carriers of X-linked genetic diseases allows potential parents not only to decide whether to have children but also to select the sex of their offspring before pregnancy or before birth.

Among the methods now available for prepregnancy and prebirth sex selection are [1] prefertilization separation of X-bearing from Y-bearing spermatozoa (through a technique that is now available although still investigational for humans), with subsequent selection for artificial insemination or for IVF; [2] preimplantation genetic diagnosis (PGD), followed by the sex selection of embryos for transfer; and [3] prenatal genetic diagnosis, followed by sex-selective abortion. The primary focus of this document is on the second method, sex selection through PGD, although the issues particular to this method overlap with the issues relevant to the others. Preimplantation genetic diagnosis is used with assisted reproductive technologies such as IVF to identify genetic disorders, but it also can provide information regarding the sex of embryos either as a by-product of testing for genetic disorders or when it is done purely for sex selection (Table 1).

As the methods of sex selection have varied throughout history, so have the motivations for it. Among the most prominent of motivations historically have been simple desires to bear and raise children of the culturally preferred gender, to ensure the economic usefulness of offspring within a family, to achieve gender balance among children in a given family, and to determine a gendered birth order.

New technologies also have served these aims, but they have raised to prominence the goal of avoiding the birth of children with sex-related genetic disorders.

Whatever its methods or its reasons, sex selection has encountered significant ethical objections throughout its history. Religious traditions and societies in general have responded with concerns varying from moral outrage at infanticide to moral reservations regarding the use of some prebirth methods of diagnosis for the sole purpose of sex selection. More recently, concerns have focused on the dangers of gender discrimination and the perpetuation of gender oppression in contemporary societies.

This document's focus on PGD for sex selection is prompted by the increasing attractiveness of prepregnancy sex selection over prenatal diagnosis and sex-selective abortion, and by the current limited availability of methods of prefertilization sex selection techniques that are both reliable and safe. Although the actual use of PGD for sex selection is still infrequent, its potential use continues to raise important ethical questions.

Central to the controversies over the use of PGD for sex selection, particularly for nonmedical reasons, are issues of gender discrimination, the appropriateness of expanding control over nonessential characteristics of offspring, and the relative importance of sex selection when weighed against medical and financial burdens to parents and against multiple demands for limited medical resources. In western societies, these concerns inevitably encounter what has become a strong presumption in favor of reproductive choice.

TABLE 1

Embryo sex identification by preimplantation genetic diagnosis for non-medical reasons.

(a) Patient is undergoing IVF and PGD.

Patient learns sex identification of embryo as *part of*, or as *a byproduct of*, PGD done for other medical reasons.

(b) Patient is undergoing IVF and PGD.

Patient requests that sex identification be *added to* PGD being done for other medical reasons.

(c) Patient is undergoing IVF, but PGD is not necessary to treatment.

Patient *requests PGD* solely for the purpose of sex identification.

(d) Patient is not undergoing either IVF or PGD (for the treatment of infertility or any other medical reason).

Patient *requests IVF and PGD* solely for the purpose of sex identification.

THE GENERAL ETHICAL DEBATE

Arguments for PGD and sex selection make two primary appeals. The first is to the right to reproductive choice on the part of the person or persons who seek to bear a child. Sex selection, it is argued, is a logical extension of this right. The second is an appeal to the important goods to be achieved through this technique and the choices it allows — above all, the medical good of preventing the transmission of sex-linked genetic disorders such as hemophilia A and B, Lesch-Nyhan syndrome, Duchenne-Becker muscular dystrophy, and Hunter syndrome. There also are perceived individual and social goods such as gender balance or distribution in a family with more than one child, parental companionship with a child of one's own gender, and a preferred gender order among one's children. More remotely, it sometimes is argued that PGD and sex selection of embryos for transfer is a lesser evil (medically and ethically) than the alternative of prenatal diagnosis and sex-selected abortion, and even that PGD and sex selection can contribute indirectly to population limitation (i.e., with this technique, parents no longer are compelled to continue to reproduce until they achieve a child of the preferred gender).

Arguments against PGD used for sex selection appeal either to what is considered inherently wrong with sex selection or to the bad consequences that are likely to outweigh the good consequences of its use. Suspicion of sex selection as wrong is lodged in the concerns identified earlier: the potential for inherent gender discrimination, inappropriate control over nonessential characteristics of children, unnecessary medical burdens and costs for parents, and inappropriate and potentially unfair use of limited medical resources for sex selection rather than for more genuine and urgent medical needs. These concerns are closely connected with predictions of negative consequences, such as risk of psychological harm to sex-selected offspring (i.e., by placing on them too high expectations), increased marital conflict over sex-selective decisions, and reinforcement of gender bias in society as a whole. Sometimes the predictions reach to dire consequences such as an overall change in the human sex ratio detrimental to the future of a particular society.

PREIMPLANTATION GENETIC DIAGNOSIS AND SEX SELECTION: JOINING THE PARTICULAR ISSUES

The right to reproductive freedom has never been considered an absolute right, certainly not if it is extended to include every sort of decision about reproduction or every demand for positive support in individuals' reproductive decisions. Still, serious reasons (e.g., the likelihood of seriously harmful consequences or the presence of a competing stronger right) must be provided if a limitation on reproductive freedom is to be justified. Hence, the weighing of opposing positions regarding PGD and sex selection depends on an assessment of the strength of the reasons given for and against it.

Preimplantation genetic diagnosis has the potential for serving sex selection in varying categories of cases, each of which raises different medical and ethical questions. Preimplantation genetic diagnosis may be done for disease prevention, or it may be done for any of the other motivations individuals have for determining the sex of their offspring. Moreover, information about the sex of an embryo may be obtained (a) as an essential part of or by-product of PGD performed for other (medical) reasons or (b) through a test for sex identification that is added to PGD performed for medical reasons. Further, (c) a patient who is undergoing IVF procedures as part of fertility treatment (but whose treatment does not require PGD for medical reasons) may request PGD solely for the purpose of sex selection, and (d) a patient who is fertile (hence, not undergoing IVF as part of treatment) may request IVF and PGD, both solely for the purpose of sex selection. Each of these situations calls for a distinct medical and ethical assessment (Table 1).

There presently is little debate over the ethical validity of PGD for sex selection when its aim is to prevent the transmission of sex-linked genetic disease. In this case, sex selection does not prefer one sex over the other for its own supposed value; it does not, therefore, have the potential to contribute as such to gender bias. And when the genetic disorder is severe, efforts to prevent it can hardly be placed in a category of trivializing or instrumentalizing human reproduction. Moreover, prepregnancy sex-selective techniques used for this purpose appear to have a clear claim on limited resources along with other medical procedures that are performed with the goal of eliminating disease and suffering.

It is less easy to eliminate concerns regarding PGD and sex selection when it is aimed at serving social and psychological goals not related to the prevention of disease. It must be recognized, of course, that individuals and couples have wide discretion and liberty in making reproductive choices, even if others object. Yet ethical arguments against sex selection appear to gain strength as the categories of potential cases descend from (a) to (d). For example, desires for family gender balance or birth order, companionship, family economic welfare, and the ready acceptance of offspring who are more "wanted" because their gender is selected may not in every case deserve the charge of unjustified gender bias, but they are vulnerable to it.

Whatever they may mean for an individual or family choice, they also, if fulfilled on a large scale through PGD for sex selection, may contribute to a society's gender stereotyping and overall gender discrimination. On the other hand, if they are expressed and fulfilled only on a small scale and sporadically (as is presently the case), their social implications will be correspondingly limited. Still, they remain vulnerable to the judgment that no matter what their basis, they identify gender as a reason to value one person over another, and they support socially constructed stereotypes of what gender means. In doing so, they not only reinforce possibilities of unfair discrimination, but they may trivialize human reproduction by making it depend on the selection of nonessential features of offspring.

Desired potential social benefits of sex selection also may appear insufficiently significant when weighed against unnecessary bodily burdens and risks for women, and when contrasted with other needs for and claims on medical resources. In particular, many would judge it unreasonable for individuals who do not otherwise need IVF (for the treatment of infertility or prevention of genetic disease) to undertake its burdens and expense solely to select the gender of their offspring. Although individuals may be free to accept such burdens, and although costs may be borne in a way that does not directly violate the rights of others, to encourage

PGD for sex selection when it is not medically indicated presents ethical problems.

More remote sorts of consequences of PGD and sex selection, both good and bad, remain too speculative to place seriously in the balance of ethical assessments of the techniques. That is, potential good consequences such as population control, and potential bad consequences such as imbalance in a society's sex ratio, seem too uncertain in their prediction to be determinative of the issues of sex selection. Even if, for example, the current rise in sex selection of offspring in a few countries suggests a correlation between the availability of sex selection methods and the concrete expression of son-preference, there can be no easy transfer of these data to other societies. This does not mean, however, that all concerns for the general social consequences of sex selection techniques regarding general gender discrimination can be dismissed.

The United States is not likely to connect sex selection practices with severe needs to limit population (as may be the case in other countries). Moreover, gender discrimination is not as deeply intertwined with economic structures in the United States as it may be elsewhere. Nonetheless, ongoing problems with the status of women in the United States make it necessary to take account of concerns for the impact of sex selection on goals of gender equality.

Moreover, the issue of controlling offspring characteristics that are perceived as nonessential cannot be summarily dismissed. Those who argue that offering parental choices of sex selection is taking a major step toward "designing" offspring present concerns that are not unreasonable in a highly technologic culture. Yet it appears precipitous to assume that the possibility of gender choices will lead to a feared radical transformation of the meaning of human reproduction. A "slippery slope" argument seems overdrawn when it is used here. The desire to have some control over the gender of offspring is older than the new technologies that make this possible. This, however, suggests that should otherwise permissible technologies for sex selection be actively promoted for nonmedical reasons — as in (b), (c), and (d) above — their threat to widely valued meanings of human reproduction may call for more serious concern than other speculative and remote negative consequences of PGD and sex selection.

Objections to PGD and sex selection on the grounds of misallocation of resources are more difficult to sustain. Questions of this sort are not so obviously relevant to systems of medical care like the one in the United States. If an individual is able and willing to pay for desired (and medically reasonable) services, there is no direct, easy way to show how any particular set of choices takes away from the right of others to basic care. Yet even here, individual and group decisions do have an impact on the overall deployment of resources for medical care and on the availability of reproductive services.

Although, as already noted, there is little controversy about the seriousness of the need to prevent genetic diseases, it is doubtful that gender preference on the basis of other social and psychological desires should be given as high a priority. The distinction between medical needs and nonmedical desires is particularly relevant if PGD is done solely for sex selection based on nonmedical preferences. The greater the demand on medical resources to achieve PGD for no other reason than sex selection, as in descending order in (b) through (d) above, the more questions surround it regarding its appropriateness for medical practice. If, on the other hand, PGD is done as part of infertility treatment, and the information that allows sex selection is not gained through the additional use of medical resources, it presumably is free of more serious problems of fairness in the allocation of scarce resources and appropriateness to the practice of medicine.

The ethical issues that have emerged in this document's concern for PGD and sex selection are in some ways particular to the uses and consequences of a specific reproductive technology. Their general significance is broader than this, however. For example, the concerns raised here provide at least a framework for an ethical assessment of new techniques for selecting X-bearing or Y-bearing sperm for IUI or IVF (ongoing clinical trial reports of which appeared while this document was being developed). Here, too, sex selection for the purposes of preventing the transmission of genetic diseases does not appear to present ethical problems. However, here also, sex selection for nonmedical reasons, especially if facilitated on a large scale, has the potential to reinforce gender bias in a society, and it may constitute inappropriate use and allocation of medical resources. Finally, although sperm sorting and IUI can entail less burden for parents, questions of the risk to offspring from techniques that involve staining and the use of a laser on sperm DNA remain under investigation.

RECOMMENDATIONS

Of the arguments in favor of PGD and sex selection, only the one based on the prevention of transmittable genetic diseases is strong enough to clearly avoid or override concerns regarding gender equality, acceptance of offspring for themselves and not their inessential characteristics, health risks and burdens for individuals attempting to achieve pregnancy, and equitable use and distribution of medical resources. These concerns remain for PGD and sex selection when it is used to fulfill nonmedical preferences or social and psychological needs. However, because it is not clear in every case that the use of PGD and sex selection for nonmedical reasons entails certainly grave wrongs or sufficiently predictable grave negative consequences, the Committee does not favor its legal prohibition. Nonetheless, the cumulative weight of the arguments against nonmedically motivated sex selection gives cause for serious ethical caution. The Committee's recommendations therefore follow from an effort to respect and to weigh ethical concerns that are sometimes in conflict — namely, the right to reproductive freedom, genuine medical needs and goals, gender equality, and justice in the distribution of medical resources. On the basis of its foregoing ethical analysis, the Committee recommends the following:

1. Preimplantation genetic diagnosis used for sex selection to prevent the transmission of serious genetic disease is ethically acceptable. It is not inherently gender biased, bears little risk of consequences detrimental to individuals or to society, and represents a use of medical resources for reasons of human health.

2. In patients undergoing IVF, PGD used for sex selection for nonmedical reasons — as in (a) through (c) above — holds some risk of gender bias, harm to individuals and society, and inappropriateness in the use and

allocation of limited medical resources. Although these risks are lower when sex identification is already part of a by-product of PGD being done for medical reasons (a), they increase when sex identification is added to PGD solely for purposes of sex selection (b) and when PGD is itself initiated solely for sex selection (c). They remain a concern whenever sex selection is done for nonmedical reasons. Such use of PGD therefore should not be encouraged.

3. The initiation of IVF with PGD solely for sex selection (d) holds even greater risk of unwarranted gender bias, social harm, and the diversion of medical resources from genuine medical need. It therefore should be discouraged.

4. Ethical caution regarding PGD for sex selection calls for study of the consequences of this practice. Such study should include cross-cultural as well as intra-cultural patterns, ongoing assessment of competing claims for medical resources, and reasonable efforts to discern changes in the level of social responsibility and respect for future generations.

NOTES AND QUESTIONS

1. *The ASRM Position.* Compare the recommendations of the ASRM Ethics Committee with regard to sex selection from 1999 (sex selection and PGD, reprinted beginning at page 298) and 2001 (preconception gender selection for nonmedical reasons, reprinted beginning at page 292). What are the fundamental differences between these two reports?

In 1999, the ASRM Ethics Committee concluded that "IVF with PGD solely for sex selection . . . should be discouraged." Three years later, in discussing preconception sex selection (i.e., sperm-sorting methods) the Ethics Committee approved gender selection for couples seeking gender variety. The most obvious reasons for these differing views on the practice of sex selection is the issue of embryo discard; ASRM disapproves of sex selection that entails embryo destruction but approves the practice for family balancing when it can be accomplished without harming existing embryos. Does this position seem sensible to you? Are there other features that distinguish pre- and post-conception gender selection that would lead you to reach different conclusions?

At least one physician practicing in the ART field studied the ASRM positions and questioned the logic and appropriateness of the Ethics Committee recommendations. Dr. Norbert Gleicher, chairman of the board of the Center for Human Reproduction (CHR), a nine-center fertility clinic in the Chicago and New York areas, wrote a letter to the chairman of the ASRM Ethics Committee expressing concerns that had been raised by CHR's institutional review board (IRB). An IRB is a voluntary group of physicians, scientists, lay people, clergy, and others who review proposed medical research protocols to ensure that the human subjects' rights and welfare are adequately protected. Since PGD was still considered experimental at the time the ASRM positions were announced, CHR asked its IRB to review and approve any use of the technology in its clinics.

The IRB found that "[i]t seemed unethical to inform the public of only one and not the other methodology of gender selection . . . [and] to offer the public access to only one and not the other technology especially because preconception gender selection was diagnostically less reliable than PGD, resulting in lower pregnancy rates per treatment cycle, and therefore was also less cost effective." In sum, the IRB "voiced the opinion that once gender selection was considered an ethically acceptable concept, patients should be informed about all the choices available and should have great discretion in the procreative decisions." Norbert Gleicher & Vishvanath Karande, *Gender Selection for Nonmedical Indications*, 78 FERTILITY & STERILITY 460, 461 (2002).

Ultimately, the ASRM reaffirmed its position that, despite the disparity in clinical success rates, preconception sex selection for gender variety could be ethically justified while PGD for nonmedical reasons should be discouraged. It explained its position that "fertilized eggs and preimplantation embryos, although not persons or moral subjects in their own right, should not be treated like any other human tissue. Rather, because of the meanings associated with their potential to implant and bring forth a new person, they deserve "special respect." On balance, the ASRM concluded, "[i]t has not yet been clearly established that a couple's desire for gender variety in offspring is sufficient to outweigh the need to show special respect to embryos." John A. Robertson, Chair, Ethics Committee, American Society for Reproductive Medicine, *Sex Selection for Gender Variety By Preimplantation Genetic Diagnosis*, 78 FERTILITY & STERILITY 463 (2002).

2. *Is PGD for Sex Selection Available?* Data about the availability and use of PGD for gender selection is not formally collected by any government agency, and thus not easily accessed. In 2008, researchers at the Genetics and Public Policy Center surveyed U.S. fertility clinics about their use of PGD, including use for sex selection. The survey found 42% of respondents offer PDG for nonmedical sex selection, with 47% of this group willing to provide the technique under all circumstances (for a first child, for example). Forty-one percent of those providing PGD for sex selection will only provide the service for family balancing. Nonmedical sex selection was performed in 9% of the PGD cycles performed by the responding clinics. *See* Susannah Baruch, David Kaufman, Kathy Hudson, *Genetic Testing of Embryos: Practices and Perspectives of US In Vitro Fertilization Clinics*, 89 FERTILITY & STERILITY 1053 (2008).

There are no laws in the U.S. either prohibiting or mandating the use of PGD for sex selection, leaving individual clinics free to generate their own policies. Suppose Mr. and Mrs. Thompson, a married couple with three girls, visit a state university-based fertility clinic to inquire about selecting a boy for their next (and last) pregnancy. The clinic director, Dr. Lee, tells the couple that the clinic's policy is to offer sperm sorting (with an 82% success rate for boys), but not to offer PGD (which has a nearly 100% success rate for gender selection). The Thompsons explain that without a "very high guarantee" of having a boy, they will avoid procreation altogether. For this reason, they ask Dr. Lee to reconsider her clinic's position, arguing that denying them PGD fails to show respect to the couple's reproductive liberty. (You guessed correctly that the Thompsons are both lawyers.) If you were counsel to the state university, what advice would you give to Dr. Lee about the clinic's stated sex selection policy?

3. *Gender Ratios.* The discussion surrounding sperm sorting and PGD for gender selection often turns to existing gender ratio disparities in places outside the United States. Universally, gender ratio disparities show a preference for boys, who outnumber girls beyond the naturally occurring ratio of about 102-106 to 100.

The President's Council on Bioethics, an advisory group appointed by President Bush in 2001, recently investigated the gender ratios in a number of countries and reported the following demographics:

The sex ratio at birth of boys to 100 girls is:

Venezuela	107.5
Yugoslavia	108.6
Egypt	108.7
Hong Kong	109.7
South Korea	110
Pakistan	110.9
Delhi, India	117
China	117
Cuba	118
Azerbaijan	120

The President's Council on Bioethics, *Beyond Therapy: Biotechnology and the Pursuit of Happiness* 61 (October 2003). The Council notes that "[a]lthough data is lacking regarding the techniques people in these countries use to produce these large shifts in the sex ratio, we suspect that sonography-plus-abortion is by far the most common." Id.

If sex selection were freely available in the United States, do you think we would see a shift in the birth ratios of boys to girls? Again, while the data is mostly anecdotal, clinics that do offer sex selection report that the vast majority of couples using sperm sorting want girls, not boys. In fact, the MicroSort trials report 945 cycles for girls compared to 291 for boys. When PGD is used, an average of 60% of couples request boys. This disparity may be due in part to the higher success rates for selecting for girls using the MicroSort sperm sorting technique; when the technology is accurate for both genders, as is the case with PGD, informal numbers suggest a U.S. preference for boys.

What is the basis for the widespread preference for boys? No doubt the answer to this complex question has its roots in history, culture, religion, economics, gender stereotyping and gender discrimination. Author Mary Carmichael investigated the male-preference phenomenon in India, a country some have referred to as "a daughterless nation." She describes in gruesome detail the gender selection process she uncovered in one region of the country:

> For years Rukmini Devi helped Indian couples in the impoverished state of Bihar choose the sex of their children. But in her decades of work, she never once used PGD. Bihar has few ultrasound machines and fewer fertility labs; many of its towns lack even basic health clinics, and most couples don't know their children's gender before birth. But boys are a

treasured commodity in Bihar, and if a couple can't choose a child's sex prenatally, they can see a dai like Devi. For 80 cents, says Devi, who is now retired, a dai will help a woman give birth. For 80 cents more, she will take a newborn girl, hold her upside down by the waist and "give a sharp jerk," snapping the spinal cord. She will then declare the infant stillborn. "Many couples insist that we get rid of the baby girl at birth," Devi says. "What can we do?"

Mary Carmichael, *No Girls, Please*, Newsweek, Jan. 26, 2004, at 50. Carmichael explains that even though Indian law prohibits the use of ultrasound to detect a fetus' gender, the practice of sex selection abortion is widespread. Even though the practice of female infanticide Carmichael reports are not known to occur in the U.S., should our law take into account the plight of girls worldwide? Or should our responses be based on U.S.-centric norms and practices?

What if a woman could learn her fetus' sex very early in the pregnancy, say at seven weeks gestation, using a simple blood test — while a medical abortion using ingested medications (as opposed to a surgical abortion) were still possible? Would this technology influence women, particularly American women, in their decisions about continuing or terminating their pregnancies? For a thoughtful piece expressing concern about the coming use of noninvasive cell-free fetal DNA testing, *see* Jaime S. King, *And Genetic Testing for All . . . The Coming Revolution in Non-Invasive Prenatal Genetic Testing*, 42 Rutgers L.J. 599 (2012).

John A. Robertson
Extending Preimplantation Genetic Diagnosis: Medical and Non-medical Uses
29 J. Med. Ethics 213 (2003)

. . . The use of medical technology to select the sex of offspring is highly controversial because of the bias against females which it usually reflects or expresses, and the resulting social disruptions which it might cause. PGD for gender selection faces the additional problem of appearing to be a relatively weak reason for creating and selecting embryos for discard or transfer.

The greatest social effects of gender selection arise when the gender of the first child is chosen. Selection for first children will overwhelmingly favour males, particularly if one child per family population policies apply. If carried out on a large scale, it could lead to great disparities in the sex ratio of the population, as has occurred in China and India through the use of ultrasound screening and abortion. PGD, however, is too expensive and inaccessible to be used on a wide scale for sex selection purposes. Allowing it to be used for the first child is only marginally likely to contribute to societal sex ratio imbalances. But its use is likely to reflect cultural notions of male privilege and may reinforce entrenched sexism toward women.

The use of PGD to choose a gender opposite to that of an existing child or children is much less susceptible to a charge of sexism. Here a couple seeks variety or "balance" in the gender of offspring because of the different rearing experiences that come with rearing children of different genders. Psychologists now recognise many biologically based differences between male and female children, including different patterns of aggression, learning, and spatial recognition, as well as hormonal differences. It may not be sexist in itself to wish to have a child or children of each gender, particularly if one has two or more children of the same gender.

Some feminists, however, would argue that any attention to the gender of offspring is inherently sexist, particularly when social attitudes and expectations play such an important role in constructing sex role expectations and behaviours. Other feminists find the choice of a child with a gender different from existing children to be morally defensible as long as "the intention and consequences of the practice are not sexist", which is plausibly the case when gender variety in children is sought. Desiring the different rearing experiences with boys and girls does not mean that the parents, who have already had children of one gender, are sexists or likely to value unfairly one or the other gender.

Based on this analysis the case is weak for allowing PGD for the first child, but may be acceptable for gender variety in a family. With regard to the first child, facilitating preferences for male firstborns carries a high risk of promoting sexist social mores. It may also strike many persons as too trivial a concern to meet shared notions of the special respect due preimplantation embryos. A proponent of gender selection, however, might argue that cultural preferences for firstborn males should be tolerated, unless a clearer case of harm has been shown. If PGD is not permitted, pregnancy and abortion might occur instead.

The case for PGD for gender variety is stronger because the risk of sexism is lessened. A couple would be selecting the gender of a second or subsequent children for variety in rearing experiences, and not out of a belief that one gender is privileged over another. Gender selection in that case would occur without running the risks of fostering sexism and hurting women.

The question still arises whether the desire for gender variety in children, even if not sexist, is a strong enough reason to justify creating and discarding embryos. The answer depends on how strong an interest that is. No one has yet marshalled the evidence showing that the need or desire for gender variety in children is substantial and important, or whether many parents would refrain from having another child if PGD for gender variety were not possible. More evidence of the strength and prevalence of this need would help in reaching a conclusion. If that case is made, then PGD for gender variety might be acceptable as well.

The ethics committee of the American Society of Reproductive Medicine (ASRM) has struggled with these issues in a series of recent opinions. It initially addressed the issue of PGD for gender selection generally, and found that it "should be discouraged" for couples not going through IVF, and "not encouraged" for couples who were, but made no distinction between PGD for gender selection of first and later children. Subsequently, it found that *preconception* gender selection would be acceptable for purposes of gender variety but not for the first child.

Perceiving these two positions to be inconsistent, a doctor who wanted to offer PGD for gender selection inquired of the ethics committee why preconception methods for gender variety, which lacked 100% certainty, were acceptable but PGD, which guaranteed that certainty, was not. Focusing only on the sexism and gender discrimination issue, the chair of the ethics committee, in a widely publicised letter, found that PGD for gender balancing would be acceptable. When the full committee reconsidered the matter, it concluded that it had not yet received enough evidence that the need for gender variety was so important in families that it justified creating and discarding embryos for that purpose. In the future if such evidence was forthcoming then PGD for gender variety might also be acceptable.

What might constitute such evidence? One source would be families with two or more children of one gender who very much would like to have another child but only if they could be sure that it would be a child of the gender opposite of existing children. Given the legitimacy of wanting to raise children of both genders, reasonable persons might find that this need outweighs the symbolic costs of creating and discarding embryos for that purpose.

Another instance would be a case in which a couple has had a girl, but now wants a boy in order to meet cultural norms of having a male heir or a male to perform funeral rituals or play other cultural roles. An IVF programme in India is now providing PGD to select male offspring as the second child of couples who have already had a daughter. Because of the importance of a male heir in India, those couples might well consider having an abortion if pregnant with a female fetus (even though illegal in India for that purpose). In that setting PGD for gender selection for gender variety appears to be justified.

Professor Robertson makes several arguments in favor of the use of sex selection for gender variety or family balancing, including the legitimate desire of parents to experience a different rearing experience, and the possibility that, absent the ability to choose their child's gender, a couple would refrain from procreating altogether. This latter argument could invoke principles of procreative liberty, if the unavailability of gender selection technology were the result of government regulations banning the practice. In the excerpt that follows, the President's Council on Bioethics discusses the connection between reproductive liberty and parental gender choice.

The President's Council on Bioethics
Beyond Therapy: Biotechnology and the Pursuit of Happiness
(October 2003) 66-68

The Limits of Liberty

. . . As we noted earlier, few policy makers or opinion leaders argue openly in favor of sex selection. Rather, the assumption is made that our most cherished ideals of individual autonomy and the right to choose preclude an unambiguous condemnation of sex selection or public policies that might curtail it. Yet this assumption is questionable.

Our society, to be sure, deeply cherishes liberty and rightfully gives a wide berth to its exercise. But liberty is never without its limits. In the case of actions that are purely self-regarding — that is, actions that affect only ourselves — society tends to give the greatest protections to personal freedom. But as we move outward, away from purely self-regarding actions to those actions that affect others, our liberty is necessarily more liable to societal and governmental oversight and restraint. Sex selection clearly does not belong in the category of purely self-regarding action. The parents' actions (their choice of a boy or a girl) are directed not only toward themselves but also toward the child-to-be.

One might argue that, since each child must be either a girl or a boy, the parents' actions in selecting the sex do not constitute much of an intrusion on the prospective child's freedom and well-being. But the binary choice among highly natural and familiar types hardly makes the choice a trivial one. And having one's sex foreordained by another is different from having it determined by the lottery of sexual union. There is thus at least a prima facie case for suggesting that the power to foreordain or control the nature of one's child's sexual identity is not encompassed in the protected sphere of inviolable reproductive liberty. It is far from clear that either the moral or the legal right to procreate includes the right to choose the sex — or other traits — of one's children.

But it is not only that sex selection affects the individual child-to-be that puts it in a class of actions fit for oversight, regulation, and (perhaps) curtailment. Sex selection, if practiced widely, can also have powerful societal effects that reach far beyond individuals and their families to the nation as a whole. The dramatic alteration in sex ratios in such countries as South Korea and Cuba bear this out. Whether or not one views the preference of individuals for sons over daughters as rational, taken together these individual preferences could and do have serious society-wide effects. The males may have diminished chances of finding an acceptable mate, while the broader society may suffer from higher crime, greater social unrest, increased incidence of prostitution, etc. — social troubles closely associated with an abnormally high incidence of men, especially unmarried men. One could argue that the choice of a male child is individually rational for parents, given the strong preference in certain cultures for males. But such individual choices may be socially costly — a case where individual parental eugenic choices do not yield a social optimum. Indeed, unrestricted sex selection offers a classic example of the Tragedy of the Commons, in which advantages sought by individuals are nullified, or worse, owing to the social costs of allowing them to everyone. In such cases, it is acceptable (and arguably necessary) for a liberal polity to place limits on individual liberty . . .

NOTES AND QUESTIONS

1. Both Professor Robertson and the President's Council note that sex selection, as it is currently practiced worldwide, reflects a strong preference for boys, confirming and contributing to bias and discrimination against women. On further reflection, the President's Council posits an alternate future for women, one in which scarcity plays to their advantage:

> Paradoxically, the anti-female bias thought by critics to be implicit in sex selection might in fact redound to the advantage of women, at least regarding marriage: their relative scarcity could give them greater selectivity, choice, and control of partners. In certain Asian countries for

example, where the ratio of boys to girls at birth has been severely skewed by sex selection, young men of marriageable age are already facing a severe shortage of young women to marry. Thus one might oppose sex selection as much for the actual harm it does to men as for the prejudice it expresses against women.

The President's Council on Bioethics, *Beyond Therapy: Biotechnology and the Pursuit of Happiness*, 66 (October 2003). The linkage between sex selection and an unbalanced sex ratio has generated much commentary, yielding a diverse field of predictions. Some feminists writers express concern that an uneven sex ratio in which males outnumber females will result in more humiliation and mistreatment of women. See, e.g., MARY ANNE WARREN, GENDERCIDE: THE IMPLICATIONS OF SEX-SELECTION (1985). Other women authors opine that a reduction in the female population will cause greater competition among men for female partners, making women more valuable and producing better treatment by the vying males. *See, e.g.*, GITA SEN & RACHEL C. SNOW, POWER AND DECISION: THE SOCIAL CONTROL OF REPRODUCTION (1994). Whether the usage of sex selection in the United States will ever be large enough to impact gender ratios is difficult to predict, but certainly the increasing use of ART in general precludes complete dismissal of the possibility.

2.   *The Legal Landscape.* The practice of sex selection, by sperm sorting or PGD, is illegal in many countries throughout the world, including Austria, Chile, Germany, Ireland, and Switzerland. See *Preimplantation Genetic Diagnosis*, 81 FERTILITY & STERILITY S38 (2004). In February 2005, the Australian National Health & Medical Research Council revised its guidelines to ban sex selection for nonmedical reasons, effectively eliminating the practice in the country. See Cathy O'Leary, *Parents Lose IVF Gender Choice*, WEST AUSTRALIAN, March 19, 2005, at 7 (reporting that hundreds of couples waiting to use sex selection will be turned away).

In England, the Human Fertilisation and Embryology Authority (HFEA), a governmental body that regulates and inspects all United Kingdom ART clinics, permits sex selection to be used only to avoid serious sex-linked disorders. The HFEA Code of Practice, which all licensed clinics must follow, provides as follows:

> [C]entres must ensure that . . . any information derived from tests on an embryo, or any material removed from it or from the gametes that produced it, is not used to select embryos of a particular sex for social reasons.

HUMAN FERTILISATION AND EMBRYOLOGY AUTHORITY CODE OF PRACTICE T88 (8th ed. 2008). The HFEA recently reviewed its policies on sex selection in light of newly emerging sperm sorting techniques and again concluded that sex selection for nonmedical reasons should be prohibited. The HFEA's conclusions were based in part on surveys in the UK which found that 80% of those surveyed did not want sex selection techniques to be made available for nonmedical reasons. See *HFEA Announces Recommendations on Sex Selection*, HFEA Press Release Archive, available at: http://www.hfea.gov.uk/PressOffice/Archive.

In the United States, sex selection is largely unregulated, leaving its availability up to individual practitioners. We have seen the ASRM issue reports discouraging the practice of sex selection for nonmedical reasons, but the voluntary organization holds no real legal sway over physicians. Do you think sex selection should be banned in the United States? If so, do you favor outlawing the technique for any reason? For nonmedical reasons? How would you define "nonmedical?" Does a parent's mental health qualify as a medical reason for seeking sex selection?

If a concern about sex selection is gender ratio imbalances, what about a regulation that allows sex selection for social reasons, but requires clinics that offer the technique perform an equal number of girl and boy procedures. Such a regulation could contain an annual reporting requirement, asking clinics to report the number of sex selection cycles performed, along with the gender ratios of those cycles. If a clinic wishes to tip its boy/girl balance, it may do so by trading girl or boy "sex selection cycles" with other clinics who are seeking a balance in favor of the opposite gender. This could result in gender imbalances in certain regions of the country, but its aim would be an even mix of genders throughout the country. Could such a regulation succeed?

B.   Choosing a Child's Genetic Make-Up

The previous section on sex selection introduced the concept that today's parents can investigate the genetic make-up of their early embryos and select embryos for further development depending on their characteristics. In the case of gender selection, one might argue that a parent is selecting *for* an embryo of the desired gender, as well as selecting *against* an embryo of the disfavored gender. Sex selection is controversial for many reasons, not the least of which is that selection *against* an embryo is often for purely social reasons, unrelated to the health of the prospective child. In this section, we turn our attention to embryo selection that is done for reasons of health. Interestingly, the health at issue is not always that of the embryo.

Recall that preimplantation genetic diagnosis (PGD) enables physicians to remove one cell from a three-day old eight-celled embryo and study its chromosomes. The PGD results can provide information in the following areas:

1) **Chromosomes** — Physicians can count and visualize the chromosomes within the cell to determine the embryo's gender (XX - girl) or (XY - boy) and to detect if the embryo has extra or missing chromosomes, a condition known as aneuploidy (pronounced \AN-yu-ploy-dee\). In some cases, an embryo with aneuploidy will fail to attach to the uterine wall or stop developing soon after attaching and miscarry. But in a few cases an embryo with an extra or missing chromosome can develop, though the child will be born with a chromosomal disorder. Examples of aneuploidic conditions include Down Syndrome (three chromosomes in Pair 21, sometime called Trisomy 21), Patau Syndrome (three chromosomes in Pair 13), Klinefelter Syndrome (a male with two X chromsomes, XXY) and Turner Syndrome (a female with only one X chromosome, XO).

If parents know that an embryo has an extra or missing chromosome, they can learn about the embryo's likelihood of survival and the disease a resulting child would face.

2) Single Gene Disorders — PGD can also be used to detect disease-causing genes that are located at specific places on a chromosome.[5] Over the past decade, scientists have learned that many diseases are caused by a single gene that is defective or mutated. Once the gene is identified and located on a chromosome, it can be viewed using PGD. Single gene disorders include cystic fibrosis, Tay Sachs disease, Huntington's disease, muscular dystrophy and sickle cell anemia.

If parents know that either gamete provider has a family history of a single-gene disorder, they can use IVF and PGD to detect embryos that inherit the deleterious gene.

3) Tissue Matching for an Existing Child — Recent advances in PGD allow physicians to determine whether an embryo is an immunological match for a sick sibling in need of compatible stem cells. Typically, in these cases an existing child suffers from leukemia or a lethal form of anemia and has failed all traditional therapies. If another child with the identical tissue type to the ill child is born, the infant's umbilical cord blood or bone marrow can be used to treat the ailing sibling. PGD tells parents whether the embryos themselves are affected with the disease (in the case of genetic disorders) and whether they are a compatible donor for the sick sibling.

PGD for tissue typing often raises the so-called "end/means" debate: Is the embryo being created and selected for its own inherent worth or merely as a means to salvage an existing child? As you read the story of one family's struggle, consider what you would do as the parent of a desperately ill child.

1. Using Preimplantation Genetic Diagnosis to Cure Illness

In 1994, Lisa and Jack Nash welcomed their first child, Molly, but shortly after their daughter's birth the couple knew there was a problem with her health. Molly was diagnosed with Fanconi Anemia, an inherited genetic disorder that leads to bone marrow failure and early forms of cancer. Many children born with the disease do not survive past their seventh birthday. As Molly neared her sixth birthday and her health began to deteriorate, Lisa and Jack decided to take a course of action that had never been tried, but offered the only chance to save their daughter's life. In 1999, the Nashes underwent in vitro fertilization, producing 15 embryos for possible implantation. The embryos were tested, using PGD, for two purposes. First, to rule out any embryos that contained the gene known to cause Fanconi Anemia, and second, to rule in only those embryos that were a perfect tissue match for Molly. The Nashes' goal was to gestate and birth a child who could serve as a stem cell donor for Molly, a treatment that provided the only hope for the girl's recovery. At least one of the embryos met these critical criteria, and the Nashes hoped for a successful pregnancy.

---

[5] The most common technique used to detect single-gene abnormalities is called polymerase chain reaction or PCR. PCR involves the isolation and amplification of short DNA fragments found in the single embryonic cell. Experts then analyze the DNA sequences to search for abnormalities associated with disorders that are known or suspected to exist in the genetic parents' family tree.

On August 29, 2000, the Nash family celebrated the birth of son Adam, whose umbilical cord blood was harvested shortly after he was born and prepared for transplant into his older sister. Weeks later, doctors at the University of Minnesota transplanted Adam's stem cells into Molly and anxiously awaited to see how she responded. By the end of the year, Molly had regained much of her strength and by January 2001 she returned to her home in Colorado. By all accounts, Molly has made a full recovery and is enjoying the life of a teen, replete with dance lessons and Girl Scouts. In fact, in early 2005 Molly made headlines for reasons unrelated to her first-in-the world treatment — she was the top-selling Girl Scout in the 2004 cookie drive, racking up sales of nearly 2,500 boxes. Molly attributed her retail acumen to a winning smile and the overall appeal of the Thin Mint. See Dan Vergano, *Custom Baby Saves A Life*, USA TODAY, Jan. 8, 2001, at 7D; Gary Massaro, *Girl Scout's Hand In Cookie-Jar Stardom*, ROCKY MOUNTAIN NEWS, Jan. 6, 2005, at 25A. The Nash family story served as the inspiration for the 2004 novel, My Sister's Keeper, by Jodi Picoult. The 2009 film version starring Cameron Diaz (as the mother struggling to save her daughter's life) grossed nearly $80 million. If you want to see both Lisa Nash and Cameron Diaz talk about their respective mother "roles," check out the Molly Nash Story on YouTube, www.youtube.com.

NOTES AND QUESTIONS

1.   The Adam Nash story is largely attributable to Yury Verlinsky, a Russian-born physician who directed the Reproductive Genetics Institute in Chicago until his death in 2009. Dr. Verlinsky pioneered the technique of testing embryos for genes that make antigens, which tell the body whether transplanted tissue is "self" or "non-self" and should be rejected. Matching antigens permits the body to accept a transplant, such as bone marrow, stem cells, or organs. When Adam was born and the unusual circumstances surrounding his conception revealed, medical ethicists weighed in on the morality of creating and testing embryos for tissue compatibility. While terms such as "spare-parts infant" and "designer baby" did occasionally surface, many ethicists gave tentative approval to the Nashs' quest largely because the treatment involved umbilical cord blood (that did not require an invasion into Adam's body) and the couple made a compelling argument that they had independently wanted another child, and wanted to be sure he or she would not inherit the same fatal genetic disease. See Bill Radford, *The Designer Baby: Right or Wrong?*, BALTIMORE SUN, Jan. 14, 2001, at 1N.

The slippery slope seems in full view here. What about a couple who needs bone marrow from an infant, a procedure that requires a large needle be inserted into the child's hip to retrieve cells?[6] How about a kidney needed for transplantation? Living

---

[6] According to a newspaper report, "That's what Abe and Mary Ayala did more than a decade ago. In a highly publicized case, the California parents conceived of a child in hopes that it could save their 16-year-old daughter Anissa, who had leukemia and desperately needed a bone marrow transplant. Unlike the [Nashs], the Ayalas were not guaranteed that the baby would be a match. Siblings have a one in four chance of being tissue compatible, compared to about a one in 20,000 chance with unrelated donors. The story ended triumphantly for the Ayalas with the birth in 1990 of Marissa, who had the same [tissue] type as her sister and who later donated bone marrow that saved her life. But some medical ethicists and others sharply criticized the family for bringing a child into the world for a utilitarian purpose. Times have changed - somewhat. In a survey last month by Johns Hopkins' Genetics and Public

donors routinely surrender kidneys, but only after being fully informed of the risks and providing unqualified consent. Should the parents who orchestrated a child's birth as a compatible tissue match be permitted to consent to organ donation on behalf of that child? If you believe PGD for tissue matching is acceptable in some situations but morally troubling in others, how would you regulate the procedure to best serve the interests of all parties involved?

2.   The tragedy of an ailing child in need of compatible tissue is sadly not uncommon, but the successful treatment of Molly Nash gave new hope to many families facing this dire scenario. Not surprisingly, a number of affected families turned to Dr. Verlinsky who reported in May 2004 that his Chicago laboratory helped create five healthy infants who could serve as stem cell donors for their ailing brothers and sisters. One of the infants was born to an English couple who traveled to Chicago after British fertility authorities (the Human Fertilisation and Embryology Authority) denied them permission to undergo the procedure in England. See *Stem-Cell Research: Chicago Lab Helps Create Five Babies to Become Future Donors*, LAW & HEALTH WEEKLY, May 29, 2004, at 742. One novel aspect of these cases was that several of the siblings suffered from leukemia, a bone marrow disease that is not thought to be the result of a genetic defect. Thus, the embryos in these families were tested for tissue-compatibility but not screened genetically for diseases. This differs from the Adam Nash situation because the Nash embryos were tested for the presence of the deleterious gene, to avoid having another child with the fatal disease. Arguably when an embryo is screened only for tissue compatibility, the benefit extends exclusively to the ailing sibling.

Are there benefits that inure to an infant conceived to save an older sibling? Perhaps the answer depends upon the outcome of the salvage therapy. If the sibling survives, a deep sense of gratitude and love (from the parents and/or the ailing sibling) may emerge. But if the sibling dies or fares poorly, will the second child feel guilt at having failed to save the family member? Will the parents anguish over the loss of the older child reflect in their rearing of the younger child? Are these potential harms to the child sufficient to deny parents access to PGD for this purpose?

The ethics surrounding the creation and testing of embryos to serve as stem cell donors are carefully considered in the reading that follows.

Susan M. Wolf, Jeffrey P. Kahn, John E. Wagner
Using Preimplantation Genetic Diagnosis to Create a Stem Cell Donor: Issues, Guidelines & Limits
31 Journal of Law, Medicine & Ethics 327 (2003)

[The authors convened an advisory group to discuss the controversial use of PGD to create a donor child who is tissue-matched with a preexisting sibling in need of stem cell transplantation. Technically, parents seek to have a child who is Human

---

Policy Center, 61 percent of 4,005 respondents said that they approved of genetically screening embryos to select one that could help an ailing sibling. But nearly as many - 57 percent - said they would not approve of the same technique to select a child's sex. Erika Niedowski, *5 Children Created to Donate Stem Cells*, Baltimore Sun, May 5, 2004, at 1A.

Leukocyte Antigen (HLA)-matched with an ailing child. HLA refers to the antigens which determine whether tissue, such as blood, organs and stem cells, will be compatible with that of an existing affected child. If the donor child is determined to be an HLA-match, at delivery stem cells from the newborn umbilical cord blood can be used to treat the affected sibling. Thus, the authors note that PGD to create a donor is not one technology, but three: IVF (to create the embryos), PGD (to test the embryos for tissue compatibility) and stem cell transplant. With these three technologies in mind, the authors provide the following analysis and recommendations.]

. . . The [Adam and Molly] Nash case illustrates the successful combination of three technologies: IVF, PGD, and stem cell transplant. However, because of the success so far of the cord blood transplant, the Nash case does not illustrate the reality that children conceived to be HLA-matched face the possibility of donation throughout their lives. The initial cord blood donation could fail for any of several reasons: inadequate cord blood cell dose, graft failure after cord blood transplant, or the recipient child experiencing a recurrence of leukemia after transplant. If cord blood transplant fails, the next step is bone morrow harvest and transplant. This, too, might not engraft or leukemia may recur, requiring yet another bone marrow transplant. Further, once an HLA-matched donor is created, the need for tissues beyond bone marrow may arise. Indeed, after bone marrow transplant, toxicities related to chemotherapy and irradiation or immunosuppressive drugs could produce organ failure involving the kidneys, liver, or other organs. Then the question would arise whether to harvest a solid organ from the donor child. The HLA-matched child created in the Nash case has thus far escaped further need for tissue or organs by his sister. However, he is quite young. He and all children created as donors face the potential of requests for donation throughout their lives . . .

PROBLEMS WITH EXISTING ANALYSES

None of the existing analyses examines in depth the potential burden to the child-to-be of serving as a lifelong donor subject to repeated tests and procedures, some involving bodily invasion, risk, and pain. To be sure, those analyses either explicitly or implicitly reject conceiving a child for solid organ harvest. However, they largely ignore the question of what limits should be placed on harvesting cord blood or, particularly, bone marrow. Nor do the analyses ask what framework we should apply in evaluating acceptable burden to the child-to-be: is the combination of IVF, PGD to create a donor, and stem cell transplant accepted treatment or should it be conducted as research with the correspondingly stricter rules regarding what risk and burden are appropriate and what consent is required? Finally, the analyses fail to address, fully what steps are necessary to address the conflict of commitment parents face in creating and then making decisions for their donor child while trying to save the older sibling. We address each of these problems to offer concrete recommendations for practice.

ANALYSIS AND RECOMMENDATIONS

Careful analysis of the problems raised by combining IVF, PGD to create a donor, and stem cell transplant suggests that PGD to create a donor is ethical only under certain conditions.

(1) Research protections should apply.

The combination of IVF, PGD to create a donor, and stem cell transplant to treat an affected sibling should currently be conducted as research rather than accepted treatment . . .

[W]hile each of the three technologies may be accepted for some indications . . . stacking them together raises questions of their combined safety and efficacy. For example, an IVF center may stretch its eligibility criteria, attempt more cycles, try to harvest more eggs per cycle, and transfer more embryos for a couple desperately trying to save a sick child. This may increase risks for the woman as well as the risks of multiple gestation for the child- or children-to-be.

Not only may IVF be conducted differently when combined with the other two technologies, but transplant may be conducted differently as well. A child created to be a donor is likely to have cord blood harvested at birth. If cord blood transplant fails, the question will immediately arise whether the donor child should undergo bone marrow harvest. Yet experience with bone marrow harvest in a neonate is minimal, in part because it is recognized to carry increased risk. In this respect, the harvesting of children conceived to be donors may be quite different from the harvesting of children not conceived in this way but who happen to be HLA-matched with a sick sibling.

Finally, we know almost nothing about the psychological impact of being conceived to serve as an HLA-matched donor and save a sibling's life. The effects on the donor child are potentially profound. Indeed, if the cord blood transplant fails or the donor child is otherwise repeatedly considered for harvest over a prolonged period of time, there may be a potential for serious effects. The potential may be all the greater if the donor child comes to resist or refuse further procedures, depending on how the family and medical team respond . . .

Combining these technologies in the context of research would render the federal rules on the protection of human subjects applicable when federal funding is involved, when an institution involved had assured the federal government that all research conducted there will comply with federal rules on human research subjects, or when Food and Drug Administration (FDA) approval is required. Both the additional protections for pregnant women, fetuses, and neonates and the additional protections for children would apply, as the protocol would extend over time through IVF, PGD, and stem cell transplant. The human subjects involved would include the recipient sibling.

The most vexing questions of research ethics here concern the donor child, who cannot either consent or assent to the IVF and PGD, and cannot consent or assent to any harvesting until many years after birth. That child's welfare may be compromised by the circumstances of conception and harvesting. The federal rules governing human subjects research in children identify four categories of approvable research . . .

[The authors discuss the first three categories, 1) research poses no greater than minimal risk, 2) research is likely to yield knowledge about the subject's disorder or condition, and 3) research will advance understanding of a serious health problem in children, and conclude the fourth category is most likely to apply to a child conceived to be a donor.]

The remaining category . . . is research involving greater than minimal risk but offering the prospect of direct benefit to the individual research subject. Analyzing the potential benefit to the donor child is complex. Part of the protocol promises medical benefit to the donor child-to-be (PGD to rule out a heritable disorder) while part does not (PGD for HLA matching plus harvest). However, the second part of the protocol may offer psychological benefit to the donor . . . [R]esearch [may be approved] on the grounds that the donor child would benefit psychologically from averting the sibling's death and consequent loss of that relationship.

As we discuss below, this prospect of future psychological benefit will be only a speculation when the protocol involving IVF, PGD to create a donor, and stem cell transplant is first proposed. Careful reevaluation of prospective benefit to the donor is essential before bone marrow harvest, in particular. But the possibility of future psychological benefit plus the medically beneficial PGD to prevent the disorder in question in the donor child-to-be is likely to justify an IRB regarding such a protocol as offering the prospect of direct benefit to the donor child.

(2) The sibling's condition should be life-threatening or seriously disabling.

PGD to create a donor imposes burdens on the woman or couple undergoing IVF and potential burdens on the child-to-be as a lifelong donor. Those burdens are only justified by significant benefit to the affected sibling. That sibling must have a medical problem that is life-threatening or seriously disabling and which, to a reasonable degree of medical certainty, is likely to be significantly ameliorated by utilizing the three technologies of IVF, PGD, and stem cell transplant. This requires seriously addressing with the couple the statistical likelihood of success in conceiving a matched donor, achieving pregnancy and healthy birth, harvesting the needed cells, and treating the sick sibling in time . . .

When PGD is used solely to create a donor and the sibling's disorder is non-heritable, then, the only possible benefit to the child-to-be will be the psychological benefit of saving the sibling . . . We are skeptical that the mere prospect of psychological benefit, without any accompanying medical benefit, is enough to justify the risks of IVF, possible risks of PGD, and clear burden of serving as a lifelong donor as described above . . .

(3) Psychological evaluation of the parents should precede IVF and PGD.

IVF plus PGD to create a donor requires independent psychological evaluation of the parents' ability to rear the donor child-to-be lovingly and without exploitation. The evaluation should be conducted by professionals who are not members of the transplant team and are not treating the affected sibling. PGD to create a donor raises the specter of the donor child being treated solely as a means rather than being loved and valued for him- or herself. The donor child is at lifelong risk of exploitation, of being told that he or she exists as an insurance policy and tissue source for the sibling, of being repeatedly subjected to testing and harvesting procedures, of being used this way no matter how severe the psychological and physical burden, and of being pressured, manipulated, or even forced over protest. The parents must intend to rear the donor child lovingly with that child's individual best interests governing all medical decisions for the child. While . . . parental motives beyond saving the affected sibling are hard to discern accurately, signs at the outset that the parents will exploit the donor child should disqualify the family.

(4) Risk to the donor child should not be increased to benefit the recipient.

Even when PGD to create a donor is acceptable, there should be no variation in IVF, gestation, delivery, or treatment of the donor child that increases risks to that child in order to benefit the affected sibling . . . Examples of variations unacceptably increasing risk are: transferring extra embryos to the woman's uterus, thereby increasing the risk of conceiving multiples with the attendant risks of prematurity and its sequelae; prolonging efforts to achieve vaginal delivery to increase the amount or quality of cord blood available for transplant, when that prolongation increases risks to the donor child; rapid umbilical cord clamping; and raising the newborn above the mother's abdomen to increase placental blood volume immediately following delivery.

(5) Psychological evaluation should precede each invasive harvesting.

Every harvesting procedure from the donor child that involves bodily invasion such as bone marrow harvest (but obviously not harvesting umbilical cord blood), must be preceded by independent psychological evaluation of the parents and donor child (when age appropriate) to assure that the parents are not exploiting the child or imposing psychological harm, that the child is adequately supported psychologically and medically, and that the child does not object. A child old enough to understand the procedure (typically approximately 7 years old) must affirmatively assent, although an IRB may assess the capacity of individual children to assent to research protocols . . .

(6) Risk or burden to the donor child should be limited before the child can decide for him- or herself.

As noted above, any risk must be justified by anticipated medical and psychological benefit to the donor child. However, the only medical benefit that derives from PGD is to rule out the disorder in question in the child-to-be and that benefit is fully realized at birth. Beyond that point, any risks or burdens imposed on the donor child are for the purpose of saving the sibling's life and the benefits to the donor are only psychological. Those benefits fail to justify much more than minimal risk or burden. Further, the risk of exploiting the donor child repeatedly before the child can maturely decide for him- or herself argues for stringent limits.

Spelling out what these limits mean in practice is challenging. It certainly seems to allow use of cord blood, as that imposes no physical risk or burden and probably little, if any, psychological risk or burden. At the other extreme is solid organ harvest under general anesthesia. Clearly that imposes substantial risk and burden, both physical and psychological. The British HFEA finds solid organ harvest in a child conceived as a donor unacceptable and we agree . . .

If conceiving a child-to-be for cord blood harvest is acceptable, but for solid organ harvest is unacceptable, that leaves the intermediate question of where conceiving for bone marrow transplant falls on the spectrum. Bone marrow harvest in children is invasive, and usually performed under general anesthesia. It involves risk of infection (albeit low), risks of general anesthesia, pain, and discomfort and may involve the risks of transfusion. Studies also indicate that the psychological burden to minors of donating bone marrow to a sibling can be significant, including guilt and a sense of responsibility for saving the sibling's life.

This suggests that each proposed bone marrow harvest of a donor child must be evaluated to determine whether the expected risk or burden to the donor will be substantially greater than minimal . . . [E]ach proposed harvest from a child not yet mature enough to consent for him- or herself should be evaluated to determine whether there is enough evidence of a positive emotional relationship between the proposed donor and recipient to ground an expectation of psychological benefit to the donor. The lack of such a relationship should render harvest unacceptable. This means that neonates, who as yet have no emotional relationship of any substance with the sibling, should not serve as bone marrow donors. Donation would have to await the development of such a relationship, even if that was too late to save the sibling. It is difficult to say at what age one might begin to see evidence of a positive emotional relationship, and the age will undoubtedly vary from case to case.

(7) The number of testing and harvesting procedures should be limited.

There should be a limit to how many times the donor child may be tested and harvested. In the Nash case, stem cell harvest from the placenta and umbilical cord worked, at least thus far. If it failed, however, the next step would be to consider bone marrow harvest. Bone marrow harvest and the battery of pre-harvest screening tests are invasive and can be psychologically burdensome and frightening to a child. If bone marrow harvest were to fail, either in the short run or long run, repeat harvest might be considered. Indeed, because the donor child was conceived as an HLA-match to the affected sibling, even solid organ transplant could be considered if the sibling's medical circumstances warranted.

The child conceived as a donor is thus vulnerable to repeated testing and harvesting, even though the long-term medical and psychological consequences of repeated testing and harvesting may not be known. That vulnerability will persist throughout childhood and, in fact, will be lifelong. While any numerical limit may appear arbitrary, we are concerned that it is excessively burdensome to the child and exploitative to subject the child to the combination of testing and harvesting more than twice before the child can make a mature and autonomous decision on further testing and harvesting him-or herself. Indeed, given the literature on the burdens of pediatric donation, it could be argued that there be a limit of one marrow harvest.

(8) The donor child should have an independent physician.

The donor child should have his or her own physician for every contemplated harvesting procedure that involves bodily invasion. That physician should not be a member of the transplant team or otherwise treating the affected sibling. It is essential that a health professional with no conflict of commitment make an independent evaluation of the donor child's medical and psychological needs . . .

(9) Harvesting should require parental permission plus ethics review.

Parental permission is necessary but not sufficient; independent review before each invasive harvesting procedure by an ethics committee or consultant is essential. There must be some body or individual charged with the responsibility of determining whether the above guidelines have been met and a proposed harvesting procedure may ethically proceed. . . . [The authors review the argument that court approval should be required in order for children to be conceived as donors, and concludes that, at this time, routine judicial review should not be required. But, the authors caution, the recommendation could be changed if data reveals a pattern of harm to donors.]

CONCLUSION

Growing demand for the combination of IVF, PGD to create a donor, and stem cell transplant suggests the need for practical guidelines. Our analysis offers guidelines providing both substantive limits and necessary procedures. The most fundamental protections we recommend are: (1) to combine these three technologies only in the context of research at present, with the attendant human subject protections and need for oversight, and (2) to safeguard the future interests of the donor child-to-be, and later the interests of the donor child. Both protections are essential to ethical conduct in the use of these technologies.

The authors give cautionary and limited approval to the practice of IVF and PGD to create a "savior sibling" to serve as a stem cell donor for an ailing brother or sister. One of the authors, John Wagner, is a physician from the University of Minnesota who treated Molly Nash with her brother's umbilical cord stem cells. The other two authors, Susan Wolf and Jeffrey Kahn, were members of the University of Minnesota's Stem Cell Ethics Advisory Board at the time Molly received her treatment. In addition to their intensive familiarity with the issues surrounding PGD and HLA-matching, the authors were motivated to produce the above guidelines by the absence of any such guidelines in the U.S. Though the ASRM and the American Medical Association have issued policy statements approving the use of PGD to prevent or avoid genetic disease, no national body has issued guidelines that govern the propriety of screening embryos solely to treat a serious disease in another person.

In contrast, the British Human Fertilisation and Embryology Authority (HFEA), the governmental regulatory body that oversees the practice of assisted conception in the UK, has been active in the debate over and regulation of PGD for tissue-matching. In December 2001 the HFEA announced that it would approve the use of PGD for HLA-matching only if the embryos conceived in the course of treatment were themselves at risk from the condition affecting the existing child; approval would not be forthcoming to create embryos solely to serve as tissue donors. In February 2002 the HFEA granted its first license to use PGD for tissue-typing to aid a family whose young son suffered from a rare genetic disorder. Soon thereafter, a group opposed to the HFEA's action filed a lawsuit challenging its authority to grant licenses for the procedure. The British Court of Appeal issued the following decision in the case.

R (ON THE APPLICATION OF QUINTAVALLE) v. HUMAN FERTILISATION AND EMBRYOLOGY AUTHORITY
Court Of Appeal (Civil Division)
[2003] Q.B. 168, EWCA Civ 667

LORD PHILLIPS OF WORTH MATRAVERS, MR.

Mr and Mrs Hashmi have five children. The fourth, a son, Zain was born with a blood disorder known as beta thalassaemia major. By the time that he was two and a half years old this had reduced him to a parlous condition, requiring him to take a daily cocktail of drugs and to submit to regular blood transfusions in hospital in order to remain alive. His life expectancy is uncertain. Mrs Hashmi had been aware that she had a genetic predisposition to producing children with this disorder and, when pregnant with Zain had undergone prenatal testing to see whether, if she carried Zain to term, he would be born with the disorder. The test failed to disclose that this was indeed the position.

Zain's condition might be cured by a transplant of stem cells from someone with matching tissue. The stem cells could be supplied from blood taken from the umbilical cord of a newborn child, or from bone marrow. The most likely source of matching tissue would be a sibling, for statistically Mrs Hashmi has one chance in four of producing a child with matching tissue, although the odds are somewhat longer of producing such a child who is not affected with beta thalassaemia major. None of Zain's three elder siblings have tissue that matches his.

Mrs Hashmi resolved to have another child, in the hope that it would have matching tissue. She conceived, but prenatal testing showed that the child would have beta thalassaemia major, so she underwent an abortion. She conceived again, and a healthy son was born, but unfortunately his tissue did not match that of Zain.

At this point Mrs Hashmi met Dr Simon Fishel, the managing and scientific director of Centres for Assisted Reproduction Ltd (CARE). CARE is the largest single provider of in vitro fertilisation (IVF) services in the United Kingdom. It provides these services at various locations both to NHS[7] and private patients. Dr Fishel told Mrs Hashmi of a procedure, at the cutting edge of technology, that had been developed at the Reproductive Genetics Institute (RGI) in Chicago in the

---

[7] The National Health Service (NHS) is the British government-sponsored universal healthcare system that funds a comprehensive range of health services - Ed.

United States and which might provide the solution to her problem. In summary, that procedure would include the following stages. (i) The fertilisation 'in vitro' of a number of eggs taken from Mrs Hashmi with sperm taken from her husband to form embryos. (ii) The removal from the developing embryo of a single cell by a biopsy. (iii) The examination of that cell using molecular genetics to see whether the embryo carried the beta thalassaemia disease. This process is commonly described as 'Pre-implantation Genetic Diagnosis' (PGD). (iv) Use simultaneously of the same process to identify whether the embryo had the same tissue type as Zain. Because this process involves examination of proteins known as human leukocyte antigens (HLA), this form of PGD is described as 'HLA typing'. I shall refer to it by the more popular phrase of 'tissue typing'. (v) Jettison of embryos found by this analysis to be either disease bearing or of a different HLA type to Zain and implantation in the womb of Mrs Hashmi of an embryo shown to be disease free and of the same HLA as Zain.

Mrs Hashmi asked Dr Fishel whether it would be possible for her to be impregnated in this country with an embryo created and selected in this way. IVF treatment can only be carried out in this country under licence issued by the appellant, the Human Fertilisation and Embryology Authority (HFEA), pursuant to the Human Fertilisation and Embryology Act 1990. For some years PGD screening against genetic disease had been carried out as part of IVF treatment licensed by the HFEA. Tissue typing had never, however, been carried out as part of such treatment and Dr Fishel considered that this procedure required express authorisation under licence from HFEA. After careful consideration of the implications, CARE applied to the HFEA for a ruling as to whether an IVF clinic could properly apply for a licence to administer treatment including tissue typing.

The HFEA announced their decision in a press release on 13 December 2001. They would be prepared in principle to grant a licence for treatment that included tissue typing, subject to a number of conditions. The HFEA decided that tissue typing should only be permitted where PGD was already necessary to avoid the passing on of a serious genetic disorder. They also decided that licences permitting PGD in conjunction with tissue typing should only be granted on a case by case basis. Such licences would only be granted subject to the following conditions. (a) The condition of the affected child should be severe or life threatening, of a sufficient seriousness to justify the use of PGD. (b) The embryos should themselves be at risk of the condition affecting the child. (c) All other possibilities of treatment and sources of tissue for the affected child should have been explored. (d) The techniques should not be available where the intended recipient is a parent. (e) The intention should be to take only cord blood for the purposes of the treatment. (f) Appropriate counselling should be given to the parents. (g) Families should be encouraged to take part in follow-up studies. (h) Embryos should not be genetically modified to provide a tissue match.

In accordance with this decision, on 22 February 2002, the HFEA granted a licence to Park Hospital operated by CARE in Nottingham to carry out IVF treatment that included PGD for 'beta thalassaemia in conjunction with HLA typing for patients known as Mr and Mrs H'.

Mr and Mrs Hashmi then made two attempts to produce a child by IVF treatment involving PGD and tissue typing. In the first IVF was effected at Park Hospital. Fifteen embryos were produced. The biopsied cells from those were then flown to RGI in Chicago for genetic analysis, while the embryos were frozen awaiting the results. Only one embryo proved to have an exact tissue match, but it carried the beta thalassaemia disease. Mr and Mrs Hashmi travelled to RGI for the second attempt. Ten embryos were produced. Two of these proved disease free and to have a tissue match with Zain. One was implanted in Mrs Hashmi, but no pregnancy resulted. Mr and Mrs Hashmi were prevented from a further attempt by the judgment that is the subject of this appeal . . .

THE CHALLENGE

The respondent, Josephine Quintavalle, acts on behalf of Comment on Reproductive Ethics (CORE). CORE is a group whose purpose is 'to focus and facilitate debate on ethical issues arising from human reproduction and, in particular, assisted reproduction'. Absolute respect for the human embryo is a principal tenet of CORE. The respondent sought and obtained permission to seek judicial review of the HFEA's decision announced on 13 December 2001. She challenged that decision on the ground that the HFEA had no power to issue a licence that permitted the use of HLA typing to select between healthy embryos. Her challenge succeeded. On 20 December 2002 Maurice Kay J [the trial judge] gave judgment in her favour, quashing the HFEA's decision (see [2003] 2 All ER 105).

Maurice Kay J gave permission to appeal against his judgment to this court because of the importance of the issue of whether tissue typing can lawfully be licensed by the HFEA. The Secretary of State for Health was concerned that the judgment has wider implications-in particular that it puts in doubt the legitimacy of the beneficial practice of PGD screening for genetic diseases. Accordingly the Secretary of State obtained permission to intervene to support the HFEA's appeal.

THE ACT

The 1990 [Human Fertilisation and Embryology] Act was passed 'to make provision in connection with human embryos and any subsequent development of such embryos; to prohibit certain practices in connection with embryos and gametes; to establish a Human Fertilisation and Embryology Authority', and for other purposes.

The following provisions of the Act are particularly material:

'2.-(1) In this Act . . .

"treatment services" means medical, surgical or obstetric services provided to the public or a section of the public for the purpose of assisting women to carry children . . .

Activities governed by the Act

3. Prohibitions in connection with embryos.-(1) No person shall-(a) bring about the creation of an embryo, or (b) keep or use an embryo, except in pursuance of a licence . . .

Scope of licences

11. Licences for treatment, storage and research.-(1) The Authority may grant the following and no other licences-(a) licences under paragraph 1 of Schedule 2 to this Act authorising activities in the course of providing treatment services, (b) licences under that Schedule authorising the storage of gametes and embryos, and (c) licences under paragraph 3 of that Schedule authorising activities for the purposes of a project of research . . .

Licence conditions

13. Conditions of licences for treatment.-(1) The following shall be conditions of every licence under para 1 of Sch 2 to this Act . . .

(5) A woman shall not be provided with treatment services unless account has been taken of the welfare of any child who may be born as a result of the treatment (including the need of that child for a father[8]), and of any other child who may be affected by the birth . . .

SCHEDULE 2

ACTIVITIES FOR WHICH LICENCES MAY BE GRANTED

Licences for treatment

(3) A licence under this paragraph cannot authorise any activity unless it appears to the Authority to be necessary or desirable for the purpose of providing treatment services . . .

Licenses for research

(2) A licence under this paragraph cannot authorise any activity unless it appears to the Authority to be necessary or desirable for the purpose of —

(e) developing methods for detecting the presence of gene or chromosome abnormalities in embryos before implantation . . .

---

[8] This provision linking the welfare of a child to the need for a father was controversial in England, especially among supporters of single and same-sex (female) parenting. The British law was amended in 2008, removing this language and replacing it with "the need for supportive parenting." -Ed.

THE ISSUES BEFORE THE JUDGE

Before Maurice Kay J two issues were canvassed. (i) Does genetic analysis of a cell taken from an embryo involve the 'use of an embryo'? (ii) Is genetic analysis for the purpose of tissue typing 'necessary or desirable for the purpose of providing treatment services'?

The first issue arose out of the submission on behalf of the HFEA that tissue typing did not require a licence because it was performed on a cell extracted from an embryo rather than the embryo itself. The HFEA accepted that the removal of the cell by a biopsy constituted 'use of an embryo', but submitted that testing the cell thereafter did not constitute such use. Mrs Quintavalle contended that tissue typing did constitute 'use of an embryo' and, in consequence, could not be carried on without a licence.

The second issue arose only if the HFEA failed on the first issue. In that event the HFEA contended that they could lawfully licence such use in that tissue typing was 'desirable for the purpose of rendering treatment services'. The HFEA argued that the relevant test was whether the activity under consideration was 'at least desirable for the overall purpose of providing fertility treatment'.

Mrs Quintavalle relied upon the definition of 'treatment services' and submitted that it could not be said that tissue typing was for the purpose of those services. The purpose of tissue typing was not to 'assist women to carry children' but to ensure that a child born to a particular woman would have tissue that was compatible with the tissue of a sibling.

THE JUDGMENT OF MAURICE KAY J

The judge held against the HFEA on both issues. There were a number of reasons why he held that tissue typing involved the use of an embryo, including the fact that it was inconceivable that Parliament intended to leave an activity such as tissue typing, which had potential for misuse, outside the control of the Act. As to the second issue he observed that tissue typing of an embryo had no impact on the ability of a woman to carry the embryo after implantation. In those circumstances it could not be said that tissue typing was 'necessary or desirable for the purpose of assisting a woman to carry a child'.

THE ISSUES BEFORE US

Mr Pannick QC[9], who appeared for the HFEA, accepted that the first issue considered by Maurice Kay J did not go to the heart of the case. He recognised that the primary object of carrying out a biopsy of each embryo was to carry out tissue typing of the cell that was removed. It was common ground that the biopsy involved 'using' the embryo. If the tissue typing was not carried out 'for the purpose of assisting a woman to carry a child', then the biopsy could not be said to be for that

---

[9] QC refers to "Queen's Counsel," a barrister appointed as counsel to the British crown. When the sovereign is a man, the term King's Counsel, KC, is used. In this case, Mr. Pannick was appointed to represent the HFEA, a government agency. - Ed.

purpose either. More broadly Mr and Mrs Hashmi's case demonstrated the true nature of treatment involving tissue typing. The primary object of the entire treatment, comprehending creation of the embryo, biopsy for PGD and tissue typing, the analysis of the cell removed by the biopsy and the implantation of the embryo, if it proved to be free of disease and a tissue match for Zain, was to produce a child whose umbilical cord would provide the stem cells which might save Zain's life. The vital question was whether this treatment was 'for the purpose of assisting a woman to carry a child'.

Mr Pannick submitted that the answer to this question was Yes. He submitted that the judge had wrongly concluded that treatment services had to have as their sole object the assistance of the physical process of producing a child. IVF coupled with PGD was a practice aimed at enabling women to have children free of hereditary diseases. Analysis of the Act, and of background material to which it was legitimate to have resort, demonstrated that treatment services extended to embrace PGD designed to prevent the implantation of embryos which would result in the birth of a children [sic] carrying genetic defects. Such screening assisted a woman to carry a child because it gave her the knowledge that the child would not be born handicapped. Without such knowledge some women who carried genetic diseases would not be prepared to have children. In the same way tissue typing would assist Mrs Hashmi to carry a child, for her wish to do so was conditional upon knowing that the birth of that child would be capable of saving the life and health of Zain.

Mr Pannick accepted that under this reasoning PGD with the object of ensuring that a child had certain characteristics for purely social reasons might also be said to be 'for the purpose of assisting women to carry children' but submitted that it was for the HFEA to control PGD to ensure that this was not used for purposes which were ethically objectionable. That accorded with the scheme of the Act. It was only practices that were unquestionably objectionable that were prohibited by the legislation. PGD for the purpose of avoiding genetic defects was not objectionable at all . . .

Mr Dingemans QC, for Mrs Quintavalle, challenged these submissions. He did not abandon the primary submission that 'treatment services' only extended to services designed to assist women in overcoming problems in conceiving and carrying a child to term. Most of his energies were, however, directed to an alternative argument. Even if PGD for the purpose of screening out genetic defects fell within the definition of 'treatment services', such a practice differed in principle from PGD screening designed to reject healthy and viable embryos because they lacked some desired characteristic. While the former might be said to assist a woman in carrying a child the latter certainly could not . . .

DISCUSSION

Maurice Kay J did not find it appropriate to consider whether the Act permits PGD screening for hereditary diseases. Mr Pannick's argument founded on this question as a stepping stone to the construction for which he contended. It seems to me not merely appropriate but necessary to consider the implications of any suggested construction on the position of screening for hereditary diseases . . .

Mr Pannick submitted that para 3(2)(b) of Sch 2 was significant. This permits the licensing of embryo research activities for the purpose of 'developing methods for detecting the presence of gene or chromosome abnormalities in embryos before implantation'. Mr Pannick argued that it would be strange if Parliament approved research to develop a method for achieving an objective which was prohibited elsewhere in the Act. The clear inference of permitting such research was that Parliament approved of PGD to avoid implantation of embryos carrying genetic defects. The phrase 'for the purpose of assisting women to carry children' and of 'suitable for that purpose' in Sch 2, para 1(1)(d) had to be read so as to embrace that activity.

I found this argument persuasive . . . Parliament chose to permit the licensing of research. It makes little sense for Parliament, at the same time, to prohibit reaping the benefit of that research, even under licence.

The question remains whether the two vital phrases 'for the purpose of assisting women to carry children' and 'designed to secure that the embryo is suitable for the purpose of being placed in a woman' are appropriate to describe the object of IVF treatment which is designed not to assist the processes of fertilisation and gestation, but to ensure that the child which is produced by those processes is healthy.

My initial reaction to the meaning of 'for the purpose of assisting women to carry children' was the same as that of Maurice Kay J. The phrase naturally suggests treatment designed to assist the physical processes from fertilisation to the birth of a child. But if the impediment to bearing a child is concern that it may be born with a hereditary defect, treatment which enables women to become pregnant and to bear children in the confidence that they will not be suffering from such defects can properly be described as 'for the purpose of assisting women to carry children'. I believe that it is appropriate to give it this meaning in order sensibly to reconcile the provisions of the Act that deal with treatment and those that deal with research. I also think that it is legitimate when deciding to adopt this construction to have regard to the fact that the more narrow alternative construction would render unlawful a practice which has been carried on for over a decade and which is patently beneficial . . .

What of the actual process of biopsy and PGD — can that properly be said to be 'designed to secure that the embryo is suitable for the purpose of being placed in a woman'? Here I agree with Mr Pannick that, once satisfied that the treatment as a whole is for the purpose of enabling a woman to carry a child, no further problem arises. The word 'suitable' takes its meaning from its context. Where the object of the treatment is to enable a woman to bear a child confident that it will not carry a hereditary defect, an embryo will only be suitable for the purpose of being placed within her if it is free of that defect. PGD is thus designed to secure that the embryo is suitable for this purpose . . .

TISSUE TYPING

I said that Mr Pannick used the question of whether the Act permitted PGD screening as a stepping stone to the construction of the Act for which he contended.

It remains to consider whether this stepping stone takes him safely to his destination.

'TREATMENT FOR THE PURPOSE OF ASSISTING WOMEN TO BEAR CHILDREN'

The discussion thus far had led me to the following conclusion. When concern as to the characteristics of any child that she may bear may inhibit a woman from bearing a child, IVF treatment coupled with PGD that will eliminate that concern can properly be said to be 'for the purpose of assisting women to carry children'. When the Act was passed women who had reason to fear that they would give birth to children with genetic defects were probably the only section of the population for whom it was envisaged that IVF treatment could be justified on this basis. No evidence suggests that the wish of a woman to bear a child in order to provide a source of stem cells for a sick or dying sibling was anticipated at that time. Such a wish is now the reality, and the case of Mr and Mrs Hashmi is not unique.

The activities that the HFEA has licensed in the case of Mr and Mrs Hashmi, are the same as those it has regularly licensed for the purpose of assisting women to bear children free of hereditary diseases: (i) creation of embryos; (ii) biopsies of the embryos; (iii) analysis of the cells removed by biopsy by the use of a DNA probe in order to identify those embryos likely to produce children with desired characteristics; and (iv) implantation of those embryos. The difference is as to the desired characteristics. That difference may be critical in determining whether or not the HFEA will decide to license the activities in question. I cannot see, however, that the difference can be critical in determining whether or not the treatment, including the PGD, is 'for the purpose of enabling women to carry children'. My conclusion is that whether the PGD has the purpose of producing a child free from genetic defects, or of producing a child with stem cells matching a sick or dying sibling, the IVF treatment that includes the PGD constitutes 'treatment for the purpose of assisting women to bear children'.

'DESIGNED TO SECURE THAT THE EMBRYO IS SUITABLE FOR THE PURPOSE OF BEING PLACED IN THE WOMAN'

Just as in the case of PGD screening for genetic defects, the meaning of 'suitable' falls to be determined having regard to its context. When the object of the treatment is to enable a woman to bear a child with a tissue type that will enable stem cells to be provided to a sick sibling, an embryo will only be suitable for the purpose of being placed within her if it will lead to the birth of a child with the tissue type in question. Accordingly I conclude that the HFEA was right to decide that the Act authorised it to licence IVF treatment with PGD for the purpose of tissue typing subject to such conditions as it considered appropriate.

CONCLUSION

IVF treatment can help women to bear children when they are unable to do so by the normal process of fertilisation. Screening of embryos before implantation enables a choice to be made as to the characteristics of the child to be born with the assistance of the treatment. Whether and for what purposes such a choice should be permitted raises difficult ethical questions. My conclusion is that Parliament has placed that choice in the hands of the HFEA. For the reasons that I have given I would allow this appeal.

NOTES AND QUESTIONS

1. *Postscript.* The British House of Lords, the highest judicial authority in the UK, affirmed the decision in this case on April 28, 2005. *Quintavalle (t/a Comment on Reproductive Ethics) v. Human Fertilisation and Embryology Authority,* [2005] UKHL 28.

2. The British Court of Appeal in *HFEA* relies in part on the fact that the Hashmis' PGD goals were twofold: to screen out embryos affected by the serious genetic disorder affecting their family and to screen for embryos that were an HLA-match for their son. The HFEA had taken the position that HLA embryo screening was only acceptable if it were secondary to screening for serious genetic disorders. Inevitably, the more difficult case arose in which parents wished to use PGD solely to select for an HLA-match:

> Michelle and Jayson Whitaker have a three-year old son, Charlie, who suffers from Diamond Blackfan Anaemia (DBA), a rare form of anaemia where the bone marrow produces few, or no, red blood cells. Symptoms are similar to other forms of anaemia and include paleness, an irregular heartbeat and heart murmurs because of the increased work the heart needs to do to keep oxygen moving round the body. The disorder can lead to irritability, tiredness and fainting and requires intensive therapy including painful daylong blood transfusions and daily injections of life-saving drugs. DBA has no cure although bone marrow transplants can help. If the Whitakers were able to have another child who would be a matching tissue type donor, then cells created by him/her could help Charlie's body to create red blood cells, giving him a 90% chance of recovery. The Whitakers requested that their doctor, Mohammed Tarranissi, be allowed to test embryos taken from Mrs Whitaker using PGD. Their case was urgent: a transplant needed to be carried out in the next 18 months to have a good chance of success. Like the Hashmis, the Whitakers claimed they wanted another baby anyway and would not view a new child *purely* as a donor infant.

> While very similar to the case of Zain Hashmi, Charlie's case differs in one important respect: the DBA from which he suffers is 'sporadic' rather than hereditary. This means that the chances of his parents having another baby with the disease are no greater than those present in the general population: five to seven per million live births. As such, there is no reason to believe that the Whitakers' embryo would have the same defect. On this basis, the HFEA rejected the Whitakers' application. The justification given was that the 'tissue typing' procedure would be performed solely to find a match for Charlie, and not in order to check whether the embryos themselves carried a genetic disorder. For the HFEA, the Whitakers' case therefore was relevantly different from the Hashmis' since, for the Hash-

mis, the procedure was in the interests of the new child as well as the interests of Zain. Whereas in the case of the Whitakers, only Charlie would directly benefit, and at some point in the future, his new brother or sister might suffer from the knowledge that she or he had been chosen, and other embryos discarded, primarily to save Charlie's life.

Sally Sheldon & Stephen Wilkinson, 'Savior Siblings: Hashmi and Whitaker, An Unjustifiable and Misguided Distinction, 12 MEDICAL LAW REV. 137 (2004). Unable to access treatment in the U.K., the Whitakers traveled to the U.S. where they enrolled in the protocol headed by Dr. Verlinsky at the Chicago Reproductive Genetics Institute. In June 2003, Jamie Whitaker was born and his umbilical cord blood was preserved for a later transplant into his brother Charlie. According to a 2004 report, cells from Jamie were transplanted into Charlie and doctors waited to see whether the procedure would prove successful. See Maxine Frith, Ruling on Embryos Clears the Way for Designer Babies, THE INDEPENDENT, July 22, 2004. In 2005, Charlie was declared "effectively cured." See Charlie Whitaker Cured by "Savior Sibling," BioNews, Aug. 22, 2005, available at: http://www.bionews.org.uk/page_12478.asp.

3.   The controversy over the Whitakers' plight continued in Britain as other similarly situated couples urged the HFEA to rethink its policy. In a further development, in July 2004 the British HFEA reversed its position on the scenario in which parents seek PGD to ensure a tissue match but do not need to screen for genetic disorders. Announcing the policy change, the HFEA's chair, Suzi Leather explained, "Faced with potential requests from parents who want to save a sick child, the emotional focus is understandably on the child who is ill. Our job is to consider the welfare of the tissue-matched child which will be born . . . Our review of the evidence does not indicate that the procedure disadvantages resulting babies compared to other IVF babies. It also shows that the risks associated with sibling to sibling stem cell donation are low and that this treatment can benefit the whole family." Maxine Frith, Ruling on Embryos Clears the Way for Designer Babies, THE INDEPENDENT, July 22, 2004. The HFEA press release on this policy change can be access at www.hfea.uk.gov.

In 2008, the British Human Fertilisation and Embryology Act was amended to explicitly authorize the use of PGD for tissue-typing. The new provision provides that licenses to ART clinics may be issued:

in a case where a person ("the sibling") who is the child of the persons whose gametes are used to bring about the creation of the embryo (or of either of those persons) suffers from a serious medical condition which could be treated by umbilical cord blood stem cells, bone marrow or other tissue of any resulting child, establishing whether the tissue of any resulting child would be compatible with that of the sibling . . .

Human Fertilisation and Embryology Act of 2008, Sch. 2, Sec. 1ZA(d), available at: http://www.legislation.gov.uk/ukpga/2008/22/schedule/2.

No doubt reasonable minds will continue to differ on the use of PGD to select tissue-compatible embryos. On the one hand, pro-life groups view the technique with disfavor because it permits healthy embryos to be discarded. "This [is] a search-and-destroy mission." said Richard Doerflinger of the U.S. Conference of Catholic Bishops. The chosen embryos "were allowed to be born so they could donate tissue to benefit someone else." *Stem-Cell Research: Chicago Labs Help Create Five Babies to Become Future Donors*, LAW & HEALTH WEEKLY, May 29, 2004, at 742. The British HFEA policy change allowing PGD for tissue-matching was met with similar sentiment by anti-abortion groups. "To attempt to create another child as a transplant source is not morally acceptable" said a spokesman for LIFE, which campaigns against abortion, cloning and other scientific procedures. "How would this child feel, for example, when he or she discovers that they were brought into the world primarily as a "spare part" for their elder brother? Human beings — particularly children — must never be used as a means to an end." Maxine Frith, *Ruling on Embryos Clears the Way for Designer Babies*, THE INDEPENDENT, July 22, 2004.

PROBLEM

You have recently been appointed as a trial judge in your jurisdiction. One of your first cases is captioned, *Center for the Concern of Early Life (CCEL) v. Young*. The case involves an unmarried couple, Maria and Edward, who have lived together for seven years, but have never taken any formal steps toward marriage. Last year Edward was diagnosed with chronic lymphocytic leukemia, a type of cancer that starts from the blood-forming cells in the bone marrow. Edward's disease is progressing, and he has failed to improve with traditional therapies. His physician has researched the possibility of a stem cell transplant, but no compatible donors can be found either within Edward's family or national stem cell banks. Maria inquires whether Edward's genetic child could be a possible stem cell donor. She learns that there is a 25% chance that Edward's offspring could be a compatible stem cell donor, from cells collected in an infant's umbilical cord and placenta following delivery.

Maria and Edward next consult with Dr. Young, a fertility doctor specializing in IVF and PGD. Dr. Young has had a few successful cases treating parents whose young children are ailing from a variety of genetic and blood-born diseases who wish to have another child with compatible tissue. He has agreed to help Edward and Maria conceive a child using IVF and then select embryos that would be a match to provide stem cells for transplantation, thus increasing the odds of a compatible donor from 25 to 100%. The couple's neighbor, Terry, is a member of the Center for the Concern of Early Life (CCEL). Terry speaks to CCEL about Edward and Maria's plans and the group immediately goes to court seeking an injunction against Dr. Young's planned activities. CCEL is asking the court to enjoin Dr. Young from using PGD to investigate the make-up of the embryos and from thereafter discarding embryos that are deemed incompatible with Edward's cell type.

How would you decide this case? What resources would you turn to reach a reasoned result? What factors and individual interests weigh most heavily in your mind? Consider drafting an opinion resolving the case.

2. Using Preimplantation Genetic Diagnosis to Avoid Illness

The previous section looked at PGD as a technology that could aid parents in finding cures for their ailing children through tissue-compatible donor siblings. We learned that this use of PGD was an offshoot or byproduct of the technique's original purpose — to screen embryos for genetic mutations or chromosomal abnormalities associated with serious illnesses. At first blush, it might seem that the intense controversy surrounding the use of PGD to *cure* illness in family members would overshadow or even quell any controversy associated with the use of PGD to *avoid* illness in children born after embryo screening. But alas, embryo screening to avoid illness generates its own set of thorny dilemmas.

The first report of successful PGD to avoid creating a child affected by a genetic disorder was published in 1989. See A.H. Handyside et al., *Biopsy of Human Preimplantation Embryos and Sexing by DNA Amplification*, 347 LANCET 49 (1989). Since then, PGD has been used to screen for such diseases as Down Syndrome, Tay Sachs, cystic fibrosis, thalassemia, sickle cell anemia, Gaucher disease and hemophilia. In many instances, these diseases cause devastating health problems for children at birth, leading parents to select against implanting affected embryos. One of the confounding factors for parents learning that one or more of their embryos is affected by a genetic disorder is that doctors cannot always predict how the disease will manifest in the individual child. For some genetic disorders, such as Down Syndrome, the range of symptoms and health problems is highly variable, meaning that some children will lead relatively healthy lives, while others will suffer a highly medicalized lifestyle.

The variable and unpredictable nature and definition of disease has raised a number of questions surrounding the use of PGD to detect illness that will or may affect the offspring born of selected embryos. Fundamental questions such as, "What is a disability?" loom large. How will PGD affect people with disabilities in our society? Can a parent affected with a disability select *for* that disability in order to create a shared culture with that child? Should a parent be able to select against an embryo with genetic markers for a disease that will not manifest until the person is an adult? Is it ethical to detect and disclose the presence of genes that are associated with a predisposition to a certain disease, but do not guarantee that the individual will develop the disease in later life? These and other questions are pondered below.

a. PGD and the Meaning of Disability

The emergence of PGD and other genetic technologies mobilized numerous groups to gather and discuss the implications of these new techniques on our society. The Genetics and Public Policy Center (GPPC) is one such group. Established at Johns Hopkins University in 2002, the GPPC released a study of PGD in January 2004, reviewing the current state of the art and presenting a range of preliminary policy options. The GPPC's goal, according to its report "is not to advocate for a single position but to make sure that policy decisions, including the decision to maintain the status quo, are undertaken with a clear-eyed understanding of their potential impact." *Preimplantation Genetic Diagnosis: A*

Discussion of Challenges, Concerns, and Preliminary Policy Options Related to the Genetic Testing of Human Embryos, Genetics & Public Policy Center 2 (Jan. 2004).

The GPPC report questions PGD's future implications for society. Specifically with respect to its impact on people with disabilities, the report poses a series of questions:

Will the availability of PGD lead to a decrease in resources and support for those living with disabilities?

Will less money be directed to finding cures for diseases that can be avoided through PGD?

Will the availability of PGD to avoid some diseases lead to a more negative societal attitude towards people with disabilities generally?

What impact does PGD have on people's experiences of both joy and sadness of life? By attempting to remove suffering from people's lives, does PGD also diminish the richness of human experience?

Does PGD foster a parental culture of conditional love for children, rather than one in which children are loved and valued for who they are, regardless of any genetic "flaws?"

Id. at 26. In response to these questions, GPPC suggests a series of options for considerations:

Option: Provide Help for People with Disabilities and Their Families

There are several policy approaches that could improve the treatment and support for people with disabilities. Such improvements could limit the possible negative effects of PGD on this community. Also, by reducing fears associated with having a disabled child, these approaches could limit the overall demand for PGD.

Government actions could include support for research into new treatments and cures for people with disabilities, anti-discrimination laws to protect the rights of people with disabilities and more support for families caring for children with disabilities and for people living with disabilities.

Arguments for:

This approach helps everyone, including people with disabilities.

Arguments against:

This approach requires additional government spending at a time when most states and the federal government are complaining of revenue shortfalls. In the past, laws dealing with discrimination against people with disabilities that in the past [sic] have been viewed as costly and burdensome on small business.

Option: Provide Prospective Parents with Counseling Opportunities

Prospective parents considering PGD may not have had a chance to reflect on some of the larger issues such as how PGD could affect the resulting child and other family members. Counseling guidelines could be developed that help prompt prospective parents to give more attention to such matters so that they may make a more informed choice.

Arguments for:

Counseling guidelines would be useful for clinicians and prospective parents and help ensure that all of the issues have been carefully considered.

Arguments against:

Prospective parents already have a great deal to think about and cope with. They could view such counseling as an unwanted intrusion into private issues.

Id. at 27.

NOTES AND QUESTIONS

1. The intersection of PGD and disabilities often raises concerns about two "Ds" — definitions and dollars. As to the latter, the GPPC report asks whether the increasing use of PGD to avoid serious illness will result in fewer resources being devoted to the study and search for cures for "avoidable" disabilities. An economic policymaker could argue that resources are better spent giving access to PGD than to funding a lifetime of health care for a seriously ill individual. Some bioethicists have expressed alarm at this possible shift of resources as a "dystopia [where] . . . people with disabilities fear they may simply be more lonely. And less money may be devoted to cures and education." *See* Amy Harmon, *The Problem With an Almost-Perfect Genetic World*, N.Y. TIMES, Nov. 20, 2005, at 4(1). Does this reasoning make sense to you? Can you think of other avoidable diseases that support or conflict with this paradigm?

A further comment on dollars for access. As with all ART, embryo screening using PGD is expensive and therefore currently only available to those who can afford the hefty price tag. We already know that IVF runs around $12,000 per cycle. PGD costs around $3,000 per cycle, adding considerably to the overall cost of access to these technologies. Since IVF is required before PGD can be performed (because the embryos must be created in the laboratory in order to study their make-up), this sophisticated screening technology will be limited to those wealthy enough to pay cash or lucky enough to have insurance coverage. For families who lack the resources to access PGD to avoid passing a genetic mutation, will they face the double whammy of crushing health care debt plus increased discrimination from a society that views the disability as preventable? For a thoughtful discussion of the intersection of disability and prenatal genetic testing see Mary A. Crossley, *Choice, Conscience, and Context*, 47 HAST. L.J. 1223 (1996).

2. *Defining Disability.* Defining and determining whether some health-related condition is a disability occupies many a lawmaker, judge, lawyer, and disability-rights advocate. Some in the disability rights community have expressed concern

that as more and more prospective parents access PGD, the definition of "disability" will broaden across society. As one scholar posited, the advent of PGD and other prenatal diagnostic techniques poses a "fear of elimination" in those living with disabilities as parents select against more and milder anomalies. *See* Suzanne Holland, *Selecting Against Difference: Assisted Reproduction, Disability and Regulation*, 30 FLA. ST. L. REV. 401 (2003). *See also* Erik Parens & Adrienne Asch, *The Disability Rights Critique of Prenatal Genetic Testing: Reflections and Recommendations*, in PRENATAL TESTING AND DISABILITY RIGHTS (Parens & Asch, eds., 2000).

Should it be up to prospective parents to define for themselves what level of function they would ideally want for their child? Not surprisingly, not all parents agree about whether a condition that diminishes a child's capacity (relative to the vast majority of other children) is in fact a disability. In some cases, even if parents agree that some condition is a disability, they may actively choose to select *for* the condition, as the story below illustrates.

In the summer of 2003, an Australian fertility clinic announced that it had used PGD to screen out embryos carrying a gene that would predispose its carriers to deafness. That announcement prompted an outcry from disabilities activists, who noted that deafness is neither life-threatening nor a certainty for those who carry the gene. Moreover, they argued that if PGD were to come into wide use for such purposes, it could reduce the deaf population and isolate a thriving culture. *See* Melissa Healy, *Fertility's New Frontier: Advanced Genetic Screening Could Help Lead to the Birth of a Healthy Baby*, L.A. TIMES, July 21, 2003, at 6(1).

In another ART story involving deafness, long-time partners Sharon and Candy sought the services of a sperm bank in order to have a child that resembled them — deaf. The sperm bank told the couple that congenital deafness is precisely the sort of condition that would eliminate a prospective donor from their ranks, thus they had no eligible donors. Determined to maximize the chances that their child would be deaf, Sharon and Candy turned to a deaf friend who agreed to serve as a donor. Six year later, the couple were parents to a daughter and a son, both deaf. See Liz Mundy, *A World of Their Own*, WASH. POST, March 31, 2002, at W22. Even though Sharon and Candy did not use PGD to select for deaf children, their story did stir emotions about the intentional diminishment of offspring using ARTs. One woman who read the couple's story in the Washington Post wrote:

> As the parent of two profoundly deaf children who hear and speak beautifully thanks to cochlear implants, I was angered by Liza Mundy's article . . . about two women who deliberately sought to have a second deaf child. My daughters never learned sign language and don't need it to communicate. Thanks to their ability to use the hearing from their implants to the maximum, they are succeeding alongside their peers in school both academically and socially, even conversing on the phone with ease.

> Sharon . . . and Candy . . . and others in the deaf culture are quick to take advantage of government-provided benefits to those with disabilities, yet claim, at the same time, that deafness is not a disability but, rather, a culture. My daughters will be able to be fully contributing members of society rather than financial burdens.

Melissa Chaikof, *Like Mother, Like Child*, Letters, WASH. POST, June 9, 2002, at W2. Another reader minced no words in sharing his views:

> That three people (I include the sperm donor) could deliberately deprive another person of a natural faculty is monstrous and cruel and reveals their basic resentment toward people who can hear. There are laws that give access to medical care for children of parents who would deny it on religious grounds. There should be similar protections for children subject to the abuse of being genetically programmed to replicate the disabilities of misguided parents.

John Sproston, *Like Mother, Like Child*, Letters, WASH. POST, June 9, 2002, at W2.

These harsh words are spoken in response to a perception that parents have intentionally harmed their children by actively seeking out a genetically based diminishment. The deaf women strongly object to the classification of deafness as a disability, arguing that it is a cultural identity, not a medical disability. They maintain they will be better parents to a deaf child than to a hearing one because they will be better able to talk to the child, to understand the child's emotions. Even accepting deafness as an identity rather than a disability, the women's critics would still argue that the limits of reproductive liberty do not permit a parent to intentionally limit a child's potential. Do you agree? If procreative liberty does not allow a parent to select for a disability, then perhaps it also requires parents to select against such disabilities whenever possible. Perhaps the same outrage expressed at the deaf women could emerge toward parents who failed to select against a genetic disease or disability. Imagine the diminished tolerance for disability in such a world.

The case of so-called "intentional diminishment" has been discussed in the context of a handful of genetically-based conditions, including deafness and dwarfism. Dwarfism, or achondroplasia, can now be detected using PGD, and reportedly parents with the syndrome have elected to screen *for* the anomaly in their quest for parenthood. *See* Darshak M. Sanghavi, *Wanting Babies Like Themselves, Some Parents Choose Genetic Defects*, N.Y. TIMES, Dec. 5, 2006, at D5.

One final story completes our discussion. Remember the Chicago-based PGD expert who pioneered the technique of screening embryos for HLA-matching to serve as stem cell donors for ailing siblings? Dr. Yury Verlinksy reported that a couple once asked him to screen their embryos for Down Syndrome so they could select *for* the affected embryos. Why, you ask? The couple explained to Dr. Verlinsky that they already had a son with Down Syndrome and they wanted to provide him a similar sibling. The doctor flatly refused to assist the couple. See Melissa Healy, *Fertility's New Frontier: Advanced Genetic Screening Could Help Lead to the Birth of a Healthy Baby*, L.A. TIMES, July 21, 2003, at 6(1).

If a parent uses PGD to birth a child with what is commonly thought to be a sensory or mobility disability, should the child have the legal right to recover damages against the parent for a diminished life? *See* Kristen Rabe Smolensky, *Creating Children with Disabilities: Parental Tort Liability for Preimplantation Genetic Interventions*, 60 HAST. L.J. 336 (2008). How about criminal prosecution? Should the parents who screen for so-called intentional diminishment prosecuted for child abuse? *See* Jacob M. Appel, *Genetic Screening and Child Abuse: Can PGS Rise to the Level of Criminality?*, 80 U.M.K.C. L. Rev. 373 (2011).

b.   PGD and Adult-Onset Diseases

The use of PGD for medical reasons is most often associated with detection of serious illnesses that will have lifelong health implications for any affected child. Diseases such as cystic fibrosis, Tay-Sachs, Down Syndrome, muscular dystrophy and hemophilia, to name a few of the genetic-based syndromes that PGD can detect, take hold from the moment of birth or very soon thereafter. As we learn more about the genetic nature of disease, we understand that many infirmities that plague the human body are predetermined by genes, even if the symptoms of the disease do not present until adulthood.

Over the past two decades, scientists have discovered the identity and chromosomal placement of many individual genes which are associated with particular disorders that do not manifest until adulthood. In some cases, the presence of the gene or a mutation in its structure means that the individual *will* develop the disease (provided the person survives into adulthood). In other cases, the gene merely predisposes the individual, meaning the affected person *may* develop the disease (but has a greater likelihood than the average person). An example of a disease certain to manifest if the gene is present is Huntington's disease, a life-threatening illness that causes degeneration of brain cells. Symptoms of Huntington's, including loss of motor control and decreased mental capacity, generally begin to appear in the third or fourth decade of life, when a person is in his or her 20s or 30s. Huntington's is an autosomal dominant disease, meaning that an affected individual has a 50% chance of passing the gene to offspring. With the discovery of the gene for Huntington's (located on the fourth chromosome), physicians can test embryos in an affected family and know for certain whether the child will eventually develop the disease.

An example of a gene that predisposes a person to disease is the gene associated with certain forms of breast cancer. BRCA1 and BRCA2 (breast cancer genes 1 and 2) are two tumor suppressor genes that, when functioning normally, help repair damage to DNA (a process that also prevents tumor development). In 1994, researchers discovered that women who carry mutations of BRCA1 or BRCA2 are at higher risk of developing both breast and ovarian cancer than women who do not have these genetic mutations. Currently, women with BRCA1 mutations account for 5% of all breast cancer cases. Though the science is still evolving, researchers believe that the presence of the BRCA 1 or 2 gene means that a woman has an 87% chance of developing breast cancer before the age of 60. Today, using PGD, a parent can learn about the presence of the breast cancer gene in embryos. A handful of reports indicate the successful use of PDG to birth children free of the BRCA anomaly. *See* Philippa Brice, *First UK Birth Following PGD for Hereditary Breast Cancer*, PGH Foundation, Jan. 9, 2009, available at: http://www. phgfoundation.org/news/4445/.

Another advance using PGD to detect adult-onset diseases came from Dr. Yury Verlinsky, the physician who helped a group of parents select for tissue-matched siblings for their ailing children. In February 2002 Dr. Verlinsky and his colleagues announced the first birth of an infant whose parents used PGD to screen for the gene that causes early-onset Alzheimer disease. In the case, a 30-year-old woman with a family history of the disease, tested positive for the mutation linked to early-onset Alzheimer's. Dr. Verlinsky tested her embryos for the presence of the mutation, described as a "predisposing gene mutation," and transferred only the unaffected embryos into the uterus. The woman gave birth to a healthy child, free of the predisposing gene. *See* Yury Verlinsky et al., *Preimplantation Diagnosis for Early-Onset Alzheimer Disease Caused By V717L Mutation*, 287 JAMA 1018 (2002). This report, and the concept of screening for adult-onset and predisposition genes, caused many to consider the ethics of such a practice. In an editorial that accompanied Dr. Verlinsky's report, the commentators analyze the case from the dual perspectives of the child and the mother. From the child's perspective, the authors express concern:

> The study by Verlinsky and colleagues . . . brings renewed concern to the issue of what does, or should, constitute ethically acceptable assisted reproduction. The authors have provided a woman with the opportunity to have a child free of an autosomal dominant form of Alzheimer disease (AD) . . . However, the mutation in her family confers onset of the disease during the fourth decade. The woman was 30 years old when the procedure was performed, which means that she will likely manifest early symptoms of AD while this child is in the early, formative childhood years. In the report on this family describing the mutation, the patient's sister was the relative in whom the mutation was first identified. One of the sister's first manifestations was difficulty in caring for her 2 children. By 5 years after the onset of symptoms, she was placed in an assisted-living facility. Much like her sister, the woman in the report by Verlinsky et al most likely will not be able to care for or even recognize her child in a few years. Analogously, women who are dying of cancer while their children are still young grieve greatly because they will not be able to see their children grow up, participate in their lives, or help protect them from harm. It is precisely these parental rights and responsibilities that are considered to be sufficiently compelling reasons for establishing an upper age limit for postmenopausal assisted reproduction. Moreover, a child living under these circumstances would be burdened by the mother's progressive and eventually profound debilitation and eventual premature demise. Of note, if this same child were orphaned, current adoption regulations would prevent this same childless couple from adopting.

Dena Towner & Roberta Springer Loewy, *Ethics of Preimplantation Diagnosis For A Woman Destined to Develop Early On-Set Alzheimer Disease*, 287 JAMA 1038 (2002). Drs. Towner and Loewy go on to critique the ethics of the mother's decision:

> . . . [T]his parent's ethical responsibility can be interpreted in at least 2 ways. One interpretation is that by resorting to selective preimplantation, the prospective parent was behaving in an ethically responsible manner by conceiving a child free of her own genetic predisposition for early-onset AD. While this is a laudable goal, it is not sufficient to satisfy this mother's ethical obligations because this interpretation is so narrow; it defines this woman's ethical responsibility solely in terms of disease prevention.

Presumably, ethical responsibility is much broader. An alternative interpretation questions the purposive choice of bringing into the world a child for whom the mother will, with near certainty, be unable to provide care. The differences between these 2 interpretations of ethical responsibility are stark, but both rest on assumptions made about reproduction — is it a privilege or is it an unquestionable and inalienable right? Is it a mere want, a deeply held desire, or a need so profound and fundamental as to trump the rights or needs of others? While it may be extremely uncomfortable to question some of the most cherished and deepest-held assumptions, not doing so risks narrowing and distorting our understanding of a situation, the range of available alternatives, and their consequences, thereby reducing the ability to craft responsive and responsible decisions.

NOTES AND QUESTIONS

1.   Do you think the woman in Dr. Verlinsky's report should have refrained from procreating altogether? After all, she knew that she was soon going to be unable to care for a child and that she would likely die during the child's minority (her affected brother died of Alzheimer's at age 39). Or do you believe she had the right to reproduce and she did so in the most responsible manner?

2.   Screening for adult-onset diseases is currently in its infancy, with only a handful of diseases detectible through PGD. But one can imagine a future in which many diseases will be detectable. The question, as later posed by Drs. Towner and Loewy, is just because we can screen for disease, should we? By increasing the "imperfections" we screen for (and presumably select against) will we grow increasingly intolerant of disease and disability in our society? Also, will research on cures and therapy be diverted to focus exclusively on detection and selection? These same questions are posed when PGD for serious lifelong illnesses is analyzed, but there is an important difference in the case of adult-onset diseases: a child born with a disease gene will enjoy decades of healthy life before any symptoms will arise, decades in which a cure or treatment could be discovered. Importantly, cures and treatments for certain diseases often give rise to therapies for other illnesses. By eradicating genetic diseases from our gene pool, are we foolishly abandoning curative medicine or are we aiding in the "natural" selection of the fittest? Should "survival of the fittest" begin with the embryo?

3.   Using Preimplantation Genetic Diagnosis to Achieve Pregnancy

The controversy surrounding PGD tends to center on its use to cure and avoid illness, but in truth these uses represent a small fraction of the overall number of embryo screenings. The most widely reported indication for PGD is infertility — more specifically, inability to achieve conception and delivery even after cycles of IVF. With the increasing popularity and use of IVF, fertility doctors have observed that certain patients fail to become pregnant, despite numerous IVF cycles and normal blood and hormone readings. A look at the embryos of these patients revealed the likely reason for their infertility: many of the embryos had aneuploidy, an extra or missing chromosome which often prevents the embryo from developing.

Researchers hypothesized that aneuploidy could explain infertility in many of their infertility patients, and thus commenced a study to investigate this hypothesis. An early study looked at three categories of patients: 1) patients with recurrent pregnancy loss (2 or more losses), 2) patients of advanced maternal age (38 years or older), and 3) patients with repeated failed IVF cycles (3 or more cycles in which no pregnancy resulted).

The embryos of the study patients were studied using PGD and the researchers' thesis was confirmed. Over half of the embryos of older woman and two-thirds of those of patients with pregnancy loss and failed cycles were chromosomally abnormal. Moreover, once the aneuploidic embryos were identified and deselected, thus allowing only chromosomally healthy embryos to be transferred, the pregnancy rates increased by nearly double. *See* Lawrence Werlin et al., *Preimplantation Genetic Diagnosis as Both a Therapeutic and Diagnostic Tool in Assisted Reproductive Technology*, 80 FERTILITY & STERILITY 467 (2003). A later study, however, yielded a contrary conclusion. In a multicenter study with far more women enrolled, researchers found that PGD did not increase but significantly reduced the rates of ongoing pregnancies and live births in women of advanced maternal age. *See* Sebastiaan Mastenbroek et al., *In Vitro Fertilization and Preimplantation Genetic Screening*, 357 NEW ENG. J. MED. 9 (2007).

Even if PGD does not boost pregnancy rates, it still gives patients insight into whether their embryos display chromosomal abnormalities. Armed with this knowledge, physicians may be able to save their patients from repeated IVF cycles by using PGD early on to diagnose the presence of aneuploidic embryos. If a couple's embryos show a high propensity toward aneuploidy, their doctor can begin dialogue about egg or sperm donation, or even adoption. But the routine use of PGD as part of infertility treatment has its own set of ethical concerns. PGD as a method of screening embryos for aneuploidy is still considered experimental, so its safety record remains in the testing phase. So far, studies indicate that children born following PGD are as healthy as other infants born in the general population, but a larger number of births may reveal hidden safety concerns. *See* Yury Verlinsky et al., *Over a Decade of Experience with Preimplantation Genetic Diagnosis: A Multicenter Report*, 82 FERTILITY & STERILITY 292 (2004) (reporting the prevalence of congenital malformations in the majority of PGD children is not different from population prevalence of 5%-6%). If PGD does become associated with a slight increase in infant birth defects, can its continued use be justified on the ground that it prevents far more birth defects than it causes?

The notion of discarding "defective" embryos still gives a start to many people. Whether because of a genetic disease, an incompatible tissue-type for an ailing child, or an abnormal number of chromosomes, the active deselection of embryos is a morally nettlesome area. In the U.S., lawmakers have grappled with these morally weighty issues, producing a smattering of laws in their wake. The legal landscape surrounding gender and genetic selection follows.

SECTION II: THE CURRENT STATE OF THE LAW

The laws governing gender and genetic selection, much like the use of PGD, are best described as sporadic and emerging. Unlike the British system in which a centralized authority uniformly regulates virtually all ART activities, the U.S. has no similar governing structure. Instead, a patchwork of federal and state laws offer guidance on the limits of embryo manipulation, a process that often accompanies gender and genetic selection. While these laws were not generally enacted with PGD or sex selection in mind, they serve as a starting place for investigating the legal landscape surrounding gender and genetic selection. The following excerpt from the Genetics & Public Policy Center summarizes the current oversight of PGD. As you read about the various legal structures in place, consider whether these same structures could be applied to all ARTs.

Genetics & Public Policy Center
Preimplantation Genetic Diagnosis: A Discussion of Challenges, Concerns, and Preliminary Options Related to the Genetic Testing of Human Embryos
7-10 (January 2004)

Federal Oversight of PGD

The federal government does not typically directly regulate the practice of medicine, leaving such oversight to the states. Nevertheless, there are a variety of mechanisms that governmental agencies use to regulate or to influence the safety and availability of health care services and medical products. These include requirements for safety and effectiveness testing, outcome reporting and oversight of clinical research. However, Congress has not explicitly authorized federal regulation of PGD.

PGD sits at the intersection of two technologies with a confusing regulatory status: assisted reproduction and genetic testing. To the degree that there is federal oversight of PGD or its component technologies, it is "derivative" — that is, it is derived from existing statutes having broader applicability. This section will briefly describe existing government oversight related to PGD. To the extent that there are gaps in oversight, new regulations or laws may be required.

Three federal agencies within the U.S. Department of Health and Human Services oversee areas related to PGD: the Centers for Disease Control and Prevention (CDC), the Food and Drug Administration (FDA) and the Center for Medicare and Medicaid Services (CMS, formerly known as the Health Care Financing Administration).

Centers for Disease Control and Prevention

CDC implements the 1992 Fertility Clinic Success Rate and Certification Act (FCSRCA). This law requires clinics that provide IVF services to report pregnancy success rates annually to the federal government. The FCSRCA requires clinics to report data concerning the type of assisted reproduction procedure used, the medical diagnosis leading to IVF treatment, the number of cycles of IVF attempted, whether fresh or frozen embryos were used, the number of embryos transferred in each cycle, the number of pregnancies achieved and the number of live births. The statute does not require clinics to report the health status of babies born as a result of the procedure or the use of diagnostic tests such as PGD . . .

Food and Drug Administration

FDA regulates drugs and devices, including those used as part of IVF treatments (such as drugs to induce ovulation and laboratory instruments used in IVF). Depending on the type of product, FDA may require submission of data from clinical studies (premarket review) and agency approval before the product may be sold.

Some of the products used by clinical laboratories to perform genetic tests are regulated as medical devices by FDA. However, most genetics laboratories develop their own tests, and FDA's jurisdiction over these so-called "home brew" tests has been a subject of debate. FDA does not currently regulate home brew tests, although it does regulate certain components that laboratories use to make them. Given the existing confusion about FDA's jurisdiction over genetic testing in general, there is uncertainty regarding its authority to regulate PGD tests.

FDA also regulates human tissues intended for transplantation. The agency's statutory authority is limited to preventing disease transmission. FDA regulations require facility registration, screening to detect infectious diseases, record keeping and the proper handling and storage of tissues. FDA can inspect tissue banks and order the recall or destruction of tissue found to be in violation of regulations. Recently, FDA has decided to extend this form of limited regulatory oversight to reproductive tissues under certain circumstances.

In addition, FDA regulates certain human tissue-based therapies as "biological products," such as tissues that are manipulated extensively or are used in a manner different from their original function in the body. However, FDA has not determined that reproductive tissues are "biological products" when used for IVF or PGD procedures and has not required premarket review for these tissues. Whether FDA has the legal authority under current statutes to take such a position, and whether it would choose to do so even if it did, is an open question.

Although FDA regulates claims a manufacturer may make about an approved product, it does not have authority to regulate the actual uses of approved products by physicians. Such decisions are considered part of medical practice. Thus, even if FDA required premarket approval for the reproductive tissue or the genetic tests used as part of PGD and limited the claims that could be made about them, the agency could not restrict the actual use of these products by PGD providers.

Center for Medicaid and Medicare Services

CMS implements the Clinical Laboratory Improvement Amendments of 1988 (CLIA). CLIA was enacted in order to improve the quality of clinical laboratory services. Although it is administered by CMS, it applies to clinical laboratories regardless of whether or not they service Medicaid and Medicare beneficiaries. CLIA defines a "clinical laboratory" as a laboratory that examines materials "derived from the human body" in order to provide "information for the diagnosis, prevention, or treatment of any disease or impairment of, or the assessment of the health of, human beings."

CLIA includes requirements addressing laboratory personnel qualifications, documentation and validation of tests and procedures, quality control standards and proficiency testing to monitor laboratory performance. CMS has not taken a position regarding whether laboratories engaged in IVF (sometimes called embryology or embryo laboratories) are "clinical laboratories" within the meaning of the statute. CMS has similarly not taken a position regarding whether laboratories that engage in the genetic analysis component of PGD are subject to regulation as clinical laboratories.[10]

The outstanding question is whether the genetic tests performed in PGD laboratories provide information that will be used to diagnose, treat or prevent disease or to assess human health. Some within the agency worry that including PGD within the definition would require CMS to take the position that an embryo meets the legal definition of a human being, although it is unclear whether this concern is well-founded since neither the agency nor any court has had occasion to formally address it. In addition, IVF providers argue that their activities constitute the practice of medicine and are not within the scope of CLIA.

If CLIA were applied and enforced with respect to laboratories performing embryo biopsy, then the laboratories would need to comply with the rules applicable to all other clinical laboratories, including those relating to personnel, record keeping, documentation, specimen handling and other quality control and assurance measures. The federal government also would have the authority to inspect PGD laboratories and review their records, and to impose sanctions on those not complying with the regulations . . .

Federal Oversight of Research

Research carried out at institutions supported with federal funds is subject to federal requirements for protecting human research subjects. These requirements also are mandatory for research to support an application to FDA for product approval. However, they are not mandatory for privately funded research (which includes research supported by foundations) that is unrelated to a request for an FDA approval, though a company or research institution may have internal guidelines that offer protections for human subjects.

As it now stands, any research on PGD techniques involving human subjects would probably fall outside federal requirements for protecting human research

---

[10] According to an updated report by the Genetics and Public Policy Center, "CMS has taken the position . . . that PGD is not covered by CLIA but rather 'is an assessment of a product and therefore falls under FDA's oversight of reproductive tissue.' Thus, laboratories that perform genetic analysis for PGD are not subject to regulation as clinical laboratories under CLIA." Susannah Baruch, David Kaufman, Kathy Hudson, *Genetic Testing of Embryos: Practices and Perspectives of US In Vitro Fertilization Clinics*, 89 Fertility & Sterility 1053, 58 (2008). - Ed.

subjects. First, there is a law against providing federal funding for research involving the creation or destruction of human embryos. Second, since FDA does not currently require premarket approval for PGD services, private research into PGD techniques that use human subjects also would fall outside the agency's purview.

State Regulation

No state has enacted laws that directly address PGD. In general, states have considerable authority to make laws and regulations that govern the practice of medicine. Some states have passed laws related to assisted reproductive technology (ART). They are mainly concerned with defining parentage, ensuring that the transfer or donation of embryos is done with informed consent or ensuring insurance coverage for fertility treatment. Some states prohibit the use of embryos for research purposes and one state, Louisiana, prohibits the intentional destruction of embryos created via IVF. For the most part, states have not assumed oversight responsibilities for fertility clinics.

For laboratories, states can create their own regulatory schemes that go beyond the federal mandates, but most states have not included laboratories that conduct IVF or PGD in their laboratory oversight duties. However, New York is in the process of developing standards for laboratories that will include oversight of the genetic tests associated with PGD.

Under the FCSRCA, CDC developed a model state program for certifying laboratories that work with human embryos. It includes standards for procedures, record keeping and laboratory personnel and criteria for inspection and certification. According to CDC, no state has formally adopted the model program . . .

Self-Regulation by Professional Organizations

Medical and scientific professional organizations present another opportunity for oversight of PGD. These groups, which generally comprise members of a particular occupation or specialty, can serve a variety of functions. They can educate members about advances in the field, develop guidelines addressing appropriate conduct or practices and impose standards of adherence that are a prerequisite for membership.

For the most part, however, such standards are voluntary, in that an individual can choose not to belong to the organization and therefore avoid the obligation to follow the standards. Professional organizations also typically do not have authority to sanction members for noncompliance. Unless the organization is specifically authorized by the federal government to act on the government's behalf in administering and enforcing government standards, actions of the professional organization do not have the force of law.

For PGD, a few different professional organizations have relevant expertise and either currently possess or could in the future develop PGD-specific guidelines or standards. For example, the American Society for Reproductive Medicine (ASRM) is a professional organization whose members are health professionals engaged in reproductive medicine. ASRM issues policy statements, guidelines and opinions regarding a variety of medical and ethical issues that reflect the thinking of the organization's various practice committees. These documents, while not binding on members, may be viewed as evidence of standards of practice in legal settings.

In 2001 ASRM issued a practice committee opinion addressing PGD stating that PGD "appears to be a viable alternative to post-conception diagnosis and pregnancy termination." It further states that while it is important for patients be aware of "potential diagnostic errors and the possibility of currently unknown long-term consequences on the fetus" from the biopsy procedure, "PGD should be regarded as an established technique with specific and expanding applications for standard clinical practice." ASRM has also issued an ethics committee opinion cautioning against the use of PGD for sex selection in the absence of a serious sex-linked disease . . .

One organization has recently formed to focus specifically on PGD. The PGD International Society (PGDIS), founded in 2003 in the United States, was created to promote PGD and to organize meetings and workshops on PGD research. PGDIS may take on additional functions in the future.

An international organization, the European Society for Human Reproduction and Embryology (ESHRE), tracks PGD outcomes on a voluntary basis, but captures primarily European data. ESHRE is an organization comprising individuals active in the field of reproductive medicine and science and is dedicated to facilitating the study and analysis of all aspects of human reproduction and embryology. ESHRE has over 4000 members, including some U.S. physicians and scientists engaged in PGD efforts . . .

NOTES AND QUESTIONS

1. *Federal Regulation of Trait Selection.* The Genetics & Public Policy Center report explains the reach of federal law governing trait selection as largely "derivative" (that is, not specific to the activity, but derived from laws having broader applicability) and "supervisory" (authorizing federal agencies to oversee certain activities in the laboratory and clinical settings), but not directly regulating the medical practices that comprise trait selection, such as sperm sorting and PGD. The lack of specific federal regulation does not mean that the federal government is absent in either the debate or the activities surrounding trait selection. As we have seen, the President's Council on Bioethics has been active in drafting reports addressing the legal, medical, social and ethical aspects of trait selection. See The President's Council on Bioethics, *Beyond Therapy: Biotechnology and the Pursuit of Happiness* (October 2003). In addition, the federal power of the purse cannot be denied. As we shall see in more detail in Chapter 9, the federal government has been largely unwilling to fund research involving human embryos, arguably shifting research and its oversight to private enterprises. Thus, even when the federal government fails to act, it can have an impact on the progress and direction of ART research.

Scholars have debated the merits of formally regulating PGD since its introduction in the ART world. As expected, views are across the board. For an argument that the federal government should create an independent agency to monitor and regulate the use of PGD, *see* Jaime King, *Predicting Probability: Regulating the Future of Preimplantation Genetic Screening*, 8 YALE J. HEALTH POL'Y L. & ETHICS 283 (2008). For an argument that regulation of PGD would negatively impact women by delineating categories of good and bad motherhood, *see* Kimberly M. Mutcherson, *Making Mommies: Law, Pre-Implantation Genetic Diagnosis, and the Complications of Pre-Motherhood*, 18 COLUM. L. GENDER & L. 313 (2008). For an argument that oversight by private medical professionals is preferable to government regulation of the technology, *see* Donna M. Gitter, *Am I My Brother's Keeper? The Use of Preimplantation Genetic diagnosis to Create a Donor of Transplantable Stem Cells for an Older Sibling Suffering From a Genetic Disorder*, 13 GEO. MASON L. REV. 975 (2006). What are your views on the role of the federal and state governments' regulation of PGD? Can you think of existing regulatory schemes that could serve as good models for regulation? How about existing models we should avoid?

What if Congress did pass a law prohibiting PGD for sex selection? Or prohibited any research that "might cause harm to human embryos?" Or outlawed PGD for tissue-typing that was not for the purpose of detecting a genetic disease in the embryo? Would these laws be valid? Recall our discussion in Chapter 2 about reproductive liberty and the right to be free from governmental interference with the "decision whether to bear or beget a child." *Eisenstadt v. Baird*, 405 U.S. 438, 453 (1972). One commentator has analyzed the potential interaction between our existing constitutional jurisprudence and laws prohibiting the use of trait selection modalities:

> Where certain fundamental rights are involved, the Court held in *Roe v. Wade* "that regulations limiting these rights may be justified only by a compelling state interest." The Court specifically noted the burdens of carrying, delivering and raising a child and concluded that a mother's interests in avoiding these burdens were significant enough to outweigh the state's interest of protecting the embryo. Therefore, it seems logical that this analysis would extend to the decision to use PGD to select for serious medical conditions that may give rise to such burdens, and that a standard of strict scrutiny would be applied to ensure that the state is "pursuing a goal important enough to warrant use of a highly suspect tool." However, the decision may be more complex because IVF separates the embryo from the womb. Therefore, if the embryo is viewed as a separate and physically discrete unit, it may be held to have rights independent of the mother. Nevertheless, this standard of strict scrutiny that the court applies when a state attempts to regulate requires a showing of a "proximate and inherently dangerous degree of harm." If such a compelling state interest does exist, the Court has stated that the restrictions that attempt to accomplish these interests must be narrowly tailored so as not to be overly inclusive.

> Supporters of prebirth selection rest their arguments on the connection between the expected characteristics of offspring and the decision of whether or not to reproduce. If PGD is used to select what is merely a preferable trait as opposed to a trait that vitally affects the decision of

whether or not to reproduce at all, then it may not be viewed within the ambit of procreative autonomy or as a fundamental right. Thus, the state may regulate to further any rational interest. This rational interest seems to exist where policy is based on the "best interests of the child" principle. Using PGD for sex selection or for selecting for nonmedical traits does not deal directly with the decision of whether an individual can reproduce, but rather it deals with the product of their decision to reproduce. Because of the Supreme Court's reluctance to recognize new rights, these types of decisions would appear to fall outside the scope of the substantive due process doctrines founded upon rights traditionally protected within our society.

Jason Christopher Roberts, *Customizing Conception: A Survey of Preimplantation Genetic Diagnosis and the Resulting Social, Ethical, and Legal Dilemmas,* 2002 DUKE L. & TECH. REV. 12, 38-39. Do you agree with this view?

2. *State Regulation of Trait Selection.* The states have been a bit more active in directly addressing the practices associated with trait selection. About half the states have enacted laws regulating research on embryos or fetuses.[11] These laws vary a great deal, with some covering research on aborted fetuses and others

---

[11] The 24 state laws are listed by June Coleman, author of *Playing God or Playing Scientists: A Constitutional analysis of State Laws Banning Embryological Procedures,* 27 Pac. L. J. 1331, 1354 (1996) as follows: Ariz.Rev.Stat.Ann. § 36-2302 (1993) (abolishing experimentation with a conceptus from an induced abortion); Ark.Code Ann. §§ 20-17-801, 20-17-802 (Michie 1991) (limiting the use of fetal tissue); Cal.Health & Safety Code §§ 25956, 25957 (West 1984) (regulating research using fetal tissue which is obtained prior to or subsequent to an abortion); Fla.Stat.Ann. § 390.001(6), (7) (West 1993) (prohibiting research on live fetuses and describing appropriate methods for disposal of fetal remains); Ind.Code Ann. § 16-34-2-6 (West Supp.1995) (criminalizing experimentation on aborted fetuses); Ky.Rev.Stat.Ann. § 436.026 (Baldwin 1993) (banning experimentation on live or viable aborted children); La.Rev.Stat.Ann. §§ 9:121-133 (West 1991) (limiting the use of any product of conception); Mass.Ann-.Laws ch. 112, § 12J (Law.Co-op.1996) (regulating the use of a live conceptus and procedures which are not conducted to determine or preserve the life or health of the conceptus); Me.Rev.Stat.Ann. tit. 22, § 1593 (West 1992) (restricting the use of a conceptus created through in vitro fertilization from the embryonic stage through the fetal stage); Mich.Comp.Laws Ann. §§ 333.2685-2692 (West 1992) (banning nontherapeutic embryological research, not to include diagnostic procedures which determine health, if the procedure substantially jeopardizes the health of the embryo or if the embryo is the subject of a planned abortion); Minn.Stat.Ann. §§ 145.421, 145.422 subd. 1, 2 (West 1992) (prohibiting research or experimentation on a conceptus when the research or experimentation is harmful to the conceptus); Mo.Ann.Stat. § 188.037 (Vernon 1983) (banning experimentation and research on fetuses prior to and subsequent to an abortion); Mont.Code Ann. § 50-20-108(3) (1991) (preventing research or experimentation on any premature, live infant, except for therapeutic purposes); Neb.Rev.Stat. §§ 28-342, 28-346 (1989) (restricting experimentation on aborted children); N.H.Rev.Stat.Ann. § 168-b:15 (1994) (limiting the maintenance of a preembryo ex utero in a noncryopreserved state to under 15 days and prohibiting the transfer of a research embryo to a uterine cavity); N.M.Stat.Ann. §§ 24-9A-1, 24-9A-3, 24-9A-5 (Michie 1994) (banning research using fetuses or embryos unless the procedure is of no significant risk to the conceptus or minimally risky and benefits the conceptus); N.D.Cent.Code §§ 14-02.2-01, 14-02.2-02 (1991) (prohibiting fetal experimentation); Ohio Rev.Code Ann. § 2919.14 (Anderson 1993) (restricting experimentation on aborted conceptus); Okla.Stat.Ann. tit. 63, § 1-735 (West 1984) (prohibiting experimentation on aborted children); 18 Pa.Cons.Stat.Ann. § 3216 (Supp.1995) (banning nontherapeutic experimentation and medical procedures on any unborn child); R.I.Gen.Laws § 11-54-1 (1994) (limiting experimentation and research on embryos and fetuses); S.D.Codified Laws Ann. § 34-23A-17 (1994) (prohibiting fetal transplantation subsequent to an abortion); Tenn.Code Ann. § 39-15- 208(a) (1991) (limiting experimentation or research on aborted fetuses without the consent from the mother); and Wyo.Stat. § 35-6-115 (1994) (describing penalties for giving away an aborted fetus for experimentation).

addressing the use of embryos for research purposes. Laws in 10 states specifically address embryos created in vitro, presumably using IVF. One state, New Hampshire, imposes minimal regulation, requiring only that the research occur prior to day 14 post-fertilization, and that any embryo donated for research not be implanted in a woman. N.H. Rev. Stat. Ann. § 168-B:15. A plain reading of the law suggests that PGD would not be barred under the New Hampshire law because a couple desiring to investigate the genetic make-up of their embryos using PGD would not be donating the embryo for research.

The remaining nine states ban research on in vitro embryos altogether. The states are: Florida, Louisiana, Maine, Massachusetts, Michigan, Minnesota, North Dakota, Pennsylvania and Rhode Island. Except in Louisiana, where the sole purpose for which an embryo may be used is human uterine implantation, the eight states that address embryo research do so in the broader context of research involving all pre-birth conceptuses. For example, Florida law provides:

> **(6) Experimentation on fetus prohibited; exception.** — No person shall use any live fetus or live, premature infant for any type of scientific, research, laboratory, or other kind of experimentation either prior to or subsequent to any termination of pregnancy procedure except as necessary to protect or preserve the life and health of such fetus or premature infant.

FLA. STAT. ANN. § 390.0111(6). Does this law prohibit PGD altogether? Does it prohibit PGD for tissue-typing when the embryo is not itself at risk for genetic disease? For a discussion of state embryo research laws, see Lori B. Andrews, *State Regulation of Embryo Stem Cell Research*, Ethical Issues in Human Stem Cell Research, A-1 (Commissioned Paper for the National Bioethics Advisory Commission, January 2000).

Consider the following three state statutes that address fetal experimentation. Is PGD prohibited under any of these statutes? Should it be?

North Dakota Century Code
Title 14. Domestic Relations and Persons
Chapter 14-02.2. Fetal Experimentation

§ 14-02.2-01 Live fetal experimentation — Penalty.

1. A person may not use any live human fetus, whether before or after expulsion from its mother's womb, for scientific, laboratory, research, or other kind of experimentation. This section does not prohibit procedures incident to the study of a human fetus while it is in its mother's womb, provided that in the best medical judgment of the physician, made at the time of the study, the procedures do not substantially jeopardize the life or health of the fetus, and provided the fetus is not the subject of a planned abortion. In any criminal proceeding the fetus is conclusively presumed not to be the subject of a planned abortion if the mother signed a written statement at the time of the study, that the mother was not planning an abortion.

2. A person may not use a fetus or newborn child, or any tissue or organ thereof, resulting from an induced abortion in animal or human research, experimentation,

or study, or for animal or human transplantation.

3. This section does not prohibit or regulate diagnostic or remedial procedures, the purpose of which is to determine the life or health of the fetus involved or to preserve the life or health of the fetus involved, or of the mother involved.

4. A fetus is a live fetus for the purposes of this section when, in the best medical judgment of a physician, it shows evidence of life as determined by the same medical standards as are used in determining evidence of life in a spontaneously aborted fetus at approximately the same stage of gestational development.

5. Any person violating this section is guilty of a class A felony.

Minn. Stat. § 145.422
Chapter 145 Public Health Provisions

145.422 Experimentation or sale

Subdivision 1. Penalty. Whoever uses or permits the use of a living human conceptus for any type of scientific, laboratory research or other experimentation except to protect the life or health of the conceptus, or except as herein provided, shall be guilty of a gross misdemeanor.

Subd. 2. Permitted acts. The use of a living human conceptus for research or experimentation which verifiable scientific evidence has shown to be harmless to the conceptus shall be permitted.

Pennsylvania Consolidated Statutes
Title 18. Crimes and Offenses
Part II, Article B. Offenses Involving Danger to the Person
Chapter 32. Abortion

18 Pa.C.S. §§ 3216 Fetal Experimentation

(a) UNBORN OR LIVE CHILD. — Any person who knowingly performs any type of nontherapeutic experimentation or nontherapeutic medical procedure (except an abortion as defined in this chapter) upon any unborn child, or upon any child born alive during the course of an abortion, commits a felony of the third degree. "Nontherapeutic" means that which is not intended to preserve the life or health of the child upon whom it is performed.

(b) DEAD CHILD. — The following standards govern the procurement and use of any fetal tissue or organ which is used in animal or human transplantation, research or experimentation:

(1) No fetal tissue or organs may be procured or used without the written consent of the mother. No consideration of any kind for such consent may be offered or given. Further, if the tissue or organs are being derived from abortion, such consent shall be valid only if obtained after the decision to abort has been made.

(2) No person who provides the information required by section 3205 (relating to informed consent) shall employ the possibility of the use of aborted fetal tissue or organs as an inducement to a pregnant woman to undergo abortion except that

payment for reasonable expenses occasioned by the actual retrieval, storage, preparation and transportation of the tissues is permitted.

(3) No remuneration, compensation or other consideration may be paid to any person or organization in connection with the procurement of fetal tissue or organs.

(4) All persons who participate in the procurement, use or transplantation of fetal tissue or organs, including the recipients of such tissue or organs, shall be informed as to whether the particular tissue or organ involved was procured as a result of either:

(i) stillbirth;

(ii) miscarriage;

(iii) ectopic pregnancy;

(iv) abortion; or

(v) any other means.

(5) No person who consents to the procurement or use of any fetal tissue or organ may designate the recipient of that tissue or organ, nor shall any other person or organization act to fulfill that designation.

(6) The department may assess a civil penalty upon any person who procures, sells or uses any fetal tissue or organs in violation of this section or the regulations issued thereunder. Such civil penalties may not exceed $5,000 for each separate violation. In assessing such penalties, the department shall give due consideration to the gravity of the violation, the good faith of the violator and the history of previous violations. Civil penalties due under this paragraph shall be paid to the department for deposit in the State Treasury and may be enforced by the department in the Commonwealth Court.

(c) CONSTRUCTION OF SECTION. — Nothing in this section shall be construed to condone or prohibit the performance of diagnostic tests while the unborn child is in utero or the performance of pathological examinations on an aborted child. Nor shall anything in this section be construed to condone or prohibit the performance of in vitro fertilization and accompanying embryo transfer.

Consider drafting a law for your state that, in your view, creates the best regulatory scheme for genetic trait selection.

SECTION III: ETHICAL AND LEGAL DEBATE SURROUNDING GENDER SELECTION

The introduction of new technologies is inevitably accompanied by commentary, both dire and praising, that explores ethical and legal aspects of the scientific advancement. We have seen some of the reactions to sex selection and genetic selection in Section 1 of this Chapter, as we have introduced each technology. What follows is a collection of academic writings exploring gender and genetic selection, concluding with a New York case in which the use of PGD is central to the parties' dispute.

A. Constitutional Analysis

Carl H. Coleman
Is There A Constitutional Right to Preconception Sex Selection?
1 Am. J. Bioethics 27 (2001)

[Professor Coleman's piece is a response to an article by Professor John Robertson entitled *Preconception Gender Selection*, 1 Am. J. Bioethics 2 (2001), in which he discusses the social consequences of preconception gender selection (PGS — for example, sperm sorting or other methods that do not involve destruction or deselection of embryos based on gender). Professor Robertson concludes "the best societal approach would, of course, be to proceed slowly, first requiring extensive studies of safety and efficacy, and then at first only permitting PGS for increasing the gender variety of offspring in particular families." Id. at 6. But, he warns, such an approach might be unavailable because "public policies that bar all nonmedical uses of PGS or restrict it to choosing gender variety in offspring could be found unconstitutional or illegal." *Id.* Professor Coleman questions this assertion.]

The ability to predict how courts will rule on constitutional challenges to governmental regulation of reproductive technologies is limited by the absence of virtually any Supreme Court precedent in the area. Although most commentators agree that the Court would recognize a right to engage in coital reproduction, at least within marriage, it has yet to confront a case in which that proposition has directly been put to the test. Whether a right to procreate would extend to noncoital reproduction is less certain, although a strong argument can be made that the use of reproductive technologies by infertile couples who otherwise could not reproduce is entitled to the same degree of protection as reproduction through sexual intercourse . . .

Governmental limitations on the use of PGS, however, would not prevent anyone from reproducing, nor would they penalize individuals for the exercise of their procreative rights. The claim that such limitations would implicate the right to procreate follows from the argument that because the ability to select offspring gender may be "essential to a couple's decision to reproduce," limitations on access to PGS may lead some people who might otherwise choose to procreate to forego reproduction entirely.

Such an expansive interpretation of procreative liberty would have significant implications. It would severely limit government's ability to regulate not only PGS, but also techniques for selecting trivial offspring characteristics like hair or eye color. More alarmingly, it might protect efforts to both "enhance" and "diminish" a child's capacities through the prenatal manipulation of genes . . . Under Robertson's framework, governmental regulation of all these technologies would be subject to heightened scrutiny whenever at least one person claimed that, without the technique, she would choose not to reproduce at all.

That the harms associated with these techniques may be "speculative or uncertain" does not mean society has no reason to be concerned. . . . [E]fforts to control offspring characteristics threaten to exacerbate social and economic inequalities, promote eugenic tendencies, and fundamentally alter the way that children are viewed . . . Trait selection poses the greatest risks when applied to characteristics that have historically been the basis for damaging stereotypes and social subordination, such as gender, skin color, and sexual orientation (assuming it becomes possible to influence this type of multifactorial trait through preconception intervention). Moreover, consider the plight of a child born of the "wrong" gender in a case where PGS fails. Robertson suggests that programs could "require that any couple or individual seeking PGS receive counseling about the risks of failure and commit to rear a child even if its gender is other than that sought through PGS." But for parents so eager to have a child of a particular gender that they would not reproduce if PGS were unavailable (which, after all, is the premise of Robertson's constitutional claim), can we really take comfort in a promise to treat the child's gender as irrelevant if things do not turn out as planned?

Given the societal stakes, as well as the relatively clean constitutional slate, we should not assume that government's authority to regulate trait selection is as limited as Robertson suggests. To the extent the Supreme Court has recognized a principle of procreative liberty, it has done so in response to limits on the *physical* ability of individuals to control whether or not they reproduce; for example, compulsory sterilization (*Skinner v. Oklahoma*, 316 U.S. 535 [1942]), laws prohibiting contraception (*Griswold v. Connecticut*, 381 U.S. 479 [1965]), or limitations on the availability of abortion (*Planned Parenthood v. Casey*, 505 U.S. 833 [1992]; and *Roe v. Wade*, 410 U.S. 113 ([1973]). That individuals may not be prevented from having children, or compelled to endure unwanted pregnancies, does not mean they have a right to engineer a child to whatever specifications they choose. . . . [T]he ability to have a child is a "basic life activity." The ability to custom design a child through "cosmetic reproductive services" is not.

Moreover, Robertson's expansive formulation of procreative liberty is difficult to reconcile with the Court's increasingly limited interpretation of reproductive rights.

The Court's recent abortion jurisprudence suggests that limits on reproductive decision making are permissible unless they place a "substantial obstacle in the path" of the individual's choice (*Planned Parenthood v. Casey*). In the context of abortion this standard has rightly been criticized as insufficiently protective of the woman's right to decide. (That right is distinguishable from decisions about trait selection, because it implicates issues of bodily autonomy and gender equality in addition to procreative liberty.) Whatever the merits of the standard, however, it is doubtful that the Court would regard limits on the ability to determine the gender of one's child a "substantial obstacle in the path" of the decision to reproduce.

That is not to say that restrictions on trait selection technologies will never raise constitutional concerns. Preventing individuals from controlling certain offspring characteristics might be functionally equivalent to physical restrictions on reproduction, because control over the characteristic would be essential to almost anyone's decision to reproduce. This would probably be the case for restrictions on techniques to avoid transmitting serious genetic disease. A right against "objectively unreasonable" restrictions on trait selection technology, however, is narrower than a right to use any technique deemed "essential" by a particular individual. Such an objective assessment of the burdens of regulation would be consistent with the Court's approach in several areas of constitutional law.

NOTES AND QUESTIONS

1.   Professor Coleman points out the lack of specific case law addressing the question of whether direct prohibitions on the use of preconception gender selection in particular, and ART in general, violate the constitutional principle of procreative liberty. By analogy, we might look to the smattering of federal cases addressing the constitutionality of abortion statutes that prohibit experimentation on an unborn child. In *Margaret S. v. Edwards*, 794 F.2d 994 (5th Cir. 1986), the court invalidated a Louisiana statute that provided in relevant part, "No person shall experiment on an unborn child . . . unless the experimentation is therapeutic to the unborn child." The problem, the court explained, is in the definition of the term "experiment":

> The plaintiffs' expert witness offered unrebutted testimony, which we find quite plausible, that physicians do not and cannot distinguish clearly between medical experiments and medical tests. As the expert witness pointed out, every medical test that is now "standard" began as an "experiment" that became standard through a gradual process of observing the results, confirming the benefits, and often modifying the technique. Thus, as the witness concluded, "we have at one end things that are obviously standard tests and [at] the other end things that are complete experimentation. But in the center there is a very broad area where diagnostic procedures of testing types overlap with experimentation procedures . . . ." Indeed, as the challenged statute itself seems to acknowledge, even medical *treatment* can be reasonably described as both a test and an experiment. This must be true whenever the results of the treatment are observed, recorded, and introduced into the data base that one or more physicians use in seeking better therapeutic methods. The whole distinction between experimentation and testing, or between research and practice, is therefore almost meaningless in the medical context. When one adds to this the fact that some innovative tests or treatments are done on fetal tissue in order to monitor the health of the mother, one can see that physicians who treat pregnant women are being threatened with an inherently standardless prohibition. We therefore think that this statute "simply has *no* core" that unquestionably applies to certain activities, *Smith v. Goguen*, 415 U.S. 566, 578, 94 S.Ct. 1242, 1249, 39 L.Ed.2d 605 (1974) (emphasis in original), and we hold that it is unconstitutionally vague.

794 F.2d at 999. Accord *Jane L. v. Bangerter*, 61 F.3d 1493 (10th Cir. 1995) (fetal experimentation ban provision of Utah statute found impermissibly vague). Do you see how this line of case law could be instructive in resolving the constitutionality of a ban on gender selection? Does your answer depend in part on whether MicroSort and other sperm sorting techniques are considered experimental?

2.   Whatever the legality of a ban on sex selection, do you believe such a prohibition could be enforced in the U.S.? The use of ultrasound to view a fetus's

gender is outlawed in India, but the sheer imbalance of birth rate gender ratios would suggest the practice is fairly widespread in that country. See Gautam N. Allahbadia, *The 50 Million Missing Women*, 19 J. ASSISTED REPRODUCTION & GENETICS 411 (2002). How would a ban on the use of MicroSort or PGD be enforced in this country?

B. Ethical Analysis

Rebecca Dresser
Cosmetic Reproductive Services and Professional Integrity
1 Am. J. Bioethics 11 (2001)

. . . Clinicians will play a pivotal role in determining the availability of [Preconception Sex Selection] PSS. Should physicians and other health professionals offer PSS for nonmedical reasons? Is this a service that falls within the realm of legitimate health care?

Definitions of health and health care are contested and imprecise. Few would argue, however, that PSS to satisfy preferences for gender variety or the gender of firstborn children falls within the definition of health care. The attempt to include PSS as simply another infertility service is strained. Helping people to have children is different from helping people to have a particular kind of child. Because infertility interferes with a basic life activity, one can reasonably argue that it merits the attention of health professionals. The inability to have a child of a particular gender presents no such interference.

Rather than being a form of health care, PSS for nonmedical reasons is like breast augmentation and other forms of cosmetic surgery. Like PSS, people strongly desire cosmetic surgery based on a hope that the intervention will enhance their psychological and social well being. Nevertheless, health insurers exclude cosmetic surgery from coverage, and this exclusion is rarely criticized.

Cosmetic surgery is regarded more as a consumer good than as a medical treatment. It is heavily promoted through advertising, which typically inflates the benefits surgical interventions will bring. Information on risks and "failure rates" is often downplayed. The same pattern is evident with PSS techniques that are currently offered.

The question is whether supplying such services is an appropriate activity for health professionals. It is difficult to distinguish between clinicians furnishing such services and hairdressers or travel agents meeting their clients' demands. In providing cosmetic surgery and PSS, clinicians act as workers in a service industry that caters to consumer preferences.

Although I applaud the move away from the "Doctor knows best" tradition, I question whether medicine should be so strongly influenced by consumer preferences. Society trusts physicians and other health professionals to define and set standards for their work. Society also subsidizes the training and infrastructure enabling them to practice their professions. In turn, clinicians assume some responsibility to use their skills and resources to meet the legitimate health needs of society.

Even if it were found to be safe and reasonably effective, PSS for nonmedical reasons would be far from risk-free. It would reinforce parental expectations that could be damaging to children of both the "right" and "wrong" genders. It would reinforce restrictive gender stereotypes. It would reinforce the same cultural beliefs that lead to female infanticide and neglect in other nations. It would reinforce the conviction that one gender would be superior and one inferior for a particular family.

Clinicians and infertility programs should give careful thought to the issues raised by offering PSS as a medical service. They ought to consider whether this is an appropriate use of their skills and resources in light of the many urgent health needs commanding their attention. They ought to consider whether they want to reinforce the attitudes and beliefs associated with gender preferences. They ought to consider the long-term effects that performing such a service could have on public respect for and trust of the medical profession. In the long run, medicine and society will be better served if professionals exclude cosmetic PSS from the activities they perform.

NOTES AND QUESTIONS

1.   Do you agree with Professor Dresser's assertion that sex selection for nonmedical reasons "is like breast augmentation and other forms of cosmetic surgery?" If so, does it follow that physicians ought not offer these services to patients who desire them, for whatever reason?

2.   One aspect of the sex selection debate focuses on usage — will the technology be used by enough parents to impact gender ratios in the U.S.? We have already seen the gender ratio disparities in other countries (mostly resulting from selective abortion), but it remains a question whether sex selection will be widely adopted in the U.S., and if so, whether the end result will be a disproportionate number of boys. We do know that ultrasonography to visualize the fetus's genitalia and elective abortion are widely available in the U.S., and we have seen no apparent shift in gender ratios as a result. But if selection can be accomplished, either preconception or preimplantation, parents may be more drawn to the technologies.

Author Rosamond Rhodes acknowledges that gender imbalance in the population may turn out to be a harm at some point, but she urges us to consider other effects of preconception sex selection (PSS) that are likely to be beneficial:

1. PSS is likely to be used by parents who want an additional child to be of a gender different from other children in the family. Without ART, "try again" has been the method to achieve that goal. PSS has the social advantage of not adding to society's overpopulation problems.

2. By helping couples achieve the gender balance they want with fewer children, PSS can benefit families by easing the economic and human burdens of providing for a large family. Today, when few enjoy the support of an extended family to help with the chores of everyday life and when both parents are typically employed outside of the home, additional children tax a family's limited resources.

3. Potential parents, that is, autonomous adults, are in the best position to assess the kind of rearing and companionship experiences that would be valuable to them. For those to whom gender makes a significant enough difference to justify PSS, the gender-selected child is likely to provide a more rewarding experience.

4. And children produced by PSS are also more likely to be attentively reared and to have a good childhood, because their parents have chosen the gender that they are more likely to nurture well.

Rosamond Rhodes, *Acceptable Sex Selection*, 1 Am. J. Bioethics 31 (2001).

If you learned that your parents used preconception sex selection to bring about your birth, what would be your reaction? Would you feel the same if the technique was PGD? What if you learned that you are the product of a failed sperm sorting attempt? Your parents hoped for and sought a child of the opposite gender, but here you are. Would this news be any different from learning your parents had hoped for a piano virtuoso or a professional baseball player?

For other views on gender selection see Mary B. Mahowald, Genes, Women, Equality 115-21 (2000); Charles Hanson, *Is Any Form of Gender Selection Ethical?*, 19 J. Assisted Reproduction & Genetics 431 (2002); E. Scott Sills, *Preimplantation Genetic Diagnosis for Elective Sex Selection, The IVF Market Economy, and the Child — Another Long Day's Journey Into Night?*, 19 J. Assisted Reproduction & Genetics 433 (2002).

SECTION IV: ETHICAL AND LEGAL DEBATE SURROUNDING GENETIC SELECTION

A. Ethical Dilemmas Surrounding Genetic Selection

The discussion about gender selection occurs in the realm of clinical reality — we have the technology to choose our children's gender through a variety of methods. Genetic enhancement, sometimes called trait selection, takes us outside the clinical reality to the futuristic and hypothetical. Current technologies do not allow parents to select for benign traits such as hair color, height, perfect pitch, intelligence and a host of qualities that are unique to the human experience. But the lack of active capability does not quell thinking about what may lie ahead. As one scientist observes:

The coming challenges of human genetic enhancement are not going to melt away; they will intensify decade by decade as we continue to unravel our biology, our nature, and the physical universe. Humanity is moving out of its childhood and into a gawky, stumbling adolescence in which it must learn not only to acknowledge its immense new powers, but to figure out how to use them wisely. The choices we face are daunting, but putting our heads in the sand is not the solution.

Gregory Stock, Redesigning Humans: Our Inevitable Genetic Future 17 (2002). Our heads fully out of the sand, we forge ahead.

Maxwell J. Mehlman
The Law of Above Averages: Leveling the New Genetic Enhancement Playing Field
85 Iowa L. Rev. 517 (2000)

. . . Genes are responsible for more than just diseases . . . In conjunction with environmental influences, they engender physical appearance, personality traits, and mental faculties such as cognition and intelligence. The same genetic testing and engineering techniques that are being developed to respond to genetic illness eventually may be employed to identify and alter a person's non-disease traits . . .

In order to comprehend how . . . societal concerns might arise, it is necessary to understand what is meant by genetic enhancement, to consider the many forms of genetic enhancements, and to predict the methods that individuals are likely to employ to acquire them. First, what is "genetic" enhancement? People employ various means in an attempt to improve themselves and their children. Their efforts may affect and may be affected — at least in part — by their genetic inheritance. For example, someone who is attractive by virtue of their genetic good fortune may find it easier to marry an attractive mate and produce attractive children. But for purposes of this paper, an enhancement is deemed "genetic" only when it is the product of biotechnological processes. These include DNA recombination to make pharmacological products, and direct manipulation of genes, such as gene insertion or deletion . . .

If the foregoing paragraph describes what is meant by "genetic" in the context of enhancement, what, then, is the meaning of "enhancement"? Not all genetic interventions are enhancements. Many, and for the time being, almost all, are aimed at treating or preventing disease. A genetic intervention is an "enhancement," however, (1) when it is undertaken for the purpose of improving a characteristic or capability that, but for the enhancement, would lie within what is generally accepted as a "normal" range for humans; or (2) when it installs a characteristic or capability that is not normally present in humans.

Genetic enhancement can occur in a number of ways. It can take the form of somatic enhancements in adults and children, pre-conception enhancement, selective abortion, embryo selection, and germ-line enhancement. Each of these will be described in turn.

Genetic enhancement may produce a *somatic enhancement effect in an adult*. A somatic effect is one that affects the non-reproductive portions of the anatomy, and therefore cannot be inherited by one's children. A classic example of a non-genetic somatic enhancement in adults is the use of drugs to improve athletic and cognitive performance. People occasionally use caffeine and nicotine to improve their concentration, and athletes long have been reported to use performance-enhancing drugs, particularly anabolic steroids, to increase muscle mass. Advances in human genetics will open the door to a new range of somatic enhancements manufactured with genetic technology. Athletes already use genetically-engineered products, like erythropoietin manufactured by recombinant DNA technology, to enhance endurance.

Another type of genetic enhancement is *somatic enhancement in children*. This type of somatic enhancement is exemplified by the reported use of genetically-engineered human growth factor in children of "normal" height. Again, because the effect is somatic, it is not genetically transferred to successive generations.

Genetic enhancement also is made possible by the development of tests to identify genetic characteristics, including non-disease traits that have genetic components. These tests create the possibility of several types of enhancement approaches related to reproductive decision-making. The first of these is *pre-conception enhancement*, in which decisions about whether or not, and with whom, to conceive a child are made on the basis of preconception genetic testing. Just as some people now test themselves to avoid conceiving a child with another person who is a "carrier" for a recessive genetic disorder, prospective mates could test themselves to determine if they are likely to produce offspring who would be desirable in terms of non-disease characteristics. Unsatisfactory test results may cause couples to refrain from marrying or conceiving, at least not without employing genetic manipulations to improve the genetic profile of the offspring. If the couple refrains from genetic manipulations, this is a passive version of enhancement. This technique would not produce a "better" child, but only enable prospective parents to avoid giving birth to a child whose genetic characteristics they deemed to be undesirable. Nevertheless, it qualifies as a genetic enhancement because one may assume that the child's characteristics would be "better" than if reproduction took place without preconception testing of the potential parents.

Enhancement via selective abortion is another passive form of genetic enhancement stemming from genetic testing. With this approach, fetuses are tested in utero and those that do not meet the parents' expectations are aborted. An alternative to selective abortion would be embryo selection for enhancement. This technique combines genetic testing with in vitro fertilization. Embryos are tested before insertion in the womb, and only embryos with advantageous characteristics are implanted.

Finally, and most dramatically, an early-stage embryo might be genetically altered prior to implantation, with DNA inserted or deleted to produce desired traits in the child. If performed at an early-enough stage of embryonic development, the alteration affects all subsequent fetal cells, including germ cells — that is, those that become eggs or sperm. This process yields germ-cell enhancement, in which genetic changes are passed on to successive generations when the enhanced individual reproduces.

It is currently impossible to be certain when these genetic enhancements will become available and how successful they will be. Moreover, there are good reasons for doubting that extensive and successful genetic enhancements are achievable. For example, it may be that somatic enhancements are accompanied by serious adverse side effects. While manipulating embryos genetically may prevent further embryonic development, it is also possible that it may create non-viable or severely impaired organisms. Altering genes that interact with other genes may have unforeseen dangers; enhancing one trait may cause the degradation of another. Finally, the effects of genetic interventions may be negated or transmuted by environmental factors.

Yet uncertainty works both ways. While the availability of some of these technologies is unlikely for several years, particularly those involving the successful genetic manipulation of embryos, there are no obvious insurmountable scientific barriers to genetic enhancement. Methods of genetic enhancement may not confer the benefits that recipients anticipate; but then again, there is a good chance that they might. What if they do? What if the new genetic technologies can significantly improve inherited traits? What might those traits be? They might comprise physical traits like beauty, stature, strength, and stamina; personality characteristics such as charm, cheerfulness, charisma, confidence, and energy; or mental capabilities, including memory, intelligence, and creativity. Ultimately, the aging process too might become subject to genetic manipulation.

These kinds of improvement will be in great demand. But how widely available will the technologies be that make them possible? The answer depends both on how many institutions and professionals are willing and able to provide enhancement services, and on the cost of such enhancements . . . Enhancements performed on embryos, including germ cell enhancement, would be costly since they necessarily impose the cost of in vitro fertilization, which currently costs an average of $37,000 per delivery, onto the cost of the genetic manipulations themselves. Moreover, these manipulations are likely to cost substantially more than the costs of in vitro fertilization (particularly when the technology is first introduced).

It is unlikely that public or private health insurance will cover the costs of genetic enhancement. This assessment seems plausible because insurance policies do not cover costs associated with cosmetic medicine, the most analogous biomedical technology currently available.

The high cost and lack of coverage by third-party payment plans does not, however, suggest that no one will gain access to genetic enhancement. Rather, it merely suggests that, if left to the forces of the marketplace, access will be limited to persons who can purchase it with their own assets. Society will thus divide into those who can afford genetic enhancements and those who can afford little, if any, just as it now divides into those who can and cannot afford cosmetic surgery, prolonged psychotherapy, or private schools.

This resulting division will give rise to two related problems. The first is the problem of *social inequality*. Enhanced individuals will achieve social success more easily than those who remain unenhanced. For example, studies show that people who are tall and physically attractive are more likely to be hired and promoted than people who are short or unattractive. Although Western democratic societies can accommodate a certain degree of inequality, the difference in prospects between the enhanced and the unenhanced could become so pronounced that serious social instability would ensue. Taken to the extreme, enhancements could be installed by manipulating germ lines, resulting in social advantages that are inherited by succeeding generations. This could eventually create a political system dominated by a genetic aristocracy, or "genobility," that possesses a lock on wealth, privilege, and power.

The second problem created by wealth-based access to genetic enhancement is the individual *unfairness* that would arise at the micro level if genetically enhanced individuals competed for scarce resources, or found themselves in conflicts of interest, with persons who were unenhanced. Genetic enhancement could confer a decisive advantage in social interactions. How should society respond to the potential unfairness of these interactions? . . .

NOTES AND QUESTIONS

1. The prospect of genetic enhancement often raises the specter of further inequality in our society because, as Professor Mehlman points out, the expensive technologies and therapies needed for enhancement would likely only be available to those already in a superior economic position. Once enhancements take hold, the economically privileged will further separate from the unenhanced whose genetic make-up places them at a disadvantage to compete for social goods. The concept of genetic enhancement and inequality is further explored in Mark Hall, *Genetic Enhancement, Distributive Justice, and the Goals of Medicine*, 39 SAN DIEGO L. REV. 669 (2002); Michael Shapiro, *The Impact of Genetic Enhancement on Equality*, 34 WAKE FOREST L. REV. 561 (1999); Cf. Daniel L. Tobey, *What's Really Wrong With Genetic Enhancement: A Second Look At Our Posthuman Future*, 6 YALE. J. L. TECH. 54 (2004) (arguing the true harm of genetic enhancement is not increased inequality, which could be solved by insuring access across income groups, but its diminution of human essence).

Professor Mehlman also acknowledges that current access to "life" enhancements such as cosmetic surgery and private schools, is uneven. When it comes to parents' desires to enhance their children, inequalities likewise reign. The phenomenon of "hyperparenting" has driven those of means to provide in-depth music training, sports coaches, private academic tutors, and college preparation programs to their children, to name but a few of the advantaging techniques available in today's market. Are genetic enhancements likely to pose a greater threat to our society than existing inequalities?

Do you hold the same views on pre-conception trait selection as you do on post-birth trait adjustments? Professor Alicia Ouellette writes about some parents' decisions to size, shape, sculpt, and mine children's bodies through the use of nontherapeutic medical and surgical interventions. Focusing on cases involving eye shaping surgery, human growth hormone, liposuction, and growth stunting, she worries that such interventions are treated as a matter of parental choice except in extraordinary cases involving grievous harm. If a parent can sculpt a child to be thinner, taller, or more Caucasian looking, can PGD for trait selection be prohibited on any principled basis? Should we focus instead on the premise that post-birth interventions are acceptable? *See* Alicia Ouellette, *Shaping Parental Authority Over Children's Bodies*, 85 IND. L. J. 955 (2010).

2. A second well-articulated objection to genetic enhancement is the potential for interference with, or diminution of, human nature. Leon Kass, Chair of the President's Council on Bioethics, explains this concern as follows:

> In a word, one major trouble with biotechnical (especially mental) "improvers" is that they produce changes in us by disrupting the normal character of human being-at-work-in-the-world, what Aristotle called *eregeia psyches*, activity of soul, which when fine and full constitutes human flourishing. With biotechnical interventions that skip the realm of intelligible meaning,

we cannot really own the transformations nor experience them as genuinely ours. And we will be at a loss to attest whether the resulting conditions and activities of our bodies and our minds are, in the fullest sense, our own as human.

Leon Kass, *Ageless Bodies, Happy Souls: Biotechnology and the Pursuit of Perfection*, THE NEW ATLANTIS 24 (Spring 2003). For further discussion of the interaction between genetic enhancement and human nature, *see* Michael J. Malinowski, *Choosing the Genetic Makeup of Children: Our Eugenics Past — Present, and Future?* 36 CONN. L. REV. 125 (2003); Michael J. Sandel, *The Case Against Perfection: What's Wrong With Designer Children, Bionic Athletes, and Genetic Engineering*, 293 ATLANTIC MONTHLY 50 (April 2004).

Francis Fukuyama, a Professor of International Political Economy and a member of the President's Council on Bioethics, writes about the "biotech revolution" and its impact on human nature in his book, *Our Posthuman Future*:

> . . . Even if genetic engineering on a species level remains twenty-five, fifty, or one-hundred years away, it is by far the most consequential of all future developments in biotechnology. The reason for this is that human nature is fundamental to our notions of justice, morality, and the good life, and all of these will undergo change if this technology becomes widespread . . .
>
> [H]uman nature is the sum of behavior and characteristics that are typical of the human species, arising from genetic rather than environmental factors . . .
>
> [A]n important reason for the persistence of the idea of the universality of human dignity has to do with what we might call the nature of nature itself. Many of the grounds on which certain groups were historically denied their share of human dignity were proven to be simply a matter of prejudice, or else based on cultural and environmental conditions that could be changed. The notions that women were too irrational or emotional to participate in politics . . . were overturned on the basis of sound, empirical science . . . [M]oral order comes from within human nature itself and is not something that has to be imposed on human nature by culture.
>
> All of this could change under the impact of future biotechnology. The most clear and present danger is that the large genetic variations between individuals will narrow and become clustered within certain distinct social groups. Today, the "genetic lottery" guarantees that the son or daughter of a rich and successful parent will not necessarily inherit the talents and abilities that created conditions conducive to the parent's success . . . But in the future, the full weight of modern technology can be put in the service of optimizing the kinds of genes that are passed on to one's offspring. This means that social elites may not just pass on social advantages but embed them genetically as well. This may one day include not only characteristics like intelligence and beauty, but behavioral traits like diligence, competitiveness, and the like . . .

What the emergence of a genetic overclass will do to the idea of universal human dignity is something worth pondering . . . [T]o the extent that [bright and successful young people] become "children of choice" who have been genetically selected by their parents for certain characteristics, they may come to believe increasingly that their success is a matter not just of luck but of good choices and planning on the part of their parents, and hence something deserved. They will look, think, act, and perhaps even feel differently from those who were not similarly chosen, and may come in time to think of themselves as different kinds of creatures. They may, in short, feel themselves to be aristocrats, and unlike aristocrats of old, their claim to better birth will be rooted in nature and not convention.

FRANCIS FUKUYAMA, OUR POSTHUMAN FUTURE: CONSEQUENCES OF THE BIOTECHNOLOGY REVOLUTION 82-3, 130, 156-57 (2002). Professor Fukuyama's assertions are considered by another pillar of the academic community, Professor Cass Sunstein, a professor at Harvard Law School currently on leave to serve in the White House Office of Information and Regulatory Affairs. He counters:

Inequality is not at the heart of Fukuyama's argument. His real claim is on behalf of "human nature." He thinks that if we understand what human nature is, we will be better equipped to approach the ethical issues raised by biotechnology. There is a sensible and important point in the background. To see it, consider Fukuyama's brief but suggestive treatment of the rights of animals. Dogs, cats, and horses should indeed have the right to be free from cruelty and neglect; and they do have that very right under state law. Still, as Fukuyama urges, no one thinks that dogs, cats, and horses should have the right to vote or to participate in literacy programs. A claim about what a dog is entitled to has everything to do with the kind of creature that a dog is. The same is true for human beings. When we think about human rights, and about what makes those rights distinctive, we can make a great deal of progress by emphasizing distinctly human characteristics.

The problem is that Fukuyama confuses this point with a very different one that has to do with what he sees as the importance, for purposes of assessing biotechnology, of "behavior and characteristics that are typical of the human species, arising from genetic rather than environmental factors." Suppose that it is "typical" for members of the human species, on the basis of genetic factors, to fear flying in airplanes, to respond with violence when insulted, or to die from cancer or heart disease after a certain age. Surely Fukuyama would not object to cultural interventions that would counteract genetic predispositions to fear of flying or to excessive violence. Surely he would not oppose efforts to alter diet so as to counteract the genetic predisposition to die from cancer or heart disease. Why, then, should anyone object to medical technologies that would take people beyond the domain of the "typical" — by, for example, screening out genetic predispositions that lead to preventable illnesses and death? Or suppose that scientists can make human beings taller, healthier, faster, stronger, and smarter than is "typical." Why, exactly, object to that? . . .

I think that Fukuyama's abstract interest in "human nature" and in what is "natural" prevents him from attending enough to what most matters: the concrete consequences, for actual human lives, of biotechnological advances. Sadness, anxiety, and aggressiveness should not be treated or screened out: bad and dark feelings are an essential part of good human lives. But if neuropharmacology can counteract crippling depression, which is far more dire than melancholy, surely it should be applauded . . . Mill was right. If science is able to make human lives healthier, longer, and better, then it is foolish to object in nature's name.

Cass Sunstein, *Keeping Up With the Cloneses*, THE NEW REPUBLIC 32 (May 6, 2002).

3.   *A Parental Duty to Use PGD?* In addition to considering the legal *right* to access PGD for genetic enhancement, scholars are debating the moral *duty* to use such technologies if and when they emerge as safe and effective. In his book, *Enhancing Evolution: The Ethical Case for Making People Better*, British bioethicist John Harris argues "it is not only feasible to use genetic technology to make people more healthy, intelligent and longer-lived, it's our moral duty to do so." Professor Harris considers that "[t]he denial of beneficial enhancements to others, whether they are our children or strangers, would be a breach of two of the most powerful moral principles, they duty to do good and the duty not to harm; whereas the consequences of that denial would leave someone more vulnerable to harm and less able to lead a healthy, fulfilling life." John Harris, ENHANCING EVOLUTION: THE ETHICAL CASE FOR MAKING PEOPLE BETTER 21 (2007). The notion of a parental duty to use PGD to maximize the health of offspring has won supporters and detractors. *See, e.g.*, Janet Malek, *Disability and the Duties of Potential Parents*, 2 ST. LOUIS J. HEALTH L & POL'Y 119 (2008) (advocating The Strong Claim that parents are morally required to use reproductive technologies to reduce the likelihood of birthing children with serious disabilities); MICHAEL SANDEL, THE CASE AGAINST PERFECTION: ETHICS IN THE AGE OF GENETIC ENGINEERING (2007) (critiquing genetic engineering as an erosion of our appreciation for natural gifts and talents; warning the ability to select a child's traits will deform parenting, harming children by transforming them into consumer projects).

The debate over the promises and perils of genetic enhancement will continue to rage, generating active dialogue among scholars, scientists, politicians and ordinary folk. From a legal perspective, a question we are confronting today is whether physicians have a duty to offer existing genetic-related medical services to patients undergoing assisted conception. In 2008, only 4% of all IVF cycles included PGD. *See* 2008 Assisted Reproductive Technology Success Rates, National Summary and Fertility Clinic Reports (Center for Disease Control and Prevention, December 2010), at 91. The next case raises the question, Does an ART physician have a duty to offer PGD to all couples undergoing IVF?

B. Legal Dilemmas Surrounding Genetic Selection

PARETTA v. MEDICAL OFFICES FOR HUMAN REPRODUCTION

Supreme Court of New York, New York County
195 Misc.2d 568, 760 N.Y.S.2d 639 (2003)

EILEEN BRANSTEIN, J. Pursuant to CPLR 3211(a)(7), defendant Medical Offices for Human Reproduction d/b/a Center for Human Reproduction (the "Center"), moves for an order dismissing the complaint of plaintiffs Josephine Paretta, Gerard Paretta and Theresa Paretta, an Infant under the Age of 14 Years by Her Parents and Natural Guardians, Josephine Paretta and Gerard Paretta, Individually. The Center urges that dismissal is warranted on the grounds that New York law does not recognize claims for "wrongful life." Defendants Dr. Steven Lindheim ("Dr. Lindheim"), New York Presbyterian Hospital s/h/a Columbia-Presbyterian Medical Center, The Trustees of Columbia University in the City of New York s/h/a Center for Women's Reproductive Care at Columbia University (the "Hospital") and Dr. Mark Sauer ("Dr. Sauer") cross-move for dismissal of the action.

Additionally, plaintiffs cross-move for summary judgment.

Background

On January 16, 1998, Josephine and Gerard Paretta ("the Parettas") sought fertility treatment from physicians affiliated with the Center and the Hospital. Dr. Sauer, one of the physicians, recommended that Mrs. Paretta undergo in-vitro fertilization using an ovum donor, and that the couple proceed in the Ovum Donor Program. Dr. Sauer allegedly further recommended that the Parettas use Mr. Paretta's sperm and "the ova of a prescreened oocyte donor." The couple agreed to proceed through the program and met with Dr. Lindheim, the program director. Dr. Lindheim provided the Parettas with detailed information about the potential oocyte donor; specifically, that she was white, a second-time donor, a heterosexual, an only child of an Irish father and English mother, a Protestant, that she was five feet six inches tall, that she had dark brown hair and brown eyes, was long necked with small eyes and ears, that she had a short thin nose, dimples and high cheekbones, and that she did not have freckles. Dr. Lindheim also allegedly told the Parettas that the donor did not have a history of mental illness or genetic diseases.

After hearing about the potential donor, the Parettas decided to use her ova. The custom and practice of the program was to screen donors for various diseases, including cystic fibrosis. "[T]he practice was to inform the patient that there was a donor or that a potential donor was a carrier, and if they elected to proceed forward, they had the option or choice to be screened to see if there was a carrier status." No one remembers ever telling the Parettas that the available donor was a carrier of cystic fibrosis and Mr. Paretta was not tested to ascertain whether he was a carrier of the disease.

Conception was successful, and on May 7, 2000, Theresa Paretta was born. Tragically, Theresa was diagnosed with cystic fibrosis, a chronic debilitating progressive genetic disease that is inherited from both parents.

For the first two months, Theresa was in intensive care. She underwent several surgeries and wore a colostomy bag for a month. According to plaintiffs, she "will have to take medication for the rest of her life * * * [and] will remain under a doctor's and/or hospital's care for the rest of her life."

On July 7, 2000 — exactly two months after Theresa's birth — Dr. Sauer wrote the Parettas:

> "I was sorry to learn of your daughter's serious illness. Your egg donor was screened for Cystic Fibrosis, and was found to be a carrier. We have no record of genetic screening in your husband. I am aware that Dr. Lindheim was your primary physician but he is no longer at Columbia University. You may wish to direct your inquiries to him at his private office in Norwalk, CT."

> "We strive to provide excellent care here, and I regret that this incident occurred. I sincerely hope that your daughter improves and that she thrives despite the illness."

In October 2000, plaintiffs commenced this action, alleging defendants committed medical malpractice when they failed to properly screen the egg and inform the Parettas that the egg tested positive for the cystic fibrosis gene. According to the complaint, the donor "was screened and tested, she was found to be a positive carrier of the [cystic fibrosis gene] and plaintiffs were never informed." The complaint further alleges that defendants were negligent in failing to test Mr. Paretta for the cystic fibrosis gene as it was only after the baby's birth that the couple learned that both the oocyte donor and Mr. Paretta carried the gene for the disease.

The Parettas, on behalf of themselves individually and Theresa, allege, among other things, that:

- "As a direct and proximate result of Defendants Lindheim and Sauer's breach of the standard of care, the Plaintiff Gerard Paretta emotionally suffers and will continue to emotionally suffer as a parent of a child affected with [cystic fibrosis] which is chronic, debilitating and painful disease for the rest of her life." . . .

- "As a result of the Defendants' breach, Plaintiffs have suffered damages representing medical, surgical, hospital costs, lost wages and/or other damages." . . .

The Center now moves for dismissal of the complaint, arguing that Theresa Paretta cannot maintain a cause of action for "wrongful life." Relying on Becker v. Schwartz, 46 N.Y.2d 401, 413 N.Y.S.2d 895, 386 N.E.2d 807 (1978), the Center contends that an infant cannot recover damages for being born with a genetic disorder. The Center further urges that the Parettas cannot maintain causes of action for emotional distress or seek compensation for lost wages as a result of caring for Theresa. Both the Hospital and Dr. Sauer cross-move for dismissal on the identical grounds . . .

Plaintiffs oppose all of defendants' motions and cross-motions, and cross-move for summary judgment. They maintain that this case is not one for "wrongful birth or wrongful life;" rather, the complaint alleges medical malpractice, negligence and lack of informed consent. The Parettas maintain that "this is also a case of negligent preconception and pre-implantation counseling.". Relying on information from the American Society For Reproduction Medicine, the Parettas argue that defendants should have conducted a pre-implantation genetic diagnosis test to ascertain whether the embryo had genetic diseases. Plaintiffs maintain that defendants were negligent in failing to test the egg, sperm and embryo before implantation . . .

Analysis

In *Becker v. Schwartz*, 46 N.Y.2d 401, 413 N.Y.S.2d 895, 386 N.E.2d 807 (1978), the Court of Appeals addressed two companion cases raising the issue of an infant's potential recovery for being born with a genetic disease . . .

The Court explained that "irrespective of the label coined, plaintiffs' complaints sound essentially in negligence or medical malpractice." . . . The Court held that regardless of the denomination of the nature of their claims, the infants could not recover because "it does not appear that [they] suffered any legally cognizable injury." . . . Because a child does not have a fundamental right to be born free of disease, the Court refused to subject the obstetricians and gynecologists to liability to the infants. "Whether it is better never to have been born at all than to have been born with even gross deficiencies," the Court stated, "is a mystery more properly left to the philosophers and the theologians."

The *Becker* Court, however, was perfectly clear in determining that the parents could recover in their own rights for damages resulting from the birth of their diseased infants . . .

Becker unquestionably is distinguishable in that, unlike here, the plaintiffs did not contend that the defendant physicians' treatment caused the abnormalities in the child. Here, by contrast, the Parettas maintain that the defendant doctors were actually responsible for Theresa's conception, had a role in her genetic composition, and combined the sperm and egg both of which carried cystic fibrosis. Theresa, however, like any other baby, does not have a protected right to be born free of genetic defects. A conclusion to the contrary, permitting infants to recover against doctors for wrongs allegedly committed during in-vitro fertilization, would give children conceived with the help of modern medical technology more rights and expectations than children conceived without medical assistance. The law does not recognize such a distinction and neither will this Court.

Likewise, *Becker* establishes that there can be no recovery for the emotional distress a parent may experience as a result of having a child with a genetic disease. There is no compelling legal authority permitting a distinction where a child has been conceived with the help of medical technology and is born with a genetic disease. This Court cannot treat the emotional distress and psychic pain suffered by parents who give birth to a sick child after in-vitro fertilization any differently from that sustained by other parents. The emotional distress experienced as a result of watching a genetically diseased child suffer, horrible as it may be, is the same regardless of how the child was conceived. It unfortunately is not compensable . . .

That plaintiffs cannot recover on Theresa's behalf and cannot recover for emotional distress or loss of services, by no means requires dismissal of the action. Indeed, *Becker* makes abundantly clear that the Parettas can pursue recovery for the pecuniary expense they have borne and continue to bear for the care and treatment of their sick infant . . . Thus, the action will go forward.

Furthermore, at this stage and on this record, the Court will not dismiss plaintiffs' allegation that they are entitled to punitive damages. Plaintiffs have alleged grossly negligent or reckless conduct, and defendants have not established that dismissal of these contentions is warranted as a matter of law . . . It is certainly possible that defendants' conduct was at the very least grossly negligent — possibly even fraudulent — and that defendants could have prevented the Parettas from having a baby with cystic fibrosis. There is evidence that defendants may have known that the egg donor was a cystic fibrosis carrier; yet, they failed to inform the Parettas or test Mr. Paretta's sperm to assess whether he too was a carrier. Had the Parettas been informed of the potential for cystic fibrosis they themselves may have chosen to have Mr. Paretta tested or may have altogether opted on using a different egg donor . . .

In sum, it is hard to ignore defendants' alleged role in Theresa's illness. Indeed, it is difficult to conceive that parents, concerned about whether the egg donor had freckles and with the size of her eyes and ears, would not have expected full disclosure of information regarding whether she carried cystic fibrosis. Thus, the Parettas will be permitted to vigorously pursue recovery.

On this record, however, the Court will not award the Parettas summary judgment. At the outset, and most important, it is well settled that application of the res ipsa loquitur doctrine as a basis for awarding summary judgment is inappropriate . . . Additionally, plaintiffs have not submitted adequate evidence establishing that they are entitled to judgment as a matter of law. Specifically, there are no affidavits from the plaintiffs or from any medical experts, leaving unresolved many factual questions that must await further determination.

Accordingly, it is ORDERED that defendants' motions and cross-motions to dismiss the action are denied except that all causes of action on behalf of Theresa Paretta are dismissed, and all causes of action for emotional distress and loss of services are dismissed . . . This constitutes the decision and order of the Court.

NOTES AND QUESTIONS

1.   The *Paretta* court makes an effort to give equal tort treatment to all parents, regardless of the manner in which their ill children were conceived. But is this fair, or possible, when the manner of the child's conception is itself the source of the tort?

2.   If you were an ART provider in New York, would you adjust your practices after the decision in *Paretta*? If you were an ART patient in any jurisdiction, would you seek a change in your treatment plan after reading the decision in *Paretta*?

Does our increasing ability to investigate and select the traits of our children signal a change in the standard of care that currently governs reproductive medicine? Is a heightened standard of care in which genetic analysis is a routine aspect of assisted conception a benefit for patients? For physicians? For society?

PROBLEM

Eve and Jose Rubell were having difficulty conceiving a child. They visited a university-based ART clinic for advice and treatment. After undergoing routine medical examinations, the Rubells learned that Eve was a carrier of Fabry disease, an X-linked recessive disorder that causes kidney failure, heart failure and an increased risk of strokes, reducing an affected person's life expectancy to age 40 or 50. Eve did not manifest the disease because in females both X-chromosomes would have to contain the anomaly. She carried the anomaly on one of her two X-chromosomes. Since Jose was not a carrier of Fabry, the couple's physician, Dr. Paulson, recommend they use IVF and PGD to maximize the health of their future child. Further, because Fabry's disease is an X-linked recessive disorder, Dr. Paulson recommended using PGD to screen the embryos' gender, selecting for female embryos only. Dr. Paulson explained, "Fabry disease is a recessive X-linked disorder, meaning it will typically only be symptomatic in boys because they have a single X-chromosome, whereas a girl born from only one affected parent will inherit only one anomalous X-chromosome."

The Rubells underwent one round of IVF and produced six embryos. Dr. Paulson conducted PGD on all six embryos and declared only two to be female, both of which carried the anomaly on only one of its X-chromosomes. Since Eve had lived a normal healthy life as a carrier of the disease, she and Jose decided to transfer both female embryos back into her uterus. The couple was overjoyed to learn Eve was pregnant, but an ultrasound at 15 weeks gestation revealed the fetus was a boy. A follow up amniocentesis contained the devastating news that their son would be born with Fabry disease. Indeed, Gabriel Rubell was later born with the disorder. The Rubells have consulted you as a legal expert in the area. What advice would you give the couple about pursing legal action against Dr. Paulson? Would you rather represent the Rubells or Dr. Paulson in this matter? Why? Which tugs at you more, your legal mind or your human heart?

Chapter 5

FAMILY LAW ISSUES IN ART: QUESTIONS OF PARENTAGE AND PARENTAL RIGHTS

Assisted conception offers the joys of parenthood to so many who, just a generation ago, could not have imagined the potential for law and medicine to combine to form family ties. We have studied the steady pace of reproductive medicine, from in vitro fertilization, to gamete donation, to genetic screening of embryos. In contrast, as is often the case, the law has lagged behind advances in medicine, reacting to each new scenario as it arises with an urgency to address the parties' dispute rather than the luxury to contemplate a comprehensive strategy. Over the past three decades, the majority of legal questions confronting ART have been in the realm of family law: Who is a parent when a child is conceived with the aid of a gamete donor? Does a woman who agrees to gestate a fetus for another couple have maternal rights once the child is born? Who are the rightful parents when an embryo is mistakenly transferred into the wrong woman's uterus? We now turn to these and other questions of parentage that occupy much of the jurisprudence surrounding ART.

SECTION I: EARLY DILEMMAS IN FAMILY LAW

A.   Determining Paternity in AID Families

STRNAD v. STRNAD
Supreme Court of New York, New York County
190 Misc. 786, 78 N.Y.S.2d 390 (1948)

GREENBERG, J. The court has assumed, for the purpose of this disposition in the light of the record and the concessions made by the defendant, that the plaintiff was artificially inseminated with the consent of the defendant and that the child is not of the blood of the defendant.

Predicated on that assumption the court concludes as follows:

(1) The defendant is entitled to rights of visitation as heretofore allowed, namely, every Sunday between the hours of 11 a. m. and 4 p. m., and during such visitations the child will be in the custody of the maternal grandmother. The additional evidence offered by plaintiff, such as it is, is not impressive and does not justify any departure from the ruling heretofore made with respect to the rights of visitation. The defendant has not been shown to be an unfit guardian; on the contrary, the evidence convinces me that the best interests of the child call for these modest visitations.

(2) The court holds that the child has been potentially adopted or semi-adopted by the defendant. In any event, in so far as this defendant is concerned and with particular reference to visitation, he is entitled to the same rights as those acquired by a foster parent who has formally adopted a child, if not the same rights as those to which a natural parent under the circumstances would be entitled.

(3) In the opinion of this court, assuming again that plaintiff was artificially inseminated with the consent of the defendant, this child is not an illegitimate child. Indeed, logically and realistically, the situation is no different than that pertaining in the case of a child born out of wedlock who by law is made legitimate upon the marriage of the interested parties.

(4) The court does not pass on the legal consequences in so far as property rights are concerned in a case of this character, nor does the court express an opinion on the propriety of procreation by the medium of artificial insemination. With such matters the court is not here concerned; the latter problem particularly is in the fields of sociology, morality and religion.

Settle findings of fact, conclusion of law and judgment on five days' notice. Appropriate exception to the plaintiff.

NOTES AND QUESTIONS

1.   The court in *Strnad* was the first to issue a written opinion on the question of parental rights and responsibilities toward a child of artificial insemination. The court's holding that "this child is not an illegitimate child" was later criticized by a 1963 case in which the Supreme Court of New York held that "the offspring of artificial insemination by a third-party donor with the consent of the mother's husband, is not the legitimate issue of the husband." *Gursky v. Gursky*, 39 Misc. 2d 1083, 242 N.Y.S.2d 406 (1963) (recall our discussion of *Gursky* in Chapter 1). Despite the different legal outcomes ("not illegitimate" v. "not legitimate" — are those truly different?), both courts did order the mother's husband to take some responsibility for the child (visitation in *Strnad*, child support in *Gursky*). If a child of AID is otherwise cared for by the mother's husband, should it matter that the child is not considered a child of the marriage?

2.   The legal battle over little Antoinette Strnad continued even after her father, Antoine, was granted visitation. Despite an order that Antoine be permitted to visit his "daughter" every Sunday between 11:00 a.m. and 4:00 p.m., Antoinette's mother, Julie, moved with the child to Oklahoma. Figuring that Julie could not meet her obligation to have Antoinette in New York City every Sunday while residing in Oklahoma, Antoine moved for an order to have his ex-wife judged in contempt of court. To no one's surprise, the court found Julie in contempt and with language reminiscent of a bygone era, it chided her for "rendering ineffectual and nugatory the provision of the decree with respect to visitation" and declared her conduct "contumacious." *Strnad v. Strnad*, 83 N.Y.S.2d 391 (1948).

PEOPLE v. SORENSEN

Supreme Court of California
68 Cal.2d 280, 66 Cal.Rptr. 7, 437 P.2d 495 (1968)

McCOMB, J. Defendant appeals from a judgment convicting him of violating section 270 of the Penal Code (willful failure to provide for his minor child), a misdemeanor.

The settled statement of facts recites that seven years after defendant's marriage it was medically determined that he was sterile. His wife desired a child, either by artificial insemination or by adoption, and at first defendant refused to consent. About 15 years after the marriage defendant agreed to the artificial insemination of his wife. Husband and wife, then residents of San Joaquin County, consulted a physician in San Francisco. They signed an agreement, which is on the letterhead of the physician, requesting the physician to inseminate the wife with the sperm of a white male. The semen was to be selected by the physician, and under no circumstances were the parties to demand the name of the donor. The agreement contains a recitation that the physician does not represent that pregnancy will occur. The physician treated Mrs. Sorensen, and she became pregnant. Defendant knew at the time he signed the consent that when his wife took the treatments she could become pregnant and that if a child was born it was to be treated as their child.

A male child was born to defendant's wife in San Joaquin County on October 14, 1960. The information for the birth certificate was given by the mother, who named defendant as the father. Defendant testified that he had not provided the information on the birth certificate and did not recall seeing it before the trial.

For about four years the family had a normal family relationship, defendant having represented to friends that he was the child's father and treated the boy as his son. In 1964, Mrs. Sorensen separated from defendant and moved to Sonoma County with the boy. At separation, Mrs. Sorensen told defendant that she wanted no support for the boy, and she consented that a divorce be granted to defendant. Defendant obtained a decree of divorce, which recites that the court retained 'jurisdiction regarding the possible support obligation of plaintiff in regard to a minor child born to defendant.'

In the summer of 1966 when Mrs. Sorensen became ill and could not work, she applied for public assistance under the Aid to Needy Children program. The County of Sonoma supplied this aid until Mrs. Sorensen was able to resume work. Defendant paid no support for the child since the separation in 1964, although demand therefor was made by the district attorney. The municipal court found defendant guilty of violating section 270 of the Penal Code and granted him probation for three years on condition that he make payments of $50 per month for support through the district attorney's office.

From the record before us, this case could be disposed of on the ground that defendant has failed to overcome the presumption that 'A child of a woman who is or has been married, born during the marriage or within 300 days after the dissolution thereof, is presumed to be a legitimate child of that marriage. This presumption may be disputed only by the people of the State of California in a criminal action brought under Section 270 of the Penal Code or by the husband or wife, or the descendant of one or both of them . . .'

[T]he only question for our determination is: Is the husband of a woman, who with his consent was artificially inseminated with semen of a third-party donor, guilty of the crime of failing to support a child who is the product of such insemination, in violation of section 270 of the Penal Code?[1] The law is that defendant is the lawful father of the child born to his wife, which child was conceived by artificial insemination to which he consented, and his conduct carries with it an obligation of support within the meaning of section 270 of the Penal Code.

Under the facts of this case, the term 'father' as used in section 270 cannot be limited to the biologic or natural father as those terms are generally understood. The determinative factor is whether the legal relationship of father and child exists. A child conceived through heterologous artificial insemination[2] does not have a 'natural father,' as that terms is commonly used. The anonymous donor of the sperm cannot be considered the 'natural father,' as he is no more responsible for the use made of his sperm than is the donor of blood or a kidney. Moreover, he could not dispute the presumption that the child is the legitimate issue of Mr. and Mrs. Sorensen, as that presumption 'may be disputed only by the people of the State of California . . . or by the husband or wife, or the descendant of one or both of them.' (Evid.Code, s 661, supra.) With the use of frozen semen, the donor may even be dead at the time the semen is used. Since there is no 'natural father,' we can only look for a lawful father.

It is doubtful that with the enactment of section 270 of the Penal Code [in 1872] and its amendments the Legislature considered the plight of a child conceived through artificial insemination. However, the intent of the Legislature obviously was to include every child, legitimate or illegitimate, born or unborn, and enforce the obligation of support against the person who could be determined to be the lawful parent. . . .

[A] reasonable man who, because of his inability to procreate, actively participates and consents to his wife's artificial insemination in the hope that a child will be produced whom they will treat as their own, knows that such behavior carries with it the legal responsibilities of fatherhood and criminal responsibility for nonsupport. One who consents to the production of a child cannot create a temporary relation to be assumed and disclaimed at will, but the arrangement must be of such character as to impose an obligation of supporting those for whose existence he is directly responsible. As noted by the trial court, it is safe to assume

---

[1] [n.1] Section 270 of the Penal Code reads: "A father of either a legitimate or illegitimate minor child who . . . willfully omits without lawful excuse to furnish necessary clothing, food, shelter or medical attendance or other remedial care for his child is guilty of a misdemeanor and punishable by a fine not exceeding one thousand dollars ($1,000) or by imprisonment in a county jail not exceeding one year, or by both such fine and imprisonment."

[2] [n.2] There are two types of artificial insemination in common use: (1) artificial insemination with the husband's semen, homologous insemination, commonly termed A.I.H. and (2) artificial insemination with semen of a third-party donor, heterologous insemination, commonly termed A.I.D. Only the latter raises legal problems of fatherhood and legitimacy. (43 ABAJ 1089, 1090.)

that without defendant's active participation and consent the child would not have been procreated.

The documentary evidence in this case consisted of the written agreement between husband and wife that the physician inseminate the wife with the sperm of a white male, and birth certificate listing defendant as the father, and a copy of the interlocutory decree of divorce. While defendant testified that he did not know the contents of the birth certificate, this testimony was not sufficient to raise a reasonable doubt that he was the father. Therefore, since, the word 'father' is construed to include a husband who, unable to accomplish his objective of creating a child by using his own semen, purchases semen from a donor and uses it to inseminate his wife to achieve his purpose, proof of paternity has been established beyond a reasonable doubt . . .

The question of the liability of the husband for support of a child created through artificial insemination is one of first impression in this state and has been raised in only a few cases outside the state, none of them involving a criminal prosecution for failure to provide. Although other courts considering the question have found some existing legal theory to hold the 'father' responsible, results have varied on the question of legitimacy. In *Gursky v. Gursky*, 39 Misc.2d 1083, 242 N.Y.S.2d 406 (Sup.Ct.1963), the court held that the child was illegitimate but that the husband was liable for the child's support because consent to the insemination implied a promise to support.

In *Strnad v. Strnad*, 190 Misc. 786, 78 N.Y.S.2d 390 (Sup.Ct.1948), the court found that a child conceived through artificial insemination was not illegitimate and granted visitation rights to the husband in a custody proceeding.

It is less crucial to determine the status of the child than the status of defendant as the father. Categorizing the child as either legitimate or illegitimate does not resolve the issue of the legal consequences flowing from defendant's participation in the child's existence. Under our statute, both legitimate and illegitimate minors have a right to support from their parents. The primary liability is on the father, and if he is dead or for any reason whatever fails to furnish support, the mother is criminally liable therefor. To permit defendant's parental responsibilities to rest on a voluntary basis would place the entire burden of support on the child's mother, and if she is incapacitated the burden is then on society. Cost to society, of course, is not the only consideration which impels the conclusion that defendant is the lawful father of the offspring of his marriage. The child is the principal party affected, and if he has no father he is forced to bear not only the handicap of social stigma but financial deprivation as well . . .

In the absence of legislation prohibiting artificial insemination, the offspring of defendant's valid marriage to the child's mother was lawfully begotten and was not the product of an illicit or adulterous relationship. Adultery is defined as 'the voluntary sexual intercourse of a married person with a person other than the offender's husband or wife.' (Civ.Code, s 93.) It has been suggested that the doctor and the wife commit adultery by the process of artificial insemination. (See 43 ABAJ 1089, 1091–1092, 1156.) Since the doctor may be a woman, or the husband himself may administer the insemination by a syringe, this is patently absurd; to consider it an act of adultery with the donor, who at the time of insemination may be a thousand miles away or may even be dead, is equally absurd. Nor are we persuaded that the concept of legitimacy demands that the child be the actual offspring of the husband of the mother and if semen of some other male is utilized the resulting child is illegitimate . . .

[W]e are not required in this case to do more than decide that, within the meaning of section 270 of the Penal Code, defendant is the lawful father of the child conceived through heterologous artificial insemination and born during his marriage to the child's mother.

The judgment is affirmed. TRAYNOR, C.J., and PETERS, TOBRINER, MOSK, BURKE and SULLIVAN, JJ., concur.

NOTES AND QUESTIONS

1.   The California Supreme Court was the first high court to rule on the rights of AID children. While previous lower courts had ruled on the legal obligations of husband's whose wives bore children through AID, the *Sorenson* court went beyond questions of a child's rights to questions of a child's status. The California court blends the concepts of "natural" father and "legal" father where AID occurs, emphasizing that a man who consents to "the production of a child" cannot escape the designation of "father" and its attendant obligations. Notice also the court's emphasis on the public policy favoring a presumption of legitimacy when a child is born during a valid marriage, concomitant with its rebuke of prior thinking that AID constitutes adultery as "patently absurd." Such "patently absurd" thinking did accompany the introduction of AID in the 1950s. For example, in 1955 the Ohio Senate contemplated a resolution that would have made AID punishable as adultery, subject to a fine of $500 or up to five years imprisonment. Though ultimately not enacted, the essence of the resolution permeated American thought on AID for nearly two decades. *See* E. Donald Shapiro & Benedene Sonnenblick, *The Widow and the Sperm: The Law of Post Mortem Insemination*, 1 J. L. & HEALTH 229, 237 (1986).

2.   Suppose the young Sorenson boy grows up and develops a taste for Black Jack. After a particularly successful weekend in Las Vegas, Master Sorensen is tragically killed while on his return to Northern California. He leaves an estate valued at $100,000. Do you think Mr. Sorensen would still deny that he is the legal father of the child? If Mr. Sorensen had continued to deny his legal obligations to the child, even after the California Supreme Court decision, should he be entitled to a share of the child's estate at death?

3.   A gender-bending version of *Sorenson* came before the Supreme Court of Tennessee in 2005. In *In Re C.K.G, C.L.G & C.L.G.*, 173 S.W.3d 714 (2005), a woman gave birth to triplets with the aid of donor eggs. Her partner of many years, an emergency room physician, provided sperm for the children's conception via IVF and agreed in writing that the couple would be the legal parents of any offspring born from the procedure. When the couple's relationship deteriorated, the father sought sole and exclusive custody of the triplets, arguing that the woman was not the children's legal mother because she lacked a genetic tie to the three youngsters.

The fact that the woman gave birth to the children was not, under Tennessee's parentage statutes, sufficient to confer maternal rights. The court acknowledged this statutory deficit, but held that under the narrow facts at issue, the birth mother was the triplets' legal mother. "We conclude that sound policy and common sense favor recognizing gestation as an important factor for establishing legal maternity." *Id.* at 729. A true analogue to *Sorenson* would have seen the mother denying parental responsibility toward the children because she lacked a genetic tie. No reported case exists in which a mother has taken such a position.

B. Early Changes in the Law

The decision in *People v. Sorensen* brought attention to the plight of AID children at risk of abandonment by fathers who were only sporadically declared legal parents by the state courts. At the time of the *Sorensen* decision in 1968, only three states had enacted laws pertaining to the status of AID children. The first statute to legitimize artificial insemination was enacted in Georgia in 1964. Ga. Code Ann. § 74-9904 provided for a conclusive presumption of legitimacy of a child born through AID when performed with the written consent of both husband and wife. It also regulated AID by permitting only licensed physicians to perform the procedure and made it a felony for anyone else to do so.

In 1967, Oklahoma enacted the second state statute to regulate artificial insemination. This statute affirmatively permitted the practice of AID by a licensed physician when so requested by a husband and wife, both of whom had to consent in writing. The statute banned the use of AID under any other circumstances, but no penalty was prescribed. Consent for the procedure had to be executed and acknowledged by the husband, wife, AID practitioner, and a judge having jurisdiction over the adoption of children. An original of the consent was to be filed with the court, which maintained confidentiality. Any child born as a result was considered legitimate. Lawmakers in Kansas enacted a third AID statute in 1968, similarly requiring written consent by the couple to be filed with the court, thereby legitimizing the born child. *See* Gaia Bernstein, *The Socio-Legal Acceptance of New Technologies: A Close Look At Artificial Insemination*, 77 WASH. L. REV. 1035 (2002).

In an attempt to unify the law across the nation and establish a national policy on the rights and liabilities of persons who utilize AID, the National Conference of Commissioners on Uniform State Laws promulgated the Uniform Parentage Act (UPA) in 1973. Like all uniform laws, the UPA is an advisory statute available for adoption by state lawmakers. The primary goal of the UPA was to guarantee substantive legal equality for all children regardless of the marital status of their parents. The status of AID children is addressed in Section 5, which provides as follows:

Uniform Parentage Act (1973)

§ 5 [Artificial Insemination]

(a) If, under the supervision of a licensed physician and with the consent of her husband, a wife is inseminated artificially with semen donated by a man not her husband, the husband is treated in law as if he were the natural father of a child thereby conceived. The husband's consent must be in writing and signed by him and his wife. The physician shall certify their signatures and the date of the insemination, and file the husband's consent with the [State Department of Health], where it shall be kept confidential and in a sealed file. However, the physician's failure to do so does not affect the father and child relationship. All papers and records pertaining to the insemination, whether part of the permanent record of a court or of a file held by the supervising physician or elsewhere, are subject to inspection only upon an order of the court for good cause shown.

(b) The donor of semen provided to a licensed physician for use in artificial insemination of a married woman other than the donor's wife is treated in law as if he were not the natural father of a child thereby conceived.

———————

As of 1998, 15 states had adopted Section 5 of the UPA or a virtually identical standard, and 15 others had enacted similar statutes that varied by eliminating the licensed physician requirement. See Marsha Garrison, *Law Making For Baby Making: An Interpretive Approach to the Determination of Legal Parentage*, 113 HARV. L.R. 835, 845-6 (2000).

As explained in the following excerpt, Section 5 of the UPA has two key elements:

First, the UPA requires that a husband consent in writing to the AID procedure in order to be treated as the "natural father" of the child. A serious problem arises in paternity disputes involving AID, because it is quite difficult to prove consent or lack thereof. The writing requirement of the UPA eliminates this problem by requiring written proof of a husband's consent to be filed with state authorities by a licensed physician. The requirement of written consent clearly indicates the intentions of the parties from the outset. However, strict statutory construction mandates that if the husband does not sign a consent form, he is not afforded the parental protections, even if he has expressed consent orally or otherwise.

Second, the UPA requires that a licensed physician perform the procedure. This requirement provides a "neutral" third party who can verify that both husband and wife agreed to the procedure. In addition, physician supervision also ensures that a woman has access to medical care during the insemination. However, because the procedure is so easy to perform, a physician may not be a necessary component of a successful insemination. Consequently, the physician supervision requirement may impose unnecessary expenses without any significant benefit, effectively forcing some couples to choose between undergoing the procedure without the assistance of a physician and losing the protection of the Act, or foregoing the procedure entirely and potentially remaining childless.

While there are rational bases for these two requirements, the potential problems are quite serious. The UPA guarantees paternity for husbands who meet both requirements; however, husbands who intend to be fathers but fail to follow the requirements have no such guarantees. The disturbing result is either that children will be deemed fatherless if either of these requirements are not met, or, alternatively, sperm donors may face paternal responsibility for children they have no intention of parenting.

Bridget R. Penick, *Give the Child a Legal Father: A Plea for Iowa to Adopt A Statute Regulating Artificial Insemination by Anonymous Donor*, 83 Iowa L. Rev. 633, 641 (1998). The UPA requirements that a husband consent in writing to AID and that a licensed physician perform the procedure, have served to settle parentage questions when a married couple reproduces using donor sperm. But what happens in cases in which neither a married couple nor a licensed physician participate in the birth of an AID child? How is the child's parentage determined under those "non-traditional" circumstances? Consider one of the first cases to address this question.

JHORDAN C. v. MARY K.
California Court of Appeal, First District
179 Cal. App. 3d 386, 224 Cal. Rptr. 530 (1986)

King, Associate Justice.

I. Holding

By statute in California a "donor of semen *provided to a licensed physician* for use in artificial insemination of a woman other than the donor's wife is treated in law as if he were not the natural father of a child thereby conceived." (Civ.Code, § 7005, subd. (b); emphasis added.) In this case we hold that where impregnation takes place by artificial insemination, and the parties have failed to take advantage of this statutory basis for preclusion of paternity, the donor of semen can be determined to be the father of the child in a paternity action.

Mary K. and Victoria T. appeal from a judgment declaring Jhordan C. to be the legal father of Mary's child, Devin. The child was conceived by artificial insemination with semen donated personally to Mary by Jhordan. We affirm the judgment.

II. Facts and Procedural History

In late 1978 Mary decided to bear a child by artificial insemination and to raise the child jointly with Victoria, a close friend who lived in a nearby town. Mary sought a semen donor by talking to friends and acquaintances. This led to three or four potential donors with whom Mary spoke directly. She and Victoria ultimately chose Jhordan after he had one personal interview with Mary and one dinner at Mary's home.

The parties' testimony was in conflict as to what agreement they had concerning the role, if any, Jhordan would play in the child's life. According to Mary, she told Jhordan she did not want a donor who desired ongoing involvement with the child, but she did agree to let him see the child to satisfy his curiosity as to how the child would look. Jhordan, in contrast, asserts they agreed he and Mary would have an ongoing friendship, he would have ongoing contact with the child, and he would care for the child as much as two or three times per week.

None of the parties sought legal advice until long after the child's birth. They were completely unaware of the existence of Civil Code section 7005. They did not attempt to draft a written agreement concerning Jhordan's status.

Jhordan provided semen to Mary on a number of occasions during a six month period commencing in late January 1979. On each occasion he came to her home, spoke briefly with her, produced the semen, and then left. The record is unclear, but Mary, who is a nurse, apparently performed the insemination by herself or with Victoria.

Contact between Mary and Jhordan continued after she became pregnant. Mary attended a Christmas party at Jhordan's home. Jhordan visited Mary several times at the health center where she worked. He took photographs of her. When he informed Mary by telephone that he had collected a crib, playpen, and high chair for the child, she told him to keep those items at his home. At one point Jhordan told Mary he had started a trust fund for the child and wanted legal guardianship in case she died; Mary vetoed the guardianship idea but did not disapprove the trust fund.

Victoria maintained a close involvement with Mary during the pregnancy. She took Mary to medical appointments, attended birthing classes, and shared information with Mary regarding pregnancy, delivery, and child rearing.

Mary gave birth to Devin on March 30, 1980. Victoria assisted in the delivery. Jhordan was listed as the father on Devin's birth certificate. Mary's roommate telephoned Jhordan that day to inform him of the birth. Jhordan visited Mary and Devin the next day and took photographs of the baby.

Five days later Jhordan telephoned Mary and said he wanted to visit Devin again. Mary initially resisted, but then allowed Jhordan to visit, although she told him she was angry. During the visit Jhordan claimed a right to see Devin, and Mary agreed to monthly visits.

Through August 1980 Jhordan visited Devin approximately five times. Mary then terminated the monthly visits. Jhordan said he would consult an attorney if Mary did not let him see Devin. Mary asked Jhordan to sign a contract indicating he would not seek to be Devin's father, but Jhordan refused.

In December 1980 Jhordan filed an action against Mary to establish paternity and visitation rights . . . In November 1982 the court granted Jhordan weekly visitation with Devin at Victoria's home.

Victoria had been closely involved with Devin since his birth. Devin spent at least two days each week in her home. On days when they did not see each other they spoke on the telephone. Victoria and Mary discussed Devin daily either in person or by telephone. They made joint decisions regarding his daily care and development. The three took vacations together. Devin and Victoria regarded each other as parent and child. Devin developed a brother-sister relationship with Victoria's 14-year-old daughter, and came to regard Victoria's parents as his grandparents. Victoria made the necessary arrangements for Devin's visits with Jhordan.

In August 1983 Victoria moved successfully for an order joining her as a party to this litigation. Supported by Mary, she sought joint legal custody (with Mary) and requested specified visitation rights, asserting she was a de facto parent of Devin

. . . Jhordan subsequently requested an award of joint custody to him and Mary.

After trial the court rendered judgment declaring Jhordan to be Devin's legal father. However, the court awarded sole legal and physical custody to Mary, and denied Jhordan any input into decisions regarding Devin's schooling, medical and dental care, and day-to-day maintenance. Jhordan received substantial visitation rights as recommended by a court-appointed psychologist. The court held Victoria was not a de facto parent, but awarded her visitation rights (not to impinge upon Jhordan's visitation schedule), which were also recommended by the psychologist.

Mary and Victoria filed a timely notice of appeal, specifying the portions of the judgment declaring Jhordan to be Devin's legal father and denying Victoria the status of de facto parent.

III. Discussion

We begin with a discussion of Civil Code section 7005, which provides in pertinent part: "(a) If, under the supervision of a licensed physician and with the consent of her husband, a wife is inseminated artificially with semen donated by a man not her husband, the husband is treated in law as if he were the natural father of a child thereby conceived. . . . [¶] (b) The donor of semen provided to a licensed physician for use in artificial insemination of a woman other than the donor's wife is treated in law as if he were not the natural father of a child thereby conceived."

Civil Code section 7005 is part of the Uniform Parentage Act (UPA), which was approved in 1973 by the National Conference of Commissioners on Uniform State Laws. (9A West's U.Laws Ann. (1979) U.Par. Act, hist. note, p. 579.) The UPA was adopted in California in 1975. (1975 stats., ch. 1244, § 11.) Section 7005 is derived almost verbatim from the UPA as originally drafted, with one crucial exception. The original UPA restricts application of the nonpaternity provision of subdivision (b) to a *"married* woman other than the donor's wife." (9A West's U. Laws Ann. (1979) U.Par. Act, § 5, subd. (b), p. 593; emphasis added.) The word "married" is excluded from subdivision (b) of section 7005, so that in California, subdivision (b) applies to all women, married or not.

Thus the California Legislature has afforded unmarried as well as married women a statutory vehicle for obtaining semen for artificial insemination without fear that the donor may claim paternity, and has likewise provided men with a statutory vehicle for donating semen to married and unmarried women alike without fear of liability for child support. Subdivision (b) states only one limitation on its application: the semen must be "provided to a licensed physician." Otherwise, whether impregnation occurs through artificial insemination or sexual intercourse, there can be a determination of paternity with the rights, duties and obligations such a determination entails.

A. *Interpretation of the Statutory Nonpaternity Provision.*

Mary and Victoria first contend that despite the requirement of physician involvement stated in Civil Code section 7005, subdivision (b), the Legislature did not intend to withhold application of the donor nonpaternity provision where semen used in artificial insemination was not provided to a licensed physician. They suggest that the element of physician involvement appears in the statute merely because the Legislature assumed (erroneously) that all artificial insemination would occur under the supervision of a physician. Alternatively, they argue the requirement of physician involvement is merely directive rather than mandatory.

We cannot presume, however, that the Legislature simply assumed or wanted to recommend physician involvement, for two reasons.

First, the history of the UPA (the source of section 7005) indicates conscious adoption of the physician requirement. The initial "discussion draft" submitted to the drafters of the UPA in 1971 did not mention the involvement of a physician in artificial insemination; . . . The eventual inclusion of the physician requirement in the final version of the UPA suggests a conscious decision to require physician involvement.

Second, there are at least two sound justifications upon which the statutory requirement of physician involvement might have been based. One relates to health: a physician can obtain a complete medical history of the donor (which may be of crucial importance to the child during his or her lifetime) and screen the donor for any hereditary or communicable diseases . . .

Another justification for physician involvement is that the presence of a professional third party such as a physician can serve to create a formal, documented structure for the donor-recipient relationship, without which, as this case illustrates, misunderstandings between the parties regarding the nature of their relationship and the donor's relationship to the child would be more likely to occur.

It is true that nothing inherent in artificial insemination requires the involvement of a physician. Artificial insemination is, as demonstrated here, a simple procedure easily performed by a woman in her own home. Also, despite the reasons outlined above in favor of physician involvement, there are countervailing considerations against requiring it. A requirement of physician involvement, as Mary argues, might offend a woman's sense of privacy and reproductive autonomy, might result in burdensome costs to some women, and might interfere with a woman's desire to conduct the procedure in a comfortable environment such as her own home or to choose the donor herself.

However, because of the way section 7005 is phrased, a woman (married or unmarried) can perform home artificial insemination or choose her donor and still obtain the benefits of the statute. Subdivision (b) does not require that a physician independently obtain the semen and perform the insemination, but requires only that the semen be "provided" to a physician. Thus, a woman who prefers home artificial insemination or who wishes to choose her donor can still obtain statutory protection from a donor's paternity claim through the relatively simple expedient of obtaining the semen, whether for home insemination or from a chosen donor (or both), through a licensed physician.

Regardless of the various countervailing considerations for and against physician involvement, our Legislature has embraced the apparently conscious decision by the drafters of the UPA to limit application of the donor nonpaternity provision to instances in which semen is provided to a licensed physician. The existence of sound justifications for physician involvement further supports a determination the Legislature intended to require it. Accordingly, section 7005, subdivision (b), by its terms does not apply to the present case. The Legislature's apparent decision to require physician involvement in order to invoke the statute cannot be subject to judicial second-guessing and cannot be disturbed, absent constitutional infirmity . . .

IV. Conclusion

We wish to stress that our opinion in this case is not intended to express any judicial preference toward traditional notions of family structure or toward providing a father where a single woman has chosen to bear a child. Public policy in these areas is best determined by the legislative branch of government, not the judicial. Our Legislature has already spoken and has afforded to unmarried women a statutory right to bear children by artificial insemination (as well as a right of men to donate semen) without fear of a paternity claim, through provision of the semen to a licensed physician. We simply hold that because Mary omitted to invoke Civil Code section 7005, subdivision (b), by obtaining Jhordan's semen through a licensed physician, and because the parties by all other conduct preserved Jhordan's status as a member of Devin's family, the trial court properly declared Jhordan to be Devin's legal father.

The judgment is affirmed.

LOW, P.J., and HANING, J., concur.

NOTES AND QUESTIONS

1. *The Role of the AID Physician.* Effective January 1, 1994, portions of the California Civil Code, including Section 7005, were repealed and replaced with equivalent provisions in the newly enacted California Family Code. Family Code Section 7613 continues former Civil Code Section 7005 without substantive change. Thus, California joins 14 other states in requiring that a physician be involved in the AID if the donor is to be treated in law "as if he were not the natural father of the child thereby conceived." Do you agree that the presence of a physician is rationally related to a finding of non-paternity on the part of a sperm donor? If Mary and Jhordan had used a physician to administer the AID, do you think Jhordan would have been less interested in pursuing his rights as Devin's legal father than he was under the stated circumstances?

2. *The Role of Spousal Consent.* The 1973 UPA accords the status of natural father to the husband of a woman who undergoes AID, so long as the couple consults a licensed physician and the man consents in writing to the procedure. The *Jhordan C.* case demonstrates the limitations of the law when a husband and a licensed physician are absent from the equation. What happens when a married woman engages a physician to perform AID, but does so without the consent of her husband? Even if you believe the law explicitly provides that the husband is not the natural father of the child, should the legal responsibility for the child fall on the

mother alone? What about the sperm donor? Does public policy in favor of caring for children override a sperm donor's right to be dismissed from the parental role?

Mrs. Shin worked for a medical office when she decided to try to conceive using artificial insemination. Though she was married, Mrs. Shin believed her boss, Dr. Kong, would be a preferred biologic father to her would-be child. Without alerting or seeking the consent of her husband, Mrs. Shin was artificially inseminated using Dr. Kong's sperm. After the child's birth, and the not-so-unexpected divorce, Mr. Shin learned of his child's true provenance and refused to provide any further support. Under the UPA, who is the child's legal father? Who should be responsible for the child's welfare? *See Shin v. Kong*, 80 Cal. App. 4th 498 (2000).

C. The Problem of Known Donors

A growing number of legal tussles reveal it is increasingly common for friends or even acquaintances to enter into AID arrangements without the aid of physicians or lawyers. Single women or lesbian partners may approach a friend or colleague and arrange for donation without clarifying the role the donor is to play in the child's life. These "known donor" scenarios can be entirely satisfactory in many cases, but sometimes the parties' expectations are unclear or dashed, causing conflict over the resulting offspring's legal parentage. In some cases, the sperm donor asserts a claim as a parent, in others the birth mother seeks to hold the donor financially responsible for the child's well-being. Courts focus on a host of factors, including any pre-conception agreements, oral or written evidence of intent and the best interest of the child. The next case teaches how very complicated these arrangements can be for all the parties involved.

FERGUSON v. McKIERNAN
Supreme Court of Pennsylvania
596 Pa. 78, 940 A.2d 1236 (2007)

Baer, J.

We are called upon to determine whether a sperm donor involved in a private sperm donation — i.e., one that occurs outside the context of an institutional sperm bank-effected through clinical rather than sexual means may be held liable for child support, notwithstanding the formation of an agreement between the donor and the donee that she will not hold the donor responsible for supporting the child that results from the arrangement. The lower courts effectively determined that such an agreement, even where bindingly formed, was unenforceable as a matter of law. Faced with this question of first impression in an area of law with profound importance for hundreds, perhaps thousands of Pennsylvania families, we disagree with the lower courts that the agreement in question is unenforceable. Accordingly, we reverse.

Former paramours Joel McKiernan (Sperm Donor) and Ivonne Ferguson (Mother) agreed that Sperm Donor would furnish his sperm in an arrangement that, by design, would feature all the hallmarks of an anonymous sperm donation: it would be carried out in a clinical setting; Sperm Donor's role in the conception would remain confidential; and neither would Sperm Donor seek visitation nor would Mother demand from him any support, financial or otherwise. At no time prior to conception, during Mother's pregnancy, or after the birth of the resultant twins did either party behave inconsistently with this agreement, until approximately five years after the twins' birth, when Mother filed a motion seeking child support from Sperm Donor. The trial court, recognizing the terms of the agreement outlined above and expressing dismay at what it found to be Mother's dishonest behavior, nevertheless found that the best interests of the twins rendered the agreement unenforceable as contrary to public policy. Thus, the court entered a support order against Sperm Donor, which the Superior Court affirmed.

The trial court found, and the record supports, the following account of the events leading up to this litigation. Sperm Donor met Mother in May 1991, when he began his employment with Pennsylvania Blue Shield, where Mother also worked. At that time, Mother was married to and living with Paul Ferguson (Husband), although whether their sexual relations continued at that point is subject to dispute. Mother was raising two children she had conceived with Husband, while he provided little if any emotional or financial support.

Later that year, Sperm Donor's and Mother's friendly relations turned intimate, and in or around November 1991 their relationship took on a sexual aspect. Mother assured Sperm Donor that she was using birth control, and the couple did not use condoms. Although Mother variously indicated to Sperm Donor that she was taking birth control pills or using injectable or implanted birth control, in fact she had undergone tubal ligation surgery in or around 1982, following the birth of her second child by Husband.

The parties continued their intimate relationship until some time in 1993, maintaining separate residences but seeing each other frequently. On more than one occasion during that span, they "broke up," only to reconcile after brief hiatuses. During the summer of 1993, however, their relationship began to flag.

Early that year, Mother had consulted a physician regarding the feasibility of reversing her tubal ligation to enable her to conceive another child. In September 1993, after learning that her tubal ligation was irreversible, Mother approached physician William Dodson at Hershey Medical Center, to discuss alternative methods of conception, specifically in vitro fertilization (IVF) using donor sperm followed by implantation of the fertilized eggs. Mother did not inform Sperm Donor of either consultation, and continued to mislead him by referring to one or more alternative methods of contraception she claimed to be using or considering using.

Toward the end of 1993, the parties' relationship had changed in character from an intimate sexual relationship to a friendship without the sexual component. At about that time, late in 1993, Mother broached the topic of bearing Sperm Donor's child. Even though Mother biologically was incapable of conceiving via intercourse due to her irreversible tubal ligation, and notwithstanding that the parties were no longer in a sexual relationship, she inexplicably suggested first that they conceive sexually. Sperm Donor, evidently unaware that the point was moot, refused. He made clear that he did not envision marrying Mother, and thus did not wish to bear a child with her.

Revising her approach, Mother then suggested that Sperm Donor furnish her with his sperm for purposes of IVF. Initially, Sperm Donor expressed his reluctance to do so. He relented, however, once Mother convinced him that she would release him from any of the financial burdens associated with conventional paternity; that she was up to the task of raising an additional child in a single-parent household and had the financial wherewithal to do so; and that, were he not to furnish his own sperm, she would seek the sperm of an anonymous donor instead.

To that end, Mother continued her consultations with Dr. Dobson at Hershey Medical Center, at least once visiting Dr. Dobson with a male companion. Although the evidence is heavily disputed in this regard, the trial court found that representations were made to Dr. Dobson that the man accompanying Mother was Husband. The trial court further found that Sperm Donor was not aware of these preliminary consultations. Moreover, most paperwork pertaining to the procedure was completed without Sperm Donor's knowledge or participation, an aspect of the case the trial court found reflective of Mother's "latent subterfuge."

On February 14, 1994, Sperm Donor traveled to Hershey Medical Center to provide a sperm sample.[3] This sample was used, in turn, to fertilize Mother's eggs, which then were implanted. The procedure succeeded, enabling Mother to become pregnant. Sperm Donor in no way subsidized the IVF procedure.

During Mother's pregnancy, Sperm Donor and Mother remained friends, visited regularly, and spoke frequently on the phone, although as noted their relationship was no longer sexual or romantic in character. The trial court found, however, that Sperm Donor attended none of Mother's prenatal examinations and did not pay any portion of Mother's prenatal expenses. Although both parties made an effort to preserve Sperm Donor's anonymity as the source of the sperm donation during the pregnancy, Mother admitted the truth to Sperm Donor's brother when he asked whether Sperm Donor was the father. Sperm Donor also admitted his own role in Mother's pregnancy to his parents when they confronted him, following their receipt of anonymous phone calls insinuating as much.

In August 1994, Mother went into labor prematurely. "In a panic," as the trial court characterized it, Mother contacted Sperm Donor and asked him to attend the birth. Believing that she had no one else to turn to, Sperm Donor joined Mother in the hospital. Even during the birth on August 25, 1994, however, Sperm Donor maintained his anonymity regarding his biological role in the pregnancy, an effort Mother affirmatively supported when she named Husband as the father on the twins' birth certificates, and reinforced by the fact that Sperm Donor neither was asked, nor offered, to contribute to the costs associated with Mother's delivery of the twins.

Regarding Sperm Donor's and Mother's post-partum interactions, the trial court found that,

> [a]fter the twins were born, [Sperm Donor] saw [Mother] and the boys on a few occasions in the hospital. Approximately two years after the births, [Sperm Donor] spent an afternoon with [Mother] and the twins while

---

[3] [n.6] Coincidentally, the paperwork for Mother's divorce from Husband was filed the same day.

visiting his parents in Harrisburg. [Sperm Donor] never provided the children with financial support or gifts, nor did he assume any parental identity. [Sperm Donor] had no further contact with either [Mother] or the children until May 1999 when [Mother] randomly obtained [Sperm Donor's] phone number[4] and subsequently filed for child support . . .

In the years after Mother gave birth to the twins and before Mother sought child support, Sperm Donor moved to Pittsburgh, met his future wife, married her, and had a child with her. Indeed, Sperm Donor's wife was pregnant with their second child when she testified in the trial court in these proceedings.

Based on this recitation of facts, the trial court found that the parties had formed a binding oral agreement prior to the twins' conception pursuant to which Sperm Donor would provide Mother with his sperm and surrender any rights and privileges to the children arising from his biological paternity in return for being released of any attendant support obligation. The parties further agreed to keep secret Sperm Donor's genetic connection to the twins. The trial court found ample evidence of the parties' intention in this regard, and determined that Sperm Donor's provision of sperm and Mother's agreement to forego any right to seek financial support from Sperm Donor constituted valid consideration as a matter of law, rendering the agreement a binding contract specifying the parties' rights and obligations.

The trial court reached this conclusion based on its determination that, "by virtue of the attendant testimony and evidence," Sperm Donor's testimony was more credible than the competing account offered by Mother. Id. at 359. "[Sperm Donor's] testimony was consistent throughout the Court's proceedings, whereas [Mother's] testimony contained numerous inconsistencies and contradictions, not to mention intentional falsehoods, fraud, and deceit involving not only [Sperm Donor] but the hospital as well." The trial court reinforced its point by highlighting numerous irregularities in Mother's testimony.

The court nevertheless found the agreement unenforceable. Citing the Superior Court's holding in Kesler v. Weniger, 744 A.2d 794, 796 (Pa.Super.2000), that "a parent cannot bind a child or bargain away that child's right to support," the court found its discretion restrained.

> [T]his Court cannot ignore and callously disregard the interests of the unheard-from third party[,] a party who without their privity to this contract renders it void. No other party, albeit a parent, can bargain away a child's support rights. Although we find the Plaintiff's actions despicable and give [sic] the Defendant a sympathetic hue, it is the interest of the children we hold most dear. Accordingly, we hold that the . . . Defendant is the legal father of the twins, and he is obligated to pay child support to the Plaintiff.

Relying on the support guidelines, based on Mother's monthly net income of

---

[4] [n.8] Although the court's characterization of the relevant interaction as "random" is not unfair, it risks being misleading. Evidently, Mother had occasion to contact Sperm Donor's office for business purposes. She discovered Sperm Donor's name and number as a consequence of that interaction, and proceeded to call him seeking support, claiming that welfare officials had pressured her to do so.

$1947.61 and Sperm Donor's monthly net income of $5262.30, the court imposed on Sperm Donor an ongoing support obligation of $1384 per month effective retroactively to January 1, 2001, with a corresponding arrear of $66,033.66 due immediately upon issuance of the order.

A panel of the Superior Court affirmed the trial court's ruling in a unanimous opinion that echoed the trial court's ruling . . .

Against this background, in which both of the lower courts found an agreement sufficiently mutual and clear to be binding, the lone question we face is as simple to state as it is vexing to answer. We must determine whether a would-be mother and a willing sperm donor can enter into an enforceable agreement under which the donor provides sperm in a clinical setting for IVF and relinquishes his right to visitation with the resultant child(ren) in return for the mother's agreement not to seek child support from the donor. In considering this pure question of law, our standard of review is de novo and the scope of our review is plenary. We begin by reviewing the thorough arguments presented by the parties.

Sperm Donor argues first that Pennsylvania law and public policy precluding parents from bargaining away a child's entitlement to child support should not preclude enforcement of an otherwise binding contract where the bargain in question occurs prior to, and indeed induces, the donation of sperm for IVF and implantation in a clinical setting. Sperm Donor urges this Court to hold that the fact that the agreement was formed months prior to conception distinguishes this case from precedent preventing parents from bargaining away a child in being's right to seek child support . . . Sperm Donor emphasizes that he provided his sperm to Mother contingent on her promise not to seek child support in the future-that the promise was, in effect, a "but for" cause of the twins' conception and birth. Sperm Donor maintains that his and Mother's shared intention "was to cloak [their] agreement in the same legal protections that an anonymous sperm donor enjoys," and that "people should be free to enter into these agreements, in the interest of allowing people access to greater . . . options concerning the areas of reproduction."

Sperm Donor contends that to uphold the Superior Court's ruling will call into question the legal status of all sperm donors, including those who donate anonymously through sperm banks. Sperm Donor buttresses his argument by reference to the Uniform Parentage Act (UPA), a proposed uniform law originally promulgated in 1973 by the American Bar Association[5] and adopted, in some form, by at least nineteen states. Sperm Donor observes that the UPA, which he acknowledges has not been adopted by this Commonwealth, does not require anonymity in the sperm donor context to protect the donor from subsequent parental responsibility and the child and parent from a donor's subsequent claim of parental privileges. Rather, the UPA provides unequivocally that "A donor is not a parent of a child conceived by means of assisted reproduction." UPA § 702. The Comment to § 702 elaborates: "The donor can neither sue to establish parental rights, nor be sued and required to support the resulting child. In sum, donors are eliminated from the

---

[5] The UPA, like all uniform state laws, was drafted and promulgated by the National Conference of Commissioners on Uniform State Laws. This is a different organization than the ABA. -Ed.

parental equation." UPA § 702 Cmt. (emphasis added). Sperm Donor argues that the Commonwealth should not concern itself with the question of anonymity if the parties to the agreement themselves are not concerned. Sperm Donor also argues that an absolute holding of parental responsibility in this case threatens other contract-based alternative reproductive arrangements, such as adoption and institutional sperm donation, since the lower court rulings both plausibly may be read to hold that any contract denying a child the support of any biological parent necessarily violates public policy.

Mother, conversely, argues that this Court should uphold the lower courts' rulings that the best interests of the child preclude enforcement of the parties' contract, contending that "there is no basis for making an exception [to the best interests approach] merely because the children at issue were conceived in a clinical setting and the agreement was made prior to their conception." She argues that if this Court rules otherwise, it will act impermissibly in place of the General Assembly and contrarily to 23 Pa.C.S. § 5102, which "mandates that without exception" all children shall be "legitimate" without regard to the marital status of their parents, and that children born out of wedlock shall enjoy all rights and privileges of children born to married parents.

We reject Mother's invocation of this section, as the matter before us is not the twins' "legitimacy" but their entitlement to Sperm Donor's support notwithstanding the contrary agreement entered into by Mother and Sperm Donor.

Mother rejects Sperm Donor's reliance on UPA § 702, emphasizing that for over thirty years the General Assembly has failed to adopt the model act. The twins, Mother argues, are Sperm Donor's offspring pursuant to § 5102, and have the same right to his support they would have if Sperm Donor and Mother had conceived by sexual intercourse. Mother observes that the General Assembly, beginning in 1975, repeatedly has considered bills purporting to elaborate on the legal relationships spawned by reproductive alternatives, but none has made it out of committee. Mother argues that the General Assembly's failure to enact these bills signals its "unwillingness . . . to adopt the UPA provision which . . . eliminates all sperm donors (except the spouse of the donee) from the 'parental equation.' " . . .

Mother's argument, for all its nuance, effectively relies on the same background principle that the lower courts found dispositive: that even mutually entered and otherwise valid contracts are unenforceable when the contracts violate clear public policy - in this case, the Commonwealth's oft-stated policy not to permit parents to bargain away their child's right to support. Notably, neither the courts below nor Mother undertake the rigorous analysis called for by our caselaw governing the enforceability of contracts supposed to violate public policy, relying instead on a tenuous analogy between the instant circumstances and those of divorce or other parenting arrangements arising in the context of sexual relationships . . .

This analogy, however, is unsustainable in the face of the evolving role played by alternative reproductive technologies in contemporary American society. It derives no authority from apposite Pennsylvania law, and it violates the commonsense distinction between reproduction via sexual intercourse and the non-sexual clinical options for conception that are increasingly common in the modern reproductive environment. The inescapable reality is that all manner of arrangements involving the donation of sperm or eggs abound in contemporary society, many of them couched in contracts or agreements of varying degrees of formality. An increasing number of would-be mothers who find themselves either unable or unwilling to conceive and raise children in the context of marriage are turning to donor arrangements to enable them to enjoy the privilege of raising a child or children, a development neither our citizens nor their General Assembly have chosen to proscribe despite its growing pervasiveness . . .

Thus, two potential cases at the extremes of an increasingly complicated continuum present themselves: dissolution of a relationship (or a mere sexual encounter) that produces a child via intercourse, which requires both parents to provide support; and an anonymous sperm donation, absent sex, resulting in the birth of a child. These opposed extremes produce two distinct views that we believe to be self-evident. In the case of traditional sexual reproduction, there simply is no question that the parties to any resultant conception and birth may not contract between themselves to deny the child the support he or she requires. In the institutional sperm donation case, however, there appears to be a growing consensus that clinical, institutional sperm donation neither imposes obligations nor confers privileges upon the sperm donor. Between these poles lies a spectrum of arrangements that exhibit characteristics of each extreme to varying degrees-informal agreements between friends to conceive a child via sexual intercourse; non-clinical non-sexual insemination; and so on.

Although locating future cases on this spectrum may call upon courts to draw very fine lines, courts are no strangers to such tasks, and the instant case, which we must resolve, is not nearly so difficult. The facts of this case . . . reveal the parties' mutual intention to preserve all of the trappings of a conventional sperm donation, including formation of a binding agreement. Indeed, the parties could have done little more than they did to imbue the transaction with the hallmarks of institutional, non-sexual conception by sperm donation and IVF. They negotiated an agreement outside the context of a romantic relationship; they agreed to terms; they sought clinical assistance to effectuate IVF and implantation of the consequent embryos, taking sexual intercourse out of the equation; they attempted to hide Sperm Donor's paternity from medical personnel, friends, and family; and for approximately five years following the birth of the twins both parties behaved in every regard consistently with the intentions they expressed at the outset of their arrangement, Sperm Donor not seeking to serve as a father to the twins, and Mother not demanding his support, financial or otherwise. That Mother knew Sperm Donor's identity, the parties failed to preserve Sperm Donor's anonymity from a handful of family members who were well acquainted with Sperm Donor and Mother alike, and Mother acted on her preference to know the identity of her sperm donor by voluntarily declining to avail herself of the services of a company that matches anonymous donors with willing mothers, reveal no obvious basis for analyzing this case any differently than we would a case involving an institutionally arranged sperm donation . . .

This Court takes very seriously the best interests of the children of this Commonwealth, and we recognize that to rule in favor of Sperm Donor in this case denies a source of support to two children who did not ask to be born into this situation. Absent the parties' agreement, however, the twins would not have been born at all, or would have been born to a different and anonymous sperm donor, who neither party disputes would be safe from a support order. Further, we cannot simply disregard the plight of Sperm Donor's marital child, who also did not ask to be born into this situation, but whose interests would suffer under the trial court's order.

The parties in this case agreed to an arrangement that to all appearances was to resemble-and in large part did resemble for approximately five years-a single-parent arrangement effectuated through the use of donor sperm secured from a sperm bank. Under these peculiar circumstances, and in considering as we must the broader implications of issuing a precedent of tremendous consequence to untold numbers of Pennsylvanians, we can discern no tenable basis to uphold the trial court's support order. Rather, we hold that the agreement found by the trial court to have been bindingly formed, which the trial court deemed nevertheless unenforceable is, in fact, enforceable.

Because we hold that the parties' agreement not to seek visitation or support is enforceable in this case, we reverse the Superior Court's order affirming the trial court's support order, and remand for further action consistent with this Opinion.

Former Justices Nigro and Newman did not participate in the decision of this case.

Chief Justice Cappy and Justice Castille join the opinion.

Justice Saylor files a dissenting opinion

Justice Eakin files a dissenting opinion.

Justice Eakin, dissenting.

I respectfully dissent from the majority's conclusion appellee can bargain away her children's right to support from their father merely because he fathered the children through a clinical sperm donation. The majority concludes this is possible because the parties intended "to preserve all of the trappings of a conventional sperm donation . . . [and] negotiated an agreement outside the context of a romantic relationship . . ." To this, I say, "So what?" The only difference between this case and any other is the means by which these two parents conceived the twin boys who now look for support. Referring to Joel McKiernan as "Sperm Donor" does not change his status-he is their father.

It is those children whose rights we address, not the rights of the parents. Do these children, unlike any other, lack the fundamental ability to look to both parents for support? If the answer is no, and the law changes as my colleagues hold, it must be for a reason of monumental significance. Is the means by which these parents contracted to accomplish conception enough to overcome that right? I think not . . .

[Parents] have no power . . . to bargain away the rights of their children. . . .

They cannot in that process set a standard that will leave their children short. Their bargain may be eminently fair, give all that the children might require and be enforceable because it is fair. When it gives less than required or less than can be given to provide for the best interest of the children, it falls under the jurisdiction of the court's wide and necessary powers to provide for that best interest.

The majority, with little citation to authority, relies on policy notions outside the record, such as "the evolving role played by alternative reproductive technologies in contemporary American society," and hypothetical scenarios concerning reproductive choices of individuals. These musings are thought-provoking, but are ultimately inapplicable to this case of enforceability of a private contract ostensibly negating a child's right to support-a contract our jurisprudence has long ago held to be unenforceable. This case has little or nothing to do with anonymous sperm clinics and reproductive technology.

Speculating about an anonymous donor's reluctance is irrelevant-there is no anonymity here and never has been. There was no effort at all to insulate the identity of the father — he was a named party to the contract! This is not a case of a sperm clinic where donors have their identity concealed. The only difference between this case and any other conception is the intervention of hardware between one identifiable would-be parent and the other . . .

This private contract involves traditional support principles not abrogated by the means chosen by the parents to inseminate the mother, and I would apply the well-settled precedent that the best interest of the children controls. A parent cannot bargain away the children's right to support. These children have a right to support from both parents, including the man who is not an anonymous sperm donor, but their father.

I would affirm the Superior Court, as the agreement here is against the public policy and thus unenforceable.

NOTES AND QUESTIONS

1. *The Updated UPA.* The *Ferguson* court notes that Pennsylvania is one of around 20 states that has not adopted the UPA provision protecting sperm donors from being held legally responsible for any offspring conceived using donated sperm. The original UPA, promulgated in 1973, was substantially revised in 2000 (and further amended in 2002), in part to reflect the enormous changes in assisted conception that had transpired in the intervening decades. The new UPA section pertaining to sperm donation, Section 702, provides: "A donor is not a parent of a child conceived by means of assisted reproduction." The old reference to a licensed physician was removed, along with language about the marital status of the woman who is inseminated. The Commissioners, in the commentary to new Section 702, explain:

> The new Act does not continue the requirement that the donor provide the sperm to a licensed physician. Further, this section of the new UPA does not limit a donor's statutory exemption from becoming a legal parent of a child resulting from ART to a situation in which the donor provides sperm for assisted reproduction by a married woman. This requirement is not

realistic in light of present ART practices and the constitutional protections of the procreative rights of unmarried as well as married women. Consequently, this section shields all donors, whether of sperm or eggs, (§ 102 (8), *supra*), from parenthood in all situations in which either a married woman or a single woman conceives a child through ART with the intent to be the child's parent, either by herself or with a man, as provided in sections 703 and 704. If a married woman bears a child of assisted reproduction using a donor's sperm, the donor will not be the father in any event. Her husband will be the father unless and until the husband's lack of consent to the assisted reproduction is proven within two years of his learning of the birth, *see* § 705, *infra*. This provides certainty of nonparentage for prospective donors.

If Pennsylvania had adopted the newest version of the UPA, including Section 702, do you think Justice Eakin would have sided with the majority opinion? If not, what argument(s) would he have made in his dissent?

2.   *More Known Donor Cases.* The highest courts in two other states, Washington and Kansas, have also tackled the question of whether a known sperm donor can be adjudged the legal parent of any resulting children. In *In the Matter of the Parentage of J.M.K. and D.R.K.*, 155 Wash. 2d 374, 119 P.3d 840 (2005), a married man who conceived children with his (unmarried) girlfriend using IVF was determined to be the offspring's legal father. The man "donated" sperm on several occasions which the woman used in two separate IVF cycles to give birth in 1998 and 2001. The court found the man's argument that he was a mere sperm donor unavailing, given he signed an affidavit of parentage and made child support payments until his wife discovered his second family. In *In the Interest of K.M.H. and K.C.H.*, 285 Kan. 53, 169 P.3d 1025 (2007), an unmarried female lawyer sought sperm from a friend, ultimately giving birth to twins. Two weeks after the twins were born, the "donor" filed a paternity action claiming he was the children's legal father. The case reached the Kansas Supreme Court, which looked to the state's statutory regime declaring "the donor of semen . . . [is] not the birth father of a child thereby conceived, unless agreed to in writing by the donor and the woman." Since the pair had entered no written agreement concerning the sperm donation, the court found the man lacking in any parental rights. Do you think the female lawyer's conduct was foresightful or merely forgetful?

3.   Your high school classmate contacts you for legal advice. She is unmarried and wants to have a child using a known sperm donor. The man she has selected is also a high school classmate who is now unmarried and living in the same city as the would-be mother. Your friend asks you to draft an agreement she can present to the donor. What questions would you ask your friend? Consider drafting the "known donor" agreement.

––––––––––

When a man is asked to provide his reproductive material for another's procreative desires, his involvement in the enterprise can be very short-lived. It is possible for him to provide his sperm and walk away entirely in a matter of moments. When a woman is asked to provide her reproductive material for another's procreative desires, her entanglement is necessarily more complex. In the case of egg retrieval, as we learned in Chapter 3, the woman's commitment lasts for at least several weeks. When a woman is asked to supply her other reproductive material — her uterus — for another's procreative desire, she must be willing to commit her resources for at least nine months, and often much longer. This arrangement in which a woman gestates a child for another is commonly referred to as a surrogate parenting agreement. In the materials that follow, consider whether the term "surrogate" is apt for these relationships that pose novel family questions.

SECTION II: BUILDING FAMILIES THROUGH SURROGATE PARENTING AGREEMENTS

A. An Introductory Case

IN THE MATTER OF BABY M
Supreme Court of New Jersey
109 N.J. 396, 537 A.2d 1227 (1988)

WILENTZ, C.J. In this matter the Court is asked to determine the validity of a contract that purports to provide a new way of bringing children into a family. For a fee of $10,000, a woman agrees to be artificially inseminated with the semen of another woman's husband; she is to conceive a child, carry it to term, and after its birth surrender it to the natural father and his wife. The intent of the contract is that the child's natural mother will thereafter be forever separated from her child. The wife is to adopt the child, and she and the natural father are to be regarded as its parents for all purposes. The contract providing for this is called a "surrogacy contract," the natural mother inappropriately called the "surrogate mother."

We invalidate the surrogacy contract because it conflicts with the law and public policy of this State. While we recognize the depth of the yearning of infertile couples to have their own children, we find the payment of money to a "surrogate" mother illegal, perhaps criminal, and potentially degrading to women. Although in this case we grant custody to the natural father, the evidence having clearly proved such custody to be in the best interests of the infant, we void both the termination of the surrogate mother's parental rights and the adoption of the child by the wife/ stepparent. We thus restore the "surrogate" as the mother of the child. We remand the issue of the natural mother's visitation rights to the trial court, since that issue was not reached below and the record before us is not sufficient to permit us to decide it *de novo*.

We find no offense to our present laws where a woman voluntarily and without payment agrees to act as a "surrogate" mother, provided that she is not subject to a binding agreement to surrender her child. Moreover, our holding today does not preclude the Legislature from altering the current statutory scheme, within constitutional limits, so as to permit surrogacy contracts. Under current law, however, the surrogacy agreement before us is illegal and invalid.

I.

FACTS

In February 1985, William Stern and Mary Beth Whitehead entered into a surrogacy contract. It recited that Stern's wife, Elizabeth, was infertile, that they wanted a child, and that Mrs. Whitehead was willing to provide that child as the mother with Mr. Stern as the father. The contract provided that through artificial insemination using Mr. Stern's sperm, Mrs. Whitehead would become pregnant, carry the child to term, bear it, deliver it to the Sterns, and thereafter do whatever was necessary to terminate her maternal rights so that Mrs. Stern could thereafter adopt the child. Mrs. Whitehead's husband, Richard, was also a party to the contract; Mrs. Stern was not. Mr. Whitehead promised to do all acts necessary to rebut the presumption of paternity under the Parentage Act. *N.J.S.A.* 9:17-43a(1), -44a. Although Mrs. Stern was not a party to the surrogacy agreement, the contract gave her sole custody of the child in the event of Mr. Stern's death. Mrs. Stern's status as a nonparty to the surrogate parenting agreement presumably was to avoid the application of the baby-selling statute to this arrangement. *N.J.S.A.* 9:3-54. Mr. Stern, on his part, agreed to attempt the artificial insemination and to pay Mrs. Whitehead $10,000 after the child's birth, on its delivery to him. In a separate contract, Mr. Stern agreed to pay $7,500 to the Infertility Center of New York ("ICNY"). The Center's advertising campaigns solicit surrogate mothers and encourage infertile couples to consider surrogacy. ICNY arranged for the surrogacy contract by bringing the parties together, explaining the process to them, furnishing the contractual form, and providing legal counsel.

The history of the parties' involvement in this arrangement suggests their good faith. William and Elizabeth Stern were married in July 1974, having met at the University of Michigan, where both were Ph.D. candidates. Due to financial considerations and Mrs. Stern's pursuit of a medical degree and residency, they decided to defer starting a family until 1981. Before then, however, Mrs. Stern learned that she might have multiple sclerosis and that the disease in some cases renders pregnancy a serious health risk. Her anxiety appears to have exceeded the actual risk, which current medical authorities assess as minimal. Nonetheless that anxiety was evidently quite real, Mrs. Stern fearing that pregnancy might precipitate blindness, paraplegia, or other forms of debilitation. Based on the perceived risk, the Sterns decided to forego having their own children. The decision had special significance for Mr. Stern. Most of his family had been destroyed in the Holocaust. As the family's only survivor, he very much wanted to continue his bloodline.

Initially the Sterns considered adoption, but were discouraged by the substantial delay apparently involved and by the potential problem they saw arising from their age and their differing religious backgrounds. They were most eager for some other means to start a family. The paths of Mrs. Whitehead and the Sterns to surrogacy were similar. Both responded to advertising by ICNY. The Sterns' response, following their inquiries into adoption, was the result of their long-standing decision to have a child. Mrs. Whitehead's response apparently resulted from her sympathy with family members and others who could have no children (she stated that she wanted to give another couple the "gift of life"); she also wanted the $10,000 to help her family . . .

Mrs. Whitehead had reached her decision concerning surrogacy before the Sterns, and had actually been involved as a potential surrogate mother with another couple. After numerous unsuccessful artificial inseminations, that effort was abandoned. Thereafter, the Sterns learned of the Infertility Center, the possibilities of surrogacy, and of Mary Beth Whitehead. The two couples met to discuss the surrogacy arrangement and decided to go forward. On February 6, 1985, Mr. Stern and Mr. and Mrs. Whitehead executed the surrogate parenting agreement. After several artificial inseminations over a period of months, Mrs. Whitehead became pregnant. The pregnancy was uneventful and on March 27, 1986, Baby M was born.

Not wishing anyone at the hospital to be aware of the surrogacy arrangement, Mr. and Mrs. Whitehead appeared to all as the proud parents of a healthy female child. Her birth certificate indicated her name to be Sara Elizabeth Whitehead and her father to be Richard Whitehead. In accordance with Mrs. Whitehead's request, the Sterns visited the hospital unobtrusively to see the newborn child.

Mrs. Whitehead realized, almost from the moment of birth, that she could not part with this child. She had felt a bond with it even during pregnancy. Some indication of the attachment was conveyed to the Sterns at the hospital when they told Mrs. Whitehead what they were going to name the baby. She apparently broke into tears and indicated that she did not know if she could give up the child. She talked about how the baby looked like her other daughter, and made it clear that she was experiencing great difficulty with the decision.

Nonetheless, Mrs. Whitehead was, for the moment, true to her word. Despite powerful inclinations to the contrary, she turned her child over to the Sterns on March 30 at the Whiteheads' home.

The Sterns were thrilled with their new child. They had planned extensively for its arrival, far beyond the practical furnishing of a room for her. It was a time of joyful celebration — not just for them but for their friends as well. The Sterns looked forward to raising their daughter, whom they named Melissa. While aware by then that Mrs. Whitehead was undergoing an emotional crisis, they were as yet not cognizant of the depth of that crisis and its implications for their newly-enlarged family.

Later in the evening of March 30, Mrs. Whitehead became deeply disturbed, disconsolate, stricken with unbearable sadness. She had to have her child. She could not eat, sleep, or concentrate on anything other than her need for her baby. The next day she went to the Sterns' home and told them how much she was suffering.

The depth of Mrs. Whitehead's despair surprised and frightened the Sterns. She told them that she could not live without her baby, that she must have her, even if only for one week, that thereafter she would surrender her child. The Sterns, concerned that Mrs. Whitehead might indeed commit suicide, not wanting under any circumstances to risk that, and in any event believing that Mrs. Whitehead would keep her word, turned the child over to her. It was not until four months later, after a series of attempts to regain possession of the child, that Melissa was returned to the Sterns, having been forcibly removed from the home where she was then living with Mr. and Mrs. Whitehead, [to] the home in Florida owned by Mary Beth Whitehead's parents.

The struggle over Baby M began when it became apparent that Mrs. Whitehead could not return the child to Mr. Stern. Due to Mrs. Whitehead's refusal to relinquish the baby, Mr. Stern filed a complaint seeking enforcement of the surrogacy contract. He alleged, accurately, that Mrs. Whitehead had not only refused to comply with the surrogacy contract but had threatened to flee from New Jersey with the child in order to avoid even the possibility of his obtaining custody. The court papers asserted that if Mrs. Whitehead were to be given notice of the application for an order requiring her to relinquish custody, she would, prior to the hearing, leave the state with the baby. And that is precisely what she did. After the order was entered, *ex parte*, the process server, aided by the police, in the presence of the Sterns, entered Mrs. Whitehead's home to execute the order. Mr. Whitehead fled with the child, who had been handed to him through a window while those who came to enforce the order were thrown off balance by a dispute over the child's current name.

The Whiteheads immediately fled to Florida with Baby M. They stayed initially with Mrs. Whitehead's parents, where one of Mrs. Whitehead's children had been living. For the next three months, the Whiteheads and Melissa lived at roughly twenty different hotels, motels, and homes in order to avoid apprehension. From time to time Mrs. Whitehead would call Mr. Stern to discuss the matter; the conversations, recorded by Mr. Stern on advice of counsel, show an escalating dispute about rights, morality, and power, accompanied by threats of Mrs. Whitehead to kill herself, to kill the child, and falsely to accuse Mr. Stern of sexually molesting Mrs. Whitehead's other daughter.

Eventually the Sterns discovered where the Whiteheads were staying, commenced supplementary proceedings in Florida, and obtained an order requiring the Whiteheads to turn over the child. Police in Florida enforced the order, forcibly removing the child from her grandparents' home. She was soon thereafter brought to New Jersey and turned over to the Sterns. The prior order of the court, issued *ex parte*, awarding custody of the child to the Sterns *pendente lite*, was reaffirmed by the trial court after consideration of the certified representations of the parties (both represented by counsel) concerning the unusual sequence of events that had unfolded. Pending final judgment, Mrs. Whitehead was awarded limited visitation with Baby M.

The Sterns' complaint, in addition to seeking possession and ultimately custody of the child, sought enforcement of the surrogacy contract. Pursuant to the contract, it asked that the child be permanently placed in their custody, that Mrs. Whitehead's parental rights be terminated, and that Mrs. Stern be allowed to adopt the child, *i.e.*, that, for all purposes, Melissa become the Sterns' child.

The trial took thirty-two days over a period of more than two months . . . [T]he bulk of the testimony was devoted to determining the parenting arrangement most compatible with the child's best interests. Soon after the conclusion of the trial, the trial court announced its opinion from the bench. 217 N.J.Super. 313, 525 A.2d 1128 (1987). It held that the surrogacy contract was valid; ordered that Mrs. Whitehead's parental rights be terminated and that sole custody of the child be granted to Mr.

Stern; and, after hearing brief testimony from Mrs. Stern, immediately entered an order allowing the adoption of Melissa by Mrs. Stern, all in accordance with the surrogacy contract. Pending the outcome of the appeal, we granted a continuation of visitation to Mrs. Whitehead, although slightly more limited than the visitation allowed during the trial . . .

On the question of best interests [of the child] — and we agree, but for different reasons, that custody was the critical issue — the court's analysis of the testimony was perceptive, demonstrating both its understanding of the case and its considerable experience in these matters. We agree substantially with both its analysis and conclusions on the matter of custody.

The court's review and analysis of the surrogacy contract, however, is not at all in accord with ours. The trial court concluded that the various statutes governing this matter, including those concerning adoption, termination of parental rights, and payment of money in connection with adoptions, do not apply to surrogacy contracts . . . It reasoned that because the Legislature did not have surrogacy contracts in mind when it passed those laws, those laws were therefore irrelevant . . . Thus, assuming it was writing on a clean slate, the trial court analyzed the interests involved and the power of the court to accommodate them. It then held that surrogacy contracts are valid and should be enforced, . . . and furthermore that Mr. Stern's rights under the surrogacy contract were constitutionally protected . . .

Mrs. Whitehead appealed. This Court granted direct certification . . .

Mrs. Whitehead contends that the surrogacy contract, for a variety of reasons, is invalid. She contends that it conflicts with public policy since it guarantees that the child will not have the nurturing of both natural parents — presumably New Jersey's goal for families. She further argues that it deprives the mother of her constitutional right to the companionship of her child, and that it conflicts with statutes concerning termination of parental rights and adoption. With the contract thus void, Mrs. Whitehead claims primary custody (with visitation rights in Mr. Stern) both on a best interests basis (stressing the "tender years" doctrine) as well as on the policy basis of discouraging surrogacy contracts. She maintains that even if custody would ordinarily go to Mr. Stern, here it should be awarded to Mrs. Whitehead to deter future surrogacy arrangements . . .

The Sterns claim that the surrogacy contract is valid and should be enforced, largely for the reasons given by the trial court. They claim a constitutional right of privacy, which includes the right of procreation, and the right of consenting adults to deal with matters of reproduction as they see fit. As for the child's best interests, their position is factual: given all of the circumstances, the child is better off in their custody with no residual parental rights reserved for Mrs. Whitehead.

Of considerable interest in this clash of views is the position of the child's guardian *ad litem*, wisely appointed by the court at the outset of the litigation . . . She . . . took the position, based on her experts' testimony, that the Sterns should have primary custody, and that while Mrs. Whitehead's parental rights should not be terminated, no visitation should . . . be allowed at least until Baby M reaches maturity . . .

II.

INVALIDITY AND UNENFORCEABILITY OF SURROGACY CONTRACT

We have concluded that this surrogacy contract is invalid. Our conclusion has two bases: direct conflict with existing statutes and conflict with the public policies of this State, as expressed in its statutory and decisional law . . .

A. Conflict with Statutory Provisions

The surrogacy contract conflicts with: (1) laws prohibiting the use of money in connection with adoptions; (2) laws requiring proof of parental unfitness or abandonment before termination of parental rights is ordered or an adoption is granted; and (3) laws that make surrender of custody and consent to adoption revocable in private placement adoptions.

(1) Our law prohibits paying or accepting money in connection with any placement of a child for adoption. N.J.S.A. 9:3-54a. Violation is a high misdemeanor. N.J.S.A. 9:3-54c. Excepted are fees of an approved agency (which must be a non-profit entity, N.J.S.A. 9:3-38a) and certain expenses in connection with child-birth. N.J.S.A. 9:3-54b.[6]

Considerable care was taken in this case to structure the surrogacy arrangement so as not to violate this prohibition. The arrangement was structured as follows: the adopting parent, Mrs. Stern, was not a party to the surrogacy contract; the money paid to Mrs. Whitehead was stated to be for her services — not for the adoption; the sole purpose of the contract was stated as being that "of giving a child to William Stern, its natural and biological father"; the money was purported to be "compensation for services and expenses and in no way . . . a fee for termination of parental rights or a payment in exchange for consent to surrender a child for adoption" . . . Nevertheless, it seems clear that the money was paid and accepted in connection with an adoption . . .

The surrogacy agreement requires Mrs. Whitehead to surrender Baby M for the purposes of adoption. The agreement notes that Mr. *and Mrs.* Stern wanted to have a child, and provides that the child be "placed" with Mrs. Stern in the event Mr. Stern dies before the child is born. The payment of the $10,000 occurs only on

---

[6] [n.4] N.J.S.A. 9:3-54 reads as follows:

a. No person, firm, partnership, corporation, association or agency shall make, offer to make or assist or participate in any placement for adoption and in connection therewith

(1) Pay, give or agree to give any money or any valuable consideration, or assume or discharge any financial obligation; or

(2) Take, receive, accept or agree to accept any money or any valuable consideration.

b. The prohibition of subsection a. shall not apply to the fees or services of any approved agency in connection with a placement for adoption, nor shall such prohibition apply to the payment or reimbursement of medical, hospital or other similar expenses incurred in connection with the birth or any illness of the child, or to the acceptance of such reimbursement by a parent of the child.

c. Any person, firm, partnership, corporation, association or agency violating this section shall be guilty of a high misdemeanor.

surrender of custody of the child and "completion of the duties and obligations" of Mrs. Whitehead, including termination of her parental rights to facilitate adoption by Mrs. Stern. As for the contention that the Sterns are paying only for services and not for an adoption, we need note only that they would pay nothing in the event the child died before the fourth month of pregnancy, and only $1,000 if the child were stillborn, even though the "services" had been fully rendered. Additionally, one of Mrs. Whitehead's estimated costs, to be assumed by Mr. Stern, was an "Adoption Fee," presumably for Mrs. Whitehead's incidental costs in connection with the adoption.

Mr. Stern knew he was paying for the adoption of a child; Mrs. Whitehead knew she was accepting money so that a child might be adopted; the Infertility Center knew that it was being paid for assisting in the adoption of a child. The actions of all three worked to frustrate the goals of the statute. It strains credulity to claim that these arrangements, touted by those in the surrogacy business as an attractive alternative to the usual route leading to an adoption, really amount to something other than a private placement adoption for money.

The prohibition of our statute is strong . . . The evils inherent in baby-bartering are loathsome for a myriad of reasons. The child is sold without regard for whether the purchasers will be suitable parents . . . The natural mother does not receive the benefit of counseling and guidance to assist her in making a decision that may affect her for a lifetime. In fact, the monetary incentive to sell her child may, depending on her financial circumstances, make her decision less voluntary . . . Furthermore, the adoptive parents may not be fully informed of the natural parents' medical history.

Baby-selling potentially results in the exploitation of all parties involved . . . Conversely, adoption statutes seek to further humanitarian goals, foremost among them the best interests of the child . . . The negative consequences of baby-buying are potentially present in the surrogacy context, especially the potential for placing and adopting a child without regard to the interest of the child or the natural mother.

(2) The termination of Mrs. Whitehead's parental rights, called for by the surrogacy contract and actually ordered by the court fails to comply with the stringent requirements of New Jersey law. Our law, recognizing the finality of any termination of parental rights, provides for such termination only where there has been a voluntary surrender of a child to an approved agency or to the Division of Youth and Family Services ("DYFS"), accompanied by a formal document acknowledging termination of parental rights, N.J.S.A. 9:2-16, - 17; N.J.S.A. 9:3-41; N.J.S.A. 30:4C-23, or where there has been a showing of parental abandonment or unfitness . . .

In this case a termination of parental rights was obtained not by proving the statutory prerequisites but by claiming the benefit of contractual provisions. From all that has been stated above, it is clear that a contractual agreement to abandon one's parental rights, or not to contest a termination action, will not be enforced in our courts. The Legislature would not have so carefully, so consistently, and so substantially restricted termination of parental rights if it had intended to allow termination to be achieved by one short sentence in a contract.

Since the termination was invalid, it follows, as noted above, that adoption of Melissa by Mrs. Stern could not properly be granted . . .

The provision in the surrogacy contract whereby the mother irrevocably agrees to surrender custody of her child and to terminate her parental rights conflicts with the settled interpretation of New Jersey statutory law. There is only one irrevocable consent, and that is the one explicitly provided for by statute: a consent to surrender of custody and a placement with an approved agency or with DYFS. The provision in the surrogacy contract, agreed to before conception, requiring the natural mother to surrender custody of the child without any right of revocation is one more indication of the essential nature of this transaction: the creation of a contractual system of termination and adoption designed to circumvent our statutes.

B. Public Policy Considerations

The surrogacy contract's invalidity, resulting from its direct conflict with the above statutory provisions, is further underlined when its goals and means are measured against New Jersey's public policy. The contract's basic premise, that the natural parents can decide in advance of birth which one is to have custody of the child, bears no relationship to the settled law that the child's best interests shall determine custody . . .

The surrogacy contract guarantees permanent separation of the child from one of its natural parents. Our policy, however, has long been that to the extent possible, children should remain with and be brought up by both of their natural parents . . .

The surrogacy contract violates the policy of this State that the rights of natural parents are equal concerning their child, the father's right no greater than the mother's . . . The whole purpose and effect of the surrogacy contract was to give the father the exclusive right to the child by destroying the rights of the mother.

The policies expressed in our comprehensive laws governing consent to the surrender of a child . . . stand in stark contrast to the surrogacy contract and what it implies. Here there is no counseling, independent or otherwise, of the natural mother, no evaluation, no warning . . .

Under the contract, the natural mother is irrevocably committed before she knows the strength of her bond with her child. She never makes a totally voluntary, informed decision, for quite clearly any decision prior to the baby's birth is, in the most important sense, uninformed, and any decision after that, compelled by a pre-existing contractual commitment, the threat of a lawsuit, and the inducement of a $10,000 payment, is less than totally voluntary. Her interests are of little concern to those who controlled this transaction.

Although the interest of the natural father and adoptive mother is certainly the predominant interest, realistically the *only* interest served, even they are left with less than what public policy requires. They know little about the natural mother, her genetic makeup, and her psychological and medical history. Moreover, not even a superficial attempt is made to determine their awareness of their responsibilities as parents.

Worst of all, however, is the contract's total disregard of the best interests of the child. There is not the slightest suggestion that any inquiry will be made at any time to determine the fitness of the Sterns as custodial parents, of Mrs. Stern as an adoptive parent, their superiority to Mrs. Whitehead, or the effect on the child of not living with her natural mother.

This is the sale of a child, or, at the very least, the sale of a mother's right to her child, the only mitigating factor being that one of the purchasers is the father. Almost every evil that prompted the prohibition on the payment of money in connection with adoptions exists here . . .

The surrogacy contract is based on, principles that are directly contrary to the objectives of our laws. It guarantees the separation of a child from its mother; it looks to adoption regardless of suitability; it totally ignores the child; it takes the child from the mother regardless of her wishes and her maternal fitness; and it does all of this, it accomplishes all of its goals, through the use of money.

Beyond that is the potential degradation of some women that may result from this arrangement. In many cases, of course, surrogacy may bring satisfaction, not only to the infertile couple, but to the surrogate mother herself. The fact, however, that many women may not perceive surrogacy negatively but rather see it as an opportunity does not diminish its potential for devastation to other women.

In sum, the harmful consequences of this surrogacy arrangement appear to us all too palpable. In New Jersey the surrogate mother's agreement to sell her child is void. Its irrevocability infects the entire contract, as does the money that purports to buy it . . .

IV.

CONSTITUTIONAL ISSUES

Both parties argue that the Constitutions — state and federal — mandate approval of their basic claims. The source of their constitutional arguments is essentially the same: the right of privacy, the right to procreate, the right to the companionship of one's child, those rights flowing either directly from the four- teenth amendment or by its incorporation of the Bill of Rights, or from the ninth amendment, or through the penumbra surrounding all of the Bill of Rights. They are the rights of personal intimacy, of marriage, of sex, of family, of procreation. Whatever their source, it is clear that they are fundamental rights protected by both the federal and state Constitutions . . . The right asserted by the Sterns is the right of procreation; that asserted by Mary Beth Whitehead is the right to the companionship of her child. We find that the right of procreation does not extend as far as claimed by the Sterns. As for the right asserted by Mrs. Whitehead, since we uphold it on other grounds (*i.e.*, we have restored her as mother and recognized her right, limited by the child's best interests, to her companionship), we need not decide that constitutional issue, and for reasons set forth below, we should not.

The right to procreate, as protected by the Constitution, has been ruled on directly only once by the United States Supreme Court. See Skinner v. Oklahoma,

316 U.S. 535, 62 S.Ct. 1110, 86 L.Ed. 1655 (forced sterilization of habitual criminals violates equal protection clause of fourteenth amendment) . . . The right to procreate very simply is the right to have natural children, whether through sexual intercourse or artificial insemination. It is no more than that. Mr. Stern has not been deprived of that right. Through artificial insemination of Mrs. Whitehead, Baby M is his child. The custody, care, companionship, and nurturing that follow birth are not parts of the right to procreation; they are rights that may also be constitutionally protected, but that involve many considerations other than the right of procreation. To assert that Mr. Stern's right of procreation gives him the right to the custody of Baby M would be to assert that Mrs. Whitehead's right of procreation does *not* give her the right to the custody of Baby M; it would be to assert that the constitutional right of procreation includes within it a constitutionally protected contractual right to destroy someone else's right of procreation.

We conclude that the right of procreation is best understood and protected if confined to its essentials, and that when dealing with rights concerning the resulting child, different interests come into play. There is nothing in our culture or society that even begins to suggest a fundamental right on the part of the father to the custody of the child as part of his right to procreate when opposed by the claim of the mother to the same child . . . Our conclusion may thus be understood as illustrating that a person's rights of privacy and self-determination are qualified by the effect on innocent third persons of the exercise of those rights . . .

V.
CUSTODY

[The court concludes that custody in the Sterns was in the best interest of the child.]

VI.
VISITATION

The trial court's decision to terminate Mrs. Whitehead's parental rights precluded it from making any determination on visitation. Our reversal of the trial court's order, however, requires delineation of Mrs. Whitehead's rights to visitation . . . We therefore remand the visitation issue to the trial court for an abbreviated hearing and determination as set forth below . . .

CONCLUSION

This case affords some insight into a new reproductive arrangement: the artificial insemination of a surrogate mother. The unfortunate events that have unfolded illustrate that its unregulated use can bring suffering to all involved. Potential victims include the surrogate mother and her family, the natural father and his wife, and most importantly, the child. Although surrogacy has apparently provided positive results for some infertile couples, it can also, as this case demonstrates, cause suffering to participants, here essentially innocent and well-intended.

We have found that our present laws do not permit the surrogacy contract used in this case. Nowhere, however, do we find any legal prohibition against surrogacy when the surrogate mother volunteers, without any payment, to act as a surrogate and is given the right to change her mind and to assert her parental rights. Moreover, the Legislature remains free to deal with this most sensitive issue as it sees fit, subject only to constitutional constraints . . .

Legislative consideration of surrogacy may also provide the opportunity to begin to focus on the overall implications of the new reproductive biotechnology — *in vitro* fertilization, preservation of sperm and eggs, embryo implantation and the like. The problem is how to enjoy the benefits of the technology — especially for infertile couples — while minimizing the risk of abuse. The problem can be addressed only when society decides what its values and objectives are in this troubling, yet promising, area.

The judgment is affirmed in part, reversed in part, and remanded for further proceedings consistent with this opinion.

For affirmance in part, reversal in part and remandment — Chief Justice WI-LENTZ and Justices CLIFFORD, HANDLER, POLLOCK, O'HERN, GARIBALDI and STEIN — 7.
Opposed — None.

NOTES AND QUESTIONS

1.   The arrangement between the Sterns and the Whiteheads may have been the first in modern memory to garner national attention, but the idea of one woman acting as a surrogate mother for another couple dates back to biblical times. Recall the story in *Genesis* in which a childless Sarah offers her handmaid, Hagar, to Abraham hoping, "it may be that I may obtain children by her." After Hagar gives birth to Abraham's son Ishmael, he sends the pair away after sensing the bad blood brewing between the birth mother and Sarah. *Genesis* 16:2, 21:14, The Holy Bible (King James Version 2000). Two generations later Jacob fathers four sons, two each with Bilhah and Zilpah, Rachel and Leah's handmaids. Sympathetic to Rachel's infertility, Jacob complies after his wife's entreat, "go in unto her, and she shall bear upon my knees, that I may also have children by her." Id. at *Genesis* 30:3. Though the exchange of money is not a part of the biblical tales, the emotionalism and family schism have a modern ring to them.

2.   The decision in *Baby M* is often cited as the seminal case in the area of surrogate parenting arrangements, but the Supreme Court of New Jersey was not the first court to rule on the validity of such agreements. Courts in at least three states had issued opinions in surrogacy cases by the time *Baby M* reached the high state court in 1988. In Michigan, two appellate courts found that surrogacy arrangements conflicted with various aspects of state law. See *Doe v. Kelley*, 106 Mich.App. 169, 307 N.W.2d 438 (1981), *cert. den.*, 459 U.S. 1183, 103 S.Ct. 834, 74 L.Ed.2d 1027 (1983) (application of sections of Michigan Adoption Law prohibiting the exchange of money to surrogacy is constitutional); Syrkowski v. Appleyard, 122 Mich.App. 506, 333 N.W.2d 90 (1983) (court held it lacked jurisdiction to issue an

"order of filiation" because surrogacy arrangements were not governed by Michigan's Paternity Act), rev'd, 420 Mich. 367, 362 N.W.2d 211 (1985) (court decided Paternity Act should be applied but did not reach the merits of the claim).

The Supreme Court of Kentucky took a somewhat different approach to surrogate arrangements. In *Surrogate Parenting Assocs. v. Commonwealth ex. rel. Armstrong*, 704 S.W.2d 209 (Ky.1986), the court held that the "fundamental differences" between surrogate arrangements and baby-selling placed the surrogate parenting agreement beyond the reach of Kentucky's baby-selling statute. The rationale for this determination was that unlike the normal adoption situation, the surrogacy agreement is entered into before conception and is not directed at avoiding the consequences of an unwanted pregnancy. Id. at 211-12. Concomitant with this pro-surrogacy conclusion, however, the court held that a "surrogate" mother has the right to void the contract if she changes her mind during pregnancy or immediately after birth. The court relied on statutes providing that consent to adoption or to the termination of parental rights prior to five days after the birth of the child is invalid, and concluded that consent before conception must also be unenforceable. Id. at 212-13.

Finally, a New York court analyzed the adoption phase of an uncontested surrogacy arrangement in *Matter of Adoption of Baby Girl, L.J.*, 132 Misc.2d 972, 505 N.Y.S.2d 813 (Sur. 1986). Although the court expressed strong moral and ethical reservations about surrogacy arrangements, it approved the adoption because it was in the best interests of the child. *Id.* at 815. The court went on to find that surrogate parenting agreements are not void, but are voidable if they are not in accordance with the state's adoption statutes. The court upheld the payment of money in connection with the surrogacy arrangement on the ground that the New York Legislature did not contemplate surrogacy when the baby-selling statute was passed. *Id.* at 817-18. Despite the court's ethical and moral problems with surrogate arrangements, it concluded that the Legislature was the appropriate forum to address the legality of surrogacy arrangements.[7]

The New Jersey court could have followed the reasoning set forth in the Kentucky or New York cases to distinguish surrogacy contracts from illegal adoption agreements on the basis that the New Jersey adoption law was drafted before the modern advent of surrogate parenting agreements. Instead, it chose to apply the plain meaning of the adoption laws to the novel parenting agreement. Do you agree that existing laws, written before the emergence of new family structures, should govern the parental status of those who venture into new familial grounds? What are the benefits of relying on existing principles to govern newly emerging family scenarios? What are the drawbacks?

3.   The New Jersey court declares commercial surrogate parenting arrangements invalid under state law because they conflict with existing laws barring payment in connection with adoptions, and because they offend public policy against baby-selling. The commercial aspects of the arrangement seem to dominate the opinion, overshadowing another element of the agreement between the Sterns and

---

[7] In 1992, the New York legislature did address the legality of surrogacy arrangements, declaring them "void and unenforceable" even when no payment is involved. N.Y. Dom. Rel. Law § 122.

the Whiteheads — intent. What role, if any, does the parties' intent play in the decision in *Baby M*? In your mind, is intent a relevant factor when adults contract to conceive a child? Is the best interest of the child served or thwarted by attention to the prospective parents' intent?

The relative supremacy of intent, biological tie and gestational connection have occupied much of the debate over determining parenthood in a surrogacy arrangement. For some, the intent of the prospective parents to bring about the birth of a child, accompanied by the lack of intent on the part of the gestational carrier to be considered the child's parent, is the most important factor in determining the legal status of parent. For others, the biological or genetic tie between the child and the surrogate cannot be dismissed in assessing what is in the best interest of the child.

A succinct discussion of the view that the intended parents should prevail as against a gestational carrier is provided by Professor John Hill:

> With the expanding popularity of the various collaborative-reproductive techniques and arrangements, including surrogate parenting, it is increasingly imperative to settle the question of parental status in collaborative-reproduction arrangements. Having considered the arguments in defense of the claims of the genetic progenitors, the gestational host, and the intended parents, it is clear why the intended parents should be considered the "parents" of the child born of the [surrogate parenting] reproductive arrangement . . .

> [T]he balance of equities favors the claims of the intended parents over those of the gestational host. The moral significance of the intended parents' role as prime movers in the procreative relationship, the preconception promise of the biological progenitors not to claim rights in the child, and the relative importance of having the identity of the parents determined from conception onward outweigh the potential harm to the gestational host in compelled relinquishment. This conclusion, of course, will not be well-regarded in all quarters. An important reason for this skepticism is that a fundamentally biological conception of parenthood is ingrained deeply in the ethos of our culture. It continues to influence our most profound intuitions concerning the nature of parenthood and parental rights.

> Nevertheless, the biological conception does not square with a number of other, equally deep, intuitions. It is not consistent with the modern understanding that parenthood is as much a social, psychological, and intentional status as it is a biological one. It also is inconsistent with the sentiment that persons are not invariably and irrevocably predisposed to a role in life — even that of parenthood — by virtue of the inexorable workings of biology. Finally, and most fundamentally, the biological conception of parenthood cannot be reconciled with the belief that other moral considerations sometimes may override claims predicated upon the biological relationship. In essence, the claims of biology cannot be deemed to trump invariably the moral claims of those who entertain no biological connection with the child.

John Lawrence Hill, *What Does It Mean to Be a "Parent"? The Claims of Biology as the Basis for Parental Rights*, 66 N.Y.U. L. REV. 353, 418-20 (1991). Other commentators who elaborate on the import of intent include Marjorie Maguire Shultz, *Reproductive Technology and Intent-Based Parenthood: An Opportunity for Gender Neutrality*, 1990 WISC. L. REV. 297; and Richard F. Storrow, *Parenthood By Pure Intention: Assisted Reproduction and the Functional Approach to Parentage*, 53 HAST. L. J. 597 (2002).

A different perspective, highlighting the import of our biological tie to our child, is given voice by Professor Randy Kandel:

> Hereditary transmission has traditionally been accorded privileged status in determining family affiliation. It is also the one facet of biological parenthood which men and women share. Feminists have critiqued the choice of genetic motherhood as both reflecting and perpetuating the dominant social patriarchy. Nonetheless, since proof of a genetic connection is sufficient to establish paternity, equal protection principles compel us to recognize the genetic mother's connection as sufficient to establish maternity.
>
> In addition, the fervent wish to raise one's genetic child, as a link to immortality or an expression of one's self, is a major reason why many people choose surrogacy rather than adoption. The genetic mother's claim to be a natural parent is compelling. The genetic parents' contribution of hereditary material determines most of the physical, mental, and temperamental qualities which the child will possess at birth. The genetic mother suffers the risky surgical removal of her eggs, often preceded by harrowing years of infertility treatments and clinicalized sexual relations which have been carefully timed to coincide with her ovulatory cycle.
>
> Yet, the gestational mother's claim is equally compelling. Apart from their intense subjective connection, the fetus and pregnant mother are elaborately linked through biochemical and hormonal interconnections; the mother provides nourishment and immunity to the fetus; the fetus uses the mother's excretory and respiratory systems. Molecular communication between the mother and fetus serves the needs of the fetus but places unique stress upon the mother, which multiplies the mother's risk of both minor pregnancy ailments and serious diseases like hypertension and diabetes.
>
> The relative biological strangeness of the fetus to the gestational mother, as compared to a woman carrying a child conceived through sexual intercourse, demands an even greater biological investment from her during the pregnancy. Accordingly, the gestational mother faces heightened risks of developing severe pregnancy complications such as infection, caesarean section, ectopic (non-uterine) pregnancy, and possibly preeclampsia and frank eclampsia. Thus, mothering the fetus is a biological hazard that places the gestational mother at risk. Further, some intrauterine experiences are remembered by the baby and affect its behavior after birth. For example, unborn babies hear, dance to, and recognize their gestational mothers' voices. Above and beyond a gestational mother's love

for the child, her investment in the fetus supports her claim to the status of natural mother.

From the perspective of biology, when the genetic mother's hereditary contribution to the child is balanced against the gestational mother's developmental contribution, both must be viewed as equally "natural" mothers. Biology, when divorced from our cultural ideology about naturalness, provides no basis for choosing only one of them . . .

Randy Frances Kandel, *Which Came First? The Mother or the Egg: A Kinship Solution to Gestational Surrogacy*, 47 RUTGERS L. REV. 165, 187-90 (1994). Professor Kandel seems to suggest a sharing arrangement between the intended parents and the gestational carrier. Do you favor this approach to parentage when a child is born via a surrogate parenting arrangement?

Both Professor Hill and Professor Kandel make their arguments in the context of a surrogacy arrangement that differs from the circumstances in *Baby M*. Recall that Mary Beth Whitehead, the surrogate in *Baby M*, supplied the egg that was fertilized by Mr. Stern's sperm. She is often referred to as a "genetic" or "traditional" surrogate. In contrast, the Hill and Kandel commentaries focus on a scenario in which the prospective parents provide the genetic material to the surrogate, who merely gestates the embryo but has no genetic tie to the resulting child. The surrogate is usually referred to as a "gestational" surrogate or carrier, to reflect her role as limited to gestating the child for nine months.

How do you think parentage designations should be made in surrogate parenting arrangements? According to intent? If so, when should intent be assessed? What if the parties change their intent at some point during the pendency of the arrangement? According to biology? If so, would it matter to you whether the surrogate was a genetic or a gestational carrier? These and other features factor into the courts' decisions when a surrogate parenting arrangement goes awry.

B. Distinguishing "Traditional" and "Gestational" Surrogacy

The modern advent of surrogate parenting arrangements can be traced to the early 1980s when commercial agencies and private attorneys began to advertise their services to match infertile couples with women willing to carry a child on their behalf. In these "early" days, the pregnancies were achieved using artificial insemination, typically with sperm supplied by the husband. This meant that the surrogate was also the genetic mother of the child, and thus she acquired the title "genetic" or "traditional" carrier. And though an intended mother may have wanted to supply the egg for the gestated embryo, the technology to make that possible was itself just being born. It was not until 1984 that scientists announced the world's first birth resulting from a donor egg, and it would take several years for the practice of retrieving eggs from one woman for implantation into another to take hold.[8] Thus, the early legal disputes involving surrogate parenting

---

[8] The practice of using the intended mother's eggs or donor eggs in surrogate parenting arrangements did indeed take hold. According to the Wall Street Journal, gestational surrogacies (in which the

arrangements involved traditional surrogacy, posing questions about the status of the genetic versus the intended mother.

1. Traditional Surrogacy

R.R. v. M.H.
Supreme Judicial Court of Massachusetts
426 Mass. 501, 689 N.E.2d 790 (1998)

WILKINS, CHIEF JUSTICE. On a report by a judge in the Probate and Family Court, we are concerned with the validity of a surrogacy parenting agreement between the plaintiff (father) and the defendant (mother). Both the mother and the father are married but not to each other. A child was conceived through artificial insemination of the mother with the father's sperm, after the mother and father had executed the surrogate parenting agreement. The agreement provided that the father would have custody of the child. During the sixth month of her pregnancy and after she had received funds from the father pursuant to the surrogacy agreement, the mother changed her mind and decided that she wanted to keep the child . . .

THE FACTS

The baby girl who is the subject of this action was born on August 15, 1997, in Leominster [Massachusetts]. The defendant mother and the plaintiff father are her biological parents. The father and his wife, who live in Rhode Island, were married in June, 1989. The wife is infertile . . . In April, 1996, responding to a newspaper advertisement for surrogacy services, they consulted a Rhode Island attorney who had drafted surrogacy contracts for both surrogates and couples seeking surrogacy services. On the attorney's advice, the father and his wife consulted the New England Surrogate Parenting Advisors (NESPA), a for-profit corporation that helps infertile couples find women willing to act as surrogate mothers. They entered into a contract with NESPA in September, 1996, and paid a fee of $6,000.

Meanwhile, in the spring of 1996, the mother, who was married and had two children, responded to a NESPA advertisement. She reported to NESPA that her family was complete and that she desired to allow others less fortunate than herself to have children. The mother submitted a surrogacy application to NESPA. The judge found that the mother was motivated to apply to NESPA by a desire to be pregnant, in order to earn money, and to help an infertile couple.

In October, Dr. Angela Figueroa of NESPA brought the mother together with the father and his wife. They had a seemingly informative exchange of information and views. The mother was advised to seek an attorney's advice concerning the surrogacy agreement. Shortly thereafter, the mother, the father, and his wife met again to discuss the surrogacy and other matters. The mother also met with a

---

carrier does not provide the egg) account for 95% of all surrogate pregnancies. See David P. Hamilton, *She's Having Our Baby: Surrogacy Is On The Rise As In Vitro Improves*, Wall St. J., Feb. 4, 2003, at D1.

clinical psychologist as part of NESPA's evaluation of her suitability to act as a surrogate. The psychologist, who also evaluated the father and his wife, advised the mother to consult legal counsel, to give her husband a chance to air his concerns, to discuss arrangements for contact with the child, to consider and discuss her expectations concerning termination of the pregnancy, and to arrange a meeting between her husband and the father and his wife. The psychologist concluded that the mother was solid, thoughtful, and well grounded, that she would have no problem giving the child to the father, and that she was happy to act as a surrogate. The mother told the psychologist that she was not motivated by money, although she did plan to use the funds received for her children's education. The mother's husband told the psychologist by telephone that he supported his wife's decision.

The mother signed the surrogate parenting agreement and her signature was notarized on November 1. The father signed on November 18. The agreement stated that the parties intended that the "Surrogate shall be inseminated with the semen of Natural Father" and "that, on the birth of the child or children so conceived, Natural Father, as the Natural Father, will have the full legal parental rights of a father, and surrogate will permit Natural Father to take the child or children home from the hospital to live with he [*sic*] and his wife." The agreement acknowledged that the mother's parental rights would not terminate if she permitted the father to take the child home and have custody, that the mother could at any time seek to enforce her parental rights by court order, but that, if she attempted to obtain custody or visitation rights, she would forfeit her rights under the agreement and would be obligated to reimburse the father for all fees and expenses paid to her under it. The agreement provided that its interpretation would be governed by Rhode Island law.

The agreement provided for compensation to the mother in the amount of $10,000 "for services rendered in conceiving, carrying and giving birth to the Child." . . . The agreement stated that no payment was made in connection with adoption of the child, the termination of parental rights, or consent to surrender the child for adoption. The father acknowledged the mother's right to determine whether to carry the pregnancy to term, but the mother agreed to refund all payments if, without the father's consent, she had an abortion that was not necessary for her physical health . . .

The judge found that the mother entered into the agreement on her own volition after consulting legal counsel. There was no evidence of undue influence, coercion, or duress. The mother fully understood that she was contracting to give custody of the baby to the father. She sought to inseminate herself on November 30 and December 1, 1996. The attempt at conception was successful.

The lawyer for the father sent the mother a check for $500 in December, 1996, and another for $2,500 in February. In May, the father's lawyer sent the mother a check for $3,500. She told the lawyer that she had changed her mind and wanted to keep the child. She returned the check uncashed in the middle of June. The mother has made no attempt to refund the amounts that the father paid her, including $550 that he paid for pregnancy-related expenses.

PROCEDURE

Approximately two weeks after the mother changed her mind and returned the check for $3,500, and before the child was born, the father commenced this action against the mother seeking to establish his paternity, alleging breach of contract, and requesting a declaration of his rights under the surrogacy agreement . . . Proceedings were held on aspects of the preliminary injunction request (now resolved) and on the mother's motion to determine whether surrogacy contracts are enforceable in Massachusetts.

On August 4, 1997, the judge entered an order directing the mother to give the child to the father when it was discharged from the hospital and granting the father temporary physical custody of the child. She did so based on her determination that the father's custody claim was likely to prevail on the merits of the contract claim, and, if not on that claim, then on the basis of the best interests of the child. The mother was granted the right to frequent visits.

On August 13, 1997, the judge reported the propriety of her August 1 order which, as we have said, was based in part on her conclusion that the surrogacy contract was enforceable . . .

DISCUSSION

1. *The governing law.* The agreement before us provided that "Rhode Island Law shall govern the interpretation of this agreement." No party has argued that Rhode Island law has any application to the issues before us . . . The child was conceived and born in Massachusetts, and the mother is a Massachusetts resident, all as contemplated in the surrogacy arrangement. The significance, if any, of the surrogacy agreement on the relationship of the parties and on the child is appropriately determined by Massachusetts law.

2. *General Laws* . . . The case before us concerns traditional surrogacy, in which the fertile member of an infertile couple is one of the child's biological parents. Surrogate fatherhood, the insemination of the fertile wife with sperm of a donor, often an anonymous donor, is a recognized and accepted procedure. If the mother's husband consents to the procedure, the resulting child is considered the legitimate child of the mother and her husband. G.L. c. 46, § 4B. Section 4B does not comment on the rights and obligations, if any, of the biological father, although inferentially he has none. In the case before us, the infertile spouse is the wife. No statute decrees the consequences of the artificial insemination of a surrogate with the sperm of a fertile husband. This situation presents different considerations from surrogate fatherhood because surrogate motherhood is never anonymous and her commitment and contribution is unavoidably much greater than that of a sperm donor.

We must face the possible application of G.L. c. 46, § 4B, to this case. Section 4B tells us that a husband who consents to the artificial insemination of his wife with the sperm of another is considered to be the father of any resulting child. In the case before us, the birth mother was married at the time of her artificial insemination. Despite what he told the psychologist, her husband was not support-ive of her desire to become a surrogate parent but acknowledged that it was her decision and her body. The husband, who filed a complaint for divorce on August 8, 1997,[9] may have simply been indifferent because he knew that the marriage was falling apart . . . It is doubtful . . . that the Legislature intended § 4B to apply to the child of a married surrogate mother. Section 4B seems to concern the status of a child born to a fertile mother whose husband, presumably infertile, consented to her artificial insemination with the sperm of another man so that the couple could have a child biologically related to the mother.

3. *Adoption statutes.* Policies underlying our adoption legislation suggest that a surrogate parenting agreement should be given no effect if the mother's agreement was obtained prior to a reasonable time after the child's birth or if her agreement was induced by the payment of money . . .

Adoptive parents may pay expenses of a birth parent but may make no direct payment to her. See G.L. c. 210, § 11A; 102 Code Mass. Regs. § 5.09 (1997). Even though the agreement seeks to attribute that payment of $10,000, not to custody or adoption, but solely to the mother's services in carrying the child, the father ostensibly was promised more than those services because, as a practical matter, the mother agreed to surrender custody of the child. She could assert custody rights, according to the agreement, only if she repaid the father all amounts that she had received and also reimbursed him for all expenses he had incurred. The statutory prohibition of payment for receiving a child through adoption suggests that, as a matter of policy, a mother's agreement to surrender custody in exchange for money (beyond pregnancy-related expenses) should be given no effect in deciding the custody of the child.

4. *Conclusion.* The mother's purported consent to custody in the agreement is ineffective because no such consent should be recognized unless given on or after the fourth day following the child's birth. In reaching this conclusion, we apply to consent to custody the same principle which underlies the statutory restriction on when a mother's consent to adoption may be effectively given. Moreover, the payment of money to influence the mother's custody decision makes the agreement as to custody void. Eliminating any financial reward to a surrogate mother is the only way to assure that no economic pressure will cause a woman, who may well be a member of an economically vulnerable class, to act as a surrogate. It is true that a surrogate enters into the agreement before she becomes pregnant and thus is not presented with the desperation that a poor unwed pregnant woman may confront. However, compensated surrogacy arrangements raise the concern that, under financial pressure, a woman will permit her body to be used and her child to be given away.

There is no doubt that compensation was a factor in inducing the mother to enter into the surrogacy agreement and to cede custody to the father. If the payment of $10,000 was really only compensation for the mother's services in carrying the child and giving birth and was unrelated to custody of the child, the agreement would not have provided that the mother must refund all compensation paid (and expenses paid) if she should challenge the father's right to custody. Nor would the agreement have provided that final payment be made only when the child is delivered to the

---

[9] This is one week before the child is born. -Ed.

father. We simply decline, on public policy grounds, to apply to a surrogacy agreement of the type involved here the general principle that an agreement between informed, mature adults should be enforced absent proof of duress, fraud, or undue influence . . .

If no compensation is paid beyond pregnancy-related expenses and if the mother is not bound by her consent to the father's custody of the child unless she consents after a suitable period has passed following the child's birth, the objections we have identified in this opinion to the enforceability of a surrogate's consent to custody would be overcome. Other conditions might be important in deciding the enforceability of a surrogacy agreement, such as a requirement that (a) the mother's husband give his informed consent to the agreement in advance; (b) the mother be an adult and have had at least one successful pregnancy; (c) the mother, her husband, and the intended parents have been evaluated for the soundness of their judgment and for their capacity to carry out the agreement; (d) the father's wife be incapable of bearing a child without endangering her health; (e) the intended parents be suitable persons to assume custody of the child; and (f) all parties have the advice of counsel. The mother and father may not, however, make a binding best-interests-of-the-child determination by private agreement. Any custody agreement is subject to a judicial determination of custody based on the best interests of the child.

The conditions that we describe are not likely to be satisfactory to an intended father because, following the birth of the child, the mother can refuse to consent to the father's custody even though the father has incurred substantial pregnancy-related expenses. A surrogacy agreement judicially approved before conception may be a better procedure, as is permitted by statutes in Virginia and New Hampshire. A Massachusetts statute concerning surrogacy agreements, pro or con, would provide guidance to judges, lawyers, infertile couples interested in surrogate parenthood, and prospective surrogate mothers . . .

A declaration shall be entered that the surrogacy agreement is not enforceable. Such further orders as may be appropriate, consistent with this opinion, may be entered in the Probate and Family Court.

So ordered.

NOTES AND QUESTIONS

1. Do you think the parties, including the attorneys, in *R.R.* were influenced by the New Jersey Supreme Court's decision in *Baby M*? From what we learn about the agreement in *R.R.*, it appears that the drafting attorneys were careful to avoid the exchange of promises that the *Baby M* court found unlawful — particularly, the surrogate's agreement to surrender custody upon birth and terminate her parental rights. Even so, the Massachusetts court read these requirements into the agreement to find that surrogate parenting arrangements violate the public policy of the state. Do you think the court was right to pierce the contract's veil to reveal what it believed to be public harms, or should the justices have permitted the private individuals to face the consequences of their bargain?

2.   The Massachusetts court takes on the aura of legislature when it sets out a six-point plan to address the enforceability of surrogate parenting contracts (points (a) through (f) in the third paragraph from the end). Which, if any, of those conditions was not satisfied in this case?

3.   The early involvement of professionals in *R.R.*, including attorneys and psychologists, proved insufficient to prevent the agreement's ultimate deterioration. Do you think that careful drafting and thorough mental health evaluations of all the parties are essential to the functionality and integrity of surrogate parenting arrangements? Consider the dispute between a traditional surrogate and a married couple in Florida. In 2006, Tom and Gwyn Lamitinas hired Stephanie Eckard to act as their traditional surrogate after the three found each other through an online website called "Surrogate Mothers Online." Using contract language adapted from the website, the couple agreed to pay Eckard to conceive and carry their child via artificial insemination. Problems in the relationship ensued and Eckard decided to keep the baby during her pregnancy. She sued Tom Lamitinas for custody and child support after a baby girl was born. A judge awarded the biologic mother full legal custody, ruling the biologic father was a mere sperm donor with no parental rights under Florida law. *See* Rene Stutzman, *Surrogate Mom Can Keep Baby, Judge Rules*, Orlando Sentinel, Oct. 11, 2007, at B1. Not surprisingly, both sides sought legal counsel after the dispute arose. Query whether the arrangement would have imploded had the parties been properly counseled prior to execution of the agreement.

4.   What are the consequences to the child of a finding that the surrogate parenting agreement is unenforceable? In both *Baby M* and *R.R.*, the court declared the contracts void, but went on to award custody to the father, with visitation rights accorded the surrogates in both cases. Presumably the father will raise the child with his wife as if the child were born to the couple. But the final step — adoption by the wife — will be unfulfilled because the surrogate, as the legal mother, has the right to refuse to surrender parental rights to the child.

Both the New Jersey and Massachusetts courts spoke at length about the need to protect the surrogate's right to have sufficient time after birth to consider her decision to surrender the child for adoption. What if a surrogate consents to the adoption within the statutory framework, but later changes her mind and seeks to withdraw her consent? See *In re Adoption of Matthew B.M.*, 232 Cal. App. 3d 1239, 284 Cal. Rptr. 18 (1991) (court denies surrogate's petition to withdraw consent to adoption 8 months after signing consent, based on best interest of the child). *See also E.A.G. v. R.W.S.*, 2010 Minn. App. Unpub. LEXIS 1091 (Minn. App.) (traditional surrogate who surrendered child to male couple/intended parents but later changed her mind deemed legal mother; biological /intended father awarded sole legal and physical custody).

What if the intended parents never take action to formalize the adoption of the child by the intended mother? If the surrogate is not making a claim for parental rights, is such a legal proceeding even necessary? In *Doe v. Doe*, 244 Conn. 403, 710 A.2d 1297 (1998), the Connecticut Supreme Court held a child born to a traditional surrogate and not formally adopted by the wife (the intended mother) was not a "child of the marriage" upon the parents' divorce. Thirteen years later, this same court held it unnecessary for an intended parent to adopt a child born to a gestational surrogate. In this later case, a male couple engaged a surrogate using one partner's sperm. The couple intended for both men to be named as parents on the resulting twins' birth certificates without having to go through a formal adoption by the nongenetic parent. The court found that Connecticut statutory law "allows an intended parent who is a party to a *valid* gestational surrogacy agreement to become a parent without first adopting the children." *Raftopol v. Ramey*, 299 Conn. 681, 12 A.3d 783 (2011) (emphasis in original). These companion Connecticut cases teach us that the law regards a woman who provides both her womb and her egg very differently from a woman who provides her womb alone. Do you agree that a traditional surrogate should presumptively be considered the child's legal mother while a gestational surrogate should not?

5.   If the infertile wife in a traditional surrogacy arrangement is considered the "intended" mother of the child, does this mean that the surrogate is the "unintended" mother of the child?

6.   Should the law treat a traditional surrogate the same way it treats a sperm donor who aids a married couple to have a child genetically related to one spouse? Is a womb donor the same as a sperm donor? Clearly the labor (quite literally) required to donate gestational services far exceeds the simple act of donating sperm. Should the law treat men and women equally with regard to their ability to donate reproductive assistance, or are there compelling reasons to distinguish between these two acts?

Recall Section (b) of the Uniform Parentage Act (1973):

(b) The donor of semen provided to a licensed physician for use in artificial insemination of a married woman other than the donor's wife is treated in law as if he were not the natural father of a child thereby conceived.

Would you favor an amendment to the UPA as follows:

(c) The donor of gestational services who undergoes artificial insemination under the supervision of a licensed physician with semen other than the donor's husband is treated in law as if she were not the natural mother of a child thereby conceived.

2.   Gestational Surrogacy

JOHNSON v. CALVERT
Supreme Court of California
5 Cal.4th 84, 19 Cal. Rptr. 2d 494, 851 P.2d 776 (1993)

PANELLI, J. In this case we address several of the legal questions raised by recent advances in reproductive technology. When, pursuant to a surrogacy agreement, a zygote[10] formed of the gametes[11] of a husband and wife is implanted in the uterus

---

[10] [n.1] An organism produced by the union of two gametes. (McGraw-Hill Dict. of Scientific and Technical Terms (4th ed. 1989) p. 783.).

[11] [n.2] A cell that participates in fertilization and development of a new organism, also known as a

of another woman, who carries the resulting fetus to term and gives birth to a child not genetically related to her, who is the child's "natural mother" under California law? Does a determination that the wife is the child's natural mother work a deprivation of the gestating woman's constitutional rights? And is such an agreement barred by any public policy of this state?

We conclude that the husband and wife are the child's natural parents, and that this result does not offend the state or federal Constitution or public policy.

Facts

Mark and Crispina Calvert are a married couple who desired to have a child. Crispina was forced to undergo a hysterectomy in 1984. Her ovaries remained capable of producing eggs, however, and the couple eventually considered surrogacy. In 1989 Anna Johnson heard about Crispina's plight from a coworker and offered to serve as a surrogate for the Calverts.

On January 15, 1990, Mark, Crispina, and Anna signed a contract providing that an embryo created by the sperm of Mark and the egg of Crispina would be implanted in Anna and the child born would be taken into Mark and Crispina's home "as their child." Anna agreed she would relinquish "all parental rights" to the child in favor of Mark and Crispina. In return, Mark and Crispina would pay Anna $10,000 in a series of installments, the last to be paid six weeks after the child's birth. Mark and Crispina were also to pay for a $200,000 life insurance policy on Anna's life.

The zygote was implanted on January 19, 1990. Less than a month later, an ultrasound test confirmed Anna was pregnant.

Unfortunately, relations deteriorated between the two sides. Mark learned that Anna had not disclosed she had suffered several stillbirths and miscarriages. Anna felt Mark and Crispina did not do enough to obtain the required insurance policy. She also felt abandoned during an onset of premature labor in June.

In July 1990, Anna sent Mark and Crispina a letter demanding the balance of the payments due her or else she would refuse to give up the child. The following month, Mark and Crispina responded with a lawsuit, seeking a declaration they were the legal parents of the unborn child. Anna filed her own action to be declared the mother of the child, and the two cases were eventually consolidated. The parties agreed to an independent guardian ad litem for the purposes of the suit.

The child was born on September 19, 1990, and blood samples were obtained from both Anna and the child for analysis. The blood test results excluded Anna as the genetic mother. The parties agreed to a court order providing that the child would remain with Mark and Crispina on a temporary basis with visits by Anna.

At trial in October 1990, the parties stipulated that Mark and Crispina were the child's genetic parents. After hearing evidence and arguments, the trial court ruled that Mark and Crispina were the child's "genetic, biological and natural" father and mother, that Anna had no "parental" rights to the child, and that the surrogacy

---

germ cell or sex cell. (McGraw-Hill Dict. of Scientific and Technical Terms, *supra*, p. 2087.)

contract was legal and enforceable against Anna's claims. The court also terminated the order allowing visitation. Anna appealed from the trial court's judgment. The Court of Appeal for the Fourth District, Division Three, affirmed. We granted review.

Discussion

Determining Maternity Under the Uniform Parentage Act

The Uniform Parentage Act (the Act) was part of a package of legislation introduced in 1975 as Senate Bill No. 347. The legislation's purpose was to eliminate the legal distinction between legitimate and illegitimate children . . . The pertinent portion of Senate Bill No. 347, which passed with negligible opposition, became part 7 of division 4 of the California Civil Code, sections 7000-7021.

Civil Code sections 7001 and 7002 replace the distinction between legitimate and illegitimate children with the concept of the "parent and child relationship." The "parent and child relationship" means "the legal relationship existing between a child and his natural or adoptive parents incident to which the law confers or imposes rights, privileges, duties, and obligations. It includes the mother and child relationship and the father and child relationship." (Civ. Code, § 7001.) . . . The "parent and child relationship" is thus a legal relationship encompassing two kinds of parents, "natural" and "adoptive."

Passage of the Act clearly was not motivated by the need to resolve surrogacy disputes, which were virtually unknown in 1975. Yet it facially applies to *any* parentage determination, including the rare case in which a child's maternity is in issue . . . Not uncommonly, courts must construe statutes in factual settings not contemplated by the enacting legislature . . . We therefore proceed to analyze the parties' contentions within the Act's framework.

These contentions are readily summarized. Anna, of course, predicates her claim of maternity on the fact that she gave birth to the child. The Calverts contend that Crispina's genetic relationship to the child establishes that she is his mother. Counsel for the minor joins in that contention . . . As will appear, we conclude that presentation of blood test evidence is one means of establishing maternity, as is proof of having given birth . . .

Civil Code section 7003 provides, in relevant part, that between a child and the natural mother a parent and child relationship "*may* be established by proof of her having given birth to the child, or under [the Act]." (Civ. Code, § 7003, subd. (1), italics added.) Apart from Civil Code section 7003, the Act sets forth no specific means by which a natural mother can establish a parent and child relationship. However, it declares that, insofar as practicable, provisions applicable to the father and child relationship apply in an action to determine the existence or nonexistence of a mother and child relationship. (Civ. Code, § 7015.) Thus, it is appropriate to examine those provisions as well.

A man can establish a father and child relationship by the means set forth in Civil Code section 7004. (Civ. Code, §§ 7006, 7004.) Paternity is presumed under that section if the man meets the conditions set forth in section 621 of the Evidence Code. (Civ. Code, § 7004, subd. (a).) The latter statute applies, by its terms, when determining the questioned paternity of a child born to a married woman, and contemplates reliance on evidence derived from blood testing. (Evid. Code, § 621, subds. (a), (b) . . .

Significantly for this case, Evidence Code section 892 provides that blood testing may be ordered in an action when paternity is a relevant fact . . . When maternity is disputed, genetic evidence derived from blood testing is likewise admissible. (Evid. Code, § 892; see Civ. Code, § 7015 . . .

Disregarding the presumptions of paternity that have no application to this case, then, we are left with the undisputed evidence that Anna, not Crispina, gave birth to the child and that Crispina, not Anna, is genetically related to him. Both women thus have adduced evidence of a mother and child relationship as contemplated by the Act. Yet for any child California law recognizes only one natural mother, despite advances in reproductive technology rendering a different outcome biologically possible.[12]

We see no clear legislative preference in Civil Code section 7003 as between blood testing evidence and proof of having given birth . . .

Because two women each have presented acceptable proof of maternity, we do not believe this case can be decided without enquiring into the parties' intentions as manifested in the surrogacy agreement. Mark and Crispina are a couple who desired to have a child of their own genes but are physically unable to do so without the help of reproductive technology. They affirmatively intended the birth of the child, and took the steps necessary to effect in vitro fertilization. But for their acted-on intention, the child would not exist. Anna agreed to facilitate the procreation of Mark's and Crispina's child. The parties' aim was to bring Mark's and Crispina's child into the world, not for Mark and Crispina to donate a zygote to Anna. Crispina from the outset intended to be the child's mother. Although the gestative function Anna performed was necessary to bring about the child's birth, it is safe to say that Anna would not have been given the opportunity to gestate or deliver the child had she, prior to implantation of the zygote, manifested her own intent to be the child's mother. No reason appears why Anna's later change of heart should vitiate the determination that Crispina is the child's natural mother.

We conclude that although the Act recognizes both genetic consanguinity and giving birth as means of establishing a mother and child relationship, when the two means do not coincide in one woman, she who intended to procreate the child-that is, she who intended to bring about the birth of a child that she intended to raise as her own-is the natural mother under California law . . .

---

[12] [n.8] We decline to accept the contention of amicus curiae the American Civil Liberties Union (ACLU) that we should find the child has two mothers. Even though rising divorce rates have made multiple parent arrangements common in our society, we see no compelling reason to recognize such a situation here. The Calverts are the genetic and intending parents of their son and have provided him, by all accounts, with a stable, intact, and nurturing home. To recognize parental rights in a third party with whom the Calvert family has had little contact since shortly after the child's birth would diminish Crispina's role as mother.

Under Anna's interpretation of the Act, by contrast, a woman who agreed to gestate a fetus genetically related to the intending parents would, contrary to her expectations, be held to be the child's natural mother, with all the responsibilities that ruling would entail, if the intending mother declined to accept the child after its birth. In what we must hope will be the extremely rare situation in which neither the gestator nor the woman who provided the ovum for fertilization is willing to assume custody of the child after birth, a rule recognizing the intending parents as the child's legal, natural parents should best promote certainty and stability for the child.

In deciding the issue of maternity under the Act we have felt free to take into account the parties' intentions, as expressed in the surrogacy contract, because in our view the agreement is not, on its face, inconsistent with public policy . . .

Anna urges that surrogacy contracts violate several social policies. Relying on her contention that she is the child's legal, natural mother, she cites the public policy embodied in Penal Code section 273, prohibiting the payment for consent to adoption of a child. She argues further that the policies underlying the adoption laws of this state are violated by the surrogacy contract because it in effect constitutes a prebirth waiver of her parental rights.

We disagree. Gestational surrogacy differs in crucial respects from adoption and so is not subject to the adoption statutes. The parties voluntarily agreed to participate in in vitro fertilization and related medical procedures before the child was conceived; at the time when Anna entered into the contract, therefore, she was not vulnerable to financial inducements to part with her own expected offspring. As discussed above, Anna was not the genetic mother of the child. The payments to Anna under the contract were meant to compensate her for her services in gestating the fetus and undergoing labor, rather than for giving up "parental" rights to the child. Payments were due both during the pregnancy and after the child's birth. We are, accordingly, unpersuaded that the contract used in this case violates the public policies embodied in Penal Code section 273 and the adoption statutes. For the same reasons, we conclude these contracts do not implicate the policies underlying the statutes governing termination of parental rights . . .

Finally, Anna and some commentators have expressed concern that surrogacy contracts tend to exploit or dehumanize women, especially women of lower economic status. Anna's objections center around the psychological harm she asserts may result from the gestator's relinquishing the child to whom she has given birth. Some have also cautioned that the practice of surrogacy may encourage society to view children as commodities, subject to trade at their parents' will.

We are all too aware that the proper forum for resolution of this issue is the Legislature, where empirical data, largely lacking from this record, can be studied and rules of general applicability developed. However, in light of our responsibility to decide this case, we have considered as best we can its possible consequences.

We are unpersuaded that gestational surrogacy arrangements are so likely to cause the untoward results Anna cites as to demand their invalidation on public policy grounds. Although common sense suggests that women of lesser means serve as surrogate mothers more often than do wealthy women, there has been no proof that surrogacy contracts exploit poor women to any greater degree than economic necessity in general exploits them by inducing them to accept lower-paid or otherwise undesirable employment. We are likewise unpersuaded by the claim that surrogacy will foster the attitude that children are mere commodities; no evidence is offered to support it. The limited data available seem to reflect an absence of significant adverse effects of surrogacy on all participants.

The argument that a woman cannot knowingly and intelligently agree to gestate and deliver a baby for intending parents carries overtones of the reasoning that for centuries prevented women from attaining equal economic rights and professional status under the law. To resurrect this view is both to foreclose a personal and economic choice on the part of the surrogate mother, and to deny intending parents what may be their only means of procreating a child of their own genes. Certainly in the present case it cannot seriously be argued that Anna, a licensed vocational nurse who had done well in school and who had previously borne a child, lacked the intellectual wherewithal or life experience necessary to make an informed decision to enter into the surrogacy contract.

Constitutionality of the Determination That Anna Johnson Is Not the Natural Mother

[Anna contends that she has a liberty interest in the companionship of the child. The court concludes that "Anna has no parental rights to the child under California law, and she fails to persuade us that sufficiently strong policy reasons exist to accord her a protected liberty interest in the companionship of the child when such an interest would necessarily detract from or impair the parental bond enjoyed by Mark and Crispina." The court rejects any assertions that Anna's constitutional rights have been infringed by a finding that she is not the natural mother of the child she gestated.]

Disposition

The judgment of the Court of Appeal is affirmed. LUCAS, C. J., MOSK, J., BAXTER, J., and GEORGE, J., concurred. ARABIAN, J., wrote a separate concurring opinion in which he concurs in the decision to find Crispina Calvert the natural mother under the Uniform Parentage Act, but "decline[s] to subscribe to the dictum in which the majority find[s] surrogacy contracts 'not . . . inconsistent with public policy.'" Instead, he argues, any such determination should be made by the legislature.

KENNARD, J., Dissenting.[13]

When a woman who wants to have a child provides her fertilized ovum to another woman who carries it through pregnancy and gives birth to a child, who is the child's legal mother? Unlike the majority, I do not agree that the determinative consideration should be the intent to have the child that originated with the woman who

---

[13] Joyce Kennard was the sole female member of the California Supreme Court at the time this case was decided. -Ed.

contributed the ovum. In my view, the woman who provided the fertilized ovum and the woman who gave birth to the child both have substantial claims to legal motherhood. Pregnancy entails a unique commitment, both psychological and emotional, to an unborn child. No less substantial, however, is the contribution of the woman from whose egg the child developed and without whose desire the child would not exist.

For each child, California law accords the legal rights and responsibilities of parenthood to only one "natural mother." When, as here, the female reproductive role is divided between two women, California law requires courts to make a decision as to which woman is the child's natural mother, but provides no standards by which to make that decision. The majority's resort to "intent" to break the "tie" between the genetic and gestational mothers is unsupported by statute, and, in the absence of appropriate protections in the law to guard against abuse of surrogacy arrangements, it is ill-advised. To determine who is the legal mother of a child born of a gestational surrogacy arrangement, I would apply the standard most protective of child welfare-the best interests of the child . . .

This "best interests" standard serves to assure that in the judicial resolution of disputes affecting a child's well-being, protection of the minor child is the foremost consideration. Consequently, I would apply "the best interests of the child" standard to determine who can best assume the social and legal responsibilities of motherhood for a child born of a gestational surrogacy arrangement.

The determination of a child's best interests does not depend on the parties' relative economic circumstances, which in a gestational surrogacy situation will usually favor the genetic mother and her spouse . . . As this court has recognized, however, superior wealth does not necessarily equate with good parenting . . .

Factors that are pertinent to good parenting, and thus that are in a child's best interests, include the ability to nurture the child physically and psychologically . . . and to provide ethical and intellectual guidance . . . Also crucial to a child's best interests is the "well recognized right" of every child "to stability and continuity." . . . The intent of the genetic mother to procreate a child is certainly relevant to the question of the child's best interests; alone, however, it should not be dispositive.

Here, the child born of the gestational surrogacy arrangement between Anna Johnson and Mark and Crispina Calvert has lived continuously with Mark and Crispina since his birth in September 1990. The trial court awarded parental rights to Mark and Crispina, concluding that as a matter of law they were the child's "genetic, biological and natural" parents. In reaching that conclusion, the trial court did not treat Anna's statutory claim to be the child's legal mother as equal to Crispina's, nor did the trial court consider the child's best interests in deciding between those two equal statutory claims. Accordingly, I would remand the matter to the trial court to undertake that evaluation.

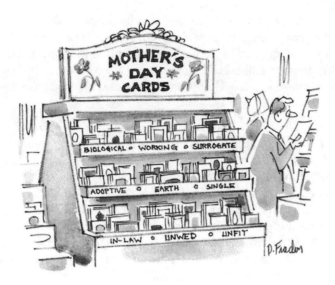

NOTES AND QUESTIONS

1. *Contested Surrogacy Cases.* The events surrounding the lawsuit in *Johnson v. Calvert*, like those in *R.R. v. M.H.* and *Baby M.*, involve a surrogate carrier who, at some point during the pregnancy, changes her mind about turning over the child to the contracting couple. These cases may give an impression that surrogate carriers frequently experience a change of heart, and that surrogate parenting arrangements are risky for all parties involved. Empirically speaking, this does not appear to be the case. According to the Organization of Parents Through Surrogacy (OPTS), there have been approximately 25,000 births through surrogate mothers in the U.S. since 1976, and only a small number have resulted in litigation. A more precise figure was reported in the *Wall Street Journal*: in the modern history of surrogate parenting arrangement, "surrogates have contested their contracts in only 24 cases over the past two decades, and intended parents have done so just 65 times." David P. Hamilton, *She's Having Our Baby: Surrogacy Is On The Rise As In Vitro Improves*, WALL ST. J., Feb. 4, 2003, at D1. A more recent analysis concludes that less than .01% of surrogacy births have resulted in court battles between the surrogate and intended parents. Elly Teman, *The Social Construction of Surrogacy Research: An Anthropological Critique of the Psychosocial Scholarship on Surrogate Motherhood*, 67 Soc. Sci. & MED. 1104 (2008).

What if a surrogate's change of heart is provoked by concern for the best interest of the child rather than an unexpected instinct to parent? When a gestational surrogate in Michigan learned shortly after giving birth to twins that the intended mother had a history of mental illness for which she continued to receive treatment, as well as a minor criminal record, the birth mother enlisted the help of law enforcement to remove the children from the intended parents' home. In the end, the twins remained with the surrogate, her husband and four other children. The twins were conceived using donor eggs and sperm. If the children had been the genetic offspring of the intended parents, would the result have been the same? *See*

Stephanie Saul, *21st Century Babies: Building a Baby, With Few Ground Rules*, NY TIMES, Dec. 13, 2009, at A1. A truly horrible ending to a surrogacy story is detailed in *Huddleston v. Infertility Center of America*, 700 A.2d 453 (Superior Ct. Pa. 1997), in which a traditional surrogate sued the agency that matched her with the genetic/intended father after he murdered the one-month old boy.

Even if the number of controversies is proportionally small, can the practice of contracting for gestational services be justified in light of the potential harm to the child when the arrangement does go awry? One might argue that the child would not have been born "but for" the surrogacy arrangement, and thus is always better off in existence, no matter what the accompanying social consequences. Alternatively, one might weigh the total harms that flow from a "failed" surrogacy arrangement, including the emotional, psychological and financial impacts incurred in varying degrees by the surrogate, the contracting couple and the child, to conclude that on balance society would be better off without this wrenching tug-of-war between prospective parents. On balance, do you find surrogate parenting arrangements socially justifiable?

2.   The rancor between Anna Johnson, the gestational carrier, and the Calverts is palpable even from the court's rather neutral description of the facts. The court mentions a letter Anna sent Mark and Crispina in July 1990 demanding the balance of the payments due her or else she would refuse to give up the child. The actual letter may give you a better sense of the highly charged atmosphere in which this case evolved:

7/23/90

Dear Chris & Mark,

I am writing you this letter to inquire if an early payment can be made of what is left to be paid of me. I would not ask if it weren't important and I feel that this is important because it deals with the well-being of the baby. The lady that owns the house in which I reside is selling it, so I must be out by the 10th of August. Since I am to be hospitalized for three weeks due to the pyleonephritis [sic] & premature contractions I need to find another place to live prior to this! Due to the complications of this pregnancy, I am unable to return to work until the delivery of this baby so my income is limited. I do not get enough from disability to make a two month rent deposit plus, the security deposit & have the telephone reconnected. I don't think you'd want your child jeopardized by living out on the street. I have looked out for this child's well being thus far, is it asking too much to look after ours?

I'm imploring nicely and trying not to be an ogre about this. But you must admit, you have not been very supportive mentally the entire pregnancy & you've showed a lack of interest unless it came to an ultrasound. I am asking you for help in paying off the final five thousand. There's only two months left & once this baby is born, my hands are free of this deal. But see, this situation can go two ways. One, you can pay me the entire sum early so I won't have to live in the streets, or two you can forget about helping me but, calling it a breach of contract & not get the baby! I don't want it to get this nasty, not coming this far, but you'd want some help too, if you had no where to go & have to worry about not only yourself but your own child & the child of someone else!!! Help me find another place & get settled in before your baby's born.

This is the only letter you will get from me. The next letter you will receive will be from my lawyers, unless I hear from you by return mail at the end of the week — 7/28/90.

Sincerely,

Anna [last name omitted]

Surrogate

Anna J. v. Mark C, 234 Cal. App. 3d 1557, 286 Cal. Rptr. 369, 372, n. 11. Mark Calvert responded to Anna Johnson's letter by filing the lawsuit at issue.

What, if anything, could the Calverts have done to prevent the adverse events that befell their surrogacy arrangement? What, if anything, could Anna Johnson have done to prevent the adverse events that befell her surrogacy arrangement?

3.   The majority opinion in *Johnson v. Calvert* relies on the concept of intent. When one woman bears a genetic relation to the child, and another gives birth, "she who intended to procreate the child — that is, she who intended to bring about the birth of a child that she intended to raise as her own — is the natural mother under California law." In *Belsito v. Clark,* 67 Ohio Misc.2d 54, 644 N.E.2d 760 (1994), the Ohio Court of Common Pleas rejects the *Johnson* intent test. The Belsitos contract with Mrs. Belsito's sister who agrees, without compensation, to gestate the couple's embryo. Prior to the child's birth, the couple petitioned the court to allow both of them to be listed on the child's birth certificate, contrary to Ohio law which records the birth mother as a child's legal mother. The court granted the couple's request, but in so doing, reviewed and rejected the reasoning set forth in the recent precedent in California.

The Ohio court worried that "intent can be difficult to prove." Id. at 62. What if, the court wondered, both the genetic and the birth mother intended to procreate and raise the child? Next, the Ohio court criticized the *Johnson* approach for discounting the similarity between surrogacy and adoption, and thereby ignoring the significant pressures that befall a gestational carrier. The intent-to-procreate test, the Ohio court warned, "does not allow for unpressured surrender of potential parental rights, nor does it provide a means to review and ensure the suitability of the gestational surrogate or her spouse as parents. . . . It is, in effect, a private adoption process that is readily subject to all the defects and pressures of such a process." Id. at 63. Instead of intent, the Ohio court turns to genetics, which it considers paramount in determining parentage. "[T]he individuals who provide the genes of [the] child are the natural parents. . . . If the genetic providers have not waived their rights and have decided to raise the child, then they must be recognized as the natural and legal parents. By formulating the law in this manner, both tests, genetics and birth, are used in determining parentage. However, they are no longer equal. The birth test becomes subordinate and secondary to genetics." Id. at 65-66.

How would the Ohio court award parentage in a case where neither woman has a genetic tie to the child? If a couple uses a donated egg to create an embryo, and then hires a gestational surrogate who later claims rights to the child, who is the legal mother in Ohio? In California? What if there is no "intended mother," just an intended father who uses a donated egg to create an embryo with the intent of becoming a single parent. Does the gestational surrogate win the status of legal mother by default? See *In re Roberto d.B.*, 399 Md. 267, 923 A.2d 115 (2007) (single father who hired egg donor and gestational surrogate won right to exclude name of "mother" on children's birth certificate); *J.F. v. D.B.*, 116 Ohio St. 3d 363, 879 N.E. 2d 740 (2007) (upholding gestational surrogacy agreement orchestrated by single father later declared sole legal parent of triplets). *But see A.G.R. v. D.R.H. & S.H.*, Docket #FD-09-1838-07 (N.J. Superior Ct 2009) (married male couple contracts with genetic father's sister to act as gestational carrier; after twins are born, trial court awards sister/surrogate parental rights, finding the intent of the parties "of no significance").

4. The decision in *Johnson v. Calvert* can be distinguished from the decision in *Baby M* on at least two important grounds: 1) Mary Beth Whitehead (*Baby M*) was a traditional surrogate who was the child's genetic mother, while Anna Johnson (*Johnson*) was a gestational surrogate with no genetic tie to the child, and 2) The New Jersey Supreme Court held that the state adoption laws governed the surrogacy arrangement, while the California Supreme Court found that "gestational surrogacy differs in crucial respects from adoption and so is not subject to the adoption statutes." Do you think factor 1 (traditional v. gestational surrogacy) is related to factor 2 (applicability of state adoption laws)?

Several commentators have focused on the interaction of these two factors, revealing different insights. One view is that:

> in gestational surrogacy cases, courts feel freer to reject an adoption default model than they do in traditional surrogacy cases where genetics and gestation are joined. Without this joining, courts can more freely grant legal weight to intention. Thus, . . . *Johnson* . . . [is] a case in which . . . "the identification and definition of mother . . . become matters of negotiable choice." . . . In [contrast], while courts in traditional surrogacy cases consider the surrogate to be the natural mother, thus necessitating compliance with adoption law for the contract to be fully performed, courts in gestational surrogacy cases, faced with greater uncertainty about the child's natural parents, are more willing to apply an intentional-parent analysis. . . . [T]hus . . . two paradigms [are] at work, a biological-parentage paradigm in traditional surrogacy cases and a presumptive-parentage paradigm in gestational surrogacy cases. This framework . . . allows for parentage to be determined completely apart from biological facts and can serve as the foundation for "a broad theory of familial relationships" that will permit policymakers to formulate "a more complicated and more malleable ideological conception of the family than existed even a few decades ago."

Richard F. Storrow, *Parenthood By Pure Intention: Assisted Reproduction and the Functional Approach to Parentage*, 53 HAST. L. J. 597, 610 (2002) (quoting from

JANET L. DOLGIN, DEFINING THE FAMILY: LAW, TECHNOLOGY, AND REPRODUCTION IN AN UNEASY AGE (1997)). Professor Storrow derives from this paradigm of biological and presumptive parentage, a hope that assisted reproduction will inspire the law to grant equal legal status to nontraditional families. *Id.* at 612. *Cf.* Radhika Rao, *Assisted Reproductive Technology and the Threat to the Traditional Family*, 47 HAST. L. J. 951 (1996) (warning that new reproductive technologies may broadly undermine the traditional family paradigm).

Do you see how the holding in *Johnson* could be favorable construed by unmarried and same-sex couples who seek legal recognition as parents of ART children?

5. To shed further light on the law's distinction between traditional and gestational surrogacy, let us revisit the jurisprudence in the state of Massachusetts. Recall in *R.R. v. M.H.* the Supreme Judicial Court held unenforceable a surrogacy agreement between a traditional surrogate who was artificially inseminated by the intended father's sperm. The court found the agreement in direct violation of existing adoption laws, which require a four-day waiting period before a new mother can consent to surrender custody of her child. Three years later, in *Culliton v. Beth Israel Deaconess Medical Center*, 435 Mass. 285, 756 N.E.2d 1133 (2001), the same Massachusetts high court reviewed a request by genetic parents for a declaration of paternity and maternity of unborn twins who were about to be born to a gestational carrier. The couple's egg and sperm had been combined, and the embryos implanted into a gestational carrier, pursuant to a surrogate parenting contract. In granting the intended parents' pre-birth order of parentage, the court distinguished its prior traditional surrogacy decision as follows:

> While this court has previously looked to the adoption statute in deciding whether to enforce a traditional surrogacy agreement, see *R.R. v. M.H.* the court did so "to assure that no economic pressure will cause a woman . . . to act as a surrogate. . . . [C]ompensated surrogacy arrangements raise the concern that, under financial pressure, a woman will permit her body to be used and her child to be given away" (emphasis added) . . . In such an arrangement, the surrogate is both the genetic mother of the child and the mother who carries the child through pregnancy and delivery. The child is thus, undisputedly, "her" child to be surrendered for adoption. Here, where it is undisputed that the plaintiffs were not donating an embryo or embryos to the gestational carrier, and that the twins have no genetic relation to the gestational carrier, the concerns are different from those at issue in *R.R. v. M.H.* Also, in these circumstances, applying the four-day waiting period of G.L. c. 210, § 2, to this gestational carrier arrangement would work unintended, and possibly detrimental, results. The duties and responsibilities of parenthood (for example, support and custody) would lie with the gestational carrier for at least four days; the gestational carrier could be free to surrender the children for adoption; and the genetic parents of the children would be forced to go through the adoption process, possibly having to wait as long as six months . . . before becoming the legal parents of the children. As is evident from its provisions, the adoption statute was not intended to resolve parentage issues arising from gestational surrogacy agreements.

Culliton v. Beth Israel Deaconess Medical Center, 435 Mass. At 290, 756 N.E.2d at 1137-38. Accord *Hodas v. Morin*, 442 Mass. 544, 814 N.E.2d 320 (2004). The court distinguishes traditional and gestational surrogacy on the basis of the woman's genetic tie to the child, and on the economic pressure brought to bear on a woman who agrees to act as a surrogate. In the case of traditional surrogacy, the economic pressure may force a woman to give up *her* child, while this same pressure in a gestational arrangement will prod her to give up *the couple's* child. Is the court abandoning its concern for the economic vulnerability of women when the child they gestate bears no genetic relation to the surrogate? Is the court right to consider the economic vulnerability of women in the context of traditional surrogacy? Did the court in *Johnson v. Calvert* consider the economic vulnerability of surrogates a controlling factor in its decision? Should it have? What about the emotional vulnerability of women who agree to act as gestational carriers? At least one court has expressed strong views on this topic, considered below.

A.H.W. v. G.H.B.
Superior Court of New Jersey
339 N.J. Super. 495, 772 A.2d 948 (2000)

KOBLITZ, P.J.F.P. [Presiding Judge, Family Part, Chancery Division]

The novel issue presented in this surrogacy matter is whether or not a court may issue a pre-birth order directing a delivering physician to list the man and woman who provided the embryo carried by a third party as legal parents on a child's birth certificate. Both the petitioning biological parents and the defendant surrogate who carried the baby agree that petitioners should be listed as the legal parents on the baby's birth certificate. However, the Attorney General's Office opposes the request of the biological parents for a pre-birth order claiming the relief is contrary to the law prohibiting surrender of a birth mother's rights until seventy-two hours after birth, and the public policy of the State of New Jersey as expressed by the New Jersey Supreme Court in *In re Baby M*, 109 N.J. 396, 537 A.2d 1227 (1988). After considering case law and statutes in other states as well as New Jersey, this Court denies plaintiffs and the defendant surrogate's request for a pre-birth order, but will issue an order which allows the petitioning biological parents' names to be placed on the birth certificate after the seventy-two hour statutory waiting period has expired but before the birth certificate must be filed [within five days of birth] . . .

FACTS

G.H.B., hereinafter "Gina," is the unmarried sister of plaintiff A.H.W., "Andrea," and the sister-in-law of P.W., "Peter." The biological parents, Andrea and Peter, entered into a gestational surrogacy contract with Gina. Gina, without financial compensation, agreed to have embryos implanted into her uterus that were created from the sperm of her brother-in-law, Peter, and the ova of her sister, Andrea. This medical procedure is commonly referred to as "ovum implantation," and permits a woman who is incapable of carrying a baby to term to have a child who is genetically related to her. The child is due to be born in about two weeks at a Bergen County hospital.

Plaintiffs filed a complaint to declare the maternity and paternity of unborn Baby A. Plaintiffs seek a pre-birth order establishing them as the legal mother and father of unborn Baby A, and placing their names on the child's birth certificate. They argue that a pre-birth order is appropriate with a gestational surrogacy.

LAW FROM OTHER STATES

Plaintiffs argue that an order should be issued pre-birth as requested because the gestational carrier has no biological link or legal rights to the fetus. In support of their position, plaintiffs cite to surrogacy procedures authorizing pre-birth orders utilized in California [*Johnson v. Calvert*, 5 Cal.4th 84, 19 Cal. Rptr.2d 494 (1993)] and Massachusetts [*Smith v. Brown*, 430 Mass. 1005, 718 N.E.2d 844 (1999)], where the courts have dealt with the issue . . .

NEW JERSEY CASE LAW

The New Jersey Supreme Court dealt with the issue of surrogate motherhood agreements in the landmark case of *In re Baby M*, 109 N.J. 396, 537 A.2d 1227 (1988) . . . The Court, in an opinion written by Chief Justice Wilentz, ruled that the surrogacy contract was void because it was contrary to public policy and in direct conflict with then existing laws. Id. at 421-22, 537 A.2d 1227. The Court found that there was "coercion of contract" because Mrs. Whitehead was forced to give up her child irrevocably prior to conception. Id. at 422, 537 A.2d 1227 . . .

PUBLIC POLICY AND STATUTES

The biological parents, Andrea and Peter, and the gestational surrogate, Gina, argue that Gina has no biological ties to the unborn child and liken the gestational carrier's role to that of an incubator. They argue that *Baby M* is distinguishable because the surrogate mother in that case was also the biological mother. While Andrea, Peter and Gina are correct that Gina will have no biological ties to the baby, their simplistic comparison to an incubator disregards the fact that there are human emotions and biological changes involved in pregnancy.

A bond is created between a gestational mother and the baby she carries in her womb for nine months. During the pregnancy, the fetus relies on the gestational mother for a myriad of contributions. A gestational mother's endocrine system determines the timing, amount and components of hormones that affect the fetus. The absence of any component at its appropriate time will irreversibly alter the life, mental capacity, appearance, susceptibility to disease and structure of the fetus forever. The gestational mother contributes an endocrine cascade that determines how the child will grow, when its cells will divide and differentiate in the womb, and how the child will appear and function for the rest of its life." *Maternal Fetal Relationships and Nongenetic Surrogates*, 33 Jurimetrics J. 387 (1993).

In this case, Gina has previously had one child and therefore had an understanding of what is involved in carrying a pregnancy to term at the time she signed the contract. The problem case will present itself when a gestational mother changes her mind and wishes to keep the newborn. This may be more likely where a gestational mother has never had a child and is unfamiliar with the emotions and biological changes involved in a pregnancy. She will not be able to predict what her feelings will be towards the child she bears. Her body will undergo significant changes and she will continue to react biologically as any other birth mother. In this case, it seems likely that the transfer of the child will occur without incident due to the close family ties of the parties and Gina's previous experience with childbirth. However, although Gina is extremely likely to surrender her rights as planned, she must not be compelled to do so in a pre-birth order.

New Jersey regulations governing the creation of birth records state that the woman who gives birth must be recorded as a parent on the birth certificate. N.J.A.C. 8:2-1.4(a). This regulation would normally necessitate that Gina's name be placed on the birth certificate along with her brother-in-law, Peter, as the father. However, all parties have agreed by written contract that Andrea and Peter's names should be placed on the birth certificate . . .

In recognition of the emotional and physical changes in the mother which occur at birth, voluntary surrenders are not valid if taken within seventy-two hours after the birth of the child. N.J.S.A. 9:3-41(e). Thus after seventy-two hours have elapsed, Gina will be able to lawfully surrender her parental rights. She will have the responsibility of making decisions for the child during this seventy-two hour period, even if her ultimate decision is to surrender her parental rights.

It is not necessary now to determine what parental rights, if any, the gestational mother may have vis-à-vis the newborn infant. That decision will have to be made if and when a gestational mother attempts to keep the infant after birth in violation of the prior agreement. Here, Gina, Peter and Andrea are closely related. The parties' detailed fifteen page agreement clearly reflects their shared intent and desired outcome for this case. Further, Gina, as Andrea's sister and Peter's sister-in-law knows the biological parents intimately and is in an excellent position to know the type of home they will provide for the child. Thus almost certainly Gina will honor the contract and surrender her rights.

CONCLUSION

. . . The attending physician who delivers Baby A should prepare a Certificate of Parentage four days after the birth of the child. This waiting period will allow Gina to surrender her parental rights after seventy-two hours and also allow a birth certificate to be issued within five days of birth. After Gina surrenders any parental rights she might have, the Certificate of Parentage shall be completed with Peter as the legal father and Andrea the legal mother. This solution represents a modification of the agreement between the parties to the least extent necessary to comply with current New Jersey statutes and the public policy concerns expressed by the Supreme Court in *Baby M.*

NOTES AND QUESTIONS

1.   Do you think Judge Koblitz, who wrote the opinion in *A.H.W.*, is a man or a woman?

2.   Do you see any potential harm in denying the intended parents' request for a pre-birth judgment naming them as legal parents upon the birth of the child? In *A.H.W.*, the court notes that the gestational carrier will have the responsibility of making decisions for the child during the first 72-hour period. Suppose the child is born severely handicapped and doctors quickly conclude that aggressive medical treatment is needed to save the child's life. What if the intended parents and the gestational carrier differ as to course of treatment? For example, doctors may offer two options for treatment that they believe to be equally beneficial; one involves a risky surgery with a resulting lifelong scar, the other relies on medication but produces significant side effects. Who should be able to make the treatment decisions on behalf of the child?

3.   Judge Koblitz refuses to authorize a pre-birth order of parentage for the intended parents because to do so would violate New Jersey law, which mandates birth mothers be given 72 hours before any voluntary surrender of a child will be deemed valid. The law, the judge explains, is in recognition of the emotional and physical changes in the mother which occur at birth. These changes, according to the judge, mean that a gestational carrier "will not be able to predict what her feelings will be towards the child she bears." This issue of the maternal-fetal bond in a surrogacy pregnancy has engendered a wide variety of viewpoints.

One concern is that a surrogate purposefully does not bond with the child in her uterus, and that lack of bonding is harmful to the child. A related concern is that surrogacy promotes the image of a woman as a birthing machine, devoid of human qualities and personal autonomy. By forcing women to overcome the natural instinct to bond with their babies, contracted pregnancy betrays women's and society's basic interests. *See, e.g.*, GENA COREA, THE MOTHER MACHINE (1985) and CHRISTINE OVERALL, ETHICS AND HUMAN REPRODUCTION (1987).

A different perspective challenges the assumption that bonding with babies is "natural" and therefore "good." One author writes:

> It would be simple-minded . . . to assume that our habits are biologically determined: our culture is permeated with pronatalist bias. "Natural" or not, whether a tendency to such attachment is desirable could reasonably be judged to depend on circumstances. When infant mortality is high or responsibility for childrearing is shared by the community, it could do more harm than good. Beware the naturalistic fallacy!

Laura M. Purdy, *Surrogate Mothering: Exploitation or Empowerment?*, in REPRO- DUCING PERSONS: ISSUES IN FEMINIST BIOETHICS 189-90 (1996). Is it helpful or harmful to women to say that maternal-fetal bonding is biologically determined? If she is "supposed" to bond and doesn't (i.e., is able to give up the child at birth) is she empowered as a person of commitment, or exploited as a gestating vessel devoid of human qualities? If she is not "supposed" to bond and does (changes her mind about surrendering the child) is she infantilized as a person unable to make decisions, or revered as the epitome of motherhood?

Yet another view of the bonding phenomenon is that gestational carriers do bond with their babies, but more as a link to the intended parents with whom the real bonding occurs. One study of traditional and surrogate carriers provides insight into the psychology of maternal-fetal bonding:

> At a practical level, surrogates have to be able to strongly disassociate themselves from the children they bear. . . . [S]ome women found it harder giving away children that were genetically linked to themselves: "Giving away a child that is half mine — I brainwashed myself so much that I never thought about it, but at the end of the day you are still giving away something that belongs to you, your flesh and blood.

Two women interviewed opted for IVF and gestational surrogacy because they felt that the baby then belonged more to the contracting couple, and it was easier for the surrogates to think of themselves simply as carriers or incubators. This attitude of distance or separation was used as a mechanism to help a woman part with the child at birth. As one woman observed,

> With your own children it is totally different. It is a joyous occasion where you share everything with your husband and your family. With surrogate pregnancy you almost cut out the family. You don't encourage the grandmother to be a grandma, and you don't start nest building and buying things for the baby. There is no comparison between the pregnancies, except that you are pregnant, only the physical symptoms.

[The study author] did not see the fragmentation of 'motherhood' as causing any difficulties with the women she interviewed. The consensus was that the social mother, the woman who raised the child, was the true mother. The surrogates interviewed placed a great deal of emphasis on nurturing as the fundamental aspect of motherhood. With 'motherhood' now defined as separable into the roles of nurturer (social) mother and biological mother, women are given a choice about motherhood. Either role can be accepted or refused, thus in deciding not to be the social nurturing mother, the value of the biological (surrogate's) contribution is minimized "while the adoptive mother's choice to nurture activates or fully brings forth motherhood."

Bryn Williams-Jones, *Commercial Surrogacy and the Redefinition of Motherhood*, 2 J. PHIL., SCIENCE & L. (2002), citing C. Snowdon, *What Makes a Mother? Interviews with Women Involved in Egg Donation and Surrogacy*, BIRTH, Vol. 21(2), p. 82, 1994. The sentiments and struggles of any particular surrogate or contracting parent are highly individualistic, but many involved in these parenting arrangements have generously shared their experiences so others could learn. A few of their stories follow.

3. Profiles in Surrogate Parenting Arrangements

The following excerpts are taken from a variety of websites that collect essays from women considering becoming a surrogate, women who are or have been surrogates, women who have donated eggs, and couples who are searching for a surrogate. In the case of the surrogates, the essays were selected to address the most frequently asked question, "How could you give up a baby at birth?"

a.   Profile of a Traditional Surrogate Mother

One Surrogate's Experience
www.surrogacy.com

I began my surrogacy one day as I was browsing the local paper. I spotted an ad from an agency searching for surrogates. My husband and I had discussed our thoughts about this before and both agreed that it was a wonderful concept, so I showed him the ad and asked him what he thought about me doing it. We already had three children of our own, and weren't planning for anymore.

We discussed it over the following days. What would our friends say? How would it affect us as a couple. What would we tell our own kids and families? And, yes, we also discussed how the money would be of help to us.

We decided to proceed with just a call. I placed the call and was asked my race, features and marital status. The agency told me that I matched up with a few of their clients, and they would get back to me. I thought okay, maybe in a few months I'll hear something. Imagine my surprise when two days later they called asking if they could give my number to a couple. I said yes, and recieved [sic] a call that evening. The couple and I talked, and then all four of us talked. They said they'd like to meet us, so they set up a time in two weeks that they would fly up.

Well, we met, talked some more, and they said they would get back to me. They called a week later and we began our journey. The agency was no longer involved. It was us and the lawyers. We began the contract agreement which took the longest. I almost decided to back out at that time; it was so stressful. I didn't want all this hassle; I just wanted to give someone the special gift of a baby. We worked it out finally, did all the testing, and began the process.

Our first try was AI [artificial insemination] with frozen sperm. It didn't work, so the next month the husband flew to the clinic and we tried again . . . this time it was successful. I was pregnant.

After about four months, they began to want different things than what the contract stated. I began to worry. If I didn't go along with what they wanted, would they drop out? I was already pregnant. What would I do with the baby? My lawyer asked them to not discuss these things with me, so they asked me to get a different lawyer. I didn't though, and after they realized that it was causing me so much strees [sic], they let up.

I realize they were just anxious for everything to go okay, but it was showing me signs of distrust, so I also began to distrust. I think I had a hard time connecting to the mother. I feel she stayed distant, maybe to keep from being hurt. This upset me because I so wanted this to be special for all of us.

Nearing my eighth month, they decided they wanted me to have the baby in a different state — a state which gave them parental rights the minute the baby was born. I again felt they didn't trust me. I told them my doctor was against me traveling. They said "try a different doctor." I was not happy with that. I had a wonderful doctor who was looking out for my well-being as along with the baby's.

I felt as though the couple didn't care what happened to me. My lawyer again stepped in and set the matter straight.

Then came time for the paternity papers. The husband didn't want to sign them until they had proof that the baby was his. We went round and round on this. We finally gave them an ultimatum — either sign and take responsibility now, or we can wait until the baby is born, put it in a foster home, and then wait for a blood test. They didn't want that anymore than I did, so he signed. I could understand their wanting to make sure the baby was theirs, but they didn't seem to understand that a test of that nature during pregnacy [sic] was a uneeded risk to the baby.

With everything settled (my lawyer finally just told them we are sticking by the contract . . . and that's that) the big day came. I was being induced, so they flew up and were present in the delivery room. About three hours later, a healthy baby girl was born. The doctor put her on my chest and I looked at her and thought "she's precious, but she's not mine", and with that, I called the mother over and said "Come and hold your baby girl."

The look that went over their faces was enough to make me forget all the trouble it had been. It was pure joy and love as they looked down at her. As I handed her to her Mommy and Daddy, I thought "okay, this is where I'll probably lose it" . . . but I didn't. It felt like the most natural thing to give her to them . . . she was theirs.

Even after all the legal mumbo-jumbo problems that arose throughout the ordeal, I will say it has been the most wonderful experience! One I may even do again. There is one thing I forgot to mention. When we decided to first do the surrogacy, we lost our best friends. It was hard for us to lose them, but worth the trade for the happiness we made happen.

It has been just over a year now — the baby just had her first birthday. I get pictures and send them pictures. We hope that one day when she is old enough, they can show her the pictures of the family that helped them make their family.

I would like to tell future surrogates to please have patience with the couple. They get the new parent jitters just like the rest of us do. And for the couple, please have trust in your surrogate. Remember, we are only trying to help you. And for both . . . communicate at all times. It will work out the best that way, with everyone knowing what the others' feelings are.

b.   Profile of a Gestational Surrogate Mother

The Experience of a Lifetime
www.surromomonline.com

I thought I knew what to expect. Choose an agency, meet a couple, get pregnant with their baby, deliver easily and live happily ever after. I was wrong! I could have NEVER, in my wildest imagination have convinced myself in the beginning of this journey that there would be times that I would question my sanity or my reasoning for why I got myself and my family into this. I thought that my motives were clear, I was 25 years old and my husband and I had decided that our family was complete so why not help someone else? It seemed simple enough. Yet, after 50 shots, 1500 miles on the car going to the doctor and a few sleepless nights, I found myself on the other end of the phone hearing "I am sorry, your count is less than five, the test is negative." I was devastated! I sat in the bathroom for hours crying and wondering what I had done? It must have been me because the doctor said that it was a perfect transfer and to expect the possibility of twins! Now this, what will I tell my IM [intended mother]? Will she believe that I did do what I was told? I did all my shots, I stayed in the bed as ordered and I followed the instructions to a tee. I remember telling John, my husband, that I could NOT do it again, I didn't care what I had agreed to in the contract, I could not go through the disappointment again. Well, needless to say, in two weeks I started the lupron again with a renewed determination that we would get pregnant and the IP's would be parents (as if I had complete control this time).

For the second transfer, we again used five embryos, and again heard the words "this is a perfect transfer, the embryo's are beautiful." So on day ten, I went in for the blood test and waited (for what seemed like forever) for the results. I called at 2:00pm as instructed only to hear, "yes, we have the results, it is negative! That was it, it HAD to be a mistake!! So I replied in my most reserved voice, are you sure? She said what is your social security number again, and after what seemed like an eternity she got back on the phone and said "I am so sorry, it is positive"! As if by my sheer will, the test had changed it's mind and was afraid of being negative. We did it! We were on our way.

We went in for the second test which showed that my levels were rising and then on to the first ultrasound where we saw one sac. I was rather disappointed again because I knew they wanted twins. They were, however, thrilled that there was at least one on the way. Our due date, December 18,1996.

The rest of the pregnancy was fairly uneventful. One small scare where I was having pre-term contractions at 34 weeks. My IM insisted on flying out to be with us for the weekend and my doctor appointment on that Monday. Then there was the constant fear toward the end that the baby would get here before the IP's [intended parents] could. But, at 39 weeks, we were ready for the induction.

My husband drove me and the kids to their hotel where the soon to be new parents were anxiously awaiting us. The babysitter was waiting for my boys in the room. So we were off. My picotin drip was started at 8:30 AM and after not much progress, my water was broke at 12 noon. By 1:00 I WANTED that epidural and got it quickly. When the time came for the birth, my husband said to the father "come here dad, you only get one chance to see your son be born". So at 2:27, after only 10 minutes of pushing, the baby (a boy) was born into his parents arms. At 7 pounds and 3 ounces, 21 inches, he was the epitome of a healthy baby. They left him in the room with us for two hours. During that time I got to personally see the parents bond with and adore their new son. I felt at such peace within myself and a very strong sense of accomplishment. They went to the nursery and I went my room while my husband went to get the kids. In that dark, peaceful room I knew that however long the journey had been, no matter how frustrating and upsetting at times it got, in that single moment of silence, it had been more than worth it.

It has been four months since the birth. Although we still talk once a week, I can feel our relationship changing. The calls are less often and shorter. The distance has began. Yet, even if we just talk once a year on the anniversary of his birth, I will never regret my choice to help them complete their family. It is still amazing to me how two strangers and their families can come together for the love of a child and family and through a journey of love, respect and laughter change each others lives forever.

c. Profile of an Intended Mother

Thoughts on Becoming a Mommy
www.surromomsonline.com

There are women that become mothers without effort, and though they are good mothers and love their children, I know that I will be better.

I will be a better mother not because of genetics, or money or that I have read better books. But because I have struggled and toiled for this child. I have longed and waited.

I have endured and planned over and over again. Like most things in life, the people who truly have appreciation are those who have struggled to attain their dreams.

I will notice everything about my child. I will take the time to watch my child sleep, explore and discover. I will marvel at this miracle everyday for the rest of my life.

I will be happy when I wake in the middle of the night to the sound of my child, knowing that I can comfort, hold and feed and that I am not waking to give myself another injection of profasi and cry tears of a broken dream — my dream will be crying for me.

I count myself as lucky in this sense, that God has given me this insight, this special vision with which I will look upon my child that my friends will not see.

Whether I parent a child I give birth to or a child God leads me to. . . . I will not be careless with my love. I will be a better mother for all that I have endured.

NOTES AND QUESTIONS

1. *The Money Issue.* The sentiments expressed by the surrogates, and by the prospective mother, focus largely on their feelings about motherhood and the children born of the contracted relationship. Noticeably absent, some would argue, is attention to the factor that truly drives surrogate parenting arrangements — money. One woman did make passing mention of the financial benefits of becoming a surrogate, but generally surrogate talk steers away from highlighting the monetary aspects of the arrangements. Why?

The cold hard facts are difficult to locate, but a good estimate is that costs for a typical surrogacy birth in the U.S. range between $75,000 and $150,000. The costs include the surrogate's fee (on average, $20,000), medical expenses (some health insurance policies explicitly exclude coverage for surrogacy pregnancies), psychological testing, legal fees, agency fees (for the brokers who match surrogates and intended parents), pregnancy-related expenses (often surrogates get a monthly allowance from the time the contract is signed), life insurance for the surrogate, plus additional fees if an egg donor is used. For a breakdown of one agency's costs estimates, *see* The Center for Surrogate Parenting, Inc., Intended Parents, Gestational Surrogacy (IVF) Estimated Costs, at http://www.creatingfamilies.com/IP/IP_Info.aspx?Type=42.

2. *The Power Issue.* The costs of surrogacy typically yield a scenario in which the intended parents are in a higher, often much higher, income bracket than the surrogate and her husband. This wealth disparity causes many, including a few of the judges who have presided over surrogacy cases, to question whether the practice is dangerously exploitative of women because it enlists poorer women to accept the burdens and risks of pregnancy based on lack of economic opportunities. Conversely, others view the prospect of women using their reproductive capacity to gain wealth as an empowering and autonomous move, one that will raise the status of women in society. The divergent views on commercial surrogacy are nicely summarized in connection with the question: Who is a mother?

> The potential ethical implications of surrogate motherhood have garnered considerable public attention, largely because the different definitions of motherhood are based on competing ethical outlooks. The argument for autonomy and choice, strongly advocated by Dr. Carmel Shalev [in her book, Birth Power: The Case For Surrogacy (1989)], maintains that women have a right to sell gestational services along with the sale of their ova and to receive payment for using their wombs. She argues that to deny women the right to do so based on concerns for their ability to consent to such a contract is patriarchal in that it questions a women's ability to make valid contracts and minimizes their full autonomy. This argument favors choice and intention as the determining factors in deciding legal motherhood. On the other end of the spectrum is the argument for protection of women from financial exploitation and the imperative to keep certain body parts or biological acts sacred, similar to the prohibition on prostitution.[14] This point of view favors using gestation or parturition as the definition of mother-hood, thereby making surrogacy arrangements less palatable since the birth mother will always be considered the legal mother.

Pamela Laufer-Ukeles, *Gestation, Work for Hire or the Essence of Motherhood? A Comparative Legal Analysis*, 9 DUKE J. GENDER, LAW & POLICY 91 (2002). Do you think the arguments about surrogacy and economics are the same for traditional surrogacy and gestational surrogacy? Is the likelihood of exploitation higher when a woman's eggs, as well as her womb, are used?

3. *Parental Change of Heart.* The case law involving surrogacy arrangements gone awry nearly always tell the tale of a surrogate changing her mind at or near the birth of the child. But, of course, the roles can be reversed. In 2001 a San Francisco couple in search of a surrogate contacted a British woman via the internet. The surrogate became pregnant with twins, and upon hearing the double

---

[14] [n.7] See Ruth Macklin, *Is There Anything Wrong with Surrogate Motherhood? An Ethical Analysis*, 16 L. Med. & Health Care 57, 62 (1988) (arguing against enforcement of surrogacy agreements because they are exploitive of poor women); Janice Raymond, *Reproductive Gifts and Gift Giving: The Altruistic Woman*, Hastings Ctr. Rep., Nov.-Dec. 1990, at 11 (arguing that even altruistic surrogacy is exploitive, in that it sets women apart as the caregiver and the breeder class).

good news, the couple asked that she terminate the pregnancy. When the surrogate refused, the couple began searching for another couple to parent the twins. Thereafter, the surrogate sued the couple for payment of her $20,000 fee, none of which had been paid previously. In the end, it is rumored that the twins were adopted by another couple. See Jessica Cohen, *Loving Family Seeks Bright, Good-Looking Egg Donor*, SUNDAY TELEGRAPH (London), Jan. 5, 2003, at 3.

This rumor, however, proved false. As reported by the attorney representing the surrogate, ". . . in the end, the court did award the twins to the original couple who appear to be currently parenting the twins, despite their rocky start. Unfortunately, the surrogate was unable to financially continue her civil suit against the couple and has not received the fees that were due to her despite the court ruling that the couple were the parents of the twins." [Correspondence to the editor dated October 21, 2004, from Theresa M. Erickson, Esq., an ART attorney then based in San Diego]

4. *Malfeasance in the Business of Surrogacy.* As previously discussed, ART in general and surrogacy in particular are big businesses involving high dollar amounts. Prospective parents pay tens and sometimes hundreds of thousands of dollars to physicians and other professionals for assistance in achieving their parental goals. Sadly, though probably not unsurprisingly, the lure of big financial payoffs has seen some ART facilitators engage in corrupt practices. Take for example, Theresa Erickson, the attorney referenced in Note 3. For years hailed as a prominent legal expert in ART with her own radio program on the subject, Ms. Erickson plead guilty to federal fraud charges in August 2011 for what is described as an international baby-selling ring. An FBI investigation revealed that Erickson and two co-conspirators solicited U.S. women to travel abroad to be implanted with donated embryos. When the women reached the second trimester of pregnancy, the trio would recruit prospective parents who were falsely told that the women were gestational carriers for other couples who had backed out of the deal. Upon a payment of $100,000 to $150,000, Erickson would submit false documents to the local court seeking a pre-birth order allowing the substitute parents to be named on the child's birth certificate. After one surrogate grew nervous because she was due to deliver with no intended parents in sight, she sought advice from another lawyer who quickly sized up the situation and notified authorities. *See* Alan Zarembo, *Scam Targeted Surrogates as Well as Couples*, L.A. TIMES, Aug. 13, 2011, available at: http://articles.latimes.com/2011/aug/13/local/la-me-baby-ring-20110814. In February 2012, Erickson was sentenced to 5 months in prison and ordered to pay a $70,000 fine.

In August 2009, clients at SurroGenesis, a Modesto, California-based surrogacy agency filed a class action lawsuit against the agency after it abruptly closed its doors shutting down access to hundreds of thousands of dollars in fees paid by hopeful parents. Dozens of expectant parents and pregnant surrogates were left without recourse for services and monies promised by the agency's owner. Finally, in 2006 a Sacramento-based surrogacy agent pleaded no contest to seven counts of grand theft and served six years in prison for duping intended parents into paying thousands of dollars for promised, but never delivered, surrogacy services. *See* Alan Zarembo & Kimi Yoshino, *Surrogacy Makes for a Perilous Path to Parenthood*, LA

Times, March 29, 2009, available at: http://articles.latimes.com/2009/mar/29/local/me-surrogate29.

5. *Public Displays of Assisted Conception.* If surrogate parenting arrangements were ever considered a matter of strict secrecy guarded within the family realm, it seems that Hollywood may be coaxing the practice out of the closet. In recent years, entertainment personalities have talked openly about their use of surrogate mothers, in glowing and grateful terms. In December 2010, pop icon Sir Elton John and his long-time partner David Furnish introduced the world to baby Zachary Jackson Levon Furnish-John, born to a California surrogate. Celebrity duo Nicole Kidman and Keith Urban announced the birth of their second daughter via gestational surrogate in December 2010, to join an older sister who arrived the old-fashioned way. Neil Patrick Harris (*How I Met Your Mother*, and for the older crowd, *Doogie Howser, M.D.*) and his partner David Burtka welcomed fraternal twins in October 2010, with each dad supplying sperm for the donor eggs that were fertilized and transferred. Surrogate mother, Michelle Ross, gave birth to Sarah Jessica Parker and Matthew Broderick's twin girls in 2009. Pop singer Ricky Martin became the single papa to twin boys with help from an egg donor and surrogate in 2008. Finally, in August 2004, famed *Frazier* star Kelsey Grammar and his wife, former Playboy model and Real Housewife of Beverly Hills Camille Donatacci, welcomed their second child through a surrogate mother. The couple's relationship later soured, perhaps after Camille confessed she needed four nannies to manage the children. She cited irritable bowel syndrome as her reason for employing a surrogate. She provided no explanation for the four nannies. For more in-depth reporting on the world of celebrity surrogacy, *see*, no kidding, TheFrisky-.com (specifically, *10 Celebs Who Are Part of the Surrogate Baby Boom*, at http://www.thefrisky.com/post/246-10-celebs-who-are-part-of-the-surrogate-baby-boom).

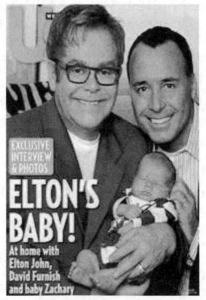

Elton John and David Furnish with baby Zachary, born in 2010

C. Statutory Responses to Surrogate Parenting Arrangements

1. Laws Regulating Surrogacy

Surrogate parenting arrangements are private agreements that touch on several areas of state law, including contract law, family law, and even criminal law. Because surrogacy arrangements raise legal questions that are largely within the realm of state law, the practice of surrogacy is regulated by the individual states, rather than by the federal government. As a result, one could say that the laws on surrogate parenting form a "checkerboard" across the country, with each state posing its own unique view of surrogate parenting arrangements. What follows is a summary of our nation's surrogacy laws, with a listing of each state's law, if any, on surrogacy contracts.

a. Individual State Laws

A significant minority of states have enacted legislation addressing surrogate parenting arrangements. At current count, 23 states and the District of Columbia have at least one statute pertaining to surrogacy. The statutes differ widely in how they regulate the practice, ranging from outright bans on all surrogacy contracts to provisions for medical and psychological screening of all parties involved. Eleven states, by statute, authorize surrogacy, with varying degrees of restrictions: Arkansas, Connecticut, Florida, Illinois, Iowa, Nevada, New Hampshire, Texas, Utah, Virginia, and West Virginia. Nine states plus the District of Columbia ban surrogacy contracts (in some cases traditional surrogacy agreements only), usually by declaring such agreements to be null and void under state law: Arizona, D.C., Indiana, Kentucky, Louisiana, Michigan, Nebraska, New York, North Dakota and Washington. The remaining states with surrogacy laws address parentage questions such as whether a parent-child relationship exists between the intended couple and the child.

State Surrogacy Laws

Alabama

Ala. Code § 26-10A-34 exempts surrogacy agreements from provisions making it a crime to sell a baby.

Alaska

There is no surrogacy law in the state.

Arizona

Ariz. Rev. Stat. Ann. § 25-218(A) bans surrogacy contracts. "No person may enter into, induce, arrange, procure or otherwise assist in the formation of a surrogate parentage contract." Two other provisions declaring the surrogate the legal mother, and her husband the legal father, were declared unconstitutional in *Soos v. Superior Court in and for County of Maricopa*, 182 Ariz. 470, 897 P.2d 1356 (1994).

Arkansas

Ark. Code Ann. § 9-10-201(b) raises the presumption that a child born to a surrogate mother is the child of the intended parents and not the surrogate.

California

There are no statutes directly regulating surrogacy, but case law approves surrogate parenting agreements as "not . . . inconsistent with public policy." *Johnson v. Calvert*, 5 Cal.4th 84, 19 Cal. Rptr. 2d 494, 851 P.2d 776 (1993).

Colorado

There is no surrogacy law in the state.

Connecticut

Conn. Gen. Stat. Ann. § 7-48a permits the intended parents under a gestational surrogacy arrangement to be named as parents on the birth certificate. The statute was amended to reflect the Connecticut Supreme Court's decision in *Raftopol v. Ramey*, 299 Conn. 681 (2011).

Delaware

There is no surrogacy law in the state.

District of Columbia

D.C. Code Ann. § 16-402(a) bans surrogacy agreements. "Surrogate parenting contracts are prohibited and rendered unenforceable in the District."

Florida

Fla. Stat. Ann. § 742.15 permits but strictly regulates surrogacy. Practice is limited to married couples, where "commissioning mother" cannot physically carry child to term, who may only reimburse a gestational surrogate for reasonable medical, legal and living expenses; if neither intended parent is genetically related to child (i.e., embryo donation), surrogate assumes parental rights and responsibilities.

Georgia

There is no surrogacy law in the state.

Hawaii

There is no surrogacy law in the state.

Idaho

There is no surrogacy law in the state.

Illinois

Il. Comp Stat. Ann., ch, 750, 45/6 recognizes parent-child relationship between genetic parents and child born to gestational surrogate. Intended parents must contribute both egg and sperm, and licensed physician must certify that child is biological child of couple and not of the surrogate and her husband.

Indiana

Ind. Code § 31-20-1-1, 2 declares surrogate parenting agreements void and unenforceable.

Iowa

Ia. Code Ann. § 710.11 exempts traditional surrogacy from the state's baby-selling laws.

Kansas

There is no surrogacy law in the state.

Kentucky

Ky. Rev. Stat. § 199.590(4) voids commercial surrogacy contracts in which woman agrees to be artificially inseminated and subsequently terminate her parental rights to child.

Louisiana

La. Rev. Stat. § 9:2713 declares surrogate mother contracts null and void; defines surrogacy as a woman's agreement, for valuable consideration, to be inseminated and relinquish rights to any resulting child.

Maine

There is no surrogacy law in the state.

Maryland

There is no surrogacy law in the state. The Maryland Attorney General opined that "surrogacy contracts that involve the payment of a fee to the birth mother are, in most instances, illegal and unenforceable under Maryland law." The AG also noted the result would be different in a gestational surrogacy case. 85 Op. Atty. Gen. No. 00-035, Dec. 19, 2000. In 2003, the Maryland Supreme Court authorized issuance of a birth certificate omitting the name of a gestational carrier and naming only the single father. In *Roberto d.B.*, 814 A.2d 570 (2003).

Massachusetts

There are no statutes directly regulating surrogacy but the state's highest court has ruled that traditional surrogacy arrangements are unenforceable, *R.R. v. M.H.* 426 Mass. 501, 689 N.E.2d 790 (1998), but gestational surrogacy arrangements are enforceable, *Culliton v. Beth Israel Deaconess Medical Center*, 435 Mass. 285, 756 N.E.2d 1133 (2001).

Michigan

Mich. Comp. Laws Ann. § 722.855 provides, "A surrogate parentage contract is void and unenforceable as contrary to public policy."

Minnesota

There is no surrogacy law in the state.

Mississippi

There is no surrogacy law in the state.

Missouri

There is no surrogacy law in the state.

Montana

There is no surrogacy law in the state.

Nebraska

Neb. Rev. Stat. Ann. § 25-21,200 declares surrogate parenthood contracts void and unenforceable.

Nevada

Nev. Rev. Stat. Ann. § 126.045 validates unpaid surrogate parenting contracts; permits payment to surrogate for "medical and necessary living expenses."

New Hampshire

N.H. Rev. Stat. § 168-B:16-21 permits unpaid surrogacy arrangements (exempting payments for medical and other pregnancy-related expenses) provided the parties receive judicial preauthorization. The law details required provisions for a valid surrogacy contract, including that the intended mother be medically unable to bear a child.

New Jersey

There is no surrogacy law in the state. Case law declares traditional surrogacy arrangements void as against state law and public policy. *In re Baby M*, 109 N.J. 396, 537 A.2d 1227 (1988).

New Mexico

New Mex. Stat. § 40-11A-801 provides that gestational agreements are not authorized or prohibited.

New York

N.Y. Dom. Rel. Law § 122 declares surrogate parenting contracts void and unenforceable; imposes civil and criminal penalties on "any other person or entity who or which induces, arranges or otherwise assists in the formation of a surrogate parenting contract for a fee."

North Carolina

There is no surrogacy law in the state.

North Dakota

N.D. Cent. Code § 14-18-01-07 declares traditional surrogate parenting contracts void; surrogate and her husband are deemed parents of any resulting child; child born to a gestational carrier is a child of the intended parents for all purposes and is not a child of the gestational carrier and the gestational carrier's husband, if any.

Ohio

There is no surrogacy law in the state. Lower court approved pre-birth judgment for intended parents whose relative acted as unpaid gestational carrier. *Belsito v. Clark*, 67 Ohio Misc.2d 54, 644 N.E.2d 760 (1994); Supreme Court of Ohio upheld gestational surrogacy contract as valid and enforceable based on principles of contract law. *J.F. v. D.B.*, 116 Ohio St. 3d 363, 879 N.E.2d 740 (2007).

Oklahoma

There is no surrogacy law in the state. The Oklahoma Attorney General concluded that a surrogate gestation contract providing for payment beyond statutory limitations to effect the adoption of a child is illegal under the state's anti-child trafficking statute. Op. Atty. Gen. No. 83-162 (Sept. 29, 1983).

Oregon

There is no surrogacy law in the state.

Pennsylvania

There is no surrogacy law in the state.

Rhode Island

There is no surrogacy law in the state.

South Carolina

There is no surrogacy law in the state.

South Dakota

There is no surrogacy law in the state.

Tennessee

Tenn. Code Ann § 36-1-102 provides, "Nothing herein shall be construed to expressly authorize the surrogate birth process in Tennessee unless otherwise approved by the courts or the general assembly."

Texas

Tex. Code Ann., Family Code § 160.754 approves gestational agreements so long as the egg is retrieved from the intended parent or a donor. The law also requires the intended parents be married to each other.

Utah

Utah Code Ann. § 78B-15-801-03 upholds gestational surrogacy agreements under certain circumstances, including the intended parents are married to each other, the intended mother is unable to bear a child on her own, all parties participate in counseling with a licensed mental health professional.

A previous law voiding surrogate parenting arrangements and declaring "the surrogate mother is the mother of the child for all legal purposes, and her husband, if she is married, is the father of the child for all legal purposes" was struck down as unconstitutional in *J.R. v. Utah*, 261 F. Supp. 2d 1268 (D. Utah 2002).

Vermont

There is no surrogacy law in the state.

Virginia

Va. Code Ann. § 20-156-160 authorizes unpaid surrogacy agreements; requires intended mother be infertile and that all parties petition the court for approval prior to performance of assisted conception.

Washington

Wash. Rev. Code § 26-26-240 declares traditional surrogate parenting contract entered into for compensation void and unenforceable as contrary to public policy. Violations of this provision are punishable as gross misdemeanors.

West Virginia

W. Va. Code § 48-22-803 exempts surrogate parenting arrangements from the state's baby-selling statute.

Wisconsin

Wisc. Code Ann. § 69.14 provides, "If the registrant of a birth certificate under this section is born to a surrogate mother, information about the surrogate mother shall be entered on the birth certificate and the information about the father shall be omitted from the birth certificate."

Wyoming

There is no surrogacy law in the state.

Compare the different approaches to surrogacy expressed in the following three state statutes:

Florida Statutes Annotated
Title XLIII. Domestic Relations
Chapter 742. Determination of Parentage

§ 742.15. Gestational Surrogacy Contract

(1) Prior to engaging in gestational surrogacy, a binding and enforceable gestational surrogacy contract shall be made between the commissioning couple and the gestational surrogate. A contract for gestational surrogacy shall not be binding and enforceable unless the gestational surrogate is 18 years of age or older and the commissioning couple are legally married and are both 18 years of age or older.

(2) The commissioning couple shall enter into a contract with a gestational surrogate only when, within reasonable medical certainty as determined by a physician licensed under chapter 458 or chapter 459:

(a) The commissioning mother cannot physically gestate a pregnancy to term;

(b) The gestation will cause a risk to the physical health of the commissioning mother; or

(c) The gestation will cause a risk to the health of the fetus.

(3) A gestational surrogacy contract must include the following provisions:

(a) The commissioning couple agrees that the gestational surrogate shall be the sole source of consent with respect to clinical intervention and management of the pregnancy.

(b) The gestational surrogate agrees to submit to reasonable medical evaluation and treatment and to adhere to reasonable medical instructions about her prenatal health.

(c) Except as provided in paragraph (e), the gestational surrogate agrees to relinquish any parental rights upon the child's birth and to proceed with the judicial proceedings prescribed under s.742.16.

(d) Except as provided in paragraph (e), the commissioning couple agrees to accept custody of and to assume full parental rights and responsibilities for the child immediately upon the child's birth, regardless of any impairment of the child.

(e) The gestational surrogate agrees to assume parental rights and responsibilities for the child born to her if it is determined that neither member of the commissioning couple is the genetic parent of the child.

(4) As part of the contract, the commissioning couple may agree to pay only reasonable living, legal, medical, psychological, and psychiatric expenses of the gestational surrogate that are directly related to prenatal, intrapartal, and postpartal periods.

Iowa Code Annotated
Title XVI. Criminal Law and Procedure
Chapter 710. Kidnapping and Related Offenses

§ 710.11. Purchase or Sale of Individual

A person commits a class "C" felony when the person purchases or sells or attempts to purchase or sell an individual to another person. This section does not apply to surrogate mother arrangements. For purposes of this section, a "surrogate mother arrangement" means an arrangement whereby a female agrees to be artificially inseminated with the semen of a donor, to bear a child, and to relinquish all rights regarding that child to the donor or donor couple.

Nebraska Revised Statutes
Chapter 25. Courts; Civil Procedure
Article 21. Surrogate Parenthood Contracts

§ 25-21,200. Contract; Void and Unenforceable: Definition.

(1) A surrogate parenthood contract entered into shall be void and unenforceable. The biological father of a child born pursuant to such a contract shall have all the rights and obligations imposed by law with respect to such child.

(2) For purposes of this section, unless the context otherwise requires, a surrogate parenthood contract shall mean a contract by which a woman is to be compensated for bearing a child of a man who is not her husband.

NOTES AND QUESTIONS

1.   The Florida surrogacy statute contains a requirement that the intended mother be physically incapable of gestating a child, or that gestation would pose a risk to the health of the intended mother or the child. Florida joins four other states, New Hampshire, Texas, Utah and Virginia, in requiring that the intended mother be infertile or unable to bear children without substantial health risks to herself or the unborn child. N.H. Rev. Stat. Ann § 168-B:17; Tex. Code Ann., Family Code § 160.756(b)(2); Utah Code Ann. § 78B-15-803; Va. Code Ann. § 20-160(8). What is the reason for this requirement? Do you agree that a commissioning woman must be infertile in order to avail herself of a surrogate parenting contract? For a thorough and thoughtful analysis of the statutory infertility requirement, see Robin Fretwell Wilson, *Uncovering the Rationale for Requiring Infertility in Surrogacy Arrangements*, 29 Am. J. Law & Med. 337 (2003).

2.   Would the following arrangements be lawful in Florida? In Iowa? In Nebraska? Which parties are most likely to be considered the lawful parents of the child in each state?

(A) Brandon and Heather are a married couple experiencing infertility. The couple has gone through three rounds of IVF and each time Heather becomes pregnant but then suffers a miscarriage early in the pregnancy. The doctors suspect the embryos are not genetically healthy and suggest the couple consider an egg donor. Brandon and Heather contract with Tracy to supply eggs to them, paying her a fee of $5,000. The couple decides to hire a surrogate to gestate the resulting embryos, formed from Tracy's eggs and Brandon's sperm. The couple agrees to pay the surrogate, Ashley, all her medical and legal expenses, as well as provide her a $10,000 budget to purchase designer maternity clothing.

(B) Todd and Bill are registered domestic partners who desire to have a child together. Todd's sister, Madison, agrees to serve as a traditional surrogate for the couple. Before she is artificially inseminated with Bill's sperm, she signs a contract agreeing to surrender the child to the couple at birth and to relinquish any parental rights as soon as the law allows.

(C) Janice is a single woman who wishes to parent a child. She had a hysterectomy at age 25, so she is not able to produce eggs or gestate a child on her own. Janice contracts with an agency to obtain embryos that are available for a fee of $8,000. Janice then contracts with a gestational carrier, Theresa, to bring the embryo to term. Theresa will be reimbursed for her medical and legal expenses only. When the child is born, Theresa and her husband claim parental rights to the child.

---

b.   Uniform Laws on Surrogacy

In addition to the individual states' responses to surrogate parenting arrangements, two uniform laws have emerged addressing the legality of such agreements. Recall that uniform laws are drafted by the National Conference of Commissioners on Uniform State Laws and are advisory in nature — meaning that they are available for adoption by each state. The first uniform law to broadly address reproductive technologies was the Uniform Status of Children of Assisted Conception Act (USCACA), promulgated in 1988. The USCACA addressed surrogacy by providing two alternatives, one that validated surrogacy contracts under prescribed circumstances, and one that declared such contracts void. The USCACA was adopted by only two states — North Dakota (adopting Alternative B, declaring surrogate parenting contracts void), and Virginia (adopting Alternative A, validating contracts which receive pre-pregnancy judicial approval).

The second uniform law addressing surrogacy came in 2000, with amendments added in 2002, when the uniform law commissioners promulgated an update of the 1973 Uniform Parentage Act. This updated law contains extensive language addressing reproductive technologies, including surrogate parenting arrangements. In a nod toward efficiency, the updated UPA withdraws the USCACA and substitutes a new article in the UPA which is modeled after the 1988 law, but incorporates only a version of Alternative A, allowing validation and enforcement of surrogacy agreements. The end result is a single uniform law pertaining to matters of assisted conception.

Below are excerpts from the two ART uniform laws.

Uniform Status of Children of Assisted Conception Act 1988

§ 1. Definitions.

In this [Act]:

(1) "Assisted conception" means a pregnancy resulting from (i) fertilizing an egg of a woman with sperm of a man by means other than sexual intercourse or (ii) implanting an embryo, but the term does not include the pregnancy of a wife resulting from fertilizing her egg with sperm of her husband.

(2) "Donor" means an individual [other than a surrogate] who produces egg or sperm used for assisted conception, whether or not a payment is made for the egg or sperm used, but does not include a woman who gives birth to a resulting child.

(3) "Intended parents" means a man and woman, married to each other, who enter into an agreement under this [Act] providing that they will be the parents of a child born to a surrogate through assisted conception using egg or sperm of one or both of the intended parents.]

(4) "Surrogate" means an adult woman who enters into an agreement to bear a child conceived through assisted conception for intended parents.

Alternative A

§ 5. Surrogacy Agreement.

(a) A surrogate, her husband, if she is married, and intended parents may enter into a written agreement whereby the surrogate relinquishes all her rights and duties as a parent of a child to be conceived through assisted conception, and the intended parents may become the parents of the child pursuant to Section 8.

(b) If the agreement is not approved by the court under Section 6 before conception, the agreement is void and the surrogate is the mother of a resulting child and the surrogate's husband, if a party to the agreement, is the father of the child. If the surrogate's husband is not a party to the agreement or the surrogate is unmarried, paternity of the child is governed by [the Uniform Parentage Act].

§ 6. Petition and Hearing for Approval of Surrogacy Agreement.

(a) The intended parents and the surrogate may file a petition in the [appropriate court] to approve a surrogacy agreement if one of them is a resident of this State. The surrogate's husband, if she is married, must join in the petition. A copy of the agreement must be attached to the petition. The court shall name a [guardian ad litem] to represent the interests of a child to be conceived by the surrogate through assisted conception and [shall] [may] appoint counsel to represent the surrogate.

(b) The court shall hold a hearing on the petition and shall enter an order approving the surrogacy agreement, authorizing assisted conception for a period of 12 months after the date of the order, declaring the intended parents to be the parents of a child to be conceived through assisted conception pursuant to the agreement and discharging the guardian ad litem and attorney for the surrogate, upon finding that:

(1) the court has jurisdiction and all parties have submitted to its jurisdiction under subsection (e) and have agreed that the law of this State governs all matters arising under this [Act] and the agreement;

(2) the intended mother is unable to bear a child or is unable to do so without

unreasonable risk to an unborn child or to the physical or mental health of the intended mother or child, and the finding is supported by medical evidence;

(3) the [relevant child-welfare agency] has made a home study of the intended parents and the surrogate and a copy of the report of the home study has been filed with the court;

(4) the intended parents, the surrogate, and the surrogate's husband, if she is married, meet the standards of fitness applicable to adoptive parents in this State;

(5) all parties have voluntarily entered into the agreement and understand its terms, nature, and meaning, and the effect of the proceeding;

(6) the surrogate has had at least one pregnancy and delivery and bearing another child will not pose an unreasonable risk to the unborn child or to the physical or mental health of the surrogate or the child, and this finding is supported by medical evidence;

(7) all parties have received counseling concerning the effect of the surrogacy by [a qualified health-care professional or social worker] and a report containing conclusions about the capacity of the parties to enter into and fulfill the agreement has been filed with the court;

(8) a report of the results of any medical or psychological examination or genetic screening agreed to by the parties or required by law has been filed with the court and made available to the parties;

(9) adequate provision has been made for all reasonable health-care costs associated with the surrogacy until the child's birth including responsibility for those costs if the agreement is terminated pursuant to Section 7; and

(10) the agreement will not be substantially detrimental to the interest of any of the affected individuals.

§ 8. Parentage Under Approved Surrogacy Agreement.

(1) Upon birth of a child to the surrogate, the intended parents are the parents of the child and the surrogate and her husband, if she is married, are not parents of the child unless the court vacates the order pursuant to Section 7(b) . . .

§ 9. Surrogacy: Miscellaneous Provisions.

(a) A surrogacy agreement that is the basis of an order under Section 6 may provide for the payment of consideration.

(b) A surrogacy agreement may not limit the right of the surrogate to make decisions regarding her health care or that of the embryo or fetus . . .

Alternative B

§ 5. Surrogate Agreements.

An agreement in which a woman agrees to become a surrogate or to relinquish her rights and duties as parent of a child thereafter conceived through assisted conception is void. However, she is the mother of a resulting child, and her husband, if a party to the agreement, is the father of the child. If her husband is not a party to the agreement or the surrogate is unmarried, paternity of the child is governed by [the Uniform Parentage Act].]

Uniform Parentage Act (approved 2000, amended 2002)

§ 801. Gestational Agreement Authorized.

(a) A prospective gestational mother, her husband if she is married, a donor or the donors, and the intended parents may enter into a written agreement providing that:

(1) the prospective gestational mother agrees to pregnancy by means of assisted reproduction;

(2) the prospective gestational mother, her husband if she is married, and the donors relinquish all rights and duties as the parents of a child conceived through assisted reproduction; and

(3) the intended parents become the parents of the child.

(b) The man and the woman who are the intended parents must both be parties to the gestational agreement.

(c) A gestational agreement is enforceable only if validated as provided in Section 803.

(d) A gestational agreement does not apply to the birth of a child conceived by means of sexual intercourse.

(e) A gestational agreement may provide for payment of consideration.

(f) A gestational agreement may not limit the right of the gestational mother to make decisions to safeguard her health or that of the embryos or fetus.

§ 802. Requirements of Petition.

(a) The intended parents and the prospective gestational mother may commence a proceeding in the [appropriate court] to validate a gestational agreement.

§ 803. Hearing to Validate Gestational Agreement.

(a) If the requirements of subsection (b) are satisfied, a court may issue an order validating the gestational agreement and declaring that the intended parents will be the parents of a child born during the term of the of the agreement.

(b) The court may issue an order under subsection (a) only on finding that:

(1) the residence requirements of Section 802 have been satisfied and the parties have submitted to the jurisdiction of the court under the jurisdictional standards of this [Act];

(2) unless waived by the court, the [relevant child-welfare agency] has made a

home study of the intended parents and the intended parents meet the standards of suitability applicable to adoptive parents;

(3) all parties have voluntarily entered into the agreement and understand its terms;

(4) adequate provision has been made for all reasonable health-care expense associated with the gestational agreement until the birth of the child, including responsibility for those expenses if the agreement is terminated; and

(5) the consideration, if any, paid to the prospective gestational mother is reasonable.

§ 809. Effect of Nonvalidated Gestational Agreement.

(a) A gestational agreement, whether in a record or not, that is not judicially validated is not enforceable.

(b) If a birth results under a gestational agreement that is not judicially validated as provided in this [article], the parent-child relationship is determined as provided in [Article] 2.

(c) Individuals who are parties to a nonvalidated gestational agreement as intended parents may be held liable for support of the resulting child, even if the agreement is otherwise unenforceable. The liability under this subsection includes assessing all expenses and fees as provided in Section 636.

NOTES AND QUESTIONS

1. What differences, if any, do you see between the Uniform Status of Children of Assisted Conception Act (1988) and the updated Uniform Parentage Act (2000 & 2002)? One way to observe any differences is to review the scenarios set out above on pages 446 and 447. How would each of the scenarios be resolved under the USCACA? The updated UPA?

2. Is legislation the best way to address the parentage of children born via assisted conception? What factors, in your mind, are most important in determining who is a parent? Can a statute be drafted with enough precision, or enough flexibility, to permit consistent application of those factors in every instance? Or are courts better arbiters when it comes to questions of parent-child relationships?

Professor Roger Dworkin compares the relative qualifications of the legislative and judicial branches to decide questions of paternity in the context of artificial insemination:

> . . . [I]n cases involving artificial insemination of unmarried and lesbian women, courts have adopted pragmatic, practical approaches that seem to make sense for the parties, while legislatures have adopted hard and fast rules that often lead to senseless results. For example, in cases involving known donors and lesbian mothers, courts have made questions of the donor's rights to custody and visitation depend upon facts such as the amount of involvement the donor has had in the life of the child; the nature of their relationship; whether the donor is paying child support; and the

mother's behavior. They have been reluctant to treat mothers' lesbian partners as "parents," but they have protected their interests by assuring that they have visitation rights, that the child is accessible to them, etc. In a messy and unpleasant situation, that is about the best one can do. The Uniform Status of Children of Assisted Conception Act, on the other hand, would simply eliminate any parental claims of the donor regardless of the facts of the particular case. That represents the triumph of ideology and the quest for certainty over good sense. Moreover, the ideology is not clear, as the drafters state that their goal is to promote the best interests of children, but in many cases cutting one parent out of a child's life is not best for that child.

Why has the common law worked so much better than legislation in dealing with legal issues raised by artificial insemination? I would suggest that the explanation lies in the fact that conduct control is not an important priority in this setting; that no social problem of magnitude is involved; that nothing that would disable judges from handling the problems exists; that sensible results are highly fact dependent; and that the issues are analogous to those with which the courts have been dealing for centuries. That is, I am not aware of anybody who thinks that artificial insemination should be prevented or strictly controlled, something courts could not do well. Artificial insemination poses no major crisis for the nation to which the law must respond. No scientific or other expertise that judges lack is needed to resolve the cases. Sound results in human relationship cases depend on the infinitely variable facts of human relationships. And issues of custody, child support, visitation, etc. are the kinds of issues courts have long known how to resolve.

The legislatures, on the other hand, have sought to impose one-size-fits-all, certain solutions on areas where certainty is not only unnecessary, but undesirable; and they have responded to imaginary problems (like the nonexistent health problems of women inseminating themselves) by ignoring the first rule of sound law making: if it ain't broke, don't fix it.

Roger B. Dworkin, *Bioethics? The Law and Biomedical Advance*, 14 HEALTH MATRIX: J. LAW-MED 43, 52-53 (2004). Do you think Professor Dworkin's thesis that case law works much better than legislation can be applied to the legality and enforcement of surrogate parenting arrangements?

3. Notice that the USCACA uses the word "surrogate" to describe a woman who enters into an agreement to bear a child through assisted conception for intended parents. Is this an appropriate term to describe the woman who gestates another's child? On the grounds that language shapes perception, the National Conference of Commissioners on Uniform State Laws considered the use of the word "surrogate" in drafting the 2000 Uniform Parentage Act. The result — a shift to the term "gestational mother." The uniform lawmakers explain the change as follows:

Article 8's replacement of the USCACA terminology, "surrogate mother," by "gestational mother" is important. First, labeling a woman who bears a child a "surrogate" does not comport with the dictionary definition of the term under any construction, to wit: "a person appointed to act in the place of another" or "something serving as a substitute." The term is especially misleading when "surrogate" refers to a woman who supplies both "egg and womb," that is, a woman who is a genetic as well as gestational mother. That combination is now typically avoided by the majority of ART practitioners in order to decrease the possibility that a genetic\gestational mother will be unwilling to relinquish her child to unrelated intended parents. Further, the term "surrogate" has acquired a negative connotation in American society, which confuses rather than enlightens the discussion.

In contrast, [the] term "gestational mother" is both more accurate and more inclusive. It applies to both a woman who, through assisted reproduction, performs the gestational function without being genetically related to a child, and a woman [who] is both the gestational and genetic mother. The key is that an agreement has been made that the child is to be raised by the intended parents. The latter practice has elicited disfavor in the ART community, which has concluded that the gestational mother's genetic link to the child too often creates additional emotional and psychological problems in enforcing a gestational agreement.

Comment by Drafters, Uniform Parentage Act (2000), Art. 8. Did the uniform lawmakers shift from the term "surrogate" to the term "gestational mother" to reflect the reality that most paid parenting agreements involve a gestational carrier — a woman who bears an embryo genetically unrelated to her — rather than a woman who is inseminated with the sperm of the intended father? Does the UPA imply a preference for gestational surrogacy by changing the key language?

2.   Constitutionality of Surrogacy Laws

J.R., M.R. AND W.K.J. v. UTAH
United States District Court, District of Utah
261 F. Supp. 2d 1268 (2002)

JENKINS, SENIOR DISTRICT JUDGE. The plaintiffs, J.R., M.R. and W.K.J., filed the instant action against the defendants under 42 U.S.C. § 1983 (2000) on March 6, 2002, seeking declaratory and injunctive relief, nominal monetary damages and attorney's fees against the defendants arising from an alleged violation of plaintiffs' federal and state constitutional rights resulting from defendants' compliance with Utah Code Ann. § 76-7-204 (1999), a Utah statute dealing with the validity and enforcement of contracts involving surrogate motherhood.

On May 7, 2002, plaintiffs filed a motion for summary judgment . . . ; on September 5, 2002, after conducting limited discovery, the defendants filed a motion for summary judgment . . . , at the same time responding to plaintiffs' earlier motion.

FACTUAL BACKGROUND

The facts in this case remain essentially undisputed.

M.R. and J.R., husband and wife, are citizens of the State of Utah, as is W.K.J., an unmarried adult woman. Unable for medical reasons to have children on their own, J.R. and M.R., entered into a written agreement with W.K.J. in February 1999 in which W.K.J. agreed to serve as a gestational carrier surrogate for a child to be conceived *in vitro* by J.R. and M.R. W.K.J. agreed to carry the implanted embryo through delivery, to have J.R. and M.R.'s names entered on the child's birth certificate as the parents of the child, and to "voluntarily surrender and waive all custody rights, if any, to the child's parents immediately upon birth of the child." . . . To that end, W.K.J. agreed to "fully cooperate with any paternity/maternity proceedings or adoption proceedings necessary to establish parentage on behalf of the Intended Parents," . . .

In consideration for W.K.J.'s services as a gestational carrier surrogate, J.R. and M.R. agree to pay a list of various expenses, including legal fees, incurred by W.K.J. in connection with her pregnancy and childbirth under the terms of the Agreement . . . They also agree to "immediately accept custody and assume full legal responsibility for the child born to [W.K.J.] pursuant to this Agreement," . . . and promise to take the child *as is* — "recognizing that the child may have genetic or congenital abnormalities."

Shortly after the making of the Agreement, viable embryos conceived *in vitro* using J.R.'s ova and M.R.'s sperm were implanted in W.K.J.'s uterus through a procedure performed in the State of California. W.K.J. carried her pregnancy to term, giving birth to twin children in January, 2000, in Salt Lake County, State of Utah. Notwithstanding the terms of the Agreement and the facts surrounding the plaintiffs' gestational surrogacy procedure, the Utah State Office of Vital Records and Statistics has declined plaintiffs' request that birth certificates be issued listing J.R. and M.R. as the parents of the two children. Instead, the existing birth certificates list W.K.J. as the mother and no one as the father. While defendant Nangle, acting as Director of that Office, has indicated that M.R. could be added to the certificates as father of the children based upon M.R. and W.K.J.'s acknowledgment, the Office would decline to remove W.K.J. and list J.R. as the mother of the children, at least "based solely on the written representations of W.K.J., M.R. and J.R. that J.R. is the biological mother of the children."

PLAINTIFFS' LEGAL THEORIES

Plaintiffs seek declaratory and injunctive relief (1) holding Utah Code Ann. § 76-7-204 (1999) unconstitutional under the Fourteenth Amendment to the United States Constitution . . . ; (2) forbidding compliance with or enforcement of Utah Code Ann. § 76-7-204 by the defendant state officers; (3) validating the plaintiffs' In Vitro/Surrogate Implantation Agreement; and (4) requiring that the Utah Office of Vital Records and Statistics issue birth certificates for the plaintiffs' children "reciting that J.R. and M.R. are the parents of the children."

Utah Code Ann. § 76-7-204 (1999) reads: (1) (a) No person, agency, institution, or intermediary may be a party to a contract for profit or gain in which a woman agrees to undergo artificial insemination or other procedures and subsequently terminate her parental rights to a child born as a result . . . (c) Contracts or agreements entered into in violation of this section are null and void, and unenforceable as contrary to public policy. (d) A violation of this subsection is a class B misdemeanor . . .

(3)(a) In any case arising under Subsection (1) or (2), the surrogate mother is the mother of the child for all legal purposes, and her husband, if she is married, is the father of the child for all legal purposes.

Plaintiffs J.R. and M.R. assert that the statute infringes upon their fundamental constitutional right to procreate by denying them the right to make an enforceable agreement to obtain the assistance of a third party in bearing children that J.R. is medically incapable of bearing on her own. If enforced according to its terms, plaintiffs argue, Utah Code Ann. § 76-7-204 effectively leaves them childless, thereby denying their right to procreate altogether. Further, the statute "[r]emov[es] the possibility that a biological mother can become the legal parent of children produced through gestational surrogacy" because it conclusively presumes the surrogate mother to be the legal parent of the child . . .

The Constitutional Right to Procreate

Counsel points to language in a series of United States Supreme Court cases indicating that "[a]n individual's right to procreate and produce a family is well established in our nation's history and traditions," and that the right to procreate represents " 'a basic liberty,' " " 'one of the basic civil rights of man . . . fundamental to the very existence and survival of the race.' " (Pltfs' Mem. at 4, 5 (quoting *Skinner v. Oklahoma ex rel. Williamson*, 316 U.S. 535, 541, 62 S.Ct. 1110, 86 L.Ed. 1655 (1942)).) . . .

The right to procreate, plaintiffs maintain, "is inextricably linked to the right to assume the role of parent to the procreated children." (*Id.* at 6.) They point to cases such as *Stanley v. Illinois*, 405 U.S. 645, 92 S.Ct. 1208, 31 L.Ed.2d 551 (1972), vindicating an unwed father's fundamental interest in the care and custody of his three children, and *Smith v. Organization of Foster Families for Equality and Reform*, 431 U.S. 816, 97 S.Ct. 2094, 53 L.Ed.2d 14 (1977), acknowledging the historical importance of biological relationships to the concept of family . . .

Gestational Surrogacy & the Right to Procreate

. . . J.R. and M.R. aver that gestational surrogacy represents their only opportunity to "bear or beget a child" that would truly be *theirs*, a true genetic and biological child of the marriage. Absent gestational surrogacy, their marriage would remain childless. Their singular opportunity to procreate through gestational surrogacy necessarily implicates their fundamental right to bear children, thereby invoking the protections of the United States Constitution and the Utah Constitution . . .

On the same basis, Plaintiffs also challenge § 76-7-204(3)(a)'s presumption that "the surrogate mother is the mother of the child for all legal purposes, and her husband, if she is married, is the father of the child for all legal purposes." If this presumption is given conclusive effect, the statute frustrates J.R. and M.R.'s exercise of their right to procreate through gestational surrogacy by denying them legal parenthood of children who are unquestionably their own . . .

Defendants' Response

Counsel for the defendants acknowledges that "[t]he ability to procreate and decisions between a man and wife relating thereto have been considered to be a fundamental right under the Due Process Clause of the United States Constitution, and that 'if privacy means anything, it is the right of the individual, married or single, to be free from unwarranted governmental intrusion into matters so fundamentally affecting a person as the decision whether to bear or beget a child.' " (Defs' Mem. at 9 (quoting *Eisenstadt v. Baird*, 405 U.S. 438, 453, 92 S.Ct. 1029, 31 L.Ed.2d 349 (1972)).) Counsel argues that § 76-7-204 does not infringe upon J.R. and M.R.'s fundamental right to procreate because that right has not yet been extended to embrace gestational surrogacy . . .

Defendants submit that state legislation such as this should not be struck down unless the finding of unconstitutionality proves to be "strictly unavoidable," . . . and that given appropriate deference, the Utah surrogacy statute should be upheld as against plaintiffs' facial or "as applied" constitutional challenge . . . The statute serves legitimate state interests in the protection of the health and well-being of surrogate mothers and the children born to them, and in avoiding the commercialization of childbirth . . .

GESTATIONAL SURROGACY & PLAINTIFFS' CONSTITUTIONAL RIGHTS

While the United States Supreme Court has not yet addressed gestational surrogacy as a constitutional matter, the Court's more recent enumeration of "certain fundamental rights and liberty interests" counsels a broader reading of those rights and interests than the defendants now suggest . . .

The question, then, is *not* one of "extending constitutional protection to an asserted right or liberty interest," or being "asked to break new ground in this field," . . . because the fundamental right to bear and raise children within the context of a marriage is already clearly established . . .

Rather, the question is whether the statute unduly burdens the exercise of that right in a fashion that demands a judicial remedy.

CONFLICT BETWEEN STATUTE AND CONSTITUTION

Where an act of the legislature comes into conflict with the command of the United States Constitution or the constitution of the state of its enactment, there is no question as to the outcome: the statute fails and the constitution prevails . . .

In the context of reproductive or procreative choice, a state law " 'which imposes an undue burden on the woman's decision' " concerning procreative matters "is unconstitutional. . . . An 'undue burden is . . . shorthand for the conclusion that a state regulation has the purpose or effect of placing a substantial obstacle in the path of a woman' " seeking to make procreative choices . . .

The question now facing this court is whether the Utah surrogacy statute unduly burdens J.R. and M.R. in the exercise of their procreative and parental rights by denying them the recognition and rights of legal parents to the care and custody of their children because the children were born through gestational surrogacy. Plaintiffs challenge the constitutionality of Utah Code Ann. § 76-7-204(2) and (3), alleging that these provisions "prevent J.R. and M.R. from legally being acknowledged as parents of their own children," even though DNA testing indicates to a presumptive certainty that "J.R. and M.R. are, respectively, the biological mother and father of the twins who are in part the subject matter of this action." . . .

Construction of Utah Code Ann. § 76-7-204(3)(a)

The Utah surrogacy statute was first enacted in 1989, following on the heels of the controversial "Baby M" litigation in the courts of the State of New Jersey. *See In re Baby M*, 109 N.J. 396, 537 A.2d 1227, 77 A.L.R.4th 1 (1988). The Legislature likely was concerned about the protection of the procreative rights of birth mothers who conceived children through artificial insemination pursuant to contracts under which they agreed in advance to forfeit their parental rights to their own genetic/biological/birth children in favor of the genetic/biological father with whom they had agreed, much like the circumstances of *Baby M* . . .

As plaintiffs point out, however, medical technology has moved beyond artificial insemination and traditional surrogacy to the viable implantation of embryos fertilized *in vitro* using ova and sperm cells from the "intended parents," *not* the surrogate birth mother. To the extent that the meaning of a statute is defined by the problem that it was designed to remedy, it may be that the Utah surrogacy statute simply did not contemplate the unique interplay of interests involved in the implantation of live embryos in the womb of a genetic stranger, in contrast to the more conventional dispute between the genetic/biological birth mother and genetic/biological father in the *Baby M* case . . .

A narrowing construction of § 76-7-204(3)(a) that would limit its application to surrogate birth mothers who have contributed their own genetics to the conception of the child would obviate the application of the statutory presumption to cases of true gestational surrogacy — such as this one — and avoid any conflict with the fundamental rights of genetic/biological parents such as J.R. and M.R . . .

[However, the statute refers to] "any case arising under Subsection (1) or (2)"; both subsections (1) & (2) refer to "a woman [who] agrees to undergo artificial insemination or *other procedures*" resulting in the birth of a child. Utah Code Ann. § 76-7-204(1), (2) (1999) (emphasis added). The "artificial insemination or other procedures" language of § 76-7-204(1) & (2) thus defines the class of persons who are affected by § 76-7-204(3)(a). Nothing in § 76-7-204 further defines the scope or expanse of the phrase "or other procedures," or indicates whether it was intended to cover gestational surrogacy or not . . .

Neither plaintiffs nor the Attorney General have suggested a narrowing construction of the statute as a means of avoiding the alleged clash of constitution and statute in this case. This court is reluctant to impose a narrowing construction *sua sponte*, at least in the absence of interpretive aids such as legislative history that support such a reading of the statute's plain language. Given its ordinary meaning, the phrase "artificial insemination *or other procedures*" appears to contemplate medical procedures beyond or in addition to the artificial insemination utilized in *Baby M*, including *in vitro* fertilization-a procedure that was available by 1989 when the statute was passed. A narrowing construction must be rejected if it "conflicts with the statutory language, . . . as it appears that it would in this instance . . .

Fundamental Rights vs. Compelling Interests

To the extent that Utah Code Ann. § 76-7-204(3)'s declaration that "the surrogate mother is the mother of the child for all legal purposes, and her husband, if she is married, is the father of the child for all legal purposes" may be read to limit or even preclude the assertion of parental rights or interests by the genetic/biological father or mother of the child, the genetic/biological parents' constitutionally protected rights have been burdened by the statute. Absent a compelling state interest justifying that burden, a finding that § 76-7-204(3) is unconstitutional as applied becomes "strictly unavoidable" if the genetic/biological parents' fundamental rights — and the constitutions that guarantee them — are to be vindicated . . .

The State's "Compelling Interests"

That gestational surrogacy implicates J.R. and M.R.'s fundamental rights does not mean that all other interests instantly give way, or that the State has nothing to say about the process. The gestational carrier surrogate is still the birth mother of the child, with at least some legally protected interests. The State asserts ongoing interests in protecting the health, safety and welfare of both the birth mother and the child born of that pregnancy, whatever the child's genetic origins may be. Indeed, defense counsel asserts that the State's legitimate — even compelling — interests include (1) protecting the best interests of the child born through gestational surrogacy; (2) avoiding complicated and unsettling custody disputes; (3) protecting the surrogate birth mother's physical health and emotional well being, and her interest in a relationship with the child she had borne; (4) preventing the exploitation of women, particularly through surrogacy-for-profit arrangements; and (5) preventing children from becoming "commodities" to be purchased and sold. (Defs' Mem. at 12-23.) . . .

"The Best Interests of the Child"

Defendants argue that "the best interest of the child [is] a sufficiently compelling interest to justify government intrusion into a person's fundamental, but qualified right to procreate," particularly when "surrogacy contracts avoid any objective determination of the best interest of the child." . . . Plaintiffs respond that § 76-7-204(3)'s conclusive presumption that the gestational surrogate (and her spouse, if any) is the legal parent of the child also "avoids any objective determination of the best interest of the child," contrary to the defendants' assertion that "those interests must be paramount." . . .

The question of "the best interests of the child" proves inescapably fact-driven. Yet § 76-7-204(3) requires *no* fact-finding to decide that it is in "the best interest of the child" in *all* instances for the gestational surrogate birth mother to be deemed the legal parent of the child — regardless of the circumstances of the genetic/biological parents who actually conceived the child — and to do so without a hearing. In every instance, it finds the fact of parenthood from the fact of childbirth. In the context of gestational surrogacy, § 76-7-204(3) serves as "an irrebuttable presumption often contrary to fact," lacking "critical ingredients of due process. . . ."

The Utah Supreme Court has already determined that under both the United States Constitution and the Utah Constitution, the Legislature may not predetermine that "the best interests of the child" alone warrant the involuntary abrogation of parental rights where there has been no adjudication of a parent's unfitness, or a showing of abandonment or substantial neglect . . .

States must "provide the parents with fundamentally fair procedures" protecting against improper termination of the parent-child relationship . . . including parent-child relationships between genetic/biological mothers and fathers and children born through gestational surrogacy. The State's concern for the "best interests of the child," however compelling it may be, cannot sustain a legislative act that would summarily rewrite the facts of parenthood to suit legislative preferences as to matters of public policy . . .

The State's Other Interests

The remaining interests asserted by the State either are not "compelling" (*e.g.*, "avoiding complicated and unsettling custody disputes"), or involve facts not presented in this case (*viz.*, exploitation of women through surrogacy-for-profit contracts, or children becoming commodities) . . .

Even assuming that the State has compelling interests in avoiding surrogacy for profit, Utah Code Ann. § 76-7-204(3)(a) cannot be said to be narrowly tailored to serve these interests because it affects *all* surrogate births, not just those entered into for profit or financial gain. No one has alleged that W.K.J.'s surrogacy was entered into for profit or gain; there is no allegation that W.K.J. has been "exploited" in some fashion, or that her interest in the children has been unfairly overborne in favor of the genetic/biological parents; and none of the uncontroverted facts of this case even hints that the two children conceived by J.R. and M.R. and borne by W.K.J. have been treated as a *commodity* (*i.e.*, "anything bought or sold; any article of commerce), by anyone. Yet defendants assert that § 76-7-204(3)(a) applies to define the parental rights of W.K.J., J.R. and M.R. no less than it would in the case of a blatant surrogacy-for-profit scheme.

Utah Code Ann. § 76-7-204(3)(a) burdens the fundamental parental rights of J.R. and M.R. by attempting to abrogate them through substitution of another legal parent, and that burden cannot be justified as serving these asserted "compelling interests," particularly where they have very little bearing upon the uncontroverted facts of this case.

Conclusive Effect & "Undue Burden"

In the context of gestational surrogacy, Utah Code Ann. § 76-7-204(3)(a) establishes a rule of substantive law that genetic/biological parents — particularly genetic/biological *mothers* who are not the birth mother — are not qualified to raise their children and declares that they will have *no* parental rights or legal relationship as a parent with the children they have conceived. It mandates that the surrogate mother "is the mother of the child for all legal purposes, and her husband, if she is married, is the father of the child for all legal purposes," to the exclusion of the child's natural parents.

In doing so, § 76-7-204(3)(a) places a substantial obstacle in the path of a woman in J.R.'s position who is seeking to make procreative choices, . . . and to bear and raise her own children, unduly burdening the exercise of her fundamental rights . . .

This blanket presumption is not narrowly tailored to serve the State's compelling interests in safeguarding the best interests of the child and the health, safety and procreative interests of the surrogate . . .

CONCLUSION

In this case, there is no genuine issue of material fact that plaintiffs J.R. and M.R. are the genetic/biological mother and father of twin children to whom plaintiff W.K.J. gave birth in January of 2002. As genetic/biological parents of children carried by a gestational carrier surrogate birth mother, J.R. and M.R. have a parent-child relationship with those children to which their fundamental constitutionally protected liberty interests apply. Utah Code Ann. § 76-7-204(3)(a) unduly burdens J.R. and M.R.'s fundamental liberty interests to the extent that it conclusively deems W.K.J. to be "the mother of the child[ren] for all legal purposes," to the exclusion of J.R. and M.R.'s "rights to conceive and raise one's children, . . . without unwarranted governmental interference.

J.R. and M.R. are entitled to declaratory relief pursuant to 42 U.S.C. § 1983 (2000) and 28 U.S.C. § 2201 (2000) in the form of a judgment that Utah Code Ann. § 76-7-204(3)(a) is unconstitutional as applied to J.R. and M.R. to the extent that it limits or precludes in any way the legal recognition or exercise of J.R. and M.R.'s fundamental rights as parents to raise the children they have conceived. By conclusively presuming W.K.J. to be "the mother of the child[ren] for all legal purposes," and thereby excluding J.R. from recognized legal motherhood of the children from and after the moment of their birth, § 76-7-204(3)(a) oversteps the limits on legislative power imposed by both the United States Constitution and the Utah Constitution in favor of the protection of fundamental liberty interests. U.S. CONST., Amends. IX, XIV; Utah Const. Art. I, §§ 7, 25 . . .

Even as it is called upon to consider new questions thrust upon it by the advent of new technology, the Legislature, no less than the court, must keep the fundamental liberty interests of the people clearly in mind . . .

IT IS ORDERED that the plaintiffs' motion for summary judgment is GRANTED IN PART as to the constitutionality of Utah Code Ann. § 76-7-204(3)(a), as applied to plaintiffs J.R. and M.R. and to the extent explained above . . .

NOTES AND QUESTIONS

1.   Judge Jenkins declares a portion of the Utah surrogacy statute unconstitutional on the ground that it unduly burdens intended parents in the exercise of their procreative and parental rights. Would the court have reached the same conclusion if the surrogate, W.K.J., was also the genetic mother of the twins? The court acknowledges that the statute was originally drafted (in 1989) to apply to traditional surrogacy, but it must now meet constitutional muster in light of changing reproductive technologies.

Is the decision in this case an incentive or a disincentive for legislatures to weigh in on questions of parentage resulting from assisted conception?

2.   *Update on Utah Surrogacy Law.* In 2005, Utah lawmakers repealed the offending surrogacy statute declared unconstitutional in *J.R.* and enacted a version of the updated Uniform Parentage Act (2000). Like Section 801 of the UPA, the new Utah law validates gestational agreements that meet certain conditions. In addition to the conditions contained in the UPA, the Utah law also requires that the gestational carriers not be receiving Medicaid or any other state assistance; that the intended parents be married (presumably to each other, though the statute does not so specify); and that the gestational carrier's eggs not be used in the procedure (thus, effectively outlawing traditional surrogacy). *See* Utah Code Ann. § 78B-15-801.

3.   Surrogacy statutes that declare the birth mother to be the legal mother of the child under any circumstances can run afoul of another constitutional parameter — equal protection. In *Soos v. Superior Court*, 182 Ariz. 470, 897 P.2d 1356 (1994), the genetic/intended parents filed for divorce while the gestational surrogate carried their triplets to term. The biological father asked the court to declare the surrogate as the legal mother, following Arizona law that provides:

> B. A surrogate is the legal mother of a child born as a result of a surrogate parentage contract and is entitled to custody of that child.
>
> C. If the mother of a child born as a result of a surrogate contract is married, her husband is presumed to be the legal father of the child. This presumption is rebuttable.

The genetic/intended mother argued that the statute unconstitutionally denied her equal protection of the laws guaranteed by the Fourteenth Amendment. The statute, she reasoned,

> allows a man to rebut the presumption of legal paternity by proving "fatherhood" but does not provide the same opportunity for a woman. A woman who may be genetically related to a child has no opportunity to prove her maternity and is thereby denied the opportunity to develop the parent-child relationship. She is afforded no procedural process by which to prove her maternity under the statute. The mother has parental interests not less deserving of protection than those of the Father. "By providing

dissimilar treatment for men and women who are thus similarly situated," the statute violates the Equal Protection Clause. (citations omitted).

Id. at 474, 897 P.2d at 1360. The court agreed, declaring the statute unconstitutional because it afforded the father a procedure for proving paternity, but did not likewise afford the mother any means by which to prove maternity, thus denying her equal protection of the laws.

If you were a legislator in Arizona who disfavored surrogate parenting contracts, how would you amend the state's surrogacy statute to meet constitutional muster? If you were a legislator in Arizona who favored surrogate parenting contracts, how would you amend the state's surrogacy statute to meet constitutional muster?

SECTION III: BUILDING FAMILIES THROUGH THE USE OF DONOR GAMETES

A.   The State of the Art in Donor Gametes

The family law dilemmas that arise in the wake of assisted conception typically share at least one commonality: the child (or children) born is a product of third-party reproduction. According to the American Society for Reproductive Medicine, the phrase "third party reproduction" refers to the use of eggs, sperm, embryos, or a uterus that are donated by a third person to enable an infertile person or couple to become parents. Thus far, we have studied the family law jurisprudence surrounding two forms of third-party reproduction — sperm donation and surrogate parenting arrangements (perhaps the more clinically accurate "uterus donation" could be adopted). We now turn to the family law dilemmas engendered by the other two forms of third-party reproduction — egg and embryo donation.

Donor eggs offer the possibility of childbearing to women whose ovaries are absent or do not reliably produce eggs capable of being fertilized. Eggs from a donor can be fertilized using in vitro fertilization or intracytoplasmic sperm injection (ICSI) in which a single sperm is injection directly into the egg to prompt fertilization. The sperm can be provided by the intended mother's husband or partner, or by a donor. Once fertilized, the embryo can be transferred into the uterus of the intended mother, or into a gestational carrier.

There are three sources for donated eggs: 1) Known donors. The intended mother may know the egg donor; she may be a close friend or relative who is willing to donate her eggs. 2) Anonymous donors. The intended mother may procure eggs through an egg donation program where she may or may not have the option of meeting the donor. Open donations are ones in which the prospective parents meet with potential egg donors. Closed or anonymous donations are ones in which the prospective parents select the egg donor from written and other materials but do not personally meet the donor. 3) IVF programs. Women undergoing IVF for treatment of their own infertility may agree to donate their excess eggs to other infertile patients.

The availability of donor eggs has never been on par with the supply of donor sperm for two main reasons. First, procuring eggs from a woman's body is far more difficult and medically dangerous than the activity surrounding sperm donation. Recall that egg retrieval requires surgery typically performed under general anesthesia. Second, whereas sperm has been successfully frozen and thawed for decades, egg freezing is only beginning to show clinical promise. Newly emerging data suggesting greater success in oocyte cryopreservation promises to increase the supply of donor eggs available for third-party reproduction. *See* Angel Petropanagos, *Reproductive "Choice" and Egg Freezing*, 156(3) ONCOFERTILITY 223 (2010). Egg banks are beginning to dot the ART landscape, boasting impressive success rates and hundreds of live births. *See* www.myeggbank.com. The American Society for Reproductive Medicine still considers egg freezing to be experimental and recommends it be offered only in connection with an approved research protocol. *See* The Practice Committee of the American Society for Reproductive Medicine and the Practice Committee of the Society for Assisted Reproductive Technology, *Ovarian Tissue and Oocyte Cryopreservation*, 90 FERTILITY & STERILITY S241 (2008).

Embryo donation involves donor eggs that have been fertilized with sperm from the egg donor's partner or with donor sperm. Embryos can be donated by a woman undergoing IVF who has satisfied her own childbearing needs and is willing to donate her remaining (often frozen) embryos. A recent addition to the area of embryo donation are religious-based embryo "adoption" agencies that facilitate placement of excess or unwanted embryos with infertile couples. One such group, the Snowflakes Embryo Adoption Program, the first embryo adoption program in the country, began matching donor embryos to infertile women in 1997 with the help of the conservative Christian group Focus on the Family. According to the group's website, www.nightlight.org, as of October 2011 Snowflakes has welcomed 280 babies born via embryo adoption. For a discussion of embryo adoption, *see* Suzanne Smalley, *A New Baby Debate: As Pro-Lifers Adopt Embryos, Critics Raise Questions*, NEWSWEEK, Mar. 24, 2003, at 53. Is there a difference between embryo donation and embryo adoption? If so, what are the differences? How do these differences affect an infertile couple who desires to gestate an embryo that is available for that purpose?

When a child is born from donor eggs, donor sperm or donor embryos, questions of parentage center on the import of genetics, gestation, intent, and the best interests of the child. As the cases that follow demonstrate, these factors do not always converge in a single individual or a single test in which parentage can be easily decided. The only certainty in the area of donor gametes is that, by all accounts, it will continue to grow in popularity. As Table 2 in Chapter 1 shows, women who use donor eggs are twice as likely to have a child through IVF than women who use their own eggs. As women continue to delay childbearing until later in life, the success of assisted conception using donor eggs will continue to draw patients, and controversy, to the practice.

B.   The State of the Law in Donor Gametes

1.   Judicial Perspectives

IN RE MARRIAGE OF BUZZANCA
California Court of Appeal, Fourth District
61 Cal. App. 4th 1410, 72 Cal. Rptr. 2d 280 (1998)

SILLS, Presiding Justice.

INTRODUCTION

Jaycee was born because Luanne and John Buzzanca agreed to have an embryo genetically unrelated to either of them implanted in a woman — a surrogate — who would carry and give birth to the child for them. After the fertilization, implantation and pregnancy, Luanne and John split up, and the question of who are Jaycee's lawful parents came before the trial court.

Luanne claimed that she and her erstwhile husband were the lawful parents, but John disclaimed any responsibility, financial or otherwise. The woman who gave birth also appeared in the case to make it clear that she made no claim to the child.

The trial court then reached an extraordinary conclusion: Jaycee had *no* lawful parents. First, the woman who gave birth to Jaycee was not the mother; the court had — astonishingly — already accepted a stipulation that neither she nor her husband were the "biological" parents. Second, Luanne was not the mother. According to the trial court, she could not be the mother because she had neither contributed the egg nor given birth. And John could not be the father, because, not having contributed the sperm, he had no biological relationship with the child. We disagree. Let us get right to the point: Jaycee never would have been born had not Luanne and John both agreed to have a fertilized egg implanted in a surrogate.

The trial judge erred because he assumed that legal motherhood, under the relevant California statutes, could *only* be established in one of two ways, either by giving birth or by contributing an egg. He failed to consider the substantial and well-settled body of law holding that there are times when *fatherhood* can be established by conduct apart from giving birth or being genetically related to a child. The typical example is when an infertile husband consents to allowing his wife to be artificially inseminated. As our Supreme Court noted in such a situation over 30 years ago, the husband is the "lawful father" because he *consented* to the procreation of the child. (See *People v. Sorensen* (1968) 68 Cal.2d 280, 284-286, 66 Cal.Rptr. 7, 437 P.2d 495.)

The same rule which makes a husband the lawful father of a child born because of his consent to artificial insemination should be applied here — by the same parity of reasoning that guided our Supreme Court in the first surrogacy case, *Johnson v. Calvert* (1993) 5 Cal.4th 84, 19 Cal.Rptr.2d 494, 851 P.2d 776 — to both husband and wife. Just as a husband is deemed to be the lawful father of a child unrelated to him when his wife gives birth after artificial insemination, so should a husband *and* wife be deemed the lawful parents of a child after a surrogate bears a biologically unrelated child on their behalf. In each instance, a child is procreated because a medical procedure was initiated and consented to by intended parents. The only difference is that in this case — unlike artificial insemination — there is no reason to distinguish between husband and wife. We therefore must reverse the trial court's judgment and direct that a new judgment be entered, declaring that both Luanne and John are the lawful parents of Jaycee.

CASE HISTORY

John filed his petition for dissolution of marriage on March 30, 1995, alleging there were no children of the marriage. Luanne filed her response on April 20, alleging that the parties were expecting a child by way of surrogate contract. Jaycee was born six days later. In September 1996 Luanne filed a separate petition to establish herself as Jaycee's mother . . . At a hearing held in March, . . . the trial court determined that Luanne was not the lawful mother of the child and therefore John could not be the lawful father or owe any support.

The trial judge said: "So I think what evidence there is, is stipulated to. And I don't think there would be any more. One, there's no genetic tie between Luanne and the child. Two, she is not the gestational mother. Three, she has not adopted the child. That, folks, to me, respectfully, is clear and convincing evidence that she's not the legal mother."

After another hearing on May 7, regarding attorney fees, a judgment on reserved issues in the dissolution was filed, terminating John's obligation to pay child support, declaring that Luanne was not the legal mother of Jaycee, and declining "to apply any estoppel proposition to the issue of John's responsibility for child support." Luanne then filed a petition for a writ of supersedeas to stay the judgment; she also filed an appeal from it. This court then granted a stay which had the effect of keeping the support order alive for Jaycee. We also consolidated the writ proceeding with the appeal . . .

DISCUSSION

The Statute Governing Artificial Insemination Which Makes a Husband the Lawful Father of a Child Unrelated to Him Applies to Both Intended Parents In This Case

Perhaps recognizing the inherent lack of appeal for any result which makes Jaycee a legal orphan, John now contends that the surrogate is Jaycee's legal mother; and further, by virtue of that fact, the surrogate's husband is the legal father. His reasoning goes like this: Under the Uniform Parentage Act (the Act), and particularly as set forth in section 7610 of California's Family Code, there are only two ways by which a woman can establish legal motherhood, i.e., giving birth or contributing genetically. Because the genetic contributors are not known to the court, the only candidate left is the surrogate who must therefore be deemed the lawful mother. And, as John's counsel commented at oral argument, if the surrogate and her husband cannot support Jaycee, the burden should fall on the taxpayers.

The law doesn't say what John says it says. It doesn't say: "The legal relationship between mother and child shall be established only by either proof of her giving birth or by genetics." The statute says "may," not "shall," and "under this part," *not* "by genetics." Here is the complete text of section 7610: "The parent and child relationship may be established as follows: [¶] (a) Between a child and the natural mother, it may be established by proof of her having given birth to the child, or under this part. [¶] (b) Between a child and the natural father, it may be established under this part. [¶] (c) Between a child and an adoptive parent, it may be established by proof of adoption."

The statute thus contains no direct reference to genetics (i.e., blood tests) at all. The *Johnson* decision teaches us that genetics is simply *subsumed* in the words "under this part." In that case, the court held that genetic consanguinity was equally "acceptable" as "proof of maternity" as evidence of giving birth. (*Johnson v. Calvert, supra,* 5 Cal.4th at p. 93, 19 Cal.Rptr.2d 494, 851 P.2d 776.)

It is important to realize, however, that in construing the words "under this part" to include genetic testing, the high court in *Johnson* relied on several statutes in the Evidence Code (former Evid.Code, §§ 892, 895, and 895.5) all of which, by their terms, only applied to paternity. . . . It was only by a "parity of reasoning" that our high court concluded those statutes which, on their face applied only to men, were also "dispositive of the question of maternity." . . .

The point bears reiterating: It was only by a parity of reasoning from statutes which, on their face, referred only to *paternity* that the court in *Johnson v. Calvert* reached the result it did on the question of *maternity.* Had the *Johnson* court reasoned as John now urges us to reason — by narrowly confining the means under the Uniform Parentage Act by which a woman could establish that she was the lawful mother of a child to texts which on their face applied only to motherhood (as distinct from fatherhood) — the court would have reached the opposite result.

In addition to blood tests there are several other ways the Act allows paternity to be established . . . A man may . . . be deemed a father under the Act in the case of artificial insemination of his wife, as provided by section 7613 of the Family Code To track the words of the statute: "If, under the supervision of a licensed physician and surgeon and with the consent of her husband, a wife is inseminated artificially with semen donated by a man not her husband, the husband is treated in law as if he were the natural father of a child thereby conceived."

As noted in *Johnson,* "courts must construe statutes in factual settings not contemplated by the enacting legislature." (*Johnson v. Calvert, supra,* 5 Cal.4th at p. 89, 19 Cal.Rptr.2d 494, 851 P.2d 776.) So it is, of course, true that application of the artificial insemination statute to a gestational surrogacy case where the genetic donors are unknown to the court may not have been contemplated by the legislature. Even so, the two kinds of artificial reproduction are *exactly* analogous in this crucial respect: Both contemplate the procreation of a child by the consent to a medical procedure of someone who intends to raise the child but who otherwise does not have any biological tie.

If a husband who consents to artificial insemination under section 7613 is "treated in law" as the father of the child by virtue of his consent, there is no reason the result should be any different in the case of a married couple who consent to in vitro fertilization by unknown donors and subsequent implantation into a woman who is, as a surrogate, willing to carry the embryo to term for them. The statute is, after all, the clearest expression of past legislative intent when the legislature did contemplate a situation where a person who caused a child to come into being had no biological relationship to the child . . .

John argues that the artificial insemination statute should not be applied because, after all, his wife did not give birth. But for purposes of the statute with its core idea of estoppel, the fact that Luanne did not give birth is irrelevant. The statute contemplates the establishment of lawful fatherhood in a situation where an intended father has no biological relationship to a child who is procreated as a result of the father's (as well as the mother's) *consent* to a medical procedure.

Luanne is the Lawful Mother of Jaycee, Not the Surrogate, and Not the Unknown Donor of the Egg

In the present case Luanne is situated like a husband in an artificial insemination case whose consent triggers a medical procedure which results in a pregnancy and eventual birth of a child. Her motherhood may therefore be established "under this part," by virtue of that consent. In light of our conclusion, John's argument that the surrogate should be declared the lawful mother disintegrates. The case is now postured like the *Johnson v. Calvert* case, where motherhood could have been "established" in either of two women under the Act, and the tie broken by noting the intent to parent as expressed in the surrogacy contract . . . The only difference is that this case is not even close as between Luanne and the surrogate. Not only was Luanne the clearly intended mother, no bona fide attempt has been made to establish the surrogate as the lawful mother.

We should also add that neither could the woman whose egg was used in the fertilization or implantation make any claim to motherhood, even if she were to come forward at this late date. Again, as between two women who would both be able to establish motherhood under the Act, the *Johnson* decision would mandate that the tie be broken in favor of the intended parent, in this case, Luanne . . .

In the case before us, we are not concerned, as John would have us believe, with a question of the enforceability of the oral and written surrogacy contracts into which he entered with Luanne. This case is not about "transferring" parenthood pursuant to those agreements. We are, rather, concerned with the consequences of those agreements as *acts* which *caused the birth* of a child . . .

In the case before us, there is absolutely no dispute that Luanne caused Jaycee's conception and birth by initiating the surrogacy arrangement whereby an embryo was implanted into a woman who agreed to carry the baby to term on Luanne's behalf. In applying the artificial insemination statute to a gestational surrogacy case where the genetic donors are unknown, there is, as we have indicated above, no reason to distinguish *between* husbands and wives. Both are equally situated from the point of view of consenting to an act which brings a child into being. Accordingly, Luanne should have been declared the lawful mother of Jaycee.

*John is the Lawful Father of Jaycee Even If Luanne Did Promise to Assume
All Responsibility for Jaycee's Care*

The same reasons which impel us to conclude that Luanne is Jaycee's lawful mother also require that John be declared Jaycee's lawful father. Even if the written surrogacy contract had not yet been signed at the time of conception and implantation, those occurrences were nonetheless the direct result of actions taken pursuant to an oral agreement which envisioned that the fertilization, implantation and ensuing pregnancy would go forward. Thus, it is still accurate to say, as we did the first time this case came before us, that for all practical purposes John caused Jaycee's conception every bit as much as if things had been done the old-fashioned way . . .

When pressed at oral argument to make an offer of proof as to the "best facts" which John might be able to show if this case were tried, John's attorney raised the point that Luanne had (allegedly, we must add) promised to assume all responsibility for the child and would not hold him responsible for the child's upbringing. However, even if this case were returned for a trial on this point (we assume that Luanne would dispute the allegation) it could make no difference as to John's lawful paternity. It is well established that parents cannot, by agreement, limit or abrogate a child's right to support.

The rule against enforcing agreements obviating a parent's child support responsibilities is also illustrated by *Stephen K. v. Roni L.* (1980) 105 Cal.App.3d 640, 164 Cal.Rptr. 618, a case which is virtually on point about Luanne's alleged promise. In *Stephen K.*, a woman was alleged to have falsely told a man that she was taking birth control pills. In "reliance" upon that statement the man had sexual intercourse with her. The woman became pregnant and brought a paternity action. While the man did not attempt to use the woman's false statement as grounds to avoid paternity, he did seek to achieve the same result by cross-complaining against the woman for damages based on her fraud.

The trial court dismissed the cross-complaint on demurrer and the appellate court affirmed. The cross-complaint was "nothing more than asking the court to supervise the promises made between two consenting adults as to the circumstances of their private sexual conduct." (*Id.* at pp. 644-645, 164 Cal.Rptr. 618.)

There is no meaningful difference between the rule articulated in *Stephen K.* and the situation here — indeed, the result applies a fortiori to the present case: If the man who engaged in an act which merely opened the possibility of the procreation of a child was held responsible for the consequences in *Stephen K.*, how much more so should a man be held responsible for giving his express consent to a medical procedure that was *intended* to result in the procreation of a child. Thus, it makes no difference that John's wife Luanne did not become pregnant. John still engaged in "procreative conduct." In plainer language, a deliberate procreator is as responsible as a casual inseminator.

CONCLUSION

Even though neither Luanne nor John are biologically related to Jaycee, they are still her lawful parents given their initiating role as the intended parents in her conception and birth. And, while the absence of a biological connection is what makes this case extraordinary, this court is hardly without statutory basis and legal precedent in so deciding. Indeed, . . . in our Supreme Court's *Johnson v. Calvert* decision, the court looked to *intent to parent* as the ultimate basis of its decision. Fortunately, as the *Johnson* court also noted, intent to parent " 'correlate[s] significantly' " with a child's best interests . . .

Again we must call on the Legislature to sort out the parental rights and responsibilities of those involved in artificial reproduction. No matter what one thinks of artificial insemination, traditional and gestational surrogacy (in all its permutations), and — as now appears in the not-too-distant future, cloning and even gene splicing — courts are still going to be faced with the problem of determining lawful parentage. A child cannot be ignored. Even if all means of artificial reproduction were outlawed with draconian criminal penalties visited on the doctors and parties involved, courts will still be called upon to decide who the lawful parents really are and who — other than the taxpayers — is obligated to provide maintenance and support for the child. These cases will not go away.

Courts can continue to make decisions on an ad hoc basis without necessarily imposing some grand scheme, looking to the imperfectly designed Uniform Parentage Act and a growing body of case law for guidance in the light of applicable family law principles. Or the Legislature can act to impose a broader order which, even though it might not be perfect on a case-by-case basis, would bring some predictability to those who seek to make use of artificial reproductive techniques. As jurists, we recognize the traditional role of the common (i.e., judge-formulated) law in applying old legal principles to new technology . . . However, we still believe it is the Legislature, with its ability to formulate general rules based on input from all its constituencies, which is the more desirable forum for lawmaking.

That said, we must now conclude the business at hand.

(1) The portion of the judgment which declares that Luanne Buzzanca is not the lawful mother of Jaycee is reversed. The matter is remanded with directions to enter a new judgment declaring her the lawful mother. The trial court shall make all appropriate orders to ensure that Luanne Buzzanca shall have legal custody of Jaycee, including entering an order that Jaycee's birth certificate shall be amended to reflect Luanne Buzzanca as the mother.

(2) The judgment is reversed to the extent that it provides that John Buzzanca is not the lawful father of Jaycee. The matter is remanded with directions to enter a new judgment declaring him the lawful father. Consonant with this determination, today's ruling is without prejudice to John in future proceedings as regards child custody and visitation as his relationship with Jaycee may develop.[15] The judgment

---

[15] [n.22] Luanne has had actual physical custody of Jaycee from the beginning. Obviously, it would be frivolous of John to seek custody of Jaycee right now in light of that fact. However, as the lawful father he certainly must be held to have the right, consistent with Jaycee's best interest, to visitation. Our decision today leaves Luanne and John in the same position as any other divorced couple with a child who has been exclusively cared for by the mother since infancy.

And while it may be true that John's consent to the fertilization, implantation and pregnancy was done as an accommodation to allow Luanne to surmount a formality, who knows what relationship he may

shall also reflect that the birth certificate shall be amended to reflect John Buzzanca as the lawful father.

(3) To the degree that the judgment makes no provision for child support it is reversed. The matter is remanded to make an appropriate permanent child support order. Until that time, the temporary child support order shall remain in effect.

Luanne and Jaycee will recover their costs on appeal. WALLIN and CROSBY, JJ., concur.

NOTES AND QUESTIONS

1. The facts in *Buzzanca* resemble a law school exam — eight adults involved in the birth of a single child, each claiming a different interest with respect to the issue of parentage. There's Luanna and John, the surrogate and her husband, the egg donor and her husband, the sperm donor and his wife. With these four couples in mind, perhaps the court was reflecting on the four possible tests for determining motherhood, summarized as follows (and containing useful citations to the legal literature):

> There have been four basic approaches used to determine motherhood in the absence of a clear natural definition. Some writers advocate contract principles which privilege the intended mother as the legal mother according to the dictates of an agreement or consent form from the egg donor. See John Lawrence Hill, *What Does It Mean to Be a "Parent"? The Claims of Biology as the Basis for Parental Rights*, 66 N.Y.U. L. Rev. 353, 419 (1991) (concluding that contractual intent provides a rule of certainty in favor of the "prime movers" of the child's conception); Richard A. Posner, *The Regulation of the Market in Adoptions*, 67 B.U. L. Rev. 59, 72 (1987) (arguing for a free market in babies and reproductive services); Marjorie Maguire Shultz, *Reproductive Technology and Intent-Based Parenthood: An Opportunity for Gender Neutrality*, 1990 Wis. L. Rev. 297, 397-98 (reasoning that contract principles further the gender-neutral goals of intention and choice in reproductive decisions).

> Others argue that the genetic mother should be considered the legal mother because the genetic contribution is the most significant. See, e.g., Ruth Macklin, *Artificial Means of Reproduction and Our Understanding of the Family*, Hastings Ctr. Rep., Jan.-Feb., 1991, at 5 (considering the various methods, including genetics, to determine the actual mother); Suzanne F. Seavello, *Are You My Mother? A Judge's Decision in In Vitro Fertilization Surrogacy*, 3 Hastings Women's L.J. 211, 211-24 (1992) (arguing for a genetics based determination); Still others claim that gestation is the most significant element of motherhood. See, e.g., Scott B.

---

develop with Jaycee in the future? Human relationships are not static; things done merely to help one individual overcome a perceived legal obstacle sometimes become much more meaningful. (See, e.g., Nicholson, Shadowlands (1990) (play based on true story of prominent British author who married American citizen in Britain in perfunctory civil ceremony to allow her to remain in country; a deeper relationship then developed).)

Rae, The Ethics of Surrogate Motherhood, Brave New Families? (1994) (arguing that the woman who gives birth to the child should be considered the legal mother of the child); Barbara Katz Rothman, Recreating Motherhood: Ideology and Technology in a Patriarchal Society (1989) (arguing that the essential maternal tie is based on carrying the child in pregnancy).

Others rely upon a "best interests of the child" standard for their final determination of which woman is the mother. *See* Martha A. Field, Surrogate Motherhood 126-60, 151-52 (1988) (arguing for a best interest test with a presumption of maternal custody in traditional surrogacy).

Pamela Laufer-Ukeles, *Gestation, Work for Hire Or The Essence of Motherhood? A Comparative Legal Analysis*, 9 Duke J. Gender, Law & Policy 91, 92 (2002). Which approach did the *Buzzanca* court select? In your mind, can the *Buzzanca* approach to determining motherhood be applied to every ART scenario in which a child's maternal parentage is disputed? How about the *Buzzanca* approach to determining fatherhood? Does that approach have universal appeal, meaning it can be used to resolve all disputes involving assisted conception and legal fatherhood?

2. The *Buzzanca* court's conclusion that the egg donor has no parental claim to Jaycee is entirely consistent with the court's ruling that the legal parents are those who intended to cause the child's conception and birth, and subsequently parent the child. In egg donor scenarios, as with artificial insemination by anonymous donor, the gamete donors do not intend to parent the resulting children. As obvious as the nonparental status of an egg donor may seem to us now, that conclusion was not always shared by parties to third-party reproduction arrangements. In *McDonald v. McDonald*, 196 A.D.2d 7, 608 N.Y.S.2d 477 (1994), twins were born to a couple using donor eggs and the husband's sperm. Though the wife carried and gave birth to the children, upon divorce her husband asked the court to declare the children "illegitimate" or, in the alternative, the legal and natural children of the husband alone. He reasoned that since the wife was not genetically related to the children, she could not be considered their legal mother.

Citing the California Supreme Court decision in *Johnson v. Calvert*, the New York Supreme Court rejected the husband's argument, finding that in a "true egg donor situation" such as the case at bar, the woman who gestates and gives birth with the intent to raise the child is the natural mother. Accord *In Re C.K.G.*, 173 S.W.3d 714 (Tenn. 2005) (unmarried couple had triplets using donor eggs and man's sperm; when couple separated man claimed children had no legal mother because egg donor waived parental rights and woman had no genetic tie to triplets. Court held woman is legal parent and the mother of the children based on intent of the parties).

3. Jack and his fiancé Ellie contract with an egg donor to create embryos using Jack's sperm. The couple further contracts with Dolores, a gestational carrier, to gestate the embryos so that the couple can become parents with her assistance. Dolores gives birth to triplets who are born prematurely and require intensive care treatment. Dolores continues to visit the children in the hospital after she is discharged and she becomes increasingly concerned that Jack and Ellie are not showing enough concern for the children, barely visiting them or asking about their progress. When the children are nearing the end of their hospital stay, Dolores

petitions the court to be declared the sole legal mother of the children. Should the court grant Dolores' petition? See *J.F. v. D.B.*, 116 Ohio St. 3d 363, 879 N.E.2d 740 (2007).

2.   Statutory Perspectives on Donor Gametes

The court in *Buzzanca* sends a clear message to the California legislature: Help! The court calls on the lawmakers to "sort out the parental rights and responsibilities of those involved in artificial reproduction." To date, no such help has been forthcoming. California, like the majority of states, has no enacted law directly addressing the parental status of those involved in collaborative reproduction (with the exception of artificial insemination by donor statutes). The few states that have ventured into this legislative morass have been aided by model or uniform laws that provide suggested language for state lawmakers to adopt. Three states' laws are excerpted below. The Texas law follows closely the Uniform Parentage Act (2000), while the Virginia code resembles the Uniform Status of Children of Assisted Conception Act (1998). The Florida law is the most comprehensive of the three, addressing the use of IVF by married couples.

Vernon's Texas Statutes and Codes Annotated
Family Code § 160.754
Title 5. The Parent-child Relationship and the Suit Affecting The Parent-child Relationship

§ 160.754. Gestational Agreement Authorized

(a) A prospective gestational mother, her husband if she is married, each donor, and each intended parent may enter into a written agreement providing that:

(1) the prospective gestational mother agrees to pregnancy by means of assisted reproduction;

(2) the prospective gestational mother, her husband if she is married, and each donor other than the intended parents, if applicable, relinquish all parental rights and duties with respect to a child conceived through assisted reproduction;

(3) the intended parents will be the parents of the child . . .

(b) The intended parents must be married to each other. Each intended parent must be a party to the gestational agreement.

(c) The gestational agreement must require that the eggs used in the assisted reproduction procedure be retrieved from an intended parent or a donor. The gestational mother's eggs may not be used in the assisted reproduction procedure.

Code of Virginia
Title 20. Domestic Relations
Chapter 9. Status of Children of Assisted Conception

§ 20-158. Parentage of child resulting from assisted conception

A. Determination of parentage, generally. — Except as provided in subsections

B, C, D, and E of this section, the parentage of any child resulting from the performance of assisted conception shall be determined as follows:

1. The gestational mother of a child is the child's mother.

2. The husband of the gestational mother of a child is the child's father . . .

3. A donor is not the parent of a child conceived through assisted conception, unless the donor is the husband of the gestational mother . . .

D. Birth pursuant to court approved surrogacy contract. — After approval of a surrogacy contract by the court and entry of an order as provided in subsection D of § 20-160, the intended parents are the parents of any resulting child . . .

E. Birth pursuant to surrogacy contract not approved by court. — In the case of a surrogacy contract that has not been approved by a court as provided in § 20-160, the parentage of any resulting child shall be determined as follows:

1. The gestational mother is the child's mother unless the intended mother is a genetic parent, in which case the intended mother is the mother.

2. If either of the intended parents is a genetic parent of the resulting child, the intended father is the child's father. However, if (i) the surrogate is married, (ii) her husband is a party to the surrogacy contract, and (iii) the surrogate exercises her right to retain custody and parental rights to the resulting child pursuant to § 20-162, then the surrogate and her husband are the parents.

3. If neither of the intended parents is a genetic parent of the resulting child, the surrogate is the mother and her husband is the child's father if he is a party to the contract. The intended parents may only obtain parental rights through adoption . . .

4. After the signing and filing of the surrogate consent and report form in conformance with the requirements of subsection A of § 20-162, the intended parents are the parents of the child and the surrogate and her husband, if any, shall not be the parents of the child.

§ 20-160. Petition and Hearing for Court Approval of Surrogacy Contracts

B. . . . The court shall enter an order approving the surrogacy contract . . . upon finding that:

. . . 9. At least one of the intended parents is expected to be the genetic parent of any child resulting from the agreement.

Florida Statutes Annotated
Title XLIII. Domestic Relations
Chapter 742. Determination of Parentage

§ 742.11. Presumed status of child conceived by means of artificial or in vitro insemination or donated eggs or preembryos

(1) Except in the case of gestational surrogacy, any child born within wedlock who has been conceived by the means of artificial or in vitro insemination is irrebuttably

presumed to be the child of the husband and wife, provided that both husband and wife have consented in writing to the artificial or in vitro insemination.

(2) Except in the case of gestational surrogacy, any child born within wedlock who has been conceived by means of donated eggs or preembryos shall be irrebuttably presumed to be the child of the recipient gestating woman and her husband, provided that both parties have consented in writing to the use of donated eggs or preembryos.

§ 742.14. Donation of eggs, sperm, or preembryos

The donor of any egg, sperm, or preembryo, other than the commissioning couple . . . , shall relinquish all maternal or paternal rights and obligations with respect to the donation or the resulting children. Only reasonable compensation directly related to the donation of eggs, sperm, and preembryos shall be permitted.

QUESTIONS

Recall that Jaycee Buzzanca is a child whose intended parents, Luanne and John, contracted with an egg donor and a sperm donor to create embryos that were implanted into a gestational carrier. Who would be Jaycee's legal mother and legal father in Texas? Virginia? Florida? Suppose that the surrogate and the egg donor each claimed to be Jaycee's legal mother. Who would be deemed the legal mother in each of these states? How about in your own state?

SECTION IV: BUILDING FAMILIES IN SAME-SEX RELATIONSHIPS

Assisted reproductive technologies, by definition, involve the separation of sexual intercourse and human conception. ART is designed to substitute for reproductive systems that are either broken (as in the case of a married couple using IVF to overcome the wife's blocked fallopian tubes) or absent (as in the case of a single woman using AID to become a parent). Thus, ART opens up the prospect of parenthood not just to those who meet the clinical definition of infertility, but to those whose family structure is something other than a heterosexual couple. Single individuals and same-sex couples can look to ART to enable them to become parents, often fulfilling a dream of biological parenthood that was simply unavailable a generation ago. But with these opportunities come controversy and legal questions over the rights and responsibilities of so-called "non-traditional" parents, particularly lesbian and gay parents. In this Section, we explore the use of ART by same-sex couples, and the emerging legal landscape that is coalescing around this growing number of families.

A.   The Prevalence of Same-Sex Parents

According to the U.S. Census Bureau, there were 646,464 same-sex couples living in the United States in 2010. Of these, 131,729 were married, while 514,735 were unmarried partners. In terms of gender breakdown, 51% of all same-sex couples are females while 49% are male. In terms of children, 111,033 or 17% of all same-sex couples are raising their own children. *See* The Williams Institute, United States Census Snapshot: 2010 (summarizing the 2010 census data on same-sex couples), available at: http://williamsinstitute.law.ucla.edu/research/census-lgbt-demographics-studies/us-census-snapshot-2010/. The 2010 figure represents about a 10% increase in the number of same-sex households from a decade earlier. According to the 2000 Census Report, the U.S. was home to 594,000 households with partners of the same sex. *See* U.S. Census Bureau, Married-Couple and Unmarried Partner Households: 2000, 1,10 (Feb. 2003) (explaining that the 2000 census cannot be compared to the 1990 census with regard to same-sex households due to changes in the editing procedures).

These census figures are considerably lower than guesstimates made outside the census process. In 1998, for example, according to writings attributable to Dr. Benjamin Spock, the legendary pediatrician and child care expert, as many as 10 million children lived with 3 million gay or lesbian parents in the United States. *See* BENJAMIN SPOCK, BABY AND CHILD CARE 685 (1998 ed.). Professor Michael Wald, citing the 1998 Census Bureau Report, pegged the number of same-sex couples in the U.S. at 1.5 million, with about 200,000 of those couples living with children. Michael S. Wald, *Same-Sex Marriage: A Family Policy Perspective*, 9 VA. J. SOC. POL. & L. 291 (2001) (citing U.S. Census Bureau, Current Population Reports, 71-73 tbl.8, v. tbl.C (March 1998 (update)).

Whatever the actual number of same-sex families, there is no dispute that gay and lesbian couples are having children through ART, so that one partner will have a genetic tie to their offspring. Women can use artificial insemination so that one partner can carry the couple's child, or both women could be involved in creating a child — one woman could donate her eggs and the other could gestate the resulting embryos. For men, genetic childbearing depends on a surrogate parenting arrangement, with a traditional surrogate agreeing to be inseminated, or a gestational carrier giving birth to a child conceived with donor eggs and one of the partner's sperm. Once the child is born, the parental relationship with the nongenetic partner depends largely on state law, a matter we take up in the cases that follow.

Before delving into the legal aspects of same-sex parenting, we pause to consider a question that often accompanies a discussion of children of gay and lesbian parents: What effect, if any, does a parent's sexual orientation have on a child? Not surprisingly, there have been a number of studies conducted to answer this question, and though interpretations of the results vary, the majority view seems to be that children of gay parents are as well off and as bad off as children of heterosexual parents. As Dr. Spock explains:

> Tests of psychological adjustment show no significant differences between the well-being of children raised by heterosexual parents and those raised by gay or lesbian parents. Like any family, what is most important for children is how loving and nurturing the parents are and whether or not the parents are aware of any special needs they may have. Since gay men and women can be as warm and caring (or as dysfunctional) as heterosexual parents, it is not surprising that the mental health of their children is comparable. These studies also show that the children of gay and lesbian parents are as likely to be heterosexual as are children growing up in more

traditional families. At the same time, these children are often more tolerant of different sexual orientations and more sensitive to minority status. Most studies show that gay and lesbian parents make a special effort to expose their children to strong role models, both male and female, both heterosexual and gay. Furthermore, sexual abuse is statistically *less* likely to happen with gay and lesbian parents. Most intrafamily sexual abuse is committed by heterosexual males.

Benjamin Spock, *Gay and Lesbian Parents*, in BABY AND CHILD CARE 685-6 (1998 ed.).

In a 2003 article, Professor Carlos Ball reviews the then most recent social science research measuring the impact of parental sexual orientation on children. He reports:

In the last two years, two important reviews of the research have been added to the growing literature in this area. The first is a report issued by the Committee on Psychosocial Aspects of Child and Family Health ("the Committee") of the American Academy of Pediatrics ("AAP"). The Committee's report reviews the research and finds that no meaningful differences exist between children raised by lesbian and gay parents and children raised by heterosexual parents. The report concludes that "parents' sexual orientation is not a variable that, in itself, predicts their ability to provide a home environment that supports children's development." The second is an essay written by sociologists Judith Stacey and Timothy Biblarz titled "(How) Does the Sexual Orientation of Parents Matter?" In their essay, Stacey and Biblarz, who are otherwise supportive of families headed by lesbians and gay men, argue that the social science research raises provocative questions about possible differences in the children studied. In particular, they note that there appear to be differences in the gender and sexual preferences and behavior of the children of lesbian and gay parents when compared to those of the children of heterosexual parents. Although the authors call for more research to be conducted, they nonetheless find it intriguing that some of the existing research (despite claims to the contrary made by the researchers themselves) raise the possibility that important and significant differences exist between the two groups of children. [citations omitted]

Carlos A. Ball, *Lesbian and Gay Families: Gender Nonconformity and the Implications of Difference*, 31 CAP. U. L. REV. 691-2 (2003) (concluding that even if further research confirms Stacey's and Biblarz's initial suggestion that there are differences in gender role conformity between the two groups of children, it does not follow that our society should as a policy matter make it more difficult for lesbians and gay men to become parents).

The question of child welfare in a same-sex household has become a key feature in the debate over marriage equality. In a handful of jurisdictions, courts have issued opinions on the constitutionality of laws that ban same-sex couples from lawfully marrying. *See, e.g., Varnum v. Brien*, 763 N.W.2d 862 (Iowa 2009); *In re Marriage Cases*, 183 P.3d 384 (Cal. 2008); *Kerrigan v. Comm'r of Public Health*, 957 A.2d 402 (Conn. 2008); *Goodridge v. Dep't Public Health*, 798 N.E.2d 941 (Mass.

2003). One of the arguments raised by opponents of same-sex marriage is that children are harmed by being raised in such a household. The Iowa Supreme Court addressed this issue in its 2009 opinion, citing to evidence produced by marriage opponents (the County which refused to issue licenses to same-sex couples) and the plaintiffs (same-sex couples seeking valid marriage licenses):

> Much of the testimony presented by the County was in the form of opinions by various individuals that same-sex marriage would harm the institution of marriage and also harm children raised in same-sex marriages. Two college professors testified that a heterosexual marriage is, overall, the optimal forum in which to raise children. A retired pediatrician challenged the accuracy of some of the medical research that concludes there is no significant difference between children raised by same-sex couples and opposite-sex couples. A clinical psychologist testified sexual orientation is not as defined and stable as race and gender and can change over time. He acknowledged, however, it is difficult to change a person's sexual orientation, and efforts to do so can be harmful to the person.
>
> The plaintiffs produced evidence to demonstrate sexual orientation and gender have no effect on children raised by same-sex couples, and same-sex couples can raise children as well as opposite-sex couples. They also submitted evidence to show that most scientific research has repudiated the commonly assumed notion that children need opposite-sex parents or biological parents to grow into well-adjusted adults. Many leading organizations, including the American Academy of Pediatrics, the American Psychiatric Association, the American Psychological Association, the National Association of Social Workers, and the Child Welfare League of America, weighed the available research and supported the conclusion that gay and lesbian parents are as effective as heterosexual parents in raising children. For example, the official policy of the American Psychological Association declares, "There is no scientific evidence that parenting effectiveness is related to parental sexual orientation: Lesbian and gay parents are as likely as heterosexual parents to provide supportive and healthy environments for children." [citation omitted] Almost every professional group that has studied the issue indicates children are not harmed when raised by same-sex couples, but to the contrary, benefit from them.

Varnum v. Brien, 763 N.W.2d at 873-74. The court held, *inter alia*, that the Iowa statute limiting civil marriage to a union between a man and a woman was not substantially related to the government goal of ensuring the optimal environment for raising children. The statute was struck down as unconstitutional.

Think about your own views on the issue of same-sex parenting. Are your views shaped by personal experiences? By your social or religious upbringing? By a review of the literature in the field? By portrayals in the media and popular culture? As individuals, our views are shaped by a variety of influences. Judges, as individuals, bring views to the bench that shape the way they perceive the cases and controversies before them. As you read the several judicial opinions in this area, think about how your views would have guided your decision-making in each case.

B. Family Law Dilemmas For Same-Sex Parents

1. Determining Paternity

C.O. v. W.S.
Court of Common Pleas of Ohio, Cuyahoga County
64 Ohio Misc. 2d 9, 639 N.E.2d 523 (1994)

PETER M. SIKORA, JUDGE.

I. Statement of Facts

Defendant, W.S., and her female partner decided that they wished to have a baby. After discussing their wish with plaintiff, C.O., and his male partner, it was agreed that plaintiff would provide the semen for defendant to conceive a child. It is undisputed that plaintiff provided the semen on one or more occasions and that defendant was impregnated with the semen other than through direct sexual intercourse. As a result of the insemination, on December 25, 1992, defendant gave birth to D.C., the subject of these proceedings. It is further agreed that plaintiff and defendant were never married to each other, and that defendant was not married during the period from the insemination to the child's birth. There is disagreement as to whether the defendant's insemination was conducted under the supervision and control of a physician.

Prior to D.C.'s birth, the parties agreed that plaintiff was to be considered a "male role model" for the child, and would be called "father." Although this agreement evidenced some intention to circumvent the artificial insemination provisions of R.C. 3111.30 *et seq.*, there is dispute between the parties as to whether it was their intention for plaintiff to have all of the rights and responsibilities of fatherhood. Plaintiff alleges that since the child's birth, defendant has refused plaintiff's requests to visit or support the child, or to participate in the child's life as his father.

On June 10, 1993, plaintiff, through counsel, filed a complaint to determine paternity, custody, support, and visitation, naming W.S. as defendant. Defendant, through counsel, filed a motion to dismiss on June 25, 1993, relying primarily on R.C. 3111.37(B), which provides:

> If a woman is the subject of a non-spousal artificial insemination, the donor shall not be treated in law or regarded as the natural father of a child conceived as a result of the artificial insemination, and a child so conceived shall not be treated in law or regarded as the natural child of the donor . . .

. . . On February 9, 1994, plaintiff filed a motion for immediate ruling on defendant's motion to dismiss, and on February 14, 1994, defendant filed a notice of joinder in plaintiff's motion. It is the purpose of this order and opinion to rule on defendant's motion to dismiss.

II. Opinion

Artificial insemination statutes are designed to provide anonymity and protection to both the donor and the mother. See *McIntyre v. Crouch* (1989), 98 Ore.App. 462, 780 P.2d 239. In furtherance of this objective, rigorous medical requirements have been included in Ohio law. For instance, a non-spousal artificial insemination must be performed by a physician or a person who is under the supervision and control of a physician (R.C. 3111.32); a complete medical history and physical examination of the donor must be obtained by a physician (R.C. 311.33[B]); and, the physician must obtain and maintain various information, statements, and records, including a statement that the donor shall not be advised as to the identity of the recipient, and that the recipient shall not be advised as to the identity of the donor (R.C. 3111.35) . . .

Even if the defendant had complied with all of the statutory medical requirements, R.C. 3111.37(B), which establishes the legal relationship between a donor and mother, would not apply to the facts of this case. The statute does not prevent a paternity adjudication where an unmarried woman solicits the participation of the donor, who was known to her, and where the donor and woman agree that there would be a relationship between the donor and child. See *In the Interest of R.C.* (Colo.1989), 775 P.2d 27; *C.M. v. C.C.* (1977), 152 N.J.Super. 160, 377 A.2d 821.

Assuming *arguendo* that R.C. 3111.37(B) does apply, the court finds that the statute is unconstitutional as applied to plaintiff and the child. Public policy supports the concept of legitimacy, and the concomitant rights of a child to support and inheritance . . . A father's voluntary assumption of fiscal responsibility for his child should be endorsed as a socially responsible action. A statute which absolutely extinguishes a father's efforts to assert the rights and responsibilities of being a father, in a case with such facts as those *sub judice*, runs contrary to due process safeguards . . .

It is, therefore, ordered that the motion to dismiss is overruled, and that the parent-child relationship between the plaintiff and the child, D.C., has been established. All other pending motions are overruled. This matter will be set for hearing on the issues of custody, visitation, and support. The court's probation department is to conduct home investigations of both plaintiff and defendant, and the court's clinic is to conduct psychological evaluations on plaintiff, his partner, the defendant, and her partner.

Judgment accordingly.

LAMARITATA v. LUCAS
District Court of Appeal of Florida, Second District
823 So.2d 316, 27 Fla. L. Weekly D1858 (2002)

BLUE, Chief Judge.

Although the parties raise numerous issues on appeal and cross-appeal, this is a simple case that can be resolved in a one-sentence opinion, to wit: Danny A. Lucas is a sperm donor, not a parent, and has no parental rights; thus the court erred in establishing a visitation schedule.

Ms. Lamaritata appeals a supplemental final judgment that grants to Mr. Lucas (1) unsupervised, overnight visitation on alternating weekends and visitation on the day after Christmas and on Father's Day; (2) telephone calls from the children when they are with their mother; and (3) the right to confer with the children's teachers and attend school events and activities . . . A brief statement of the pertinent facts was set forth in this court's prior opinion.

D.A.L. (donor) and L.A.L. (recipient) entered into a contract whereby the donor would provide sperm to recipient with the expectation that she would become pregnant through artificial insemination and deliver offspring. The agreement provided that if childbirth resulted, the donor would have no parental rights and obligations associated with the delivery, and both parties would be foreclosed from establishing those rights and obligations by the institution of an action to determine the paternity of any such child or children. Notwithstanding the clear language of the contract, after the recipient gave birth to twin boys the donor filed an action in circuit court seeking to establish paternity and an award of those rights associated with it. In defense of the action, the recipient alleged that the contract barred such an action, that section 742.14, Florida Statutes (1997), disallowed sperm donors any parental rights, and that the donor was not in fact the biological father of the children. *L.A.L. v. D.A.L.*, 714 So.2d 595, 596 (Fla. 2d DCA 1998). This court quashed the order for paternity testing and directed the circuit court to proceed in a manner consistent with this court's opinion.

In the opinion, after considering the express language of section 742.14, Florida Statutes (1997),[16] this court held: "Should the trial court decide that this statute is constitutionally applicable to the facts in the underlying litigation, the donor, whether or not he is scientifically determined to be the biological parent of these boys, will be foreclosed from all parental rights, including his access to the children." 714 So.2d at 596 (emphasis added). Likewise, after considering the express language of the parties' contract, this court held that "if the clear intent of the parties to this agreement is enforced by the trial court," Mr. Lucas waived his right to institute a paternity proceeding.

In an attempt to avoid application of the statute, Mr. Lucas now argues that he is not a sperm donor. Sperm donor is not defined in the statute. The contract, however, calls Mr. Lucas "donor" and indicates that sperm is the only donation required of him. Thus we easily conclude that Mr. Lucas qualifies as a sperm donor.

We just as easily reject Mr. Lucas's argument that he and Ms. Lamaritata constitute a "commissioning couple." Commissioning couple is defined in the statute as "the intended mother and father of a child who will be conceived by means of assisted reproductive technology using the eggs or sperm of at least one of the intended parents." § 742.13(2). There are no facts to show that Mr. Lucas and Ms. Lamaritata have any type of relationship that would fall under the rubric of

---

[16] [n.2] Section 742.14 provides in pertinent part: "The donor of any egg, sperm, or preembryo, other than the commissioning couple or a father who has executed a preplanned adoption agreement under s. 63.212, shall relinquish all maternal or paternal rights and obligations with respect to the donation or the resulting children."

"couple." Further, they did not commission or contract to jointly raise the children as mother and father. Rather, they joined forces solely for the purpose of artificially inseminating Ms. Lamaritata, an intent clearly set forth in the parties' contract.

A person who provides sperm for a woman to conceive a child by artificial insemination is not a parent. Both the contract between the parties and the Florida statute controlling these arrangements provide that there are no parental rights or responsibilities resulting to the donor of sperm . . . If the sperm donor has no parental rights, the sperm donor is a nonparent, a statutory stranger to the children.

Even though the parties entered into subsequent stipulations, purportedly to give visitation rights to this nonparent, we conclude that agreement is not enforceable. There are numerous Florida cases holding that nonparents are not entitled to visitation rights . . . Therefore, pursuant to the contract's severability clause, we sever the unenforceable portion of the contract purporting to give visitation rights to Mr. Lucas.

The sperm donor here has no legal parental rights, and this case should have been dismissed after our prior opinion. Accordingly, we reverse the supplemental final judgment and remand to the trial court for the entry of a final judgment declaring that Mr. Lucas has no enforceable parental rights.

Reversed and remanded with directions.

GREEN and COVINGTON, JJ., Concur.

NOTES AND QUESTIONS

1. Compare the outcomes in *C.O. v. W.S.* and *Lamaritata v. Lucas.* What factors account for the different holdings? Legal factors? Factual differences between the two case scenarios? Perhaps the passage of time?

2. Recall our discussion of *Jhordan C. v. Mary K.* 179 Cal. App. 3d 386, 224 Cal. Rptr. 530 (1986) in Section 1(B). The California court declared a sperm donor to be the resulting child's legal father because the mother failed to obtain sperm through a licensed physician, as required by state law. The ruling in *C.O.* demonstrates that courts continue to strictly apply the statutory medical requirements in order for the status of "nonparent" to attach to the donor. What if a married woman undergoes physician-administered donor insemination, and in a later divorce action her husband disclaims paternity of the child on the grounds that the consent form he signed was not properly certified by the physician, as required by state law? Should the court treat the husband as the child's father, despite this lack of technical compliance with the statute? See *Alexandra S. v. Pacific Fertility Medical Center*, 55 Cal. App. 4th 110, 64 Cal. Rptr.2d 23 (1997).

3. The court in *C.O.* declares the Ohio AID statute unconstitutional as applied to the sperm donor and the child. The court fails to specify which constitutional provision, state or federal, is violated. Judge Sikora supports his finding with the rationale that public policy favors legitimacy and a child's right to support and

inheritance. What possible constitutional infirmities could the judge have had in mind?

4.   Is it possible for a woman to be declared the father of children born through donor insemination? In *Karin T. v. Michael T.*, 127 Misc. 2d 14, 484 N.Y.S.2d 780 (1985), Michael, born Marlene, dressed as a man and married Karin. During the "marriage" (so-quoted as New York did not recognize same-sex marriage at the time the case was decided), two children were born to Karin following donor insemination. In both instances, Michael signed an agreement prior to the inseminations declaring that any children born from the procedure would be considered his own legitimate offspring. When the couple split up, Michael disclaimed any responsibility for the children, arguing that as a female she, biologically, could not be considered a parent. The court disagreed. Looking to the agreement, the court declared Michael a parent for having "brought forth these offspring as if done biologically." Id. at 19, 484 N.Y.S.2d at 784. Did the court consider Michael a father or a mother?

For a discussion of the law surrounding the rights of transgendered parents, *see* COURTNEY JOSLIN & SHANNON MINTNER, LESBIAN, GAY, BISEXUAL AND TRANSGENDER FAMILY LAW (database updated June 2011).

5.   The cases resolving questions of paternity in AID scenarios typically involve single or lesbian women in which the court can choose between naming the donor as the father, or declaring that the donor has no parental rights. Most of the reported cases involve men seeking legal rights (and willing to accept legal responsibilities) toward the child that resulted from their sperm donation. Occasionally, a mother seeks to hold a donor legally responsible for her AID children. In *Jacob v. Shultz-Jacob*, 923 A.2d 473 (Pa. 2007), the court found that a sperm donor was an "indispensable party" to a child custody battle involving two women, one of whom he had aided in birthing two children. When a trial court awarded the biological mother monthly child support from her ex-partner, the latter attempted to join the sperm donor in an effort to defray her financial obligations. The court found the donor's prior financial and emotional support of the children sufficient to order his continued monetary involvement. Think the case is odd? There's more. The sperm donor died just weeks before the court issued its opinion, leaving his estate lawyers scratching their heads. *See Sperm Donor Ordered to Pay Child Support*, POST-GAZETTE, May 10, 2007, available at: http://www.post-gazette.com/pg/07130/784968-100.stm.

While the above Pennsylvania case was mostly about money, it indirectly raises the question of whether a non-biological same-sex partner can be considered the legal parent of a child born into or raised during the relationship. The right to be considered a legal parent can be important both during and after a same-sex relationship. Consider the following cases.

Adoption of Tammy
Supreme Judicial Court of Massachusetts
416 Mass. 205, 619 N.E.2d 315 (1993)

GREANEY, Justice. In this case, two unmarried women, Susan and Helen, filed a joint petition in the Probate and Family Court Department under G.L. c. 210, § 1 (1992 ed.) to adopt as their child Tammy, a minor, who is Susan's biological daughter. Following an evidentiary hearing, a judge of the Probate and Family Court entered a memorandum of decision containing findings of fact and conclusions of law. Based on her finding that Helen and Susan "are each functioning, separately and together, as the custodial and psychological parents of [Tammy]," and that "it is the best interest of said [Tammy] that she be adopted by both," the judge entered a decree allowing the adoption. . . . We transferred the case to this court on our own motion. We conclude that the adoption was properly allowed under G.L. c. 210.

We summarize the relevant facts as found by the judge. Helen and Susan have lived together in a committed relationship, which they consider to be permanent, for more than ten years. In June, 1983, they jointly purchased a house in Cambridge. Both women are physicians specializing in surgery. At the time the petition was filed, Helen maintained a private practice in general surgery at Mount Auburn Hospital and Susan, a nationally recognized expert in the field of breast cancer, was director of the Faulkner Breast Center and a surgical oncologist at the Dana Farber Cancer Institute. Both women also held positions on the faculty of Harvard Medical School.

For several years prior to the birth of Tammy, Helen and Susan planned to have a child, biologically related to both of them, whom they would jointly parent. Helen first attempted to conceive a child through artificial insemination by Susan's brother. When those efforts failed, Susan successfully conceived a child through artificial insemination by Helen's biological cousin, Francis. The women attended childbirth classes together and Helen was present when Susan gave birth to Tammy on April 30, 1988. Although Tammy's birth certificate reflects Francis as her biological father, she was given a hyphenated surname using Susan and Helen's last names.

Since her birth, Tammy has lived with, and been raised and supported by, Helen and Susan. Tammy views both women as her parents, calling Helen "mama" and Susan "mommy." Tammy has strong emotional and psychological bonds with both Helen and Susan. Together, Helen and Susan have provided Tammy with a comfortable home, and have created a warm and stable environment which is supportive of Tammy's growth and over-all well being. Both women jointly and equally participate in parenting Tammy, and both have a strong financial commitment to her. During the work week, Helen usually has lunch at home with Tammy, and on weekends both women spend time together with Tammy at special events or running errands. When Helen and Susan are working, Tammy is cared for by a nanny. The three vacation together at least ten days every three to four months, frequently spending time with Helen's and Susan's respective extended families in California and Mexico. Francis does not participate in parenting Tammy and does not support her. His intention was to assist Helen and Susan in having a child, and he does not intend to be involved with Tammy, except as a distant relative. Francis signed an adoption surrender and supports the joint adoption by both women.

Helen and Susan, recognizing that the laws of the Commonwealth do not permit them to enter into a legally cognizable marriage,[17] believe that the best interests of Tammy require legal recognition of her identical emotional relationship to both women . . . Susan indicated . . . that she has no reservation about allowing Helen to adopt. Apart from the emotional security and current practical ramifications which legal recognition of the reality of her parental relationships will provide Tammy, Susan indicated that the adoption is important for Tammy in terms of potential inheritance from Helen. Helen and her living issue are the beneficiaries of three irrevocable family trusts. Unless Tammy is adopted, Helen's share of the trusts may pass to others . . .

Over a dozen witnesses, including mental health professionals, teachers, colleagues, neighbors, blood relatives and a priest and nun, testified to the fact that Helen and Susan participate equally in raising Tammy, that Tammy relates to both women as her parents, and that the three form a healthy, happy, and stable family unit . . .

The Department of Social Services (department) conducted a home study in connection with the adoption petition which recommended the adoption, concluding that "the petitioners and their home are suitable for the proper rearing of this child." Tammy's pediatrician reported to the department that Tammy receives regular pediatric care and that she "could not have more excellent parents than Helen and Susan." A court-appointed guardian ad litem, Dr. Steven Nickman, assistant clinical professor of psychiatry at Harvard Medical School, conducted a clinical assessment of Tammy and her family with a view toward determining whether or not it would be in Tammy's best interests to be adopted by Helen and Susan. Dr. Nickman considered the ramifications of the fact that Tammy will be brought up in a "non-standard" family. As part of his report, he reviewed and referenced literature on child psychiatry and child psychology which supports the conclusion that children raised by lesbian parents develop normally . . . Dr. Nickman concluded that "there is every reason for [Helen] to become a legal parent to Tammy just as [Susan] is," and he recommended that the court so order. An attorney appointed to represent Tammy's interests also strongly recommended that the joint petition be granted.

Despite the overwhelming support for the joint adoption and the judge's conclusion that joint adoption is clearly in Tammy's best interests, the question remains whether there is anything in the law of the Commonwealth that would prevent this adoption. The law of adoption is purely statutory, . . . and the governing statute, G.L. c. 210 (1992 ed.), is to be strictly followed in all its essential particulars . . . The primary purpose of the adoption statute, particularly with regard to children under the age of fourteen, is undoubtedly the advancement of the best interests of the subject child . . . With these considerations in mind, we

---

[17] On May 17, 2004 Massachusetts became the first U.S. state to issue valid marriage licenses to same-sex couples, following the Supreme Judicial Court's decision in *Goodridge v. Department of Public Health*, 440 Mass. 309, 798 N.E.2d 941 (2003) finding that the limitation of protections, benefits and obligations of civil marriage to individuals of opposite sexes lacked rational basis and violated state constitutional equal protection principles. -Ed.

examine the statute to determine whether adoption in the circumstances of this case is permitted.

1. The initial question is whether the Probate Court judge had jurisdiction under G.L. c. 210 to enter a judgment on a joint petition for adoption brought by two unmarried cohabitants in the petitioners' circumstances. We answer this question in the affirmative.

There is nothing on the face of the statute which precludes the joint adoption of a child by two unmarried cohabitants such as the petitioners. Chapter 210, § 1, provides that "[a] person of full age may petition the probate court in the county where he resides for leave to adopt as his child another person younger than himself, unless such other person is his or her wife or husband, or brother, sister, uncle or aunt, of the whole or half blood." Other than requiring that a spouse join in the petition, if the petitioner is married and the spouse is competent to join therein, the statute does not expressly prohibit or require joinder by any person. Although the singular "a person" is used, it is a legislatively mandated rule of statutory construction that "[w]ords importing the singular number may extend and be applied to several persons" unless the resulting construction is "inconsistent with the manifest intent of the law-making body or repugnant to the context of the same statute." G.L. c. 4, § 6 (1992 ed.). In the context of adoption, where the legislative intent to promote the best interests of the child is evidenced throughout the governing statute, and the adoption of a child by two unmarried individuals accomplishes that goal, construing the term "person" as "persons" clearly enhances, rather than defeats, the purpose of the statute. . . .

While the Legislature may not have envisioned adoption by same-sex partners, there is no indication that it attempted to define all possible categories of persons leading to adoptions in the best interests of children. Rather than limit the potential categories of persons entitled to adopt (other than those described in the first sentence of § 1), the Legislature used general language to define who may adopt and who may be adopted. The Probate Court has thus been granted jurisdiction to consider a variety of adoption petitions . . .

In this case all requirements in [the adoption statute] are met . . . Adoption will not result in any tangible change in Tammy's daily life; it will, however, serve to provide her with a significant legal relationship which may be important in her future. At the most practical level, adoption will entitle Tammy to inherit from Helen's family trusts and from Helen and her family under the law of intestate succession . . . to receive support from Helen, who will be legally obligated to provide such support . . . , to be eligible for coverage under Helen's health insurance policies, and to be eligible for social security benefits in the event of Helen's disability or death . . .

Of equal, if not greater significance, adoption will enable Tammy to preserve her unique filial ties to Helen in the event that Helen and Susan separate, or Susan predeceases Helen . . . As the case law and commentary on the subject illustrate, when the functional parents of children born in circumstances similar to Tammy separate or one dies, the children often remain in legal limbo for years while their future is disputed in the courts . . . Adoption serves to establish legal rights and responsibilities so that, in the event that problems arise in the future, issues of custody and visitation may be promptly resolved by reference to the best interests of the child within the recognized framework of the law . . . There is no jurisdictional bar in the statute to the judge's consideration of this joint petition. The conclusion that the adoption is in the best interests of Tammy is also well warranted . . .

3. We conclude that the Probate Court has jurisdiction to enter a decree on a joint adoption petition brought by the two petitioners when the judge has found that joint adoption is in the subject child's best interests. We further conclude that, when a natural parent is a party to a joint adoption petition, that parent's legal relationship to the child does not terminate on entry of the adoption decree.

4. So much of the decree as allows the adoption of Tammy by both petitioners is affirmed. So much of the decree as provides in the alternative for the adoption of Tammy by Helen and the retention of rights of custody and visitation by Susan is vacated.

So ordered.

LIACOS, C.J., WILKINS, J, AND ABRAMS, J concur.

NOLAN, Justice (dissenting).

I write separately in dissent only because I do not agree with the sentiments expressed by my brother Lynch in the first few sentences of his dissent. His dissent is otherwise a faultless analysis of our existing jurisprudence to which I subscribe.

LYNCH, Justice (dissenting, with whom O'CONNOR, Justice, joins).

At the outset I wish to make clear that my views are not motivated by any disapproval of the two petitioners here or their life-style. The judge has found that the petitioners have provided the child with a healthy, happy, stable family unit. The evidence supports the judge's findings. Nor is my disagreement with the court related to the sexual orientation of the petitioners. I am firmly of the view that a litigant's expression of human sexuality ought not determine the outcome of litigation as long as it involves consenting adults and is not harmful to others. However, the court's decision, which is inconsistent with the statutory language, cannot be justified by a desire to achieve what is in the child's best interests. Indeed, those interests can be accommodated without doing violence to the statute by accepting the alternative to joint adoption suggested by the Probate Court judge . . . ; that is, permitting Helen to adopt Tammy while allowing Susan to retain all her parental rights and obligations . . .

The court concludes that the Probate and Family Court has jurisdiction to grant a joint petition for adoption by two unmarried cohabitants because they meet the statutory requirements of G.L. c. 210, § 1, and it is in the child's best interests to be adopted by both . . . The court has also interpreted the statute as permitting a biological parent of full age to petition for the adoption of his or her own child . . . There is, however, nothing in the statute indicating a legislative intent to allow two or more unmarried persons jointly to petition for adoption . . .

The court opines that the use of the singular form "a person" in the first sentence of the statute should not be construed as prohibiting joint petitions by unmarried persons because such an interpretation would not be in the best interests of the child . . . [W]hether the petition be singular or joint, has nothing to do with the best interests of the child. The court's reasoning . . . amounts to a tacit agreement with this position. Furthermore, on examining § 1 as a whole, I find no inconsistent use of the singular form from the first sentence that "[a] person . . . may . . . adopt . . . another person younger than himself," to the final sentence pertaining to nonresidents who wish to adopt. Throughout the section, the singular is preserved. The only time a second petitioner is contemplated is where the initial petitioner has a living, competent spouse. There is nothing in the statute to suggest that joint petitions other than by spouses are permitted.

A biological mother may petition alone for the adoption of her child. Helen also meets the statutory requirements and may petition alone for the adoption of Tammy with Susan's consent . . . Despite the admirable parenting and thriving environment being provided by these two unmarried cohabitants for this child, the statute does not permit their joint petition for adoption of Tammy.

NOTES AND QUESTIONS

1. Dr. Susan Love and Dr. Helen Cooksey continued their prestigious medical careers after finalizing the adoption of their daughter. The family moved to Los Angeles in the early 1990s, where Susan joined the faculty of the UCLA School of Medicine and founded the Revlon/UCLA Breast Center. She is the author of *Dr. Susan Love's Breast Book*, a comprehensive patient guidebook on the diagnosis and treatment of breast cancer. In 1996, Susan retired from surgery in order to direct the Susan Love MD Breast Cancer Research Foundation. Susan's career as a surgeon may not necessarily have been her first calling. In 1968, according to the National Women's History Project, Susan briefly entered the convent.

After the family moved to L.A., Helen continued her general surgery practice at the Jeffrey Goodman Special Care Clinic of the Los Angeles Gay and Lesbian Center. In February 2004, the couple availed themselves of a brief opportunity provided by the Mayor of San Francisco for same-sex partners to marry. Susan and Helen's wedding announcement appeared in the *New York Times* on February 22, 2004. On August 12, 2004, the California Supreme Court declared the roughly 4,000 marriages of gay and lesbian couples conducted in San Francisco "void from their inception and a legality nullity." *Lockyer v. City and County of San Francisco*, 33 Cal. 4th 1055, 17 Cal. Rptr. 3d 225 (2004). Determined, the couple (re)married in July 2008, during the brief period between the California Supreme Court's decision in *In re Marriage Cases*, 43 Cal. 4th 757, 76 Cal. Rptr. 683 (2008) invalidating the state's ban on same-sex marriage and the November 2008 passage of Proposition 8, a voter-approved initiative reinstating the ban.

2. *Adoption by Same-Sex Partners.* The Massachusetts Supreme Judicial Court was the second American appellate court to sanction adoption by a same-sex partner. In *Adoptions of B.L.V.B. and E.L.V.B*, 160 Vt. 368, 628 A.2d 1271 (1993) the Vermont Supreme Court authorized the nation's first co-parent adoption by a birth mother's lesbian partner, holding that a same-sex partner may adopt without

terminating the birth mother's parental rights. At last count, 18 U.S. states and the District of Columbia now permit second-parent adoption by same-sex couples based on either state statute or a ruling by the state's appellate court. The jurisdictions are California, Colorado, Connecticut, Delaware, the District of Columbia, Florida, Illinois, Indiana, Iowa, Maine, Massachusetts, Nevada, New Hampshire, New Jersey, New York, Oregon, Pennsylvania, Vermont and Washington. In eight other states, trial courts have granted second-parent adoptions to same-sex couples, but the states' high courts or legislatures have yet to sanction the practice. These states are Alabama, Alaska, Hawaii, Maryland, Minnesota, New Mexico, Rhode Island and Texas. In contrast, two states — Mississippi, and Utah — bar same-sex partners from adopting. See Human Rights Campaign, Parenting Laws: Second Parent Adoption, available at: http://www.hrc.org/files/images/general/2nd_Parent_ Adoption.pdf.

The path from prohibition to legalization of adoption by same-sex couples can be traced through Florida's evolving law. In 1977, the Dade County Metropolitan Commission passed an ordinance prohibiting discrimination against homosexuals in the areas of employment, public accommodations and housing. Outraged, pop singer Anita Bryant led a campaign to repeal the ordinance and replace it with a statewide law prohibiting adoption by and marriage between homosexuals. The adoption prohibition remained law for more than 30 years, winning support from a federal appeals court in 2005. *See Lofton v. Secretary of Department of Children and Family Services*, 358 F.3d 804 (11th Cir. 2004), *cert. denied*, 125 S.Ct. 869 (2005) (upholding constitutionality of Florida prohibition on adoption of children by "practicing" homosexuals). The ban was finally struck down as unconstitutional by a Florida court of appeal in 2010. *See Florida Dept. Children & Families v. Adoption of X.X.G*, 45 So.3d 79 (2010) (finding the statutory exclusion served no rational purpose and violated the equal protection clause of the state constitution).

3.   One of the primary justifications given the Massachusetts court by Susan and Helen to permit the co-parent adoption was the need to establish Tammy's rights as a lawful heir of Helen. If Helen adopts Tammy, she is treated as Helen's issue for purposes of intestate succession. This may mean that if Helen does not subsequently marry or have any other children, Tammy will be Helen's sole heir if she dies intestate, that is, without having made a valid will.

Assume that neither Susan nor Helen execute a valid will, and Susan dies intestate in California in 2000. Since Susan was not married at the time of her death, her sole heir would be her issue (children, grandchildren, etc.). See Cal. Probate Code § 6402. Will Tammy be entitled to inherit Susan's property under California law, which provides as follows:

a) An adoption severs the relationship of parent and child between an adopted person and a natural parent of the adopted person unless both of the following requirements are satisfied:

(1) The natural parent and the adopted person lived together at any time as parent and child, or the natural parent was married to or cohabiting with the other natural parent at the time the person was conceived and died before the person's birth.

(2) The adoption was by the spouse of either of the natural parents or after the death of either of the natural parents.

Cal. Probate Code § 6451. Can you see how Tammy may fail to qualify as her own birth mother's child for purposes of inheritance? See Laura M. Padilla, *Flesh of My Flesh But Not My Heir: Unintended Disinheritance*, 36 BRANDEIS J. FAM. L. 219 (Sp. 1997-98).

4. The case law on surrogate parenting arrangements teaches us that legal motherhood can be established either by giving birth or by having a genetic connection with the child. We know that a woman who gives birth to a child will not necessarily be deemed the legal mother if the egg donor intended to bring about the child's birth, as was the result in *Johnson v. Calvert*, 5 Cal.4th 84, 93, 19 Cal.Rptr.2d 494, 851 P.2d 776 (1993). A newly emerging technology allows doctors to transplant one woman's ovarian tissue into another woman in order to assist the transplantee's reproductive capacity. Yes, really. See Crystal Phend, *Ovarian tissue Transplantation Works Despite Genetic Differences, MedPage Today (Aug. 2, 2007)*, available at: http://www.medpagetoday.com/OBGYN/Infertility/6321; Cheryl Wittenauer, *Patient Is Sick and Thrilled About It; Woman Who Received Transplanted Ovarian Tissue Is Pregnant*, CHARLOTTE OBSERVER, Oct. 16, 2004, at 19A. What if a birth mother receives ovarian tissue from another woman and then gives birth to a child? Who is the child's mother according to the law established in *Johnson v. Calvert*? How about in your state?

Who is the legal mother when both the birth mother and the egg donor intend to bring about the child's conception and birth? The Golden State brings us yet another family law conundrum.

K.M. v. E.G.
Supreme Court of California
37 Cal. 4th 130, 33 Cal. Rptr. 3d 61, 117 P.3d 673 (2005)

MORENO, J.

We granted review in this case . . . to consider the parental rights and obligations, if any, of a woman with regard to a child born to her partner in a lesbian relationship.

In the present case, we must decide whether a woman who provided ova to her lesbian partner so that the partner could bear children by means of in vitro fertilization is a parent of those children. For the reasons that follow, we conclude that Family Code section 7613, subdivision (b), which provides that a man is not a father if he provides semen to a physician to inseminate a woman who is not his wife, does not apply when a woman provides her ova to impregnate her partner in a lesbian relationship in order to produce children who will be raised in their joint home. Accordingly, when partners in a lesbian relationship decide to produce children in this manner, both the woman who provides her ova and her partner who bears the children are the children's parents.

FACTS

On March 6, 2001, petitioner K.M. filed a petition to establish a parental relationship with twin five-year-old girls born to respondent E.G., her former lesbian partner. K.M. alleged that she "is the biological parent of the minor children" because "[s]he donated her egg to respondent, the gestational mother of the children." E.G. moved to dismiss the petition on the grounds that, although K.M. and E.G. "were lesbian partners who lived together until this action was filed," K.M. "explicitly donated her ovum under a clear written agreement by which she relinquished any claim to offspring born of her donation."

On April 18, 2001, K.M. filed a motion for custody of and visitation with the twins.

A hearing was held at which E.G. testified that she first considered raising a child before she met K.M., at a time when she did not have a partner. She met K.M. in October, 1992 and they became romantically involved in June 1993. E.G. told K.M. that she planned to adopt a baby as a single mother. E.G. applied for adoption in November, 1993. K.M. and E.G. began living together in March, 1994 and registered as domestic partners in San Francisco.

E.G. visited several fertility clinics in March, 1993 to inquire about artificial insemination and she attempted artificial insemination, without success, on 13 occasions from July, 1993 through November, 1994. K.M. accompanied her to most of these appointments. K.M. testified that she and E.G. planned to raise the child together, while E.G. insisted that, although K.M. was very supportive, E.G. made it clear that her intention was to become "a single parent."

In December, 1994, E.G. consulted with Dr. Mary Martin at the fertility practice of the University of California at San Francisco Medical Center (UCSF). E.G.'s first attempts at in vitro fertilization failed because she was unable to produce sufficient ova. In January, 1995, Dr. Martin suggested using K.M.'s ova. E.G. then asked K.M. to donate her ova, explaining that she would accept the ova only if K.M. "would really be a donor" and E.G. would "be the mother of any child," adding that she would not even consider permitting K.M. to adopt the child "for at least five years until [she] felt the relationship was stable and would endure." E.G. told K.M. that she "had seen too many lesbian relationships end quickly, and [she] did not want to be in a custody battle." E.G. and K.M. agreed they would not tell anyone that K.M. was the ova donor.

K.M. acknowledged that she agreed not to disclose to anyone that she was the ova donor, but insisted that she only agreed to provide her ova because she and E.G. had agreed to raise the child together. K.M. and E.G. selected the sperm donor together. K.M. denied that E.G. had said she wanted to be a single parent and insisted that she would not have donated her ova had she known E.G. intended to be the sole parent.

On March 8, 1995, K.M. signed a four-page form on UCSF letterhead entitled "Consent Form for Ovum Donor (Known)." The form states that K.M. agrees "to have eggs taken from my ovaries, in order that they may be donated to another woman." After explaining the medical procedures involved, the form states on the third page: "It is understood that I waive any right and relinquish any claim to the donated eggs or any pregnancy or offspring that might result from them. I agree that the recipient may regard the donated eggs and any offspring resulting therefrom as her own children." The following appears on page 4 of the form, above K.M.'s signature and the signature of a witness: "I specifically disclaim and waive any right in or any child that may be conceived as a result of the use of any ovum or egg of mine, and I agree not to attempt to discover the identity of the recipient thereof." . . .

E.G. testified she received the . . . form . . . in a letter from UCSF dated February 2, 1995, and discussed the consent form . . . with K.M. during February and March. E.G. stated she would not have accepted K.M.'s ova if K.M. had not signed the consent form, because E.G. wanted to have a child on her own and believed the consent form "protected" her in this regard.

K.M. testified to the contrary that she first saw the ovum donation consent form 10 minutes before she signed it on March 8, 1995. K.M. admitted reading the form, but thought parts of the form were "odd" and did not pertain to her, such as the part stating that the donor promised not to discover the identity of the recipient. She did not intend to relinquish her rights and only signed the form so that "we could have children." Despite having signed the form, K.M. "thought [she] was going to be a parent."

Ova were withdrawn from K.M. on April 11, 1995, and embryos were implanted in E.G. on April 13, 1995 . . . The twins were born on December 7, 1995. The twins' birth certificates listed E.G. as their mother and did not reflect a father's name. As they had agreed, neither E.G. nor K.M. told anyone K.M. had donated the ova, including their friends, family and the twins' pediatrician. Soon after the twins were born, E.G. asked K.M. to marry her, and on Christmas Day, the couple exchanged rings.

Within a month of their birth, E.G. added the twins to her health insurance policy, named them as her beneficiary for all employment benefits, and increased her life insurance with the twins as the beneficiary. K.M. did not do the same.

E.G. referred to her mother, as well as K.M.'s parents, as the twins' grandparents and referred to K.M.'s sister and brother as the twins' aunt and uncle, and K.M.'s nieces as their cousins. Two school forms listed both K.M. and respondent as the twins' parents. The children's nanny testified that both K.M. and E.G. "were the babies' mother."

The relationship between K.M. and E.G. ended in March, 2001 and K.M. filed the present action. In September, 2001, E.G. and the twins moved to Massachusetts to live with E.G.'s mother.

The superior court granted E.G.'s motion to dismiss finding, in a statement of decision, "that [K.M.] . . . knowingly, voluntarily and intelligently executed the ovum donor form, thereby acknowledging her understanding that, by the donation of her ova, she was relinquishing and waiving all rights to claim legal parentage of any children who might result from the *in vitro* fertilization . . . [K.M.]'s testimony on the subject of her execution of the ovum donor form was contradictory and not always credible . . .

". . . By voluntarily signing the ovum donation form, [K.M.] was donating genetic material. Her position was analogous to that of a sperm donor, who is treated as a legal stranger to a child if he donates sperm through a licensed physician and surgeon under Family Code section 7613[, subdivision] (b). The Court finds no reason to treat ovum donors as having greater claims to parentage than sperm donors. . . .

The Court of Appeal affirmed the judgment, ruling that K.M. did not qualify as a parent "because substantial evidence supports the trial courts factual finding that *only* E.G. intended to bring about the birth of a child whom she intended to raise as her own." . . . Having concluded that the parties intended at the time of conception that only E.G. would be the child's mother, the court concluded that the parties actions following the birth did not alter this agreement. The Court of Appeal concluded that if the parties had changed their intentions and wanted K.M. to be a parent, their only option was adoption.

We granted review.

DISCUSSION

K.M. asserts that she is a parent of the twins because she supplied the ova that were fertilized in vitro and implanted in her lesbian partner, resulting in the birth of the twins. As we will explain, we agree that K.M. is a parent of the twins because she supplied the ova that produced the children, and Family Code section 7613, subdivision (b) . . . which provides that a man is not a father if he provides semen to a physician to inseminate a woman who is not his wife, does not apply because K.M. supplied her ova to impregnate her lesbian partner in order to produce children who would be raised in their joint home . . .

In *Johnson v. Calvert* (1993) 5 Cal.4th 84, 87, 19 Cal.Rptr.2d 494, 851 P.2d 776, we determined that a wife whose ovum was fertilized in vitro by her husband's sperm and implanted in a surrogate mother was the "natural mother" of the child thus produced. We noted that the UPA [Uniform Parentage Act] states that provisions applicable to determining a father and child relationship shall be used to determine a mother and child relationship "insofar as practicable." . . . We relied, therefore, on the provisions in the UPA regarding presumptions of paternity and concluded that "genetic consanguinity" could be the basis for a finding of maternity just as it is for paternity . . . Under this authority, K.M.'s genetic relationship to the children in the present case constitutes "evidence of a mother and child relationship as contemplated by the Act . . .

The Court of Appeal in the present case concluded, however, that K.M. was not a parent of the twins, despite her genetic relationship to them, because she had the same status as a sperm donor. Section 7613(b) states: "The donor of semen provided to a licensed physician and surgeon for use in artificial insemination of a woman other than the donor's wife is treated in law as if he were not the natural father of a child thereby conceived." In *Johnson*, . . . we observed that "in a true 'egg donation' situation, where a woman gestates and gives birth to a child formed from the egg of another woman with the intent to raise the child as her own, the birth mother is the natural mother under California law." We held that the statute did not apply under the circumstances in *Johnson*, because the husband and wife in

Johnson did not intend to "donate" their sperm and ova to the surrogate mother, but rather "intended to procreate a child genetically related to them by the only available means."

The circumstances of the present case are not identical to those in *Johnson*, but they are similar in a crucial respect; both the couple in *Johnson* and the couple in the present case intended to produce a child that would be raised in their own home. In *Johnson*, it was clear that the married couple did not intend to "donate" their semen and ova to the surrogate mother, but rather permitted their semen and ova to be used to impregnate the surrogate mother in order to produce a child to be raised by them. In the present case, K.M. contends that she did not intend to donate her ova, but rather provided her ova so that E.G. could give birth to a child to be raised jointly by K.M. and E.G. E.G. hotly contests this, asserting that K.M. donated her ova to E.G., agreeing that E.G. would be the sole parent. It is undisputed, however, that the couple lived together and that they both intended to bring the child into their joint home. Thus, even accepting as true E.G.'s version of the facts (which the superior court did), the present case, like *Johnson*, does not present a "true 'egg donation' " situation. K.M. did not intend to simply donate her ova to E.G., but rather provided her ova to her lesbian partner with whom she was living so that E.G. could give birth to a child that would be raised in their joint home. Even if we assume that the provisions of section 7613(b) apply to women who donate ova, the statute does not apply under the circumstances of the present case . . .

We are faced with a . . . compelling situation, because K.M. and E.G. were more than "friends" when K.M. provided her ova, through a physician, to be used to impregnate E.G.; they lived together and were registered domestic partners. Although the parties dispute whether both women were intended to be parents of the resulting child, it is undisputed that they intended that the resulting child would be raised in their joint home. Neither the Model UPA, nor section 7613(b) was intended to apply under such circumstances . . .

K.M.'s genetic relationship with the twins constitutes evidence of a mother and child relationship under the UPA . . . and . . . section 7613(b) does not apply to exclude K.M. as a parent of the twins. The circumstance that E.G. gave birth to the twins also constitutes evidence of a mother and child relationship. Thus, both K.M. and E.G. are mothers of the twins under the UPA.

It is true we said in *Johnson* that "for any child California law recognizes only one natural mother." But as we explain in the companion case of *Elisa B. v. Superior Court, supra*, 37 Cal.4th 108, 119, 33 Cal.Rptr.3d at 53, 117 P.3d at 666-667, this statement in *Johnson* must be understood in light of the issue presented in that case; "our decision in *Johnson* does not preclude a child from having two parents both of whom are women." . . .

[A] child can have two mothers. Thus, this case differs from *Johnson* in that both K.M. and E.G. can be the children's mothers. Unlike in *Johnson*, their parental claims are not mutually exclusive. K.M. acknowledges that E.G. is the twins' mother. K.M. does not claim to be the twins' mother *instead of* E.G., but *in addition to* E.G., so we need not consider their intent in order to decide between them. Rather, the parentage of the twins is determined by application of the UPA. E.G. is the twins' mother because she gave birth to them and K.M. also is the twins' mother because she provided the ova from which they were produced . . .

The superior court in the present case found that K.M. signed a waiver form, thereby "relinquishing and waiving all rights to claim legal parentage of any children who might result." But such a waiver does not affect our determination of parentage. Section 7632 provides: "Regardless of its terms, an agreement between an alleged or presumed father and the mother or child does not bar an action under this chapter." (See *In re Marriage of Buzzanca, supra*, 61 Cal.App.4th 1410, 1426, 72 Cal.Rptr.2d 280 ["It is well established that parents cannot, by agreement, limit or abrogate a child's right to support." A woman who supplies ova to be used to impregnate her lesbian partner, with the understanding that the resulting child will be raised in their joint home, cannot waive her responsibility to support that child. Nor can such a purported waiver effectively cause that woman to relinquish her parental rights.

In light of our conclusion that section 7613(b) does not apply and that K.M. is the twins' parent (together with E.G.), based upon K.M.'s genetic relationship to the twins, we need not, and do not, consider whether K.M. is presumed to be a parent of the twins under section 7611, subdivision (d), which provides that a man is presumed to be a child's father if "[h]e receives the child into his home and openly holds out the child as his natural child."

DISPOSITION

The judgment of the Court of Appeal is reversed.

GEORGE, C.J., BAXTER and CHIN, JJ, concur.

Dissenting Opinion by KENNARD, J.

Unlike the majority, I would apply the controlling statutes as written. The statutory scheme for determining parentage contains two provisions that resolve K.M.'s claim to be a parent of the twins born to E.G. Under one provision, a man who donates sperm for physician-assisted artificial insemination of a woman to whom he is not married is not the father of the resulting child. (Fam.Code, § 7613, subd. (b).) Under the other provision, rules for determining fatherhood are to be used for determining motherhood "[i]nsofar as practical." (*Id.*, § 7650.) Because K.M. donated her ova for physician-assisted artificial insemination and implantation in another woman, and knowingly and voluntarily signed a document declaring her intention *not* to become a parent of any resulting children, she is not a parent of the twins . . .

Here it is "practicable" to treat a woman who donates ova to a licensed physician for in vitro fertilization and implantation in another woman, in the same fashion as a man who donates sperm to a licensed physician for artificial insemination of a woman to whom he is not married. Treating male and female donors alike is not only practicable, but it is also consistent with the trial court's factual finding here that K.M. intended "to donate ova to E.G." so that E.G. would be the sole mother of a child born to her . . .

The majority's desire to give the twins a second parent is understandable and laudable. To achieve that worthy goal, however, the majority must rewrite a statute and disregard the intentions that the parties expressed when the twins were conceived. The majority amends the sperm-donor statute by inserting a new provision making a sperm donor the legal father of a child born to a woman artificially inseminated with his sperm whenever the sperm donor and the birth mother *"intended that the resulting child would be raised in their joint home,"* even though both the donor and birth mother also intended that the donor *not* be the child's father. Finding nothing in the statutory language or history to support this construction, I reject it. Relying on the plain meaning of the statutory language, and the trial court's findings that both K.M. and E.G. intended that E.G. would be the only parent of any children resulting from the artificial insemination, I would affirm the judgment of the Court of Appeal, which in turn affirmed the trial court, rejecting K.M.'s claim to parentage of the twins born to E.G.

Dissenting Opinion by WERDEGAR, J.

The majority determines that the twins who developed from the ova K.M. donated to E.G. have two mothers rather than one. While I disagree, as I shall explain, with that ultimate conclusion, I agree with the majority's premise that a child can have two mothers . . .

I cannot agree with the majority that the children in this case do in fact have two mothers. Until today, when one woman has provided the ova and another has given birth, the established rule for determining disputed claims to motherhood was clear: we looked to the intent of the parties. "[I]n a true 'egg donation' situation, where a woman gestates and gives birth to a child formed from the egg of another woman with the intent to raise the child as her own, the birth mother is the natural mother under California law." (*Johnson, supra,* 5 Cal.4th 84, 93, fn. 10, 19 Cal.Rptr.2d 494, 851 P.2d 776.) . . .

[T]o apply *Johnson's* intent test to the facts of this case necessarily leads to the conclusion that E.G. is a mother and K.M. is not. That E.G. intended to become the mother — and the only mother — of the children to whom she gave birth is unquestioned. Whether K.M. for her part also intended to become the children's mother was disputed, but the trial court found on the basis of conflicting evidence that she did not. We must defer to the trial court's findings on this point because substantial evidence supports them. K.M. represented in connection with the ovum donation process, both orally and in writing, that she did not intend to become the children's mother, and consistently with those representations subsequently held the children out to the world as E.G.'s but not her own. Thus constrained by the facts, the majority can justify its conclusion that K.M. is also the children's mother only by changing the law . . .

Perhaps the best way to understand today's decision is that we appear to be moving in cases of assisted reproduction from a categorical determination of parentage based on formal, preconception manifestations of intent to a case-by-case approach implicitly motivated at least in part by our intuitions about the children's best interests. We expressly eschewed a best interests approach in *Johnson, supra,* 5 Cal.4th 84, 19 Cal.Rptr.2d 494, 851 P.2d 776, explaining that it "raises the repugnant specter of governmental interference in matters implicating our most fundamental notions of privacy, and confuses concepts of parentage and custody." (*Id.*, at p. 93, fn. 10, 19 Cal.Rptr.2d 494, 851 P.2d 776.) This case, in which the majority compels E.G. to accept K.M. as an unintended parent to E.G.'s children, in part because of E.G.'s and K.M.'s sexual orientation and the character of their private relationship, shows that *Johnson's* warning was prescient. Only legislation defining parentage in the context of assisted reproduction is likely to restore predictability and prevent further lapses into the disorder of ad hoc adjudication.

NOTES AND QUESTIONS

1.   This case is a cautionary tale about the role of intent in ART parentage disputes. The egg "donor," K.M., argues that she intended to be a parent to any offspring born by her then-partner, E.G., and therefore should be considered the girls' mother. Further, she explains that initially she believed she did not have to adopt the girls because she was their genetic, and therefore their legal, mother. Only when her relationship with E.G. turned south did she begin to contemplate a formal adoption to solidify her rights. The birth mother, E.G., argues it was the couple's intent that she serve as the sole parent, a sentiment backed up by the egg donor agreement, which contained language waiving the egg donor's parental rights to any child born of the donation. Notice that the majority and dissenting opinions express very different views on the parties' intent, views that are at the heart of each jurists' holding.

The question arises: When and how should intent be measured? If K.M. did not intend to legally parent the children at the time of her donation, should she be held to that intent? If she changes her mind, should her initial expression of intent govern? Should the best interest of the child standard be used to determine parentage, regardless of prior expressions of intent? Or should parentage be established by agreement of the parties, regardless of statutory presumptions detailing who is a legal parent?

These questions arose when a lesbian couple separated and disputed the parental rights toward a child born during their relationship. One woman conceived the child through donor insemination. Before the birth, the partners obtained a pre-birth order indicating both women would be the child's mothers. In addition, the birth certificate reflected their joint parental status. The couple split two years later, at which point the birth mother challenged the very pre-birth order she had sought, arguing the court lacked jurisdiction to determine parentage based on the parties' agreement. In a companion case to *K.M. v. E.G.*, the California Supreme Court disagreed, holding that the biological mother was estopped from attacking the validity of a judgment to which she had stipulated. *Kristine H. v. Lisa R.*, 37 Cal. 4th 156, 33 Cal. Rptr. 3d 81, 117 P.3d 690 (2005).

Justice Moreno, who authored the decisions in *K.M.* and *Kristine H.*, seems to take a different view of the impact signed pre-birth pledges have on later challenges to parenthood. Both cases involve plaintiffs trying to disavow legal documents each signed agreeing to future parental rights (or lack thereof). In *Kristine H.*, Justice Moreno holds the birth mother to a stipulation of joint parental rights that she and her then partner procured during Kristine's pregnancy. In *K.M.*, he disregards the plain language of the egg donor contract that K.M. signed, waiving all rights to any resulting child. Are these decisions, issued on the same day, consistent? Perhaps the answer lies in how well the parties understood the legal baggage each was agreeing to carry. Do you think the plaintiffs had an equally good understanding of the document each signed? In *Kristine H.*, a pregnant woman asked a court to name her female partner as a co-parent to her unborn child. Intentionality seems clear.

In *K.M.*, the egg donor is presented with a lengthy and technical legal document prior to undergoing a surgical procedure to retrieve her eggs. She claims the document provided her inadequate notice of the fact she was surrendering her parental rights. Have you ever signed a contract without fully reading every word? Are you at all sympathetic to the idea that K.M. likely did not read the egg donation contract, and did not intend to sign away her parental rights at the time of her donation? One scholar argues that fertility clinics do a disservice when they present their patients with a single legal document, often entitled "Consent Form," that combines an acknowledgment of informed consent for treatment with a directive for the disposition of eggs and embryos. Patients undergoing fertility treatment, including aspiration of eggs for donation, are largely focused on the risks from the procedure, and will not necessarily focus on the other major portion of the long document — the language regarding legal rights to any resulting offspring. In fact, there is ample evidence that patients often sign such documents with little or no appreciation of their content. See Ellen A. Waldman, *Disputing Over Embryos: Of Contract and Consents*, 32 ARIZ. ST. L. J. 897 (2000) (suggesting that patients receive separate documents pertaining to informed consent and disposition of frozen or unused embryos).

Postscript. The reasoning and holding in *K.M.* was adopted by a Florida court presented with a similar fact scenario. Lesbian partners had a child when one woman supplied the eggs and the other gestated the embryo in their shared reproductive plan. After the couple broke up, the birth mother argued that state law denies any parental rights to gamete donors, and that the ex-partner had waived her parental rights when she signed the standard egg donation form at the fertility clinic. The court disagreed, finding that the consent form did not serve as a waiver of parental rights and that existing state law requiring egg donors to relinquish all maternal rights to a resulting child violate the genetic mother's constitutionally protected parental rights to the child. *T.M.H.* v. *D.M.T.*, 2011 WL 6437247 (Fla. App. 5 Dist.).

2. *Second-Parent Adoptions.* The legal dispute in *K.M. v. E.G.* could have been avoided if K.M. formally adopted the girls after their birth. Perhaps the couple investigated the law surrounding second-parent adoption in California and found it far from settled. In fact, it was not until after the parties filed their petitions with the court that the law on second-parent adoption was clarified in the state. In *Sharon S. v. Superior Court*, 31 Cal. 4th 417, 2 Cal. Rptr. 3d 699, 73 P.3d 554 (2003), the California Supreme Court held that second-parent adoptions are valid under the state's independent adoption laws, and that a birth parent need not relinquish parental rights in order for the adoption to proceed.

The need for second-parent adoption by the nonbiologic parent in a same-sex couple depends upon the legal status accorded that couple under state law. In the (as of early 2012) seven jurisdictions that recognize same-sex marriage, no adoption is required if the child is born during the marriage. In other states, civil union or domestic partner laws may likewise permit a child born of the recognized relationship to be considered the child of both partners, regardless of any genetic tie to the nonbiologic parent. For example, the California Domestic Partnership law, codified in Family Code Section 297.5(d), provides: "The rights and obligations of registered domestic partners with respect to a child of either of them shall be the same as those of spouses. The rights and obligations of former or surviving registered domestic partners with respect to a child of either of them shall be the same as those of former or surviving spouses." Essentially, this means that second-parent adoptions by registered domestic partners are not necessary, as a second parent will automatically be a legal parent if the child is born while the domestic partnership is in effect.

3.   *Conflict of Law Issues.* Holly and Cheri live in Vermont before the state recognized same-sex marriage. In 1998 the couple adopted a son born in Mississippi. The family lived in Vermont, but Holly and Cheri wanted to obtain an amended copy of their son's birth certificate from the State of Mississippi, reflecting that the women were his legal parents. When a clerk at the Mississippi Bureau of Health Statistics noticed that both parents' names were female, the birth certificate issuance was halted. With the aid of Lambda Legal Defense and Education Fund, an advocacy group for gay and lesbian individuals, Holly and Cheri sued the Bureau to issue a birth certificate naming both women as their child's parents. A judge ruled in the couple's favor, reasoning that nothing in the state's law required two parents to be of different sexes. *See* Anne Wallace Allen, *Lesbian Couple Prevails in Mississippi Adoption Suit*, SUN HERALD, Mar. 20, 2003, at 8. Mississippi has since outlawed adoption by gay couples. See Miss. Code Ann. § 93-17-3 ("adoption by couples of the same gender is prohibited").

Holly and Cheri's story reminds same-sex couples that the shifting and varying state of the law across our country may mean a parentage judgment in one state will not necessarily be honored in another state. As states diverge on questions of gay adoption, same-sex marriage, and second-parent adoption, couples are advised to familiarize themselves with their own state's law, as well as laws in a state they may someday call home. For a thorough discussion of conflict of law concerns in same-sex family structures, *see* Deborah L. Forman, *Interstate Recognition of Same-Sex Parents in the Wake of Gay Marriage, Civil Unions and Domestic Partnerships*, 46 B.C.L. REV. 1 (2005).

SECTION V: MISHAPS IN THE LABORATORY: THE CHILDREN OF ART GAMETE MIX-UPS

A.   Defining the Problem

The children of reproductive technologies often begin their lives in a laboratory, after a successful mixing of sperm and eggs. The location of conception outside the female body may raise questions about the "naturalness" of assisted reproduction,[18] but a more practical concern centers on the opportunities for mishaps — human errors in which eggs, sperm or embryos reach an unintended destination. Mishaps can arise from negligence or intentional conduct. The consequences of such mistakes can result in a woman's egg being paired with the wrong sperm, or vice versa, with the resulting embryo gestated by an unknowing mother-to-be. Human error can lead to one couple's embryo being mistakenly implanted into another woman's uterus. Once children are born of human errors involving gametes, disputes abound as to the rightful parentage of these offspring.

The most notorious tale of laboratory malfeasance occurred in Orange County, California in the mid-1990s. On May 16, 1995, the University of California at Irvine (UCI) filed a lawsuit against the three physician directors of its prestigious and lucrative Center for Reproductive Health, alleging various improprieties in the research conducted at the fertility clinic. In the weeks following this first public disclosure of possible malfeasance at the facility, allegations against the three physician directors were dramatically expanded to include misappropriation of patient eggs and embryos. In essence, the doctors were accused of taking eggs and embryos that had been retrieved from patients and implanting them into other patients without either woman's knowledge or consent. The UCI clinic was promptly closed, but subsequent lawsuits and investigations revealed that at least 15 children were born of these illicit transfers, some thought to be from the embryos of couples who were unsuccessful in their own efforts to reproduce. The "egg scandal" engendered more than 100 lawsuits, costing California taxpayers $24 million to cover the costs of settlements with the injured couples. *See* Kimi Yoshino, *UCI Settles Dozens of Fertility Suits*, L.A. TIMES, Sept. 11, 2009, available at: http://articles.latimes.com/2009/sep/11/local/me-uci-fertility11.

In all likelihood, the affected parties will never know exactly what happened during the nine years that the UCI fertility clinic operated because two of the physicians fled the country when the allegations began to unfold. Dr. Ricardo Asch, a revered pioneer in the infertility field, fled to his native Mexico City where he is said to be directing a fertility clinic. Dr. Jose Balmaceda took refuge in Chile, his country of origin, and likewise continues to offer reproductive medical services. The third physician, Dr. Sergio Stone, remained in his native United States and was convicted of federal charges of mail fraud, stemming from his practice of fraudulently billing insurance companies. He was sentenced to four years' probation and fined $71,000, while his co-conspirators, thought to be the actual perpetrators of the egg theft, remain at large, the subject of federal criminal indictments. The scandal spawned numerous reports and commentaries, ultimately yielding two reporters from the local Orange County Register a Pulitzer Prize in 1996. You can read about the events in *Stealing Dreams: A Fertility Clinic Scandal* by Mary Dodge and Gilbert Geis (Northeastern University Press 2004).

Inevitably the courts were called upon to resolve disputes between the parents who gave birth to the children, fully believing them to be their genetic offspring, and

---

[18] Such concerns have been raised by the President's Council on Bioethics. In their 2004 report, the Council warned that human manipulation of the early stages of human life diminish regard for the "naturalness" and awe-inspiring power of the procreative process. The President's Council on Bioethics, Reproduction and Responsibility: The Regulation of New Biotechnologies 18 (March 2004).

the couples whose embryos were misappropriated for reasons that remain a mystery. Only one case reached the appellate level, though at least two others were filed by couples who believed themselves to be the genetic parents of another family's children. Both sides' anguish seems palpable in the case that follows.

B. Judicial Perspectives on Gamete Mix-Ups

1. The Case of Physician Malfeasance

PRATO-MORRISON v. DOE

California Court of Appeal, Second District
103 Cal. App. 4th 222, 126 Cal. Rptr. 2d 509 (2002)

VOGEL, J. Donna Prato-Morrison and Robert Morrison engaged the services of a fertility clinic, to no avail, and ultimately abandoned their efforts to conceive, believing their unused genetic materials would be destroyed. When the clinic later became the target of an investigation into its widespread misuse of genetic materials, the Morrisons (along with many others) sued the clinic and later settled their claims for an undisclosed amount of money. The Morrisons, "wondering whether [they have] a genetic child or children in the world," then embarked on a campaign to intrude into the lives of another fertility clinic family (Judith and Jacob Doe) who might have innocently received Donna Morrison's genetic material. The Morrisons filed a complaint in which they asked the court to determine whether they are the genetic parents of the Does' twin daughters (now almost 14 years old) and, if so, to grant custody of the children (who know nothing about this claim and who have no reason to question their parentage) to the Morrisons. Although the Morrisons later withdrew their request for custody, they continued their efforts to compel blood tests and obtain the right to visit the twins.

The Does sought protective orders and moved to quash the Morrisons' complaint. When the Morrisons were unable to present any admissible evidence to establish a connection between their genetic material and the fertility services received by the Does, the trial court granted the Does' motion to quash and dismissed the Morrisons' complaint. The Morrisons appeal, claiming the trial court should have either admitted their inadmissible evidence or otherwise concluded that the Morrisons' curiosity justified a further intrusion into the Does' lives. We reject the Morrisons' claims and affirm. We hold that the Morrisons' evidence was properly excluded, and that they have not shown any link at all to the Does' daughters. We also hold that, assuming a genetic connection between the Morrisons and the twins, the best interests of the children dictate the result reached by the trial court.

Facts

A.

In 1988, Donna Prato-Morrison and Robert Morrison were fertility clinic patients of the Center for Reproductive Health (CRH) at the University of California at Irvine (UCI). As part of the *in vitro* fertilization process, the

Morrisons' eggs and sperm were entrusted to CRH with the intent that the resulting embryos would produce the child they hoped to conceive. No pregnancy was achieved and the Morrisons ultimately abandoned their efforts on the assumption that any remaining genetic material would be destroyed by CRH.

B.

In the mid-1990s, UCI learned there had been medical and other improprieties at CRH. An investigation ensued, and findings were made that "egg stealing" had occurred — "human eggs were taken from one patient and implanted in another without the consent of the donor." (*Stone v. Regents of University of California* (1999) 77 Cal.App.4th 736, 740 [92 Cal.Rptr.2d 94].) The Morrisons (and many others) sued CRH, UCI, and the doctors involved in the "egg stealing." The Morrisons' case was settled by the payment of money — but only after the Morrisons learned through the discovery process that their genetic material might not have been destroyed, that Judith and Jacob Doe (who were also patients of the CRH fertility clinic) *might have* (without the Does' knowledge) received the Morrisons' eggs, sperm, or embryos, and that (in December 1988) Judith Doe had given birth to twin daughters, Ida and Rose. The Morrisons claim they are the twins' genetic parents.

C.

In 1996, the Morrisons filed a "complaint to establish parental relationship," naming the Does as defendants, alleging that the Morrisons are the "biological and legal parents" of the twins, and asking for custody, visitation rights, and an award of attorney's fees. Between 1996 and 1999, the Morrisons attempted to obtain blood tests and DNA samples from the twins but the Does refused to provide them and these "negotiations" ultimately failed.

In 1999, the Morrisons filed an amended complaint in which they abandoned their quest for custody but reasserted their demands for blood tests and for visitation. At the Morrisons' request, a hearing was set to determine the Morrisons' right (1) to obtain DNA tests and (2) to have a mental health professional appointed to help determine "the commencement, frequency, degree of contact or visitation" the Morrisons should have with the twins . . .[19]

---

[19] [n.1] In a declaration filed in October 1999, the Does' lawyer told the court the Morrisons are both employed as sheriff's deputies in Northern California; that the Morrisons' lawyer had told him that the Morrisons had engaged private investigators to locate and investigate the Does and their family, to engage in "surveillance" of the Does and the twins, to photograph the twins, and to obtain private information about the Does' home, their treatment of the twins, and the details of the twins' "home and school situations." According to the Does' lawyer, his conversations with the Morrisons' lawyer "were punctuated by thinly veiled threats that [the Morrisons] would reveal their claims to [the twins] . . . even if their parents opposed such disclosures. The message was clear that if [the Does] were unwilling to introduce [the Morrisons] into the children's lives, that the litigation process would inevitably bring the matter to the children's attention. [¶] . . . [¶] My conversations with [the Morrisons' lawyer] led me to believe that [Donna Morrison] is obsessed with the notion that [the Does' children] are 'theirs,' and that she [is] willing and able to contact the children directly." *The Morrisons have never suggested that this description of their conduct is false or exaggerated.*

In April 2000, the Does asked the trial court (1) to seal the records of this case; (2) to issue protective orders "to ensure the privacy of the children in this potentially high-profile litigation, and to preclude deliberate or accidental disclosure of the existence of this litigation and the [Morrisons'] claims . . . to the children"; and (3) to quash the Morrisons' petition on the grounds (among others) that (a) the Does are the "presumed natural and legal parents" of the twins, and (b) the Morrisons lacked standing to pursue a parentage action or to compel blood or DNA testing . . .

In support of their motions, the Does submitted declarations establishing that since 1983 they have lived together continuously as husband and wife, that in addition to the twins they have two older children . . . , and that the twins were conceived because the Does had "actively tried to conceive with medical assistance, intending to use Jacob's sperm and anonymously and voluntarily donated ova." Judith Doe "became pregnant by [her] husband," gave birth to the twins, and remains a "full time mother." . . . When Judith Doe gave birth to the twins, the Does "knowingly and joyously received the twins into [their] home and family. [They] have adored [the twins and have] reared them in [the Does'] culture and religion . . ." The Does "are the only parents that Ida and Rose have ever known." The Does objected to the release of any medical information to the Morrisons, pointed out that the Morrisons' claims had caused "great emotional stress" to the Does, and said the introduction of the Morrisons into the Does "family life would be a monstrous intrusion."

In opposition to the Does' motion to quash, the Morrisons claimed they had standing to pursue this action because Donna Morrison is "a genetic mother." To prove this point, the Morrisons submitted a copy of a 1996 letter from UCI to the Morrisons and a copy of an unauthenticated "redacted copy" of one handwritten page of "the seven page Teri Ord donor/recipient list in which" Donna Morrison's name appeared . . . The Does objected to the Morrisons' "evidence," pointing out that the unauthenticated list contained privileged information and did not connect the Morrisons to the Does or to anyone, genetically or otherwise.

D.

At a hearing held in June 2000, the family law court sustained the Does' objections to the Morrison's evidence and found that the Morrisons had failed to establish their status as "interested parties" entitled to pursue a parentage action. The court nevertheless continued the matter to afford the Morrisons an opportunity to present additional evidence.

As "additional evidence," the Morrisons submitted an unredacted copy of the handwritten list and a declaration from Teri Ord — who stated that she was employed from 1986 through and including 1988 by AMI Medical Center as an "I[n] V[itro] F[ertilization] Biologist" in charge of "the embryology lab at that facility." In that capacity, she states, she "participated" in "transfers of genetic materials obtained by the doctors [at UCI] from fertility patients. [¶] According to laboratory records, Donna [Morrison] was an infertility patient at AMI . . . between March and May 1988, as was [Judith Doe]." Ord stated that, based on information contained in other clinical and laboratory records, she prepared the handwritten document in *1995* to show that, "between March and May of *1988*, patient '[Judith Doe]' received sixteen eggs from patient '[Donna Morrison].' Twenty-one eggs were extracted from [Donna Morrison], and five transferred into [Donna Morrison's] own fallopian tubes. The remaining sixteen were transferred to [Judith Doe]," and the notations next to Judith Doe's name show that "a twin pregnancy resulted." (Italics added.) . . .

The Does objected to Ord's declaration and compilation as hearsay, and on the ground that it violated the Does' physician-patient privilege and their right to reproductive privacy. In October 2000, the family law court sustained the Does' evidentiary objections and granted their motion to quash. In April 2001, the court dismissed the Morrisons' action. The Morrisons appeal from the order of dismissal.

Discussion

I.

(1a) The Morrisons contend their evidence is sufficient to establish Donna Morrison's status as the genetic mother and, therefore, her standing to pursue a parentage action. We disagree.

(2) "Any interested person may bring an action to determine the existence or nonexistence of a mother and child relationship" (§ 7650), but an unrelated person who is not a genetic parent is not an "interested person" within the meaning of section 7650 . . . The threshold question, therefore, is whether Ord's declaration and handwritten list were properly excluded by the trial court. If so, there is no evidence at all to suggest that Donna Morrison is the twins' genetic mother, or that either of the Morrisons is otherwise related to the twins.

The declaration and list were properly excluded as inadmissible hearsay that does not satisfy the requirements of the business records exception to the hearsay rule. As Ord concedes in her declaration, the list was compiled from other, non-identified clinical and laboratory records, and she does not attempt to establish her personal knowledge of the information stated on her list . . . She does not say she was a percipient witness to the transfers of genetic material, or that she made the entries in the original records. She admits the list was not made at or near the time of the events it purports to describe, but was in fact made almost eight years later. She offers no clue as to *why* the list was made. By Ord's own admission, her sources of information and method and time of preparation show a lack of trustworthiness and defeat the Morrisons' contention that the list comes within the business records exception to the hearsay rule . . . Since Ord's declaration and list were properly excluded and since there is no other evidence suggesting a genetic link between the Morrisons and the Does' twins, the Morrisons had no standing to pursue their parentage action.

II.

(3) The Morrisons contend they should be allowed to "discover" whether the twins were born "as a result of the theft of their genetic materials," and that their

rights as alleged biological parents ought to trump the Does' rights as presumed parents. We disagree.

The Morrisons' "rights" were vindicated when they accepted an undisclosed amount of money to resolve their lawsuit against CRH, UCI, and the individuals involved in the misuse of the Morrisons' genetic materials. The rights still at issue are not the Morrisons' rights. They are the rights of the Does and their twins to be free from the interference of strangers who have no standing to pursue their demands for blood tests or visitation rights, and the Morrisons cannot alter the focus of this issue by characterizing the Does' rights as mere privacy interests that may, under appropriate circumstances, give way to greater rights . . .

(4) The trial court found, and we agree, that the dismissal of this action is in the best interests of the children. More to the point, we conclude that, had the Morrisons presented proof of a genetic link to the twins sufficient to establish their standing to pursue a parentage action, it would not be in the best interests of the twins to have the Morrisons intrude into their lives, or to be subjected to the blood tests and "mental health" evaluation suggested by the Morrisons. Because the twins are now almost 14 years old, their relationship with their presumed parents is considerably more palpable than the possibility of a new relationship with a previously unknown biological parent, and the Morrisons will not be allowed to disrupt the Does' "family in order to satisfy the [alleged] biological [parents'] unilateral desire, however strong, to turn their genetic connection into a personal relationship." . . .

Simply put, the social relationship established by the Does and their daughters is more important to the children than a genetic relationship with a stranger.[20]

Disposition

The order of dismissal is affirmed. The Does are awarded their costs of appeal.

SPENCER, P. J., and ORTEGA, J., concurred.

NOTES AND QUESTIONS

1. The *Prato-Morrison* court offers both a procedural and a substantive rationale for denying the plaintiffs' request to discover whether they have a genetic tie to the defendants' twin daughters. First, the court excludes as hearsay a written record compiled by Teri Ord, the fertility clinic's biologist in charge of the embryology lab. The record, produced in 1995, documents that the Morrison eggs were implanted in Mrs. Doe in 1988. The court questions the veracity of the document because it was compiled seven years after the alleged events. Why do you

---

[20] [n.10] We join the chorus of judicial voices pleading for legislative attention to the increasing number of complex legal issues spawned by recent advances in the field of artificial reproduction. Whatever merit there may be to a fact-driven case-by-case resolution of each new issue, some overall legislative guidelines would allow the participants to make informed choices and the courts to strive for uniformity in their decisions. (*In re Marriage of Buzzanca* (1998) 61 Cal.App.4th 1410, 1428-1429 [72 Cal.Rptr.2d 280, 77 A.L.R.5th 775]; *Johnson v. Calvert*, 5 Cal.4th at p. 101.)

think Teri Ord compiled the document in 1995?

The court also declares it in the children's best interest not to be subjected to testing to learn their true genetic identity. Do you agree with the court's conclusion that these teenage girls are better off not knowing that their parents may not be their genetic ancestors? Can you imagine a scenario where revealing the genetic truth would be in the children's best interest? What if one of the girls was in need of a kidney or a stem cell transplant to save her life. Do you think the court would have excluded the Teri Ord written record showing a possible link to the Morrisons if the Does had been the ones requesting genetic testing? What if the Morrisons had refused to be tested, saying their own disappointment in not having children will only be renewed if they are forced to interact with the Doe family? See *McFall v. Shimp*, 10 Pa. D. & C.3d 90 (1978) (court refused to compel cousin to submit to testing for bone marrow compatibility with relative); *In re Geroge*, 630 S.W.2d 614 (Mo. Ct. App. 1982) (court refused to open adoption records for leukemia patient after natural father refused to be tested).

2.   Was the court's decision based on the age of the twins? If the switched eggs had been discovered when Mrs. Doe was pregnant, would the result have been to deny the Morrisons any rights to learn the genetic identity of the girls?

3.   The court suggests that any damage the Morrisons suffered was addressed by the damage award they received from UCI and the Center for Reproductive Health. Do you agree? What other methods of injury compensation could be used to address the harms in a case such as this one?

4.   The court is sympathetic to the privacy needs of the Does and their girls, perhaps because they are viewed as innocent victims of the physicians' nefarious deeds. But aren't the Morrisons equally innocent victims in this case? Does the court portray the Morrisons as equal victims of the egg scandal?

Suppose the Does were not so innocent, and had orchestrated to steal Mrs. Morrison's eggs because they were told she had high-quality eggs that were likely to implant. If the Does' theft was discovered years later, when the girls were teenagers, would the court deny the Morrisons any right to discover the genetic identity of the girls? What if the theft was discovered when Mrs. Doe was still pregnant?

Proximity of the mix-up discovery to the birth of a child may play a role in swaying a court's decision, as this next case demonstrates.

2. Cases of Physician Negligence

ROBERT B. v. SUSAN B.
California Court of Appeal, Sixth District
109 Cal. App.4th 1109, 135 Cal. Rptr. 2d 785 (2003)

ELIA, J. At the center of this parentage action is two-year-old Daniel B., who was born to appellant Susan B., a single woman, after a fertility clinic implanted embryos belonging to Robert and Denise B. into Susan. The trial court ruled that Susan is Daniel's mother and Robert is his father. Denise was dismissed for lack of standing.

Both Susan and Denise appeal. Susan contends that the court erred by failing to apply Family Code section 7613, subdivision (b) to preclude Robert's paternity claim. Denise contends that the court improperly dismissed her because she had standing as an "interested person" under section 7650. We find no error and affirm the judgment.

Background

In May 2000 respondents Robert and Denise B. contracted with an anonymous ovum donor to obtain the donor's eggs for fertilization with Robert's sperm. The contract reflected the intent of the contracting parties that Robert and Denise would be the parents of any children produced from the resulting embryos.

Meanwhile, Susan went to the same fertility clinic with the intent of purchasing genetic material from "two strangers who would contractually sign away their rights" so that "there would be no paternity case against her, ever." She therefore contracted with the clinic for an embryo created from anonymously donated ova and sperm.

About 13 embryos were produced for Robert and Denise. In June 2000 some of them were implanted in Denise's uterus. Through an apparent clinic error, Susan received three of these embryos. When she became pregnant, Susan believed that the child she was carrying was the result of the anonymous donation procedure for which she had contracted. In February 2001, ten days apart, Susan gave birth to Daniel and Denise gave birth to Daniel's genetic sister, Madeline.

In December 2001 the fertility physician informed Robert and Denise that "a mistake had occurred," in that the clinic had "inadvertently" implanted some of Robert and Denise's embryos in Susan's uterus, resulting in Daniel's birth. Robert and Denise promptly sought contact with Daniel. Susan was initially receptive, but after the three adults and two children met, she refused to relinquish custody, and Robert and Denise brought this parentage action.

Over Susan's opposition the trial court determined that Robert had standing to bring a paternity action under section 7630, subdivision (c), and it ordered genetic testing. After receiving the test results, the court declared Robert to be the father of Daniel.

The court next took up the question of Denise's standing . . . The court . . .

dismissed Denise with prejudice. The court noted that Susan was the gestational mother and that Denise had no genetic connection with Daniel, and it concluded that "there really is only one mother in this case at this point." Any contractual rights Denise had were to embryos, "but now what we're talking about is a live person, not an embryo." The court then proceeded to hear the issues regarding custody and visitation. Temporary custody was awarded to Susan, with temporary visitation to Robert.

Discussion

1. *Susan's Appeal*

On appeal, Susan challenges the court's paternity order. Seeking a liberal construction of section 7613, subdivision (b) (section 7613(b)), Susan contends that Robert must be deemed a sperm donor in order to protect "the integrity of [her] single parent family unit." Any other result, she argues, would contravene the Legislature's intent to preserve the "procreative rights of unmarried women," unfairly burden her with a situation she had done her best to prevent, and impair "Daniel's established constitutional right to maintain a stable, permanent placement." . . .

We need not go beyond the language of section 7613(b) to resolve Susan's claim. This provision states: "The donor of semen provided to a licensed physician and surgeon for use in artificial insemination of a woman other than the donor's wife is treated in law as if he were not the natural father of a child thereby conceived." As the trial court recognized, the plain meaning of the statutory language does not permit the application Susan urges. A "donor" is simply a person who gives, presents, or contributes. (Compact Edition of the Oxford Dict. (1971) p. 599, Col. 3; Amer. Heritage Dict. (3d ed.1997) p. 411.) In order to be a donor under section 7613(b) a man must provide semen to a physician for the purpose of artificially inseminating "a woman other than the donor's wife." It is uncontested that Robert did not provide his semen for the purpose of inseminating anyone other than Denise. On the contrary, the consent form he signed indicated that the unused embryos were to be frozen and stored "for the exclusive use" of him and Denise. Consequently, section 7613(b) is inapplicable in these circumstances . . .

2. *Denise's Appeal*

Denise contends that she should be accorded standing as an "interested person" within the meaning of Family Code section 7650. She seeks an opportunity to show that Susan colluded with the fertility clinic to obtain the embryo and/or that she herself is the "intended" mother of Daniel.

Section 7650 permits "[a]ny interested person [to] bring an action to determine the existence or nonexistence of a mother and child relationship. Insofar as practicable, the provisions of this part [the Uniform Parentage Act] applicable to the father and child relationship apply." On its face, this provision does not restrict the standing of alleged mothers to those who are genetically or gestationally related to the child.

Two appellate courts, however, have refused to recognize a biologically *unrelated* woman as an "interested person" under section 7650. Addressing a former lesbian partner's attempt to obtain recognition of her parental status for purposes of custody or visitation, the Third District stated: "Here, there is no . . . statutory standing. As a person unrelated to [the child], [the partner] is not an 'interested person' and, therefore, may not drag West [the genetic and gestational mother] into the courts, under the Uniform Parentage Act, on the issue of visitation with West's daughter." *West v. Superior Court* (1997) 59 Cal.App.4th 302, 306, 69 Cal.Rptr.2d 160.) . . . In *Prato-Morrison v. Doe* (2002) 103 Cal.App.4th 222, 126 Cal.Rptr.2d 509, a husband and wife suspected unauthorized use of their genetic material for another couple, who had used the same clinic and thus became the parents of twins. Responding to the plaintiff wife's assertion of standing, the appellate court quoted the "interested person" language of section 7650 and then added, "but an unrelated person who is not a genetic parent is not an 'interested person' within the meaning of section 7650." (*Id.* at p. 229, 126 Cal.Rptr.2d 509.) Because the wife was unable to offer admissible evidence of a genetic relationship to the twins (who were by then almost 14 years old), she had no standing to pursue a parentage action . . .

Denise's attempt to show that she was entitled to assert her own parental status as Daniel's *intended* mother must fail. The concept of "intended mother" is employed only as a tie-breaker when two women have equal claims by "genetic consanguinity" and childbirth. (*Johnson v. Calvert*, 5 Cal.4th at pp. 92-93, 19 Cal.Rptr.2d 494, 851 P.2d 776.) Thus, in *Johnson v. Calvert*, the Supreme Court explained that where Anna Johnson had agreed to bear the genetic child of the plaintiffs, both Johnson (the surrogate) and Crispina Calvert (the genetic mother) had equal claims. Because the child would not have existed but for the surrogacy agreement, the tie was broken in favor of Calvert, the intended mother under the contract. There is no tie here, however, because Denise has neither a gestational nor a genetic relationship to Daniel, whereas Susan does.[21]

. . . We must conclude, therefore, that the trial court properly declared Robert to be Daniel's father and Susan to be Daniel's mother under sections 7630 and 7610 respectively. The court's ruling comported with this state's interest "in establishing paternity for all children" (§ 7570), recognized the valid claims of gestational mothers, and adhered to the Supreme Court's determination that there can be only one natural mother under California law.

---

[21] [n.7] Moreover, even if we were to invoke the concept of intended mother here, which party would qualify? Both — and neither. Susan intended to be the mother of the child created from an embryo implanted in her uterus that day at the clinic — but not *that* embryo, not one belonging to someone else. Indeed, her intent was to obtain an embryo created entirely from the egg and sperm of anonymous donors. Denise intended to be the mother of the child created from this very embryo — but not at that time, and she did not intend for another woman to bear the child.

Disposition

The judgment is affirmed. The parties shall bear their own costs on appeal. We concur: RUSHING, P.J., and MIHARA, J.

NOTES AND QUESTIONS

1. Why did the court order genetic testing in *Robert B. v. Susan B.* but refuse to allow such testing in *Prato-Morrison v. Doe*?

2. *Postscript.* In 2004, Susan B. reached a $1 million settlement with the doctor who performed the IVF procedure in which she was given the wrong embryo. Part of her anger likely arose from the fact that she was not notified about the mix-up until a year after her son's birth, and even then *not* from her doctor, but from the Medical Board of California, which had been investigating the clinic where the procedure took place. In April 2005, the Medical Board revoked the responsible doctor's license, after testimony revealed that he had been informed by his embryologist of the mistaken implantation about 10 minutes after it happened. During his license revocation hearing, the doctor conceded that Susan's right to know that the wrong embryo had been implanted "trumped his anxiety over the harm disclosure would unleash." See Katherine Seligman, *License Revoked For Embryo Mix-Up*, S.F. CHRON., March 31, 2004, at B4.

3. Recall the facts in *Buzzanca v. Buzzanca*. A married couple contracts with an egg donor, a sperm donor and a gestational surrogate in order to have a child. After Jaycee Buzzanca is born, her parents' divorce and Mr. Buzzanca claims there are no children of the marriage since neither spouse bears a genetic or gestational relation to the child. The court declares husband and wife Jaycee's lawful parents because they consented to a medical procedure that they intended to result in the birth of a child. Is Robert's wife, Denise, akin to Mrs. Buzzanca? After all, she consented to a medical procedure (mixing of her husband's sperm with a donor egg) that she intended to result in the birth of a child? Or is *Buzzanca* distinguishable from the facts in *Robert B*?

What if Denise were the egg donor in this case? In all likelihood, she wanted to provide the eggs for her child, but her infertility prevented her from doing so. Does the holding in the case discriminate against the infertile? If the embryo mistakenly implanted in Susan B. bore a full genetic relationship to Robert and Denise, would the case be decided the same?

4. We are not told the race or ethnic origin of Robert, Denise or Susan. Would a difference in the race of the parties lead to a different result when the gametes are mistakenly switched? Consider the next case.

PERRY-ROGERS v. FASANO
Supreme Court of New York, Appellate Division, First Department
715 N.Y.S.2d 19 (2000)

SAXE, J.

This appeal concerns a tragic mix-up at a fertility clinic through which a woman became a "gestational mother" to another couple's embryo, when the embryo was mistakenly implanted into the wrong woman's uterus. Since a determination of the issues presented may have far-ranging consequences, we attempt here to ensure that our holding is appropriately limited.

FACTS

In April, 1998, plaintiffs Deborah Perry-Rogers and Robert Rogers began an in vitro fertilization and embryo transfer program with the In Vitro Fertility Center of New York. However, in the process, embryos consisting entirely of the Rogerses' genetic material were mistakenly implanted into the uterus of defendant Donna Fasano, along with embryos from Ms. Fasano's and her husband's genetic material. It is undisputed that on May 28, 1998 both couples were notified of the mistake and of the need for DNA and amniocentesis tests. The Rogerses further allege, and the Fasanos do not deny, that the Fasanos were unresponsive to the Rogerses' efforts to contact them.

On December 29, 1998, Donna Fasano gave birth to two male infants, of two different races. One, a white child, is concededly the Fasanos' biological child, named Vincent Fasano. The other, initially named Joseph Fasano, is a black child, who subsequent tests confirmed to be the Rogerses' biological son, now known as Akeil Richard Rogers.

The Fasanos took no action regarding the clinic's apparent error until the Rogerses, upon discovering that Ms. Fasano had given birth to a child who could be theirs, located and commenced an action against them.

PROCEDURAL HISTORY OF THE LITIGATION

On March 12, 1999, the Rogerses commenced a Supreme Court action against the Fasanos as well as the fertility clinic and its doctors. As against the medical defendants, the complaint alleged medical malpractice and breach of contract; as against the Fasanos, it sought a declaratory judgment declaring the rights, obligations and relationships of the parties concerning Akeil.

On April 1 and April 2, 1999, DNA testing was conducted. The results of the test, issued on April 13, 1999, established that the Rogerses were the genetic parents of Akeil. However, according to Ms. Perry-Rogers, the Fasanos agreed to relinquish custody of Akeil to the Rogerses only upon the execution of a written agreement, which entitled the Fasanos to future visitation with Akeil. Ms. Perry-Rogers states that during the period between Akeil's birth on December 29, 1998 and May 10, 1999, the Fasanos only permitted her two brief visits with Akeil, and that she felt compelled to sign the agreement in order to gain custody of her son. The agreement, executed April 29, 1999, contains a visitation schedule providing for visits one full weekend per month, one weekend day each month, one week each summer, and alternating holidays. The agreement also contained a liquidated damages clause, providing that a violation of the Fasanos' visitation rights under the agreement would entitle them to $200,000.

On May 5, 1999 the Fasanos signed affidavits acknowledging that the Rogerses were the genetic parents of the infant, and consenting to the entry of a final order of custody of the child in favor of the Rogerses and to an amendment of the birth certificate naming the Rogerses as the biological and legal parents of the infant. On May 10, 1999, the Fasanos turned over custody of Akeil to the Rogerses, and the following day, May 11, 1999, counsel for the parties signed a stipulation discontinuing with prejudice the plenary action as against the Fasanos.

Despite the discontinuance, by order to show cause dated May 25, 1999, . . . the Rogerses served a petition seeking a declaratory judgment against the Fasanos, naming the Rogerses as Akeil's legal and biological parents, granting them sole and exclusive custody, and permitting them to amend the birth certificate to reflect Akeil's biological heritage. Their application made no mention of the April 29, 1999 visitation agreement. The Fasanos submitted no opposition to the application, and the court granted the application without opposition in a decision dated June 7, 1999, directing settlement of an order.

The Fasanos then sought vacatur of the June 7, 1999 decision on the grounds that the Rogerses had failed to inform the court of the April 29, 1999 agreement, which they contended was a condition precedent to the signing of an order. The Fasanos proposed, in the alternative, a counter order which specifically acknowledged the visitation agreement . . .

The Rogerses assert that over the next few months, the IAS court issued oral "visitation orders" in apparent reliance upon the visitation agreement, and directed that a full forensic psychological evaluation of the parties and their infants be conducted by two sets of mental health experts. On January 14, 2000, the IAS court granted the Fasanos visitation with the child every other weekend.

The Rogerses now challenge the court's January 14, 2000 visitation order. For their part, the Fasanos appeal from the order . . . giving the Rogerses custody of the child . . .

SUBJECT MATTER JURISDICTION AND STANDING

The Rogerses suggest that the Supreme Court lacks subject matter jurisdiction over this dispute because the Fasanos are "genetic strangers" to Akeil. We decline to dispose of the Fasanos' claim on this basis alone. The Supreme Court of the State of New York has subject matter jurisdiction over petitions for custody and visitation pursuant to both the Domestic Relations Law and the Family Court Act.

This is not to say that the Fasanos necessarily have standing to seek visitation with Akeil. However, on this issue we will not simply adopt the Rogerses' suggestion that no gestational mother may ever claim visitation with the infant she carried, in view of her status as a "genetic stranger" to the infant. In recognition of current reproductive technology, the term "genetic stranger" alone can no longer be enough to end a discussion of this issue . . .

Until recently, there was no question as to who was a child's "natural" mother. It was the woman in whose uterus the child was conceived and borne . . . It was only with the recent advent of in vitro fertilization technology that it became possible to divide between two women the functions that traditionally defined a mother, at least prenatally. With this technology, a troublesome legal dilemma has arisen: When one woman's fertilized eggs are implanted in another, which woman is the child's "natural" mother?

Although the technology is still fairly new, several cases have been decided that focus on competing claims to child custody arising out of the use of in vitro fertilization technology. These cases are not dispositive here, since visitation rights rather than custody is at issue. However, they contain analysis that provides important background for the issues raised on this appeal.

In *Johnson v. Calvert*, 5 Cal.4th 84, 19 Cal.Rptr.2d 494, 851 P.2d 776, *cert. denied* ,510 U.S. 874, 114 S.Ct. 206, 126 L.Ed.2d 163, a surrogate mother, unrelated genetically to the child she had carried, declined to give the child to its genetic parents upon its birth, as had been agreed in a surrogacy contract. While "recogniz[ing] [both] genetic consanguinity and giving birth as a means of establishing a mother and child relationship," the California Supreme Court concluded that when the two means do not coincide in one woman, she who intended to procreate the child — that is, she who intended to bring about the birth of a child that she intended to raise as her own — is the natural mother under California law . . .

It is apparent from the foregoing cases that a "gestational mother" may possess enforceable rights under the law, despite her being a "genetic stranger" to the child. Given the complex possibilities in these kind of circumstances, it is simply inappropriate to render any determination solely as a consequence of genetics.

Parenthetically, it is worth noting that even if the Fasanos had claimed the right to custody of the child, application of the "intent" analysis . . . would — in our view — require that custody be awarded to the Rogerses. It was they who purposefully arranged for their genetic material to be taken and used in order to attempt to create their own child, whom they intended to rear.

STANDING TO SEEK VISITATION

To establish their claim that the Fasanos lack standing, the Rogerses focus upon the strict limits of New York statutory and case law regarding who may seek visitation. Under New York statutory law, the only people who have the right to seek visitation are parents (Domestic Relations Law §§ 70, 240), grandparents (Domestic Relations Law §§ 71, 240) and siblings related by whole or half-blood (Domestic Relations Law § 72). The Rogerses rely on the proposition that because the statutes must be strictly construed, they must be interpreted to preclude the Fasanos from within their framework. Specifically, they suggest that by their act of ceding Akeil to the Rogerses, the child's genetic parents, the Fasanos have surrendered any conceivable right to the parental status necessary to claim visitation rights.

We agree that under the circumstances presented, the Fasanos lack standing under Domestic Relations Law § 70 to seek visitation as the child's parents. However, this is not because we necessarily accept the broad premise that in *any* situation where a parent, possessed of that status by virtue of having borne and given birth to the child, acknowledges another couple's entitlement to the status of parent by virtue of their having provided the genetic materials that created the child, the birth parent automatically gives up all parental rights.

Rather, we recognize that in these rather unique circumstances, where the Rogerses' embryo was implanted in Donna Fasano by mistake, and where the Fasanos knew of the error not long after it occurred, the happenstance of the Fasanos' nominal parenthood over Akeil should have been treated as a mistake to be corrected as soon as possible, *before the development of a parental relationship.* It bears more similarity to a mix-up at the time of a hospital's discharge of two newborn infants, which should simply be corrected at once,[22] than to one where a gestational mother has arguably the same rights to claim parentage as the genetic mother. Under such circumstances, the Fasanos will not be heard to claim the status of parents, entitled to seek an award of visitation.

Additionally, the Fasanos' child, Vincent, is not a sibling "by whole or half-blood" with the right to proceed under Domestic Relations Law § 71, since the statute makes no reference to "gestational siblings." . . .

APPLICABILITY OF A "BEST INTERESTS" APPROACH

The Fasanos argue that determination at this point of the parties' respective rights regarding Akeil would be premature, in view of the preliminary procedural posture of this case. Indeed, there has been neither testimony nor even joinder of issue. Nevertheless, in this instance, we conclude that a determination on the law may, and indeed must, be made at this time. While there may well be occasions where a dispute between gestational and genetic parents requires a full evidentiary "best interests" hearing to ensure that the child's interests are fully protected, this is *not* such a case.

The only facts needed for this determination are those that are clearly established on this meager record: (1) plaintiffs are the genetic parents of the child, Akeil Rogers, and are concededly entitled to custody of him; (2) defendant Donna Fasano is the child's "gestational mother", having given birth to him after being implanted by mistake with the fertilized embryo of plaintiffs, (3) the parties were made aware of the mistake by the medical facility prior to the birth of the child, and

---

[22] [n.2] If a hospital mix-up is discovered right away, there should be no question that it must be corrected at once; although, in circumstances where years have passed before the error is discovered, courts might consider some arrangement other than a simple change of custody (*compare, Twigg v. Mays*, 1993 WL 330624 [Fl.Cir.Ct. No. 88-4489-CA-01] [switch discovered after 10 years, change of custody denied]; *Pope v. Moore*, 261 Ga. 253, 403 S.E.2d 205 [1991] [mistake discovered after 4 years, genetic mother awarded visitation, denied custody]; *see generally*, Note, *What's Best for Babies Switched at Birth? The Role of the Court, Rights of Nonbiological Parents, and Mandatory Mediation of the Custodial Agreements*, 21 Whittier L.Rev. 315).

(4) in the process of working out the transfer of Akeil to plaintiffs, the Fasanos and the Rogerses entered into an agreement providing for visitation.

In other circumstances, inquiry may be appropriate as to whether a psychological bond exists which should not be abruptly severed, and if so, what living arrangements would be in the child's best interests. For instance, when a child has been born into and raised as a part of a family for an extended period of time, a basis may be presented for directing custody with one family and visitation to another.

We are also cognizant that a bond may well develop between a gestational mother and the infant she carried, before, during and immediately after the birth . . . and that indeed, here, the parties' visitation agreement itself proclaimed the existence of a bond between the two infants. Nevertheless, the suggested existence of a bond is not enough under the present circumstances.

In the present case, any bonding on the part of Akeil to his gestational mother and her family was the direct result of the Fasanos' failure to take timely action upon being informed of the clinic's admitted error. Defendants cannot be permitted to purposefully act in such a way as to create a bond, and then rely upon it for their assertion of rights to which they would not otherwise be entitled.

Nor may the parties' visitation agreement form the basis for a court order of visitation. "[A] voluntary agreement * * * will not of itself confer standing upon a person not related by blood to assert a legal claim to visitation or custody" . . .

Accordingly, the order of the Supreme Court, New York County (Diane Lebedeff, J.), entered February 2, 2000, which granted defendants visitation with the infant Joseph Fasano, now known as Akeil Richard Rogers, should be reversed, on the law, without costs, and the application for an order of visitation denied . . .

All concur.

Leslie Bender
Genes, Parents, and Assisted Reproductive Technologies: ARTs, Mistakes, Sex, Race, & Law
12 Colum. J. Gender & L. 1, 33–36(2003)

What really is at issue in the *Perry-Rogers v. Fasano* case is the degree to which genetics ought to define parenthood in our era of assisted reproductive technologies. The court makes false stabs at the issue, but ultimately only grazes it, instead resting its decision on a shaky finding of no standing. Had it granted the Fasanos standing as parents (at a minimum, had it granted Donna Fasano standing as a mother), the court would have been required to decide the contested visitation claim based on a "best interests of the child" analysis, according to New York law. Since the parties reached an agreement about visitation that included a specific paragraph clearly acknowledging the importance of the child's continued relationship with the Fasanos, the court had a mutually agreed upon basis regarding Joseph/Akeil's best interests. This case was easier than it could have been if the parties had not already worked out the transfer of custody or visitation agreement.

The end result imposed by the court, with each set of parents ending up with one twin, suggests a Solomonic split-the-baby decision, but unlike Solomon's story, in this case the split ostensibly helps the parents, rather than kills the baby (although it "kills the twins"). But to look at this case as one about two children who are equally divided among two sets of parents distorts the analysis. This case is about one of the children only, about Joseph/Akeil. The parents had worked out a more Solomon-like decision than the court. In their visitation agreement, each set of parents got a piece of the child's time and affection, and the child got the benefit of both couples' love, time, and attention. In the court's resolution, the child is no longer "split" between the couples, but the child is also no longer the beneficiary of both families' attention and love. The child loses all connection to his birth parent and twin sibling, despite their ardent desire for further contact. The child's interests seem to have been subordinated to some grander principle, though that principle is not articulated. Paradoxically, Joseph/Akeil was deprived of his birth family and sibling in the easier case where the court only had to decide about visitation, not primary physical and legal custody, and the parties had negotiated a plan in advance . . . The Appellate Division decision touches on some of the deeper issues and implications of the case in its standing analysis. In a footnote it acknowledges that in some cases both the gestational and genetic mothers may be parents for "certain purposes." In the text the court indicates that it will not let genetics be its sole guide . . .

The court's subconscious or silent preference for genetics over gestation prevails, regardless of any rhetoric it uses to the contrary. Finding the Fasanos had no standing was the same as finding that the Rogerses were the sole and appropriate parents. The genetic parents win completely. No other parents could even come before the court to argue for the legitimacy of their claims. Certainly the court realized that its resolution foreclosed the Fasanos from visitation, and therefore foreclosed them from having any relationship with their child . . . [T]he injustice of this decision is compounded because the court makes this decision based on a procedural analysis rather than a substantive one.

We need reasoned opinions on the substantive issues of this case. These issues include genetic essentialism, a gendered analysis of motherhood, and even more submerged issues of the role of race and class in family disputes arising from the use of ARTs. General issues about the reconceptualization of legal parenthood in a post-ART age loom large in this case. The court has an obligation to explain why even though it acknowledges the bonds between a pregnant woman and her fetus, it ignores those bonds entirely in reaching its decision. If the court denies its reliance on biological determinism, or "genetic essentialism," but reaches a result only explainable by genetic ties, it needs to be explicit about its reasoning. At a minimum the court must explain why it preferred genetic evidence of family status over biological (gestational), cultural notions of family and kinship. This "no standing" decision fails miserably in explaining its rationale and the result of completely cutting off the child from his birth family.

NOTES AND QUESTIONS

1.   Professor Bender's piercing and meticulous analysis of the *Perry-Rogers v. Fasano* case is well worth the read. She critiques the New York court on several grounds, including its reliance on form over substance, its dismissiveness toward

Mrs. Fasano's prenatal bonding with both boys, and its understated, almost underhanded, reliance on the race of the child, leading her to conclude, "The court's race-based assumptions may have skewed its decision and caused the unjust result in the case." 12 COLUM. J. GENDER & L. at 39 (2003). Those "race-based assumptions," Professor Bender later explains, can be culled from the court's virtually blaming Mrs. Fasano for bonding with both babies in utero and immediately after their birth, as if to suggest that a woman "ought" not bond with a child of a different race.

Do you agree that the court fixated on form (in this case, standing) in order to avoid a discussion of substance (priority of race, genetics and gestation)? If the court had reached the issue of the best interest of the child, how do you think it would have ruled? How should it have ruled? *See* Cynthia R. Mabry, *"Who Is My Real Father? The Delicate Task of Identifying a Father and Parenting Children Created from an In Vitro Mix-Up*, 18 NAT'L BLACK L. J. 1 (2004) (discussing the psychological and cultural challenges that confront biracial families formed via embryo mix-ups).

2.   In January 2003 the British High Court of Justice heard a similar case involving mixed-race twins born to a white woman following a "mistake" in the laboratory. Two couples, Mr. and Mrs. A, a white couple, and Mr. and Mrs. B, of West Indian origin, sought treatment at a British fertility clinic. Physicians retrieved eggs from Mrs. A and mistakenly mixed them with sperm from Mr. B. Mrs. A became pregnant and gave birth to twins; she is the genetic mother of the twins and tests confirm that Mr. B was the genetic father. The court expressed its intent to leave the twins with the couple who gave birth to and is raising them, Mr. and Mrs. A. The ruling, however, also found that Mr. B is the twins' legal father, requiring Mr. A to adopt them if he is to become their legal father. *The L Teaching Hospitals NHS v. Mr. A*, 2003 WL 270761 (High Court of Justice Queens Bench Division).

Compare the holdings in *Prato-Morrison v. Doe, Robert B. v. Susan B., Perry-Rogers v. Fasano*, and *The L Teaching Hospitals NHS v. Mr. A.* Can you articulate a common theme or principle in these cases? Do you believe a common theme or principle should govern gamete mix-up cases?

3.   A 2009 Ohio case of embryo mix-up garnered much media attention and praise for a birth mother who, "in a remarkable act of generosity," agreed to give up the child she knew from the beginning was not her genetic child. When Carolyn Savage, a mother of three children, was told she was pregnant following an IVF cycle, she was also told the embryo belonged to another couple. Carolyn and husband Sean gave up their hopes of having a fourth child, telling the genetic parents they were willing to continue the pregnancy and hand over the child. When a boy was born in September 2009, the baby, as well as book manuscripts from both sets of parents, were delivered as promised. *See* Kristen Criswell, *Savages Use Baby Mix-Up Journey to Help Others*, TOLEDO FREE PRESS, Feb. 27, 2011, available at http://www.toledofreepress.com/tag/logan-savage-morell/. The Savages welcomed twin girls into their family in August 2011, born with the help of a gestational carrier.

C. Legislative Perspectives on Gamete Mix-Ups

The law governing negligent or criminal conduct in the provision of ART services is largely derived from judicial decisions, i.e., common law. Federal and state lawmakers have been mostly silent in response to the theft and innocent mistakes that have devastated families; these victims are left to pursue their claims through negligence and malpractice actions against the responsible physicians and fertility clinics. Tort, family, and criminal law all offer methods of redress when gametes have been tampered with, and we have seen each of these areas of law invoked in response to the isolated, but tragic, cases when gamete mix-ups produce anguished consequences.

In California, home to the notorious UCI Center for Reproductive Health, lawmakers responded to the alleged malfeasance of Drs. Asch, Balmaceda, and Stone by enacting a law designed to deter and punish tampering with gametic material. Senate Bill 1555, enacted on September 25, 1996, adds Section 367g to the Penal Code, and provides as follows:

California Penal Code
Part 1. Of Crimes and Punishments

§ 367g. Assisted reproduction technology; unauthorized use or implantation of sperm, ova, or embryos; violation; penalty

(a) It shall be unlawful for anyone to knowingly use sperm, ova, or embryos in assisted reproduction technology, for any purpose other than that indicated by the sperm, ova, or embryo provider's signature on a written consent form.

(b) It shall be unlawful for anyone to knowingly implant sperm, ova, or embryos, through the use of assisted reproduction technology, into a recipient who is not the sperm, ova, or embryo provider, without the signed written consent of the sperm, ova, or embryo provider and recipient.

(c) Any person who violates this section shall be punished by imprisonment in the state prison for three, four, or five years, by a fine not to exceed fifty thousand dollars ($50,000), or by both that fine and imprisonment.

(d) Written consent, for the purposes of this section, shall not be required of men who donate sperm to a licensed tissue bank.

A brief history of this law may explain why other states have not followed California's lead by enacting similar legislation.

> . . . The original impetus for this bill came when prosecutors in Orange County declared they could not charge the UCI physicians under existing California law because no statute covered "egg theft." The bill's sponsor, Senator Tom Hayden, explained through an aide that the state's theft and embezzlement statutes could not be used because both "would have to assign a value to the embryos." In fact, California's embezzlement statute contains no valuation language, merely declaring that, "[e]mbezzlement is

the fraudulent appropriation of property by a person to whom it has been intrusted." Clearly, if the physicians took eggs and embryos from patients without their consent and implanted them in other patients or used them for research, they would be guilty of embezzlement. What likely concerned prosecutors in bringing embezzlement charges was not the problem of placing a value on the stolen property, but rather the idea of calling this potential human life "property" as required by the statute.

Prosecutors were likely similarly concerned with charging the doctors under California's theft statute, which does contain valuation of property language. Penal Code Section 487 states that grand theft is committed "[w]hen the . . . personal property taken is of a value exceeding four hundred dollars ($400)." Charging the UCI directors with grand theft would have meant declaring the patient's eggs and embryos "personal property" and attaching a monetary value to something not traded on the open market. Such declaration, Senator Hayden worried, "seemed morally offensive [because it was] to say this material of life was property."

In my mind, such skittishness on the part of prosecutors was both unwarranted and unwise. First, while I acknowledge the legitimate debate over the appropriate characterization of human embryos — persons or property — such moral conundrums need not be debated or resolved when criminal conduct of the nature alleged is at issue. Doctors at UCI were entrusted with the patients' gametic material that they are accused of fraudulently appropriating, presumably for their own benefit (higher pregnancy success rates to advertise and attract more patients, personal edification for having achieved more pregnancies, advanced research agenda). Such conduct should not go unpunished in the name of moral labeling. When patients undergo IVF and other forms of ART, they know that for a time their eggs and resulting embryos will be under the control of their doctor and other clinic personnel. This recognition alone includes a sense that gametic material has dispositional, transportable, and protectable qualities that aptly place it in the realm of property. No disrespect or moral underclassing need follow such an acknowledgment. Instead, any malfeasance in the handling of such material should be susceptible to the type of redress used to punish those who invade the dispositional rights of others.

If UCI patients were robbed of the opportunity to control the disposition of their embryos, theft and embezzlement seem well suited to address this reprehensible conduct. The newly enacted California law, specifically aimed at failure to obtain consent to use sperm, ova, and embryos, may not carry the same semantic weight as long-standing property crimes. Juries would likely understand what it means to steal embryos, but might struggle to understand the nature of the consent process surrounding reproductive technologies. Since the gravamen of the new crime is the failure to obtain the patient's signature on a written consent form, prosecutors may find themselves trying to explain the doctrine of informed consent to juries when patients claim that their signatures were procured without sufficient disclosures. A prosecution under these circumstances is essentially a claim of lack of informed consent converted from a negligence calculus into a criminal action. Surely patients are not well served when they, via prosecutors, must prove beyond a reasonable doubt that their fertility specialist failed to properly inform them about the risks and alternatives to a proposed therapy. Heightening the burden of proof on what can be construed as an informed consent claim is certainly not in the best interest of patients . . .

In addition to worries about weighing in on the embryo as person/property debate, another stated concern of prosecutors was placing a monetary value on the eggs and embryos taken. How ironic that prosecutors were afraid to value the very thing that doctors had no problem valuing to procure. It is estimated that a single cycle of IVF can cost up to $10,000, and patients often undergo multiple cycles before a pregnancy is achieved. Again, without deciding on the moral status of the embryos, prosecutors could have easily charged doctors with stealing property (in its grandest sense) worth over $400. Procurement value alone was far in excess of the stated statutory minimum and thus could have relieved the district attorney from having to specifically value the embryos themselves.

In the end, the only ones to benefit from the prosecutors' interpretation of penal law were the UCI doctors who will likely escape criminal prosecution for their "egg stealing" conduct. Thus, the concern over labeling and its symbolic significance robbed numerous patients of the right to redress from the criminal justice system. Lawmakers may feel satisfied that the new law will deter such outrageous conduct in the future. But fertility doctors probably considered themselves susceptible to criminal theft and embezzlement charges before prosecutors denied their applicability to embryos. Obviously these criminal laws did nothing to deter the alleged misappropriation. Query whether a more specific criminal statute will have any more of an impact on such premeditated conduct.

Judith F. Daar, *Regulating Reproductive Technologies: Panacea or Paper Tiger?*, 34 HOUS. L. REV. 609, 646-9 (1997). Do you agree with Professor Daar that additional, specific laws will not necessarily deter criminal or even negligent conduct surrounding ART? Are existing laws sufficient to give redress to children and families harmed by the wrongful conduct of physicians and others who misappropriate gametes? Consider drafting a comprehensive bill that addresses the rights and liabilities of parties affected by gamete misappropriation.

Chapter 6

LIFE AFTER DEATH: POSTMORTEM REPRODUCTION

The cycle of life in which a person is born, reproduces, and then dies has reigned over all of human history, creating a reliable expectation that those who choose to bear offspring will do so within the course of their lifetime. Scientific advances in the waning years of the twentieth century offered the potential for rearranging this cycle of life, allowing children to be born long after their genetic parents have departed the earthly world. Posthumous or postmortem reproduction refers to the birth of a child after the death of the gamete provider, either the man who provided the sperm or the woman who provided the egg, or possibly both.[1] Increasingly, postmortem reproduction is gender neutral, meaning that both men and women can become "parents" after their own death. The main advance that makes birth after death possible is cryopreservation, or freezing, of the necessary ingredients of reproduction. Today it is possible to freeze and subsequently thaw viable sperm, eggs, and embryos, so that an individual's genetic child can be born years, decades, or even centuries after the progenitor has passed.[2]

---

[1] A brief note about language. While the terms posthumous and postmortem are often used interchangeably to describe the birth of a child after a parent's death, a slight clarification may be useful. Posthumous refers to events that occur after death while postmortem is used to describe activities that are carried on after death. For purposes of our discussion in this Chapter, posthumous reproduction refers to the birth of a child after the death of one or both of the gamete providers. Posthumous reproduction involves a child who is conceived and in utero during the lifetime of a gametic parent but born after that parent's death. Postmortem conception refers to the conception or gestation and birth of a child after the death of one or both of the gamete providers. Postmortem conception can be accomplished by freezing sperm, eggs or embryos during the lifetime of the gamete provider(s), and then thawing and implanting any resulting embryo after death. Sperm and eggs may also be retrieved from the gamete provider shortly after the person's death, and any resulting child born of that process would be considered a postmortem conception child.

[2] Let us clarify that cryopreservation of gametes should not be confused with cryonics — freezing the human body after death. According to Alcor Life Extension Foundation, cryonics is "the science of using ultra-cold temperature to preserve human life with the intent of restoring good health when technology becomes available to do so . . . [It is] "hea speculative life support technology that seeks practice of using cold to preserve the human life in a state that will be viable and treatable by future medicine. It is expected that future medicine will include mature nanotechnology, and the ability to heal at the cellular and molecular levels of a person who can no longer be supported by ordinary medicine. The goal is to carry the person forward through time, for however many decades or centuries might be necessary, until the preservation process can be reversed, and the person restored to full health." Alcor operates a facility in Scottsdale, Arizona, offering clients full body preservation for $120200,000 and neuropreservation (freezing of the brain and skull) for $580,000. To date, no human has ever been revived from temperatures far below freezing, but Alcor and its supporters believe that future technology will be available to reverse the cryonics process and revive the human subject. The Scottsdale facility currently houses 59106 cryopatients, including baseball legend Ted Williams whose 2002 death and instructions for cryopreservation sparked objections from family members who preferred the more traditional cremation

Postmortem reproduction raises questions large and small. Big-picture ethical concerns loom large over the practice of purposefully creating children who will never know their genetic parent. Just because we can have children far into the future, should we embrace or guard against the practice? What effect will postmortem reproduction have on children and families? Practical concerns arise as well, including questions about the legal parentage and inheritance rights of children born after the death of a genetic parent. Is the child considered a lawful heir of the parent, entitled to share in the decedent's long-closed estate? Before delving into the ethics and family law conundrums surrounding postmortem reproduction, we first investigate the current state of the ART of birth after death.

SECTION I: THE POSSIBILITIES FOR POSTMORTEM REPRODUCTION

Birth after death can be accomplished by freezing sperm, eggs, or embryos when they are viable, maintaining them in a frozen state in a manner that preserves their structure and function, and thawing the material so as to restore their capacity to become a new human being. Over the past 60 years, the freezing, storing, and thawing process has yielded successful pregnancies and births beginning in the 1950s with the first report of a pregnancy using frozen sperm. Thirty years later, Australian scientists reported the world's first pregnancy from a frozen embryo, and today researchers are increasingly optimistic about the prospects of cryopreserving eggs for future use, a technique that until very recently had been viewed as technically out of reach.

Currently the vast majority of gametes are retrieved while the progenitor is still alive, but we are quickly approaching the next frontier in postmortem reproduction — postmortem retrieval of sperm and eggs. More than a handful of births have been reported using sperm retrieved from a man who has been declared dead, and while there are no verified reports of postmortem egg retrieval and birth, no technophile can doubt this possibility is on the horizon. The history and details of each technology sets the stage for the legal controversies that have or inevitably will follow.

A. Freezing Sperm

1. Sperm Retrieval During Life

a. Sperm Freezing — Past and Present

Scientists first began to contemplate the possibility of freezing and thawing semen in the mid-nineteenth century. Reportedly in 1866, an Italian scientist named Montegazza was the first to envision banks for frozen human sperm. He suggested that "a man dying on a battlefield may beget a legal heir with his semen

---

route for the dearly departed slugger. See *Cryonics Firm Ordered to Release Records*, Bos. Globe, Oct. 14, 2004, at B2.

frozen and stored at home."[3] The first major scientific breakthrough in sperm cryopreservation came in 1949 when A.S. Parkes and two British scientists developed a method of using a syrupy substance known as glycerol to protect semen from injury during freezing. The process was further refined in 1953 by Dr. Jerome K. Sherman, an American pioneer in sperm freezing. Dr. Sherman introduced a simple method of preserving human sperm using glycerol, but he combined this with a slow cooling of sperm, and storage with solid carbon dioxide as a refrigerant. As a result of this research, the first successful human pregnancy with frozen sperm was reported in 1953. *See* R. Bunge & J. Sherman, *Fertilizing Capacity of Frozen Human Spermatazoa*, 172 NATURE 767 (1953).

Early advances in sperm cryopreservation coincided, coincidentally, with advances in space travel. In 1962, famed Harvard law professor W. Barton Leach wed the emerging technologies of sperm banking and space exploration in an article appearing in the American Bar Association Journal. In *Perpetuities in the Atomic Age: The Sperm Bank and the Fertile Decedent*, 48 A.B.A.J. 942 (1962), Professor Leach wondered whether the new phenomenon of sperm banks, created to protect the issue of astronauts from mutations caused by ionizing radiation in outer space, posed a threat to every first year law student's favorite doctrine, the Rule Against Perpetuities. If sperm could be preserved for long periods, would a resulting child, born long after her father's death, vest in interest in a testamentary gift within a "life in being" plus twenty-one years, as required by the dreaded common law rule? Perhaps shunned as science fiction at the time, Professor Leach's hypothetical became a reality in 1977 when an Australian newspaper reported that a widow had given birth to a child using her dead husband's frozen sperm. *See* Kristine S. Knaplund, *Postmortem Conception and a Father's Last Will*, 46 ARIZ. L. REV. 91, 92 (2004) (citing a report in the *Sydney Morning Herald*, July 12, 1977).[4]

Commercial sperm banks were first established in the early 1970s. Initially, clientele were men facing voluntary or medically indicated sterilization. Freezing sperm before vasectomy or radiation therapy was a way of preserving future fertility, should the donor wish to pursue parenthood at some later point. An early concern of men depositing sperm to preserve their fertility was the question of longevity. How long could sperm be frozen before it lost its ability to fertilize a woman's egg? At least a generation, according to recent reports. In 2002, a woman in Manchester, England, gave birth after undergoing in vitro fertilization using sperm that had been frozen for 21 years. The woman's husband had been diagnosed with testicular cancer when he was 17 years old. Before undergoing treatment, he deposited five vials of sperm that were cryopreserved for later use.

---

[3] This quote is reported by Sonia Fader in Sperm Banking: A Reproductive Resource (1993), reproduced in www.cryobank.com. The history of sperm banking in this paragraph is largely derived from Ms. Fader's work.

[4] This first known posthumously conceived child was Milo Casali, son of Kim Casali, the celebrated artist behind the "Love Is" cartoons published in newspapers across the world. Milo's birth in 1977, 17 months after his father's death from testicular cancer, was announced by an illustration of the "Love Is" girl, pushing a baby carriage with the words inside reading "Proudly Presenting Milos Roberto. Parents: Kim and the late Roberto (posthumously by artificial insemination)." See Natasha Courtenay-Smith, *A Baby Born 17 Months After His Father Died*, Daily Mail, Oct. 27, 2004.

In 2009, a Charlotte, North Carolina couple tied the English record, welcoming a baby girl conceived using sperm banked for 21 years. These cases represent the current record for sperm preservation and live birth, but barriers to much lengthier intervals seem flimsy indeed. See Jenny Hope, *21 Today — Baby's Amazing Journey From Father's Sperm In The 1970s*, DAILY TELEGRAPH, May 26, 2004, at 11; *IVF Baby Born From 21 Year-Old Sperm, Ties World Record* (April 9, 2009), available at: http://www.prnewswire.com/news-releases/ivf-baby-born-from-21-year-old-frozen-sperm-ties-world-record-61787767.html.[5]

The popularity of sperm cryopreservation is reflected in the growing number of sperm banks and freezing facilities. According to the Centers for Disease Control, in 1988, 74% of fertility clinics reported offering sperm cryopreservation; by 2009 a full 100% of clinics offered this service to their patients. Moreover, previous doubts about the effectiveness of frozen sperm, compared to fresh sperm, have been put to rest. A 2004 study revealed that fresh and frozen sperm were equally effective in producing healthy embryos and successful pregnancies when used in IVF cycles. Researchers compared IVF outcomes over a 10-year period and concluded that fresh and frozen sperm produced equivalent results, prompting the study authors to hail the use of frozen sperm for its convenience and ability to avoid "the risk of a failure to obtain sperm on the day of oocyte retrieval." *Data Shows No Difference In IVF Outcomes With Fresh vs. Frozen Sperm*, LAW & HEALTH WEEKLY, June 5, 2004, at 185.

b.   Emerging Legal Disputes Over Frozen Sperm

Lifetime retrieval of frozen sperm for lifetime use by the donor poses little concern, as the freezing process merely interrupts the progenitor's procreative process. Inter vivos storage and use of frozen sperm is bordered on both ends of the time spectrum by the gamete provider's intent to become a parent. A man who deposits sperm for safekeeping expresses an intent to maintain the option of future parenthood, and that intent is further manifested when the donor withdraws the sperm for thaw and introduction to a desired partner's eggs. But what happens if the donor dies before he can direct the disposition of his frozen sperm? Can a surviving spouse or girlfriend claim ownership of the sperm based on a presumed intent that the donor made the deposit in order for his beloved to birth his future child? What about the rights of the donor's surviving mother or father who deeply desire to become a grandparent to their deceased child's child? Does the act of depositing sperm carry an implicit consent to become a parent posthumously?

The first case to bring the question of postmortem sperm disposition to the legal front unfolded in France in 1984. Alain Parpalaix was diagnosed with cancer in 1981, depositing his sperm at the government-run Centers for the Study and Conservation of Sperm (CECOS) to preserve his future fertility. On December 23,

---

[5] In addition to concerns about longevity of viable sperm, men using sperm banking to preserve their fertility may worry that an equipment malfunction could rob them of future offspring. Such a tragic case did unfold in England in the summer of 2001. The semen of some 300 men, mostly cancer patients, was put at risk when a faulty freezer partially defrosted the hospital's sperm bank. Several patients sued the hospital for damages, though it remains unclear whether the sperm is suitable for future use. See Lucy Bannerman, *Patients Sue Over Sperm Bank Flaw*, The Herald, Feb. 12, 2004, at 7.

1983, 26 year-old Alain married his girlfriend Corrine and died two days later. Alain's widow attempted to obtain his sperm, but CECOS refused to surrender the gametic material, prompting Corrine to sue for possession. The French court focused on intent, giving priority to the donor's prior instructions. The problem for Corrine was that Alain had not left any explicit instructions regarding disposition, forcing the court to search out other evidence of the donor's intent. Alain's parents and widow testified as to the decedent's desire to procreate posthumously, persuading the court that the decedent had a strong desire for his wife to be the mother of their child. Ultimately, the court ordered CECOS to turn over the sperm to Corrine's chosen physician, but to no avail — the widow's attempts at insemination failed to produce a child. The Parpalaix case is reported and discussed in E. Donald Shapiro & Benedene Sonnenblick, *The Widow and the Sperm: The Law of Post-Mortem Insemination*, 1 J.L. & Health 229 (1987).

The legal dilemma of postmortem sperm disposition made its way to the U.S. in the early 1990s, calling upon several courts to resolve the question of ownership once the donor passed on.

HALL v. FERTILITY INSTITUTE OF NEW ORLEANS
Court of Appeal of Louisiana, Fourth Circuit
647 So. 2d 1348 (1994)

Waltzer, J.

STATEMENT OF THE CASE

Mary Alice Hall ("Executrix" hereinafter), the duly appointed testamentary executrix of the Succession of her son, Barry S. Hall, sued the Fertility Institute of New Orleans ("Institute" hereinafter) for a declaratory judgment declaring Hall's frozen semen on deposit with the Institute to be Succession property; alternatively asking that the material be destroyed; and for temporary, preliminary and ultimately permanent injunctive relief preventing the release of the material absent a court order. The trial court preliminarily enjoined the Institute from releasing the material.

Christine C. St. John intervened, alleging ownership of the material pursuant to a formal written act of donation executed by Hall on 29 November 1992, claiming to be an indispensable party to the litigation, and seeking dissolution of the preliminary injunction . . .

On 4 March 1994, the trial court granted St. John's motion to dissolve the preliminary injunction and temporarily restrained the parties from taking any action with respect to the genetic material. An evidentiary hearing was held on the Executrix' motion for a preliminary injunction, following which the trial court entered judgment in favor of the Executrix and against St. John and the Institute, prohibiting St. John from taking possession, directly or indirectly, of Hall's frozen sperm . . . From that judgment, St. John appeals. We affirm.

STATEMENT OF FACTS

Hall died on 29 October 1993 of metastatic cancer. He was survived by a son, his sole heir under a will dated 18 September 1993. Following diagnosis of his disease, Hall and St. John on 13 January 1992 consulted Dr. Richard Dickey of the Institute, according to St. John's affidavit, to discuss the effects of contemplated chemotherapy on Hall's ability to father children and to find out about preserving his sperm deposits for St. John's artificial insemination at a later date. According to Dickey's deposition, sperm deposits were taken and tests thereon were made from January through 13 March 1992, totalling 15 vials. The doctor saw St. John last on 5 February, at which time preparations for beginning an insemination cycle were started. On 17 March 1992, St. John notified Dickey that she would not pursue further attempts at pregnancy for at least three months. There was no further contact by Hall or St. John with the Institute or Dr. Dickey, and the vials of Hall's sperm remain on deposit at the Institute. St. John was billed for and paid the Institute's 1992 storage fee.

On 29 November 1992, Hall and St. John executed an Act of Donation before St. John's law partner, Michael Guarisco, by which Hall purported to convey his interest in his frozen semen deposits to St. John, in consideration of his "love and affection" for her. On 25 October 1993, Hall executed a living will . . . appointing St. John as his health care agent . . . Hall's sister, Donna Hall-Whitlock witnessed the living will, declaring her belief that Hall was of sound mind at that time.

Only affidavit and deposition evidence was taken at the hearing on the motion for a preliminary injunction. In affidavits, the moderator and four members of a Cancer Support Group/Wellness Group in which Hall participated prior to his death said Hall had told them he could not marry St. John because of his illness, but had deposited sperm in order that she could have the option to bear a child by him. The notary who executed Hall's will declared by affidavit that on the occasions when he met with Hall in August and September of 1993, Hall was lucid and competent . . . Hall's primary care physician declared by affidavit that on all occasions that she met with Hall or spoke with him by telephone, "he appeared coherent and capable of making rational decisions."

Michael Hall, Hall's only child, provided an affidavit asserting his wish, as next of kin, to bury all his father's remains, including the semen deposits. Michael asserted his belief that had Hall wished to father children by St. John, Hall would have married her, impregnated her before undergoing treatment, or allowed her to be artificially inseminated while he was alive. He also declared the extreme emotional upset, embarrassment and anger he suffers at the prospect of posthumous creation of blood relatives.

Hall's sister, Donna Hall-Whitlock, signed an affidavit declaring . . . "toward the end", Hall was not responsible for his actions, was heavily sedated against pain and at all times under St. John's dominant influence. Donna also stated that she, her sister and her mother were Hall's primary caretakers during the two years of his illness, and that St. John disclaimed responsibility for Hall. Donna said Hall told her the semen deposit was intended for use when he finished treatment and was cured. She also said that had Hall wished to marry and have a family with St. John he would have done so. The affidavits of Hall's sister, Martha, and of his mother are similar in content.

While the record does not contain the trial court's reasons for judgment, we conclude that the judgment reflects the trial judge's determination, based on the conflicting affidavit evidence, that a preliminary injunction should issue to preserve the status quo until the issue of Hall's competency and intention could be determined in a full trial on the merits.

STANDARD OF REVIEW

. . . We find no merit in the Executrix' arguments that the authentic act of donation should be set aside for reasons of public policy, and reject the notion that St. John's proposed artificial insemination would be *contra bonos mores* in this State. Similarly, we are not called upon to address the constitutional propriety of artificial insemination *in vitro* or *in utero*, or the question of posthumous reproduction set out with great erudition in the *amicus curiae* brief filed herein. The sole issue relevant to disposition of the instant case is the validity *vel non* of the authentic act of donation that purports to convey to St. John the decedent's fifteen vials of sperm now on deposit with the Institute. If it is shown at trial that decedent was competent and not under undue influence at the time the act was passed, the frozen semen is St. John's property, and she has full rights to its disposition.

Applying this analysis to the facts of this case, we conclude that the trial court did not abuse its "great discretion" in granting a preliminary injunction to the Executrix herein . . .

We have examined the consequences should preliminary injunctive relief be denied, and find the potential consequences to constitute irreparable harm. Should St. John be allowed to obtain Hall's sperm deposits during the pendency of this action, one or more embryos could well come into existence. Depending on the length of time the matter requires prior to final conclusion, the possible development of human beings is such a serious consequence that the irreparable nature of the risk at issue is clear. The emotional damage to the decedent's mother and Executrix should the donation prove to have been illegally obtained and children sired against the wishes of her dead son is obvious and cannot be compensated adequately. Further, the determination of the validity of the act of donation should be made without the influence of the existence of embryos or an actual pregnancy.

The determination of the validity of the Act of Donation is a factual issue that must be determined by a full trial on the merits, particularly where the preliminary injunction hearing produced conflicting affidavit and deposition evidence on this issue. The Executrix, representing the Succession, is the proper party to claim and preserve succession assets, and presents a *prima facie* entitlement to possession of the frozen material. Her likelihood of prevailing on the merits will depend on the validity of the act of donation, a mixed question of fact, addressing Hall's competency and intent, and of law, under the applicable statutes. We find it reasonable that the trial court apparently concluded that the Executrix presented a *prima facie* case that the Act of Donation was invalid. Among the factors raised by the deposition and affidavits touching the issue of donative intent are the following:

1. Evidence that Hall deposited his sperm prior to undergoing chemotherapy, the effects of which could damage the sperm cells, in order that he might father a healthy child after his own recovery from his disease.

2. Hall left nothing to St. John under his will. The trial court is thus asked to conclude that Hall intended to father a posthumous child but not to provide for its welfare from his resources. The record does not contain evidence of either *inter vivos* arrangements by decedent for the benefit of posthumous children or the lack of necessity of those arrangements for other reasons.

3. St. John advised Dr. Dickey that plans for her impregnation were no longer immediate and neither Hall nor St. John had further contact with the Institute.

4. St. John and the decedent apparently chose not to begin the insemination process prior to his death, when there would be no question of the legality of the action. Had Hall intended to father a child even were he to die of his disease, would he not have wished to begin the process during his life in order to avoid the publicity and acrimony that have attended the posthumous conception process?

5. The Act of Donation was procured through the offices of St. John's law partner, rather than through a disinterested attorney. The Executrix may be able to prove at trial her allegations that the decedent was sufficiently ill and dependent upon St. John at the time the act was executed that he was not aware that it was an unconditional donation or did not freely give his consent thereto.

Any of these illustrative concerns could form a basis for the trial court's belief that the Act of Donation might be proven at trial to be invalid, and serve as a foundation for his discretionary grant of preliminary injunctive relief. We express no opinion on the preponderance of the evidence that will be adduced at a full trial on the merits, but we believe that the trial judge did not abuse his discretion in preserving the status quo pending that trial . . .

CONCLUSION

We find no abuse of the trial court's discretion in the decision to maintain the status quo while a full and complete determination of the validity of the act of donation may be made without the possible complication and distraction of the existence of human embryos or more developed offspring.

Affirmed.

JONES, J. and WARD, J. Concur.

NOTES AND QUESTIONS

1. If you were a juror presiding at the trial in this case, for whom would you find? Do you believe the preponderance of the evidence supports Christine St. John's claim that Barry Hall fully and competently expressed his intent to give her

control of his sperm for posthumous use?

Do you agree with the court that posthumous reproduction via frozen sperm is not against public policy? Whose interests are served by permitting a woman to give birth to a man's child after he has died? Whose interests are harmed?

2. There are several reasons why a man might want to bank frozen sperm, including preserving fertility in the face of cancer treatment, as a reserve prior to vasectomy, or in anticipation of IVF so that sperm is available on the day of egg retrieval. Increasingly, men who are in the military are encouraged to visit the sperm bank before they deploy into harm's way. Overseas the soldiers risk death, or impaired fertility due to exposure to chemical or biological weapons. See Valerie Alvord, *Some Troops Freeze Sperm Before Deploying*, USA Today, Jan. 27, 2003, at 1A. In a nod to our men in uniform, many sperm banks offer a "military discount" to servicemen, significantly reducing the cost of sperm retrieval, preparation and storage. On a tight budget, these savings can be significant, considering the cost for freezing a single specimen can run as high as $250, plus an additional annual fee of $330 for storage. See www.cryobank.com.

3. The *Hall* case bears some factual similarity to a California case that was winding its way through the court system at about the same time. On October 30, 1991, William Kane, aged 48, committed suicide at the Mirage Hotel in Las Vegas, leaving behind a note for the management reassuring them he had no complaints with the hotel. In the month before his death, Kane deposited 15 vials of sperm at the California Cryobank in Los Angeles, with written instructions authorizing the sperm bank to release the specimens to Deborah Hecht, his 38-year-old girlfriend. In addition, Kane's will specifically bequeathed the sperm to Hecht. When Hecht sought release of the vials, she was confronted by Kane's adult children who bitterly opposed their father's paramour in her pursuit to give birth to their half-sibling.

In a 1993 opinion, the California Court of Appeal reversed a trial court order directing Kane's executor to destroy all of the decedent's sperm. The court found that Kane had an interest in the sperm which falls within the broad definition of property, and thus could be the subject of a bequest. In addition, like the court in *Hall*, the California court concluded that public policy does not prohibit artificial insemination of a single woman, nor does it preclude an unmarried woman from engaging in posthumous conception. Ultimately, the court deferred to what it believed to be Kane's clear intent that Hecht should have access to his sperm for purposes of posthumous reproduction. *Hecht v. Superior Court*, 16 Cal. App. 4th 836, 20 Cal. Rptr. 2d 275 (1993). *Compare In re Estate of Kievernagal*, 166 Cal. App. 4th 1024, 83 Cal. Rptr. 3d 311, (Cal. Ct. App. 2008) (denying widow's request for distribution of late husband's frozen sperm because he checked "discard in event of death" on consent form; sperm was not part of husband's estate for purposes of asset distribution).

Despite this ruling, the children continued their litigation to deny Hecht the sperm, represented by their attorney-mother, Kane's first wife. Finally in 1996, the court dismissed all the children's claims and ordered all 15 vials distributed to Hecht, the named beneficiary. 50 Cal. App. 4th 1289, 59 Cal. Rptr. 2d 222 (1996). Perhaps the Kane family had more in mind than the vigorous pursuit of their claim; by the time Hecht received the sperm she was nearing 42, considered "AMA" (advanced maternal age) in fertility circles. Reportedly upon receiving the vials, she exclaimed "I have sperm and I'm going to get preggers now," adding, "We're going in vitro, and I'm excited." Carla Hall, *Lover Wins Custody of Dead Man's Sperm*, L.A. TIMES, Feb. 25, 1997, at A1. There is no record of Hecht having given birth.

Michael H. Shapiro
Illicit Reasons and Means for Reproduction: On Excessive Choice and Categorical and Technological Imperatives
47 Hast. L. J. 1081, 1127 (1996)

Posthumous Reproduction Through Use of Gametes

There are several mechanisms for posthumous production: obtaining and saving gametes or embryos while the genetic parents are alive; harvesting gametes after their sources are dead; and maintaining the bodies of dead pregnant women . . . What one thinks of posthumous reproducing may depend not only on analysis of the reasons gamete sources or others have for doing so, and on the circumstances involved, but on the precise mechanism used.

There are situations in which we would be hard pressed to establish that preservation of gametes for posthumous reproduction is selfish or irresponsible. A standard example would be a soldier going off to war. If there is something unpleasantly egotistical about this, it is not so awful that it should be discouraged. From the standpoint of the soldier's mate, there is little to be said for the idea that he or she is selfish for wanting a child formed in part by the departed soldier. But, to get to the obvious point, what of the late Mr. Kane and Ms. Hecht, who wished to use his stored sperm? Mr. Kane's children accused him of selfishness. To wish for fatherhood after one's death is "egotistic and irresponsible," according to Mr. Kane's survivors.

Once again, a presumption of selfishness or irresponsibility makes little sense. For one thing, the deceased may have wished to make Ms. Hecht, his significant other, happy. If her desire to have a child by him rather than by anyone else was at the time irrational, so be it; wanting to reproduce . . . is not the place to look for exemplars of rational behavior. If he wanted to make her happy, why is this either selfish or irresponsible? If he thought posthumous reproduction was a way of extending his own existence, the same question applies. If the thought is foolish, it is not necessarily illegitimate.

Perhaps it is selfish because it imposes unacceptable risks on the child: a single-parent household, only one provider, and a world that thinks her origins are bizarre. It seems even worse if the dead parent disliked the idea of caring for children. One may concede that there are risks here, but that these risks are unacceptable is another matter. I am aware of neither facts nor theory that would clearly show such reproduction to be bad for anyone, including the resulting children. It is quite possible to seriously doubt one's parenting skills but think it beneficial to have offspring after death — to make the prospective mother happy, to transmit an excellent genome, or, again, to extend one's being. When we consider some of the questionable reasons for having children while we are alive (everybody else does it? carrying on the family name?), posthumous parenthood seems less odd, less like tampering with death. Moreover, any instabilities concerning property distributions could easily be ameliorated by legislation regulating posthumous claims. Section 4 of the Uniform Status of Children of Assisted Conception Act, for example, deals with this problem by providing that a fertile decedent "is not a parent of the resulting child."

This is not to say that there is a strong constitutional liberty interest in this form of procreation. Critics rightly analyze it by referring to the split between biological reproduction and the ordinarily expected benefits of companionship of one's children. Few people would value reproduction if their children were snatched and raised by the State in some version of Plato's Republic. This would be mere "abstract parenthood," parenthood without responsibility — the ultimate delegation of parenthood to others. There is a large gap between the genetic forebear and his personal connection with the children. Being a dead forbear is not what "parenting" is about and fails to take parenthood seriously — or so one might say. So why defer to such a preference for procreation without connection?

But this is an incomplete account. There are different possible circumstances for posthumous parenting through saved gametes. If the decedent had a personally known, living parent-to-be in mind (as did Kane), his preference seems less abstract and bizarre than, say, pursuing "immortality" by saving gametes for anyone to use, even eons after one's own death. Perhaps present happiness is elevated when one believes that a loved one will raise one's child. And the intended surviving parent has her/his own liberty interest at stake, which is likely to be more highly rated under the Constitution than the decedent's.

It appears, then, that Mr. Kane's plans were far from irrational, however unusual they were. He had already experienced the companionship of his prior children and apparently wished to help promote the same enjoyment for Ms. Hecht. This case is not about losing your child to the state or to anyone else. It is not about child abandonment; nor is it about any classic form of irresponsibility. One can imagine cases in which we would be right to ascribe selfishness or irresponsibility to someone who wishes to reproduce posthumously, but round condemnations of such plans, once again, make no sense.

Ms. Hecht, of course, did not plan to be a posthumous parent. Is there any basis for ascribing selfishness, irresponsibility, or any other category of illicitness to her? She may be a single parent, at least at first — but so what? Her child will likely be advised of his or her origins — but so what? As the court pointed out, there was no relevant policy against reproduction by single women, and whatever the incremental risks involved, no compelling case for interdiction is apparent.

Compare Hecht v. Kane-like situations with harvesting the gametes of the recently dead. Imagine, for example, a young man killed before he is able to reproduce. If there were indications that he was likely to attempt reproduction with a specific woman (the clearest case would be if he were married or engaged to her), would she have a reasonable claim for requesting a sperm harvest? What about his parents, who may wish for grandchildren?

There may be many important reasons why sperm might be sought for postmortem fatherhood. It may be that partners had long promised one another to have children; that goal may have been a sustaining feature of the relationship. In other instances, having a child may not honor any specific promise to the brain dead partner, but it might serve as a meaningful way for a surviving partner to honor the nature of the previous relationship, whether this relation was formalized in marriage or not.

I suppose one could argue that wanting a memento of a dead loved one is perfectly rational — depending on the memento and its future. But to reproduce for the purpose of designating a living person as nothing but a "memento" is an example of selfishness, irresponsibility, objectification, and using someone solely as a means, rather than treating them as an end. It is fine to view children as chips off living blocks (or blocks who actually had a hand in nurturing them), but not acceptable to use a child as a photograph. This reflects pathological obsession with the memory of the dead, and the remedy is Prozac, not reproduction.

The arguments against posthumous reproduction are vulnerable, however. The risks to the child are not well established, and in any event, the alternative is nonexistence. More, the very descriptions offered may be question-begging: who says that the children are mere mementos, living photographs, used only as a sort of homage to the dead? What would this mean? Neither the motivation nor the means seem obviously illicit in any of the senses mentioned earlier. Unless one relies on rigid authoritative postulates such as cultural norms of certain sorts, the case for condemnation seems weak.

Have any risks been overlooked, after all? Apart from financial matters, prior children of the deceased may not want their emotional lives complicated by new siblings, especially if they dislike the intended live parent. But they might also welcome other children of their dead parent and cultivate a relationship with them. In any case, how should we rate the surviving children's preferences? Should posthumous gamete use rest on what these children prefer? Should a former wife's wishes count? Does the risk that a posthumous child will become a public charge or menace outweigh the decedent's wishes? Perhaps the risks of single parenting, whatever they are, are amplified by posthumous reproduction, and should be taken only when they are justified — as where the parent of an existing fetus is dying. But is it fair to limit the chance for posthumous parenthood to dying persons?

More generally: will the occasional "unnatural" practice of posthumous artificial insemination or inovulation erode important social values? Reproduction that straddles life and death seems to challenge the worth of an institution favoring optimal child rearing by both a mother and father, preferably within a marriage entailing a "hands on" personal commitment and bond. Challenging this ideal, one might argue, will propel us into social chaos. To run that risk evidences both selfishness and irresponsibility.

It seems unlikely, however, that the occasional practice of posthumous reproduction will lead us to social chaos. In any case, the risk is sufficiently speculative that attributions of selfishness or irresponsibility seem extravagant.

Professor Shapiro's poignant analysis raises some of the same issues we considered in Chapter 3 in connection with postmenopausal reproduction. Both practices pull reproduction away from the "norm" and invite balancing of rights (to procreate) and harms (to offspring). Arguable, postmortem reproduction becomes the more ethically complex practice when ambiguities about the donor's consent present. While consent to procreate may be inferred from a man who made deposits at a sperm bank prior to death, such consent is not as easily inferred when no such lifetime actions were taken. Can it be said that a man who expressed no intent to procreate during life is an appropriate subject for parenthood after death? With this question in mind, we next consider the practice of postmortem sperm retrieval — harvesting sperm from a dead man.

2. Sperm Retrieval After Death

The posthumous disposition of frozen sperm can usually be resolved by reference to the written or oral instructions left by the donor, or even by reference to the donor's conduct surrounding the specimen donations. What if the donor is already dead when the sperm is retrieved? In recent years, scientists have learned that sperm can survive a man's death for up to 36 hours, making postmortem sperm retrieval a realistic possibility. Moreover, postmortem sperm has proved viable, aiding in the conception and birth of a small, but growing number of children.

Postmortem sperm retrieval was first reported in 1980 by Dr. Cappy Rothman, the current director of the California Cryobank. See C.M. Rothman, *A Method for Obtaining Viable Sperm in the Postmortem State*, 34 FERTILITY & STERILITY 512 (1980). Between 1980 and 1995, researchers reported a total of 82 requests at 40 facilities across the United States for sperm retrieval from a man declared legally dead. See Susan Kerr, *Post-Mortem Sperm Procurement: Is It Legal?*, 3 DEPAUL J. HEALTH CARE L. 39, 45 (1999). So common are these requests, some institutions have issued written policies surrounding requests for postmortem sperm retrieval. *See, e.g.*, New York Hospital Guidelines for Consideration for Requests for Postmortem Sperm Retrieval, available at: https://www.cornellurology.com/resources/guidelines/. There are several methods for posthumous sperm removal, including electroejaculation, microsurgical epididymal sperm aspiration (MESA) in which a syringe is placed in the epididymal tubule to aspirate sperm, and testicular sperm extraction (TSE) in which the entire testes are removed for sperm retrieval in the laboratory. See Frances R. Batzer, Joshua M. Hurwitz, & Arthur Caplan, *Postmortem Parenthood and the Need for a Protocol With Posthumous Sperm Procurement*, 79 FERTILITY & STERILITY 1263 (2003).

The first case of posthumous sperm retrieval to garner international attention involved Diane Blood, a British woman whose young husband developed meningitis and died suddenly in 1995. Immediately before and after his death, sperm was retrieved from Mr. Blood at Mrs. Blood's request. The problem arose when Mrs. Blood sought to use the specimens. Prevailing British law, the 1990 Human Fertilisation and Embryology Act, established government guidelines to safeguard the interests of the resulting child in such unique and difficult cases. The British Court of Appeal ruled that insemination could not take place in the United Kingdom without Mr. Blood's written consent, but Mrs. Blood could proceed with treatments outside the UK. *Regina v. Human Fertilisation and Embryology Authority*, [1999] Fam. 151 (Court of Appeal). Eventually, Diane Blood was inseminated in Belgium and she is now the mother of two sons, Liam born in 1998 and Joel in 2002. See Anne Marie Owens, *Babies From Beyond the Grave*, NAT'L. POST, Sept, 28, 2004, at A1.

A California woman became the first American to give birth using sperm retrieved from her dead husband. Gaby Vernoff had sperm removed from her husband's body 30 hours after his death, and stored the specimens for 15 months before trying to conceive. After the bereavement period, Vernoff underwent IVF with ICSI (in which the sperm is injected directly into the egg) and gave birth to a daughter, Brendalynn, in 1999. Vernoff filed a lawsuit in federal court in 2004 after the Social Security Administration ruled that Brendalynn Vernoff was not eligible for her genetic father's survivor benefits because she was not a child of the deceased under state law. See Lindsay Fortado, *Born Into Legal Limbo: Kids Conceived Posthumously Are Winning In Court*, 26 NAT'L. L. J. 1 (2004). A federal appeals court affirmed the SSA denial of benefits, reasoning that the decedent was not the child's "natural father" under California law. *Vernoff v. Astrue*, 568 F.3d 1102 (9th Cir. 2009). In Section 2, *infra*, we take a closer look at inheritance and other economic issues that plague postmortem conceived children.

Postmortem reproduction in general raises questions about the parental status of the gamete provider (Is the sperm donor the legal parent of the posthumously born child?) and the inheritance rights of the child (Is the child a lawful heir of the sperm donor under state intestate succession law?). Postmortem sperm retrieval adds an additional factor — the donor's consent to have sperm removed after death. If the man left no evidence that he wanted to father children, or had been outspoken in his desire to *not* become a father, could a physician accommodate a wife or girlfriend's request to procure his sperm after death? What if the request came from a man's mother or sister who wished for her beloved son or brother to "live on" through a child? If the donor and the donee were not married or intimate with one another, should retrieval be automatically ruled out? These and other questions are considered in the commentary that follows.

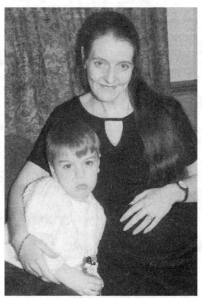

Diane Blood with son Liam, expecting son Joel
February 2002

Carson Strong
Ethical and Legal Aspects of Sperm Retrieval After Death
or Persistent Vegetative State
27 J. Law, Medicine & Ethics 347 (1999)

. . . Some have put forward the view that postmortem sperm retrieval and insemination should not be performed without explicit prior consent . . . Something close to this view is accepted as a matter of policy in the United Kingdom, where the Human Fertilisation and Embryology Act forbids the storage of sperm after death without the man's prior written consent . . .

What seems to underlie the view that explicit consent is necessary is a concern to respect previously alive persons and, specifically, to be respectful to their dead bodies. A potential for disrespect arises from at least two features of postmortem sperm retrieval: the physical manipulation and the reproductive implications. Sperm retrieval involves physical manipulations that penetrate the dead man's body. In our culture, it is considered disrespectful to the dead to do things to their bodies to which they would have objected when alive . . . Although the concern about reproductive implications has not been articulated thoroughly, for now we can say at least this much: it is disrespectful to previously alive persons to use their gametes for reproductive purposes to which they would have objected. Because respect for the previously alive person includes respect for that person's autonomy, any disrespect that might otherwise be involved in postmortem sperm retrieval is removed if the person autonomously gave explicit prior consent.

My main thesis is that the ethics of postmortem sperm retrieval is not as straightforward as these advocates of explicit prior consent think. Although requiring explicit prior consent might initially appear ethically sound, it involves a problem that needs to be addressed. Specifically, in other areas of medicine where decisions must be made in the absence of explicit prior consent, it is recognized as respectful of patient autonomy to make decisions in accordance with the reasonably inferred wishes of the patient. Consider, for example, decisions about whether to procure organs from brain-dead patients who have not signed donor cards or previously discussed organ donation with their physicians. In such circumstances, it is possible to respect the autonomy of the previously alive person when it can be ascertained what that person would have wanted. Family members might be asked whether the patient had ever expressed a desire to donate organs after death. If it can reasonably be inferred that the patient would approve of organ donation, then removal of organs for transplantation would be respectful of his autonomy.

Similar considerations seem to apply to postmortem sperm retrieval when explicit prior consent is absent. If it is reasonable to infer that the previously alive person would approve of sperm retrieval and insemination, then carrying out such procedures would be respectful of that person's autonomy . . .

I am only claiming that reasonably inferred consent provides a basis for respecting patient autonomy — and not that reasonably inferred consent makes postmortem sperm retrieval ethically justifiable. The fact that autonomy is respected does not in itself make the retrieval justifiable; additional arguments are needed to support that claim . . .

Is freedom to procreate (or not procreate) after death valuable?

Let us begin by considering situations in which persons have explicitly stated their autonomous wishes concerning procreation after death, whether those wishes be for or against such procreation. We can suppose that the patient gave an unrevoked written or verbal statement of wishes to health care professionals. We want to consider what reasons might exist for respecting a person's wishes in this type of case . . .

Let us begin with the scenario in which the man states that he wants his sperm to be used. [What are] some of the reasons for valuing freedom to procreate[?] First, such use of sperm could involve participation in the creation of a person. Such participation can be meaningful to individuals for a variety of reasons. Some might attach importance to the idea of bringing into being an individual who develops self-consciousness. For others, the significance of participating in the creation of a person might be religious . . . [I]t is reasonable to say that a man can participate in the creation of a person even though the insemination occurs after death. After all, the man can take actions when alive that will cause the insemination to occur, and it is his sperm that would be used. Admittedly, the man would not know whether the attempt to create a person would be successful. Nevertheless, the plan to accomplish it and the hope that the plan succeeds could be meaningful to a person and could contribute to self-identity.

Second, a plan to procreate after the death of one member of a couple can be an affirmation of mutual love and acceptance. There have been cases in which postmortem procreation has been planned and has had this sort of special meaning for the couple . . . Such plans can contribute to self-identity and self-fulfillment.

Third, some value procreation because it provides a link to future persons. There may be various ways in which such a link could have personal meaning. For some, it may be important to play a role in the continuation of humanity. For others, having a family line that continues may have significance. Such a link to the future can be created even though conception occurs after one's death. Although the man would not know whether the link actually occurred, the plan to create it could have personal significance and contribute to self-identity.

Thus, persons can give significant reasons for valuing procreation after death. Because such reasons can be given, freedom to attempt such procreation deserves at least some degree of respect . . .

A second possibility is that a man would state a wish not to procreate after death. Although some of the main reasons for valuing freedom not to procreate in the ordinary context do not apply to postmortem procreation, at least one can; namely, the desire to avoid bringing a child into being in circumstances the person considers undesirable for rearing. Some men might be opposed to creating a child when they would be unable to participate in rearing, as in postmortem procreation. It should be acknowledged that freedom not to procreate after death has less impact on one's life than freedom not to procreate during one's lifetime. Thus, the argument for respecting freedom not to procreate when alive is stronger than the argument for respecting freedom not to procreate after death. Nevertheless, avoiding procreation after death can be important to some persons, and this gives the argument for respecting those decisions some degree of strength . . .

When is postmortem sperm retrieval and insemination defensible?

. . . [I]magine a scenario in which a wife requests [postmortem sperm retrieval] in opposition to a man's reasonably inferred desire that they not be performed. For example, family members other than the wife might give a convincing account that the man would not want postmortem retrieval. In this type of situation, a conflict arises between the wife's freedom to procreate and the previously existing man's freedom not to procreate . . . [T]he wife's freedom to procreate is comparable in strength to freedom to procreate in the ordinary scenario; . . . freedom not to procreate posthumously is less important than freedom not to procreate in the ordinary context. If one relied only on these arguments, one would conclude that the wife's wishes should prevail. However, additional considerations exist, and they strongly support giving priority to the man's freedom. First, the retrieval would involve physical manipulations that penetrate the dead man's body; as pointed out, it is disrespectful to the dead to do things to their bodies to which they would have objected when alive. Second, other avenues for procreating would be available to the wife; she could find another partner or use donor sperm, for example. For these reasons, retrieval would not be ethically justifiable if it were reasonable to infer that the man would object. Even if the wife has legal authority to make decisions concerning disposition of his body, ethically, that authority ought not extend to include a right to have sperm removed from his body against his wishes.

A more common scenario involves a wife requesting retrieval when neither the man's approval nor disapproval can reasonably be inferred. In these circumstances, the question is whether her freedom to procreate should prevail despite an absence of the man's reasonably inferred consent. It can be argued that retrieval should not be performed in this type of situation as well. Near the outset, I stated that it is disrespectful to previously alive persons to use their gametes for reproductive purposes to which they would have objected. Based on the above discussion, we can state the following, more encompassing, ethical rule: a person's gametes, and preembryos created with those gametes, should not be used for procreative purposes without the person's explicit or reasonably inferred consent. The retrieval and insemination in question would violate this rule . . .

NOTES AND QUESTIONS

1.   Professor Strong's view that postmortem sperm retrieval can be justified if the decedent left explicit prior consent *or* reasonably inferred consent has drawn dissenters. Some criticize the concept of "reasonably inferred consent" as too vague, making it impossible for physicians to judge whether a lifetime expression or lack of expression can be inferred as consent to postmortem retrieval. See Gladys B. White, *Commentary: Legal and Ethical Aspects of Sperm Retrieval*, 27 J. LAW, MED. & ETHICS 359 (1999). Critics of the "reasonably inferred consent" standard would much prefer a requirement of explicit prior consent of the man, so as to minimize the impact of emotional and biased testimonials from grieving family members.

Other critics take exception to Professor Strong's assertion that the freedom to procreate after death can be meaningful during a person's life and should thus be respected in the form of posthumous sperm retrieval. The experiences that make reproduction a valued freedom — conception, gestation, birth, and rearing — would be lost on a predeceased parent, thus cannot be used to support a right to posthumous procreative liberty. See John Robertson, *Posthumous Reproduction*, 69 Ind. L. J. 1027 (1994); John A. Gibbons, *Who's Your Daddy? A Constitutional Analysis of Post-Mortem Insemination*, 14 J. CONTEMP. HEALTH L. & POL'Y 187 (1997).

A final controversial point is Professor Strong's analogy to solid organ harvesting, such as when family members consent to have the kidneys, lungs, hearts or livers removed from their dying or deceased relative. In most states, the Uniform Anatomical Gift Act allows next of kin to consent to the retrieval of organs and tissues after death, unless there is evidence that the decedent would not have consented. Is Professor Strong's analogy to solid organ donation apt? Is retrieving sperm for insemination the same as harvesting organs for transplantation? For a thorough analysis distinguishing posthumous reproduction from organ procurement and transplantation, see Anne Reichman Schiff, *Arising From the Dead: Challenges of Posthumous Procreation*, 75 N.C. L. REV. 901 (1997).

2.   *Requests by Parents and Partners.* Most of the academic literature on the merits and ethics of postmortem sperm retrieval focuses on requests by the dead man's wife. In fact, increasingly requests for these services are being made by the deceased's parent (typically the mother) and nonspousal partner (a fiancee or girlfriend). The story of Daniel Christy is both tragic and typical. At the age of 23,

Daniel was gravely injured in a motorcycle accident in his home state of Iowa. While on life support, his fiancee asked that his sperm be retrieved so she could fulfill their plans to have a family in the future. Daniel's parents supported this posthumous reproductive plan and the threesome brought the issue to a local judge who ruled that the state's Anatomical Gift Act permitted the parents to consent to the retrieval. *See* Martha Neil, *Iowa Judge OKs Sperm Donation by Dying Man*, ABA JOURNAL (Sept. 14, 2007). *See also* Joel Greenberg, *In Life a Soldier, In Death a Father?* CHI. TRIBUNE (Jan. 29, 2007) (detailing legal journey of Israeli mother who sued to use sperm retrieved from her son after being killed by a sniper while on military patrol; court permitted mother to seek out an egg donor and gestational carrier to give birth to her grandchild).

Anecdotal reports suggest that requests for postmortem sperm retrieval far exceed subsequent requests for its use. Cappy Rothman, medical director at the California Cryobank and author of the first academic paper describing postmortem sperm retrieval, reveals that in a span of 30 years, he has performed approximately 50 retrievals, with only two wives requesting and successfully using the salvaged gametes. *See* Eric Laborde, Jay Sandlow & Robert E. Brannigan, *Postmortem Sperm Retrieval*, 32(5) J. ANDROLOGY (Sept./Oct. 2011).

3. The American Society for Reproductive Medicine considered the implications of postmortem reproduction in 1997 and again in 2004, urging its member physicians and fertility clinics to have patients complete consent forms that stipulate the disposition of gametes and embryos after death. When patients fail to leave instructions, or when the surviving spouse seeks to use gametes or embryos that the decedent explicitly declined to authorize for posthumous reproduction, the ASRM counsels:

> Programs are urged to insist that donors make their wishes known. If no decision on disposition after death has been made, one would expect that in most instances this would preclude any posthumous use.

> A request by a husband or wife for use of stored gametes or embryos to override a prior denial of posthumous reproduction by the deceased spouse should not be honored. A spouse's request that sperm or ova be obtained terminally or soon after death without the prior consent or known wishes of the deceased spouse need not be honored.

Ethics Committee of the American Society for Reproductive Medicine, *Posthumous Reproduction*, 82 FERTILITY & STERILITY S260 (2004). How do you interpret the ASRM position on reasonably inferred consent?

A different, arguably more flexible, approach to postmortem sperm retrieval is offered by a group of physicians and bioethicists:

> Posthumous sperm procurement may be performed if written documentation from the deceased authorizing the procedure is available. If such documentation is not present, proof from a nonbenefiting party, such as a physician, may be presented in support of the request. Reasonable effort should be made to obtain support or objections from other family members. Because reasonably inferred consent is difficult to determine, a judicial order may be required.

Frances R. A, Joshua M. Hurwitz, & Arthur Caplan, *Postmortem Parenthood and the Need for a Protocol With Posthumous Sperm Procurement*, 79 FERTILITY & STERILITY 1263 (2003).

Suppose a urologist is called upon to retrieve sperm from a 30-year-old man who has been in a coma for three years. The man's mother explains that her son talked enthusiastically about someday becoming a father before a diving accident left him in his debilitated state. The mother pledges that she will not use the sperm if her son dies, but only wants to preserve his fertility should he regain consciousness. How should the doctor respond? According to Professor Strong? According to the ASRM? According to Drs. Batzer, Hurwitz and Caplan?

4. Kathy and Russell are a married couple undergoing treatment for infertility at the American Fertility Center (AFC), under the supervision of Dr. Ramirez. The couple just completed an unsuccessful cycle of IVF and they are about to begin their second attempt. One week before the treatment is scheduled to begin, Russell telephones Dr. Ramirez to say that he feels his marriage is "on the rocks" and he is uncertain about continuing the IVF treatments.

Russell makes an appointment to speak personally with Dr. Ramirez the next day, but tragically he is killed in an automobile accident that evening. Late into the night, Dr. Ramirez receives a call from Dr. Nguyen, a urologist who has been contacted by Kathy. Dr. Nguyen explains that Kathy has asked her to retrieve sperm from Russell, explaining that his intent to become a parent is evidenced by the couple's ongoing treatment at AFC. Dr. Nguyen says that she has the technical expertise to retrieve viable sperm from Russell, but she is seeking confirmation from Dr. Ramirez that his patient would have consented to such action. Advise Dr. Ramirez.

B. Freezing Eggs: Retrieval During Life and After Death

The process of freezing and thawing a woman's eggs is a relatively new and emerging technology. While sperm and embryos have been successfully cryopreserved for years, eggs proved more difficult to freeze because they contain a significant amount of water, causing damaging ice crystals to form at low temperatures. Much of the early research on egg freezing was conducted by Italian scientists in the early 1990s, but the research has become more global in the ensuing years. New techniques focus on a process known as vitrification, in which eggs are cooled and dehydrated at a rapid rate to minimize damage to the cell structures. Today it is estimated that around 2,000 children have been born from frozen eggs worldwide, about 400 of them in the United States. *See* Alison Motluk, *Growth of Egg Freezing Blurs 'Experimental' Label*, 476 NATURE 382 (Aug. 2011), available at: http://www.nature.com/news/2011/110823/full/476382a.html.

Women elect to freeze their eggs for two primary reasons — fertility preservation and delayed reproduction. For women, and even girls, diagnosed with diseases that require life-saving but fertility-destroying treatment (such as some chemo-therapeutic agents and radiation), retrieving and freezing eggs prior to undergoing medical therapy can stave off infertility in the future. Success with egg freezing in the face of a sterilizing medical therapy means that women who face such treatments can preserve their fertility without having to pair their eggs with sperm in order to create an embryo, which was previously the only way to insure a future opportunity for genetic parenthood. Single women, for example, can now wait until they marry or find a chosen male partner before creating an embryo for implantation.[6]

Egg freezing is also an option for women who wish to delay childbearing but maximize their chance for a successful conception and pregnancy by preserving their gametes at a younger, more viable stage. While physicians are cautiously optimistic about the science of egg freezing, they stress that women who use the technology to preserve younger eggs for later childbearing should be aware of the risks. The pregnancy rates are still lower than with fresh eggs, and the costs are unaffordable for many women. A business enterprise called Extend Fertility, operates centers in eight cities across the U.S., offering prospective clients "the opportunity to effectively slow their biological clocks." The price for this decelerated tick tock? Clients should be prepared to spend $10,000 to $15,000 for one treatment cycle, plus $500 annually for frozen storage fees.[7] Of course, no guarantees are made on the condition of the eggs once thawed. The hope of the business' backers is that women interested in delaying childbearing will be willing to pay the fee as an insurance policy against later infertility. Recognizing the potential for egg freezing to create false hopes and mislead the general public, the American Society for Reproductive Medicine warns that oocyte cryopreservation, "should not be currently either marketed or offered as a means to defer reproductive aging." *See* The Practice Committee of the American Society for Reproductive Medicine and the Practice Committee of the Society for Assisted Reproductive Technology, *Ovarian Tissue and Oocyte Cryopreservation*, 90 FERTILITY & STERILITY S241 (2008).

To date, all known instances of egg freezing and subsequent thawing have involved women or girls who were alive at the time their gametes were harvested. As we discovered in reviewing sperm retrieval, science has advanced to the point where a man's gametes can be successfully retrieved after his death and used by his spouse or partner (or parent) in a later IVF cycle. Is the same true for postmortem retrieval of a woman's eggs? Can a husband, partner or parent ask a surgeon to remove a deceased woman's eggs (or portion of her ovary containing developing oocytes) and expect that she can become a genetic mother posthumously? The

---

[6] Fertility preservation techniques for women facing cancer treatment can involve the removal and freezing of a portion of the ovary prior to chemotherapy or radiation. Once the patient recovers and is ready to reproduce, the ovarian tissue is thawed and grafted under the remaining ovary. This technique has proved successful, allowing cancer survivors to conceive healthy children "the old-fashioned way." *See* Helen Pearson, *Frozen ovary Restores Fertility*, 26 DISCOVER 27 (Jan. 2005).

[7] Tipping the other end of the mercenary scale is a nationwide program called Sharing Hope, which offers discounts on fertility preservation treatments for cancer patients facing gamete-damaging therapy. The program provides discounted egg, sperm and embryo freezing and storage services at 15 fertility clinics and sperm banks nationwide. Sharing Hope founders, a group named Fertile Hope, started the program after learning that insurance companies often do not cover fertility-preservation treatments because patients do not qualify as infertile (failure to conceive after one year of unprotected intercourse) until after their treatment is over, when the damage is often irreversible. The Lance Armstrong Foundation is providing funding for the administration of the Sharing Hope program. See Amy Dockser Marcus, *Prices Cut for Fertility Preservation*, Wall St. J., Sept. 28, 2004, at D6.

answer is probably. In August 2011, the parents of a 17-year-old Israeli girl killed while crossing a street asked surgeons to remove and freeze their daughter's eggs for future use. Under Israeli law, the parents were forced to seek a court order authorizing the oocyte retrieval. The court granted the parents' request and the surgery was performed. The eggs remain in frozen storage awaiting possible thaw and fertilization. *See* Dan Even, *Dead Woman's Ova Harvested After Court Okays Family Request*, HAARETZ, Aug. 8, 2011.

In the U.S., a similar request for oocyte retrieval from the family of a 36-year-old woman who suddenly fell ill on a transatlantic flight was declined. The hospital cited medical, ethical and legal reasons for refusing to offer the procedure in that case. *See* David Greer, Aaron Styer, Thomas Toth, Charles Kindregan, Javier Romero, *Case 21-2010: A Request for Retrieval of Oocytes from a 36 Year-Old Woman with Anoxic Brain Injury*, 363 NEW ENG. J. MED. 276 (2010). If the U.S. physicians had agreed to harvest the woman's eggs after she died, and then fertilized them with the sperm retrieved postmortem, the world would welcome the first child to be conceived using the egg and sperm of two predeceased parents. Technically, the capability for birth of such a child exists. In 2007, a California woman gave birth to the world's first baby conceived using both frozen egg and frozen sperm. *See Orange County Woman Makes History by Giving Birth to the Nation's First Frozen Egg/Frozen Sperm Baby*, BIOTECH WEEK 385 (Apr. 25, 2007).

PROBLEM

Dr. Michael Soules, Director of the Division of Reproductive Endocrinology at the University of Washington, recalls the night he received a telephone call from a 21-year-old woman whose 19-year-old sister was brain dead 12 hours after a motor vehicle accident. Curious why the woman would call him at such a time, she explained the family's wish that the sister's ovaries be harvested and her eggs preserved. "I want to keep a part of my sister so she will continue to live," lamented the woman. See Michael R. Soules, *Commentary: Pasthumous Harvesting of Gametes — A Physician's Perspective*, 27 J. LAW, MED. & ETHICS 362 (1999).

Suppose Dr. Soules was able to harvest the sister's ovaries and preserve her eggs for later use. Two years later the mother calls and asks to have the eggs thawed in preparation for fertilization. The sperm will be provided by a family friend and the embryo will be gestated by the sister, who is unmarried. The child will be raised by the mother, who would be the child's grandmother. Should Dr. Soules comply with the family's request? If not, what rationale should he provide to the family?

C. Freezing Embryos

The ability to freeze and thaw embryos drew scientific attention shortly after the introduction of in vitro fertilization in the late 1970s. The first pregnancy resulting from a frozen embryo was reported in Australia in 1983. *See* Alan Tounson & Linda Mohr, *Human Pregnancy Following Cryopreservation, Thawing and Transfer of an Eight-Cell Embryo*, 305 NATURE 707 (1983). A year later, the first live birth from a frozen and thawed embryo was reported. Today, embryo cryopreservation is a routine part of IVF treatment, as typically a couple produces more embryos than can reasonably be implanted in any single cycle. Freezing preserves embryos for future cycles, enabling women to attempt pregnancy without having to repeat the egg retrieval process. Though pregnancy rates using frozen embryos are lower than rates using fresh embryos (35.2% for frozen compared to 47.2% for fresh embryos in women under age 35, as reported by the CDC in 2011), the success rate is still substantial enough for individuals and couples to utilize the freezing and thawing technology in their quest for reproduction.

The process of embryo cryopreservation is described in nice detail by Professors Sharona Hoffman and Andrew Morriss:

> Cryopreservation of embryos involves a complex, multi-step process. First, a sequence of drugs is used to induce the maturation of multiple follicles so that several eggs, or oocytes, can be retrieved from the woman. Just prior to ovulation, the eggs are removed in a minor surgical procedure called ultrasound-guided transvaginal aspiration. While an ultrasound transducer provides images of the reproductive organs, a needle is inserted through the vaginal wall and into a developed ovarian follicle. The fluid inside the follicle is withdrawn together with the egg it contains, and the procedure is repeated for each follicle, utilizing the initial vaginal puncture.

> After retrieval, eggs are examined in the laboratory to determine their level of maturity and optimal time for fertilization. The oocytes are then placed in a tissue-culture medium where they remain undisturbed for two to twenty-four hours prior to fertilization.

> Semen is obtained from the male partner and is processed so that a concentrated sample can be introduced into individual culture dishes, each containing medium and one egg. After a day, the oocyte is examined to determine whether fertilization has occurred, and, if it has, the cell is an embryo, and it is stored in a nutrient culture medium that is placed in a warm incubator.

> Embryos are frozen on the second or third day after oocyte retrieval, when they have divided into four to eight cells. Prior to freezing, the cells' liquid interior is replaced with a cryoprotectant solution so that the embryos are protected from the formation of damaging ice crystals. Embryos are then placed in straws that contain a very small amount of fluid and are slowly frozen, using computerized machines. The straws are stored in canisters that are kept frozen with liquid nitrogen. Prior to implantation, the storage straws are gradually warmed, the cryoprotectants are removed, and the embryos are cultured for about a day.

Sharona Hoffman & Andrew P. Morriss, *Birth After Death: Perpetuities and the New Reproductive Technologies*, 38 GA. L. REV. 575, 595-60 (2004).

An indication of the success and attraction of cryopreservation are the large numbers of embryos currently held in frozen storage. In 2003, it was estimated that some 400,000 embryos were housed in sub-zero facilities in the United States alone. See Rick Weiss, *400,000 Human Embryos Frozen in U.S.: Number at Fertility Clinics Is Far Greater Than Previous Estimates, Survey Finds*, WASH. POST, May 8,

2003, at A10. Though no formal subsequent count has been undertaken, the fact that 150,000 cycles of IVF are performed every year in the U.S. suggests the number of frozen embryos has grown in the past decade. Inevitably, like taxes, the progenitors of these embryos will die, some leaving no instructions as to the disposition of this potential future generation. If the woman dies, can the man hire a gestational carrier to gestate the couple's embryos? If a man dies, can the woman implant the embryos without any prior written authority from the man? If both parents/ progenitors die, can the embryos be adopted by another couple? If the embryos are gestated, are the resulting children heirs of their genetic parents?

The only known case to test the limits of posthumous reproduction using frozen embryos in which both gamete providers had died occurred about 30 years ago. In 1983, Los Angeles residents Elsa and Mario Rios were killed in a plane crash in the mountains over Chile, leaving two frozen embryos in storage in Australia. The couple died intestate, meaning they had not made a will naming the beneficiaries of their estate. Mr. Rios' adult son from a prior marriage openly contested the notion that the embryos be given an opportunity to be born, and perhaps assert rights against his father's estate, valued at approximately seven million dollars. In Australia, the Waller Committee, a government-appointed task force charged with studying the legal, social, and ethical issues arising from in vitro fertilization, was asked to investigate the questions regarding the Rios frozen embryos. The Waller Committee determined it would be proper to destroy the embryos, as the embryos had no independent legal rights. Subsequently, legislators of the state of Victoria, Australia, passed a law requiring that the embryos be made available for implantation in surrogates, and then, after birth, be placed for adoption.

In 1985, the matter was resolved in the United States when the Los Angeles Superior Court ruled that any children born from the frozen embryos would be barred from staking any legal claim to the Rios estate. Though the court cleared the way for embryo adoption, there is no evidence that the Rios embryos were ever adopted or gestated. See Thomas D. Arado, *Frozen Embryos and Divorce: Technological Marvel Meets the Human Condition*, 21 N. ILL. L. REV. 241 (2001); Kate W. Lyon, *Babies on Ice: The Legal Status of Frozen Embryos Involved In custody Disputes During Divorce*, 21 WHITTIER L. REV. 695 (2000); Andrea Michelle Siegel, *Legal Resolution to the Frozen Embryo Dilemma*, 4 J. PHARMACY & LAW 43 (1994); Bruce L. Wilder, *Assisted Reproduction Technology: Trends and Suggestions for the Developing Law*, 18 J. AM. ACAD. MATRIMONIAL L. 177 (2002).

The Rios case brings to light the numerous legal challenges posed by posthumous reproduction. Questions of parentage — is the deceased gamete provider a legal parent to the posthumous offspring — can hinge on such factors as consent to posthumous reproduction during lifetime, marital status of the surviving spouse at the birth of a posthumous child, and compliance with existing laws determining parenthood. Once parentage is established, ancillary issues relating to financial and other benefits arise. If a posthumous child is considered a lawful heir of the decedent, how and when should the decedent's estate be distributed? These and other legal issues are considered below.

SECTION II: LEGAL DILEMMAS IN POSTMORTEM REPRODUCTION

A. Family Law Questions: Who Is A Parent?

The question of who is a parent is largely resolved by state law, a jurisprudential system that could inevitably create a veritable "checkerboard" of tests and standards when it comes to determining the lawful parent of a posthumous child. In the absence of specific laws governing posthumous reproduction, and there are only a handful of such laws enacted to date, family court judges called upon to determine legal parentage will be forced to interpret existing law, written without consideration of the rapidly developing technologies that allow birth to occur long after death.

In most states, a posthumous child would be considered the lawful child of a man whose sperm was used only if: 1) the man was married to the child's mother at the time of death, and 2) the child was born within 300 days after the man's death. See Uniform Parentage Act § 204 (2002) (providing that a child born within 300 days of death of the husband is presumed to be the child of the husband). As you can quickly discern, this standard was designed to accommodate a pregnancy that was ongoing at the time of a married man's death. The 300-day limitation seemingly rules out lawful paternity for a child whose mother waited months or years after a husband died to attempt a pregnancy using frozen sperm, as the child would not be born within the requisite 10-month period. Moreover, the UPA presumption of posthumous paternity is silent on the legal fate of a child born to a single woman who gives birth after the death of a male partner.[8]

Questions of legal parentage are often related to money — obligations to pay child support, inheritance, life insurance and Social Security death benefits. But the inclusion of a dead husband or partner can play a significant symbolic and emotional role in the lives of the posthumous family. Recall the story of Diane Blood, the British woman who waged a court battle in England to obtain possession of the vials of sperm procured *after* her young husband died. See *supra* Section 1(A)(2). Mrs. Blood did eventually gain access to the sperm and became the mother of two sons, born four years apart, the youngest child born seven years after his father's death in 1995. After her second son's birth, Mrs. Blood sought to have her late husband named as "Father" on the children's birth certificate. Under prevailing British law, a deceased parent could not be included on the child's birth certificates; the slot had to be left blank. For Mrs. Blood, it was important for her sons to be recognized as full-blood brothers, and to have her late husband acknowledged as the boys' father. In September 2003 she won the right to include her husband's name on the legal documents when the British Parliament enacted the Human Fertilisation and Embryology (Deceased Father) Act, which creates parameters for deceased parents to be included on their children's birth

---

[8] The UPA does provide for parental designation of an unmarried man who "for the first two years of the child's life . . . reside[s] in the same household with the child and openly [holds] out the child as his own. UPA § 204(a)(5). Obviously, a man who dies before his genetic child is conceived or born cannot fulfill the requirements of this section.

certificates. See Wesley Johnson, *Widow Wins Right to Register Sons From Her Dead Husband*, BIRMINGHAM POST, Dec. 2, 2003, at 6.

The designation of a deceased person as a parent can also play an important role in the financial stability of a posthumous child, as this next case illustrates.

IN RE ESTATE OF KOLACY
Superior Court of New Jersey, Chancery Division
753 A.2d 1257 (2000)

STANTON, A.J.S.C. On March 31, 2000, I delivered an oral opinion declaring that Amanda Kolacy and Elyse Kolacy, three year old girls who are residents of New Jersey, are the heirs of their father William Kolacy, even though they were born eighteen months after his death. This opinion supersedes my earlier oral opinion.

The plaintiff in this action is Mariantonia Kolacy. She has brought this action to obtain a declaration that her two children, Amanda and Elyse, have the status of intestate heirs of her late husband, William J. Kolacy. Because this action involves a claim that one or more statutes of the State of New Jersey are unconstitutional, the Attorney General of New Jersey was notified of the action and has appeared through a Deputy Attorney General to defend the constitutionality of the state statutes involved.

On February 7, 1994, William J. Kolacy and Mariantonia Kolacy were a young married couple living in Rockaway, New Jersey. On that date, William Kolacy was diagnosed as having leukemia and he was advised to start chemotherapy as quickly as possible. He feared that he would be rendered infertile by the disease or by the treatment for the disease, so he decided to place his sperm in the Sperm and Embryo Bank of NJ. On the morning of February 8, 1994, William Kolacy and Mariantonia Kolacy harvested his sperm and Mariantonia Kolacy delivered it to the sperm bank. Later that day, the chemotherapy began. After the chemotherapy had been in progress for one month, a second harvesting of sperm occurred and was placed in the sperm bank.

Unfortunately, William Kolacy's leukemia led to his death at the age of 26 on April 15, 1995. He died domiciled in New Jersey. On April 3, 1996, almost a year after the death of William Kolacy, plaintiff Mariantonia Kolacy authorized the release of his sperm from the Sperm and Embryo Bank of NJ to the Center for Reproductive Medicine and Infertility at Cornell University Medical College in New York City. An IVF fertilization procedure uniting the sperm of William Kolacy and eggs taken from Mariantonia Kolacy was performed at the Center. The procedure was successful and the embryos which resulted were transferred into the womb of Mariantonia Kolacy. Twin girls, Amanda and Elyse, were born to Mariantonia Kolacy on November 3, 1996. The births occurred slightly more than eighteen months after the death of William Kolacy . . .

. . . [T]he plaintiff states her reasons for bringing this action as follows:

"7. The Social Security Administration has denied dependent benefits to Amanda and Elyse Kolacy contending they are not children of a deceased worker. On

November 16, 1999 Administrative Law Judge Richard L. De Steno upheld the denial of benefits in a written decision.

8. Section 216 of the Social Security Act provides, *inter alia*, that '[c]hild's insurance benefits can be paid to a child who could inherit under the State's intestate laws.'

9. Plaintiff seeks a declaration that her daughters, posthumously conceived utilizing the late William J. Kolacy's stored sperm, are among the class of persons who are his intestate heirs so as to pursue her claim for child's insurance benefits on behalf of the decedent's children under the Social Security Act."

Plaintiff is currently pursuing her claims and those of the children through appellate process within the Social Security Administration, and, if necessary, will eventually litigate them in the federal courts. In bringing this action in the Superior Court, the plaintiff is attempting to obtain a state court ruling which will be helpful to her in pursuing her federal claims before a federal administrative agency and before the federal courts . . .

[Th]e interpretation of New Jersey statutes and the determination of what New Jersey law is are primarily the responsibility of New Jersey courts. Federal courts routinely look to state courts for authoritative rulings with respect to state law . . . In the case before me, a proper determination of what New Jersey law is will not necessarily be dispositive of the rights of plaintiff and the children under federal law, and it would not be appropriate for a state court to intrude into federal adjudicatory processes. On the other hand, it would clearly be unfortunate for those federal adjudicatory processes to reach a result based in part upon an incorrect determination by federal tribunals of New Jersey law. Accordingly, even if this action is viewed primarily as an adjunct to claims asserted in federal proceedings, it is appropriate for me to interpret New Jersey statutory law as it applies to Amanda and Elyse Kolacy . . .

There are no New Jersey decisions dealing with the central issue presented in this case — whether Amanda and Elyse Kolacy, conceived after the death of their biological father and born more than eighteen months after his death, qualify as his heirs under state intestate law. I have not been able to find any American appellate court decisions dealing with that central issue.

Counsel have discussed at some length N.J.S.A. 3B:5-8, which is the New Jersey statute dealing with after born heirs. That statute provides as follows: "Relatives of the decedent conceived before his death but born thereafter inherit as if they had been born in the lifetime of the decedent" . . .

A brief discussion of elementary estate law concepts is appropriate at this point. When a person dies, whether he dies leaving a will or whether he dies intestate, there is a real life need and a legal need to determine which persons are entitled to take his estate, and when that determination is made the general policy is to deliver to those persons rather promptly the property to which they are entitled. Thus, the identity of people who will take property from a decedent has traditionally been determined as of the date of the decedent's death.

However, there have long been exceptions to the rule that the identity of takers from a decedent's estate is determined as of the date of death. Those exceptions are based on human experience going back to time immemorial. We have always been aware that men sometimes cause a woman to become pregnant and then die before the pregnancy comes to term and a child is born. It has always been routine human experience that men sometimes have children after they die. To deal fairly with this reality, decisional law and statutory law have long recognized that it is appropriate to hold the process of identifying takers from a decedent's estate open long enough to allow after born children to receive property from and through their father . . .

The ability to remove sperm and eggs from human beings and to preserve their viability by storing them for long periods of time at low temperatures makes it possible for children to come into existence as the genetic and biological offspring of a father or of a mother who has long since been dead. My impression is that it is now possible to preserve the viability of human genetic material for as long as ten years. It is likely that the time will be extended in the future. The evolving human productive technology opens up some wonderful possibilities, but it also creates difficult issues and potential problems in many areas. It would undoubtedly be useful for the Legislature to deal consciously and in a well informed way with at least some of the issues presented by reproductive technology . . .

As I look at N.J.S.A. 3B:5-8 and other statutory provisions dealing with intestate succession, I discern a basic legislative intent to enable children to take property from their parents and through their parents from parental relatives. Although the Legislature has not dealt with the kind of issue presented by children such as Amanda and Elyse, it has manifested a general intent that the children of a decedent should be amply provided for with respect to property passing from him or through him as the result of a death. It is my view that the general intent should prevail over a restrictive, literal reading of statutes which did not consciously purport to deal with the kind of problem before us.

Given that general legislative intent, it seems to me that once we establish, as we have in this case, that a child is indeed the offspring of a decedent, we should routinely grant that child the legal status of being an heir of the decedent, unless doing so would unfairly intrude on the rights of other persons or would cause serious problems in terms of the orderly administration of estates.

I note that after born children who come into existence because of modern reproductive techniques pose special challenges to society and to our legal system. Historically, after born children were conceived and in their mother's womb at the time of a decedent's death and they could be counted on to appear no later than approximately nine months after that death. Now they can appear after the death of either a mother or a father and they can appear a number of years after that death. Estates cannot be held open for years simply to allow for the possibility that after born children may come into existence. People alive at the time of a decedent's death who are entitled to receive property from the decedent's estate are entitled to receive it reasonably promptly. It would undoubtedly be both fair and constitutional for a Legislature to impose time limits and other situationally described limits on the ability of after born children to take from or through a parent. In the absence of legislative provision in that regard, it would undoubtedly be fair and constitutional for courts to impose limits on the ability of after born children to take in particular cases.

In our present case, there are no estate administration problems involved and there are no competing interests of other persons who were alive at the time of William Kolacy's death which would be unfairly frustrated by recognizing Amanda and Elyse as his heirs. Even in situations where competing interests such as other children born during the lifetime of the decedent are in existence at the time of his death, it might be possible to accommodate those interests with the interests of after born children. For example, by statutory provision or decisional rule, payments made in the course of routine estate administration before the advent of after born children could be treated as vested and left undisturbed, while distributions made following the birth of after born children could be made to both categories of children . . .

The ability to cause children to come into existence long after the death of a parent is a recently acquired ability for human society. There are probably wise and wonderful ways in which that ability can be used. There are also undoubtedly some special problems that the exercise of that ability might pose. There are, I think, ethical problems, social policy problems and legal problems which are presented when a child is brought into existence under circumstances where a traditionally normal parenting situation is not available. One would hope that a prospective parent thinking about causing a child to come into existence after the death of a genetic and biological parent would think very carefully about the potential consequences of doing that. The law should certainly be cautious about encouraging parents to move precipitously in this area.

I accept as true Mariantonia Kolacy's statement that her husband unequivocally expressed his desire that she use his stored sperm after his death to bear his children. She did, in fact, use his sperm to bear his children. Some may question the wisdom of such a course of action, but one can certainly understand why a loving and caring couple in the Kolacys' position might choose it. Be all that as it may, once a child has come into existence, she is a full-fledged human being and is entitled to all of the love, respect, dignity and legal protection which that status requires. It seems to me that a fundamental policy of the law should be to enhance and enlarge the rights of each human being to the maximum extent possible, consistent with the duty not to intrude unfairly upon the interests of other persons. Given that viewpoint, and given the facts of this case, including particularly the fact that William Kolacy by his intentional conduct created the possibility of having long-delayed after born children, I believe it is entirely fitting to recognize that Amanda and Elyse Kolacy are the legal heirs of William Kolacy under the intestate laws of New Jersey.

NOTES AND QUESTIONS

1. Do you agree with Justice Stanton that existing New Jersey law limiting heirship to children conceived before death but born thereafter, manifests a "basic legislative intent" to enable children to take property from their parents, regardless of the date of their birth?

The court suggests that reasonable limits could be placed on the ability of posthumous children to inherit from deceased parents, but encourages the Legislature to enact fully formed guidelines. If you were a state legislator asked to draft such a law, what factors would you consider in determining posthumous heirship? What reasonable limitations would you place on the inheritance rights of posthumously born children?

2. Amanda and Elyse stand to inherit nothing from their father's estate because he left no assets at his death. If Mr. Kolacy likewise left no Social Security benefits for his wife and offspring, would there be any reason for Mrs. Kolacy to pursue a designation of heirship for her daughters?

3. The New Jersey court accepts as true Mrs. Kolacy's statement that her husband expressed his desire that *she* use his stored sperm posthumously to bear his children. Does this amount to a directed donation to his widow for her exclusive use, or does it give Mrs. Kolacy the right to dispose of the sperm as she sees fit? What if, for example, she wanted to donate the sperm to a relative or friend? Would William Kolacy be the posthumously conceived child's father in that case? See The American Medical Association Council on Ethical & Judicial Affairs, *Code of Medical Ethics: Current Opinions* § E-2.04 (2003) (advocating that if a donor leaves no instructions, it is reasonable for the remaining partner to use the sperm, but not to donate the sperm to anyone else).

Suppose William Kolacy was a wealthy single man who feared dying childless after a cancer diagnosis. If Mr. Kolacy visits his local sperm bank, makes deposits, indicates on a written record that he wishes to become a father posthumously, and makes a provision in his will for any future children born of his sperm, can the sperm bank release his sperm to a woman who wishes to bear the Kolacy heir? If such an heir is born, how should Mr. Kolacy's estate be distributed?

4. *The Future of Posthumous Reproduction.* Mariantonia Kolacy is one of around 100 widows who have petitioned the Social Security Administration for an award of benefits on behalf of children conceived and born posthumously using their deceased husband's sperm. In the main, the SSA has taken the position that these children are not entitled to benefits under the federal law because the term "child" is defined therein by reference to the child's eligibility to inherit from the predeceased father under the prevailing state law on intestate succession. The case and notes that follow trace the history and current controversy over the rights of posthumous ART-conceived children to enjoy the same property rights as children conceived within their parents' lifetime. You may be surprised to learn our journey will take us all the way to the U.S. Supreme Court.

For a discussion of the earliest cases involving posthumously conceived children and property rights, *see Girl to Get Benefits in Death of Father Before Conception*, N.Y. TIMES, March 12, 1996, at A13; Helene S. Shapo, *Matters of Life and Death: Inheritance Consequences of Reproductive Technologies*, 25 HOFSTRA L. REV. 1091, 1159 (1997); Ronald Chester, *Freezing the Heir Apparent: A Dialogue on Postmortem Conception, Parental Responsibility, and Inheritance*, 33 HOUS. L. REV. 967, 988-93 (1996).

B. Probate Law: Awarding Inheritance Rights and Death Benefits

WOODWARD v. COMMISSIONER OF SOCIAL SECURITY
Supreme Judicial Court of Massachusetts
435 Mass. 536, 760 N.E.2d 257 (2002)

MARSHALL, C.J. The United States District Court for the District of Massachusetts has certified the following question to this court . . .

"If a married man and woman arrange for sperm to be withdrawn from the husband for the purpose of artificially impregnating the wife, and the woman is impregnated with that sperm after the man, her husband, has died, will children resulting from such pregnancy enjoy the inheritance rights of natural children under Massachusetts' law of intestate succession?"

We answer the certified question as follows: In certain limited circumstances, a child resulting from posthumous reproduction may enjoy the inheritance rights of "issue" under the Massachusetts intestacy statute. These limited circumstances exist where, as a threshold matter, the surviving parent or the child's other legal representative demonstrates a genetic relationship between the child and the decedent. The survivor or representative must then establish both that the decedent affirmatively consented to posthumous conception and to the support of any resulting child. Even where such circumstances exist, time limitations may preclude commencing a claim for succession rights on behalf of a posthumously conceived child. Because the government has conceded that the timeliness of the wife's paternity action under our intestacy law is irrelevant to her Federal appeal, we do not address that question today . . .

I

The undisputed facts and relevant procedural history are as follows. In January, 1993, about three and one-half years after they were married, Lauren Woodward and Warren Woodward were informed that the husband had leukemia. At the time, the couple was childless. Advised that the husband's leukemia treatment might leave him sterile, the Woodwards arranged for a quantity of the husband's semen to be medically withdrawn and preserved, in a process commonly known as "sperm banking." The husband then underwent a bone marrow transplant. The treatment was not successful. The husband died in October, 1993, and the wife was appointed administratrix of his estate.

In October, 1995, the wife gave birth to twin girls. The children were conceived through artificial insemination using the husband's preserved semen. In January, 1996, the wife applied for two forms of Social Security survivor benefits: "child's" benefits under 42 U.S.C. § 402(d)(1) (1994 & Supp. V 1999), and "mother's" benefits under 42 U.S.C. § 402(g)(1) (1994).

The Social Security Administration (SSA) rejected the wife's claims on the ground that she had not established that the twins were the husband's "children" within the meaning of the Act.[9] In February, 1996, as she pursued a series of appeals from the SSA decision, the wife filed a "complaint for correction of birth record" in the Probate and Family Court against the clerk of the city of Beverly, seeking to add her deceased husband as the "father" on the twins' birth certificates. In October, 1996, a judge in the Probate and Family Court entered a judgment of paternity and an order to amend both birth certificates declaring the deceased husband to be the children's father . . .

The wife presented the judgment of paternity and the amended birth certificates to the SSA, but the agency remained unpersuaded. A United States administrative law judge, hearing the wife's claims de novo, concluded, among other things, that the children did not qualify for benefits because they "are not entitled to inherit from [the husband] under the Massachusetts intestacy and paternity laws." The appeals council of the SSA affirmed the administrative law judge's decision, which thus became the commissioner's final decision for purposes of judicial review. The wife appealed to the United States District Court for the District of Massachusetts, seeking a declaratory judgment to reverse the commissioner's ruling . . .

II

A

We have been asked to determine the inheritance rights under Massachusetts law of children conceived from the gametes of a deceased individual and his or her surviving spouse. We have not previously been asked to consider whether our intestacy statute accords inheritance rights to posthumously conceived genetic children. Nor has any American court of last resort considered, in a published opinion, the question of posthumously conceived genetic children's inheritance rights under other States' intestacy laws.[10]

---

[9] [n.4] . . . As stated in the certification order, the wife's "appeal centers on only one possible basis for eligibility, which is that under SSA regulations the children are eligible if they would be treated as [the husband's] natural children for the disposition of his personal property under the Massachusetts law of intestate succession. See 42 U.S.C. §§ 402(d)(3) and 416(h)(2)(A); 20 C.F.R. § 404.355(a)(1); 20 C.F.R. § 404.361(a)."

[10] [n.9] We are aware of only two cases that have addressed, in varying degrees, the question before us. In *Hecht v. Superior Court*, 16 Cal.App.4th 836, 20 Cal.Rptr.2d 275 (1993), the California Court of Appeal considered, among other things, whether a decedent's sperm was "property" that could be bequeathed to his girl friend. Id. at 847, 20 Cal.Rptr.2d 275. In answering in the affirmative, the court noted, in dicta and without elaboration, that, under the provisions of California's Probate Code, "it is unlikely that the estate would be subject to claims with respect to any such children" resulting from insemination of the girl friend with the decedent's sperm. Id. at 859, 20 Cal.Rptr.2d 275. *In Matter of Estate of Kolacy*, 332 N.J.Super. 593, 753 A.2d 1257 (2000), the plaintiff brought a declaratory judgment action to have her children, who were conceived after the death of her husband, declared the intestate heirs of her deceased husband in order to pursue the children's claims for survivor benefits with the Social Security Administration. A New Jersey Superior Court judge held that, in circumstances where the decedent left no estate and an adjudication of parentage did not unfairly intrude on the rights of others or cause "serious problems" with the orderly administration of estates, the children would be entitled to inherit under the State's intestacy law. Id. at 602, 753 A.2d 1257.

This case presents a narrow set of circumstances, yet the issues it raises are far reaching. Because the law regarding the rights of posthumously conceived children is unsettled, the certified question is understandably broad. Moreover, the parties have articulated extreme positions. The wife's principal argument is that, by virtue of their genetic connection with the decedent, posthumously conceived children must *always* be permitted to enjoy the inheritance rights of the deceased parent's children under our law of intestate succession. The government's principal argument is that, because posthumously conceived children are not "in being" as of the date of the parent's death, they are *always* barred from enjoying such inheritance rights.

Neither party's position is tenable. In this developing and relatively uncharted area of human relations, bright-line rules are not favored unless the applicable statute requires them. The Massachusetts intestacy statute does not. Neither the statute's "posthumous children" provision, see G.L. c. 190, § 8, nor any other provision of our intestacy law limits the class of posthumous children to those in utero at the time of the decedent's death. Cf. La. Civ.Code Ann. art. 939 (West 2000) ("A successor must exist at the death of the decedent"). On the other hand, with the act of procreation now separated from coitus, posthumous reproduction can occur under a variety of conditions that may conflict with the purposes of the intestacy law and implicate other firmly established State and individual interests. We look to our intestacy law to resolve these tensions.

B

We begin our analysis with an overview of Massachusetts intestacy law. In our Commonwealth, the devolution of real and personal property in intestacy is neither a natural nor a constitutional right. It is a privilege conferred by statute . . .

Section 1 of the intestacy statute directs that, if a decedent "leaves issue," such "issue" will inherit a fixed portion of his real and personal property, subject to debts and expenses, the rights of the surviving spouse, and other statutory payments not relevant here. See G.L. c. 190, § 1. To answer the certified question, then, we must first determine whether the twins are the "issue" of the husband.

The intestacy statute does not define "issue." However, in the context of intestacy the term "issue" means all lineal (genetic) descendants, and now includes both marital and nonmarital descendants . . .

Turning to "issue" who are the nonmarital children of an intestate, the intestacy statute treats different classes of nonmarital children differently based on the presumed ease of establishing their consanguinity with the deceased parent. A nonmarital child is presumptively the child of his or her mother and is entitled by virtue of this presumption to enjoy inheritance rights as her issue. G.L. c. 190, § 5. However, to enjoy inheritance rights as the issue of a deceased father, a nonmarital child, in the absence of the father's acknowledgment of paternity or marriage to the mother, must obtain a judicial determination that he or she is the father's child. G.L. c. 190, § 7 . . .

The "posthumous children" provision of the intestacy statute, G.L. c. 190, § 8, is yet another expression of the Legislature's intent to preserve wealth for consanguineous descendants. That section provides that "[p]osthumous children shall be considered as living at the death of their parent." The Legislature, however, has left the term "posthumous children" undefined . . .

The Massachusetts intestacy statute thus does not contain an express, affirmative requirement that posthumous children must "be in existence" as of the date of the decedent's death. The Legislature could surely have enacted such a provision had it desired to do so. Cf. La. Civ.Code Ann. art. 939 (effective July 1, 1999) (West 2000) ("A successor must exist at the death of the decedent"). See also N.D. Cent.Code Ann. 14-18-04 (Michie 1997) ("A person who dies before a conception using that person's sperm or egg is not a parent of any resulting child born of the conception"). We must therefore determine whether, under our intestacy law, there is any reason that children conceived after the decedent's death who are the decedent's direct genetic descendants . . . may not enjoy the same succession rights as children conceived before the decedent's death who are the decedent's direct genetic descendants . . .

The question whether posthumously conceived genetic children may enjoy inheritance rights under the intestacy statute implicates three powerful State interests: the best interests of children, the State's interest in the orderly administration of estates, and the reproductive rights of the genetic parent. Our task is to balance and harmonize these interests to effect the Legislature's over-all purposes.

1. First and foremost we consider the overriding legislative concern to promote the best interests of children . . . Repeatedly, forcefully, and unequivocally, the Legislature has expressed its will that all children be "entitled to the same rights and protections of the law" regardless of the accidents of their birth. G.L. c. 209C, § 1. See G.L. c. 119, § 1 . . . Among the many rights and protections vouchsafed to all children are rights to financial support from their parents and their parents' estates . . .

Posthumously conceived children may not come into the world the way the majority of children do. But they are children nonetheless. We may assume that the Legislature intended that such children be "entitled," in so far as possible, "to the same rights and protections of the law" as children conceived before death. See G.L. c. 209C, § 1.

2. However, in the context of our intestacy laws, the best interests of the posthumously conceived child, while of great importance, are not in themselves conclusive. They must be balanced against other important State interests, not the least of which is the protection of children who are alive or conceived before the intestate parent's death. In an era in which serial marriages, serial families, and blended families are not uncommon, according succession rights under our intestacy laws to posthumously conceived children may, in a given case, have the potential to pit child against child and family against family. Any inheritance rights of posthumously conceived children will reduce the intestate share available to children born prior to the decedent's death. See G.L. c. 190, § 3(1). Such considerations, among others, lead us to examine a second important legislative purpose: to provide certainty to heirs and creditors by effecting the orderly, prompt, and accurate administration of intestate estates.

The intestacy statute furthers the Legislature's administrative goals in two principal ways: (1) by requiring certainty of filiation between the decedent and his issue, and (2) by establishing limitations periods for the commencement of claims against the intestate estate. [The court later notes that paternity actions must be brought within one year of death under the intestacy laws.] . . .

[T]he limitations question is inextricably tied to consideration of the intestacy statute's administrative goals. In the case of posthumously conceived children, the application of the one-year limitations period of G.L. c. 190, § 7 is not clear; it may pose significant burdens on the surviving parent, and consequently on the child. It requires, in effect, that the survivor make a decision to bear children while in the freshness of grieving. It also requires that attempts at conception succeed quickly. Cf. Commentary, Modern Reproductive Technologies: Legal Issues Concerning Cryopreservation and Posthumous Conception, 17 J. Legal Med. 547, 549 (1996) ("It takes an average of seven insemination attempts over 4.4 menstrual cycles to establish pregnancy"). Because the resolution of the time constraints question is not required here, it must await the appropriate case, should one arise.

3. Finally, the question certified to us implicates a third important State interest: to honor the reproductive choices of individuals. We need not address the wife's argument that her reproductive rights would be infringed by denying succession rights to her children under our intestacy law. Nothing in the record even remotely suggests that she was prevented by the State from choosing to conceive children using her deceased husband's semen. The husband's reproductive rights are a more complicated matter . . .

The prospective donor parent must clearly and unequivocally consent not only to posthumous reproduction but also to the support of any resulting child . . .

This two-fold consent requirement arises from the nature of alternative reproduction itself. It will not always be the case that a person elects to have his or her gametes medically preserved to create "issue" posthumously. A man, for example, may preserve his semen for myriad reasons, including, among others: to reproduce after recovery from medical treatment, to reproduce after an event that leaves him sterile, or to reproduce when his spouse has a genetic disorder or otherwise cannot have or safely bear children. That a man has medically preserved his gametes for use by his spouse thus may indicate only that he wished to reproduce after some contingency while he was alive, and not that he consented to the different circumstance of creating a child after his death. Uncertainty as to consent may be compounded by the fact that medically preserved semen can remain viable for up to ten years after it was first extracted, long after the original decision to preserve the semen has passed and when such changed circumstances as divorce, remarriage, and a second family may have intervened . . .

As expressed in our intestacy and paternity laws, sound public policy dictates the requirements we have outlined above. Legal parentage imposes substantial obligations on adults for the welfare of children . . . Where conception results from a third-party medical procedure using a deceased person's gametes, it is entirely consistent with our laws on children, parentage, and reproductive freedom to place the burden on the surviving parent (or the posthumously conceived child's other legal representative) to demonstrate the genetic relationship of the child to the decedent and that the intestate consented both to reproduce posthumously and to support any resulting child.

C

It is undisputed in this case that the husband is the genetic father of the wife's children. However, for the reasons stated above, that fact, in itself, cannot be sufficient to establish that the husband is the children's legal father for purposes of the devolution and distribution of his intestate property. In the United States District Court, the wife may come forward with other evidence as to her husband's consent to posthumously conceive children. She may come forward with evidence of his consent to support such children. We do not speculate as to the sufficiency of evidence she may submit at trial . . .

III

For the second time this term, we have been confronted with novel questions involving the rights of children born from assistive reproductive technologies. See Culliton v. Beth Israel Deaconess Med. Ctr., 435 Mass. 285, 756 N.E.2d 1133 (2001). As these technologies advance, the number of children they produce will continue to multiply. So, too, will the complex moral, legal, social, and ethical questions that surround their birth. The questions present in this case cry out for lengthy, careful examination outside the adversary process, which can only address the specific circumstances of each controversy that presents itself. They demand a comprehensive response reflecting the considered will of the people.

In the absence of statutory directives, we have answered the certified question by identifying and harmonizing the important State interests implicated therein in a manner that advances the Legislature's over-all purposes. In so doing, we conclude that limited circumstances may exist, consistent with the mandates of our Legislature, in which posthumously conceived children may enjoy the inheritance rights of "issue" under our intestacy law. These limited circumstances exist where, as a threshold matter, the surviving parent or the child's other legal representative demonstrates a genetic relationship between the child and the decedent. The survivor or representative must then establish both that the decedent affirmatively consented to posthumous conception and to the support of any resulting child. Even where such circumstances exist, time limitations may preclude commencing a claim for succession rights on behalf of a posthumously conceived child. In any action brought to establish such inheritance rights, notice must be given to all interested parties.

NOTES AND QUESTIONS

1. The court in *Woodward* can be praised for setting forth a three-part test clarifying the requirements for a posthumous child to be considered the decedent's child for purposes of inheritance. Before the Massachusetts court stepped in to create the parameters of: 1) genetic tie, 2) affirmative consent to posthumous reproduction, and 3) affirmative consent to support, decisions about heirship were made on an ad hoc, case-by-case basis. Conversely, the trilogy of standards have

garnered some criticism, aimed largely at the vague and ill-defined requirement for "affirmative consent."

Professor Ronald Chester worries that "leaving the definition of 'affirmative consent' unclear will lead to needless confusion and litigation." He wonders, for example, whether a court would accept only "objectively verifiable evidence of affirmative consent" or would consider passing comments of the decedent's desire to reproduce posthumously as sufficient under the Massachusetts standard. See Ronald Chester, *Posthumously Conceived Heirs Under A Revised Uniform Probate Code*, 38 REAL PROP., PROBATE & TRUST J. 727, 734 (2004). Instead, Professor Chester recommends states adopt a requirement that a prospective parent "consent in a record" to the posthumous reproduction. He further urges abandonment of the requirement that a decedent consent to support any resulting child, arguing it will be the rare individual who has the foresight to authorize posthumous support, a concept not commonly explored when sperm donations are made.

2. Suppose Warren Woodward died testate, leaving a will that provided a portion of his estate to "my future children born of the frozen sperm I have left for my beloved wife Lauren." Would the Social Security Administration have rejected Mrs. Woodward's claim for survivor benefits for her daughters if she filed the will as an attachment to her SSA request?

3. *Post-Woodward Decisions.* Several state courts have grappled with the same questions presented to the high court in Massachusetts since that court set forth its three-part test for determining the inheritance rights of postmortem conception children. In *Khabbaz v. Commissioner*, 155 N.H. 798, 930 A.2d 1180 (2007), the Supreme Court of New Hampshire held that a child conceived and born via artificial insemination after her father's death was not eligible to inherit as a surviving issue under that state's intestacy law. The court reasoned that intestacy was limited to issue who "survive" the decedent, requiring a child to be alive at the time of the parent's death. *Accord Finley v. Astrue*, 372 Ark. 103, 270 S.W.3d 849 (2008).

In a ruling mirroring the result in *Woodward* and calling on the legislature to enact comprehensive legislation to "resolve the issues raised by advances in biotechnology," the Surrogate's Court in New York held that trust language benefitting the settlor's "issue" and "descendants" included a predeceased son's posthumously children conceived. *In re Martin B*, 841 N.Y.S.2d 207 (2007) is the first reported case to consider the rights of posthumously conceived grandchildren to take under a preexisting trust. The trust at issue was established in 1969, long before the settlor (or the drafting attorney) could have imagined the birth of posthumously conceived grandchildren. Was the court right to construe the trust language in light of contemporary technologies, or should the trustee be instructed to follow the meaning of "issue" at the time the trust was created?

4. *The Rule Against Perpetuities.* Leaving property in a will or trust to unborn children can evoke the wrath of the infamous Rule Against Perpetuities, a deceptively short common law property rule: No interest is good unless it must vest, if at all, not later than twenty-one years after some life in being at the creation of the interest. *See* JOHN CHIPMAN GRAY, THE RULE AGAINST PERPETUITIES § 201 (4th ed. 1942). The Rule evolved from judicial efforts during the seventeenth century to limit control of title to real property by the dead hand of landowners reaching into future

generations. The guiding principle behind the Rule is it is socially undesirable for property to be inalienable for an unreasonable period of time. The Rule operates to prospectively void any property interest that *might* fail to vest in a grantee within the perpetuities period — lives in being plus 21 years.

The notion of "lives in being" was traditionally limited to persons living at the time the interest was created. If the interest is created in a will, then the lives in being are those who survive the testator at the time of death. But as *Woodward* and *Kolacy* demonstrate, a child born long after the death of a father can gain legal status as the decedent's issue for purposes of inheritance. Suppose a testator's will leaves property "to my grandchildren upon reaching the age of 21." Ordinarily, the interests in the grandchildren are considered valid because under prevailing reproductive standards they will vest (reach 21) within 21 years of the death of their parents, the testator's children (i.e., the lives in being). Suppose this testator also left a vial of frozen sperm, which his wife uses to give birth 10 years after his death. If the posthumous child is considered a lawful child of the testator, is she also considered a life in being for purposes of the Rule? If so, any interest given to the posthumously born child's issue (the grandchildren of the testator) could vest long after all the *actual* lives in being plus 21 years, thus casting doubt on the validity of the interest under the common law Rule. These and other mind-twisting scenarios are considered in Sharona Hoffman & Andrew P. Morriss, *Birth After Death: Perpetuities and the New Reproductive Technologies*, 38 GA. L. REV. 575, 595-60 (2004).

Posthumously Conceived Children and the U.S. Supreme Court

The court in *Woodward* makes only faint mention of the statutory provisions in the Social Security Act that the federal agency relies upon to determine a posthumously conceived child's eligibility for survivor benefits. The Act, enacted in 1939 — long before freezing future lives was a contemplated reality — has lately served a pivotal role in a very modern dilemma. The Massachusetts court references Sections 402(d) and 416(h) in footnote 4, explaining that these sections instruct the Social Security Administration to award benefits only if a child would be treated as the deceased wage earner's heir under the prevailing state law of intestate succession. As we shall see in Section III, most states do not include posthumously conceived children as intestate takers, thus the SSA has routinely denied claims made on behalf of this class of children.

Once the SSA denies a claim for benefits, the disappointed claimant (typically the mother on behalf of her child) is entitled to request a hearing before an Administrative Law Judge. If the ALJ affirms the denial of benefits, a claimant can seek judicial review in the United States District Court. The appeal route thereafter is the usual process available in federal court — appeal to the Circuit Court of Appeals and then petition of certiorari to the United States Supreme Court.

Such was the path of Karen Capato. In 1999, shortly after her wedding, Karen's new husband Robert was diagnosed with esophageal cancer. Prior to undergoing chemotherapy that was predicted to render him sterile, Robert deposited several vials of semen at a local Florida sperm bank. After his death in 2002, Karen used the sperm in a successful in vitro fertilization cycle, giving birth to twins 18 months after the demise of their biological father. Mrs. Capato soon applied to the Social Security Administration for surviving child's insurance benefits based on her deceased husband's earnings record.

The SSA denied the twins' benefits, reasoning that the posthumously conceived pair failed to qualify as "children" under the Social Security Act. The agency looked to Section 416(h) of the Act — the same section relied upon in *Woodward* — which incorporates the state's laws on intestate succession to determine a child's eligibility for survivor benefits. Since Florida law, which governed, did not recognize the twins as Robert's children for purposes of inheritance, the SSA denied benefits. Following affirmance by an ALJ and the District Court, the Third Circuit reversed, finding that the twins were the "undisputed biological children" of the deceased wage earner and thus entitled to SSA benefits. The appeals court relied on Section 416(e) which defines "child" broadly to include "the child or legally adopted child of an individual." Since the twins were the biological children of the wage earner, no further inquiry into alternative definitions of "child" was necessary. The court dismissed the intestacy test, set forth in Section 416(h), deeming it applicable only as a secondary standard when the child's status is in doubt. (*Astrue v. Capato*, 631 F.3d 626 (3d Cir. 2011)).

Capato joined three other federal Court of Appeals decisions involving virtually identical fact scenarios. The Third Circuit case aligned with a Ninth Circuit decision (*Gillett-Netting v. Barnhart*, 371 F.3d 593 (9th Cir. 2004)), but clashed with cases from the Fourth and Eighth Circuits upholding the SSA's denial of benefits (*Schafer v. Astrue*, 641 F.3d 49 (4th Cir. 2011); *Beeler v. Astrue*, 651 F.3d 954 (8th Cir. 2011)). This even split in the federal circuits made the case ripe for high court review, generating little surprise when the Supreme Court granted the SSA Commissioner's petition for certiorari in November 2011. Oral arguments in the case were heard on March 19, 2012. On May 21, 2012, a unanimous Supreme Court reversed the 3rd Circuit in *Capato*, siding with the SSA's more limited interpretation of the Social Security Act. Writing for the Court, Justice Ginsburg concluded that the federal agency's "reading is better attuned to the statute's text and its design to benefit primarily those supported by the deceased wage earner in his or her lifetime." Reference to state intestacy laws, the Court held, better fulfills the core purpose of the federal law to "provide . . . dependent members of [a wage earner's] family with protection against the hardship occasioned by [the] loss of [the insured's] earnings" *Astrue v. Capato*, 132 S. Ct. 2021 (2102) (internal citations omitted).

The Supreme Court's ruling does not mean that children conceived postmortem will never be entitled to social security benefits, rather that their eligibility depends upon the intestacy law in the state in which their deceased parent was domiciled. These laws are complex and varied. The next Section details the various legal schemes that govern the legal status and rights of postmortem conception children.

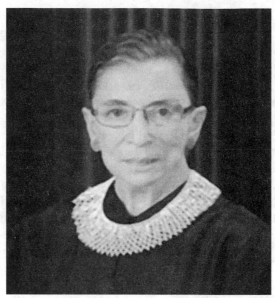

Justice Ruth Bader Ginsburg

SECTION III: STATUTORY FRAMEWORKS FOR EVALUATING THE RIGHTS OF POSTMORTEM CONCEPTION CHILDREN

The legal issues surrounding postmortem conception and reproduction are beginning to gain the attention of lawmakers. To date, about one-quarter of the states have enacted laws that address the parentage and inheritance rights of children conceived and born after the death of a parent. As we have seen in cases such as *Woodward* and *Kolacy*, if a legal dilemma arises involving a postmortem conception child, absent specific legislation a court will extrapolate from existing laws to resolve a scenario that was never contemplated by the body that enacted the statute. But as the practice of birth after the death of a parent becomes more widespread, lawmakers may continue to take up the issues in order to provide clarity within their borders. If a legislative body does decide to enact governing standards, there are ample models of legislative schemes to study for guidance. Groups such as the American Bar Association, the National Conference of Commissioners on Uniform State Laws, and the American Law Institute (drafters of the Restatements of the Law) have promulgated model laws available for adoption or modification in any state.

The two main questions that a state statutory scheme must address are: 1) Does a parent-child relationship exist between a postmortem conception child and the decedent parent, and 2) Is the postmortem conception child an heir of the genetic parent, entitled to inherit from the decedent's estate? These questions of family and probate law are related, as a finding of a parent-child relationship serves as the basis for awarding inheritance rights.[11] Typically, state family law codes address the question of parent-child relationship, while probate and estate laws govern inheritance, often referring to the family code to answer the foundational question of parentage. Many of the states' family and probate codes are derived from two uniform laws originally drafted nearly 40 years ago — the Uniform Parentage Act, originally promulgated in 1973 and updated in 2000 and 2002, and the Uniform Probate Code, first appearing in 1969 and most recently updated in 2008. These codes provide a starting point for exploring the statutory schemes surrounding posthumous reproduction.

A.   Uniform Laws Governing Postmortem Reproduction

1.   The Uniform Parentage Act

Section 707. Parental Status of Deceased Individual (as amended in 2002)

> If an individual who consented in a record to be a parent by assisted reproduction dies before placement of eggs, sperm, or embryos, the deceased individual is not a parent of the resulting child unless the deceased individual consented in a record that if assisted reproduction were to occur after death, the deceased individual would be a parent of the child.

Comment:

> Absent consent in a record, the death of an individual whose genetic material is subsequently used either in conceiving an embryo or in implanting an already existing embryo into a womb ends the potential legal parenthood of the deceased. This section is designed primarily to avoid the problems of intestate succession which could arise if the posthumous use of a person's genetic material leads to the deceased being determined to be a parent. Of course, an individual who wants to explicitly provide for such children in his or her will may do so.

---

[11] It may be that even if a posthumously conceived/born child is deemed an heir for inheritance purposes, that child will not inherit from the deceased father under the state's laws of intestate succession. In all jurisdictions in this country, the surviving spouse is the first taker of a decedent's estate. The spouse's share varies in each jurisdiction, and in some cases the spouse may inherit the entire estate. For example, Cal. Prob. Code § 6401(a) provides that the intestate share of the surviving spouse is *the* one-half of the community property that belongs to the decedent. This gives the surviving spouse *all* of the couple's community property because each spouse owns one-half of the community property during life. If a man dies owning only community property, it would all pass to the surviving spouse, nothing would remain to pass to his issue.

In every jurisdiction, after the spouse's share is set aside, children and issue of the deceased children take the remainder of the property to the exclusion of everyone else. Thus, a posthumously conceived child could potentially inherit from the decedent parent if the estate does not all pass to the surviving spouse. See Jesse Dukeminier, Robert Sitkoff & Stanley M. Johanson, James Lindgren, Wills, Trusts, and Estates 8672-73 (68th ed. 20009).

NOTES AND QUESTIONS

1. The 2002 Uniform Parentage Act provision on posthumous reproduction is taken from Section 4(b) of the 1988 Uniform Status of Children of Assisted Conception Act, which provides: "An individual who dies before implantation of an embryo, or before a child is conceived other than through sexual intercourse, using the individual's egg or sperm, is not a parent of the resulting child." Do you see any differences between the 1988 and 2002 proposed laws? If so, what do you think accounts for these differences?

2. Seven state legislatures have adopted the language contained in Section 707 of the Uniform Parentage Act, requiring some written record of the deceased individual's desire to become a parent after death. As originally amended in 2000, the UPA referred to a "spouse who dies before placement of eggs . . ." The 2002 version replaced "spouse" with "individual" in an effort to equalize the treatment of marital and nonmarital children. Four of the states adopting UPA Section 707 have incorporated the marriage-neutral 2002 version, while three states retain the 2000 version applying only to spouses. See Colo. Rev. Stat. § 19-4-106(8) (enacted in 2003, adopting 2000 version of the UPA); Del. Code Ann., ti. 13, § 8-707 (enacted in 2003, adopting 2000 version); N.D. Cent. Code § 14-20-65 (enacted in 2005, adopting 2002 version); Tex. Fam. Code Ann. § 160.707 (Vernon 2004) (enacted in 2001, adopting the 2000 version); Utah Code Ann. § 78B-15-707 (enacted in 2005, adopting the 2000 version); Wash. Rev. Code § 26.26.730 (revised in 2011 to update to 2002 language); Wyo. Stat. Ann. § 14-2-907 (enacted in 2003, adopting the 2002 version).

Virginia law also addresses the question of posthumous parentage, providing as follows:

> Death of spouse. — Any child resulting from the insemination of a wife's ovum using her husband's sperm, with his consent, is the child of the husband and wife notwithstanding that, during the ten-month period immediately preceding the birth, either party died.
>
> However, any person who dies before in utero implantation of an embryo resulting from the union of his sperm or her ovum with another gamete, whether or not the other gamete is that of the person's spouse, is not the parent of any resulting child unless (i) implantation occurs before notice of the death can reasonably be communicated to the physician performing the procedure or (ii) the person consents to be a parent in writing executed before the implantation.

Va. Code Ann. § 20-158(B) (2004). In Virginia, if a married man dies, leaving sperm and written permission to release the vials to his widow, would the resulting child be considered a child of the husband if she were born, say, three years later?

3. In the majority of states where lawmakers have not enacted specific legislation addressing the parentage of posthumous children, judges could still be called upon to resolve disputes involving children conceived after a genetic parent has died. What sources of law could a judge look to in the absence of explicit law on the topic of postmortem conception?

In most states, paternity can be proven after the alleged father's death by clear and convincing evidence. Suppose a widow gives birth using frozen sperm two years after her husband's death, but vows never to tell her son about his conception because she fears he will be confused and distraught at knowing his father died long before he was born. She plans to tell her son he was conceived using donor sperm obtained from a local sperm bank. The child's grandmother (the husband's mother) fears a more sinister motive — inheritance. Under the prevailing state law, a widow must share the decedent's estate with the decedent's issue. If the grandmother brings an action for declaration of paternity on the son's behalf (assuming she has standing to bring such an action and the statute of limitations has not run), what would constitute clear and convincing evidence of the late husband's paternity? Would a record of his deposits at the sperm bank, along with a record showing the wife was inseminated with that sperm suffice? What evidence might the wife offer to counter the written record of deposit and insemination? Ultimately, the only sure way to determine parentage may be to exhume the father's body. Would a court be likely to order such a drastic measure? See *Alexander v. Alexander*, 42 Ohio Misc. 2d 30, 537 N.E.2d 1310 (1988); *In re Estate of Janis*, 157 Misc. 2d 999, 600 N.Y.S.2d 416 (1993).

2. The Uniform Probate Code

The Uniform Probate Code was originally promulgated in 1969 and revised several times, including in 1990 and again in 2008. Major portions of the UPC have been adopted in about one-third of states, with other states adopting more limited parts of the suggested law. In 1969, the thought of posthumous conception was not even a twinkle in a prospective father's eye, thus the code was silent on the matter. But the notion that a child could be born after his father's death, or at least within nine months of his father's death, was well within the drafters' contemplation. To account for the child of a pregnant widow, the UPC provides:

Section 2-108. Afterborn Heirs.

Relatives of the decedent conceived before his death but born thereafter inherit as if they had been born in the lifetime of the decedent.

In 1990, Section 2-108 of the UPC was revised to provide as follows:

An individual in gestation at a particular time is treated as living at that time if the individual lives 120 hours or more after birth.

In 2008, Section 2-108 was deleted and moved to Section 2-104 as follows:

An individual in gestation at a decedent's death is deemed to be living at the decedent's death if the individual lives 120 hours after birth. If it is not established by clear and convincing evidence that an individual in gestation at the decedent's death lived 120 hours after birth, it is deemed that the individual failed to survive for the required period.

NOTES AND QUESTIONS

1. Why do you think the uniform law commissioners revised the UPC provision on afterborn heirs in 1990? Why did the commissioners again rewrite the language regarding afterborn heirs in 2008? Does the 1990 change increase or decrease the opportunity for an afterborn child to inherit from the decedent parent? How about the 2008 change? Do either of the changes even affect a child conceived after her father's death using frozen sperm?

2. *The Updated UPC and the Rights of Postmortem Conception Children.* Keep in mind that the UPC is primarily concerned with inheritance and testamentary rights, rather than more generalized rights of ART-conceived children. Still, the code does recognize the growing number of families that rely on ART for family formation, and has been updated to reflect those family scenarios in more recent versions. After all, as previously noted, inheritance rights do flow from a legally recognized parent-child relationship, thus it makes sense for a probate code to firmly establish under what circumstances those relationships lawfully arise.

In 2008, the UPC adopted several provisions that address the parental status, and thus the inheritance rights of postmortem conception children. Sections 2-120 and 2-121 address the rights of posthumously conceived children to be treated as "in gestation" for purposes of Section 2-104, reprinted above. Take a look at the language:

Uniform Probate Code Section 2-120(k)

If, under this section, an individual is a parent of a child of assisted reproduction who is conceived after the individual's death, the child is treated as in gestation at the individual's death for purposes of Section 2-104(a)(2) if the child is:

(1)   in utero not later than 36 months after the individual's death; or

(2)   born not later than 45 months after the individual's death.

Uniform Probate Code Section 2-121(h)

If, under this section, an individual is a parent of a gestational child who is conceived after the individual's death, the child is treated as in gestation at the individual's death for purposes of Section 2-104(a)(2) if the child is:

(1)   in utero not later than 36 months after the individual's death; or

(2)   born not later than 45 months after the individual's death.

At first blush, the only difference between these two sections is the exchange of "child of assisted reproduction" in Sec. 2-120 for "gestational child" in Sec. 2-121. But Professor Kristine Knaplund has carefully analyzed these and other sections of the 2008 UPC to reveal that a postmortem child's legal status under the code will vary according to her parent's sex and marital status. Digging deeply into the UPC language, Professor Knaplund concludes that the following seemingly identical scenarios would obtain different legal outcomes:

Two married heterosexual couples are in a car crash. The husband of couple #1 dies instantly, as does the wife of couple #2. At the hospital, at their spouses' requests, doctors are able to retrieve Husband #1's (H1) sperm and Wife #2's (W2) ova for cryopreservation. Two years later, Wife #1 (W1) uses her dead husband's frozen sperm to become pregnant; Husband #2 (H2) uses his dead wife's frozen ova and arranges to have a baby with a gestational carrier. Will the predeceased spouses be the parents of the resulting children, conceived and born years after their deaths? . . .

For couple #1, as long as they were married with no divorce proceedings pending at the time of the car crash, UPC § 2-120 presumes that H1 is the father of the child even though his sperm was retrieved after his death . . . Couple #2, on the other hand, does not benefit from any presumption that W2 was the child's mother. UPC § 2-121 raises the presumption of parentage for W2 only if she deposited her ova before she died. Thus, for W2 to be named as the parent of the child, we need either her written consent or clear and convincing evidence that she wanted to have children conceived and born after her death.

Kristine S. Knaplund, *The New Uniform Probate Code's Surprising Gender Inequities*, 18 Duke J. Gender Law & Policy 335 (2011). In her article, Professor Knaplund lauds the UPC drafters for addressing the rights of posthumously conceived children, but suggests several sensible language changes that would equalize the treatment of children conceived under such dire circumstances.

3.   Another source of guidance for lawmakers is the Restatement of the Law (Third) — Property: Wills & Donative Transfers § 2.5, pertaining to the designation of a parent/child relationship. The Restatement takes a more liberal view of posthumous reproduction than the UPC, suggesting that:

. . . to inherit from the decedent, a child produced from genetic material of the decedent by assisted reproductive technology must be born within a reasonable time after the decedent's death in circumstances indicating that the decedent would have approved of the child's right to inherit. A clear case would be that of a child produced by artificial insemination of the decedent's widow with his frozen sperm. If the AIH procedure occurs after the husband's death, and if the child is born within a reasonable time after the husband's death, the child should be treated as the husband's child for purposes of inheritance *from* the husband. Once conceived, such a child is the husband's and wife's child for all purposes of inheritance by, from, or through an intestate decedent who dies thereafter.

Restatement (Third) of Property: Wills & Donative Transfers § 2.5 cmt. l (1999). The Restatement's use of the language "reasonable time" after death, and "circumstances indicating that the decedent would have approved of the child's right to inherit" seem to reflect a presumption in favor of inheritance for posthumous children, in contrast to the strict necessity of a record or clear and convincing evidence proving intent required by the UPC. Which position do you favor, a presumption in favor of rights if the decedent left frozen sperm or eggs, or a presumption against inheritance rights unless the decedent left a written record of intent?

B. Emerging Laws Governing the Rights of Posthumous Children

The uniform laws discussed in Section 3(A) provide lawmakers with suggested language that can be modified or adopted on a state-by-state basis. Alternatively, a state legislature can draft its own language, creating a statutory structure that suits the unique perspective of its citizens. The need for legislative action may arise when a particular case gains media or judicial attention. Such was the case in California when a widow used sperm extracted 30 hours *after* her husband died in an accident. Recall the case of Gaby Vernoff, discussed in Section (1)(A)(2), who gave birth four years after her husband's death. When the Social Security Administration denied her claim for survivor benefits on behalf of her daughter, a local lawmaker became interested in the matter of posthumous reproduction and inheritance rights. In February 2004, Assembly Member Tom Harman introduced A.B. 1910, dubbed the "dead dads" bill, which would grant inheritance rights to children who are conceived within one year after a parent dies. During the legislative process, the one-year time frame was increased to two years, giving a surviving spouse more time to contemplate using the decedent's gametic material. The bill passed the California legislature and was signed by Governor Schwarzenegger on September 24, 2004 (with slight amendments passed into law in 2005).

The new California law is a good example of the complexity of legal aspects of postmortem reproduction. The law makes changes to four areas of the state's massive statutory code structure — it amends the Family Law Code, the Health & Safety Code, the Insurance Code, and the Probate Code. The parameters for recognizing a postmortem child's rights to inherit from the deceased parent are set out in the Probate Code provisions:

California Probate Code
Chap. 3 Identity of Heirs

Section 249.5 is added to the Probate Code, to read:

249.5. For purposes of determining rights to property to be distributed upon the death of a decedent, a child of the decedent conceived and born after the death of the decedent shall be deemed to have been born in the lifetime of the decedent, and after the execution of all of the decedent's testamentary instruments, if the child or his or her representative proves by clear and convincing evidence that all of the following conditions are satisfied:

(a) The decedent, in writing, specifies that his or her genetic material shall be used for the posthumous conception of a child of the decedent, subject to the following:

(1) The specification shall be signed by the decedent and dated.

(2) The specification may be revoked or amended only by a writing, signed by the decedent and dated.

(3) A person is designated by the decedent to control the use of the genetic

material . . .

(c) The child was in utero using the decedent's genetic material and was in utero within two years of the date of issuance of a certificate of the decedent's death or entry of a judgment determining the fact of the decedent's death, whichever event occurs first. This subdivision does not apply to a child who shares all of his or her nuclear genes with the person donating the implanted nucleus as a result of the application of somatic nuclear transfer technology commonly known as human cloning.

NOTES AND QUESTIONS

1. *Will Substitute?* Notice the California law addresses two different aspects of testamentary disposition. First, the law determines whether a postmortem conception child is a lawful heir of the decedent, and second, the law spells out how "genetic material" can be effectively passed at the decedent's death. This second scenario looks a lot like the passage of property at death, something that would require a valid will or will substitute. Probate Code Section 249.5 requires that the decedent sign and date a written directive designating a beneficiary to control the use of his or her genetic material. Though sounding rather formal, this writing falls short of the requirements for a valid will set forth in Cal. Probate Code Section 6110 (a writing signed by the testator and two witnesses present at the same time the testator signs the will). Do you think that a person's directive to distribute his or her reproductive material after death should meet the same standards as that person's directive to distribute his or her real and personal property after death? Which type of asset — and assurances about its proper handling — would be more important to a decedent?

2. Can a woman seek to have her husband's sperm retrieved *after* he has died, under the above California law? If so, will the posthumous child be considered a child of the decedent?

3. What is the relevance of the law's provision deeming a posthumous child who meets the statutory requirements, "born in the lifetime of the decedent, and after the execution of all of the decedent's testamentary instruments." This envisions a scenario in which the decedent makes a will, dies, and then becomes a parent to a child for inheritance purposes. Do you think it likely under these circumstances that a decedent would include in his will a bequest for his posthumously conceived child or children? If the decedent dies with a will that does not name any posthumously conceived child, does this mean such a child receives no interest in the deceased parent's estate? Not necessarily.

Nearly every state has a statute protecting children from unintentional disinheritance by a parent. These statutes are known as "pretermitted child statutes." Though they vary widely in structure, the general idea behind pretermission statutes is to award a share of the testator's estate to a child born after the execution of the will. The statutes are based on the presumption that the testator did not mean to disinherit the child, but rather neglected to update the will following the child's birth. A pretermitted child is often awarded an intestate share of the estate, which in many states can be as much as half of the estate in which a spouse survives.

The newly added section of the California Probate Code appears to contemplate that a posthumously conceived child could be considered pretermitted, as the child would necessarily be born "after the execution of all of the decedent's testamentary instruments," in a case where the decedent executed testamentary instruments during lifetime. How would the interaction of the pretermitted child statute and the posthumous heir statute affect the decedent's other children, born in the decedent's lifetime and before any testamentary instruments were executed?

Let's meet a family and find out. Harry married Paula in 1983 and the couple had two children, Jonathan and Rachel. Then Harry met Sally. He divorced Paula and married Sally in 1995. In 2005 Harry executes a will leaving his entire estate to Sally. Harry and Sally try to conceive but have difficulty. They seek the services of the local fertility clinic, where Harry banks sperm for future treatments, signing an authorization for Sally to use his sperm at any time, including after his death. The written authorization is witnessed by the patient coordinator at the fertility clinic. In 2010 Harry is killed in a plane crash. In 2012 Sally gives birth to Aaron and Sara, twins conceived using Harry's frozen sperm.

In addition to Probate Code § 249.5, consider the following statutes:

> **Probate Code § 21620. . . .** [I]f a decedent fails to provide in a testamentary instrument for a child of decedent born or adopted after the execution of all of the decedent's testamentary instruments, the omitted child shall receive a share in the decedent's estate equal in value to that which the child would have received if the decedent had died without having executed any testamentary instrument.

> **Probate Code § 6401(c)(3)(A). . . .** [T]he intestate share of the surviving spouse . . . is . . . one-third of the intestate estate . . . where the decedent leaves more than one child.

> **Probate Code § 6402(a). . . .** [T]he intestate estate not passing to the surviving spouse . . . passes . . . to the issue of the decedent.

How will Harry's estate be distributed under California law? Under the law in your state? Do you see the potential for family disharmony once Harry's estate is distributed? For a discussion of the problem of pretermission and posthumous reproduction, see James E. Bailey, *An Analytical Framework for Resolving the Issues Raised by the Interaction Between Reproductive Technology and the Law of Inheritance*, 47 DePaul L. Rev. 743, 792 (1998).

4. At least one other state has contemplated the problem of a posthumous child being considered pretermitted under the state's existing probate code. Florida law provides:

> A child conceived from the eggs or sperm of a person or persons who died before the transfer of their eggs, sperm, or preembryos to a woman's body shall not be eligible for a claim against the decedent's estate unless the child has been provided for by the decedent's will.

Fla. Stat. Ann. § 742.17. Thus, Florida law seems to makes posthumous children ineligible to inherit from their parent's estate either by intestacy or by pretermission. What if a Florida testator writes a will that states, "I wish to acknowledge any future child I may have from the sperm I have deposited with the Florida Sperm Bank." Has this child been "provided for" by the decedent's will? If so, would the child be eligible to take a share of the estate under Florida's pretermission statute?

C. Model Laws and Task Force Reports

A final source of model legislation can be found in materials issued by commissioned studies and volunteer organizations such as the American Bar Association. For the most part, these sources of law have tended to disfavor posthumous conception (unless explicitly agreed to by the decedent), both as a reproductive practice and as a means of establishing a parent/child relationship between the decedent and the offspring. Two groups' recommendations are briefly set forth below — the ABA and the New York State Task Force on Life and the Law, a group created by state executive order in 1985 and charged with recommending policy on a host of issues, including assisted reproductive technologies.

1. The ABA Model Act

In 2008, the American Bar Association House of Delegates approved and adopted the Model Act Governing Assisted Reproduction. The work was the result of many years of study and drafting by the ABA Section of Family Law, Committee on the Law of Genetic and Reproduction Technology. The Model Act covers many of the practices discussed throughout the book, including postmortem conception. Sections 205 and 501 apply directly to the subject at hand:

Model Act Governing Assisted Reproduction Section of Family Law, American Bar Association

Section 205. Collection of Gametes or Embryos From Preserved Tissue or From Deceased or Incompetent Persons

1. Gametes or embryos shall not be collected from deceased or incompetent individuals or from preserved tissues unless consent in a record was executed prior to death or incompetency by the individual from whom the gametes or embryos are to be collected or the individual's authorized fiduciary who has express authorization from the principal to so consent.

2. In the event of an emergency where the required consent is alleged but unavailable and where, in the opinion of the treating physician, loss of viability would occur as a result of delay, and where there is a genuine question as to the existence of consent in a record, an exception is permissible.

3. If gametes or embryos are collected pursuant to paragraph 2 of this Section, transfer of gametes or of an embryo is expressly prohibited unless approved by a Court. Absence of a record as described in Paragraph 1 shall constitute a presumption of non-consent.

4. Any individual or entity not acting in accordance with this Section may be subject to civil and/or criminal liability as provided in law.

Section 501. Parental Rights and Obligations Under Embryo Agreements

(f) Following the death of an intended parent who has previously consented in a record to posthumous use of cryopreserved gametes and/or embryos, the surviving intended parent may discard, donate, or use the embryos for his/her own parenting purposes. An individual born as a result of embryo transfer after the death of an intended parent or gamete provider is not the child of that gamete provider or intended parent unless the deceased individual consented in a record that if assisted reproduction were to occur after death, the deceased individual would be a parent of the child.

QUESTIONS

What conduct is unlawful under the ABA Model Act? Under Section 205(4) what are the penalties for unlawful conduct under this law? If a woman uses sperm retrieved from her dead husband without his written consent, is she committing an unlawful act? Is the physician who assists her in the retrieval? How about the physician who performs the insemination?

2. The New York State Task Force on Life and the Law

In April 1998 the Task Force issued a comprehensive and well-researched report titled "Assisted Reproductive Technologies: Analysis and Recommendations for Public Policy." Ably administered by its Executive Director, Carl Coleman, the Task Force met regularly for several years, deliberating on each recommendation contained in the Report. A few of the many recommendations pertain to posthumous reproduction.

Chapter 10. Retrieval of Gametes Without Consent

> Gametes should generally not be retrieved without informed consent. New York should enact legislation prohibiting the retrieval of gametes from deceased persons or living individuals incapable of providing informed consent, unless the individual consented to the retrieval of gametes under the particular circumstances, in writing, when able to do so, or the person seeking to retrieve the gametes establishes extraordinary circumstances in a judicial proceeding.

Chapter 12. Children Conceived or Gestated After a Parent's Death

> New York should adopt the [Uniform Status of Children of Assisted Conception Act's] provision that "an individual who dies before implantation of an embryo, or before a child is conceived other than through sexual intercourse, using the individual's egg or sperm, is not a parent of the resulting child."

QUESTIONS

The NY Task Force, like the ABA, recommends resort to a court of law should a party wish to retrieve (NYTF) or transfer (ABA) gametes without consent from the deceased person. Would such a judicial proceeding place an undue burden on a grieving spouse, causing him or her to abandon the quest to procreate using the decedent's gametes? Perhaps both professional groups had another scenario in mind — celebrity gamete hunting. If gametes could easily be retrieved from a deceased person, imagine the crowds that would assemble for a chance at parenthood using John F. Kennedy Jr.'s sperm or Princess Diana's egg. Clearly scenarios in which strangers seek to obtain the gametes of those they admire from a distance is appropriately placed in the hands of the judiciary.

Chapter 7

ART AND DIVORCE: DISPUTES OVER FROZEN EMBRYOS

The events and emotions surrounding procreation are typically positive, often joyous, as parents anticipate and prepare to welcome their beloved children. Reproduction using ART can imbue this same euphoric sentiment in prospective parents whose sense of wonder and gratitude may be even sharper after struggling to overcome infertility at great personal and financial expense. While the use of ART can bring joy to parents and families, it also has the unique capacity to wreak havoc on those whose journey to parenthood has detoured into the laboratory. Unlike natural conception, with its certain and rigid time frame between intercourse and birth, assisted conception introduces an element of uncertainty into the procreative formula. Once embryos are formed in the laboratory, they can be cryopreserved — frozen — for use in the future. Much can transpire in the lives of the expectant parents from conception to gestation. Death of one or both spouses,[1] malfunction in the storage facility, spontaneous pregnancy in the woman, or a change of heart in the couple's desire to become parents can dramatically alter the original plan for each embryo to be implanted amid a hopeful expectation of pregnancy. Of all of the possible unforeseen contingencies, by far the most common is the schism that plagues nearly one in every two marriages — divorce. The plight of frozen embryos upon marital dissolution has become a not-too-uncommon occurrence, generating law and commentary worthy of study.

Before launching into our discussion of ART and divorce, let's take a brief look at some of the other unplanned events that can derail a frozen embryo's preplanned destination. The science of cryopreservation, while enormously important for preserving, enabling, and extending procreative possibilities, remains a technique that is subject to human and technological error. When an embryo is damaged or destroyed while in frozen storage, parents, physicians, and judges are asked to grapple with questions of liability and compensation. Ultimately, these actors confront the same query we pondered in Chapter 1: What is the nature and status of an unimplanted embryo? The answer to this foundational question can clear the path for resolving the frozen embryo dispute that dashed the parties' hopes and dreams for parenthood.

---

[1] The birth of a child conceived before but born after the death of a genetic parent — posthumous reproduction — is discussed in Chapter 6.

SECTION I: THE POPULARITY AND FRAILTY OF EMBRYO CRYOPRESERVATION

The science of embryo cryopreservation[2] is now decades old, as the first live births from frozen embryos were reported in Australia in 1984 and in the United States in 1986. In the intervening decades, the use of ART has grown exponentially, due in no small measure to the ability to freeze embryos for use in multiple cycles. Thus, logically, one can deduce that in the past nearly 30 years, a supply of embryos has accumulated in our nation's fertility clinic freezers. Curious about the number of embryos in frozen storage in the U.S., the Society for Assisted Reproductive Technology (SART) teamed with research giant RAND to calculate this figure in the early part of the twenty-first century. The team surveyed all 430 ART practices in the U.S., asking a host of questions ranging from the facility's use of cryopreservation to the number of embryos currently being stored at the facility. The results indicated a total of nearly 400,000 embryos in frozen storage in the U.S., twice the number that had previously been speculated. See David I. Hoffman, et al., *Cryopreserved Embryos in the United States and their Availability for Research*, 79 FERTILITY & STERILITY 1063 (2003).

By all accounts, the number of embryos in frozen storage has continued to grow. According to Dr. Robert Nachtigall, a researcher at the University of California, San Francisco, about 50,000 new frozen embryos are accumulating each year in the U.S. *See* John Schieszer, *Couples' Feelings Mixed About Extra Embryos*, Reuters Health Information, Oct. 14, 2003. For many couples, especially those who have successfully concluded fertility treatments, the future of their frozen embryos presents a wrenching dilemma. To learn more about his patients' views, Dr. Nachtigall conducted a survey among 26 couples who had conceived, but had frozen embryos in storage, asking about their future plans for disposition. Only nine couples had decided what to do — four intended to donate their embryos to research, three planned disposal, one wanted to donate to another couple, and one planned to have another child. The remaining 17 couples had made no decision about their embryos future; presumably the embryos would remain in frozen storage until a decision was reached.

Another aspect of Dr. Nachtigall's survey touched on the couple's view of these eight-cell entities. When asked about their concept of the embryos' status, some of the couples reported they viewed the frozen embryos as living beings capable of discomfort and suffering. Others saw the embryos as children with interests that must be considered. Still others viewed the embryos as family members, genetic or psychological insurance, or symbolic reminders of past infertility. Finally, some couples looked upon their frozen embryos as something that could be used in the future as part of a potential medical therapy for their current children.

---

[2] Cryopreservation is defined as the "[m]aintenance of the viability of excised tissues or organs at extremely low temperatures. Stedman's Medical Dictionary 416 (26th ed. 1995). Typically embryos are cryopreserved in a special storage tank, in individual straws suspended in liquid nitrogen at negative 196 degrees centigrade. The liquid nitrogen tanks are equipped with automatic fill detectors and alarm systems to prevent, as much as is humanly possible, any mishaps that could cause the embryos to thaw.

A more recent survey of patient attitudes toward their cryopreserved embryos found the same mix of uncertainty and angst among contemporary frozen embryo holders. In 2007, more than 1,000 fertility patients were questioned about their disposition preferences. While 54% expressed an interest in using the embryos for their own reproductive purposes, among the patients who did not desire more children, 41% of this group considered donation to research, 16% were willing to consider donating their embryos to another couple, while 12% contemplated thaw and discard. In many instances, there was a mismatch between patient preferences and the availability of these preferences — in particular the options to donate to research or to other couples for reproduction — prompting the survey authors to conclude, "the results of this study emphasize the need for intensive restructuring of the informed consent process for infertility treatment that involves embryo cryopreservation." Anne Drapkin Lyerly et al., *Fertility Patients' Views About Frozen Embryo Disposition: Results of a Multi-Institutional U.S. Survey*, 93(2) FERTILITY & STERILITY 499 (2010).

When a couple or an individual agrees to place embryos in frozen storage, there is an expectation that the embryos will be available for whatever disposition the depositor chooses. But not every embryo that is frozen is available for use upon thaw. About 35% of frozen embryos do not survive the freeze-thaw process, and of those that do survive, only about 35% will survive to the blastocyst (5-day) stage. These losses are expected, and should be part of the disclosure of information given to patients who elect to freeze their embryos. Some losses, however, are unexpected and thus can cause great pain and suffering to prospective parents who relied on their fertility clinic to assiduously guard their future offspring. What remedy, if any, should be available when frozen embryos are negligently or intentionally destroyed? The case law is slim, but extant.

FRISINA v. WOMAN AND INFANT HOSPITAL OF RHODE ISLAND
Superior Court of Rhode Island
2002 R.I. Super. LEXIS 73 (2002)

GIBNEY, J. These matters are before the Court on the motion of defendant Women and Infants Hospital of Rhode Island (hereinafter "defendant" or "Hospital") for summary judgment pursuant to Super. R. Civ. P. 56. The plaintiffs — David and Carol Frisina, George and Susan Doyle, and Robert and Vickie Lamontagne — have filed timely objections to the defendant's motion.

Facts/Travel

Each of the three cases brought against the defendant involves certain incidents that occurred at the Hospital's In Vitro Fertilization (hereinafter "IVF") Clinic. The plaintiffs were all evaluated, and eventually accepted into, the Hospital's IVF Program.

In January 1992, Plaintiff Carol Frisina became a patient of the Endocrinology-Fertility Unit within the Department of Obstetrics and Gynecology at the Hospital . . . In August 1992, Plaintiff Carol Frisina underwent a fresh cycle transfer by which a number of her eggs were harvested and fertilized. Of the thirteen eggs that were successfully fertilized four were transferred to Plaintiff Carol Frisina in the first attempt at conception. The nine remaining embryos were frozen for future use. This initial transfer proved unsuccessful. In June 1993, the Frisinas were treated at the Hospital in preparation for the second attempt at conception using the previously frozen embryos. However, the Frisinas were informed that of the nine frozen embryos from the August 1992 process, only three were available. Moreover, the three frozen embryos were not successfully thawed or suitable for transfer. On July 24, 1995, the Frisinas brought suit against the Hospital for the loss and destruction of their embryos . . .

[Plaintiff Vickie Lamontagne alleges that after undergoing an IVF cycle which produced seven embryos, defendant lost two of her embryos, neither of which were ever found. Plaintiff Susan Doyle alleges that defendant informed her that five embryos frozen at the IVF Clinic had been inadvertently destroyed when the Hospital moved its facility. All three plaintiffs sued the defendant Hospital for the loss or destruction of their embryos.]

In their complaints, the plaintiffs have asserted three theories of recovery: medical malpractice, bailment, and breach of contract. In all three counts, the plaintiffs contend that they have "suffered severe trauma and emotional anguish, pain and suffering." . . . Before this Court is defendant's motion for summary judgment which is premised on the argument that although these matters present unique issues — the legal status of human pre-embryos, the duties owed to such pre-embryos and their progenitors, and the damages which may flow from their loss or destruction — the plaintiffs have nonetheless failed to state a claim upon which relief may be granted. The defendant contends that, as a matter of law, plaintiffs cannot recover damages for emotional harm based upon alleged loss of the pre-embryos; that it would be unfair and illogical to allow plaintiffs greater rights with respect to a frozen pre-embryo than with respect to a non-viable fetus; that Rhode Island law does not permit recovery for emotional harm resulting from alleged negligent conduct where plaintiffs have not suffered actual or threatened physical harm and have not witnessed physical injury inflicted on a relative; that as a matter of law plaintiffs cannot recover damages for emotional harm resulting from the loss of personal property whether as a result of breach of contract or negligence; and, finally, that plaintiffs' complaints should be dismissed because plaintiffs were specifically informed of, consented to and expressly assumed the risk of any loss or damage to the frozen pre-embryos. In turn, the plaintiffs advance a number of arguments in opposition to the summary judgment motion . . .

Negligent Infliction of Emotional Distress

. . . The Rhode Island Supreme Court first recognized liability for negligent infliction of emotional distress in *D'Ambra v. United States*, 114 R.I. 643, 338 A.2d 524 (1975) . . . The court set out the elements of a claim for negligent infliction of emotional distress when it wrote that "a party must (1) be a close relative of the victim, (2) be present at the scene of the accident and be aware that the victim is being injured, and (3) as a result of experiencing the accident, suffer serious emotional injury that is accompanied by physical symptomatology."

The defendant contends that plaintiffs cannot succeed on a claim for negligent infliction of emotional distress because plaintiffs fail to meet all of the required elements of the claim. The plaintiffs argue that their cases represent issues of first impression that do not fall within the ambit of prior decisions rendered by the Supreme Court . . .

A. Pre-embryos as Victims

First, the defendant argues that since pre-embryos are not considered persons within the meaning of the law, pre-embryos cannot be victims and the first element of a negligent infliction of emotional distress claim cannot be met. To arrive at this conclusion, the defendant relies on the court's holding in *Miccolis v. Amica Mutual Insurance Co.*, 587 A.2d 67, 71 (R.I.1991), that a nonviable fetus is not a "person" within the meaning of the wrongful death statute. Defendant contends that through such a holding, the court also precluded recovery for "damages for loss of society and companionship." (Def.'s Mem. of Law at 8.) Thus, defendant argues that where the court has barred recovery for emotional harm relating to the death of a nonviable fetus, it is logical that the court would also preclude recovery for emotional harm relating to the loss of pre-embryos. *Id.*

Despite the "long period of time that IVF has been used and the number of couples who seek its miracles each year," there is a dearth of both statutory authority and case law regarding pre-embryos. [citation omitted] Although a majority of the decided cases deal with disputes regarding custody of the frozen pre-embryos, which is not at issue in the instant case, an examination of these cases is nonetheless warranted because they reveal the legal status accorded to pre-embryos. The first case to consider the disposition of frozen pre-embryos in an action for dissolution of a marriage was *Davis v. Davis*, 842 S.W.2d 588 (Tenn. 1992) . . . The court held that under Tennessee law pre-embryos could not be considered "persons." In addition, the court held that any interest that Mr. and Mrs. Davis may have in the pre-embryos is not a "true property interest . . . [but] they do have an interest in the nature of ownership, to the extent that they have decision-making authority concerning disposition of the preembryos." *Id.* at 597. Thus the court concluded that "preembryos are not, strictly speaking, either 'persons' or 'property,' but occupy an interim category that entitles them to special respect because of their potential for human life." *Id.* . . .

Finally, a leading expert in the field has written that "[i]f negligent loss of an embryo is not covered under wrongful death statutes, it may be difficult to fashion a remedy. There is no way to show that particular embryos would have been implanted and gone to term."[3]

B. Plaintiffs Were Not Present at the Scene

The defendant next argues that the plaintiffs would fail to meet the second prong of the negligent infliction of emotional distress test because the plaintiffs were not

---

[3] [n.12] *See* John A. Robertson, *Reproductive Technology and Reproductive Rights: In the Beginning The Legal Status of Early Embryos*, 76 Va. L.Rev. 437, 460 n. 61 (1990) (Citations omitted.)

present and did not witness the loss or destruction of the embryos. See *Marchetti v. Parsons*, 638 A.2d 1047,1052 (R.I.1994) . . . The plaintiffs concede that because they did not witness the actual destruction or injury to the embryos "under traditional tort standards . . . [they] find themselves outside the scope of compensable emotional harm." (Pls. Mem. of Law at 10.) However, the plaintiffs contend that "the knowledge by the putative parents that loss or destruction of embryos entrusted to an IVF Clinic has wrongfully occurred must suffice to expose the Clinic to liability for its wrongful conduct." *Id.*

C. Physical Symptomatology Requirement

Finally, the defendant maintains that the plaintiffs did not suffer any actual or threatened physical harm due to the emotional anguish they experienced. In *Reilly v. United States*, 547 A.2d 894 (R.I.1988), the Rhode Island Supreme Court followed the majority of jurisdictions when it imposed the requirement that "a plaintiff must suffer physical symptomatology to recover damages for negligent infliction of emotional distress." The Court continues to adhere to its physical symptomatology requirement . . .

Thus, the current state of Rhode Island law with respect to the required elements for a claim of negligent infliction of emotional distress appears to present an insurmountable obstacle for the plaintiffs . . . [D]efendant's motion for summary judgment with respect to this claim must be granted.

Emotional Distress based on Loss of Personal Property

The plaintiffs also allege in Counts II and III that they have suffered the "loss of irreplaceable property." The defendant contends that there are no Rhode Island cases permitting an award of damages for emotional distress from the loss of property based on breach of contract or negligence . . .

This Court finds that the plaintiffs are seeking to recover for the physical loss of their pre-embryos rather than for the loss of the possibility of achieving pregnancy as claimed by the defendant. Moreover, the Court finds merit in the argument raised by plaintiffs that recovery for damages for emotional distress based on the "loss of irreplaceable property," the loss of their pre-embryos, is permissible under the Rhode Island Supreme Court's holding in *Hawkins v. Scituate Oil*, 723 A.2d 771 (R.I.1999) . . . Accordingly, defendant's motion for summary judgment on the issue of damages for emotional harm due to the loss of irreplaceable property must be, and, is denied.

Assumption of Risk

The final argument raised by the defendant is that the plaintiffs assumed the risk of any loss or damage to the frozen pre-embryos as evidenced by their execution of certain documents. A document entitled "INFORMED CONSENT: *IN VITRO* FERTILIZATION (In Connection with Pre-Embryo Freezing)" was signed by each of the plaintiffs. This form contained language stating that although the Hospital may proceed with due care, there were twelve events which could nonetheless prevent pregnancy, including that "a laboratory accident may result in loss or damage to the fertilized egg(s) or pre-embryo(s)." Also, each of the plaintiffs signed another document entitled "INFORMED CONSENT AND CONTRACT FOR EMBRYO FREEZING," which contained the following language:

> "3. Husband and Wife acknowledge, understand and agree that despite the Hospital, its physicians and its employees proceeding with due care, it is possible that a laboratory accident in the Hospital may result in loss or damage to one or more of said frozen embryos."

. . . Plaintiffs maintain, however, that they were "NOT asked to, nor did they assume the risk that their embryos might be destroyed because of the failure of those participating in the IVF program to exercise due care for the safety of the embryos." (Pl.'s Mem. of Law at 21.) Rather, the plaintiffs contend that they accepted only the risk of a laboratory accident that could occur despite the defendant's due care . . .

In the cases at bar, each of the plaintiffs during his or her deposition testimony admits to having been presented with the informed consent documents and signing those documents, which contain the provision that damage or loss to the embryos may result due to a laboratory accident. However, it appears that plaintiffs interpreted the exculpatory clauses differently than defendant as evidenced by the following exchange during Susan Doyle's deposition:

Q: So you understood when you signed this form that you were accepting the risk that a laboratory accident could cause loss or damage to the fertilized eggs or pre-embryos, correct?

Mr. Oliviera: Objection.

A: I signed accepting that if there was an accident, it would be a careful accident, not an accident of carelessness or sloppiness. That's what I initialed and what I signed.

Q: Does it say something in this form that you can point me to about a careful accident, not a sloppy accident?

A: Well, in the form — would you repeat your question, please?

Mr. Oliviera: Read it back please. (Last question read.)

A: To me a careful accident — to answer your question, I'm sorry. There is no description as what a careful accident and what a careless accident is on this form.

Q: Okay. And when you signed this form or at anytime before you signed this form, you didn't tell somebody that you understood the form to only refer to a so-called careful accident, as opposed to a sloppy accident, did you?

A: I'm sorry. Would you repeat that.

Q: Before you signed this form, you didn't tell anybody that you understood this to only be referring to a so-called careful accident, did you?

A: I don't recall.

Q: You have no recollection of saying that, do you?

A: No.

Q: Now, can you tell me, ma'am, what a careful accident is, as compared to a sloppy accident?

A: M-hm. (Affirmative.) Yes. A careful accident is one, I believe, that is an act of God. A careless or a sloppy accident is one of human error.

Q: And where did you develop that understanding?

A: It's common sense. (Dep. on August 2, 2000 at 56-57.)

Plaintiffs understood the exculpatory clauses in the informed consent documents to mean that where the defendant acted with due care and a laboratory accident nonetheless occurs the defendant would be absolved of liability for loss or destruction of their pre-embryos. Plaintiffs did not construe the exculpatory clauses to excuse the defendant from liability where loss or destruction of their pre-embryos resulted from defendant's negligence, such as the loss of pre-embryos during the clinic's relocation to a new facility . . .

Accordingly, defendant's motion for summary judgment on its defense of assumption of risk is denied.

Conclusion

Summary judgment will be granted when this Court finds that there are no genuine issues of material fact and the moving party is entitled to judgment as a matter of law . . . [T]his Court finds there is no genuine issue of material fact as to plaintiffs' allegation of negligent infliction of emotional distress. However, this Court finds that genuine issues of material fact exist with respect to plaintiffs' claim of emotional distress due to breach of contract and defendant's assumption of risk defense. Therefore, defendant's motion for summary judgment is granted in part and denied in part. Counsel shall submit an appropriate order and judgment for entry.

MILLER v. AMERICAN INFERTILITY GROUP OF ILLINOIS, S.C.
Appellate Court of Illinois
386 Ill.App.3d 141, 325 Ill. Dec. 298, 897 N.E.2d 837 (2008)

FROSSARD, J.

This case appears before us on interlocutory appeal pursuant to Supreme Court Rule 308 (155 Ill.2d R. 308) to consider the question certified by the circuit court. In 2000, plaintiffs Alison Miller and Todd Parrish underwent attempted *in vitro* fertilization (IVF) at defendant American Infertility Group of Illinois, S.C., d/b/a The Center for Human Reproduction Illinois (Center). The defendant Center, however, did not cryopreserve the resulting blastocyst for future use . . .

In 2003, plaintiffs and Todd Parrish as special administrator of the estate of Baby

Miller–Parrish filed a three-count amended complaint that set forth negligence, battery and breach of contract causes of action. Each count sought recovery of damages under the Wrongful Death Act (740 ILCS 180/0.01 *et seq.* (West 2002)). Specifically, the complaint alleged that: an IVF performed on January 7, 2000, resulted in nine viable embryos, one of which developed into a healthy blastocyst that was to be cryopreserved for future implantation; on or about January 13, 2000, defendant failed to properly cryopreserve the blastocyst; and plaintiffs were not informed of the failed cryopreservation until June 21, 2000, when they contacted defendant to have their blastocyst transferred to another center.

Defendant filed a motion to dismiss pursuant to section 2–615 of the Illinois Code of Civil Procedure (735 ILCS 5/2–615 (West 2002)), arguing that the Wrongful Death Act did not create a cause of action for the loss of a blastocyst created by IVF and not yet implanted within the IVF patient's uterus. Specifically, defendant argued that section 2.2 of the Wrongful Death Act applied only to the loss of a fetus, *i.e.*, an intrauterine pregnancy.

Section 2.2 of the Wrongful Death Act provides, in pertinent part:

> "The state of gestation or development of a human being when an injury is caused, when an injury takes effect, or at death, shall not foreclose maintenance of any cause of action under the law of this State arising from the death of a human being caused by wrongful act, neglect or default." 740 ILCS 180/2.2 (West 2006).

Initially, the circuit court granted defendant's motion and dismissed plaintiffs' wrongful death claims. Ultimately, however, the circuit court granted plaintiffs' second motion to reconsider and reinstated their wrongful death claims, holding that a "pre-embryo is a 'human being' within the meaning of Sec. 2.2 of the Wrongful Death Act and that a claim lies for its wrongful destruction whether or not it is implanted in its mother's womb." . . . The circuit court denied defendant's motion to reconsider that ruling, but certified the following question for review on interlocutory appeal:

> "Does Section 2.2 of the Illinois Wrongful Death Act (740 ILCS 180/2.2) allow a cause of action or recovery under the Act for loss of an embryo created by *in vitro* fertilization that has not been implanted into the mother?"

For the reasons that follow, we answer the certified question in the negative.

ANALYSIS

. . . The Wrongful Death Act provides for recovery for the death of a person by a wrongful act. 740 ILCS 180/1 (West 2006). As a requirement for a wrongful death action, the decedent must have had the potential, at the time of death, to maintain an action for personal injury against the defendant . . .

The parties dispute the meaning of the phrase "state of gestation or development of a human being," and the term *human being* is not defined in the Wrongful Death Act. We cannot discern the drafters' intent from the plain language of the statute alone. Consequently, we will go outside the language of section 2.2 and examine its legislative history . . .

[T]he questions or concerns raised by other legislators during the debates [on the bill that became the current law] concerned *in utero* pregnancies . . . There was no mention of *in vitro* fertilization during the legislative debates . . . The purpose of section 2.2 was simply to eliminate the distinction between a viable and a nonviable fetus.

Because the Wrongful Death Act is in derogation of common law, the court cannot extend the reach of the statute to embrace situations not within the intent of the legislature. The Wrongful Death Act has never been interpreted to apply to situations involving the *in vitro* fertilization process and cryopreservation of blastocysts or pre-embryos. Such a cause of action could only come about through legislative action, not judicial pronouncement.

Thus, it is clear that the legislature's intent in enacting section 2.2 of the Wrongful Death Act was to extend the cause of action to pregnancies in the mother's body regardless of whether the fetus was viable or nonviable. Therefore, we answer *no* to the certified question that asked whether section 2.2 of the Wrongful Death Act allowed a cause of action or recovery under the Act for loss of an embryo created by *in vitro* fertilization that has not been implanted into the mother . . .

Plaintiffs also argue that the legislature's use of the term *development* in the phrase "the state of gestation or development of a human being" of section 2.2 of the Wrongful Death Act demonstrates the legislature's intent to extend wrongful death actions to whatever beings might develop outside the purview of gestation, and necessarily includes beings created by *in vitro* fertilization. Plaintiffs note that when the legislature deleted the terms *dependency, capacity* and *disability* from the original bill, it kept the terms *gestation* and *development.* Citing the rules of statutory construction, plaintiffs argue that *development* must not be interpreted in a manner that renders it superfluous.

Plaintiffs' argument is not persuasive. Senator Rhoads clarified that the proposed legislation "only talked . . . about a state of gestation and not other stages of development." 81st Ill. Gen. Assem., Senate Proceedings, May 9, 1979, at 57 (statements of Senator Rhoads). Moreover, the statutory terms *gestation* and *development* are not redundant. The legislative debates established that the intent of the bill was confined to permit a cause of action under the Wrongful Death Act for the nonviable fetus still in a state of gestation where the pre-existing law already addressed situations involving the viable fetus still in a state of gestation and the born-alive infant at any stage of development. *Gestation* refers to the *in utero* fetus, whereas *development* refers to the live-born fetus or infant.

CONCLUSION

For the foregoing reasons, we answer the certified question in the negative. Section 2.2 of the Wrongful Death Act does not allow a cause of action or recovery under the Act for the loss of an embryo created by *in vitro* fertilization that has not been implanted into the mother. We remand the cause to the circuit court.

FITZGERALD SMITH, P.J. and TULLY, J, concur.

NOTES AND QUESTIONS

1. *Tort and Compensation Rules.* In *Frisina*, the plaintiffs pursue tort claims against the IVF Clinic for the alleged "loss and destruction of their embryos." By denying the IVF Clinic's motion for summary judgment on the claims of emotional distress based on loss of the embryos, the court allows the plaintiffs to proceed to trial to prove up this theory of recovery. If the plaintiffs' succeed in proving emotional distress based on the loss of their irreplaceable property, how should the damages be measured?

Damages awarded to compensate for loss or destruction of property are typically based on market value — what a willing buyer would pay a willing seller for the goods. In this case, as one scholar opined, "[f]ixing a market value for eggs or embryos is difficult as well as unsettling." Judith D. Fischer, *Misappropriation of Human Eggs and Embryos and the Tort of Conversion*, 32 LOY. L.A. L. REV. 384, 419 (1999). Do you agree? If pressed, how would you determine the market value of a human embryo?

Professor John Robertson suggests the parties negotiate the market value of the embryos in advance, noting that:

> [S]ome remedy for negligent destruction or disposition of embryos seems justified. Legal concepts of tort and property may have to evolve to take care of this situation. A practical solution would be to have the couple and the program or storage bank set liquidated damages for negligent loss of embryos in the initial storage contract. A sum based on the cost of creating the embryo plus a percentage for emotional damages might be a reasonable basis for most losses, and should be no more offensive than similar provisions in accident or life insurance policies.

John A. Robertson, *Ethical and Legal Issues in Cryopreservation of Human Embryos*, 47 FERTILITY & STERILITY 371, 379-80 (1987). The notion of a preconception agreement that is negotiated between the intended parents and the fertility clinic seems a good idea in theory. Does the excerpted deposition testimony from one of the plaintiffs in *Frisina* give you pause as to the effect a prior agreement would have in practice?

2. *Wrongful Death and Embryo Personhood.* The plaintiffs in *Miller* elevate their tort claims against the medical facility by alleging wrongful death — an action typically used to compensate family members whose loved one dies at the negligent hand of another — rather than framing their loss in traditional destruction of property or emotional distress causes of action. The court in *Miller* joins at least one other appellate court in dismissing a wrongful death claim against a fertility clinic charged with embryo loss. In *Jeter v. Mayo Clinic Arizona*, 211 Ariz. 386, 121 P.3d 1256, 467 Ariz. Adv. Rep. 5 (2005), the court dismissed the claim finding that three-day-old fertilized human eggs are not "persons" for purposes of the state's wrongful death statute.

In recent years, several states have considered adopting so-called personhood laws, either by legislative enactment or popular vote in those jurisdictions with mechanisms for direct democracy (voting on propositions). A typical example is Virginia House Bill No. 1, introduced in early 2012. If enacted, the law would establish that "the life of each human being begins at conception" and would grant to "unborn children" all rights, privileges and immunities available to other persons in the Commonwealth of Virginia. If Virginia, or any other state, passed a personhood law, what impact, if any, would such a law have on the practice of reproductive medicine? Would plaintiffs in embryo destruction cases be guaranteed recovery if they were able to prove breach of a duty of care toward their frozen embryos? Would embryo cryopreservation even be an option for IVF patients in personhood states?

3. *Intentional Destruction of Embryos.* Should damages for loss or destruction of embryos be greater if the defendant's conduct is intentional, rather than negligent? In *Del Zio v. Columbia Presbyterian Hospital*, 1978 U.S. Dist. LEXIS 14450, a supervising physician at a New York hospital learned that a colleague had succeeded in creating a "test tube embryo" for the plaintiffs, a novel and groundbreaking accomplishment in 1973. The physician objected to the procedure and intentionally removed the test tube and its contents from the incubator, believing that the "experiment should be stopped." The embryo was destroyed, causing the Del Zios substantial mental and emotional suffering. A jury awarded Mrs. Del Zio $50,000 for intentional infliction of emotional distress. In an ironic twist, the Del Zio trial was held in the summer of 1978, coinciding with the July 21 birth of Louise Brown, the world' first "test tube baby." Recall that Louise Brown and the doctors who assisted her conception through in vitro fertilization, were located in England. Perhaps the events in *Del Zio* offer some insight into why the perfection of IVF took place across the Atlantic.

Today, if a physician intentionally destroys an embryo without the permission of the gamete providers, can he or she be held criminally liable? See Cal. Penal Code 367g.

4. *Longevity of Frozen Embryos.* Cryopreservation techniques continue to improve, pushing the time between conception and gestation further into the future. To date, the longest successful embryo cryopreservation period is 20 years, accomplished in 2010 when a New York couple welcomed a baby boy conceived and frozen in 1990. The embryo was originally created by another couple undergoing IVF, and then later donated to the New York couple for their reproductive use. *See* Mara Hvistendahl, *Baby Born From 20-year Old Frozen Embryo*, (Oct. 11, 2010), available at: http://www.popsci.com/science/article/2010-10/baby-born-20-year-old-frozen-embryo.

A lot can happen in 20 years. In the case of couples who undergo IVF and cryopreservation, one of the most common events that changes the embryos' destiny is the couple's divorce. When a couple divorces, they no longer have a shared intent to conceive and rear a child together. Thus, the fate of frozen embryos becomes a major issue in the dissolution of the couple's marriage. The cases the follow track the development of the jurisprudence surrounding frozen embryo disputes.

SECTION II: THE LEGAL LANDSCAPE SURROUNDING FROZEN EMBRYO DISPUTES

A. An Introductory Case

DAVIS v. DAVIS
Supreme Court of Tennessee
842 S.W.2d 588 (1992)

[We have met Junior and Mary Sue Davis on two previous occasions, once in Chapter 1 when we studied the legal status of the human embryo, and again in Chapter 2 when we explored the right of procreational autonomy. Recall that the Davis' underwent seven cycles of IVF, all having failed to produce a child. Their final attempt yielded seven embryos that were frozen for later use. Shortly after the embryos were frozen the couple filed for divorce. The issue that dominated the couple's divorce action was the disputed custody of the frozen embryos. Junior preferred to see the embryos discarded, while Mary Sue wanted to donate them to another childless couple. At the time the embryos were frozen, the Davis' did not indicate what was to happen to the embryos in the event of divorce. They provided no written or oral instructions to the fertility clinic, thus the matter landed in the court system.

In the portion of the *Davis* opinion reprinted in Chapter 1, the Tennessee Supreme Court evaluated the biologic, legal and moral status of the 3-day-old embryos, concluding that they "are not, strictly speaking, either "persons" or "property," but occupy an interim category that entitles them to special respect because of their potential for human life." The Chapter 2 *Davis* excerpt details the court's view of ART as a form of reproduction due the same constitutional protections afforded natural conception. The court acknowledges that ART "centers on the two aspects of procreational autonomy — the right to procreate and the right to avoid procreation." With these rights seen as equally compelling, the court next tackles the resolution of the dispute between Junior and Mary Sue. The court's inquiry begins with an assessment of contracts that gamete providers could enter into prior to freezing their resulting embryos. Even though the Davis' did not enter into such an agreement, the court recognized its role in making a decision for future scenarios.]

DAUGHTREY, J.

V. *The Enforceability of Contract*

Establishing the locus of the decision-making authority in this context is crucial to deciding whether the parties could have made a valid contingency agreement prior to undergoing the IVF procedures and whether such an agreement would now be enforceable on the question of disposition. Under the trial court's analysis, obviously, an agreement of this kind would be unenforceable in the event of a later disagreement, because the trial court would have to make an ad hoc "best interest of the child" determination in every case. In its opinion, the Court of Appeals did not address the question of the enforceability of prior agreements, undoubtedly because that issue was not directly raised on appeal. Despite our reluctance to treat a question not strictly necessary to the result in the case, we conclude that discussion is warranted in order to provide the necessary guidance to all those involved with IVF procedures in Tennessee in the future — the health care professionals who administer IVF programs and the scientists who engage in infertility research, as well as prospective parents seeking to achieve pregnancy by means of IVF, their physicians, and their counselors.

We believe, as a starting point, that an agreement regarding disposition of any untransferred preembryos in the event of contingencies (such as the death of one or more of the parties, divorce, financial reversals, or abandonment of the program) should be presumed valid and should be enforced as between the progenitors. This conclusion is in keeping with the proposition that the progenitors, having provided the gametic material giving rise to the preembryos, retain decision-making authority as to their disposition.[4]

At the same time, we recognize that life is not static, and that human emotions run particularly high when a married couple is attempting to overcome infertility problems. It follows that the parties' initial "informed consent" to IVF procedures will often not be truly informed because of the near impossibility of anticipating, emotionally and psychologically, all the turns that events may take as the IVF process unfolds. Providing that the initial agreements may later be modified *by agreement* will, we think, protect the parties against some of the risks they face in this regard. But, in the absence of such agreed modification, we conclude that their prior agreements should be considered binding.

It might be argued in this case that the parties had an implied contract to reproduce using *in vitro* fertilization, that Mary Sue Davis relied on that agreement in undergoing IVF procedures, and that the court should enforce an implied contract against Junior Davis, allowing Mary Sue to dispose of the preembryos in a manner calculated to result in reproduction. The problem with such an analysis is that there is no indication in the record that disposition in the event of contingencies other than Mary Sue Davis's pregnancy was ever considered by the parties, or that Junior Davis intended to pursue reproduction outside the confines of a continuing marital relationship with Mary Sue. We therefore decline to decide this case on the basis of implied contract or the reliance doctrine.[5]

We are therefore left with this situation: there was initially no agreement between the parties concerning disposition of the preembryos under the circumstances of this case; there has been no agreement since; and there is no formula in

---

[4] [n.20] This situation is thus distinguishable from that in which a couple makes an agreement concerning abortion in the event of a future pregnancy. Such agreements are unenforceable because of the woman's right to privacy and autonomy. *See Planned Parenthood v. Danforth*, 428 U.S. 52, 96 S.Ct. 2831, 49 L.Ed.2d 788 (1976) (invalidating written consent of spouse as a pre-requisite to abortion).

[5] [n.21] We also point out that if the roles were reversed in this case, it is highly unlikely that Junior Davis could force transfer of the preembryos to Mary Sue over her objection. Because she has an absolute right to seek termination of any resulting pregnancy, at least within the first trimester, ordering her to undergo a uterine transfer would be a futility. Ordering donation over objection would raise the other constitutional problems discussed in Section VI [reprinted in Chapter 2].

the Court of Appeals opinion for determining the outcome if the parties cannot reach an agreement in the future . . .

VII. *Balancing the Parties' Interests*

Resolving disputes over conflicting interests of constitutional import is a task familiar to the courts. One way of resolving these disputes is to consider the positions of the parties, the significance of their interests, and the relative burdens that will be imposed by differing resolutions . . . In this case, the issue centers on the two aspects of procreational autonomy — the right to procreate and the right to avoid procreation. We start by considering the burdens imposed on the parties by solutions that would have the effect of disallowing the exercise of individual procreational autonomy with respect to these particular preembryos.

Beginning with the burden imposed on Junior Davis, we note that the consequences are obvious. Any disposition which results in the gestation of the preembryos would impose unwanted parenthood on him, with all of its possible financial and psychological consequences. The impact that this unwanted parenthood would have on Junior Davis can only be understood by considering his particular circumstances, as revealed in the record.

Junior Davis testified that he was the fifth youngest of six children. When he was five years old, his parents divorced, his mother had a nervous break-down, and he and three of his brothers went to live at a home for boys run by the Lutheran Church. Another brother was taken in by an aunt, and his sister stayed with their mother. From that day forward, he had monthly visits with his mother but saw his father only three more times before he died in 1976. Junior Davis testified that, as a boy, he had severe problems caused by separation from his parents. He said that it was especially hard to leave his mother after each monthly visit. He clearly feels that he has suffered because of his lack of opportunity to establish a relationship with his parents and particularly because of the absence of his father.

In light of his boyhood experiences, Junior Davis is vehemently opposed to fathering a child that would not live with both parents. Regardless of whether he or Mary Sue had custody, he feels that the child's bond with the non-custodial parent would not be satisfactory. He testified very clearly that his concern was for the psychological obstacles a child in such a situation would face, as well as the burdens it would impose on him. Likewise, he is opposed to donation because the recipient couple might divorce, leaving the child (which he definitely would consider his own) in a single-parent setting.

Balanced against Junior Davis's interest in avoiding parenthood is Mary Sue Davis's interest in donating the preembryos to another couple for implantation. Refusal to permit donation of the preembryos would impose on her the burden of knowing that the lengthy IVF procedures she underwent were futile, and that the preembryos to which she contributed genetic material would never become children. While this is not an insubstantial emotional burden, we can only conclude that Mary Sue Davis's interest in donation is not as significant as the interest Junior Davis has in avoiding parenthood. If she were allowed to donate these preembryos, he would face a lifetime of either wondering about his parental status or knowing about his parental status but having no control over it. He testified quite clearly that if these preembryos were brought to term he would fight for custody of his child or children. Donation, if a child came of it, would rob him twice — his procreational autonomy would be defeated and his relationship with his offspring would be prohibited.

The case would be closer if Mary Sue Davis were seeking to use the preembryos herself, but only if she could not achieve parenthood by any other reasonable means. We recognize the trauma that Mary Sue has already experienced and the additional discomfort to which she would be subjected if she opts to attempt IVF again. Still, she would have a reasonable opportunity, through IVF, to try once again to achieve parenthood in all its aspects — genetic, gestational, bearing, and rearing.

Further, we note that if Mary Sue Davis were unable to undergo another round of IVF, or opted not to try, she could still achieve the child-rearing aspects of parenthood through adoption. The fact that she and Junior Davis pursued adoption indicates that, at least at one time, she was willing to forego genetic parenthood and would have been satisfied by the child-rearing aspects of parenthood alone.

VIII. *Conclusion*

In summary, we hold that disputes involving the disposition of preembryos produced by *in vitro* fertilization should be resolved, first, by looking to the preferences of the progenitors. If their wishes cannot be ascertained, or if there is dispute, then their prior agreement concerning disposition should be carried out. If no prior agreement exists, then the relative interests of the parties in using or not using the preembryos must be weighed. Ordinarily, the party wishing to avoid procreation should prevail, assuming that the other party has a reasonable possibility of achieving parenthood by means other than use of the preembryos in question. If no other reasonable alternatives exist, then the argument in favor of using the preembryos to achieve pregnancy should be considered. However, if the party seeking control of the preembryos intends merely to donate them to another couple, the objecting party obviously has the greater interest and should prevail.

But the rule does not contemplate the creation of an automatic veto, and in affirming the judgment of the Court of Appeals, we would not wish to be interpreted as so holding. For the reasons set out above, the judgment of the Court of Appeals is affirmed, in the appellee's favor. This ruling means that the Knoxville Fertility Clinic is free to follow its normal procedure in dealing with unused preembryos, as long as that procedure is not in conflict with this opinion. Costs on appeal will be taxed to the appellant.

REID, C.J., and DROWOTA, O'BRIEN and ANDERSON, JJ., concur.

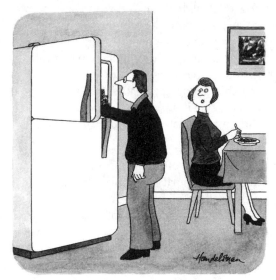

"Don't knock over the frozen embryos."

NOTES AND QUESTIONS

1.   For all practical purposes, the dispute between Junior and Mary Sue Davis came to an end on June 10, 1993 when Junior Davis picked up the frozen embryos at the Tennessee fertility clinic, took them home and disposed of them. See **Mark Curriden, *Embryos End: Biological "Dad" Gets "Custody"*, 79 A.B.A.J. 42 (1993).** When questioned about the method of disposal, Mr. Davis would not say what he did with the embryos, but added, "I don't think I have done anything wrong with the way I disposed of them."

2.   *The Davis Legacy.* The three-part test for resolving frozen embryo disputes set out by the Tennessee Supreme Court has shaped the decision of virtually every subsequent court to consider similar dissolution controversies. Though not necessarily adopted verbatim by each court, the *Davis* test has figured prominently in every case involving the disposition of frozen embryos upon divorce. In your mind, which test presents the most logical and fair approach to resolving the disposition of disputed embryos: 1) the preferences of the progenitors, 2) prior agreements concerning disposition, and 3) balancing the parties' interests, favoring procreation avoidance when the other party has a reasonable means of achieving parenthood by other means? A brief look at each prong may aid in your analysis.

a. The Preference of the Progenitors. Searching for accord in the preferences of the progenitors is often a futile exercise — if the progenitors agreed about the disposition of their embryos, they wouldn't be in court in the first place. But clearly the *Davis* court had scenarios in mind in which the preferences of the progenitors could be used to resolve a dispute over embryo disposition. Can you imagine such a scenario? (*Hint:* The litigants would not be the progenitors themselves.)

Another aspect of the first *Davis* prong worth pondering is the scope of the term "progenitor." According to the Merriam-Webster Dictionary, a "progenitor" is "a direct ancestor: forefather; originator, precursor." The term implies a direct genetic link, meaning a progenitor is one who supplies the gamete (sperm or egg) for the embryo. Does this mean that, under *Davis*, if a couple employs a gamete donor, the spouse who is not genetically related to the embryo will not be considered a progenitor? If so, does this prong give the spouse who *did* contribute a gamete exclusive right to control disposition, as he or she would be the only "progenitor" whose preference could be manifested? Do you think the *Davis* test contemplates such an outcome?

b. Prior Agreements. As a case of first impression, *Davis* was carefully watched by fertility clinics, the vast majority of which instituted some type of written agreement regarding disposition of frozen embryos to be signed by the intended parents. Yet, as we shall see, the existence of a preconception contract does not always keep the parties out of court, nor does a written agreement always serve to settle the couple's dispute by its clear and unambiguous language. An embryo disposition contract, even if presumed valid (as the *Davis* court suggested), will still be subject to attacks common to all contract disputes. Objections to enforcement could stem, for example, from the capacity of the parties to enter into an agreement, the clarity of the terms, or the public policy of enforcing the contract terms.

One possible method of enhancing the enforceability of a preconception agreement would be to seek judicial approval of the contract before the embryos are formed. Pre-fertilization judicial approval has been suggested by two law professors who urge that such approval can serve two purposes: 1) to evaluate the integrity of the contract itself, including the intent of the parties to enter into an agreement, the precise meaning of the contract terms, and the contingencies not provided for by the precise contract terms; and 2) to determine whether the jurisdiction will be willing to enforce such a contract if properly executed. Infirmities in the contract can be repaired before any dispute arises, often at a time when couples are still unified in their desires regarding parenthood. See Howard Fink & June Carbone, *Between Private Ordering and Public Fiat: A New Paradigm for Family Law Decision-Making*, 5 J.L. & FAM. STUD. 1, 67-69 (2003).

Another approach to shore up the validity of embryo disposition agreements would be to treat them the same as written instruments disposing of a person's property at death, i.e., wills. A preconception contract could be deemed valid only if it was in writing, signed by the intended parents, and signed by two competent witnesses — all requirements that mirror the elements of a valid will. Compare the purposes of a will with those of an embryo disposition agreement. Do the ritual and evidentiary functions that serve the testamentary instrument fulfill the same goals of a preconception agreement?

c. Balancing Interests, Avoiding Forced Procreation. The third *Davis* prong urges courts to balance the interests of the parties, favoring the party wishing to avoid procreation "assuming that the other party has a reasonable possibility of achieving parenthood by means other than use of the preembryos in question." Leaving for later the issue of procreation avoidance as a legal and policy option, let's focus on the court's admonition that the party wishing to use the disputed embryos for procreation look instead to other options for "achieving parenthood." Though this provision is written in gender-neutral terms, in practical reality the opportunities for parenthood other than by existing embryos is typically far more difficult for women than for men.

As succinctly stated by one scholar, "For women, age is the enemy of fertility." Ellen Waldman, *The Parent Trap: Uncovering the Myth of "Coerced Parenthood" In Frozen Embryo Disputes*, 53 Am. U.L. Rev. 1021, 1054 (2004). Professor Waldman reviews the medical literature showing that as a woman ages, her chances of producing viable eggs and sustaining a pregnancy to term diminish to the point of near impossibility as she approaches 50. This fertility cool down is not similarly experienced by men, who can produce viable sperm well into their later years. Thus, for women who undergo fertility treatment, cryopreservation "serves as partial insurance . . . Secure in the knowledge that the embryos exist for future use, their owners need not take additional precautions such as freezing eggs or retrieving additional eggs for fertilization with anonymous donors." Id. at 1055.

The *Davis* court also seems to suggest that the party wishing to procreate could achieve parenthood by turning to adoption. Again, in reality, the difficulties, risks and costs in achieving parenthood through adoption are well-documented, especially for "non-traditional" parents such as older, single individuals. Id. at 1056-559; See generally W. Feigelman & A. Silverman, *Single Parent Adoption*, in The Handbook for Single Adoptive Parents (1997); Christine Adamec & William L. Pierce, The Encyclopedia of Adoption (1991); National Committee For Adoption, Adoption Factbook: United States Date, Issues, Regulations and Resources (1989).

Warts and all, *Davis* is foundational to the law surrounding frozen embryo disputes, an area of law that continues to expand, helped along by the increasing popularity of ART and cryopreservation, and the ironically stable statistic that roughly 50% of all marriages end in divorce. See Centers for Disease Control, National Marriage and Divorce Rate Trends (2000-2010), available at http://www.cdc.gov/nchs/nvss/marriage_divorce_tables.htm.

The *Davis* progeny, like one's own children, each possess unique characteristics that distinguish and endear them to all interested parties. The cases are grouped according to the principle that seemed to guide the result in each instance. As you read each case, see if you agree with the designation accorded the court's decision.

B. The Contract Approach

KASS v. KASS
Court of Appeals of New York
91 N.Y.2d 554, 673 N.Y.S.2d 350, 696 N.E.2d 174 (1998)

[The trial court opinion in this case is reprinted in Chapter 2.]

Kaye, C.J. Although *in vitro* fertilization (IVF) procedures are now more than two decades old and in wide use, this is the first such dispute to reach our Court. Specifically in issue is the disposition of five frozen, stored pre-embryos, or "pre-zygotes," created five years ago, during the parties' marriage, to assist them in having a child. Now divorced, appellant (Maureen Kass) wants the pre-zygotes implanted, claiming this is her only chance for genetic motherhood; respondent (Steven Kass) objects to the burdens of unwanted fatherhood, claiming that the parties agreed at the time they embarked on the effort that in the present circumstances the pre-zygotes would be donated to the IVF program for approved research purposes. Like the two-Justice plurality at the Appellate Division, we conclude that the parties' agreement providing for donation to the IVF program controls. The Appellate Division order should therefore be affirmed.

Facts

. . . Beginning in March 1990, appellant underwent the egg retrieval process five times and fertilized eggs were transferred to her nine times. She became pregnant twice — once in October 1991, ending in a miscarriage and again a few months later, when an ectopic pregnancy had to be surgically terminated.

Before the final procedure, for the first time involving cryopreservation, the couple on May 12, 1993 signed four consent forms provided by the hospital . . . [The first two forms provided informed consent for the IVF procedure, explaining the risks and benefits of the procedure, and notifying the parties it was necessary to make an informed decision regarding disposition of unused embryos.]

The "Additional Consent Form for Cryopreservation," a seven-page, single-spaced typewritten document, is also in two parts. The first, "INFORMED CONSENT FORM NO. 2: CRYOPRESERVATION OF HUMAN PRE-ZYGOTES," provides:

"III. *Disposition of Pre-Zygotes.*

"We understand that our frozen pre-zygotes will be stored for a maximum of 5 years. We have the principal responsibility to decide the disposition of our frozen pre-zygotes. Our frozen pre-zygotes will not be released from storage for any purpose without the written consent of *both* of us, consistent with the policies of the IVF Program and applicable law. In the event of divorce, we understand that legal ownership of any stored pre-zygotes must be determined in a property settlement and will be released as directed by order of a court of competent jurisdiction. Should we for any reason no longer wish to attempt to initiate a pregnancy, we understand that we may determine the disposition of our frozen pre-zygotes remaining in storage. . . .

"The possibility of our death or any other unforeseen circumstances that may result in neither of us being able to determine the disposition of any stored frozen pre-zygotes requires that we now indicate our wishes. THESE IMPORTANT DECISIONS MUST BE DISCUSSED WITH OUR IVF PHYSICIAN AND OUR WISHES MUST BE STATED (BEFORE EGG RETRIEVAL) ON THE AT-TACHED ADDENDUM NO. 2-1, STATEMENT OF DISPOSITION. THIS STATEMENT OF DISPOSITION MAY BE CHANGED ONLY BY OUR SIGN-ING ANOTHER STATEMENT OF DISPOSITION WHICH IS FILED WITH THE IVF PROGRAM" (emphasis in original).

The second part, titled "INFORMED CONSENT FORM NO. 2 — ADDENDUM

NO. 2-1: CRYOPRESERVATIONSTATEMENT OF DISPOSITION," states: "We understand that it is IVF Program Policy to obtain our informed consent to the number of pre-zygotes which are to be cryopreserved and to the disposition of excess cryopreserved pre-zygotes. *We are to indicate our choices by signing our initials where noted below.*

"1. We consent to cryopreservation of all pre-zygotes which are not transferred during this IVF cycle for possible use . . . by us in a future IVF cycle. . . .

"2. In the event that we no longer wish to initiate a pregnancy or are unable to make a decision regarding the disposition of our stored, frozen pre-zygotes, we now indicate our desire for the disposition of our pre-zygotes and direct the IVF program to (choose one): . . .

"(b) Our frozen pre-zygotes may be examined by the IVF Program for biological studies and be disposed of by the IVF Program for approved research investigation as determined by the IVF Program" (emphasis in original).

On May 20, 1993, doctors retrieved 16 eggs from appellant, resulting in nine pre-zygotes. Two days later, four were transferred to appellant's sister, who had volunteered to be a surrogate mother, and the remaining five were cryopreserved. The couple learned shortly thereafter that the results were negative and that appellant's sister was no longer willing to participate in the program. They then decided to dissolve their marriage. The total cost of their IVF efforts exceeded $75,000.

With divorce imminent, the parties themselves on June 7, 1993 — barely three weeks after signing the consents — drew up and signed an "uncontested divorce" agreement, typed by appellant, including the following:

"The disposition of the frozen 5 pre-zygotes at Mather Hospital is that they should be disposed of [in] the manner outlined in our consent form and that neither Maureen Kass[,] Steve Kass or anyone else will lay claim to custody of these pre-zygotes."

On June 28, 1993, appellant by letter informed the hospital and her IVF physician of her marital problems and expressed her opposition to destruction or release of the pre-zygotes.

One month later, appellant commenced the present matrimonial action, requesting sole custody of the pre-zygotes so that she could undergo another implantation procedure. Respondent opposed removal of the pre-zygotes and any further attempts by appellant to achieve pregnancy, and counterclaimed for specific performance of the parties' agreement to permit the IVF program to retain the pre-zygotes for research, as specified in ADDENDUM NO. 2-1. By stipulation dated December 17, 1993, the couple settled all issues in the matrimonial action except each party's claim with respect to the pre-zygotes, which was submitted to the court for determination. While this aspect of the case remained open, a divorce judgment was entered on May 16, 1994 . . .

Supreme Court granted appellant custody of the pre-zygotes and directed her to exercise her right to implant them within a medically reasonable time. The court reasoned that a female participant in the IVF procedure has exclusive decisional authority over the fertilized eggs created through that process, just as a pregnant woman has exclusive decisional authority over a nonviable fetus, and that appellant had not waived her right either in the May 12, 1993 consents or in the June 7, 1993 "uncontested divorce" agreement.

While a divided Appellate Division reversed that decision (235 AD2d 150), all five Justices unanimously agreed on two fundamental propositions. First, they concluded that a woman's right to privacy and bodily integrity are not implicated before implantation occurs. Second, the court unanimously recognized that when parties to an IVF procedure have themselves determined the disposition of any unused fertilized eggs, their agreement should control.

The panel split, however, on the question whether the agreement at issue was sufficiently clear to control disposition of the pre-zygotes. According to the two-Justice plurality, the agreement unambiguously indicated the parties' desire to donate the pre-zygotes for research purposes if the couple could not reach a joint decision regarding disposition. The concurring Justice agreed to reverse but found the consent fatally ambiguous . . .

We now affirm, agreeing with the plurality that the parties clearly expressed their intent that in the circumstances presented the pre-zygotes would be donated to the IVF program for research purposes.

Analysis

A. *The Legal Landscape Generally.* . . . In the past two decades, thousands of children have been born through IVF, the best known of several methods of assisted reproduction. Additionally, tens of thousands of frozen embryos annually are routinely stored in liquid nitrogen canisters, some having been in that state for more than 10 years with no instructions for their use or disposal . . . As science races ahead, it leaves in its trail mind-numbing ethical and legal questions . . .

In the case law, only *Davis v. Davis* (842 SW2d 588, 604 [Tenn 1992], *cert denied sub nom. Stowe v. Davis*, 507 US 911) attempts to lay out an analytical framework for disputes between a divorcing couple regarding the disposition of frozen embryos . . . Having declared that embryos are entitled to "special respect because of their potential for human life" (842 SW2d at 597, *supra,*) *Davis* recognized the procreative autonomy of both gamete providers, which includes an interest in avoiding genetic parenthood as well as an interest in becoming a genetic parent. In the absence of any prior written agreement between the parties — which should be presumed valid, and implemented — according to *Davis*, courts must in every case balance these competing interests, each deserving of judicial respect. In *Davis* itself, that balance weighed in favor of the husband's interest in avoiding genetic parenthood, which was deemed more significant than the wife's desire to donate the embryos to a childless couple . . .

Proliferating cases regarding the disposition of embryos, as well as other assisted reproduction issues, will unquestionably spark further progression of the law. What is plain, however, is the need for clear, consistent principles to guide parties in protecting their interests and resolving their disputes, and the need for particular care in fashioning such principles as issues are better defined and appreciated. Against that backdrop we turn to the present appeal.

B. *The Appeal Before Us.* Like the Appellate Division, we conclude that disposition of these pre-zygotes does not implicate a woman's right of privacy or bodily integrity in the area of reproductive choice; nor are the pre-zygotes recognized as "persons" for constitutional purposes (*see, Roe v. Wade*, 410 US 113, 162; *Byrn v. New York City Health & Hosps. Corp.*, 31 NY2d 194, 203, *appeal dismissed* 410 US 949). The relevant inquiry thus becomes who has dispositional authority over them. Because that question is answered in this case by the parties' agreement, for purposes of resolving the present appeal we have no cause to decide whether the pre-zygotes are entitled to "special respect" (*cf., Davis v. Davis*, 842 SW2d 588, 596-597, *supra; see also*, Ethics Comm of Am Fertility Socy, *Ethical Considerations of the New Reproductive Technologies*, 46 Fertility & Sterility 1S, 32S [Supp 1 1986]).

(1) Agreements between progenitors, or gamete donors, regarding disposition of their pre-zygotes should generally be presumed valid and binding, and enforced in any dispute between them . . . Indeed, parties should be encouraged in advance, before embarking on IVF and cryopreservation, to think through possible contingencies and carefully specify their wishes in writing. Explicit agreements avoid costly litigation in business transactions. They are all the more necessary and desirable in personal matters of reproductive choice, where the intangible costs of any litigation are simply incalculable. Advance directives, subject to mutual change of mind that must be jointly expressed, both minimize misunderstandings and maximize procreative liberty by reserving to the progenitors the authority to make what is in the first instance a quintessentially personal, private decision. Written agreements also provide the certainty needed for effective operation of IVF programs . . .

While the value of arriving at explicit agreements is apparent, we also recognize the extraordinary difficulty such an exercise presents. All agreements looking to the future to some extent deal with the unknown. Here, however, the uncertainties inherent in the IVF process itself are vastly complicated by cryopreservation, which extends the viability of pre-zygotes indefinitely and allows time for minds, and circumstances, to change. Divorce; death, disappearance or incapacity of one or both partners; aging; the birth of other children are but a sampling of obvious changes in individual circumstances that might take place over time.

These factors make it particularly important that courts seek to honor the parties' expressions of choice, made before disputes erupt, with the parties' over-all direction always uppermost in the analysis. Knowing that advance agreements will be enforced underscores the seriousness and integrity of the consent process. Advance agreements as to disposition would have little purpose if they were enforceable only in the event the parties continued to agree. To the extent possible, it should be the progenitors — not the State and not the courts — who by their prior directive make this deeply personal life choice.

Here, the parties prior to cryopreservation of the pre-zygotes signed consents indicating their dispositional intent. While these documents were technically provided by the IVF program, neither party disputes that they are an expression of their own intent regarding disposition of their pre-zygotes. Nor do the parties contest the legality of those agreements, or that they were freely and knowingly made. The central issue is whether the consents clearly express the parties' intent regarding disposition of the pre-zygotes in the present circumstances. Appellant claims the consents are fraught with ambiguity in this respect; respondent urges they plainly mandate transfer to the IVF program.

The subject of this dispute may be novel but the common-law principles governing contract interpretation are not. Whether an agreement is ambiguous is a question of law for the courts . . . Ambiguity is determined by looking within the four corners of the document, not to outside sources . . . And in deciding whether an agreement is ambiguous courts "should examine the entire contract and consider the relation of the parties and the circumstances under which it was executed. . . ." [citation omitted].

Applying those principles, we agree that the informed consents signed by the parties unequivocally manifest their mutual intention that in the present circumstances the pre-zygotes be donated for research to the IVF program.

The conclusion that emerges most strikingly from reviewing these consents as a whole is that appellant and respondent intended that disposition of the pre-zygotes was to be their joint decision. The consents manifest that what they above all did not want was a stranger taking that decision out of their hands. Even in unforeseen circumstances, even if they were unavailable, even if they were dead, the consents jointly specified the disposition that would be made. That sentiment explicitly appears again and again throughout the lengthy documents. Words of shared understanding — "we," "us" and "our" — permeate the pages. The overriding choice of these parties could not be plainer: *"We have the principal responsibility to decide the disposition of our frozen pre-zygotes. Our frozen pre-zygotes will not be released from storage for any purpose without the written consent of both of us, consistent with the policies of the IVF Program and applicable law"* (emphasis added).

That pervasive sentiment — both parties assuming "principal responsibility to decide the disposition of [their] frozen pre-zygotes" — is carried forward in ADDENDUM NO. 2-1:

"In the event that we . . . are unable to make a decision regarding disposition of our stored, frozen pre-zygotes, we now indicate our desire for the disposition of our pre-zygotes and direct the IVF Program to . . .

"Our frozen pre-zygotes may be examined by the IVF Program for biological studies and be disposed of by the IVF Program for approved research investigation as determined by the IVF Program."

Thus, only by joint decision of the parties would the pre-zygotes be used for implantation. And otherwise, by mutual consent they would be donated to the IVF program for research purposes.

The Appellate Division plurality identified, and correctly resolved, two claimed ambiguities in the consents. The first is the following sentence in INFORMED CONSENT NO. 2: "In the event of divorce, we understand that legal ownership of any stored pre-zygotes must be determined in a property settlement and will be released as directed by order of a court of competent jurisdiction." Appellant would instead read that sentence: "In the event of divorce, we understand that legal ownership of any stored pre-zygotes must be determined by a court of competent jurisdiction." That is not, however, what the sentence says. Appellant's construction ignores the direction that ownership of the pre-zygotes "must be determined in a property settlement" — words that also must be given meaning, words that connote the parties' anticipated agreement as to disposition. Indeed, appellant and respondent did actually reach a settlement stipulation, reserving only the issue of the pre-zygotes (the subject of their earlier consents).

Additionally, while extrinsic evidence cannot *create* an ambiguity in an agreement, the plurality properly looked to the "uncontested divorce" instrument, signed only weeks after the consents, to *resolve* any ambiguity in the cited sentence. Although that instrument never became operative, it reaffirmed the earlier understanding that neither party would alone lay claim to possession of the pre-zygotes.

Apart from construing the sentence in isolation, the plurality also read it in the context of the consents as a whole. Viewed in that light, we too conclude that the isolated sentence was not dispositional at all but rather was "clearly designed to insulate the hospital and the IVF program from liability in the event of a legal dispute over the pre-zygotes arising in the context of a divorce" (235 AD2d at 160). To construe the sentence as appellant suggests — surrendering all control over the pre-zygotes to the courts — is directly at odds with the intent of the parties plainly manifested throughout the consents that disposition be only by joint agreement . . .

As they embarked on the IVF program, appellant and respondent — "husband" and "wife," signing as such — clearly contemplated the fulfillment of a life dream of having a child during their marriage. The consents they signed provided for other contingencies, most especially that in the present circumstances the pre-zygotes would be donated to the IVF program for approved research purposes. These parties having clearly manifested their intention, the law will honor it.

Accordingly, the order of the Appellate Division should be affirmed, with costs.

JUDGES TITONE, BELLACOSA, SMITH, LEVINE, CIPARICK and WESLEY concur.

NOTES AND QUESTIONS

1. *The Contract Approach to Frozen Embryo Disputes.* The court in *Kass* is outspoken in its support for the presumptive validity and enforceability of preconception agreements — written documents signed by a couple undergoing infertility treatment in which the man's sperm and the woman's egg are combined to form embryos that are frozen for later use. The court's praise for such agreements references several perceived attributes — written agreements avoid costly litigation (present company presumably excluded), they minimize misunderstandings and maximize procreative liberty by authorizing the progenitors to make a personal decision about whether to reproduce in the future, and they provide certainty for the orderly administration of a fertility clinic. Were all, or any, of these benefits achieved in this case? If not, why not?

2. *Recent Support for the Contract Approach.* The number of appellate cases dealing with embryo disposition upon divorce has slowed considerably in recent years. Of the handful of reported cases, at least two favor the contract approach adopted in *Davis* and *Kass*. In *Roman v. Roman*, 193 S.W.3d 40 (Ct. App. Tex. 2006), the court upheld a preconception agreement calling for discard of the couple's embryos upon divorce, remarking "the public policy of this State would permit a husband and wife to enter voluntarily into an agreement, before implantation, that would provide for an embryo's disposition in the event of a contingency, such as divorce, death, or changed circumstances." In *In the Marriage of Dahl*, 222 Or. App. 572, 194 P.3d 834 (2008), the court praised the contract approach, upholding an agreement that it interpreted to give the wife decision-making authority over the couple's frozen embryos in the event the parties were unable to reach a mutual decision. The appellate court approved Mrs. Dahl's decision to discard the embryos over her ex-husband's objection that they "are life" and should be given the chance "to develop their full potential as human beings."

What do you think accounts for the slowdown in reported appellate decisions on embryo disposition? The answer does not lie in a slowdown in the use of ART, as noted in Chapter 1. Perhaps the spate of litigation in the 1990s encouraged more clinics and patients to carefully contemplate the use of embryo agreements? Maybe, but concerns about the value and enforceability of embryo agreements persist.

3. *Critiquing the Contract Approach.* The contract approach to preconception agreements has been criticized on three major grounds. First, commentators argue that a system of per se validation of contracts relating to the disposition of human embryos is flawed, citing several factors that make automatic enforcement problematic. Second, the *Kass* court has been criticized for its interpretation of the contract signed by Maureen and Steven Kass. If the court's interpretation of the Kass contract is flawed, the argument goes, the decision itself delegitimizes the very principle it purports to advance. Third, some argue the very fact that agreements are contested, and sometimes abrogated, proves their inherent unreliability. Basically, the argument is that the agreements aren't worth the paper they are written on when a dispute arises. Let's take a closer look at each of these critiques.

a. *Problems with the Per Se Validation of Contracts Approach.* The contract approach to resolving frozen embryo disputes is criticized as flawed for three main reasons: 1) the parties lack informed consent when they sign preconception agreements, 2) automatic enforcement does not permit a party's change of heart to prevail, even when the new position is reasonable and nonpunitive toward the objecting spouse, and 3) enforcing preconception agreements is against public policy which disfavors forced procreation. Again, each reason is briefly set out below.

1. *Informed Consent.* Contracts can be daunting, especially for those in the throes of the inherent, inevitable, and often overwhelming stress that fertility treatment engenders. Legal documents, by habit and perhaps even by necessity, are complex to the untrained eye, often to the point of tempting the brightest among us to "sign on the dotted line" without absorbing even the major themes contained therein. Preconception agreements for the disposition of frozen embryos, by all accounts, suffer the same intimidation factor that plagues other important agree-

ments, leading patients and their spouses to affix a signature without fully comprehending the contents of the document. This problem of informed assent is compounded by the fact that most embryo disposition agreements are drafted as part of the fertility clinic's overall "Informed Consent Forms." Recall in *Kass* that the couple signed four "consent forms" — two that provided informed consent for the IVF procedure, and two that dealt with the cryopreservation and disposition of embryos. Embedding disposition agreements into medical informed consent forms has been deemed unwise for several reasons:

> First, the forms used to secure informed consent rarely inspire the rich deliberative process that informed consent jurisprudence envisions. Patients are generally loathe to fully consider the risks involved in medical treatment. When the medical service sought is infertility treatment, careful attention to the content of the informed consent forms is even more unlikely. Text imported into these forms will likely be glossed over as patients erect cognitive barriers to the thoughtful consideration of undesirable outcomes.

> Second, even if patients were inclined to treat informed consent documents with more attention than they frequently do, dispositional agreements should not be imported into them because the agreements treat different subject matter. The considerations associated with determining what should be done with excess embryos are separate and unrelated to those associated with determining if a desired medical treatment is worth the danger it creates. The disjunction between the thrust of informed consent documents and dispositional agreements, when combined with the one-sided nature of these agreements, raise unconscionability concerns.

Ellen A. Waldman, *Disputing Over Embryos: Of Contract and Consents*, 32 ARIZ. ST. L. J. 897, 940 (2000). Professor Waldman suggests that patients receive separate documents pertaining to informed consent and disposition of frozen or unused embryos. Having a separate disposition agreement, she argues, would at least give couples an opportunity to focus exclusively on the anticipated future of disputed embryos without the backdrop of technical medical terminology.

Look back at the consent forms signed by Mr. and Mrs. Kass. Do these forms strike you as clear and understandable? Do you think the Kasses were aware that they signed at least two provisions pertaining to disposition of frozen embryos? Can you find the disposition provisions? Which does the court rule should prevail? Which do you think should prevail?

2. Change of Heart. Preconception embryo disposition agreements are signed at one point in time in order to direct the parties' conduct at a future point in time. By design, they lock in the position of the parties; absent mutual agreement to modify the original contract, preconception agreements are unfriendly to one party's change of heart about the disposition of embryos. For Professor Carl Coleman, the inability to change one's mind about reproduction is incompatible with the constitutional protections surrounding procreative choice. He argues "the widespread support for a contractual solution to questions surrounding the disposition of frozen embryos is misguided. Rather than promoting procreative liberty, requiring couples to make binding decisions about the future disposition of their frozen embryos undermines a central aspect of procreative freedom — the right to make contemporaneous decisions about how one's reproductive capacity will be used." Instead of enforcing preconception agreements, "the law should protect both partners' interest in making contemporaneous reproductive decisions by treating the right to control the disposition of one's frozen embryos as an inalienable right — one that cannot be relinquished irrevocably until a disposition decision actually is carried out. Carl H. Coleman, *Procreative Liberty and Contemporaneous Choice: An Inalienable Rights Approach to Frozen Embryo Disputes*, 84 MINN. L. REV. 55, 56-58 (1999).

Under Professor Coleman's calculus, preconception agreements could never be enforced when the parties disagree about disposition of embryos, because one party's change of heart is tantamount to an assertion of an inalienable (i.e., nonwaivable) right to control his or her procreative future. Decisions about disposition must be made in the present, for the present, rather than in the past, for the future. Cf. John A. Robertson, *Precommitment Strategies for Disposition of Frozen Embryos*, 50 EMORY L. J. 989, 1027 (2001) (arguing nonenforcement of preconception agreements will frustrate the reproductive freedom that parties gain by entering into agreements; reliance on knowingly and intelligently made contracts is essential for individuals to plan for the consequences of participating in IVF).

If courts were unwilling to enforce preconception agreements when one party has a change of heart regarding procreation, would this judicial action doom the drafting of all such agreements? Are there any situations in which a court would enforce a prior agreement, even when a party has a change of heart? Imagine, for example, a spouse who has a change of heart about paying the annual storage fee.

3. Procreation Avoidance. Enforcing prior embryo disposition agreements can have the effect of "forcing" one party to become a genetic parent against his or her wishes. If the *Kass* court had awarded Maureen the remaining embryos and she gave birth to a child, Steven would be the child's genetic father, with support obligations likely to follow. If Maureen did not force Steven to contribute sperm during the IVF process, why is she viewed as forcing parenthood on him at a later time? Why does public policy elevate a person's right to avoid procreation over an objecting party's right to engage in reproduction when frozen embryos are in dispute?

b. *Problems With the New York Court's Analysis.* In addition to concerns over the per se enforcement of preconception contracts, commentators have struggled with the reasoning and result advanced by the New York Court of Appeal in *Kass*. As one author argues, presumed validity does not guarantee presumed clarity:

> Contracts that are presumptively valid are not necessarily presumptively clear and unambiguous. In the event of a dispute between parties, even the most carefully drafted agreement may come under a judge's scrutiny. A judge will inevitably confront at least two different interpretations of the plain meaning of the document. Even if such a judge purportedly applies the plain meaning rule to the instrument, one judge's plain meaning is another's ambiguity. In other words, to hold that a contract must be enforced does not guarantee that the remedy will be

obvious or forthcoming from the document. The parties still must look to the judge's interpretation of the instrument should they choose to litigate the dispute.

This problem of contract interpretation arose in the case that initially adopted the presumed validity standard. In *Kass v. Kass*, Maureen and Steven Kass signed four consent forms prior to undergoing their final IVF attempt. At least two of the forms provided the Kasses with the opportunity to direct the disposition of any frozen embryos should the couple come to disagree about the future of their gametic material. In one form, entitled "Informed Consent Form No. 2: Cryopreservation of Human Pre-Zygotes," the couple signed off on the following language: "In the event of divorce, we understand that legal ownership of any stored pre-zygotes must be determined in a property settlement and will be released as directed by order of a court of competent jurisdiction." In an addendum to this informed consent form, the couple also signed their names to the following instructions:

In the event we no longer wish to initiate a pregnancy or are unable to make a decision regarding the disposition of our stored, frozen pre-zygotes, we now indicate our desire for the disposition of our pre-zygotes and direct the IVF program to (choose one): . . . (b) Our frozen pre-zygotes may be examined by the IVF Program for biological studies and be disposed of by the IVF Program for approved research investigation as determined by the IVF Program.

Thus, the Kasses' forms contained at least two directives in the event of a disagreement: one giving jurisdiction to a court, the other authorizing donation for research purposes. As might be expected in the litigation, Maureen Kass argued that the consent forms were "fraught with ambiguity," while Steven Kass urged that they "plainly mandate[d] transfer to the IVF program." After citing to a series of common law cases dealing with contract interpretation, a unanimous New York Court of Appeals declared that the consent forms "unequivocally manifest[ed]" the parties' mutual intention that the embryos be donated for research. The court reasoned that the consent forms, read as a whole, indicated a shared intent that any disposition be made as a joint decision of the parties and that no party alone could lay claim to the embryos. The court further discounted the form's language that specifically called for a court to resolve any dispute in the event of divorce. The court stated that such language was "clearly designed to insulate the hospital and the IVF program from liability in the event of a legal dispute over the pre-zygotes arising in the context of a divorce."

It is startling that all seven members of a highly respected state supreme court found no ambiguity in the forms signed by the Kasses. How could language addressing vague circumstances — "[we] are unable to make a decision regarding the disposition of our [embryos]" — have been deemed unequivocally superior to language addressing the specific circumstances that had transpired? On the day that the Kasses signed the consent forms, they expressly indicated that should they divorce, a court of competent jurisdiction would direct the disposition of their frozen embryos as part of a larger property settlement. Presumably, a court would have the opportunity to learn firsthand what the parties intended when they signed the four consent forms. Nowhere did the divorce scenario language mention hospital liability, nor were the Kasses pursuing a claim against the hospital. Moreover, in the end, the court's decision was contrary to the very rationale it advanced. Although the court spoke of its desire to allow joint decision making by the parties, it ultimately allowed Steven Kass to gain unilateral control over the embryos. Maureen Kass probably did not intend that her husband would be able to override her desire to implant the embryos; therefore, a finding that this was her clearly expressed intent seems highly suspect.

The lesson from *Kass* is that the doctrine of presumed enforceability still entails some degree of contract interpretation, which, by definition, gives courts tremendous leeway in designing embryo dispositions. If a court of competent jurisdiction in New York had heard the Kass embryo matter, it may very well have sided with Steven Kass and recommended donation. Presumably, such a court would decide the case after hearing all the evidence surrounding the signing of the consent forms, and, perhaps it would also balance the interests of the parties in light of their written words.

Judith F. Daar, *Assisted Reproductive Technologies and the Pregnancy Process: Developing An Equality Model to Protect Reproductive Liberties*, 25 Amer. J. Law & Med. 455, 470-71 (1999). Professor Daar suggests, in essence, that the decision in *Kass* was result-oriented, rather than process-oriented; the court wanted to reach a result (procreation avoidance) and did so by interpreting broad contract doctrine to support that desired result. Assuming arguendo that assertion is true, is it problematic?

c. *Problems with Legal Uncertainties Surrounding Agreements.* The fact that divorcing couples have litigated the meaning and validity of their prior agreements, and the varying responses that courts (and, as we shall see, legislatures) have provided has prompted commentators to question that value of these agreements to the parties and to the practice of reproductive medicine. If patients and ART practitioners rely on the enforceability of these agreements only to have them disregarded, misinterpreted or abrogated by a court, it is no surprise to see these ART stakeholders question the value of investing time and resources into these often lengthy complicated forms. Professor Deborah Forman suggests an abandonment approach:

> Standardized clinic consent forms signed prior to treatment present a particularly poor vehicle for ascertaining and expressing the parties' intentions either at that point in time or projecting into the future. Nor is the process surrounding use of the forms or their content likely to improve sufficiently to justify reliance on them. Physicians have neither the incentive nor the expertise to ensure embryo dispositions related to divorce have resulted from careful thought and accurately reflect the parties' preferences. Legal uncertainties and myriad variations in life circum-

stances would make drafting even a customized contract between the parties challenging. A standardized form simply cannot hope to accomplish the task, nor should it pretend to.

Consequently, to avoid the illusion of certainty and the potential for misplaced reliance, clinic consent forms should be drafted to make clear that disputes between the progenitors in the event of divorce or comparable change in relationship status will be decided by a court or other binding alternative dispute resolution process if the parties cannot reach agreement at that time. The forms can, and should, inform the parties that disputes have arisen in the context of divorce and invite them to seek legal counsel to answer any questions they may have. Statutes like California's that currently require health care providers to provide disposition forms should likewise be modified, if necessary, to eliminate any apparent requirement that the parties select a disposition choice in the event of relationship break down or divorce.

Deborah L. Forman, *Embryo Disposition and Divorce: Why Clinic Consent Forms Are Not the Answer*, 24 J. Am. Acad. Matrimonial Lawyers 57 (2011). Do you agree with Professor Forman that clinic consent forms as currently constituted should be abandoned and that parties should simply be warned that any dispute over embryos will be decided by a judicial process? Would such a bare reliance on third-party decision-makers (judges, mediators, arbitrators) invite or discourage divorcing couples to fight over their frozen embryos?

4. *Implied Contracts.* As every first year law student learns in Contracts, a valid contract can be express or implied. In *Kass* the contract was obviously express, and in *Davis* the contract was obviously absent. Or was it? Perhaps an implied contract was formed. The Restatement (Second) of Contracts § 2(1) (1979) provides that an implied contract is an enforceable contract and is found when a party makes "a manifestation of intention to act or refrain from acting in a specified way . . . [so as] to justify a promisee in understanding that a commitment has been made." Do a husband and wife who seek out fertility treatment and agree to procure and freeze embryos for later use manifest an intent to procreate? If so, would one spouse be justified in relying on the other's manifestation of intent to procreate in seeking control of disputed embryos? See Tanya Feliciano, *Davis v. Davis: What About Future Disputes?*, 26 Conn. L. Rev. 305 (1993) (arguing it is "easy" to find an implied contract between two parties who attempt IVF: participation in IVF program is conduct that reasonably leads to the assumption that both parties have committed to reproduction). The court in *Davis v. Davis* considered and summarily dismissed the argument that the parties entered an implied contract to reproduce, citing an absence of evidence that the parties ever considered a contingency other than Mrs. Davis' pregnancy within the confines of marriage. Does this reasoning in *Davis* rule out the possibility for a successful claim based on implied contract by a party wishing to use frozen embryos to procreate against the wishes of a former spouse or partner?

LITOWITZ v. LITOWITZ
Supreme Court of Washington
146 Wash. 2d 514, 48 P.3d 261 (2002)

[This case is also reprinted, in part, and discussed in Chapter 3.]

SMITH, J. Petitioner Becky M. Litowitz seeks review of a decision of the Court of Appeals, Division Two, which affirmed an order of the Thurston County Superior Court in favor of Respondent David J. Litowitz in a dissolution action in which Respondent was awarded two cryopreserved preembryos. The Court of Appeals affirmed the trial court and awarded the preembryos to Respondent. This court granted review. We reverse . . .

STATEMENT OF FACTS

On February 27, 1982 Petitioner Becky M. Litowitz and Respondent David J. Litowitz were married. Respondent adopted Petitioner's two children from a previous marriage. On July 15, 1980, prior to their marriage, Petitioner and Respondent had a child together, Jacob Litowitz. Shortly after Jacob was born Petitioner Litowitz had a hysterectomy leaving her unable to produce eggs or to naturally give birth to a child.

Petitioner and Respondent decided to have another child through *in vitro* fertilization. They sought the services of the Center for Surrogate Parenting, Loma Linda University Gynecology and Obstetrics Medical Group, in Loma Linda, California. Five preembryos were created with eggs received from an egg donor. The eggs were fertilized by Respondent Litowitz' sperm. Three of the five preembryos were implanted in a surrogate mother, producing a female child, M., who was born January 25, 1997. The two remaining preembryos were cryopreserved and stored in the clinic in Loma Linda, California.

Petitioner and Respondent entered into a contract in Beverly Hills, California with the egg donor. The contract was signed by Petitioner Becky M. Litowitz on March 20, 1996, by Respondent David J. Litowitz on March 21, 1996 and by the egg donor, J.Y., and her husband, E.Y., on April 1, 1996. The contract defined Petitioner as the "Intended Mother" and Respondent as the "Natural Father." The "Intended Mother" and "Natural Father" are further defined as the "Intended Parents." The egg donor contract provided in part:

PARAGRAPH 13

All eggs produced by the Egg Donor pursuant to this Agreement shall be deemed the property of the Intended Parents and as such, the Intended Parents shall have the sole right to determine the disposition of said egg(s). In no event may the Intended Parents allow any other party the use of said eggs without express *written* permission of the Egg Donor.

Respondent and Petitioner entered into two contracts with the Loma Linda Center for Fertility and In Vitro Fertilization in Loma Linda, California. One, a consent and authorization for preembryo cryopreservation (freezing) following *in vitro* fertilization, dated March 25, 1996, provided for freezing the preembryos. The other was an agreement and consent for cryogenic preservation (short term), dated March 25, 1996.

The consent and authorization for preembryo cryopreservation contract stated in part:

LEGAL STATUS AND DISPOSITIONAL CHOICES

. . . We agree that because both the husband and wife are participants in the cryopreservation program, that any decision regarding the disposition of our pre-embryos will be made by mutual consent. In the event we are unable to reach a mutual decision regarding the disposition of our pre-embryos, we must petition to a Court of competent jurisdiction for instructions concerning the appropriate disposition of our pre-embryos.

We are aware that for a variety of reason [sic], (e.g. our choice, death of both of us, our achieving our desired family size) one or more pre-embryos may remain frozen and will not be wanted or needed by us. *By this document, we wish to provide the Center with our mutual direction regarding disposition of our pre-embryos upon the occurrence of any one of the following four (4) events or dates:*

A. The death of the surviving spouse or in the event of our simultaneous death.

B. In the event we mutually withdraw our consent for participation in the cryopreservation program.

C. *Our pre-embryos have been maintained in cryopreservation for five (5) years after the initial date of cryopreservation unless the Center agrees, at our request, to extend our participation for an additional period of time.*

D. The Center ceases its *in vitro* fertilization and cryopreservation program.

At the earliest of the above-mentioned events or dates, we authorize and request that one of the following options be utilized for the disposition of our pre-embryos remaining in cryopreservation:

(1) That our pre-embryos be donated to another infertile couple (who shall remain unknown to all parties concerned), selected by the attending physician and/or the medical director of the Program, in which case we would relinquish any and all claim of maternal and/or paternal right to the donated pre-embryos;

(2) That our pre-embryos be donated for approved research and/or investigation;

(3) *That our pre-embryos be thawed but not allowed to undergo further development;*

> (4) That our pre-embryos be disposed of in accordance with the best judgement [sic] of the professional staff of the Center. [emphasis added]

Petitioner and Respondent indicated their "desire for the ultimate disposition of [their] pre-embryos" by writing in longhand in the space provided on the contract "# 3 — That our pre-embryos be thawed but not allowed to undergo further development." Following that statement and the signatures of the Litowitzes, the contract stated, "We agree that this option selection is binding upon us until such time as it is changed, in writing, by our joint direction."

Petitioner and Respondent separated before their daughter, M., was born.[6] In the dissolution proceedings in the Pierce County Superior Court, Respondent on October 21, 1998 indicated his wish to put the remaining preembryos up for adoption. In those proceedings Petitioner on October 26, 1998 indicated her wish to implant the remaining preembryos in a surrogate mother and bring them to term. On December 11, 1998 the trial court, the Honorable Waldo F. Stone, awarded the preembryos to Respondent David J. Litowitz based upon the "best interest of the child." The order signed by Judge Stone provided in part:

> DISPOSITION OF PREEMBRYOS: This court makes the following decision awarding the preembryos to father in the best interest of the child. If this child is brought into the world here in Tacoma or Federal Way, Washington the alternatives are not in the child's best interest. In the first alternative the child would be a child of a single parent. That is not in the best interest of a child that could have an opportunity to be brought up by two parents. In the second alternative, the child may have a life of turmoil as the child of divorced parents. Also, both parties here are old enough to be the grandparents of any child, and that is not an ideal circumstance. The court awards the preembryos to Father with orders to use his best efforts for adoption to a two-parent, husband and wife, family outside the State of Washington, considering the egg donor in that, as Father is required.[7]

On December 11, 1998, Judge Stone also issued an order staying the order on preembryos and the restraining order on Petitioner. The order prevented Petitioner from removing or in any way altering the status of the preembryos until final judgments including "any and all appeals" are entered in the action . . .

In affirming the trial court, the Court of Appeals concluded the contracts signed by Petitioner and Respondent in California did not require Respondent to continue with their family plan to have another child and that Respondent's right not to procreate compelled the court to award the preembryos to him.

On November 16, 2000 Petitioner Becky M. Litowitz sought review by this court which was granted on April 12, 2001.

---

[6] The Litowitz divorce was likely not a friendly parting of the ways. In another part of the opinion, David asks the court to consider allowing him to submit additional evidence to the trial court relating to Becky's drug use and testimony regarding a report that his ex-wife paid a third party to have him killed. The Washington Supreme Court denied this request. - Ed.

[7] [n.28] . . . The characterization of frozen preembryos as "children" is of dubious legal or scientific correctness. However, it is of no consequence to our determination in this case.

DISCUSSION
CONTRACTUAL ISSUES

This is the first case in which this court has been asked to resolve a dispute over disposition of frozen preembryos in a dissolution action. There is limited case law in other jurisdictions involving disputes over disposition of frozen preembryos. We have identified cases addressing the issue from the highest courts of Tennessee, Massachusetts, New York and New Jersey . . .

[The court reviews the decisions in *Davis v. Davis*, 842 S.W.2d 588 (Tenn. 1992); *Kass v. Kass*, 91 N.Y.2d 554, 673 N.Y.S.2d 350, 696 N.E.2d 174 (1998); *A.Z. v. B.Z.*, 431 Mass. 150, 725 N.E.2d 1051 (2000); and *J.B. v. M.B.*, 170 N.J. 9, 783 A.2d 707 (2001). Each of these cases is reprinted and discussed in this Chapter. - Ed.]

This case involves a dispute over frozen preembryos between Petitioner, who is not a progenitor, and Respondent, who is a progenitor. In the four cases cited from Tennessee, Massachusetts, New York and New Jersey, one party to each dispute contributed the egg and the other party contributed the sperm. They were all progenitors. In this case Petitioner did not produce the eggs used to create the preembryos. She has no biological connection to the preembryos and is not a progenitor. Any right she may have to the preembryos must be based solely upon contract . . .

It is obvious that Petitioner and Respondent have not reached a mutual decision regarding disposition of the preembryos. Because they have not, it is appropriate for the courts to determine disposition of the preembryos under the cryopreservation contract . . .

The cryopreservation contract, signed March 25, 1996, provided for disposition of the Litowitzes' two remaining preembryos. They unequivocally chose the option "[t]hat [their] pre-embryos be thawed but not allowed to undergo further development." The contract provided that when the preembryos had been cryopreserved for five years after the initial date of cryopreservation, the "preembryos would be thawed but not allowed to undergo any further development" unless the Litowitzes requested participation for an additional period of time and the Center agreed. The record does not indicate the exact date the remaining preembryos were frozen. However, the cryopreservation contract was signed by the Litowitzes on March 25, 1996. More than five years have passed since that date. The probable date of implantation of the three preembryos actually used was April 20, 1996 [based on the date of birth of the couple's child, M, who resulted from the same IVF cycle that produced the disputes frozen embryos. - Ed.]. More than five years have passed since that date. Neither Petitioner nor Respondent claims extension of the contract beyond five years. Under the five-year termination provision of the cryopreservation contract, the Center is directed by the Litowitzes to thaw the preembryos and not allow them to develop any further. There is nothing in the record to indicate whether the two preembryos still exist . . .

The Court of Appeals correctly concluded the egg donor contract . . . did not prevent Respondent from donating the preembryos to another couple. The court indicated Respondent would not need written permission from the egg donor to donate the preembryos because the egg donor contract only required written permission for transfer of the donated eggs. The court correctly observed that the eggs no longer existed as they were identified in the egg donor contract because they were later fertilized by Respondent's sperm and their character was then changed to preembryos. The Court of Appeals did not rule on the rights of the egg donor under the egg donor contract because that matter has not been before the court at any stage of these proceedings. Even if it were, it is doubtful that the egg donor would have a remaining contractual right once the eggs have been fertilized and become preembryos.

Petitioner Becky M. Litowitz argues . . . she has a constitutional right to custody and companionship of a child . . . Petitioner has not cited sufficient authority to support her argument . . .

SUMMARY AND CONCLUSIONS

. . . We base our decision in this case solely upon the contractual rights of the parties under the preembryo cryopreservation contract with the Loma Linda Center for Fertility and In Vitro Fertilization dated March 25, 1996. Under that contract Petitioner and Respondent gave direction to the Loma Linda Center for disposition of the remaining preembryos resulting from fertilization of five eggs they acquired under the egg donor contract. They directed that the remaining preembryos be "thawed out but not allowed to undergo further development" and disposed of when the preembryos "have been maintained in cryopreservation for five (5) years after the initial date of cryopreservation unless the Center agree[d], at [the Litowitzes'] request, to extend [their] participation for an additional period of time." The record does not indicate whether the two cryopreserved preembryos are still in existence. Neither Petitioner nor Respondent has requested an extension of their contract with the Loma Linda Center. Under terms of the contract, then, the remaining preembryos would have been thawed out and not allowed to undergo further development five years after the initial date of cryopreservation, which by simplest calculation would have occurred on March 24, 2001 . . .

We reverse the decision of the Court of Appeals, Division Two.

ALEXANDER, C.J., JOHNSON, MADSEN (result only), SMITH, IRELAND, BRIDGE AND OW-ENS, JJ., concur.

CHAMBERS, J. (concurring and writing separately to suggest the matter be remanded so the trial court can consider the contract in light of equity and public policy).

SANDERS, J. (dissenting).

The majority contends the cryopreservation contract controls the disposition of the preembryos . . . But even if so, I posit that the contractual text does not support the majority's disposition, but rather the trial court's.

The contract states in pertinent part:

We agree that because both the husband and wife are participants in the cryopreservation program, that any decision regarding the disposition of our pre-embryos will be made by mutual consent. *In the event we are unable to reach a mutual decision regarding the disposition of our pre-embryos, we must petition to a Court of competent jurisdiction for instructions concerning the appropriate disposition of our pre-embryos.*

Pet'r's Ex. 410, at 3 (Cryopreservation Contract) (emphasis added). The contractual provision vested the trial court with exclusive discretion to determine an appropriate disposition of the preembryos upon request but absent the agreement of the parties.

I however posit this provision of the contract is applicable because the parties *were* unable to come to a mutual decision, and *did* petition a court for an appropriate disposition of their preembryos, strictly in accordance with this clause of the contract. In the reasonable exercise of its contractually vested discretion — and the majority does not claim that discretion was abused — the trial court adopted the "best interests of the child" criterion and awarded the preembryos to David Litowitz. Nevertheless, the majority bases its reversal on the mistaken conclusion that the next clause of the contract dictates a different result. That clause provides:

. . . By this document, we wish to provide the Center with our mutual direction regarding disposition of our pre-embryos *upon the occurrence of any one of the following four (4) events or dates:*

A. The death of the surviving spouse or in the event of our simultaneous death.

B. In the event we mutually withdraw our consent for participation in the cryopreservation program.

C. Our pre-embryos have been maintained in cryopreservation for five (5) years after the initial date of cryopreservation unless the Center agrees, at our request, to extend our participation for an additional period of time.

D. The Center ceases it's [sic] *in vitro* fertilization and cryopreservation program.

At the earliest of the above-mentioned events or dates, we authorize and request that one of the following options be utilized for the disposition of our pre-embryos remaining in cryopreservation:

. . .

(3) That our pre-embryos be thawed but not allowed to undergo further development [selected option].

Id. (emphasis added); majority at 268.

This provision is facially inapplicable because its stated contingencies concern either a *mutual* decision not to produce a child (B, C), the death of both parties (A), or impossibility (D), none of which is present here. Nevertheless, with the unerring precision of a moth to the flame, the majority seizes upon the third contingency, ignoring the mutuality of decision implicit in the phrase "at *our* request." *Id.*

(emphasis added).

Its errant reliance on, and misinterpretation of, this provision is further aggravated when the majority gives *no effect* to the previous relevant and operative provision. *See, e.g., McDonald v. State Farm Fire & Cas. Co.*, 119 Wash.2d 724, 734, 837 P.2d 1000 (1992) (courts should interpret the contract in a way that gives effect to each provision). Thus the majority defeats the plain meaning of the first paragraph by divesting the trial court of the authority contractually and exclusively vested in it to resolve disputes of this kind.

Even if one were to apply the second paragraph, carelessly setting aside the former operative provision and ignoring the mutual consent implicit in the third contingency, the contract *still* would not support the majority's outcome because the contractual time period was tolled by the timely commencement of this litigation as a matter of law . . .

This contract was signed and the cryopreservation began in the spring of 1996. The dissolution proceeding commenced only two years later and included a timely request that the court provide a timely disposition of the preembryos. The proceeding culminated in a dissolution order dated December 11, 1998. That by today more than five years has passed since the cryopreservation commenced is irrelevant because the judicial action which provided for the disposition of the preembryos was commenced well within the five-year window thereby tolling the contracted period of limitations . . .

This agreement stated exactly what the parties intended in the event they could not agree on the disposition of their preembryos: let the court decide. Provisions whereby parties agree to resort to resolution by courts or arbitrators in the event of disagreement are routinely enforced . . .

One thing the parties obviously did not intend was to destroy the whole object of the contract, the preembryos, simply because this litigation was prolonged beyond five years after the initial date of cryopreservation while the parties were patiently waiting for appropriate court "instructions concerning the appropriate disposition of [their] pre-embryos," *nor has either party even argued for that unimagined result.* But the majority's disposition apparently calls for the destruction of unborn human life even when, or if, both contracting parties agreed the preembryos should be brought to fruition as a living child reserving their disagreement over custody for judicial determination. Thus the majority denies these parties that option left by Solomon in lieu of chopping the baby in half. The wisdom of Solomon is nowhere to be found here.

The trial court's decision to strive for a result in the best interest of the potential child was certainly at least one reasonable way to effectuate the intent of the parties. There may have been others, but I cannot fault a trial court that recognized the fundamental purpose and objective of the contract and dealt with the prospect a child would be born, the future of which was of paramount concern and profound responsibility. Even if we were to disagree with the trial court, it was the trial court's discretion to exercise, not ours.

I would therefore affirm the trial court's resolution by ordering David Litowitz to donate the preembryos to a couple suitable to raise the child.

NOTES AND QUESTIONS

1. *Post Script.* The Litowitz battle did not end with the "required thaw" suggested by the court. Instead, "[a]fter the Washington decision, the embryos remained stored in a California facility, and the fight over them moved there. Now, under a legal agreement, the embryos are expected to be offered to another patient, whose identity won't be divulged. The result works for all sides, said Roland Bainer, attorney for Loma Linda University Gynecology and Obstetrics Medical Group, which stored the embryos. 'Becky . . . gets the satisfaction of knowing that the embryos have a chance to become human life,' he said. 'David Litowitz has that satisfaction, as well as the knowledge he won't be made a parent against his will. And, hopefully some patient out there gets the chance to have a child.' Had they been destroyed, Becky Litowitz would have been devastated. She said she spent $1 million on the fight. 'I did it because of my core belief that life begins at conception,' she said." Cathy Kightlinger, *Couples Fight Over Custody of Embryos*, INDIANAPOLIS STAR, July 11, 2004, at A1.

2. The Washington Supreme Court, much like the New York Court of Appeals in *Kass v. Kass*, scrutinizes the language of the lengthy contracts signed by the parties prior to undergoing IVF and embryo cryopreservation. The *Litowitz* court finds language supporting the destruction of the frozen embryos, over the objection of both spouses. As you read the facts of the case, do you believe Becky and David Litowitz intended for the Loma Linda IVF clinic to destroy their frozen embryos at the five-year mark? As you read the contract language, did you, as a trained legal expert, reach the conclusion that the IVF clinic was obligated to thaw the embryos if it had not received instructions directing otherwise from the couple?

3. *Legal Malpractice?* Does either Becky or David Litowitz have a malpractice claim against their respective attorneys for not alerting them to the five-year automatic thaw provision in the contract? The couple's divorce proceedings were heard in 1998, only two years after the embryos had been placed in frozen storage. Did their attorneys fail to exercise reasonable care by not alerting them of the need to notify the IVF clinic about continuing to store the frozen embryos? If so, what are the appropriate damages for such negligence?

4. *Rights of ART Siblings.* In an embryo dispute, the court takes into account the arguments of the intended parents, but tends to disregard the sentiments of all other parties. The Washington court made it clear that the egg donor had no place in the litigation, as any interest she had disappeared when the sperm penetrated the eggs and the embryos were formed. Other than the intended parents and the gamete donors, do any other parties have an interest in the outcome of these disputes? What about M, the Litowitz's daughter? Does she have any right to the companionship of her full sibling? For a discussion of the rights of sibling association in the context of the child dependency system (for example, when a parent's rights are terminated due to abuse or neglect), see William W. Patton & Sara Latz, *Severing Hansel from Gretel: An Analysis of Siblings' Association Rights*, 48 U. MIAMI L. REV. 745 (1994).

5. The existence of a preconception agreement in a frozen embryo dispute arguably facilitates resolution of the conflict, either by the IVF facility, the parties' attorneys, or a court. If expression of the parties' intent plays such an essential role

in resolving embryo disputes, should states require that every party to a cryo-preservation agreement execute a written expression of disposition intent? Florida is one state that has taken this legislative leap.

Florida Statutes Annotated
Title XLIII. Domestic Relations
Chapter 742. Determination of Parentage

§ 742.17. Disposition of eggs, sperm, or preembryos; rights of inheritance

A commissioning couple and the treating physician shall enter into a written agreement that provides for the disposition of the commissioning couple's eggs, sperm, and preembryos in the event of a divorce, the death of a spouse, or any other unforeseen circumstance.

(1) Absent a written agreement, any remaining eggs or sperm shall remain under the control of the party that provides the eggs or sperm.

(2) Absent a written agreement, decisionmaking authority regarding the disposition of preembryos shall reside jointly with the commissioning couple.

(3) Absent a written agreement, in the case of the death of one member of the commissioning couple, any eggs, sperm, or preembryos shall remain under the control of the surviving member of the commissioning couple.

If a law similar to the Florida statute had been in place in Tennessee when the Mary Sue and Junior Davis first began treatment for their infertility, would it have changed the outcome in that case? Does mandating that a couple sign a disposition agreement avoid litigation, or does it provide another basis on which the parties can disagree?

C.   The Public Policy Approach

A.Z. v. B.Z.
Supreme Judicial Court of Massachusetts
431 Mass. 150, 725 N.E.2d 1051 (2000)

COWIN, J. We transferred this case to this court on our own motion to consider for the first time the effect of a consent form between a married couple and an in vitro fertilization (IVF) clinic (clinic) concerning disposition of frozen preembryos. B.Z., the former wife (wife) of A.Z. (husband), appeals from a judgment of the Probate and Family Court that included, inter alia, a permanent injunction in favor of the husband, prohibiting the wife "from utilizing" the frozen preembryos held in cryopreservation at the clinic. The probate judge bifurcated the issue concerning the disposition of the frozen preembryos from the then-pending divorce action. The wife appeals only from the issuance of the permanent injunction. On February 8, 2000, we issued an order affirming the judgment of the Probate and Family Court. The order stated: "It is ordered that the permanent injunction entered on the docket on March 25, 1996 in Suffolk County Probate Court (Docket No. 95 D 1683 DV) be, and the same hereby is, affirmed. Opinion or opinions to follow." This opinion states the reasons for that order.

1. *Factual background* . . .

a. *History of the couple.* The husband and wife were married in 1977. For the first two years of their marriage they resided in Virginia, where they both served in the armed forces. While in Virginia, they encountered their first difficulties conceiving a child and underwent fertility testing. During their stay in Virginia the wife did become pregnant, but she suffered an ectopic pregnancy,[8] as a result of which she miscarried and her left fallopian tube was removed.

In 1980, the husband and wife moved to Maryland where they underwent additional fertility treatment. The treatment lasted one year and did not result in a pregnancy. In 1988, the wife was transferred to Massachusetts and the husband remained in Maryland to continue his schooling. After arriving in Massachusetts, the wife began IVF treatments at an IVF clinic here. At first the husband traveled from Maryland to participate in the treatments. In 1991, he moved to Massachusetts.

Given their medical history, the husband and wife were eligible for . . . IVF . . .

They underwent IVF treatment from 1988 through 1991. As a result of the 1991 treatment, the wife conceived and gave birth to twin daughters in 1992. During the 1991 IVF treatment, more preembryos were formed than were necessary for immediate implantation, and two vials of preembryos were frozen for possible future implantation.

In the spring of 1995, before the couple separated, the wife desired more children and had one of the remaining vials of preembryos thawed and one preembryo was implanted. She did so without informing her husband. The husband learned of this when he received a notice from his insurance company regarding the procedure. During this period relations between the husband and wife deteriorated. The wife sought and received a protective order against the husband under G.L. c. 209A. Ultimately, they separated and the husband filed for divorce.

At the time of the divorce, one vial containing four frozen preembryos remained in storage at the clinic. Using one or more of these preembryos, it is possible that the wife could conceive; the likelihood of conception depends, inter alia, on the condition of the preembryos which cannot be ascertained until the preembryos are thawed. The husband filed a motion to obtain a permanent injunction, prohibiting the wife from "using" the remaining vial of frozen preembryos.

b. *The IVF clinic and the consent forms.* In order to participate in fertility treatment, including GIFT and IVF, the clinic required egg and sperm donors (donors) to sign certain consent forms for the relevant procedures. Each time before removal of the eggs from the wife, the clinic required the husband and wife in this case to sign a preprinted consent form concerning ultimate disposition of the

---

[8] [n.6] An ectopic pregnancy is one that occurs outside the uterus, the normal locus of pregnancy. Stedman's Medical Dictionary 488 (25th ed.1990). In this case, the pregnancy occurred in and ruptured the fallopian tube, requiring surgery to remove it.

frozen preembryos. The wife signed a number of forms on which the husband's signature was not required. The only forms that both the husband and the wife were required to sign were those entitled "Consent Form for Freezing (Cyropreservation) of Embryos" (consent form), one of which is the form at issue here.

Each consent form explains the general nature of the IVF procedure and outlines the freezing process, including the financial cost and the potential benefits and risks of that process. The consent form also requires the donors to decide the disposition of the frozen preembryos on certain listed contingencies: "wife or donor" reaching normal menopause or age forty-five years; preembryos no longer being healthy; "one of us dying;" "[s]hould we become separated"; "[s]hould we both die." Under each contingency the consent form provides the following as options for disposition of the preembryos: "donated or destroyed — choose one or both." A blank line beneath these choices permits the donors to write in additional alternatives not listed as options on the form, and the form notifies the donors that they may do so. The consent form also informs the donors that they may change their minds as to any disposition, provided that both donors convey that fact in writing to the clinic . . .

c. *The execution of the forms.* Every time before eggs were retrieved from the wife and combined with sperm from the husband, they each signed a consent form. The husband was present when the first form was completed by the wife in October, 1988. They both signed that consent form after it was finished. The form, as filled out by the wife, stated, inter alia, that if they "[s]hould become separated, [they] both agree[d] to have the embryo(s) . . . return[ed] to [the] wife for implant." The husband and wife thereafter underwent six additional egg retrievals for freezing and signed six additional consent forms, one each in June, 1989, and February, 1989, two forms in December, 1989, and one each in August, 1990, and August, 1991. The August, 1991, consent form governs the vial of frozen preembryos now stored at the clinic.

Each time after signing the first consent form in October, 1988, the husband always signed a blank consent form. Sometimes a consent form was signed by the husband while he and his wife were traveling to the IVF clinic; other forms were signed before the two went to the IVF clinic. Each time, after the husband signed the form, the wife filled in the disposition and other information, and then signed the form herself. All the words she wrote in the later forms were substantially similar to the words she inserted in the first October, 1988, form. In each instance the wife specified in the option for "[s]hould we become separated," that the preembryos were to be returned to the wife for implantation.

2. *The Probate Court's decision.* The probate judge concluded that, while donors are generally free to agree as to the ultimate disposition of frozen preembryos, the agreement at issue was unenforceable because of "change in circumstances" occurring during the four years after the husband and wife signed the last, and governing, consent form in 1991: the birth of the twins as a result of the IVF procedure, the wife's obtaining a protective order against the husband, the husband's filing for a divorce, and the wife's then seeking "to thaw the preembryos for implantation in the hopes of having additional children." The probate judge

concluded that "[n]o agreement should be enforced in equity when intervening events have changed the circumstances such that the agreement which was originally signed did not contemplate the actual situation now facing the parties." In the absence of a binding agreement, the judge determined that the "best solution" was to balance the wife's interest in procreation against the husband's interest in avoiding procreation. Based on his findings, the judge determined that the husband's interest in avoiding procreation outweighed the wife's interest in having additional children and granted the permanent injunction in favor of the husband.

3. *Legal background.* While IVF has been available for over two decades and has been the focus of much academic commentary, there is little law on the enforceability of agreements concerning the disposition of frozen preembryos. Only three States have enacted legislation addressing the issue. See Fla. Stat. Ann. § 742.17 (West 1997) (requiring couples to execute written agreement for disposition in event of death, divorce or other unforeseen circumstances); N.H.Rev.Stat. Ann. §§ 168-B:13 thru 168-B:15, 168-B:18 (1994 & Supp.1999) (requiring couples to undergo medical examinations and counseling and imposing a fourteen-day limit for maintenance of ex utero prezygotes); La.Rev.Stat. Ann. §§ 9:121-9:133 (1991) (providing that "prezygote considered 'juridical person' that must be implanted[,]" *Kass v. Kass*, 91 N.Y.2d 554, 563, 673 N.Y.S.2d 350, 696 N.E.2d 174 [1998]).

Two State courts of last resort, the Supreme Court of Tennessee and the Court of Appeals of New York, have dealt with the enforceability of agreements between donors regarding the disposition of preembryos and have concluded that such agreements should ordinarily be enforced . . .

4. *Legal analysis.* This is the first reported case involving the disposition of frozen preembryos in which a consent form signed between the donors on the one hand and the clinic on the other provided that, on the donors' separation, the preembryos were to be given to one of the donors for implantation. In view of the purpose of the form (drafted by and to give assistance to the clinic) and the circumstances of execution, we are dubious at best that it represents the intent of the husband and the wife regarding disposition of the preembryos in the case of a dispute between them. In any event, for several independent reasons, we conclude that the form should not be enforced in the circumstances of this case.

First, the consent form's primary purpose is to explain to the donors the benefits and risks of freezing, and to record the donors' desires for disposition of the frozen preembryos at the time the form is executed in order to provide the clinic with guidance if the donors (as a unit) no longer wish to use the frozen preembryos. The form does not state, and the record does not indicate, that the husband and wife intended the consent form to act as a binding agreement between them should they later disagree as to the disposition. Rather, it appears that it was intended only to define the donors' relationship as a unit with the clinic.

Second, the consent form does not contain a duration provision. The wife sought to enforce this particular form four years after it was signed by the husband in significantly changed circumstances and over the husband's objection. In the absence of any evidence that the donors agreed on the time period during which the consent form was to govern their conduct, we cannot assume that the donors intended the consent form to govern the disposition of the frozen preembryos four years after it was executed, especially in light of the fundamental change in their relationship (i.e., divorce).

Third, the form uses the term "[s]hould we become separated" in referring to the disposition of the frozen preembryos without defining "become separated." Because this dispute arose in the context of a divorce, we cannot conclude that the consent form was intended to govern in these circumstances. Separation and divorce have distinct legal meanings. Legal changes occur by operation of law when a couple divorces that do not occur when a couple separates. Because divorce legally ends a couple's marriage, we shall not assume, in the absence of any evidence to the contrary, that an agreement on this issue providing for separation was meant to govern in the event of a divorce.

The donors' conduct in connection with the execution of the consent forms also creates doubt whether the consent form at issue here represents the clear intentions of both donors. The probate judge found that, prior to the signing of the first consent form, the wife called the IVF clinic to inquire about the section of the form regarding disposition "upon separation": that section of the preprinted form that asked the donors to specify either "donated" or "destroyed" or "both." A clinic representative told her that "she could cross out any of the language on the form and fill in her own [language] to fit her wishes." Further, although the wife used language in each subsequent form similar to the language used in the first form that she and her husband signed together, the consent form at issue here was signed in blank by the husband, before the wife filled in the language indicating that she would use the preembryos for implantation on separation. We therefore cannot conclude that the consent form represents the true intention of the husband for the disposition of the preembryos.

Finally, the consent form is not a separation agreement that is binding on the couple in a divorce proceeding pursuant to G.L. c. 208, § 34. The consent form does not contain provisions for custody, support, and maintenance, in the event that the wife conceives and gives birth to a child. See G.L. c. 208, § 1A; C.P. Kindregan, Jr. & M.L. Inker, Family Law and Practice § 50.3 (2d ed.1996). In summary, the consent form is legally insufficient in several important respects and does not approach the minimum level of completeness needed to denominate it as an enforceable contract in a dispute between the husband and the wife.

With this said, we conclude that, even had the husband and the wife entered into an unambiguous agreement between themselves regarding the disposition of the frozen preembryos, we would not enforce an agreement that would compel one donor to become a parent against his or her will.[9] As a matter of public policy, we conclude that forced procreation is not an area amenable to judicial enforcement. It is well-established that courts will not enforce contracts that violate public policy

---

[9] [n.22] That is the relief sought by the wife in this case. We express no view regarding whether an unambiguous agreement between two donors concerning the disposition of frozen preembryos could be enforced over the contemporaneous objection of one of the donors, when such agreement contemplated destruction or donation of the preembryos either for research or implantation in a surrogate. We also recognize that agreements among donors and IVF clinics are essential to clinic operations. There is no impediment to the enforcement of such contracts by the clinics or by the donors against the clinics, consistent with the principles of this opinion.

. . . While courts are hesitant to invalidate contracts on these public policy grounds, the public interest in freedom of contract is sometimes outweighed by other public policy considerations; in those cases the contract will not be enforced . . . To determine public policy, we look to the expressions of the Legislature and to those of this court . . .

The Legislature has already determined by statute that individuals should not be bound by certain agreements binding them to enter or not enter into familial relationships. In G.L. c. 207, § 47A, the Legislature abolished the cause of action for the breach of a promise to marry. In G.L. c. 210, § 2, the Legislature provided that no mother may agree to surrender her child "sooner than the fourth calendar day after the date of birth of the child to be adopted" regardless of any prior agreement.

Similarly, this court has expressed its hesitancy to become involved in intimate questions inherent in the marriage relationship. *Doe v. Doe*, 365 Mass. 556, 563, 314 N.E.2d 128 (1974). "Except in cases involving divorce or separation, our law has not in general undertaken to resolve the many delicate questions inherent in the marriage relationship. We would not order either a husband or a wife to do what is necessary to conceive a child or to prevent conception, any more than we would order either party to do what is necessary to make the other happy." *Id.*

In our decisions, we have also indicated a reluctance to enforce prior agreements that bind individuals to future family relationships. In *R.R. v. M.H.*, 426 Mass. 501, 689 N.E.2d 790 (1998), we held that a surrogacy agreement in which the surrogate mother agreed to give up the child on its birth is unenforceable unless the agreement contained, inter alia, a "reasonable" waiting period during which the mother could change her mind. *Id.* at 510, 689 N.E.2d 790 . . .

We glean from these statutes and judicial decisions that prior agreements to enter into familial relationships (marriage or parenthood) should not be enforced against individuals who subsequently reconsider their decisions. This enhances the "freedom of personal choice in matters of marriage and family life." *Moore v. East Cleveland*, 431 U.S. 494, 499, 97 S.Ct. 1932, 52 L.Ed.2d 531 (1977), quoting *Cleveland Bd. of Educ. v. LaFleur*, 414 U.S. 632, 639-640, 94 S.Ct. 791, 39 L.Ed.2d 52 (1974).

We derive from existing State laws and judicial precedent a public policy in this Commonwealth that individuals shall not be compelled to enter into intimate family relationships, and that the law shall not be used as a mechanism for forcing such relationships when they are not desired. This policy is grounded in the notion that respect for liberty and privacy requires that individuals be accorded the freedom to decide whether to enter into a family relationship . . .

In this case, we are asked to decide whether the law of the Commonwealth may compel an individual to become a parent over his or her contemporaneous objection. The husband signed this consent form in 1991. Enforcing the form against him would require him to become a parent over his present objection to such an undertaking. We decline to do so.

Judith F. Daar
Frozen Embryo Disputes Revisited: A Trilogy of Procreation-Avoidance Approaches
29 J. Law. Med. & Ethics 197, 198-99 (2001)

. . . [In *A.Z. v. B.Z.* the] Massachusetts Supreme Judicial Court affirmed the permanent injunction issued by the probate court but did not follow the lower court's reasoning. Instead, the court offered several independent reasons for its holding, each tied to the specific facts in the case.

First, the court concluded that the August 1991 consent form governing the embryos in dispute did not state that the couple intended the form to act as a binding agreement between them should they later disagree as to the disposition. Rather, the court argued, the agreement "was intended only to define the donors' relationship as a unit with the clinic."

This interpretation seems an illogical departure from the very purpose of contractual agreements, i.e., to anticipate and govern the future conduct of the parties. An agreement which reads, "should we separate, then return the embryos to the wife," is by its plain language anticipatory. The language cannot reasonably be construed to apply only to the contemporaneous status of the couple, as they were not separated at the time they executed the agreement. The court was silent, moreover, as to the exact language that "define[s] the donors' relationship as a unit with the clinic." In the context of the language provided, the only unit defined is the unity of the husband and wife in their agreement that remaining embryos should be made available to the wife in the event of divorce.

Second, the high court incorporated the trial court's rationale of "changed circumstances" to invalidate the agreement. The court emphasized that the agreement was signed four years before the dispute occurred, during which time the couple experienced a "fundamental change in their relationship" (i.e., divorce). The court then translated this change in marital status into a vitiation of the couple's intent to dispose of the embryos as indicated in the agreement.

But this analysis, like the court's first rationale, disregards the very purpose of consensual agreements, which is to anticipate future contingencies. The agreement at issue here expressly provided for the very change in circumstance that the court interpreted as invalidating the couple's consent. This portion of the opinion clearly warns future couples undergoing infertility treatment that even their most painstaking efforts to prospectively resolve future contingencies may not be honored in the face of overwhelming public policy concerns.

The court's third rationale seems to reject the time-honored plain-meaning rule governing the interpretation of contracts. Specifically, the court found that the phrase "[s]hould we become separated" in referring to the disposition of the frozen embryos was not intended to apply in the context of divorce. Rather, the court speculated that because separation and divorce have distinct legal meanings, the couple was limiting its disposition intentions to separation only. In its defense, the court cited several cases dealing with the difference in disposition of property upon separation and divorce.

While separation and divorce do have distinct legal meanings in the context of marital property distribution, nowhere did the court suggest that its overall decision was grounded in principles of property division. In fact, the court carefully avoided labeling the embryos as property, as have other courts confronting the disposition dilemma. Logic dictates, moreover, that the couple did intend to include divorce in their reference to separation. Divorce is the ultimate separation of a married couple, and there is no indication that the couple intended the agreement to apply only to the interim period between marriage and final separation upon divorce.

Next, the Supreme Judicial Court questioned whether the consent form represented the true intent of the husband who signed all but one of the forms in blank, allowing his wife to fill in the language indicating that any disputed embryos would be given to her. The trial court provided slightly more description as to the signing process, noting that the husband was present when the wife filled in and signed the first consent form. At that time, the court explained, "[t]he couple discussed how comfortable they were with the decision." Presumably, the couple was indeed comfortable with the decision, since instead of revisiting the disposition question, they relied on their previous expressions of intent.

In its decision, the high court made much of the fact that the consent form at issue was signed by the husband in blank and later filled in by the wife. In fact, the court translated this into a lack of intent as to disposition of the embryos. There is no evidence, however, that at the time the final consent form was signed, the husband lacked the intent to dispose of any disputed embryos in the same way as in the six prior agreements. If anything, his conduct supports a continued desire to reiterate his previous expressions of intent. At any time during the three years in which the seven forms were signed, he could have revoked his consent or elected a different disposition. His failure to make any such change is a strong indication of assent to his original choice, not a revocation thereof . . .

After much discussion about the form and substance of the agreement in this case, the court disclosed that the true basis for its decision was grounded not in contract law, but in public policy. Even if presented with an airtight unambiguous agreement as to embryo disposition, the court admitted, "we would not enforce an agreement that would compel one donor to become a parent against his or her will." Thus, procreation avoidance is the true principle that emerges from *A.Z.* Stressing the preeminence of public policy, the court emphasized its prior reluctance to enforce agreements that would have the effect of binding individuals to future family relationships. These historically prohibited agreements include surrogate parenting agreements] and contracts containing a promise to abandon a marriage. In this case, the court viewed enforcement of the embryo contract as a violation of A.Z.'s liberty and privacy, since it would force an unwanted relationship between A.Z. and his would-be future child.

Treating the husband in A.Z. as a reluctant and even non-consenting prospective parent is simply inconsistent with both the facts of the case as well as the prevailing law in this area. Factually, A.Z. consented to the prospect of future parenthood when he agreed, over a three-year period, to fully participate in the couple's infertility treatment. Treatment for infertility contemplates no goal other than becoming a parent in the future. It is true that the technology of assisted reproduction does yield the possibility of delayed parenthood amid changed circumstances, a sometimes unfortunate but highly foreseeable outcome for which solutions have been proposed. It cannot be said, however, that A.Z. did not contemplate or consent to the prospect of future parenthood.

Taking issue with A.Z.: forced parenthood a reality under the law

In its legal analysis, the Supreme Judicial Court stressed that "forced procreation is not an area amenable to judicial enforcement." This statement is not entirely correct. Under long-standing constitutional principles, courts can force unwanted parenthood on individuals whose actions result in procreation. In *Planned Parenthood v. Danforth*, [428 U.S. 52 (1976)] and again in *Planned Parenthood v. Casey*, [505 U.S. 833 (1992)] the Supreme Court established that once a woman is pregnant, her male partner cannot legally force her to have an abortion, nor can he prevent her from terminating her pregnancy if she so chooses. Control of the early embryo rests with the female, who can choose to continue the pregnancy to term and pursue legal remedies for support against the non-consenting male.

Even under state law principles, forced parenthood is a reality. For example, in *Roni D. v. Stephen K.*, [105 Cal. App. 3d 640 (1980)] Stephen sued Roni in tort for falsely representing that she was taking birth control pills. In reliance on that representation, Stephen engaged in sexual intercourse with Roni, from which act a child was born. In denying Stephen's tort claims, the court noted his voluntary participation in the procreation process, suggesting that the time for deciding against parenthood is before sperm leaves the body, not afterward. Stephen's actions resulted in forced parenthood, just as the couple in A.Z. contemplated that their actions could lead to procreation and parenthood. The only difference between the scenarios (representations regarding birth control aside) is that of natural versus assisted reproduction. In *A.Z.*, the court allowed the fortuity of technology to excuse the husband's responsibility for the consequences of his actions. Such a result seems particularly egregious when the parties unequivocally contracted for a particular result.

Finally, deference to an original "intent to parent" in the face of a subsequently objecting parent is also seen clearly in the related area of surrogate parenting arrangements. In states that recognize surrogacy as a valid method of creating families, courts look to the parties' intent to determine — and at times compel — parenthood. In *In re Marriage of Buzzanca*, [61 Cal. App. 4th 1410 (1998)] a case that offers many parallels to *A.Z.*, a husband and wife entered into a surrogacy agreement that resulted in the birth of a child. The child, conceived using a donor egg and donor sperm, was gestated by a surrogate, a woman who carried the child for the intended parents. Shortly before the child was born, the couple separated. The husband thereafter disclaimed any responsibility, financial or otherwise, for the child, arguing that he was not the legal or biological father. Saying bluntly that the child "never would have been born had not [the intended parents] both agreed to have a fertilized egg implanted in a surrogate," the court disagreed and imposed the financial responsibilities of fatherhood on the husband.

Analogies to the law and policy of surrogate parenting arrangements, like those to abortion, are obviously strained by the reality that in frozen embryo disputes, the all important interests of a child or growing fetus are absent. It seems logical, however, to expand these developed doctrines to include forced parenthood in embryo disputes as a corollary principle. If intent to parent is honored in the case of an unborn child conceived and gestated pursuant to a valid contract, this same principle should be given equal consideration when a child is merely conceived, since the intent to parent has been expressed by the voluntary surrender of gametes.

NOTES AND QUESTIONS

1. *An A.Z. Reprise.* One of the more unusual aspects of *A.Z.* was the wife's unilateral attempt to become pregnant using one of the couple's frozen embryos. To many observers' surprise, the wife succeeded in coaxing the IVF clinic to thaw and implant the embryo without her husband's knowledge or consent. The husband only learned of his estranged wife's actions via a routine mailing from his health insurance company, a chance transmittal that initiated the lengthy lawsuit. While initially viewed as unique, a recent lawsuit reveals that a virtually identical scenario took place at another Massachusetts fertility clinic at roughly the same time the wife in *A.Z.* secured her disputed embryo.

In December 1995 Meredith McLeod made a solo visit to a Boston IVF clinic where she underwent an embryo transfer using two thawed embryos created with donor eggs and her estranged husband's sperm. When she learned she was pregnant, she informed her soon-to-be ex-husband, who described the revelation as a "devastating nightmare." After his daughter was born, Richard Gladu sued the Boston clinic for breach of contract, arguing the consent form he signed for earlier treatments did not extend to his wife's unilateral use of their remaining embryos. See John Ellement & Thanassis Cambanis, *Ex-Husband Sues Clinic Over Birth of Daughter*, Boston Globe, Jan. 15, 2004, at B1. In February 2004 a jury awarded the father $108,000, representing $98,000 for the costs of raising his daughter and $10,00 for emotional distress. *See* ObGyn & Reprod. Weekly, *Legal Issues; Man Gets $108,000 from Fertility Clinic for Breach of Contract*, Feb. 16, 2004, at 27.

2. The decision in *A.Z. v. B.Z.* was much anticipated in the ART world because it was the first case to involve a written contract that explicitly awarded frozen embryos to one of the parties in the event of divorce. The two previous state high court opinions — *Davis v. Davis* (Tennessee 1992) and *Kass v. Kass* (New York 1998) — strongly favored enforcement of preconception agreements, so many wondered whether a court would enforce such an agreement if it meant that one party could become a parent against his or her wishes. The Massachusetts court turned away from the contract toward the more ethereal concept of public policy.

Does the ruling in *A.Z.* mean that preconception agreements are unenforceable in the state of Massachusetts? The court addresses this issue in footnote 22 of the case, leaving lingering the question of which, if any, IVF-related agreements would be enforced in the state. A group of researchers from the University of Michigan pondered the result in *A.Z.* in an effort to create a framework for disposition agreements that would be universally enforced. The group concluded that there are five "desirable characteristics" that should be included in every disposition contract:

1) Agreements should be unambiguous and comprehensive. Couples should consider all possible circumstances under which disposition could occur (death, divorce, separation, disease, aging, incapacity, disappearance, . . .) and should include all options for disposition (destruction, donation for gestation or research, transfer, continued storage, . . .).

2) All contract provisions should be consistent with public policy. [This may require the parties to seek judicial pre-approval of a disposition agreement as public policy is often a common law concept accessible only via a conversation with the court.]

3) The duration of the agreement should be clear. [Recall the *Litowitz* dispute was resolved by reference to a time limit in the written agreement.]

4) Abundant contact information should be included, to enable the clinic to reach the parties at a later date.

5) The rights and responsibilities of all parties should be made clear. If the parties abandon their embryos, the clinic should disclose its policy on transferring or discarding the cryopreserved material.

Timothy G. Schuster, Kathryn Hickner-Cruz, Dana A. Ohl, Edward Goldman & Gary D. Smith, *Legal Considerations for Cryopreservation of Sperm and Embryos*, 80 FERTILITY & STERILITY 61 (2003). Is this a comprehensive list of drafting rules for IVF clinics and their patients? What additions and/or deletions would you suggest to a couple contemplating IVF and embryo cryopreservation?

3. *The California Approach.* California lawmakers considered how patients in the numerous Golden State fertility clinics could best be served by preconception agreements. As a result, the California Health & Safety Code was amended to include the following mandate:

§ 125315. Information to be provided to fertility treatment patients.

(a) A physician and surgeon or other health care provider delivering fertility treatment shall provide his or her patient with timely, relevant, and appropriate information to allow the individual to make an informed and voluntary choice regarding the disposition of any human embryos remaining following the fertility treatment . . .

(b) . . . When providing fertility treatment, a physician and surgeon or other health care provider shall provide a form to the male and female partner, or the individual without a partner, as applicable, that sets forth advanced written directives regarding the disposition of embryos. This form . . . shall provide, at a minimum, the following choices for disposition of the embryos based on the following circumstances: . . .

(3) In the event of separation or divorce of the partners, the embryos shall be disposed of by one of the following actions:

(A)   Made available to the female partner.

(B)   Made available to the male partner.

(C)   Donation for research purposes.

(D)   Thawed with no further action taken.

(E)   Donation to another couple or individual.

(F)   Other disposition that is clearly stated.

CAL. HEALTH & SAFETY CODE § 125315 (2004). If the couple in *A.Z. v. B.Z.* resided in, and received their fertility treatment in California, would the case have been resolved the same way? Does the fact that California law allows a couple to elect to turn over unused embryos to one spouse mean that procreation avoidance is not the public policy of the State of California?

4.   *Public Policy Outside the U.S.* In the United States, public policy is typically a concept reserved to state lawmakers and the people they represent. What is best for, accepted, sanctioned or condoned in any particular state can be shaped by history, politics, demographics, and a host of variables that converge to create a jurisdiction's unique personality. These variations in public policy can be seen across nations, where differing public policies can produce different outcomes in similar cases. Such an observation can be made about a 1996 Israeli Supreme Court decision involving a dispute over frozen embryos. Though the facts were quite similar to the situation in *A.Z.*, the Israeli Court's sensibility about the governing public policy was distinct.

In *Nachmani v. Nachmani*, a childless Israeli couple agreed to undergo IVF and then to contract with a surrogate in California to bear their child, because the wife could neither gestate nor carry the fetus to term. The couple did not sign an agreement with the IVF clinic regarding disposition of the embryos, although they did sign a surrogacy agreement. The wife, Ruthi, went through medical treatments to extract eggs, which were the last eggs she could produce. Eleven eggs were fertilized with her husband's sperm and frozen for future implantation. The couple then separated. Danni, the husband, subsequently lived with another woman, and had two children in that relationship.

Ruthi requested that the clinic release the frozen pre-embryos to her so that she could arrange for a surrogate mother, but Danni opposed the request and the clinic refused to release the pre-embryos. Ruthi then initiated litigation to obtain them. She was successful in the district court where the judge, seeming reproachful of Danni, held that he had breached his contract with his wife. Like a husband whose wife becomes pregnant from intercourse, the judge ruled, Danni could not withdraw his agreement to have a child once the fertilization had gone forward.

A five-judge panel of the Supreme Court of Israel reversed the trial court, upholding Danni's fundamental right not to be forced to be a parent. The court stated that just as it could not force parenthood on a woman, it could not force it upon a man when the couple had used technology. The couple's agreement was unenforceable because its performance as originally contemplated was impossible. Until the embryos were implanted, the couple's joint agreement was required at every stage.

The Supreme Court reheard the case as a panel of eleven justices and, in a 7-4 decision, reversed the five-justice panel and awarded the fertilized eggs to Ruthi. Each justice wrote a separate decision. The majority viewed this case as one to which no statutes or precedents applied, and looked primarily to principles of justice and morality, and to the paramount value of life, rather than to contract law. Some of the majority justices stressed that successful implantation of the fertilized eggs was Ruthi's only chance to become a mother of biologically-related children. According to one of the justices, the majority relied on a number of concepts including a balancing analysis, an "absolute approach to justice," requiring a decision in favor of creating life, and an understanding of justice as "that which does the least harm," requiring a decision in favor of Ruthi because the harm of denying her a chance of parenthood would be greater than the harm to Danni. The balancing analysis took account of all of the relevant circumstances of the case, comparing the parties' good faith defense of their rights, the point at which Danni decided to contest Ruthi's access to the pre-embryos, Ruthi's reliance on Danni's representations, and her lack of available alternatives to achieve genetic parenthood. The justices decided that the harm to Ruthi in denying her the chance to be a biological mother was greater than the harm to Danni of becoming a parent against his wishes.

Helen S. Shapo, *Frozen Pre-Embryos and the Right to Change One's Mind*, 12 DUKE J. COMP. INT'L L. 75 (2002). What factors, in your mind, account for the differences in public policy between the U.S. and Israel when it comes to "forced parenthood"? Why, in the context of disputed frozen embryos, is "forced childlessness" an accepted public policy in the U.S. while "forced procreation" is not?

5. *Gender Neutrality Revisited.* After our discussion of *Davis v. Davis* in Section 2, we explored whether a policy of procreation avoidance is gender neutral, hearing from scholars who argue that without existing frozen embryos, it is far more difficult for women to become genetic parents than their male counterparts. (See Note 2, subpart c). This question of gender neutrality in the disposition of frozen embryos can also be evaluated from the perspective of feminist theory which posits that "neutral standards serve only to reinforce the status quo or to further subordinate women." Tracey S. Pachman, *Disputes Over Frozen Preembryos & The "Right Not To Be A Parent"*, 12 COL. J. GENDER & L. 128, 133-34 (2003), citing JUDITH A. BAER, OUR LIVES BEFORE THE LAW 120 (1999) ("[N]eutral principles, consistently applied, will ultimately reinforce the status quo."); MARTHA ALBERTSON FINEMAN, FEMINIST THEORY IN LAW: THE DIFFERENCE IT MAKES, IN GENDER AND AMERICAN LAW 53, 58 (Karen J. Mashkle ed., 1997) ("[G]ender neutrality may ultimately be as oppressive to the interests of women as was the creation of differences."); Catharine A. MacKinnon, *Difference and Dominance*, in FEMINISM UNMODIFIED 32-45 (1987), reprinted in MARY BECKER ET AL., FEMINIST JURISPRUDENCE 108-16 (2001) ("Gender neutrality is . . . simply the male standard.").

Ms. Pachman notes that in virtually every case involving disputed embryos, the "gender neutral" policy has resulted in the female partner being denied the right and opportunity to become a parent via the frozen embryos. This outcome, she argues, is hardly gender neutral. In addition, she focuses on the imbalance of physical effort that the male and female partner must devote to each IVF cycle.

"[A]lthough it appears to be gender-neutral, the application of the right not to be a parent in preembryo dispute cases effectively discriminates against women by failing to recognize contributions and rights of women in the IVF procedure . . . [T]he arbitrary decision to focus on the future benefits and burdens of parenthood, rather than the past contributions to the couples' efforts to achieve parenthood, devalues the enormous contributions of women to the IVF procedure and thereby discriminates against women in preembryo disputes." Id. at 128-29.

Should the contribution each party makes to the IVF process be taken into account when the resulting embryos become disputed? Is a "sweat equity" policy any more gender neutral than a policy of "procreation avoidance"?

Should the parties' motivation in undergoing IVF be relevant to any dispute that arises subsequently? What if a married couple undergoes treatment in order to preserve one spouse's fertility in the face of cancer treatment (which can render the patient infertile)? In a subsequent divorce action, should the infertile spouse's request for use of the embryos be honored as that person's only opportunity to achieve biological parenthood? *See Reber v. Reiss*, 42 A.3d 1131 (Pa. Super. 2012).

What if a divorcing couple is engaged in role reversal, with the wife asking the court to order the embryos destroyed and the husband seeking to use the embryos to bring about the birth of his child in the future? Though such cases are rare, a couple in New Jersey presented this conundrum in the next case.

J.B. v. M.B.
Supreme Court of New Jersey
170 N.J. 9, 783 A.2d 707 (2001)

PORITZ, C.J. In this case, a divorced couple disagree about the disposition of seven preembryos that remain in storage after the couple, during their marriage, undertook in vitro fertilization procedures. We must first decide whether the husband and wife have entered into an enforceable contract that is now determinative on the disposition issue. If not, we must consider how such conflicts should be resolved by our courts . . .

A

J.B. and M.B. were married in February 1992. After J.B. suffered a miscarriage early in the marriage, the couple encountered difficulty conceiving a child and sought medical advice from the Jefferson Center for Women's Specialties. Although M.B. did not have infertility problems, J.B. learned that she had a condition that prevented her from becoming pregnant. On that diagnosis, the couple decided to attempt in vitro fertilization at the Cooper Center for In Vitro Fertilization, P.C. (the Cooper Center) . . .

The Cooper Center's consent form describes the procedure:

IVF [or in vitro fertilization] will be accomplished in a routine fashion: that is, ovulation induction followed by egg recovery, insemination, fertilization, embryo development and embryo transfer of up to three or four embryos in the stimulated cycle. With the couple's consent, any "extra" embryos beyond three or four will be cryopreserved according to our freezing protocol and stored at -196 C. Extra embryos, upon thawing, must meet certain criteria for viability before being considered eligible for transfer. These criteria require that a certain minimum number of cells composing the embryo survive the freeze-thaw process. These extra embryos will be transferred into the woman's uterus in one or more future menstrual cycles for the purpose of establishing a normal pregnancy. The physicians and embryologists on the IVF team will be responsible for determining the appropriate biological conditions and the timing for transfers of cryopreserved embryos.

. . . Before undertaking in vitro fertilization in March 1995, the Cooper Center gave J.B. and M.B. the consent form with an attached agreement for their signatures. The agreement states, in relevant part:

I, J.B. (patient), and M.B. (partner), agree that all control, direction, and ownership of our tissues will be relinquished to the IVF Program under the following circumstances:

1. A dissolution of our marriage by court order, unless the court specifies who takes control and direction of the tissues. . . .

B

The in vitro fertilization procedure was carried out in May 1995 and resulted in eleven preembryos. Four were transferred to J.B. and seven were cryopreserved. J.B. became pregnant, either as a result of the procedure or through natural means, and gave birth to the couple's daughter on March 19, 1996. In September 1996, however, the couple separated, and J.B. informed M.B. that she wished to have the remaining preembryos discarded. M.B. did not agree.

J.B. filed a complaint for divorce on November 25, 1996, in which she sought an order from the court "with regard to the eight frozen embryos." In a counterclaim filed on November 24, 1997, M.B. demanded judgment compelling his wife "to allow the (8) eight frozen embryos currently in storage to be implanted or donated to other infertile couples." J.B. filed a motion for summary judgment on the preembryo issue in April 1998 alleging, in a certification filed with the motion, that she had intended to use the preembryos solely within her marriage to M.B. She stated:

Defendant and I made the decision to attempt conception through in vitro fertilization treatment. Those decisions were made during a time when defendant and I were married and intended to remain married. Defendant and I planned to raise a family together as a married couple. I endured the in vitro process and agreed to preserve the preembryos for our use in the context of an intact family.

J.B. also certified that "[t]here were never any discussions between the Defendant and I regarding the disposition of the frozen embryos should our marriage be dissolved."

M.B., in a cross-motion filed in July 1998, described his understanding very differently. He certified that he and J.B. had agreed prior to undergoing the in vitro fertilization procedure that any unused preembryos would not be destroyed, but would be used by his wife or donated to infertile couples. His certification stated:

> Before we began the I.V.F. treatments, we had many long and serious discussions regarding the process and the moral and ethical repercussions. For me, as a Catholic, the I.V.F. procedure itself posed a dilemma. We discussed this issue extensively and had agreed that no matter what happened the eggs would be either utilized by us or by other infertile couples. In fact, the option to donate [the preembryos] to infertile couples was the Plaintiff's idea. She came up with this idea because she knew of other individuals in her work place who were having trouble conceiving.

M.B.'s mother, father, and sister also certified that on several occasions during family gatherings J.B. had stated her intention to either use or donate the preembryos.

The couple's final judgment of divorce, entered in September 1998, resolved all issues except disposition of the preembryos. Shortly thereafter, the trial court granted J.B.'s motion for summary judgment on that issue. The court found that the reason for the parties' decision to attempt in vitro fertilization — to create a family as a married couple — no longer existed. J.B. and M.B. had become parents and were now divorced. Moreover, M.B. was not infertile and could achieve parenthood in the future through natural means. The court did not accept M.B.'s argument that the parties undertook the in vitro fertilization procedure to "create life," and found no need for further fact finding on the existence of an agreement between them, noting that there was no written contract memorializing the parties' intentions. Because the husband was "fully able to father a child," and because he sought control of the preembryos "merely to donate them to another couple," the court concluded that the wife had "the greater interest and should prevail."

The Appellate Division affirmed . . .

C

M.B. contends that the judgment of the court below violated his constitutional rights to procreation and the care and companionship of his children. He also contends that his constitutional rights outweigh J.B.'s right not to procreate because her right to bodily integrity is not implicated, as it would be in a case involving abortion. He asserts that religious convictions regarding preservation of the preembryos, and the State's interest in protecting potential life, take precedence over his former wife's more limited interests. Finally, M.B. argues that the Appellate Division should have enforced the clear agreement between the parties to give the preembryos a chance at life . . .

J.B. argues that the Appellate Division properly held that any alleged agreement between the parties to use or donate the preembryos would be unenforceable as a matter of public policy. She contends that New Jersey has "long recognized that individuals should not be bound by agreements requiring them to enter into family relationships or [that] seek to regulate personal intimate decisions relating to parenthood and family life." J.B. also argues that in the absence of an express agreement establishing the disposition of the preembryos, a court should not imply that an agreement exists. It is J.B.'s position that requiring use or donation of the preembryos would violate her constitutional right not to procreate. Discarding the preembryos, on the other hand, would not significantly affect M.B.'s right to procreate because he is fertile and capable of fathering another child.

LifeNet, Inc. (LifeNet) and the American Civil Liberties Union of New Jersey, the American Society for Reproductive Medicine, and RESOLVE, a National Infertility Association (ACLU *Amici*), have participated as *amici curiae* before the Appellate Division and now before this Court. LifeNet urges the Court not to allow destruction of the preembryos. The ACLU *Amici* argue that, although agreements governing disposition of preembryos should be presumed to be enforceable, agreements compelling implantation violate public policy by forcing parenthood on the non-consenting donor. The ACLU *Amici* argue further that in the absence of an agreement the right not to procreate should, in general, outweigh the right to procreate.

II

M.B. contends that he and J.B. entered into an agreement to use or donate the preembryos, and J.B. disputes the existence of any such agreement. As an initial matter, then, we must decide whether this case involves a contract for the disposition of the cryopreserved preembryos resulting from in vitro fertilization. We begin, therefore, with the consent form provided to J.B. and M.B. by the Cooper Center . . . That form states, among other things:

> The control and disposition of the embryos belongs to the Patient and her Partner. You will be asked to execute the attached legal statement regarding control and disposition of cryopreserved embryos.

The attachment, executed by J.B. and M.B., provides further detail in respect of the parties' "control and disposition":

> I, J.B. (patient), and M.B. (partner) agree that all control, direction, and ownership of our tissues will be relinquished to the IVF Program under the following circumstances: 1. A dissolution of our marriage by court order, unless the court specifies who takes control and direction of the tissues, or

> 2. In the event of death of both of the above named individuals, or unless provisions are made in a Will, or

> 3. When the patient is no longer capable of sustaining a normal pregnancy, however, the couple has the right to keep embryos maintained for up to two years before making a decision [regarding a] "host womb" or

> 4. At any time by our/my election which shall be in writing, or

> 5. When a patient fails to pay periodic embryo maintenance payment.

The consent form, and more important, the attachment, do not manifest a clear intent by J.B. and M.B. regarding disposition of the preembryos in the event of "[a] dissolution of [their] marriage." Although the attachment indicates that the preembryos "will be relinquished" to the clinic if the parties divorce, it carves out an exception that permits the parties to obtain a court order directing disposition of the preembryos . . . Clearly, the thrust of the document signed by J.B. and M.B. is that the Cooper Center obtains control over the preembryos unless the parties choose otherwise in a writing, or unless a court specifically directs otherwise in an order of divorce . . .

Here, the parties have agreed that on the dissolution of their marriage the Cooper Center obtains control of the preembryos unless the court specifically makes another determination. Under that provision, the parties have sought another determination from the court.

M.B. asserts, however, that he and J.B. jointly intended another disposition. Because there are no other writings that express the parties' intentions, M.B. asks the Court either to remand for an evidentiary hearing on that issue or to consider his certified statement. In his statement, he claims that before undergoing in vitro fertilization the couple engaged in extensive discussions in which they agreed to use the preembryos themselves or donate them to others. In opposition, J.B. has certified that the parties never discussed the disposition of unused preembryos and that there was no agreement on that issue.

We find no need for a remand to determine the parties' intentions at the time of the in vitro fertilization process. Assuming that it would be possible to enter into a valid agreement at that time irrevocably deciding the disposition of preembryos in circumstances such as we have here, a formal, unambiguous memorialization of the parties' intentions would be required to confirm their joint determination. The parties do not contest the lack of such a writing. We hold, therefore, that J.B. and M.B. never entered into a separate binding contract providing for the disposition of the cryopreserved preembryos now in the possession of the Cooper Center.

III

In essence, J.B. and M.B. have agreed only that on their divorce the decision in respect of control, and therefore disposition, of their cryopreserved preembryos will be directed by the court . . . Without guidance from the Legislature, we must consider a means by which courts can engage in a principled review of the issues presented in such cases in order to achieve a just result. Because the claims before us derive, in part, from concepts found in the Federal Constitution and the Constitution of this State, we begin with those concepts.

A

Both parties and the ACLU *Amici* invoke the right to privacy in support of their respective positions. More specifically, they claim procreational autonomy as a fundamental attribute of the privacy rights guaranteed by both the Federal and New Jersey Constitutions. Their arguments are based on various opinions of the United States Supreme Court that discuss the right to be free from governmental interference with procreational decisions. See *Eisenstadt v. Baird*, 405 U.S. 438, 453, 92 S.Ct. 1029, 1038, 31 L.Ed.2d 349, 362 (1972); *Griswold v. Connecticut*, 381 U.S. 479, 485-86, 85 S.Ct. 1678, 1682, 14 L.Ed.2d 510, 515-16 (1965); *Skinner v. Oklahoma*, 316 U.S. 535, 541, 62 S.Ct. 1110, 1113, 86 L.Ed. 1655, 1660 (1942) . . .

Those decisions provide a framework within which disputes over the disposition of preembryos can be resolved. In *Davis* [*v. Davis*], for example, a divorced couple could not agree on the disposition of their unused, cryopreserved preembryos. 842 S.W.2d at 589. The Tennessee Supreme Court balanced the right to procreate of the party seeking to donate the preembryos (the wife), against the right not to procreate of the party seeking destruction of the preembryos (the husband) . . . The court held that the scales "[o]rdinarily" would tip in favor of the right not to procreate if the opposing party could become a parent through other reasonable means.

B

We agree with the Tennessee Supreme Court that "[o]rdinarily, the party wishing to avoid procreation should prevail." Here, the Appellate Division succinctly described the "apparent" conflict between J.B. and M.B.:

> In the present case, the wife's right not to become a parent seemingly conflicts with the husband's right to procreate. The conflict, however, is more apparent than real. Recognition and enforcement of the wife's right would not seriously impair the husband's right to procreate. Though his right to procreate using the wife's egg would be terminated, he retains the capacity to father children.

. . . In other words, M.B.'s right to procreate is not lost if he is denied an opportunity to use or donate the preembryos. M.B. is already a father and is able to become a father to additional children, whether through natural procreation or further in vitro fertilization. In contrast, J.B.'s right not to procreate may be lost through attempted use or through donation of the preembryos. Implantation, if successful, would result in the birth of her biological child and could have life-long emotional and psychological repercussions . . . Her fundamental right not to procreate is irrevocably extinguished if a surrogate mother bears J.B.'s child. We will not force J.B. to become a biological parent against her will.

C

The court below "conclude[d] that a contract to procreate is contrary to New Jersey public policy and is unenforceable." 331 N.J.Super. at 234, 751 A.2d 613. That determination follows the reasoning of the Massachusetts Supreme Judicial Court in *A.Z. v. B.Z.*, wherein an agreement to compel biological parenthood was deemed unenforceable as a matter of public policy. 431 Mass. 150, 725 N.E.2d 1051, 1057-58 (2000) . . .

As the Appellate Division opinion in this case points out, the laws of New Jersey also evince a policy against enforcing private contracts to enter into or terminate familial relationships . . .

Enforcement of a contract that would allow the implantation of preembryos at some future date in a case where one party has reconsidered his or her earlier acquiescence raises similar issues. If implantation is successful, that party will have been forced to become a biological parent against his or her will. We note disagreement on the issue both among legal commentators and in the limited case law on the subject. *Kass*, supra, held that "[a]greements between progenitors, or gamete donors, regarding disposition of their prezygotes should generally be presumed valid and binding, and enforced in a dispute between them. . . ." 673 N.Y.S.2d 350, 696 N.E.2d at 180. Yet, as discussed above, the Massachusetts Supreme Judicial Court as well as our Appellate Division have declared that when agreements compel procreation over the subsequent objection of one of the parties, those agreements are violative of public policy . . .

We recognize that persuasive reasons exist for enforcing preembryo disposition agreements. Both the *Kass* and *Davis* decisions pointed out the benefits of enforcing agreements between the parties . . . We also recognize that in vitro fertilization is in widespread use, and that there is a need for agreements between the participants and the clinics that perform the procedure. We believe that the better rule, and the one we adopt, is to enforce agreements entered into at the time in vitro fertilization is begun, subject to the right of either party to change his or her mind about disposition up to the point of use or destruction of any stored preembryos.

The public policy concerns that underlie limitations on contracts involving family relationships are protected by permitting either party to object at a later date to provisions specifying a disposition of preembryos that that party no longer accepts. Moreover, despite the conditional nature of the disposition provisions, in the large majority of cases the agreements will control, permitting fertility clinics and other like facilities to rely on their terms. Only when a party affirmatively notifies a clinic in writing of a change in intention should the disposition issue be reopened. Principles of fairness dictate that agreements provided by a clinic should be written in plain language, and that a qualified clinic representative should review the terms with the parties prior to execution. Agreements should not be signed in blank, as in *A.Z.*, *supra*, 725 N.E.2d at 1057, or in a manner suggesting that the parties have not given due consideration to the disposition question. Those and other reasonable safeguards should serve to limit later disputes.

Finally, if there is disagreement as to disposition because one party has reconsidered his or her earlier decision, the interests of both parties must be evaluated . . . Because ordinarily the party choosing not to become a biological parent will prevail, we do not anticipate increased litigation as a result of our decision. In this case, after having considered that M.B. is a father and is capable of fathering additional children, we have affirmed J.B.'s right to prevent implantation of the preembryos. We express no opinion in respect of a case in which a party who has become infertile seeks use of stored preembryos against the wishes of his or her partner, noting only that the possibility of adoption also may be a consideration, among others, in the court's assessment.

IV

Under the judgment of the Appellate Division, the seven remaining preembryos are to be destroyed. It was represented to us at oral argument, however, that J.B. does not object to their continued storage if M.B. wishes to pay any fees associated with that storage. M.B. must inform the trial court forthwith whether he will do so;

otherwise, the preembryos are to be destroyed. The judgment of the Appellate Division is affirmed as modified.

VERNIERO, J., concurring.

I join in the disposition of this case and in all but one aspect of the Court's opinion. I do not agree with the Court's suggestion, in *dicta*, that the right to procreate may depend on adoption as a consideration . . .

I also write to express my view that the same principles that compel the outcome in this case would permit an infertile party to assert his or her right to use a preembryo against the objections of the other party, if such use were the only means of procreation. In that instance, the balance arguably would weigh in favor of the infertile party absent countervailing factors of greater weight. I do not decide that profound question today, and the Court should not decide it or suggest a result, because it is absent from this case.

JUSTICE ZAZZALI joins in this opinion.

For Affirmance as Modified CHIEF JUSTICE PORITZ and JUSTICES STEIN, COLEMAN, LONG, VERNIERO, LA VECCHIA, ZAZZALI

NOTES AND QUESTIONS

1. *A Third Approach?* The New Jersey Supreme Court adopts the rule, "to enforce agreements entered into at the time in vitro fertilization is begun, subject to the right of either party to change his or her mind about disposition up to the point of use or destruction of any stored preembryos."[10] Is this rule a contract approach? Is it a public policy approach? Is it something else?

Perhaps the test in *J.B. v. M.B.* can be classified as a balancing test. This characterization is largely based on the court's proposal that when one party objects to an originally agreed-upon disposition, there is a need for judicial intervention in the form of balancing the interests of the parties. Specifically, the court in *J.B.* concludes, "if there is disagreement as to disposition because one party has reconsidered his or her earlier decision, the interests of both parties must be evaluated." This evaluation resembles the balancing test first suggested by the Tennessee Supreme Court in *Davis v. Davis.*

The balancing test has been criticized for being little more than a default to

---

[10] A word about "change of mind." Surveys of couples with stored frozen embryos suggest a penchant for change of heart and mind at some point during the storage period. According to the American Society for Reproductive Medicine, in a study of couples with frozen embryos: 'Of the 41 couples that had recorded both a pre-treatment and post-treatment decision about embryo disposition, only 12 (29%) kept the same disposition choice.' What Do Patients Want to Do with Excess Embryos?, Am. Soc. Reprod. Med. Bull., Oct. 17, 2001, at http://www.asrm.org/Washington/Bulletins/vol3no37.html, as cited in Sara D. Petersen, *Dealing With Cryopreserved Embryos Upon Divorce: A Contractual Approach Aimed At Preserving Party Expectations*, 50 UCLA L. REV. 1065, 1090, n. 156 (2003).

procreation avoidance. As one commentator explains, "The premise of the balancing test . . . is flawed. The spouses in these cases do not have equivalent interests. The fundamental right to procreate does not include the right to have the preembryos implanted, while the fundamental right to avoid procreation does include the right to oppose implantation. The inequality of the spouses' interests makes it nearly impossible for the spouse desiring implantation to prevail. Christina C. Lawrence, Note, *Procreative Liberty and the Preembryo Problem: Developing a Medical and Legal Framework to Settle the Disposition of Frozen Embryos*, 52 Case Western Res. L. Rev. 721, 738 (2002).

Does the New Jersey Supreme Court give any indication how it would balance the interests of the parties in the more common gender scenario — where the infertile wife sought the embryos for a last chance at genetic parenthood? What factors would weigh in such a balance?

2. *A Fourth Approach?* In December 2003 the Iowa Supreme Court became the sixth state high court to weigh in on the disposition of disputed frozen embryos. In *In Re Marriage of Witten*, 672 N.W.2d 768 (Iowa 2003), a wife sought custody of frozen embryos created with her egg and the sperm of her soon-to-be ex-husband. The court found that the agreements signed by the couple prior to IVF did not explicitly deal with the question of disposition upon divorce, thus the "contract approach" was unavailable. The court rejected the balancing test, because it "simply substitutes the court as decision maker." Id. at 783. As for public policy, the court described Iowa judicial decisions and statutes as reflecting "respect for the right of individuals to make family and reproductive decisions based on the current views and values." Id. at 782.

From this public policy flowed a fourth approach to resolving embryo disputes — contemporaneous mutual consent. Based largely on the work of Professor Carl Coleman in his 1999 article, *Procreative Liberty and Contemporaneous Choice: An Inalienable Rights Approach to Frozen Embryo Disputes*, 84 Minn. L. Rev. 55, the Iowa court adopts a requirement of contemporaneous mutual consent, which dictates that "no transfer, release, disposition, or use of the embryos can occur without the signed authorization of both donors. If a stalemate results, the status quo would be maintained." 672 N.W.2d at 783. The practical effect of this approach is that embryos are stored indefinitely unless both parties can agree to their use or destruction.

3. Arthur and Tamara are a married couple about to undergo IVF at the OSU Fertility Clinic in Columbus, Ohio. The couple has enlisted the aid of an egg and a sperm donor, as both Arthur and Tamara were unable to produce viable gametes. The egg was supplied by Tamara's sister, Grace. The sperm was supplied by an anonymous donor, selected from the sperm bank located at OSU. Tamara has a healthy uterus, thus she is planning to carry the embryo to term. Before the embryos are transferred to Tamara, the couple signs a number of consent forms, including a form entitled "Disposition of Frozen Embryos" The form provides as follows:

> In the event wife (Tamara) and husband (Arthur) divorce or physically separate for a period exceeding six months, the embryos in frozen storage are to be disposed as follows:

(Fill in your mutual preference)

Arthur and Tamara discuss their wishes for their embryos and decide that if they divorce, they would want the embryos returned to Grace, the egg donor, so that she could gestate her own biologic child. Grace agrees that if she is ever awarded the embryos, she will implant them and treat any resulting child as her own. The couple scribes, "The embryos are to be given to Grace for implantation in her uterus."

Arthur and Tamara successfully undergo IVF, and a son is born to the happy couple. Seven embryos are frozen for later use. Five years go by and the couple begins to experience marital discord. Ultimately, Arthur and Tamara divorce and the feuding over the frozen embryos begins. Tamara wants the embryos turned over to her sister, according to the terms of the consent form. Arthur objects, saying he does not want his son's full sibling to be raised in a separate household. He would prefer that the embryos be donated for research.

How is the Ohio court likely to rule in this case? Which approach — contract, public policy, balancing, contemporaneous mutual consent — do you believe the court should adopt? What result is the court likely to obtain under each of these approaches?

D.   The Question of Parental Rights

To date, every U.S. divorcing couple who has fully litigated their embryo dispute has ultimately received the same dispensation from the court: If one spouse objects to becoming a parent to any child born of the disputed embryos, the other spouse is barred from accessing the frozen embryos for purposes of implantation. Such a monolithic edict precludes judicial discussion of the parental rights of a gamete provider who objected to the use of disputed embryos, but whose spouse managed to access the eight-celled embryos and cause the birth of a child. Would a person who objected to the use of the embryos still be considered a parent to the resulting child, or would the objection act as a waiver of parental rights? Though not exactly on point, the next case gives a sense of how courts might react generally to "the objecting ex-spouse."

IN RE O.G.M.
Court of Appeals of Texas
988 S.W.2d 473 (1999)

Eric Andell, Justice.

The trial court rendered summary judgment for the appellee, Donald McGill, on the issue of paternity of a child born through *in vitro* fertilization. In three points of error, the appellant, Mildred McGill Schmit, complains the trial court erred by denying her summary judgment motion, granting McGill's motion, and refusing to grant her attorney's fees. We affirm.

Facts

Donald McGill (McGill) married Mildred McGill Schmit (Schmit) in 1976. After having three children, Schmit underwent tubal ligation. In 1994, Schmit and McGill sought the services of an assisted reproduction clinic in an effort to create another child through *in vitro* fertilization (IVF) . . .

During the couple's marriage, Schmit unsuccessfully attempted the IVF procedure several times using her ova and McGill's sperm. The couple executed an informed consent form wherein they agreed that in the event of divorce, they would dispose of the pre-embryos according to both of their wishes. When Schmit and McGill were divorced in 1996, the clinic was storing four of their frozen pre-embryos. Their divorce decree did not address the disposition of the pre-embryos. Three months post-divorce, McGill accompanied Schmit to the assisted reproduction clinic where Schmit attempted the IVF procedure again. The parties claim they orally agreed as to McGill's rights to any child resulting from the procedure. However, Schmit claims McGill donated the pre-embryos to her, while McGill claims they agreed he would be the father.

Because the IVF procedure was successful this time, Schmit gave birth to baby O.G.M. in June 1997. Three months later, McGill filed a paternity suit and Schmit answered. Both parties then moved for summary judgment on the issue of paternity. The trial court granted McGill's motion and denied Schmit's. After a six day trial, a jury appointed Schmit O.G.M.'s sole managing conservator and McGill O.G.M.'s possessory conservator. McGill is also possessory conservator of the parties' other minor child.

I. Discussion

This is a case of first impression without any statutory or precedential guidance. Because of the complexity of potential legal issues arising from the *in vitro* fertilization procedure, we will give deference to the Texas Legislature to enact legislation deciding the rights of parties involved in the *in vitro* fertilization process. Accordingly, we will frame our issue as narrowly as possible.

We are deciding whether a biological father should be denied paternity to a child born through *in vitro* fertilization from a frozen pre-embryo conceived during marriage but implanted into the biological mother after divorce.

II. Summary Judgment Motions

In points of error one and two, Schmit complains the trial court erred by granting McGill's summary judgment motion, and by denying Schmit's summary judgment motion . . .

C. Does the Artificial Insemination Statute Control?

In Schmit's summary judgment motion, she alleges the artificial insemination statute controls any parental rights to O.G.M. because the artificial transfer of an embryo to her uterus is analogous to artificial sperm transfer from a donor. See Tex.

Fam.Code Ann. § 151.101.[11] Schmit contends the legislature intended to provide a method for women to have children without fear of paternity claims by biological fathers. As a result, Schmit contends that no presumptions of paternity exist, and McGill is not O.G.M.'s father.

The legislative history of section 151.101 does not make any reference to the *in vitro* fertilization procedure. Webster's dictionary defines artificial insemination as the introduction of semen into the uterus or oviduct by other than natural means. MERRIAM-WEBSTER'S COLLEGIATE DICTIONARY 106 (10th ed.1995). The *in vitro* fertilization procedure which produced O.G.M. involved removing ova from Schmit, fertilizing her ova with McGill's semen in a lab procedure, freezing a portion of the resulting pre-embryos, and later implanting a pre-embryo into Schmit's uterus. Schmit does not cite any authority holding that IVF is the same as artificial insemination. We find Family Code section 151.101 entitled "Artificial Insemination" inapplicable to the facts of this case.

D. Does the Parties' Intent Control a Court's Determination of Parentage?

Schmit contends the courts have uniformly looked at intent in assisted conception cases. In support, Schmit cites *In the Interest of R.C.*, 775 P.2d 27 (Colo.1989), *McDonald v. McDonald*, 196 A.D.2d 7, 608 N.Y.S.2d 477 (1994), and *Johnson v. Calvert*, 5 Cal.4th 84, 19 Cal.Rptr.2d 494, 851 P.2d 776 (Ca.1993), for the proposition that the parties' intent is a relevant consideration to a court's determination of parentage. We find Schmit's reliance misplaced. In *R.C.*, a semen donor, who was never married to the child's mother, sought paternity to a child conceived through artificial insemination. 775 P.2d at 28. The court held that a statute extinguishing rights to children born through artificial insemination does not apply to a known semen donor; and the parties' agreement and subsequent conduct is relevant in determining the donor's parental rights. 775 P.2d at 35. In *McDonald*, a married woman who gave birth to a child created from *donated* ova and her husband's sperm divorced her husband and sought maternity adjudication. 196 A.D.2d at 8-9, 608 N.Y.S.2d 477. The court found her to be the "natural mother." 196 A.D.2d at 9, 608 N.Y.S.2d 477. In *Johnson*, a husband and wife sought parental rights to a child born from a surrogate mother. 851 P.2d at 777. The court found the surrogate mother was not the natural mother. 851 P.2d at 782. None of these cases deal with a biological father seeking paternal rights to a child born from his ex-wife through IVF from pre-embryos conceived during marriage. We find these cases to be inapplicable to the case at bar.

E. Summary

At the summary judgment hearing, the following evidence was before the trial court: (1) McGill is O.G.M's biological father; (2) McGill was named O.G.M.'s father

---

[11] Section 151.101, "Artificial Insemination" provides:

(a) If a husband consents to the artificial insemination of his wife, any resulting child is the child of both of them. The consent must be in writing and must be acknowledged.

(b) If a woman is artificially inseminated, the resulting child is not the child of the donor unless he is the husband. - Ed.

on her birth certificate; (3) McGill filed a statement of paternity; (4) the pre-embryos were conceived while McGill was married to Schmit; (5) McGill consented to Schmit's implantation of pre-embryos created with the her ova and his semen; (6) McGill was present when the IVF procedure took place; (7) McGill pays child support for O.G.M.; (8) Schmit was unmarried at the time O.G.M. was born; (9) there was no writing setting out the parties' agreement regarding rights and obligations to O.G.M.; and (10) depriving McGill of paternity rights would bastardize O.G.M.

We find, as a matter of law, the evidence was sufficient to support the rendition of summary judgment. Accordingly, we find no error in the trial court's rendition of summary judgment in McGill's favor . . .

We affirm the trial court's judgment.

NOTES AND QUESTIONS

1.   Would the result in *O.G.M.* be the same (genetic father granted paternity) if McGill had objected to being named the child's father? In all likelihood, the answer is yes.

The general family law principle applied by courts is that people who engage in sexual intercourse are presumed to consent to procreation. As explained by Professor Marsha Garrison, "courts have uniformly imposed parental responsibilities on . . . those who had been tricked into fathering a child [for example, by the woman falsely representing she was on birth control]; they have refused to honor nonpaternity agreements whether made before or after the child's conception." Marsha Garrison, *Law Making For Baby Making: An Interpretive Approach to the Determination of Legal Parentage*, 113 Harv. L.R. 835, 860 (2000).

Arguably, by extension, any person who participates in a medical procedure designed to assist in conception is presumed to consent to the birth of any resulting child. Is this the standard that courts apply in frozen embryo disputes? If not, can an argument be made that courts are treating fertile and infertile individuals differently when it comes to reproductive rights and responsibilities? Could such disparate treatment be considered a violation of an infertile individual's guarantee of equal protection? For a fuller discussion of this argument see Judith F. Daar, *Assisted Reproductive Technologies and the Pregnancy Process: Developing An Equality Model to Protect Reproductive Liberties*, 25 Amer. J. Law & Med. 455 (1999).

2.   *Statutory Relief From Post-Divorce Parenthood.* A handful of states, including Texas, have enacted statutes providing that if gametes or embryos are placed after a couple's divorce, the former spouse will not be considered the legal parent of the resulting child. Texas Family Code § 160.706 provides:

> If a marriage is dissolved before the placement of eggs, sperm, or embryos, the former spouse is not a parent of the resulting child unless the former spouse consented in a record kept by a licensed physician that if assisted reproduction were to occur after a divorce the former spouse would be a parent of the child.

This statute was enacted in 2001, after *O.G.M.* was decided. If the law had been in place at the time the case went to trial, what result would have obtained?

3.   Recall Arthur and Tamara from Note 3 on page 631. Suppose Tamara wins in her quest to transfer the embryos to her unmarried sister Grace, who gives birth to a daughter. Who are the child's legal parents? Can Arthur make a viable argument that he is not the girl's legal father? Can Tamara make a viable argument that she *is* the child's legal mother?

SECTION III: THE PROBLEM OF EXCESS AND ABANDONED EMBRYOS

The previous section details the travails of couples who are engaged in bitter battles over the disposition of frozen embryos. These disputes often end up in court because fertility clinics are unable or unwilling to mediate a solution acceptable to both spouses. From the perspective of a fertility clinic, it is far better to allow a court to decide the disposition of disputed embryos, than to make a decision that would undoubtedly unleash the wrath, and the attorney, of the losing party. Though well-publicized, spousal disputes over frozen embryos are few in number compared to the number of embryos that remain in frozen storage for long periods, often long after their progenitors have fulfilled their dreams of parenthood. These excess embryos are typically not the subject of dispute between the progenitors, but nevertheless pose dilemmas for the personnel charged with their continued maintenance and care.

Embryos that remain in frozen storage can meet this fate for a variety of reasons. Patients can choose to keep their embryos frozen in perpetuity because they do not wish to use, discard or donate them. Maintaining embryos in a frozen state is an active, voluntary choice that some couples make, and though financially costly, allows them to defer a decision about ultimate disposition well into the future.

Conversely, embryos can remain in frozen storage because their progenitors have either intentionally or unintentionally failed to stay in contact with the storage facility. As we noted at the beginning of this chapter, it is estimated that at least 400,000 embryos reside in frozen storage in the U.S. Approximately 4% of these embryos, or 16,000, remain in storage because the facility lacks specific instructions from the progenitors as to their disposition. These embryos are often considered "abandoned" because, by all accounts, their owners have demonstrated no intent to return or reclaim their reproductive products. When the gamete providers cannot be located for clarification, storage facilities are forced to maintain the embryos in frozen storage at their own expense, or discard the abandoned embryos, perhaps at their own peril of having a couple reappear after a long absence and demand return of their embryos.

Whether the result of informed choice or unintentional abandonment, the growing use of ART and the improving state of cryopreservation make the dilemma of excess and abandoned embryos of current and future concern.

A. Excess Embryos and Patient Choice

Today virtually every ART clinic requires that couples, or individuals, sign a consent form indicating their disposition preferences in a variety of contingent circumstances. A study revealed that 338 of 340 responding ART practices required all patients to indicate in writing "what is to be done with the frozen embryos in the event that no one is able to make a decision." David I. Hoffman, et al., *Cryopreserved Embryos in the United States and Their Availability for Research*, 79 FERTILITY & STERILITY 1063, 1066 (2003). Virtually all consent forms allow patients to choose from the following four options:

1) Donate the embryos for research

2) Discard the embryos after a designated time frame

3) Maintain the embryos in frozen storage

4) Donate the embryos to another couple or individual.

Each choice engenders its own set of issues, not all of which will be obvious to the couple or individual undergoing fertility treatment. A brief description of each choice is in order.

1. Donate the Embryos for Research

This choice raises two main concerns: 1) what type of research is being authorized, and 2) does the relevant state law allow such research?

a. Type of Research

The question of "type of research" is a relatively new question, coming on the scene with the discovery of embryonic stem cells in the late 1990s as a potential source of therapy for human diseases. We explore the medical, legal and ethical parameters of embryonic stem cell research in Chapter 9. Suffice it to say for purposes of our current discussion, that couples undergoing IVF can now consider donating unwanted embryos to scientific laboratories that will grow their embryos to the blastocyst stage (about five-days post-fertilization) and then extract cells from the core of the embryo for further study. These inner cells contained in the early embryo are known as stem cells, because they are "pluripotent," meaning they have the potential to develop into any cell of the human body, and thus may be used to replace damaged cells in ailing patients.

Patients can also elect to donate their unused embryos for research into infertility and IVF. The embryos can be used to study the ways in which the gametes and early embryo develop so that methods of in vitro fertilization and implantation can be improved for future fertility patients.

If a patient elects the "research" option, should she and her partner be given the option to further designate the type of research the embryo will be used for? Or should the type of research be left up to the fertility clinic? In at least one state, patients undergoing infertility treatment must be given the option of donating unwanted embryos to research, and if this option is selected, they must be informed about the type of research the embryos will support.

California Health & Safety Code § 125315 provides:

(c) A physician and surgeon or other health care provider delivering fertility treatment shall obtain written consent from any individual who elects to donate embryos remaining after fertility treatments for research. For any individual considering donating the embryos for research, to obtain informed consent, the health care provider shall convey all of the following to the individual:

(1) A statement that the early human embryos will be used to derive human pluripotent stem cells for research and that the cells may be used, at some future time, for human transplantation research.

(2) A statement that all identifiers associated with the embryos will be removed prior to the derivation of human pluripotent stem cells.

(3) A statement that donors will not receive any information about subsequent testing on the embryo or the derived human pluripotent cells.

(4) A statement that derived cells or cell lines, with all identifiers removed, may be kept for many years.

(5) Disclosure of the possibility that the donated material may have commercial potential, and a statement that the donor will not receive financial or any other benefits from any future commercial development.

(6) A statement that the human pluripotent stem cell research is not intended to provide direct medical benefit to the donor.

(7) A statement that early human embryos donated will not be transferred to a woman's uterus, will not survive the human pluripotent stem cell derivation process, and will be handled respectfully, as is appropriate for all human tissue used in research.

———————

Do you think a consent form that contained this required disclosure language would make a couple more or less likely to select the research option? Can a patient in California direct her embryos to IVF research, or does the statute limit research using donated embryos from IVF clinics to embryonic stem cell research?

b.   State Law Prohibitions on Embryo Research

The question of whether an embryo may be donated for research is largely a matter of state law. Couples who wish to donate their unused embryos for research should consult with the fertility clinic as to whether such disposition is permitted under the state's relevant statutes. Laws in at least two states — Louisiana and Kentucky — would appear to limit donation for research purposes. Louisiana Revised Statutes § 129, entitled "Destruction" provides:

A viable in vitro fertilized human ovum is a juridical person which shall not be intentionally destroyed by any natural or other juridical person or through the actions of any other such person.

Donation for research in Louisiana would be prohibited by statute if the research involved the intentional destruction of the embryo. Clearly, embryonic stem cell research (as it is currently practiced) would violate the Louisiana law because the act of extracting the inner stem cells does result in the demise of the embryo. If IVF research could be performed without the intentional destruction of the embryo, perhaps it would be permitted under state law. To the extent that current research practices do result in the destruction of the embryo, donation would not be a permitted option for fertility patients in Louisiana.

Kentucky law regulates the use of public funds for reproductive services, including in vitro fertilization. Chapter 311, Section 311.715 of the Kentucky Revised Statutes provides:

> Public medical facilities may be used for the purpose of conducting research into or the performance of in-vitro fertilization as long as such procedures do not result in the intentional destruction of a human embryo.

Like Louisiana, Kentucky prohibits the intentional destruction of embryos, but the Kentucky law is limited in scope to activities at public facilities. The Kentucky statute seems to suggest that IVF research could be carried out without destroying the embryo, and to the extent that such research is carried out, it may be carried out in state-funded medical facilities in the state. Presumably private medical facilities are free to conduct research, even if such activities involve the intentional destruction of the embryos. Thus patients being treated at private clinics could choose to donate their unused embryos to research, while those receiving care at public facilities would be more limited.

2.   Discard the Embryos After a Designated Time Frame

Fertility clinics are generally empowered to create their own policies regarding the discard of unwanted embryos (absent state law directing otherwise). Clinics are free to decide whether they are willing to freeze extra embryos, and if so, whether they are willing to destroy such embryos at the request of patients. A recent survey of 217 fertility clinics across the country revealed the following picture of clinic practices:

-   Nearly all clinics were willing to permanently preserve embryos in frozen storage

-   15% of clinics were unwilling to dispose of frozen embryos

-   3% of clinics were unwilling to freeze excess embryos (meaning all were implanted or donated at the time of creation)

-   2% returned thawed embryos to the patients

David B. Caruso, *Clinics Vary Widely in Embryo Disposal*, CHARLOTTE OBSERVER, Sept. 19, 2004, at 10A (reporting on a study conducted at the University of Pennsylvania and Rutgers University). Extrapolating from these figures, we can see that a majority of clinics are willing to discard frozen embryos at the request of patients. The methods of discard varied widely across clinics, from performing a quasi-religious ceremony for each embryo, to barring patients from being in the room when the thaw occurs, to giving patients the tiny straws containing their embryos to take home.

Recall in *Litowitz v. Litowitz* the court determined that the consent form signed by Becky and David Litowitz allowed the fertility clinic to thaw the couple's embryos after five years. Though the embryos ultimately were not destroyed, the case instructs that clinics may include discard language in their consent forms, which can be viewed as self-executing. The consent form in *Litowitz* required the couple to contact the clinic if discard was not desired, thus the onus for keeping the embryos in frozen storage resided with the couple.

If you were counsel to a fertility clinic, would you advise your client to adopt similar language for its consent forms? Is it a good idea to place the burden of communication on the couple? If a couple fails to communicate with the clinic to request an extension of the storage agreement, should the clinic proceed to thaw the embryos without making any effort to contact the patient and/or the patient's partner?

3.   Maintain the Embryos in Frozen Storage

As noted above, nearly all fertility clinics are willing to maintain embryos in frozen storage indefinitely. Even so, resource issues do present. For some clinics, cost and space constraints are causing a reevaluation of the policy of perpetual preservation. If a couple stops paying the annual storage fee, the clinics typically see themselves as having little choice but to absorb the cost of maintaining and storing the embryos [more on the issue of abandoned embryos in Section B, infra]. Though the fee for frozen embryo storage is relatively small, about $300 per year, if the number of patients who fail to pay this fee mounts, clinics could face financial difficulties. The natural response, in all probability, would be to increase fees for other couples or other services to make up for the shortfall.

Smaller clinics also confront space limitations, finding they can no longer maintain the liquid nitrogen tanks that house the embryos on site of their cramped quarters. Indeed, an entrepreneurial business offering long-term embryo storage has emerged to meet the needs of over-flowing fertility clinics. ReproTech Ltd. of Roseville, Minnesota, has developed off-site storage facilities that service fertility clinics in much the same way traditional storage facilities assist law firms and corporations who lack space for their documents and files. Programs that employ these off-site facilities typically offer patients the option of transferring their frozen embryos to the remote site. Inherent in any move is the risk that the embryos will be damaged in transport, a risk that should be allocated and insured against before any transfer is undertaken.

4.   Donate the Embryos to Another Couple

Embryo Donation. Embryo donation allows couples to transfer their excess embryos to other couples or individuals who are unable to conceive on their own. In recent years, the term "embryo adoption" has crept into the ART lexicon, suggesting the emergence of a separate and distinct practice involving the voluntary surrender of unwanted embryos. Though disagreement as to terminology remains, it is probably fair to declare that embryo donation and embryo adoption are distinct practices, distinguished primarily according to the intermediary who facilitates the transfer from the genetic parents to the parent or parents who intend to gestate and raise the child.

When a couple elects to donate an embryo, typically the fertility clinic will facilitate the transfer to an existing or future patient. According to the U.S. Centers for Disease Control, 58% of all U.S. fertility clinics offer donor embryos to infertile couples. In the main, embryo donation is an anonymous system, in that the donor and recipient couple do not meet. The donee couple can peruse the clinic's catalog of available embryos, searching the characteristics of the donor couple in order to select an embryo that fulfills the intended parents' aspirations for their child. This process gives the donee couple control over the selection, with the donor couple often uninvolved in the process once the decision to relinquish their embryo is made.

The number of couples willing to donate embryos for others' use is fairly small, for reasons that relate to the potential existence of full-blood siblings to the donor couple's existing child or children. A donated embryo could, and in fact is designed to, result in the birth of full genetic sibling to an existing child. If the donation is anonymous, a later encounter by the full-blood siblings could result in unknowing incest and the birth of children affected by genetic disorders related to consanguinity. A 2003 study looking at the disposition of excess embryos confirms that donation is exceedingly rare. Only 1% of the study patients surveyed donated their leftover embryos for implantation by another infertile couple. *See* Katheryn D. Katz, *Snowflake Adoptions and Orphan Embryos: The Legal Implications of Embryo Donation*, 18 WISC. WOMEN'S LAW J. 179, 189 (2003). A more recent study found the number of willing donors rose to 16% among couples who had satisfied their own reproductive desires. *See* Anne Drapkin Lyerly et al., *Fertility Patients' Views About Frozen Embryo Disposition: Results of a Multi-Institutional U.S. Survey*, 93(2) FERTILITY & STERILITY 499 (2010).

Embryo Banks? People who agree to donate their excess embryos to other couples or individuals are often lauded as altruistic and empathic, surrendering a part of themselves for the benefit of others. Would this same adulation be visited upon someone who procured sperm and egg from willing donors and then created embryos for "donation" to interested wannabe parents? This idea of an embryo bank, where individuals and couples can make "deposits" of their gametes for use by prospective parents, has raised a few eyebrows. In 2007, entrepreneur Jennalee Ryan opened the Abraham Center of Life in San Antonio, where clients could order up embryos from stocked eggs and sperm based on the progenitor's race, education, appearance, and other characteristics. The price of a made-to-order embryo was less than what the "customer" would have paid for separately procuring an egg donor and a sperm donor — with all its attendant medical and transaction costs. While some condemned this world's first human embryo bank as an unethical commodification of "mail-order children," others observed that "people are already choosing sperm and egg donors in separate transactions. Combining them doesn't pose any new major ethical problems." Rob Stein, *'Embryo Bank' Stirs Ethics Fears*, WASH. POST, Jan 6, 2007. The Abraham Center of Life closed in May 2007, a few months after opening.

Embryo Adoption. Embryo adoption is a relatively new disposition option, popularized in large measure by the Snowflakes Embryo Adoption Program run by

Nightlight Christian Adoptions. Founded in 1997 with the help of the conservative Christian group Focus on the Family, Snowflakes seeks to mimic traditional adoption by matching donors and recipients on the same basis that adoption agencies place children. According to the Snowflakes website, the organization, "provides the same safeguards that the traditional adoption process offers. The genetic family knows that the family they have chosen to parent their child has been screened for a criminal history and child abuse record, as well as received education about how to parent an adoptee. The genetic parents have the peace of mind of having handpicked a family to raise their genetic child. They also have the opportunity to have contact with the adopting family to whatever extent both families are comfortable." www.snowflakes.org. As of December 2011, Snowflakes report on its website that 283 babies have been born as a result of their program. A spokesman for Nightlife Christian Adoptions estimates that over 3,000 babies have been born via embryo adoption in general. *See Embryo Adoption Becoming the Rage*, THE WASH. TIMES, Apr. 19, 2009.

The use of the term "embryo adoption" has caused some concern in both the adoption and the ART communities. From the perspective of traditional adoption, "adoption law does not and cannot really apply to donating embryos because many state statutes specifically invalidate biological parents' consent to adoption that is given prior to childbirth . . . It logically follows that because embryos are not children, adoption statutes cannot apply to their donation." Charles P. Kingregan, Jr. & Maureen McBrien, *Embryo Donation: Unresolved Legal Issues in the Transfer of Surplus Crypreserved Embryos*, 49 VILL. L. REV. 169 (2004) (suggesting the laws governing gestational surrogacy arrangements are more suited to embryo transfer than traditional adoption law); Compare Paul C. Redman & Lauren Fielder Redman, *Seeking a Better Solution for the Disposition of Frozen Embryos: Is Embryo Adoption the Answer?*, 35 TULSA L.J. 583 (2000) (favoring an adoption approach to the disposition of excess embryos); Olga Batsedis, *Embryo Adoption: A Science Fiction or an Alternative to Traditional Adoption?*, 41 FAM. CT. REV. 565 (2003) (concluding embryo adoption is an "effective alternative to traditional adoption"). While Snowflakes acknowledges that its practice is not recognized by current adoption laws, it uses the same steps and similar forms to those used in traditional adoption, in the "hope that instead of creating a new set of laws, the current laws for adoption will simply be expanded to include embryos."

If adoption laws were applied to embryo transfers, reproductive rights advocates worry that such a move would symbolize the demise of reproductive liberty in both the abortion and infertility context. If embryos are treated the same as children for purposes of adoption, "[c]arried to its logical extreme, an embryo protective position supports a ban on [abortion and] all assisted reproductive technologies that involve fertilization outside the human body." Katz, *supra* at 194. Again, Snowflakes is up front about its views on the status of the embryo. "[W]e recognize the personhood of embryos; we treat them as precious pre-born children, not property to be transferred."

The Snowflakes program began to receive governmental financial backing in 2002 when the U.S. Department of Health and Human Services released $1 million in grants to launch embryo adoption awareness campaigns. About half of the grant money was awarded to Snowflakes, which pledged to use the funds to produce

11,000 embryo adoption videos for distribution to the public, medical community and news media. *See* Andis Robeznieks, *Researchers Ponder Best Use of 400,000 Stored Embryos*, AM. MED. NEWS, June 16, 2003, at 13. Since 2002, the federal government has continued its funding of an embryo adoption awareness campaign, allocating over $4 million in fiscal years 2009 and 2010. The allocation fell to $2 million in 2011. In March 2012, DHHS announced that the Embryo Adoption Awareness Campaign would be discontinued in 2013, owing to limited interest and a very small pool of repeat grant applicants.

Embryo transfers, whether anonymous and clinic-sponsored or open and religiously based, still represent a fraction of the dispositions that couples select for their excess embryos. Along with orders for discard, permanent frozen storage and donation to research as possible dispositions, embryo transfers round out the range of options that patients select among when deciding the future of their soon-to-be frozen embryos. But, as we have seen in the case of divorce, patients can change their minds about a once favored disposition, leaving fertility clinics uncertain about their continuing duty to support the frozen material. This uncertainty is greatest when patients exit the scene, leaving no forwarding address and no clue as to their wishes for their potential progeny. The problem of abandoned embryos rounds out our discussion of disposition dilemmas.

B.   Excess Embryos and Lack of Patient Choice: The Problem of Abandonment

The dilemma of abandoned frozen embryos gained worldwide attention in the summer of 1996 when officials at fertility clinics across Great Britain removed about 3,300 embryos from frozen storage and allowed the frozen material to thaw and die. The fertility personnel were not making a political statement, but rather following British law which requires the destruction of frozen embryos after a specified period of time. The Human Fertilisation and Embryology Act, enacted in 1990, governs and regulates the use of reproductive technologies in Great Britain. Section 14 of the HFEA provides:

> (1) The following shall be conditions of every licence authorising the storage of gametes or embryos —
>
> (c) that no gametes or embryos shall be kept in storage for longer than the statutory storage period and, if stored at the end of the period, shall be allowed to perish . . .
>
> (4) The statutory storage period in respect of embryos is such period not exceeding five years as the licence may specify.

The HFEA was implemented on August 1, 1991. In preparation for the mandated thaw on August 1, 1996, fertility clinics attempted to contact donor couples to provide notice and for clarification of their wishes. The law allows an extension of storage for up to 10 years if both gamete providers consented in writing. Despite attempt by certain religious groups to intervene, and over the objection of several women who were unable to obtain the written permission of their male partner (one had become mentally incompetent and the other was an anonymous sperm donor who could not be located), the clinics proceeded to follow the law and destroy several thousand embryos that had languished in frozen storage for half a decade. For a further account of the British experience see Heidi Forster, *The Legal and Ethical Debate Surrounding the Storage and Destruction of Frozen Human Embryos: A Reaction to the Mass Disposal in Britain and the Lack of Law in the United States*, 76 WASH. L. Q. 759 (1998). In 2008, the HFEA was amended to extend the storage limitation to 10 years.

As the above-referenced law review article indicates, the U.S. has no formal law on the preservation or destruction of frozen embryos. To date, fertility clinics have been reluctant to destroy embryos, even those that can be confidently classified as "abandoned" — circumstances in which the gamete donors have renounced any claim to their potential progeny. Fertility clinics with embryos whose progenitors have failed to pay storage fees and failed to communicate with the clinic despite the latter's good faith efforts to make contact, face at least two dilemmas — when can embryos be classified as abandoned, and when, if ever, can a clinic discard abandoned embryos?

The American Society for Reproductive Medicine, a professional organization comprised of reproductive technology specialists, first considered the issue of abandoned embryos in July 1996. ASRM revisited the issue in 2004, essentially affirming the prior guidance it had provided to its member clinics. The ASRM position follows.

Disposition of Abandoned Embryos

Couples undergoing in vitro fertilization who consent to cryopreservation of embryos usually state in writing their wishes regarding future disposition of cryopreserved embryos in writing. In some cases, however, couples have not stated their wishes and cannot be contacted to make their wishes known, which poses a problem for programs faced with continued storage of the couples' embryos.

Because of the uncertainties that exist in such a situation, programs should require each couple contemplating embryo storage to give written instruction concerning disposition of embryos in the case of death, divorce, separation, failure to pay storage charges, inability to agree on disposition in the future, or lack of contact with the program. The cryopreservation consent form should state specifically that the program may dispose of embryos if no contact with the program has occurred for a specified period, and the couple has not kept the program informed of their current address and telephone number. A couple may jointly agree at a later time to alter any advance directions for disposition of embryos by submission of a new set of written directions for disposition of stored embryos.

In cases in which written directions for disposition of embryos does not exist, a program will be faced with continued storage or disposal of embryos. At present, the law does not give clear guidance on this issue, though it is reasonable to assume that the law will treat the embryos, after a certain passage of time, as abandoned. In the face of legal uncertainty, some programs might prefer to continue storage indefinitely. Other programs will find the risk of liability to be acceptable and dispose of embryos after a lengthy passage of time and unsuccessful efforts to contact the couple.

As an ethical matter, a program should be free to dispose of embryos after a passage of time that reasonably suggests that the couple has abandoned the embryos. A program's willingness to store embryos does not imply an ethical obligation to store them indefinitely. A couple that has not given written instruction for disposition, has not been in contact with the program for a substantial period of time, and has not provided a current address and telephone number cannot reasonably claim injury if the program treats the embryos as abandoned and disposes of them.

The Ethics Committee finds that it is ethically acceptable for a program to consider embryos to have been abandoned if more than five years have passed since contact with a couple, diligent efforts have been made by telephone and registered mail to contact the couple at their last known address, and no written instruction from the couple exists concerning disposition. In implementing this standard, a program should make diligent efforts to contact the couple at the last known address both by telephone and registered mail, return receipt requested.

If a program reasonably determines under this standard that embryos have been abandoned, the Ethics Committee concludes that the program may dispose of the embryos by removal from storage and thawing without transfer. In no case without prior consent, should embryos deemed abandoned be donated to other couples or be used in research.

The Ethics Committee of the American Society for Reproductive Medicine, *Disposition of Abandoned Embryos*, 82 FERTILITY & STERILITY S253 (2004).

NOTES AND QUESTIONS

1.   The ASRM position was originally adopted in July 1996, just days before the British law was scheduled to take effect. No doubt American fertility clinics were pressing their leaders for guidance on the policy across the pond. Despite the ASRM's pronouncement that a program may dispose of embryos left without contact in frozen storage for five years, to date no U.S. fertility clinic has publicly acknowledged availing itself of the suggested policy. *See* Shari Roan, *On the Cusp of Life, and of Law*, L.A. TIMES, Oct. 6, 2008 (quoting Dr. Richard Paulson, fertility specialist at University of Southern California on unilateral embryo discard by clinics. "To my knowledge, no one in the United States has ever done that," he says. "We're all paranoid that a couple will show up the next day and say they want their embryos"). *See also* Judith Graham, *Fertility Clinics Face Tough Call; Crowded Labs Feel Pressure to Discard Unwanted Embryos*, CHICAGO TRI., Sept. 12, 2004, at 1 (pegging the number of abandoned embryos in frozen storage at 20,000 nationwide).

2.   Risa and Veejay Patel were overjoyed at the birth of their twin daughters in 2005. The girls were conceived at the Northeast Fertility Center (NFC) through an IVF cycle in which 10 embryos were produced. Six of those embryos remain in frozen storage at NFC. When the couple underwent treatment, they signed a consent form indicating, "[I]n the event our embryos have not been used for five years, NFC has our permission to discard the embryos according to the standard procedures used for this process." In 2010 the Patels stopped paying the annual

storage fee of $300 and despite numerous attempts to contact the couple, NFC has been unsuccessful in locating or communicating with them. Despite the Patels failure to pay the fees and respond to registered letters from NFC, each December the couple sends a holiday card to the clinic, featuring a photo of their growing daughters. No return address appears on the letter, only a message of yuletide cheer accompanies the mailing.

NFC seeks your advice as to how to proceed. Space and financial considerations lead NFC to favor thawing the Patels' embryos. Would you advise NFC to thaw the embryos according to the 2005 consent form signed by the couple? According to the ASRM policy?

What if the Patels suddenly reappear in 2012 and demanded return of their embryos? If NFC still retained possession of the embryos and refused to turn them over until the storage fees were paid in full, can the couple secure a court order forcing the clinic to immediately return the embryos? Consider the next case.

YORK v. JONES
United States District Court, Eastern District of Virginia
717 F. Supp. 421 (1989)

CLARKE, DISTRICT JUDGE. This matter comes before the Court on a Motion to Dismiss filed by defendants Howard W. Jones, Jr., M.D. (Dr. Jones), Suheil J. Muasher, M.D. (Dr. Muasher) and the Medical College of Hampton Roads (Medical College) pursuant to Rule 12(b)(6) of the Federal Rules of Civil Procedure. The plaintiffs have responded, the parties have waived oral argument, and the Motion is therefore ripe for disposition.

Introduction

The plaintiffs' Complaint in this case raises an issue of first impression in the rapidly developing field of human reproductive technology. The plaintiffs, Steven York, M.D. and Risa Adler-York (the Yorks), are the progenitors of the cryopreserved human pre-zygote (the pre-zygote) at issue in this case. The plaintiffs seek the release and transfer of the pre-zygote from the defendant The Howard and Georgeanna Jones Institute For Reproductive Medicine (Jones Institute) in Norfolk, Virginia to the Institute for Reproductive Research at the Hospital of the Good Samaritan located in Los Angeles, California. The defendants have refused to consent to an inter-institutional transfer of the pre-zygote.

This matter was originally brought before the Court on plaintiffs' Petition for a Temporary Restraining Order and Preliminary Injunction. On June 9, 1989, the Court held an evidentiary hearing on plaintiffs' request for a preliminary injunction. The Court found that the plaintiffs had failed to establish that any irreparable harm would befall either the pre-zygote or the Yorks during the relatively short period of time required to bring this matter to trial. Accordingly, the Court denied the Motion for Preliminary Injunction.

The plaintiffs' Complaint in this matter is in four counts: breach of contract (Count I); quasi-contract (Count II); detinue (Count III) and 42 U.S.C. § 1983

(Count IV). The plaintiffs seek declaratory, injunctive and compensatory relief . . .

The plaintiffs have made the following factual allegations in their Complaint. The plaintiffs were married in 1983 and have been attempting to achieve a pregnancy since 1984. Because of damage to Mrs. York's remaining Fallopian tube, the Yorks are unable to achieve a pregnancy through normal coital reproduction. The plaintiffs were advised that through *in vitro* fertilization, plaintiffs would be able to become the parents of their own genetic child . . . In the spring of 1986, plaintiffs consulted with Drs. Jones and Kreiner at the Jones Institute in Norfolk, Virginia in order to determine whether they were viable candidates for the *in vitro* fertilization (IVF) program, known as the Vital Initiation of Pregnancy (VIP) program. The Yorks were accepted into the IVF program and signed VIP Consent Form No. 6B . . . Consent Form 6B stated, and Dr. Kreiner assured the Yorks, that the expectation of pregnancy is about 20 percent after the transfer of one fertilized mature egg, about 28 percent after the transfer of two fertilized mature eggs and about 38 percent after the transfer of three fertilized mature eggs. At the time the Yorks entered the IVF program in Norfolk, they were residents of New Jersey. During the course of treatment, the Yorks moved to California.

The Yorks returned to the Jones Institute on four separate occasions to undergo the *in vitro* fertilization process . . . None of these *in vitro* fertilization attempts resulted in pregnancy. Prior to the attempt in May 1987, the plaintiffs signed a form entitled "Informed Consent: Human Pre- Zygotes Cryopreservation" (Cryopreservation Agreement) . . . The consent form outlined the procedure for cryopreservation or freezing of pre-zygotes and detailed the couple's rights in the frozen pre-zygote.

The Cryopreservation Agreement explained that the cryopreservation procedure is available in the event more than five pre-zygotes are retrieved during the IVF treatment . . . After signing the Agreement, the plaintiffs underwent the IVF process on May 17, 1987. On May 27, 1987, Dr. Kreiner removed six eggs from Mrs. York and fertilized those eggs with Dr. York's sperm, creating six embryos. On May 29, 1987, five embryos were transferred to Mrs. York's uterus. The remaining embryo, which is the subject of this litigation, was cryogenically preserved in accordance with the procedures outlined in the Cryopreservation Agreement.

In May of 1988, a year after the pre-zygote was frozen, the Yorks sought to have the pre-zygote transferred from the Jones Institute in Norfolk, Virginia to the Institute for Reproductive Research at the Hospital of the Good Samaritan in Los Angeles, California. At the Los Angeles clinic, Dr. Richard Marrs would thaw the embryo and insert it in Mrs. York through *in vitro* fertilization.[12] The plaintiffs consulted two embryologists to arrange for proper cryogenic support in order to successfully transport the embryo. The plaintiffs planned to have Dr. York personally retrieve the embryo from Norfolk and transport it to California by

---

[12] Is the court's terminology correct? In vitro fertilization refers to the fertilization of an egg by a sperm "in glass" or in a laboratory petri dish. The procedure the court is referring to is embryo transfer, which takes place about three days after the embryo has formed. Typically, embryos are grown in the laboratory for three days until they reach the eight-cell stage. At that point, they are either transferred into a woman's uterus or frozen for later use. -Ed.

commercial airliner. The pre-zygote would be housed in a biological dry shipper during the flight.

On May 28, 1988, the Yorks wrote Dr. Muasher and indicated their intent to retrieve and transfer the pre-zygote. By letter dated June 13, 1988, Dr. Muasher, writing on behalf of the Jones Institute, refused to allow such a transfer. On June 18, 1988, Dr. Richard Marrs, on behalf of the Yorks, sought consent to transfer the pre-zygote from physicians at the Jones Institute. By letter dated August 9, 1988, Dr. Jones refused to approve the transfer of the frozen pre-zygote.

Breach of Contract

The plaintiffs allege that the defendants' continued dominion and control over the frozen pre-zygote is contrary to the language of the Cryopreservation Agreement . . . The pertinent provision of the Cryopreservation Agreement provides:

> We may withdraw our consent and discontinue participation at any time without prejudice and we understand our pre-zygotes will be stored only as long as we are active IVF patients at The Howard and Georgeanna Jones Institute For Reproductive Medicine or until the end of our normal reproductive years. We have the principle responsibility to decide the disposition of our pre-zygotes. Our frozen pre-zygotes will not be released from storage for the purpose of intrauterine transfer without the written consents of us both. In the event of divorce, we understand legal ownership of any stored pre-zygotes must be determined in a property settlement and will be released as directed by order of a court of competent jurisdiction. Should we for any reason no longer wish to attempt to initiate a pregnancy, we understand we may choose one of three fates for our pre-zygotes that remain in frozen storage. Our pre-zygotes may be: 1) donated to another infertile couple (who will remain unknown to us) 2) donated for approved research investigation 3) thawed but not allowed to undergo further development.

The defendants argue that plaintiffs' proprietary rights in the pre-zygote are limited to the "three fates" enumerated in this provision because there is no established protocol for the inter-institutional transfer of pre-zygotes.

The Court begins its analysis by noting that the Cryopreservation Agreement created a bailor-bailee relationship between the plaintiffs and defendants. While the parties in this case expressed no intent to create a bailment, under Virginia law, no formal contract or actual meeting of the minds is necessary. *Morris v. Hamilton*, 225 Va. 372, 302 S.E.2d 51, 52 (1983). Rather, all that is needed "is the element of lawful possession however created, and duty to account for the thing as the property of another that creates the bailment. . . ." *Crandall v. Woodard*, 206 Va. 321, 143 S.E.2d 923, 927 (1965). The essential nature of a bailment relationship imposes on the bailee, when the purpose of the bailment has terminated, an absolute obligation to return the subject matter of the bailment to the bailor. 8 Am.Jur.2d Bailments § 178 (1980). The obligation to return the property is implied from the fact of lawful possession of the personal property of another. Id.

In the instant case, the requisite elements of a bailment relationship are present.

It is undisputed that the Jones Institutes' possession of the pre-zygote was lawful pursuant to the Cryopreservation Agreement. The defendants also recognized their duty to account for the pre-zygote by virtue of a paragraph in the Cryopreservation Agreement purporting to disclaim liability for any injury to the pre-zygote. Finally, the defendants consistently refer to the pre-zygote as the "property" of the Yorks in the Cryopreservation Agreement. Although the Cryopreservation Agreement constitutes a bailment contract, the Agreement is nevertheless governed by the same principles as apply to other contracts . . .

The Court notes the Cryopreservation Agreement should be more strictly construed against the defendants, the parties who drafted the Agreement. *Winn v. Aleda Construction Co.*, 227 Va. 304, 315 S.E.2d 193, 195 (1984). The defendants have defined the extent of their possession interest as bailee of the pre-zygote by the following provision of the Agreement: "We may withdraw our consent and discontinue participation at any time without prejudice and we understand our pre-zygote will be stored only as long as we are active IVF patients at the [Jones Institute] . . . ." The testimony at the hearing on plaintiffs' Motion for Temporary Injunction and the briefs submitted by the plaintiffs make it clear that plaintiffs wish to terminate their relationship with the Jones Institute and continue treatment at the fertility clinic in Los Angeles, California.

The defendants have further defined the limits of their possessory interest by recognizing the plaintiffs' proprietary rights in the pre-zygote. The Agreement repeatedly refers to "our pre-zygote," and explicitly provides that in the event of a divorce, the legal ownership of the pre-zygote "must be determined in a property settlement" by a court of competent jurisdiction. The Agreement further provides that the plaintiffs have "the principal responsibility to decide the disposition" of the pre-zygote and that the pre-zygote will not be released from storage without the written consent of both plaintiffs. The Court finds that the inference to be drawn from these provisions of the Cryopreservation Agreement is that the defendants fully recognize plaintiffs' property rights in the pre-zygote and have limited their rights as bailee to exercise dominion and control over the pre-zygote.

The defendants take the position that the plain language of the Cryopreservation Agreement limits the plaintiffs' proprietary right to the pre-zygote to the "three fates" listed in the Agreement: (1) donation to another infertile couple; (2) donation for approved research; and (3) thawing. The Court finds, however, that the applicability of the three fates is limited by the following language, "Should we [the Yorks] for any reason no longer wish to initiate a pregnancy, we understand we may choose one of three fates for our pre-zygotes that remain in frozen storage." The allegations of plaintiffs' Complaint, and the entire thrust of this litigation, suggest that plaintiffs continue to desire to achieve pregnancy. The Agreement does not state that the attempt to initiate a pregnancy is restricted to procedures employed at the Jones Institute. The "three fates" are therefore inapplicable to the case at bar.

For the reasons stated herein, the Court finds that Count I of plaintiffs' Complaint states a claim upon which relief can be granted. Count II is pled in the alternative alleging an action based on quasi-contract. Accordingly, defendants' Motion to Dismiss Counts I and II are DENIED . . .

[The Court also denies defendants' Motion to Dismiss Counts III and IV.]

IT IS SO ORDERED.

NOTES AND QUESTIONS

1. Why did Drs. Jones and Muasher refuse to allow the Yorks' frozen embryo to be transported to California? If the Virginia doctors were worried about damage to the embryo in transport, would a release signed by the Yorks absolving the doctors of any and all liability, have persuaded them to relent on their refusal?

2. If the Yorks had received treatment in New Orleans, rather than Norfolk, would the Louisiana doctors been permitted under state law to release and transport the cryopreserved embryo to another state? To another clinic within the state borders? The relevant law in Louisiana provides:

> An in vitro fertilized human ovum is a biological human being which is not the property of the physician which acts as an agent of fertilization, or the facility which employs him or the donors of the sperm and ovum. If the in vitro fertilization patients express their identity, then their rights as parents as provided under the Louisiana Civil Code will be preserved. If the in vitro fertilization patients fail to express their identity, then the physician shall be deemed to be temporary guardian of the in vitro fertilized human ovum until adoptive implantation can occur. A court in the parish where the in vitro fertilized ovum is located may appoint a curator, upon motion of the in vitro fertilization patients, their heirs, or physicians who caused in vitro fertilization to be performed, to protect the in vitro fertilized human ovum's rights.

La. Rev. Stat. § 9:126. Is it possible for an embryo to be considered abandoned in Louisiana? How long must the IVF patients "fail to express their identity" before "adoptive implantation" can occur?

PROBLEM

The Missouri Reproductive Center (MRC) is an ART provider located near St. Louis. During the 1990s and early 2000s MRC had a large patient base, providing IVF and cryopreservation services to hundreds of patients. In 2007 the Center's business started to decline due in large measure to a competing clinic that opened in the same area. By 2012, MRC was forced to declare bankruptcy and close its doors. The Center contacted all of its patients who had embryos in frozen storage. Most patients arranged to have their embryos transferred to another storage facility, but 20 patients did not respond to the many attempts MRC made to alert the couples to their bankrupt status. These same 20 couples have failed to pay their annual storage fees for at least two years, and have been out of touch with MRC for an equal length of time.

The medical director of MRC, Dr. Baldwin, has been told by the bankruptcy trustee that the facility will be locked and all power will be turned off in 30 days. This includes the electricity that powers the fill mechanism on the liquid nitrogen tanks, risking the possibility that the tanks will warm to room temperature and thaw the embryos contained therein. Dr. Baldwin has contacted every fertility clinic in the state to ask for assistance, but each facility has been unwilling to take in the embryos, claiming an inability to absorb the costs of long-term storage. What are Dr. Baldwin's alternatives at this point? How would you advise him to proceed?

Chapter 8

REGULATING REPRODUCTIVE TECHNOLOGIES

The provision of ART services has at its core the practice of medicine, an activity largely relegated to the auspices of state government. States regulate the practice of medicine, including the practice of reproductive medicine, in a variety of ways, including licensure of physicians and certification of hospitals and other medical facilities. While ART bears similarities to other medical practices in which drugs are prescribed or surgeries are administered to correct bodily malfunctions, the practice of assisted conception raises unique scenarios that often fall outside the ambit of routine regulatory schemes. For this reason, regulating the practice of reproductive medicine is a complex and often controversial task. Laws that dictate the ways in which a physician can treat an infertile patient can affect the patient's reproductive autonomy, on the rights of third parties who act as gamete donors or gestational carriers, and on the health and well-being of children born of the proposed treatment. The myriad individuals affected by the practice of reproductive medicine has produced a cacophony of viewpoints and strategies on how to best serve the physicians, patients and children of ART.

The world of ART regulation is seen through many lenses. Physicians who must comply with reporting and disclosure requirements that are unique to reproductive medicine may view these obligations as unnecessary, even oppressive and discriminatory, while some patient advocates see ART as an unregulated, laissez-faire practice best described as "the wild west of medicine."[1] Whether ART regulation is truly on the frontier or under the tight control of regulators will be left to your judgment. To make that judgment, you will need to know who can, who has, and who might regulate the practice of ART medicine. A layout of the current regulatory scheme, its supporters and critics, will guide you along the way.

---

[1] Even more colorful phraseology has been used to describe the regulation of ART. Brooks A. Keel, professor of obstetrics and gynecology and associate dean for research at the University of Kansas School of Medicine in Wichita proffered, "A woman gets more regulatory oversight when she gets a tattoo than when she gets IVF." R. Alta Charo, a professor of law at the University of Wisconsin and a member of President Clinton's National Bioethics Advisory Commission put it this way, "We have in many respects far better protections for hamsters than for human fertility patients." Rick Weiss, *Fertility Innovation or Exploitation? Regulatory Void Allows for Trial — and Error — Without Patient Disclosure Rules*, WASH. POST, Feb. 9, 1998, at A1.

SECTION I: THE LEGAL LANDSCAPE FOR ART: AN INTRODUCTION

A. The Goals of Regulation

Judith F. Daar
Regulating Reproductive Technologies: Panacea or Paper Tiger?
34 Hous. L. Rev. 609, 637-8 (1997)

The term "regulation" raises the specter of the imposition of laws or legal infrastructures on the interaction between and among targeted actors. The field of reproductive medicine is comprised of two categories of actors — providers of reproductive services, including physicians and their support staff, and consumers, including patients and their support network. This network can include spouses and significant others, as well as third parties willing to assist in the reproduction process such as egg donors or womb donors, a.k.a. surrogate mothers. The juxtaposition of providers and consumers provides opportunity for regulation to occur at three levels. First, regulation can focus exclusively on the providers who render the ART services. Regulation in this area might include licensure of ART personnel, certification of ART facilities, reporting requirements for all aspects of initiated procedures, including patient demographics and pregnancy success rates, and standardization of clinical techniques. The goal behind regulation aimed at providers would be to assure quality and uniformity in the practice of reproductive medicine.

Regulating practitioners could also mean limiting the availability of certain ART techniques, or restricting ART to certain patient populations. For example, lawmakers could conclude that because invasive modalities such as IVF and GIFT have a low success rate among women over age forty, doctors should be prohibited from offering these services to older patients. Regulation aimed at achieving this degree of social control is most unlikely to appear given our country's laissez-faire approach to procreative and medical decision-making. Additionally, reproductive medicine doctors would be in the right to question why their practices should be subject to intensive scrutiny and regulation, while their colleagues in other specialties face no such oversight.

Second, regulation can be geared at the relationship between providers and consumers. These laws would focus primarily on the interaction between doctors and patients. For example, state laws could be drafted to require word-specific, written informed consent for any ART procedure. Or laws could be designed to sanction misconduct in the practice of reproductive medicine, such as egg or embryo theft. This body of regulation would be geared toward creating and maintaining a fair, open, and balanced relationship between doctors and patients.

And third, regulation could focus strictly on the rights and obligations of patients and other parties availing themselves of ART services. These laws would speak, for example, to the familial status of children born of ART or to the validity of contracts between and among these parties . . .

NOTES AND QUESTIONS

1.   The regulation of an industry as large and diverse as the infertility industry will necessarily take on many different facets and goals. Professor Daar suggests viewing the regulation of ART in relational terms — regulations can be aimed at the relationship between practitioners and a high quality of care, between practitioners and patients, and between patients and third parties who assist in conception. This third category has already been addressed in Chapter 3, looking at the statutes and case law governing the rights and liabilities of gamete donors and gestational carriers, and Chapter 5, which reviews the parentage of ART offspring in the context of existing family laws. The goal herein is to evaluate the first two categories by investigating the structures and rules that govern the provision of ART services to patients.

What are the ways in which the law could interact with the practice of reproductive medicine? If you were a physician, how could the law assist you in providing high-quality medical services to your patients? If you were a patient, how could the law aid you in obtaining the best possible infertility treatment?

2.   *Defining Regulatory Goals.* Regulatory schemes are often constructed to achieve a set of desired goals. Professor Helen Alvare suggests that existing ART laws can be characterized as attempts to fulfill the following goals:

> . . . to facilitate transactions in gametes and embryos by allowing the reassignment of parental rights from biological donors to intending parent(s); to prevent the transmission of some diseases; to prevent fraud on customers and promote truth in advertising; and to provide some protection for human embryos.

Helen M. Alvare, *The Case for Regulating Collaborative Reproduction: A Children's Rights Perspective*, 40 HARV. J. LEG. 1 (2003). Other commentators have suggested that the primary goal of ART regulation should be to promote and ensure the safety and effectiveness of the medical technologies utilized, with an eye toward the health of both patients and children. *See, e.g.,* Yaniv Heled, *The Regulation of Genetic Aspects of Donated Reproductive Tissue: The Need for Federal Regulation*, 11 COL. SCI. & TECH. L. REV. 243(2010) (urging the Food and Drug Administration to create a regulatory framework requiring screening and testing of reproductive tissue donors for genetic diseases); Lars Noah, *Assisted Reproductive Technologies and the Pitfalls of Unregulated Biomedical Innovation*, 55 FLA. L. REV. 603 (2003) (calling on the FDA to consider restricting or withdrawing fertility drugs used to induce ovulation due to the high number of multiple pregnancies, which pose harm to women and offspring); Jennifer L. Rosato, *The Children of ART (Assisted Reproductive Technology): Should the Law Protect Them From Harm?*, 57 UTAH L. REV. 57, 62 (2004) (advocating a system of state and federal reform whose "overall goal would be to provide the children of ART needed protection from known harms."). What goals do you believe ART regulation should seek to achieve? Are any of these goals mutually exclusive, in that one can only be achieved at the expense of the other? If so, how would you prioritize your goals?

3.   *Stakeholder Views on Regulation.* Interestingly, if not ironically, published literature suggests that the two groups most affected by government regulation of

ART — doctors and patients — both disfavor additional regulatory action by lawmakers. The physicians' view is gleaned from a survey conducted by the American Association for the Advancement of Science (AAAS). In 2002, the AAAS surveyed some 370 fertility clinics to solicit their views about the possibility of additional oversight by one federal agency, the Food and Drug Administration. The respondents overwhelmingly disfavored additional oversight, citing a number of reasons for this view. Several clinics feared the FDA's intervention would compromise future health benefits for patients by imposing unnecessary restraint on the progress of medical science. Others questioned the agency's competence to regulate fertility clinics, declaring that the "FDA's expertise in this particular area is nonexistent." Many of the clinics were in agreement that existing self-regulation by fertility professionals was sufficient to maintain high ethical and clinical practice in the field. See Mark S. Frankel, *A View from the Field on Food and Drug Administration Regulation: Report of a 2002 Survey of U.S. Fertility Clinics*, 79 FERTILITY & STERILITY 1060 (2003) (concluding the survey responses reflect "deep scorn" for the FDA).

The fact that physicians shun additional regulation is hardly surprising, but one might expect to see patients welcoming government intervention aimed at protecting their health and that of their offspring. But at least one statement from the nation's oldest and largest organization representing individuals with infertility, RESOLVE, suggests that patients strongly disfavor increased regulation and oversight by government authorities. In a letter dated October 2, 2003 to the President's Council on Bioethics,[2] RESOLVE responded to the Council's draft recommendations to ratchet up federal regulation. The infertility group noted "no widespread consumer outcry for increased scrutiny" of ART, and "no groundswell of discontent from infertile patients that they lack the necessary information to make informed decisions about building their families with medical help." Instead, the patient group perceived additional reporting and disclosure requirements as "an example of ART being singled out from other medical treatments . . . while the [additional] requirements will increase clinics' administrative costs and therefore raise the cost of obtaining infertility treatment." Finally, RESOLVE bristled at the prospect of government interference with the private area of reproduction, concluding, "Proposals that would outlaw family building treatments for many individuals and couples desirous of having children do not advance dignity or accord the respect." Vicki Baldwin, Chair of the Board of Directors, RESOLVE, in letter to Leon R. Kass, Chair of the President's Council on Bioethics.

If doctors and patients oppose increased regulation, should lawmakers continue to pursue methods of increased oversight and administration of fertility practices? Are there any other interests that could be served by increased regulation?

---

[2] The President's Council on Bioethics was an executive level advisory panel created by President George W. Bush on November 28, 2001, by means of Executive Order 13237. In 2002, the Council took up the topic of ART regulation, in which it accepted public comment on a series of published draft recommendations. The Council issued its final report in March 2004 entitled, "Reproduction and Responsibility: The Regulation of New Biotechnologies." The President Bush-appointed Council was disbanded by President Barack Obama in June 2009. In November 2009, President Obama signed Executive Order 13521 establishing his own Presidential Commission for the Study of Bioethical Issues. Information about presidential bioethics commissions can be found at www.bioethics.gov.

B. The Current State of Regulation

Before delving into the substance of our current regulatory scheme governing ART, we pause to take note of the depth and diversity of action and approaches that government intervention can take. As noted by the President's Council on Bioethics in its report on ART regulation:

> [I]t is necessary to bear in mind the range and variety of activities that may be properly deemed regulation for purposes of this inquiry. Regulation comes in myriad forms, from various sources, with widely differing results. Regulation can include a variety of mechanisms, ranging from legal prohibition and statutory obligations to mere monitoring and data collection. Methods of enforcement range from criminal prosecution to mere hortatory suggestion. Even information-gathering can serve as a kind of cautionary regulatory function. It signals to practitioners in the field that society is paying attention and has a stake in the underlying activity. In addition, the source of regulation can be governmental (with the coercive power of the state as the principal mechanism for implementation) or nongovernmental (where market forces and peer evaluation are the chief means of implementation).

President's Council on Bioethics, *Reproduction and Responsibility: The Regulation of New Biotechnologies* 11 (2004). With this caveat in mind, the Council goes on to classify the current regulatory landscape of ART as a "patchwork, with authority divided among numerous sources of oversight." *Id.* at 75. Those sources can be roughly divided into five categories: 1) direct regulation by the federal government, 2) indirect regulation by the federal government, 3) direct regulation by state governments, 4) indirect regulation by state governments, and 5) self-regulation by the fertility industry. A brief description of each category follows.

1. Direct Regulation by the Federal Government

The only federal law to directly and explicitly regulate the provision of infertility services is The Fertility Clinic Success Rate and Certification Act of 1992, 42 U.S.C. § 263a-1 et seq., ("the Act"). The Act was born out of a concern that fertility clinics were misleading prospective patients about pregnancy success rates in an era when reporting of such data was completely voluntary.[3] The Act contains two essential components. First, the Act requires standardized reporting of pregnancy success rates to the Secretary of Health and Human Services through the CDC, which data is in turn made available to the public. The goal of the Act's reporting provisions is to provide consumers with reliable and accurate information about individual clinics'

---

[3] The bill which became the Fertility Clinic Success Rate and Certification Act was introduced into the 102d Congress by Representative Ron Wyden (D-Oregon) as H.R. 3940. The hearings on the bill featured witnesses who testified to the misleading advertising practices employed by some fertility clinics. Congressman Henry Waxman (D-California), Chair of the House Subcommittee on Health and the environment, noted that couples are often misled about ART success rates because some clinics use criteria such as the number of eggs retrieved, number of eggs fertilized, or number of embryo transfers to tout success, rather than the number of live births. To combat such deception, the Act was designed to standardize reporting. See Fertility Clinic Services: Hearing before Subcomm. on Health and the Env't of the House Comm. On energy and Commerce, 102 Cong., 2d Sess. 1-2.

pregnancy and "take home baby" success rates. As a result of the Act, the vast majority of ART clinics in the U.S. annually report their success rates and a host of other data to the CDC which publishes a comprehensive report detailing national statistics, as well as specific information about each reporting clinic. See Centers for Disease Control, 2009 Assisted Reproductive Technologies Success Rates: National Summary and Fertility Clinics Reports, National Summary Table (2011), available at http://www.cdc.gov/art/. (The 2009 data is not available until 2011 because surveyors must wait for 9 months after the December 2009 cycles have been administered to calculate the number of babies born as a result of treatment provided in calendar year 2009.).

One criticism of the Act's reporting requirement is the lack of any real penalty surrounding nonreporting. If a clinic fails to report, the Act simply requires that the name of the nonreporting clinic be included in the annual report. This "shaming" technique is drawn from Section 263a-5 of the Act:

> The Secretary, through the Centers for Disease Control, shall not later than 3 years after October 24, 1992, and annually thereafter publish and distribute to the States and the public —
>
> (1) (A) pregnancy success rates reported to the Secretary under section 263a-1(a)(1) of this title and, in the case of an assisted reproductive technology program which failed to report one or more success rates as required under such section, the name of each such program and each pregnancy success rate which the program failed to report.

42 U.S.C. § 236a-5. On average, about 10% of all U.S. fertility clinics do not report their success rates to the CDC, and thus find themselves listed as nonreporters in the annual report. Query how the CDC is aware that a clinic is providing service if it fails to report its clinical outcomes to the federal authorities? One way may be by clinic patients who contact the CDC, as per the agency's request set out in the annual report. "Consumers who are aware of a clinic that was in operation in [year of report] but is not included in the lists of either reporting or nonreporting clinics in this report are encouraged to contact us with the complete name, mailing address, and telephone number of the clinic" entreats the CDC. Alas, nonreporters beware your well-informed and civic-minded consumers.

A second part of the Act empowers the CDC to develop a model program for certification of embryo laboratories that can be adopted by each state. The CDC issued the final version of the model certification program in 1999, but to date no state has adopted the program into its regulatory scheme. Thus, federal regulation of ART can be described as an active reporting requirement and a dormant certification program.

This sparse law in the U.S. can be contrasted with comprehensive regulatory schemes in place in other countries. In the United Kingdom, for example, the provision of all ART services is regulated under the Human Fertilisation and Embryology Act ("HFEA"), which empowers a centralized agency to license and oversee every clinic that offers assisted conception. In addition to establishing a system of licensure, the HFEA authorizes limits on the provision of services to all U.K. patients. Examples of HFEA limitations include a cap on the number of embryos that can be transferred to the uterus in a single cycle, and outlawing of preimplantation genetic diagnosis for purposes of nonmedical sex selection. In March 2004 the Canadian Parliament adopted the British model with passage of the Assisted Human Reproduction Act, a comprehensive piece of legislation regulating the provision of ART services in that country. The law was challenged as exceeding the legislative authority of the Canadian Parliament to rest regulation of ART in federal, rather than provincial (state-like) hands. After six years of litigation, in December 2010 the Supreme Court of Canada struck down several key features of the law, leaving much of the regulatory authority in the hands of provincial authorities. In many ways, Canadian regulation of ART now more resembles that of its neighbor to the south rather than its mother country.

2.   Indirect Regulation by the Federal Government

Indirect regulation refers to statutes and federal agencies that are not explicitly aimed at or authorized to regulate fertility services, but that indirectly oversee or capture the practice of reproductive medicine within their jurisdiction. The most prominent example of such an indirect federal law is the Clinical Laboratories Improvement Amendments of 1988, 42 U.S.C. § 263a, ("CLIA"), providing for federal certification of clinical laboratories. CLIA applies to laboratories engaged in the "examination of materials derived from the human body" for purposes of disease diagnosis, prevention or treatment. While CLIA authorizes federal authorities to maintain quality control over clinical labs, the law is unclear as to whether it applies to embryology labs essential to IVF and other ART practices. In an effort to clarify CLIA's application to ART, in 1999 the American Board of Bioanalysis, which advocates on behalf of lab directors, brought suit to compel the Department of Health and Human Services to apply CLIA to all ART laboratories. The suit was dismissed for lack of plaintiff's standing, leaving the question of CLIA's relationship to ART unclear.

The American Society for Reproductive Medicine has since clarified CLIA's role in ART in a 2010 monograph entitled, "Oversight of Assisted Reproductive Technologies." According to ASRM, "[l]ab tests used in the diagnosis of infertility, such as semen and blood analysis, are covered by CLIA. The procedures performed in embryology labs, which are not considered diagnostic, do not fall under CLIA's mandate." Thus, much of what drives reproductive medicine — embryo formation and transfer — is not covered under federal law designed to ensure quality laboratory testing. The ASRM monograph on ART regulation can be found at http://www.asrm.org/Oversight_of_ART/.

A second federal authority that is indirectly involved with the regulation of ART is the Food and Drug Administration, an agency that regulates drugs, devices and biologics that are marketed in the U.S. The FDA is primarily responsible for ensuring the safety and efficacy of products over which it has jurisdiction. Until somewhat recently, the FDA did not insert itself into the regulation of ART, perhaps because the materials used in assisted conception are not easily defined as drugs, devices or biologics.[4] However, in 2001 that FDA announced its intent to strictly

---

[4] A biologic is defined as "any virus, therapeutic serum, toxin, anti-toxin, vaccine, blood, blood

regulate a new and controversial practice — ooplasm transfer, in which a woman's egg is injected with cytoplasm from a donor egg. Cytoplasm is the material that surrounds the egg cell nucleus (but does not include the nucleus) and can be used to "boost" the ability of older eggs to fertilize and implant in the uterus. The procedure was successful in aiding women who experienced recurrent ART failure, but became controversial when researchers discovered that children born via ooplasm transfer contained genetic material from three people — the genetic mother who supplied the egg, the genetic father who supplied the sperm, and the egg donor whose cytoplasm contained mitochondrial DNA that was passed to the babies. The FDA considered this practice a clinical investigation and required any facilities offering ooplasm transfer to submit an Investigational New Drug application to the agency, a cumbersome process that resulted in abandonment of the infertility treatment by U.S. ART clinics.

In May 2005 the FDA again extended its oversight of ART, issuing regulations that increase testing requirements for donated human tissue, including eggs and sperm. The new regulations require tissue banks to test donors and donated tissues for a host of infectious diseases including HIV, hepatitis, and syphilis. In addition, tissue banks are now required to ask donors a series of questions to determine their risk factors for particular diseases. Thus, while the new regulations are not aimed exclusively or directly at ART clinics, they do have an impact on the practice of reproductive medicine when donor gametes are used.

Finally, a third federal agency that has dabbled at the edges of ART regulation is the Federal Trade Commission. The FTC, among other tasks, is charged with promoting truth in advertising in interstate commerce. Since 1991, the FTC has won several cease-and-desist agreements over deceptive advertising claims by fertility clinics. These clinics exaggerated success rates in promotional brochures and flyers, inflating their "take home baby" rate in some instances by nearly 100%. See Trip Gabriel, *High-Tech Pregnancies Test Hope's Limit*, N.Y. TIMES, Jan 7, 1996, at 1. Presumably the Fertility Clinic Success Rate and Certification Act, which standardizes reporting of pregnancy success rates, is designed to directly address the truth in advertising problem by creating industry-wide reporting parameters.

3. Direct Regulation by State Governments

In previous Chapters we have noted a variety of state laws that have an impact on assisted conception. These laws range in scope from mandates for the provision of infertility insurance coverage (Chapter 3), to the regulation of research on embryos (Chapter 4), to the statutory responses to surrogate parenting arrangements (Chapter 5), to the plight of postmortem conception children as heirs of their parent's estate (Chapter 6), to the requirement that couples sign a contract designating the disposition of frozen embryos (Chapter 7). These statutory schemes show the breadth and scope of assisted conception's interaction with the law, as the process of conceiving, gestating, and raising a child are of the utmost concern to lawmakers striving to institute public policy protecting the welfare of society. But none of the specific laws we have studied can be considered a comprehensive scheme

---

component or derivative, allergenic product or analogous product, applicable to the prevention, treatment or cure of diseases or injuries to humans." 42 U.S.C. § 262(i).

regulating the provision of ART services — that is, the delivery of medical and other services that enable infertile individuals to procreate.

Instead, direct regulation of the provision of ART services is seen in a handful of state laws that each focus on a single aspect of the multifaceted field of assisted conception. A few of the state regulatory laws are listed below.

Louisiana imposes professional standards on all ART practitioners, requiring that all clinics and their medical directors adhere to guidelines for IVF issued by professional organizations, specifically naming the American Fertility Society (which since changed its name to the American Society for Reproductive Medicine) and the American College of Obstetricians and Gynecologists. La. Rev. Stat. Ann. § 9:128.

New Hampshire probably has the most comprehensive legislation of any state when it comes to regulating the health and safety of ART participants. State law requires all women undergoing IVF or artificial insemination, all gamete donors, and all gestational carriers to undergo a medical evaluation and be deemed "medically acceptable" before treatment can be administered. The state also requires intended parents enlisting a gestational carrier to undergo genetic counseling, if the surrogate is 35 or older. Presumably, these provisions are designed to maximize the health of the ART offspring, as well as that of the participating adults. N.H. Rev. Stat. Ann. §§ 168-B:13, 168-B:16, 168-B:19.

Pennsylvania law focuses largely on reporting by ART clinics. State law requires all ART clinics make publicly available reports on the location and personnel of each clinic, as well as the number of eggs fertilized, discarded and implanted at any given site. This statute is part of the state's abortion statute and is presumably contained therein to monitor the disposition of embryos in the reproductive medicine setting. 18 Pa. Cons. Stat. Ann. § 3213(e).

Virginia law explores informed consent, requiring all ART patients to sign a disclosure form indicating the treating clinic's success rate for the particular procedure the patient is undergoing. The statute specifies the information that each clinic must provide, including pregnancy rates and rates of live births per treatment cycle. The law does not require that physicians disclose the risks, benefits and alternatives of treatment, the traditional calculus comprising medical informed consent, though presumably such disclosure would be required under other state law provisions. Va. Code Ann. § 54.1-2971.1.

4. Indirect Regulation by State Governments

At its core, the provision of ART services is the practice of medicine. As such, it is subjected to the same regulatory schemes that oversee the practice of medicine generally. State law plays an important, almost exclusive, role in regulating the practice of medicine and thus, indirectly regulates the practice of reproductive medicine.

States regulate the practice of medicine in two broad ways: 1) by a network of licensing and credentialing requirements, and 2) by tort law. The first of these categories arises from the state's police power, which enables state governments to protect the health, safety and general welfare of its citizens. States regulate the practice of medicine by, for example, requiring physicians to be licensed by state medical boards; these boards are authorized to discipline doctors who violate quality standards of care or commit unprofessional acts. In addition, states are involved in credentialing (also referred to as "accrediting") hospitals, clinics, and other health care facilities to ensure that the delivery of health care services is of the highest possible quality.

Credentialing, however, is often linked to the health care facility's ability to receive funds from the federal government through its Medicare program. Since Medicare generally covers individuals aged 65 and older, typically ART clinics do not receive such funds. However, the annual report by the CDC on the status of ART clinics reveals that a substantial number of U.S. clinics do receive accreditation by one or more credentialing authorities, including the prominent Joint Commission on Accreditation of Healthcare Organizations. In 2009, for example, 93% of all U.S. ART laboratories were accredited. See Centers for Disease Control, 2009 Assisted Reproductive Technologies Success Rates: National Summary and Fertility Clinics Reports, National Summary Table (2011), available at http://www.cdc.gov/art/ ARTReports.htm.

State tort law is largely the product of private litigation. Patients who are aggrieved by the acts and omissions of their doctors can access relief by instituting lawsuits seeking money damages. Appellate courts that review these cases help shape the common law rules that set standards of care for activities such as the practice of medicine. If an ART patient is unhappy with the treatment she received, she can file suit against her doctor and clinic for such state law claims as negligence, misrepresentation, fraud, and lack of informed consent. The ability of the tort system to effectively regulate the fertility industry is much debated, with some arguing that the imposition of damage awards and the threat of litigation incentivize physicians to deliver quality care, while others see malpractice litigation having little deterrent effect on medical incompetency. *Compare* John A. Robertson, *Assisted Reproductive Technology and the Family*, 47 HAST. L.J. 911, 921 (1996) ("The current system of malpractice law, medical licensure, and professional standards, despite its defects, already provides some incentives to assure good, quality care, and it can easily be modified to provide more.") *with* Lars Noah, *Assisted Reproductive Technologies and the Pitfalls of Unregulated Biomedical Innovation*, 55 FLA. L. REV. 603, 634 (2003) (describing the threat of tort liability as "clumsy," having "at best a fairly modest deterrent effect").

The impact of tort litigation on the practice of medicine has been widely debated, with central themes focusing on whether private lawsuits improve patient safety, reduce medical error or establish appropriate standards of care. One oft-expressed concern is that the ease of filing private lawsuits causes doctors to practice "defensive medicine." The practice of defensive medicine means that doctors order more tests and consult more subspecialists than is medically optimal for the patient in order to protect themselves from legal liability. Survey data bears out this relationship between patient access to the legal system and physician behavior. In a 2009 survey of obstetricians and gynecologists, 60% responded they had made one or more changes to their practices as a result of the risk or fear of professional liability claims or litigation. *See* Jeffrey Klagholz and Albert L. Strunk, *2009 ACOG Survey on Professional Liability Results*, available at: http://www.acog.org/

departments/dept_notice.cfm?recno=4&bulletin=4899.

The percentage of physicians who self-report practicing defensive medicine is even higher in other fields, with 93% of some subspecialists confirming their behavior is affected by the threat of litigation. *See* David M. Studdert, Michelle M. Mello, William M. Sage, *Defensive Medicine Among High-Risk Specialist Physicians in a Volatile Malpractice Environment*, 293 JAMA 2609 (2005) (noting doctors in fields like ob/gyn, emergency medicine, neurosurgery and others reported a rate of 93% for practice of defensive medicine). While debate continues over whether the practice of defensive medicine improves or reduces the quality of patient care, it seems reasonable to conclude that private lawsuits affect physician behavior as much, if not more, than formal regulation and industry guidelines.

What would the practice of defensive medicine entail in ART? Do you think infertility specialists are more concerned about being sued for transferring too many embryos and producing a multiple pregnancy or transferring too few embryos and producing no pregnancy?

5. Self-Regulation by the Fertility Industry

The major ART industry group to regulate the provision of ART services is the American Society for Reproductive Medicine (ASRM), and its affiliate organization the Society for Assisted Reproductive Technology (SART), based in Birmingham, Alabama. The ASRM is a voluntary professional organization, founded in 1944, whose mission statement provides:

> ASRM is a multidisciplinary organization for the advancement of the art, science, and practice of reproductive medicine. The Society accomplishes its mission through the pursuit of excellence in education and research and through advocacy on behalf of patients, physicians, and affiliated health care providers. The Society is committed to supporting and sponsoring educational activities for the lay public and continuing medical education activities for professionals who are engaged in the practice of and research in reproductive medicine.

Available at www.asrm.org. To fulfill its mission, ASRM publishes the work of its several committees, including the Practice Committee (suggesting guidelines for ART practices, including the number of embryos transferred in IVF, gamete and embryo donation, egg and embryo cryopreservation, ICSI, and PGD), and the Ethics Committee (assessing and making recommendations on newly emerging ethical dilemmas in ART such as the use of sex selection, the disclosure to offspring of their conception via gamete donation and the provision of services to HIV-infected individuals.). ASRM requires that all its members comply with all the organization's standards issued through its committees. Compliance is monitored through an on-site validation process, conducted in conjunction with the CDC and its annual survey of ART clinic statistics (described above in Section 1, Direct Regulation by the Federal Government).

The problem with self-regulation, it can be argued, is the lack of any real enforcement if suggested guidelines are not followed. Professor Jennifer Rosato summarizes the problem as follows:

[T]he current system of self-regulation does not effectively curtail harmful and unethical ART practices . . . [E]xisting enforcement mechanisms are ineffective. On-site validations of laboratories only occur every three years, which is too infrequent to assess practices in such a quickly evolving field. Further, compliance with the standards is voluntary and not every program is a member of ASRM. The penalty for noncompliance is removal from group membership, but violators are still free to offer services to willing parents. As a result, non-reporters can still build a lucrative fertility practice without any effective oversight.

Jennifer L. Rosato, *The Children of ART (Assisted Reproductive Technology): Should the Law Protect Them From Harm?*, 57 UTAH L. REV. 57, 67-8 (2004).

ART self-regulation in general and the ASRM guidelines on embryo transfer limits in particular came under intense scrutiny in early 2009 when Nadya Suleman, dubbed the so-called "Octomom" gave birth to octuplets following IVF in which 12 embryos were transferred. Ms. Suleman's physician, Michael Kamrava, was eventually stripped of his medical license by the California Medical Board and expelled from ASRM for violating the Society's practice standards (which advised patients' in Ms. Suleman's age group receive 1-2 embryos per transfer). *See* Rita Rubin, *"Octomom" Doctor Expelled From Fertility Group*, USA TODAY, Oct. 19, 2009, available at: http://www.usatoday.com/news/health/2009-10-18-octomom-doctor-fertility_N.htm. Do these measures strike you as a sufficient response to Dr. Kamrava's clear violation of industry standards? Would it matter to you to know that Ms. Suleman fully supported her physician throughout his legal ordeals?

NOTES AND QUESTIONS

1. *ART Across the Pond.* The lack of comprehensive regulation in the U.S. is often contrasted with the British system, in which a single governmental agency, the Human Fertilisation and Embryology Authority (HFEA), regulates assisted reproduction in the United Kingdom. The HFEA inspects and licenses all UK clinics providing IVF, donor insemination or the storage of eggs, sperm or embryos. Similar to the ASRM, the HFEA publishes a Code of Practice which gives guidelines about the proper conduct of ART activities, but unlike the voluntary professional organization, the HFEA has authority to revoke the licenses of clinics whose practices fall outside the scope of licensed activities.

Could a governmental authority such as the HFEA exist and flourish in the U.S.? Are there other models of comprehensive federal regulatory authority in the U.S. that policymakers could look to in forming such a body? Are there differences between the U.S. and the UK that might impede comprehensive oversight of the type that has seemingly worked well across the pond for more than two decades (the HFEA was established in 1991 following the passage of the Human Fertilisation and Embryology Act of 1990)? For a proposal that the U.S. create a federal entity similar to the British HFEA, *see* Erik Parens & Lori P. Knowles, *Reprogenetics and Public Policy: Reflections and Recommendations*, 33 HAST. CEN. RPT. S1 (July 2003) (proposing a federal Reprogenetics Technologies Board with authority for policy-making and licensing).

2. *Modern Calls for Comprehensive Reform.* The legal and bioethical literature is rich with debate over the state of ART regulation. Some scholars take a directed approach, setting forth specific reforms in particular areas. *See, e.g.*, Deborah Spar & Anna M. Harrington, *Building a Better Baby Business*, 10 MINN. J.L. SCI. & TECH. 41 (2009) (suggesting four reforms, including increased access to clinic information, registration of gamete donor identities and increased insurance coverage for IVF). Other authors take a broad approach, suggesting systemic reforms to the provision and monitoring of ART. For example, one comprehensive proposal reads as follows:

> What we propose consists of a set of ethical guiding principles, a series of prohibited and regulated activities, and a new regulatory institution. In the enabling legislation, Congress would spell out the ethical principles it considers indispensable to inform the operation of the newly established regulatory agency, identify which activities should be taken off the table up front and which can be performed under suitable regulatory oversight, and establish in some detail the structure of the new regulatory institution.

Franco Furger & Francis Fukuyama, *A Proposal for Modernizing the Regulation of Human Biotechnologies*, 37 HAST. CEN. RPT. 16 (2007). *See also* Naomi R. Cahn, Test Tube Families: Why the Fertility Market Needs Legal Regulation (2009). Still other writers argue the current patchwork of direct, indirect and self-regulation are sufficiently protective of ART stakeholder interests. *See, e.g.*, John A. Robertson, *The Virtues of Muddling Through*, 37 HASTINGS CEN. RPT. 29 (2007) (advocating allowing "our mixed public-private regulatory system, with its strong common law tradition, handle [ART] nonsystematically, as it has for years"); Judith Daar, *Federalizing Embryo Transfers: Taming the Wild West of Reproductive Medicine*, 23 COLUMBIA J. GENDER & L. 257 (2012) (rejecting calls for a federal law limiting embryo transfers in response to the Octomom births).

3. *Drafting Challenges.* Lawmakers often face a difficult balancing act when trying to draft regulatory legislation. On the one hand, the regulation needs to be sufficiently detailed and comprehensive to avoid unwanted conduct escaping the statute's reaches, but at the same time the scheme should avoid overreaching into unintended areas, thus disrupting legitimate practices in its wake.

To evaluate this problem of balance, let us review one state's approach to ART regulation, the New Hampshire statute mentioned above. The New Hampshire law on "In Vitro Fertilization and Preembyo Transfer," provides in relevant part:

> In vitro fertilization and preembryo transfer shall be performed in accordance with rules adopted by the department of health and human services and shall be available only to a woman:

> I. Who is 21 years of age or older;

> II. Who has been medically evaluated and the results, documented in accordance with rules adopted by the department of health and human services, demonstrate the medical acceptability of the woman to undergo the in vitro fertilization or preembryo transfer procedure;

III. Who receives counseling pursuant to RSA 168-B:18, and provides written certification of the counseling and evaluation to the health care provider performing the in vitro fertilization or preembryo transfer procedure; and

IV. Whose husband, if the recipient is married, receives appropriate counseling, pursuant to RSA 168-B:18, and:

(a) Successfully completes the medical evaluation, if he is the gamete donor in the in vitro fertilization or preembryo transfer procedure;

(b) Provides written certification of the nonmedical counseling and any evaluation to the health care provider performing the in vitro fertilization or preembryo transfer procedure; and

(c) Indicates, by a writing, acceptance of the legal rights and responsibilities of parenthood for any resulting child, unless the husband contributes his sperm for the in vitro fertilization or preembryo transfer procedure.

N.H. Rev. Stat. § 168-B:13. What purpose does this statute serve? Does it advance the state's interest in protecting the health, safety and welfare of the people of New Hampshire? If you were a person experiencing infertility in, say, Concord (the state's capital) you could receive treatment in the state's only ART clinic, located in Lebanon (near Dartmouth College), or you could travel the same 60-ish miles to access several facilities in the Boston area. If the travel time were the same to the New Hampshire and Massachusetts clinics, which would you chose? Would the fact that Massachusetts has no law requiring medical and other counseling in order to access ART services be meaningful to you?

If you were a physician licensed to practice medicine in both New Hampshire and Massachusetts, in which state would you chose to establish a practice in reproductive medicine? Does the New Hampshire law make an ART practice more or less attractive to physicians?

SECTION II: IS (INCREASED) ART REGULATION NECESSARY?

The prospect of increased regulation of any activity raises questions about benefit and harm — who will benefit from added government involvement and who may potentially be harmed by such action? Increased regulation of ART typically evokes claims that four groups will benefit if the government exercises greater oversight and control over reproductive medicine — ART patients, ART offspring, ART physicians and society.[5] The last of these groups, society, may benefit when the other three are better off, thus we can assume that any collective benefit

---

[5] A fifth group — gamete donors and gestation carriers — are also essential stakeholders in ART whose interests would be impacted by increased regulation. Regulatory efforts applied to these third-party participants are treated in Chapter 3 and Chapter 5. In particular, consider revisiting the discussion of statutory mandates to provide informed consent in advertising to egg donors (beginning at page 222) and prosecution of surrogacy agents and agencies that commit fraud or other financial malfeasances negatively impacting gestational carriers (beginning at page 437).

experienced by patients, children and doctors will inure to society at large. Let us explore the potential benefits and possible accompanying harms that could attach to increased regulation of ART from the perspective of those most likely to be affected by the reach of government authority.

A. Protecting ART Patients

Patients who undergo treatment for infertility can potentially be harmed at different stops along the road between diagnosis and the delivery of a baby. In any woman's journey, she could encounter a host of unscrupulous actors, including an ART clinic whose false advertising promoting inflated success rates draws her into the facility, a less-than-forthcoming physician who fails to inform her about the risks associated with drug-induced ovulation induction, a clinic-wide policy that does not require sperm be tested for certain genetic diseases, a nefarious laboratory technician who switches the embryos she intends to use with that of another couple, an over-eager doctor who assures her that implanting six embryos will guarantee her a successful outcome, and an absent-minded laboratory assistant who fails to refill the liquid nitrogen tanks causing the frozen embryos contained therein to thaw. How, if at all, could each of these disasters be averted by regulation?

1. Luring Patients: False Advertising and Deceptive Statements

KARLIN v. IVF AMERICA, INC.
Court of Appeals of New York
93 N.Y.2d 282, 690 N.Y.S.2d 495, 712 N.E.2d 662 (1999)

CHIEF JUDGE KAYE.

In order to ensure an honest marketplace, the General Business Law prohibits all deceptive practices, including false advertising, "in the conduct of any business, trade or commerce or in the furnishing of any service in this state" (General Business Law § 349[a]; § 350; Governor's Approval Mem., L. 1970, ch. 43, 1970 McKinney's Session Laws of N.Y., at 3074). This appeal requires us to determine whether plaintiffs can maintain an action against defendants operating an *in vitro* fertilization (IVF) program for deceptive practices and false advertising under General Business Law §§ 349 and 350, or are instead limited to a claim for medical malpractice based on lack of informed consent. We hold that plaintiffs have properly stated causes of action under these consumer protection statutes, and are not precluded from pursuing those claims because the alleged misrepresentations relate to the provision of medical services.

Facts

In 1987, plaintiffs Jayne and Kenneth R. Karlin sought evaluation and treatment from defendants' IVF program. The IVF procedure involves removal of multiple eggs from a woman's ovaries, fertilization of the eggs outside her body and transfer of the fertilized eggs to her uterus in an attempt to impregnate her (*see, Kass v. Kass*, 91 N.Y.2d 554, 557, 673 N.Y.S.2d 350, 696 N.E.2d 174). Over the course of 2 ½ years, Mrs. Karlin completed seven IVF cycles at defendants' clinic but did not become pregnant.

In 1990, the Federal Trade Commission (FTC) charged IVF America and related entities (IVF America) with deceptively advertising and promoting its program, finding the following statements typical of representations in their promotional materials:

> "1. 'LIKELY TREATMENT OUTCOMES . . . Our experience indicates that when a patient at an IVF [America] Program completes four IVF treatment cycles, the chance of giving birth is about 50%. * * * If *25* women begin a total of *100* IVF cycles . . . About *13* (or about 50%) of the women give birth to *18* babies' (emphasis in original) * * *.

> "2. '[M]ore than 28% of the couples who complete a cycle of treatment are becoming pregnant' * * *.

> "3. '[O]ne out of three couples who complete a cycle of treatment is becoming pregnant.' "

According to the FTC, these statements were misleading because women who participate in IVF America's treatment program "consisting of four IVF cycles have considerably less than a 50 percent chance of giving birth," and women who participate in IVF America's treatment program "consisting of one IVF cycle have considerably less than a 28 to 33 percent chance of becoming pregnant." By consent decree dated December 31, 1990, IVF America agreed to cease and desist from misrepresenting success rates, and also agreed in the future to disclose the basis used for calculating the percentage of patients who have become pregnant or given birth.

In February 1993, however, the ABC News program "20/20" televised an investigative report on the IVF industry in which IVF America employees were shown informing prospective patients that after four to six cycles, IVF America had pregnancy success rates "between 60 to 80 percent." The report also showed an IVF America representative telling a seminar participant that there are "[a]bsolutely not" any long-term effects of the IVF procedure. This report prompted New York City's Department of Consumer Affairs to charge IVF America with violations of the City's Consumer Protection Law. As part of a settlement reached in April 1993, IVF America agreed to refrain both from marketing its services using unsubstantiated pregnancy success rates and from stating that IVF procedures posed no adverse health risks.

The following year, plaintiffs commenced this action alleging that defendants engaged in fraudulent and misleading conduct by disseminating false success rates and misrepresenting health risks associated with IVF. In particular, plaintiffs claim that defendants "exaggerated success rates, excluding certain subsets of failed treatment procedures, emphasizing numerically false and misleading overall success rates and conceal[ing] and misrepresent[ing] significant health risks, high miscarriage rates and excessive neonatal deaths and abnormalities of infants even if a birth resulted from the treatment rendered by defendants."

Supreme Court dismissed all of plaintiffs' causes of action except those alleging unfair and deceptive trade practices in violation of General Business Law § 349, false advertising in violation of General Business Law § 350 and lack of informed consent in violation of Public Health Law § 2805-d . . . On appeal, the Appellate Division dismissed plaintiffs' General Business Law §§ 349 and 350 claims, categorically refusing to apply "the consumer fraud statutes to the providers of medical services" in order to prevent what the court perceived as "a drastic change in basic tort law where the Legislature has not explicitly expressed its intent to effect such a change" . . .

After the case returned to Supreme Court, defendants successfully moved for summary judgment on the sole remaining claim — for lack of informed consent — on the ground that it was time-barred. Plaintiffs then moved for leave to appeal to this Court, seeking review of the two earlier, nonfinal Appellate Division orders . . . [T]he Appellate Division order dismissing plaintiffs' General Business Law §§ 349 and 350 claims and affirming the dismissal of five other claims does necessarily affect the final judgment. Thus, we may review this order.

We now conclude that plaintiffs may pursue their General Business Law §§ 349 and 350 claims, and accordingly modify the Appellate Division order brought up for review and the judgment appealed from by denying defendants' motion to dismiss these two causes of action.

Analysis

Pursuant to General Business Law § 349(a), it is unlawful to perform "[d]eceptive acts or practices in the conduct of *any* business, trade or commerce or in the furnishing of *any* service in this state" (emphasis added). The scope of General Business Law § 350 is equally broad, prohibiting the promulgation of "[f]alse advertising in the conduct of *any* business, trade or commerce or in the furnishing of *any* service in this state" (emphasis added). Advertising is "false" if it "is misleading in a material respect" (General Business Law § 350-a [1]).

These statutes on their face apply to virtually all economic activity, and their application has been correspondingly broad . . .

A blanket exemption for providers of medical services and products is contrary to the plain language of the statutes. Such an exemption is also contrary to legislative history, as supporters of the consumer protection bills recognized that consumers of medical services and products might be particularly vulnerable to unscrupulous business practices . . .

Notwithstanding defendants' procrustean efforts to cast plaintiffs' deceptive acts and false advertising claims as malpractice claims for lack of informed consent, plaintiffs have clearly alleged conduct beyond the purview of Public Health Law § 2805-d [statute regulating informed consent]. Plaintiffs do not merely charge that "the person providing the professional treatment" failed to disclose certain pertinent information "to the patient" . . . Rather, they claim that defendants' "promotional materials, advertisements, slide presentations * * * and so-called 'educational' seminars" contained misrepresentations that had the effect of "deceiving and misleading members of the public." Nor are plaintiffs' claims limited, as defendants urge, to information provided by defendants "during the course of their medical treatment at the Program." On the contrary, plaintiffs assert that before they started any course of treatment, defendants "deceptively lured" plaintiffs and others, including physicians who refer patients to the IVF America programs, by "deceiving and misleading" them . . .

Defendants' alleged multi-media dissemination of information to the public is precisely the sort of consumer-oriented conduct that is targeted by General Business Law §§ 349 and 350 . . . By alleging that defendants have injured them with consumer-oriented conduct "that is deceptive or misleading in a material way," plaintiffs have stated claims under General Business Law §§ 349 and 350 even though the subject of the conduct was *in vitro* fertilization . . .

Defendants' concern that allowing plaintiffs to sue doctors for deceptive consumer practices and false advertising may cause a tidal wave of litigation against doctors is misplaced. Because plaintiffs bringing a claim under the consumer protection statutes must demonstrate an impact on consumers at large — something that a physician's treatment of an individual patient typically does not have — these statutes will not supplant traditional medical malpractice actions. Furthermore, as this Court has already observed, the possibility of excessive litigation under the consumer protection statutes is avoided by our "adoption of an objective definition of deceptive acts and practices, whether representations or omissions, limited to those likely to mislead a reasonable consumer acting reasonably under the circumstances" (*Oswego Laborers' Local 214 Pension Fund v. Marine Midland Bank, supra*, 85 N.Y.2d, at 26, 623 N.Y.S.2d 529, 647 N.E.2d 741) . . .

Accordingly, the judgment appealed from and the order of the Appellate Division brought up for review should be modified, with costs to plaintiffs, by denying defendants' motion to dismiss the first and second causes of action and, as so modified, affirmed.

JUDGES BELLACOSA, SMITH, LEVINE, CIPARICK, WESLEY and ROSENBLATT concur.

NOTES AND QUESTIONS

1. The Karlins paved the way for New York patients to use general consumer protection laws to battle deceptive claims by ART clinics. Bringing suit under the New York General Business Law represents a broadening of patients' options, because the statute of limitations for bringing suit under this statute is six years, compared to two and a half years under the state's medical malpractice law.

Why didn't the Karlins bring an action for malpractice against IVF America?

2. The defendant ART clinic, IVF America, was no stranger to regulation. In 1990, the Federal Trade Commission imposed a cease and desist order on IVF to end its misleading advertising in which pregnancy success rates were substantially inflated; IVF also agreed to disclose its system for calculating success rates, a transparency designed to give patients accurate information about a clinic's practices. But three years later, IVF was at it again. Exposed by a popular (translation — highly watched) television news magazine for the same deceptive

practices, IVF was sanctioned by local New York City authorities and again promised to clean up its act.

If existing federal, state, and local consumer protection laws are not able to thwart the likes of IVF America's advertising practices, would additional regulation be more effective in curbing these deceptive practices? If you were the Attorney General of your state, charged with protecting the consuming public's health, safety, and welfare, what law(s) would you want to see enacted to assist you in your role as protector?

2.   Lack of Informed Consent

In addition to truth in advertising, patients also have the right to be informed about the treatment options available and to make an informed choice about accepting or declining any given treatment. This doctrine of informed consent is largely a state law doctrine which can evolve from state common law, or as in New York, be codified by state legislatures. Recall the NY Public Health Law § 2805-d, mentioned in *Karlin*, which sets forth the requirements for informed consent in the state: "[A] person providing the professional treatment or diagnosis . . . [must] disclose to the patient such alternatives thereto and the reasonably foreseeable risks and benefits involved as a reasonable medical . . . practitioner under similar circumstances would have disclosed, in a manner permitting the patient to make a knowledgeable evaluation."

Exactly what information would satisfy this standard when IVF services are offered? The American Society for Reproductive Medicine has published guidelines for ART practitioners on the substance and parameters of informed consent. Drafted by the ASRM Practice Committee, the Report provides in relevant part:

Elements to Be Considered in Obtaining Informed Consent for ART
86(4) Fertility & Sterility S272 (2006)

A Practice Committee Opinion

All informed consents must be in writing, signed by all participating parties, and properly witnessed. In addition to information about chance of success and financial obligations, the following issues should be addressed in the process of obtaining consent. It is also important that couples be provided full information concerning alternative procedures available to manage their specific infertility problems, including procedures that are not performed by the treating center, as well as non-medical options such as adoption and non-treatment. Couples must be informed about the federal reporting requirements. Couples must also be informed through consent forms that de-identified cycle-specific data will be provided to the federal government.

I. IVF, GIFT, and ZIFT

A. Description of procedure including:

1. Use of medications including ovulation induction agents, luteal support, antibiotics, etc.

2. Use of monitoring including laboratory tests and ultrasound

3. Collection of sperm

4. Oocyte retrieval

5. Fertilization in the laboratory (IVF and ZIFT) or in the fallopian tubes (GIFT)

6. Monitoring of early pregnancy

B. Barriers to successful pregnancy including:

1. Poor response to ovulation induction agents

2. Unsuccessful oocyte retrieval

3. Abnormal oocytes

4. Inability to produce semen specimens or acquire sperm of sufficient quality or quantity

5. Failure of fertilization

6. Abnormal embryo development

7. Difficult or failed embryo transfer

8. Failure of implantation

9. Loss or damage to oocytes or embryos

C. Success rates and complications of pregnancy including:

1. Factors which affect pregnancy rates

2. Risks of multiple pregnancies, spontaneous abortion, ectopic pregnancies, stillbirths, and congenital abnormalities

D. Possible risks associated with the following procedures:

1. Blood drawing

2. Ovulation induction agents including allergic reactions, injections, hyperstimulation, multiple births, and association with ovarian cancer

3. Antibiotic administration

4. Oocyte retrieval or tubal transfer

5.   Laboratory and clinical handling of gametes and embryos

6.   Embryo transfer

E. Disposition of oocytes and embryos including:

1.   Option to attempt fertilization and/or freeze unused embryos

2.   Discarding of unused oocytes and low quality or abnormal embryos

The Committee Report goes on to suggest informed consent guidelines for cryopreservation of embryos, oocyte donation, microoperative procedures (including ICSI), and embryo donation.

As you can see, there is a lot of ground to cover when an individual or couple undergoes treatment using IVF. Should states or even the federal government develop a standardized consent form to be provided every patient so that all patients have equal access to uniform information about the medical treatment? Would uniform standards of informed consent increase patient protection? For a critique of governmental and ASRM efforts to draft uniform consent forms for adoption by individual clinics, *see* Deborah L. Forman, *Embryo Disposition and Divorce: Why Clinic Consent Forms Are Not the Answer*, 24 J. Am. Acad. Matrimonial Lawyers 57 (2011).

3.   Treatment Errors: Negligence, Theft, and Fraud

A patient can be harmed in the course of receiving infertility treatment in several ways. She can fail to become pregnant because her doctor acted in a negligent manner; she can become pregnant with three or more fetuses, a medically dangerous situation which places her and her babies at risk; she can be the subject of switched gametes or embryos, in which egg, sperm or embryos are misdirected and produce a child whose genetic make-up differs from that intended by the patient. To date, these scenarios have been governed mainly by state tort and criminal law. The question for our current consideration is "Should lawmakers increase regulation of the delivery of infertility medical services, and if so, how?"

If a patient is harmed by the negligent practice of reproductive medicine, she can bring an action for malpractice against her physician and the fertility clinic. But according to Professor Lars Noah, only a handful of reported cases raise tort claims against fertility doctors or fertility clinics, and what's more, plaintiffs rarely succeed when cases are brought. Lars Noah, *Assisted Reproductive Technologies and the Pitfalls of Unregulated Biomedical Innovation*, 55 Fla. L. Rev. 603, 635 (2003), citing *Doolan v. IVF America, Inc.*, 2000 Mass. Super. LEXIS 581 (Mass. Super Ct. 2000) (rejecting tort claim brought on behalf of child born with cystic fibrosis against fertility clinic for negligence in genetic testing of IVF embryos before implantation); *Morgan v. Christman*, 1990 U.S. Dist. LEXIS 12179 (D. Kan. 1990) (permitting patient who gave birth to quadruplets to proceed with negligence and informed consent claims against doctor who prescribed fertility drug without disclosing risk of multiple pregnancy).

Recall in Chapter 5 we looked at several cases in which clinics mixed up gametes, resulting in patients gestating a child who was the genetic child of another intended parent. The cases we reviewed involved family law questions — who is the legal parent of a child whose gametes were mistakenly switched by fertility clinic personnel? In addition to the family law suits, a number of the parties involved in the gamete and embryo cases brought malpractice actions against the treating clinics. In September 2004, the Perry-Rogers, a black couple whose embryo was mistakenly implanted in a white woman who gave birth to twins, one black and one white, settled a lawsuit against the embryologist who admitted the mistake. The terms of the settlement remain sealed, but future patients can hope that the publicity and payout surrounding this high profile case will have a positive step toward preventing such mix-ups in the future. *See* Helen Peterson, *Hatch Deal in Embryo Mixup*, DAILY NEWS, Sept. 14, 2004, at 6. See also *Experts Troubled by Case of Woman Who Said She Was Given Wrong Sperm*, WOMAN'S HEALTH WEEKLY, Aug. 5, 2004, at 99 (detailing lawsuit against infertility doctor by woman mistakenly inseminated with sperm of another man, instead of her fiancé).

The largest and most notorious incident of gamete and embryo malfeasance occurred at the University of California Irvine Center for Reproductive Health in the early 1990s, where three physicians allegedly (no trial on the merits was ever held) took eggs and embryos from unsuspecting patients and transferred them to other patients, without any woman's knowledge or consent. Because two of the physicians fled the country shortly after the revelations surfaced, little is officially known about the goings-on at the fertility center, but many of the affected couples and individuals brought suit against UCI for its role in the scandal. Eventually, the University settled more than 100 suits, paying out $24 million in damages to bring an end to the massive litigation. (The case is discussed in more detail in Chapter 5, beginning at page 499.)

For some California lawmakers, the UCI fertility clinic scandal represented the predictable fallout from a lack of regulation of the reproductive medicine industry. To fill the regulatory void, the Legislature enacted Penal Code Section 367g, which provides, in relevant part, "It shall be unlawful for anyone to knowingly use sperm, ova, or embryos in assisted reproduction technology, for any purpose other than that indicated by the sperm, ova, or embryo provider's signature on a written consent form." Violation of this penal code statute is punishable by a minimum three-year prison term and a $50,000 fine. In the time since the law took effect, no similarly large-scale embryo switching has taken place, but at least one fertility clinic mistakenly implanted the wrong embryos in a patient seeking treatment at the same time as another couple, three of whose embryos wound up in an unintended uterus. No criminal charges were ever filed against the responsible individuals, suggesting the switch was not done "knowingly", but rather negligently. See *Robert B. v. Susan B.*, 109 Cal. App.4th 1109, 135 Cal. Rptr. 785 (2003) (reprinted in Chapter 5, beginning at page 506.)

If negligent conduct can in fact be curtailed by some combination of tort litigation and increased oversight and reporting requirements, then perhaps a more detailed system for tracking and storing gametes and embryos is in order. But if a physician or other clinic employee is bent on nefarious activity, can a law really prevent such conduct? When gamete and embryo switching moves from the negligent to the criminal, how can the law best protect patients, children and society from the damage that flows from an individual's knowing and intentional misconduct? Again, a single, infamous case leaps out as demonstrative.

In 1992 Dr. Cecil Jacobson, a fertility specialist in Virginia, was convicted of 52 counts of fraud and perjury for telling patients they were pregnant when they were not, and for using his own semen to impregnate women who went to him for what they believed was an anonymous sperm donation program. Prosecutors in the case maintained that Dr. Jacobson may have fathered more than 70 children from patients who sought treatment at his fertility clinic. He was sentenced to five years in prison without parole and ordered to pay $116,000 in fines. *See* Robert F. Howe, *Citing Cruel Lies by Jacobson, Judge Gives Him 5 Years, Fine*, WASH. POST, May 9, 1992, at D1. If a law similar to the California penal code cited above had been in place at the time Dr. Jacobson was operating his clinic, do you think the malfeasance he committed would have been thwarted? Is the threat of criminal prosecution a deterrent to a physician who is determined, for whatever reason, to misdirect gametes and embryos? If not, what else can the law do?

4. Protecting Patient Health

Women who undergo IVF face two major health hazards. First, they can experience side effects and complications from the medical procedure itself, including ovarian hyperstimulation and possible ovarian rupture from the powerful drugs administered to stimulate the ovaries to produce multiple eggs, infection from the surgical egg retrieval process, and a possible increased risk of future cancers associated with long-term use of fertility drugs. Even if an IVF cycle goes smoothly, the woman is a great risk for having a multiple pregnancy, the second major health hazard facing ART patients. In 2009, around one-third of all ART pregnancies involved multiple fetuses — twins, triplets, or greater. As we learned in Chapter 1, multiple pregnancy poses risk to both mother and babies, with the risks rising as the number of fetuses increases. Multiple pregnancy-related maternal complications include pre-term labor, hypertension, hemorrhage, anemia, premature delivery, and postpartum blood transfusions. Infants face long-term health problems associated with premature birth and low birth weight, including respiratory problems, cerebral palsy, and learning disabilities.

The high rate of multiple pregnancy is considered by some a necessary side effect of existing infertility treatment, while others argue that transferring more than one, or perhaps two embryos back into a woman's uterus poses an unacceptable hazard to women and offspring. Compare Tarum Jain et al., *Trends in Embryo-Transfer Practice and in Outcomes of the Use of Assisted Reproductive Technology in the United States*, 350 NEW ENG. J. MED. 1639 (2004) (reporting that twin rate has remained constant, but rate of high-order multiples has declined, following decrease in number of embryos transferred per cycle) and Francois Olivennes, *Double Trouble: Yes a Twin Pregnancy Is an Adverse Outcome*, 15 HUM. REPROD. 1663 (2000) (acknowledging triplet and higher order pregnancies are a major adverse outcome of ART) with Gladys B. White & Steven R. Leuthner, *Infertility Treatment and Neonatal Care: The Ethical Obligation to Transcend Specialty Practice in the Interest of Reducing Multiple Births*, 12 J. CLINICAL ETHICS 223 (2001) (calling birth of three of more infants an unacceptable hazard of infertility treatment).

An obvious solution to the problem of multiple birth is to limit the number of embryos that a doctor can transfer in any ART cycle. This approach has been adopted in a number of other countries including Germany, Denmark, Norway, Spain and Switzerland, which limit implantations to two or three embryos per cycle. *See* Howard W. Jones, Jr. & Jean Cohen, *IFFS Report Surveillance '07*, 87 FERTILITY & STERILITY S20 (Supp. 1 2007). An even more restrictive law is in place in the United Kingdom, which sets a two-embryo limit for most ART cycles. THE HUMAN FERTILISATION & EMBRYOLOGY AUTHORITY, CODE OF PRACTICE (8th Edition), revised in March 2009, provides:

Limits on Egg and Embryo Transfer

7.4 The centre should not transfer more than three eggs or two embryos in any treatment cycle if:

a) the woman is to receive treatment using her own eggs, or embryos created using her own eggs (fresh or cryopreserved), and

b) the woman is aged under 40 at the time of transfer.

7.5 The centre should not transfer more than four eggs or three embryos in any treatment cycle if:

a) the woman is to receive treatment using her own eggs, or embryos created using her own eggs (fresh or cryopreserved), and

b) the woman is aged 40 or over at the time of transfer.

7.6 If a woman is to receive treatment using donated eggs or embryos, or embryos created with donated eggs, the centre should not transfer more than three eggs or two embryos in a treatment cycle. This is regardless of the procedure used and the woman's age at the time of transfer.

Could a similar law restricting embryo transfers to two or three per ART cycle be enacted in the United States? If so, would the law be enacted by Congress or by individual states? One scholar proposes that such a law could and should be adopted in the individual states. Professor Jennifer Rosato urges that states limit the number of embryos implanted to no more than three per cycle. She defends against the inevitable and vociferous opposition by patients and doctors that is likely to accompany such a law by arguing:

The patients will argue that their rights to procreate and to parent are being infringed. The doctors will argue that such a limitation is too restrictive and prevents them from making an informed medical determination based on a myriad of factors that sometime warrant implantation of more than three embryos. The limit is also subject to additional criticisms; for instance, that it is not based on empirical evidence and, more generally, that lawmakers should not be in the practice of legislating medicine.

In the end, however, none of these arguments should be considered persuasive enough to outweigh the interests of the children of ART. The harm caused by multiples is well-documented, and self-regulation has been ineffective in reducing the number of multiples caused by ART. The limit of three is based on sound public policy and is already being modeled by countries that have shown their commitment to reducing multiples.

Jennifer L. Rosato, *The Children of ART (Assisted Reproductive Technology): Should the Law Protect Them From Harm?*, 57 UTAH L. REV. 57, 87 (2004). *But see* Norbert Gleicher & David Barad, *Twin Pregnancy, Contrary to Consensus, Is a Desirable Outcome in Infertility*, 91 FERTILITY & STERILITY 2426 (2009) (arguing that the medical consensus that twin births from ART are a negative outcome to be avoided is flawed).

There are many published studies looking at the success of ART treatment using only a single embryo transfer. In a recent study published in the *New England Journal of Medicine*, researchers compared pregnancy success rates using double embryo transfers (transferring two embryos back to a woman's uterus) and single embryo transfers performed during two cycles. Women who received a single embryo and failed to give birth were offered a second cycle in which another embryo would be transferred. Initially, the two-embryo approach yielded a higher success rate — 43.4% for the two embryo group v. 29.6% for the single embryo transfers. But when the subsequent cycle was performed, the pregnancy success rates became closer, as 38.8% of the "single" group gave birth. Importantly, the rate of multiple birth was dramatically different, with only 0.8 of the single transfer group having a multiple birth, compared to 33.1 of the two embryo transfer group. *See* Owen K. Davis, *Elective Single-Embryo Transfer — Has Its Time Arrived?*, 351 NEW ENG. J. MED. 2440 (2004).

Given the substantial reduction of multiple birth using single embryo transfers,[6] could a state impose a "one embryo" limit on ART clinics as a way of protecting the health, safety, and welfare of patients and prospective offspring receiving care in the state? Is such a limitation reasonably related to this compelling state interest? Is the limitation narrowly tailored to achieve the governmental objective of protecting health? What other means could a state employ to reduce or eliminate the rate of multiple births that result from ART treatment?

Perhaps another approach can be found in the area of clinic reporting. In recent years, ART physicians have focused increasing attention on the incidence of multiple births, at least as indicated by a blossoming medical literature devoted to the problem. Researchers have even concocted an acronym to describe the desired outcome in an ART cycle — BESST (birth emphasizing a successful singleton at term). In 2004, Canadian researchers proposed that ART providers report the delivery of single, term gestation, live babies as a measure of treatment success. Premature babies, and multiple births would not be considered a "success," but rather a complication of ART treatment. *See* Jason K. Min, Sue A. Breheny, Vivien MacLachlan & David L. Healy, *What Is the Most Relevant Standard of Success in*

---

[6] Single embryo transfer would not eliminate the incidence of multiple pregnancy because of the incidence of monozygote twinning, meaning that a single embryo splits into two at the earliest stages of development producing "identical" twins. *See* KI Aston, CM Peterson, DT Carrell, *Monozygote Twinning Associated with Assisted Reproductive Technologies: A Review*, 136(4) Reproduction 377-86 (2008) (reporting that identical twin pregnancies occur at a significantly higher rate following IVF compared with the natural incidence).

Assisted Reproduction? The Singleton, Term Gestation, Live Birth Rate Per Cycle Initiated: The BESST Endpoint for Assisted Reproduction, 19 HUMAN REPRODUCTION 3 (2004).

If BESST is adopted, reported success rates will appear to decline, because they will not include the birth of twins, triplets and higher order multiple births. Arguably the rates will reflect the outcome that most infertility patients seek — the birth of a healthy single baby. Or do they? Surveys of infertility patients reveal that many patients prefer more than one child at a time, with nearly all favoring twins as a clinical outcome. *See* W.A. Grobman et al., *Patient Perceptions of Multiple Gestations: An Assessment of Knowledge and Risk Aversion*, 185(4) AM. J. OBSTETRICS & GYNECOLOGY 920-4 (2001); Mary D'Alton, *Infertility and the Desire for Multiple Births*, 81 FERTILITY & STERILITY 523 (2004) (noting 20% of women surveyed preferred multiple birth, 94% seeking twins).

B. Protecting ART Offspring

Any comprehensive, or even limited, regulatory scheme addressing the infertility industry would undoubtedly focus on the welfare of children born of ART. The British law regulating ART specifically provides, "A woman shall not be provided with treatment services unless account has been taken of the welfare of any child who may be born as a result of the treatment, . . . and of any other child who may be affected by the birth." Human Fertilisation & Embryology Act of 1990, Sec. 13(5). The suggested regulatory schemes addressing multiple births are aimed at protecting the health of ART children, a full third of whom are born along with siblings and thus face increased health problems. How else can the law protect the children of ART? At least one family sought legal redress for harm to their child as a result of assisted conception. Let us assess how responsive the legal system was to their claim.

DOOLAN v. IVF AMERICA (MA), INC.
Superior Court of Massachusetts
2000 Mass. Super. LEXIS 581, 12 Mass. L. Rep. 482 (2000)

CRATSLEY, J. This matter comes before this Court on defendants' motion for summary judgment on each of plaintiff Thomas Doolan's negligence claims . . . as well as on each of plaintiffs John and Laureen Doolan's loss of consortium claims . . . pursuant to Mass.R.Civ.P. 56. Based on an examination of the record and the arguments of counsel heard on September 25, 2000, and for the reasons set forth below, the defendants' motion for summary judgment is *ALLOWED* . . .

Pursuant to the summary judgment record, the undisputed material facts are as follows:

In 1993, plaintiff Laureen Doolan gave birth to her first child, Samantha, who was born afflicted with cystic fibrosis. Laureen and her husband, plaintiff John Doolan, subsequently learned that they were both carriers of a cystic fibrosis gene mutation known as Delta F-508. Mr. and Mrs. Doolan wished to have another child, but they wanted some assurance that their second child would not have cystic fibrosis.

In 1996 Mr. and Mrs. Doolan agreed to participate in a series of procedures conducted jointly by the co-defendants[7] that were designed to provide the Doolans with a degree of certainty that their second child would not be afflicted with cystic fibrosis. In November 1996 defendant Ronald Carson, Ph.D. ("Dr. Carson"), the Scientific and Laboratory Director at defendant MPD, harvested a series of Mrs. Doolan's eggs, fertilized the eggs with Mr. Doolan's sperm in vitro, and prepared the resulting embryos for genetic testing. A cell from each of the resulting ten embryos was then retrieved by MPD, whereupon the cells were sent to defendant Genzyme Corporation ("Genzyme").

In December 1996 Genzyme tested the ten cells to ascertain which embryos were (1) afflicted with, (2) carriers of, or (3) free of the cystic fibrosis gene mutation, Delta F-508. In a letter dated December 23, 1996, defendant Katherine Klinger, Ph.D. ("Dr. Klinger"), the Vice President of Science at Genzyme, advised MPD that Embryo No. 7 was free of the cystic fibrosis gene mutation and suitable for implantation. As a result of this finding, Mr. and Mrs. Doolan decided to have MPD implant Embryo No. 7 into Mrs. Doolan on March 10, 1997.

On November 21, 1997, Mrs. Doolan gave birth to her son, minor plaintiff Thomas Doolan. Shortly after Thomas' birth, it was discovered that he did, in fact, suffer from cystic fibrosis and that his condition was due to the Delta F-508 genetic mutation. All three plaintiffs assert claims arising out of (1) MPD's and Dr. Carson's alleged negligence in implanting an embryo that contained the cystic fibrosis gene mutation, and (2) Genzyme's and Dr. Klinger's alleged negligence in advising MPD that Embryo No. 7 was free of the Delta F-508 gene mutation and therefore was suitable for implantation.

DISCUSSION . . .

B. Minor Plaintiff Thomas Doolan's Negligence Claim

The almost universal rule in this country is that a physician is not liable to a child who was born because of the physician's negligence. *Viccaro v. Milunsky*, 406 Mass. 777, 783 (1990). Courts have generally referred to claims alleging that the physician negligently failed to inform the child's parents of the possibility of their bearing a severely defective child, thereby preventing a parental choice to avoid the child's birth, as "wrongful life" cases. *Payton v. Abbott Labs*, 386 Mass. 540, 557-58 (1982), citing *Phillips v. United States*, 508 F.Supp. 537, 538 n. 1 (D.S.C.1980). The Massachusetts Supreme Judicial Court (SJC) has reasoned that granting the minor plaintiff a cause of action in wrongful life cases would require a comparison of the relative monetary values of existence and nonexistence, a task that is beyond the competence of the judicial system. *Payton* at 559 . . .

The holding in *Viccaro* [rejecting wrongful life claim of child born with a genetic

---

[7] [n.3] Defendants IVF America (MA), Inc., MPD Medical Associates (MA), P.C., d/b/a Reproductive Science Center of Boston, and Integramed America, Inc. are related entities and will be referred to as "MPD."

disorder after physician erroneously told parents they were not carriers] is clearly applicable to this case, where it is undisputed that Thomas Doolan would never have been born were it not for the defendants' alleged negligence in testing and/or implanting Embryo No. 7. Plainly put, Thomas Doolan asserts that the defendants' alleged negligence denied his parents the opportunity to choose not to conceive and give birth to him . . .

Perhaps sensing the tenuous nature of his "wrongful life" claim under the holding in *Viccaro*, minor plaintiff Thomas Doolan asserts that his negligence claim against the defendants is not a "wrongful life" claim, but rather it is a pre-conception tort, and as such it is not foreclosed under Massachusetts law. Unlike "wrongful life" claims, which the holding in *Viccaro* expressly bars, the SJC has yet to address the viability of pre-conception tort claims. *See McNulty v. McDowell*, 415 Mass. 369, 373 (1993).

An analysis of the context in which other jurisdictions have recognized pre-conception tort claims serves only to re-enforce this Court's conclusion that Thomas Doolan's claim is one for "wrongful life." The Supreme Court of Indiana has defined pre-conception torts as those cases which allege a defendant's tortious conduct as the cause of abnormalities in infants that would otherwise have been born normal and healthy. *Walker v. Rinck*, 604 N.E.2d 591, 594 (Ind.1992). In *Walker*, the Supreme Court of Indiana upheld a child's cause of action for pre-conception tort where the defendant physician failed to administer RhoGAM injections to the minor plaintiffs' mother, who had Rh-negative blood. *Id.* at 592. The defendant's failure to administer RhoGAM during Mrs. Walker's first pregnancy resulted in her blood developing antibodies that caused her three later-conceived children to be born with serious defects. *Id.* Since the three minor plaintiffs would have been born normal and healthy were it not for the defendant's negligence in failing to provide Mrs. Walker with RhoGAM injections during her first pregnancy, the Supreme Court of Indiana upheld their cause of action for pre-conception tort. *Id.* at 594 . . .

In . . . *Rinck* . . . , the negligence of the defendant caused the minor plaintiff to be born with severe defects, when he/she would have otherwise been born healthy. In this case, however, there is no such causal connection between the alleged negligence of the defendants and the injuries actually suffered by Thomas Doolan. The minor plaintiff has not alleged that any of the defendants did anything to directly cause Thomas Doolan to be afflicted with the Delta F-508 gene mutation. Stated otherwise, there is no way Thomas Doolan could ever have been born without cystic fibrosis. Therefore, given the way other jurisdictions have interpreted the pre-conception tort, it is evident that this case does not fall within its scope . . .

C. John and Laureen Doolan's Claims for Loss of Consortium

Plaintiffs John and Laureen Doolan advance two arguments in support of their claims for loss of consortium. The plaintiffs first argue that M.G.L. c. 231, § 85X creates a cause of action for parents seeking to recover for the loss of consortium of a dependent child. Section 85X provides:

> The parents of a minor child or an adult child who is dependent on his parents for support shall have a cause of action for loss of consortium of the

child who has been seriously injured against any person who is legally responsible for causing such injury.

The plain language of the preceding section indicates that the plaintiffs may only recover for the loss of consortium of Thomas Doolan against any person who is legally responsible for causing such injury. Plaintiffs have failed to put forth any evidence suggesting that the defendants are legally responsible for causing Thomas Doolan to be born afflicted with cystic fibrosis. This analysis is similar to that found in Section B, regarding Thomas Doolan's own negligence claims . . . Therefore, this Court holds as a matter of law that M.G.L. c. 231, § 85X does not confer a cause of action for loss of consortium on the plaintiffs, John and Laureen Doolan.

The second argument made by the plaintiffs in support of their loss of consortium claims asks this Court to undertake an analysis in the realm of the hypothetical. Mr. and Mrs. Doolan assert that were it not for the alleged negligence of the defendants, they would currently be raising a boy named Thomas, and that this child would not be afflicted with cystic fibrosis. Since this hypothetical "healthy" Thomas Doolan would be more likely to be able to offer society and companionship to his parents for the duration of their lifetimes than would the actual Thomas Doolan, plaintiffs reason that they have a cause of action for loss of consortium.

Plaintiffs' argument fails for two reasons. First, the extent of any loss of consortium damages for a child that was never born would be far too speculative to uphold plaintiffs' cause of action. For example, the jury would have to consider the quality of the relationship plaintiffs might have had with their hypothetical son in assessing Mr. and Mrs. Doolan's loss of consortium damages. Furthermore, plaintiffs' assertion that this hypothetical Thomas Doolan would have been "healthy" discounts the possibility that he might have been afflicted with another type of birth defect or long term illness . . .

ORDER

For the reasons stated herein, it is *ORDERED* that defendants' motion for summary judgment is ALLOWED . . .

NOTES AND QUESTIONS

1. *Tort as Regulation?* Does the denial of Thomas's claim for recovery mean that ART practitioners are free to commit negligence in the creation and testing of human embryos, because they owe no legal duty of care to any child born as a result of their conduct? Certainly not. Parents who utilize the services of ART professionals can recover for the expenses incurred in caring for a sick or disabled child, and may also be able to seek punitive damages in some instances. See *Paretta v. Medical Offices for Human Reproduction*, 195 Misc. 2d 568, 760 N.Y.S.2d 639 (2003) (reprinted in Chapter 4 beginning on page 365). But *Doolan* is instructive for demonstrating the parameters (some might say, limitations) of our current tort system as a mechanism for addressing the harm to ART children.

Suppose a court agreed to recognize preconception torts and claims for wrongful life on behalf of ART children. Could the court justify its continued refusal to recognize such tort claims brought by naturally conceived children on the grounds that the assisted conception itself was the source of the negligence? What effect would recognition of wrongful life claims have on the practice of ART in that state? Would it make ART safer for children? Would it make ART less available and more expensive for adults? If you answered "yes" to both previous questions, is the result a reasonable compromise?

2. *Human Subject Research.* The field of ART is a relative newcomer to the practice of medicine, raising questions about whether the techniques employed should be considered experimental. If ART is experimental, should the children produced by this medical research be protected as human research subjects?

The federal government exercises enormous control over medical research through a gigantic network of agencies, regulations, and guidelines. The scope of federal prowess over medical research might lead one to conclude that IVF and other ART techniques are closely scrutinized because they often involve experimentation, as evidenced by the several novel techniques to emerge from the field in recent years, including preimplantation genetic diagnosis (PGD), ooplasm transfer (in which an older egg is injected with cytoplasm of a younger egg to enhance fertilization), and ICSI (in which the sperm is injected directly into the egg). In fact, federal regulators have little or no authority to oversee developments and experimentation in ART for two primary reasons.

First, the scope of federal authority is generally tied to the disbursement of federal funds to researchers or healthcare institutions. The Department of Health and Human Services (HHS), and the National Institutes of Health (NIH) have issued extensive regulations and policies that must be adhered to by researchers who either receive federal funds directly, or who work at institutions that receive any federal funds (for example, virtually all hospitals receive federal funds through the Medicare program). Few, if any, ART practitioners receive funding directly from the federal government, and many infertility clinics are free-standing medical practices, and thus are unaffiliated with a hospital or other healthcare institution that receives federal funding. Thus, the reach of federal rules governing medical experimentation typically does not extend to most ART practices.

A second reason that ART is not regulated in the same manner as other medical research has to do with the patient population that is the subject of experimentation. Federal law protects "human subjects" by requiring that all research involving human subjects be reviewed, approved, and monitored by an institutional review board (IRB), an independent ethical body charged with upholding the best interest of research subjects. See 45 C.F.R. 46.107. Research that does not involve human subjects is not subject to IRB review and approval. When a physician seeks to improve IVF by, for example, experimenting with the temperature of the culture medium in which the early embryos grow, who is the subject of that experiment? Is it the woman who is hoping to become pregnant or is it the embryo? If it is the women, what type of medical research is being performed on her? If it is the embryo, is this very early form of life a human subject within the meaning of federal law? To date, human embryos that are outside the body have never been treated as "human subjects" under federal research guidelines, thus most ART research travels without any oversight by federal authorities.

To combat both real and perceived concerns that advances in reproductive medicine are the result of unethical and potentially harmful experimentation involving patients and embryos, many clinics have sought out IRB approval, either by hiring a private IRB or asking a proximate hospital board to review the clinic's proposed research project. In at least one instance, the former method — enlisting a private IRB — raised even more concerns when it was revealed that all five members of the group had a personal relationship with the physicians who proposed the research. Three of the IRB members were the clinic's own doctors, one member was the clinic director's administrative secretary, and the fifth was a close friend of one of the clinic's doctors. *See* Rick Weiss, *Fertility Innovation or Exploitation? Regulatory Void Allows for Trial — and Error — Without Patient Disclosure Rules*, Wash. Post, Feb. 9, 1998, at A1.

3.   *Parental Views Toward Harm to ART Offspring.* The goal of protecting ART children from harm through increased regulation has a rather odd array of supporters and detractors. Medical ethicists, governmental commissions, and some academic commentators have favored banning or restricting certain ART practices because of potential or even proven risk of harm to resulting offspring. In contrast, even when increased risk of health hazards are verifiable, prospective parents seem undeterred in their quest to procreate, railing against any proposed restrictions on access to available technology. A recent example of this clash between "observers" and "participants" can be seen through the research on the most widely used from of assisted conception — IVF. A 2004 study found that children conceived by IVF are nine times as likely to have a rare disorder called Beckwith-Wiedermann Syndrome (BWS) as those conceived naturally. BWS can make certain parts of the body, such as the tongue, grow larger than normal, and it increases the risk of certain cancers. When asked about the impact of this study on patients considering IVF, one embryologist surmised that would-be parents will not be deterred, adding, "Patients will still be prepared to take that risk and have a higher chance of pregnancy." Cathy Holding, *IVF Raises Risk of Birth Defect*, New Scientist, Aug. 14, 2004, at 11.

Should prospective parents be given the option of utilizing a technology that presents a ninefold risk of producing a child with a serious, albeit not universally life-threatening, disease? In terms of absolute numbers, BWS was found to occur in 1 in every 4,000 IVF births. Compare this scenario to one in which a pediatric drug produced a serious side effect in 1 of every 4,000 users. Would the FDA intervene and order the drug withdrawn from the market? Should a parent who believes his or her child is aided by the drug be permitted to continue using the drug, even after it is taken off the market (perhaps the parent stockpiled the drug before the recall)? If the child develops the serious side effect from taking the drug, could the District Attorney consider prosecuting the parent for child abuse? How, if at all, is the continued use of IVF in light of data that suggests harm to offspring different from post-birth harms that are attributable to parent conduct?

4.   Is harm to offspring a compelling reason to ban certain forms of assisted conception? If procreative liberty is a protected and fundamental right, could lawmakers meet the standard of "narrowly tailored to meet a compelling state interest" in banning the use of a reproductive technique that posed a risk of harm to the children born therefrom? Would the ban also have to include reproduction by

individuals whose genetic make-up poses a risk of transmission of a genetic disease? For a discussion of the duty of parents to shield their children from preventable harms, see, e.g., THOMAS H. MURRAY, THE WORTH OF A CHILD (1996); MELINDA ROBERTS, CHILD VERSUS CHILDMAKER: FUTURE PERSONS AND PRESENT DUTIES IN ETHICS AND THE LAW (1998); John A. Robertson, *Procreative Liberty and Harm to Offspring in Assisted Reproduction*, 30 AM. J. LAW & MED. 7 (2004).

C.   Protecting ART Physicians

The lack of a comprehensive ART regulatory scheme may appear, at first blush, an entirely favorable system for practitioners who enjoy total freedom to practice reproductive medicine untethered by burdensome and time-consuming external rules and requirements. As we have seen, the practice of reproductive medicine is not entirely unregulated. ART providers must report their pregnancy success rates to the federal government (though the penalties for nonreporting seem soft); a smattering of federal agencies, including the FDA and FTC, exercise some oversight over certain ART practices; reproductive medicine doctors are held to the same standards as other physicians as far as licensing and malpractice are concerned; a few states regulate access to ART through screening requirements and reporting mandates. But is the overall freedom to practice without established boundaries necessarily a good thing for ART physicians? Would greater regulation produce an overall benefit for providers?

1.   Enhancing Public Confidence

One argument, that increased regulation would offer greater protection to ART physicians than the current system, stems from the empiric assumption that increased oversight would weed out untrained, unethical, and unprofessional practitioners. If the so-called "bad apples" could be identified without sweeping out some of the "good apples," then the upstanding practitioners would be better off in terms of reputation in the community for a high standard of practice. The counterargument to the proposition that greater regulation breeds greater public confidence may be best summed by continuing the apple metaphor, "One bad apple can spoil the whole bunch." If a single practitioner is bent on malfeasance even in the face of tight oversight, the entire industry may suffer a loss of reputation as a result. The tale of Dr. Fielding is instructive.

Dr. Paul Fielding was a British doctor charged with creating fake embryos and pretending to implant them in patients' wombs, then taking payments for each procedure carried out. He worked as the head embryologist for several fertility clinics, where he is accused of creating duplicate plugs (to resemble embryos) and straws (where the embryos are frozen) in order to generate extra "embryos" that he could then charge patients to transfer. At least eight women underwent a sham surgery as part of Dr. Fielding's elaborate plan, a plan hatched out of the doctor's "horrendous" financial position. See Nicola Woolcock, *Indebted Doctor Accused of Faking Embryo Implants*, DAILY TELEGRAPH, Nov. 27, 2002, at A15.

The instructive aspect of the Fielding case is that it occurred in England, a country well-known for its comprehensive regulation of ART. Each fertility clinic is subject to routine inspection, in which a clinic's success rates for frozen embryo transfers are reviewed. It turns out that regulators in England failed to visit one of the clinics where Dr. Fielding worked, and a regulator who did visit another site failed to follow up on the fact that there were no pregnancies using frozen embryos for a three-year period. *See* Shelley Jofre, *Focus Babymakers: Part Three The Debate; The Lack of Regulation Really Shocked Me*, INDEPENDENT ON SUNDAY, July 6, 2003, at 17 (noting Dr. Fielding was jailed for his conduct). Tales such as the Fielding debacle, though rare, can have a pervasive and lasting effect, forcing patients and lawmakers to rethink the benefits and mechanisms of regulation.

2. Authorizing Treatment Denials

A second argument for increased regulation is to give practitioners greater flexibility in declining to treat certain patients. How, you may wonder, are doctors better off if regulations decrease the population of patients they can treat? The answer envisions a system in which physicians are spared having to make the morally difficult decision of whether to provide ART services to an individual who may present a risk of harm to a child born of the treatment. Bright-line rules that determine who can and who cannot receive infertility treatment may be a welcome shield for some physicians who struggle personally and professionally when a patient of questionable parenting skills seeks assistance with conception. Other doctors may view such restrictions as professionally intrusive and dangerously paternalistic, depriving infertile patients the right to reproduce freely enjoyed by all fertile members of society.

The Ethics Committee of the American Society for Reproductive Medicine studied the parameters of the debate over the provision of ART services in the face of possible harm to offspring, producing the following Ethics Opinion.

The Ethics Committee of the American Society for Reproductive Medicine
Child-Rearing Ability and the Provision of Fertility Services
92 Fertility & Sterility 864 (2009)

. . . Providers of infertility services are sometimes faced with patients who do not appear to be well-situated to provide good care for children. Treating them may lead to the birth of a child who is reared by parents who are psychologically unstable, who abuse drugs, who may abuse the child or the other parent, or present other risks to the well-being of the child. Predictions about parental child-rearing ability, however, are not easily made, and personnel in fertility programs may not be well-situated to make them. This poses an ethical dilemma in which clinicians must weigh the potential interests of offspring against the needs and desires of infertile patients. The aim of this statement is to provide guidance to fertility programs in such circumstances. It addresses the question of whether clinicians may — or must — provide services to persons whom they suspect may not be good child-rearers, or whether they have an ethical obligation not to provide these services. It also discusses the extent to which a physician's own moral views of minimally acceptable childrearing may appropriately be taken into account in deciding whether to accept a patient for infertility treatment.

THE NATURE OF THE DILEMMA

. . . With the growth of fertility programs and increased access for many people in the population, a wide variety of individuals now seek infertility treatment, including subcategories of patients for whom questions of child-rearing ability might legitimately arise. Many programs have had treatment requests from patients that raise such questions, for example, from persons who have a history of psychiatric illness, substance abuse, or ongoing physical or emotional abuse in relationships. Some patients or their partners may also have a history of perpetrating child or spousal abuse, or they present other factors that lead fertility programs to question whether they are likely to cause significant harm to a future child. In addition, persons with disabilities are increasingly seeking fertility services. While most disabilities do not impair child- rearing ability, there are some situations in which questions about child-rearing ability of persons with severe disabilities could reasonably arise . . .

Fertility programs . . . are not totally removed from social and psychological assessment of patients. Many programs require patients to spend time with a counselor to ensure that patients can handle the stresses of treatment. They may also ask patients for a social or psychological history. Such assessments have become routine for IVF and for procedures involving the use of donor gametes or surrogacy. Even though fertility programs do not seek specifically to assess parenting ability, pre-treatment evaluation of patients might reveal potential problems, such as uncontrolled psychiatric illness, a history of child or spousal abuse, or drug abuse. In such situations some programs and providers may be reluctant to proceed with treatments, either out of concern about their role in bringing about a situation that is not beneficial to the child or because of fears of legal liability. At the same time they may feel that they are not competent to make such predictions and should not be required to do so. They may also feel that it is necessary to respect the right of persons to have children if they choose and to avoid charges of unlawful or improper discrimination in withholding services from them.

The problem is complicated because many interests are implicated in such dilemmas. The interest of future children in having a healthy home environment and minimally competent rearing parents must be reconciled with the interest of infertile persons in receiving the treatment services they need to reproduce and the provider's own sense of moral responsibility in deciding what patients to treat.

RECONCILING THE INTERESTS

We analyze below the interests of offspring, infertile persons, and providers of fertility services. Recognizing that it is difficult to reach optimal solutions for all situations, we believe that fertility programs should be attentive to serious child-rearing deficiencies in their patients, and if they have a substantial, non-arbitrary basis for thinking that parents will provide inadequate child-rearing, they should be free to refuse to provide treatment services to such patients. Because of the difficulty of making such judgments reliably, however, clinicians should deny services on the basis of inadequate child-rearing abilities only after investigation shows that there is a substantial basis for such judgments. In reaching such conclusions, it is imperative that they not engage in unjustified discrimination.

However, we do not believe that fertility providers are morally obligated to refuse services in all cases in which questions of inadequate child-rearing arise. Such judgments may be very difficult to make reliably. Also, given the great importance of procreation, infertile persons should not be denied services without good reason after an assessment jointly made by members of the treatment team. Programs may adopt a policy that they will provide fertility services to all persons who medically qualify except when significant harm to future children is likely . . .

PROVIDER AUTONOMY

An important difference between reproduction by fertile and infertile persons is that fertile individuals do not need the help of physicians to conceive or get pregnant. Persons who seek the assistance of a physician to reproduce necessarily implicate the physician in the outcome that they seek. Requests for reproductive assistance thus also raise the question of whether physicians are obligated to treat all patients who seek their services. Although a strong ethic urges physicians to treat all persons in need, physician and professional autonomy is also an important value. Ordinarily, physicians are free to decide whether to enter into a doctor — patient relationship with a patient, and once in it, whether, with adequate notice to the patients, to terminate that relation. Unless the conditions of their employment require otherwise, physicians providing fertility services are generally free not to provide those services to individuals as they choose, subject only to federal and state laws against unjustified discrimination on the grounds of race, religion, ethnicity, or disability. Physicians faced with individuals or couples whom they have strong reasons to believe may be seriously deficient child-rearers may have very good reasons for choosing not to treat them. Precisely because fertility services could produce a child, physicians may reasonably believe that they have a moral responsibility for the situation of the resulting child and choose not to help bring about such an outcome. If they take that view and do not discriminate on the basis of disability or other impermissible factor, they may take the welfare of resulting children into account in deciding whether to provide services.

By the same token, some providers may believe that they have an obligation to treat all patients who would benefit from medical treatment and should not be required to make assessments of a patient's child-rearing abilities or other child welfare issues. This too is a reasonable position, except when significant harm to a future child is likely. Physicians and providers with this treatment philosophy should be free to accept persons for treatment as long as they have a reasonable basis for thinking that the child will not suffer significant harm from being born in those circumstances. Professional autonomy thus has two aspects. It entitles physicians to choose *not to treat* persons whom they think will be inadequate child-rearers (as long as they comply with anti-discrimination laws). It also generally entitles them *to treat* such patients if they choose.

RECOMMENDATIONS

Offspring welfare is a valid consideration that fertility programs may take into account in selecting patients and providing services as long as they do not discriminate on the basis of disability or other impermissible factor. However, it does not follow that they are morally obligated to withhold such services, except when significant harm to future children is likely. Physician autonomy entitles physicians to provide medical services if they choose, but they are not usually obligated to do so. While practitioners and clinics may — except in the case of impermissible discrimination — make their own moral decisions about whether to accept individuals as patients, their decisions should be based on empirical evidence, not stereotype or prejudice. For example, they should not assume that a history of social or psychological problems or serious disability automatically disqualifies someone from being a capable rearing parent.

Such assessments need careful inquiry and should be dependent on empirical facts. To aid in the process fertility programs should develop explicit policies and procedures for handling such situations. Written policies might address such matters as the information and evaluation that will be required of potential patients and what conditions would preclude medical treatment for infertility (e.g., uncontrolled psychiatric illness, substance abuse, on-going physical or emotional abuse, or a history of perpetrating physical or emotional abuse). Programs should also establish a procedure for making such assessments when questions about the child-rearing adequacy of prospective parents arise. This might involve evaluation by a mental health worker and consideration by psychological or other consultants culminating in a group assessment or review prior to a final determination.

NOTES AND QUESTIONS

1. *The Ethical Continuum.* The ASRM Ethics Opinion is intended to aid ART practitioners in establishing inclusion and exclusion criteria for treating patients, by establishing the ethical boundaries within which each clinic should strive to operate. The ethical continuum seems to have the following end points: All exclusion criteria are ethically acceptable except those that discriminate on the basis of disability or other impermissible factor. All inclusion criteria are ethically acceptable except when significant harm to future children is likely.

Do these end points strike you as sensible? Are they understandable from a clinical perspective? Imagine you are counsel for an established fertility clinic with a diverse patient population — diverse in terms of age, race, sexual orientation, disability, and psychological health. The medical director tells you she wants to establish guidelines within the ASRM ethical parameters, with an eye toward providing as wide a range of services as possible. What research would you conduct in order to prepare these guidelines? Consider taking a crack at drafting these guidelines.

2. *The Role of Self-Regulation.* The ASRM recommendations are aspirational, rather than mandatory. Could a governmental regulatory authority adopt these guidelines into law without running the risk of a court declaring the enactment void for vagueness? If the government does not adopt rules that protect ART children from harm (including the harm of being born), is self-regulation by the fertility industry a sufficient mechanism for protecting offspring?

3. *Adoption v. Natural Conception.* The provision of ART services often finds itself placed somewhere in between the regulatory-free practice of natural concep-

tion and the regulatory-heavy institution of adoption. Should ART services be treated more like natural conception in which prospective parents are free to make child-bearing decisions free of any governmental interference, or should government seize the opportunity, as it does in adoption, to protect the welfare of children by assessing the adults' ability to care for the child? In adoption, such assessment is made by conducting home studies, requiring parents attend educational classes, and performing psychological screening to determine child-rearing ability. Screening for ART parental suitability could include these measures, as well as testing for genetic and infectious diseases that could be passed to offspring. If such measures were adopted, who would conduct the required screening?

4. *Disability Discrimination?* In November 1999 a Colorado fertility clinic refused to continue providing fertility treatment to Kijuana Chambers, a single woman who was blind. Ms. Chambers had undergone several unsuccessful artificial insemination procedures before a new doctor stopped her treatment, citing the patient's poor hygiene, lack of a partner, family or other support system, and emotional outbursts. The doctor explained she felt morally obligated to be sure her patient could raise a child before aiding her in that endeavor.

Kijuana Chambers sued the fertility clinic under the federal Americans With Disabilities Act, claiming the only reason the physician stopped treating her was because she was blind. The ADA prohibits discrimination in the provision of health care on the basis of a disability; blindness is a disability under the federal law. Before the trial, Ms. Chambers sought treatment at another fertility clinic where she became pregnant and later gave birth to a daughter on January 1, 2001.

The jury found against the plaintiff, concluding that the fertility clinic did not discriminate against her because she was blind. See Karen Abbott, *Mom Loses Discrimination Suit*, Rocky Mountain News, Nov. 22, 2003, at 19A. Does the outcome of this case give any indication of how patients are likely to fare when they challenge denials of treatment by fertility clinics? *But see North Coast Women's Care Medical Group, Inc. v. San Diego County Superior Court*, 44 Cal. 4th 1145, 189 P.3d 959 (2008) (upholding right of lesbian patient to pursue antidiscrimination claim against physicians who denied service based on religious beliefs), reprinted in Chapter 3 beginning at page 256.

SECTION III: PROPOSED REGULATORY SCHEMES

Over the past decade a number of law and policy-oriented groups have studied the state of ART regulation, and proposed changes and additions to existing structures. In 1998, the New York State Task Force on Life and the Law published a comprehensive report titled, *Assisted Reproductive Technologies: Analysis and Recommendations for Public Policy.* The nearly 500-page report concludes with numerous legislative and regulatory recommendations, suggesting changes in state law on matters ranging from parental rights and responsibilities when children are conceived using donor gametes to certification and licensure of embryo laboratories. Another thorough review has been undertaken by the American Bar Association, Section of Family Law, Committee on the Law of Genetic and Reproduction Technology. The ABA formally adopted the Model Act Governing Assisted Reproductive Technology in 2008. In its preface, the Model Act aspires to "provide . . . a flexible framework that will serve as a mechanism to resolve contemporary controversies, to adapt to the need for resolution of controversies that are envisioned but that may have not yet occurred, and to guide the expansion of ways by which families are formed." The Model Act's twelve articles deal with a range of ART issues, including informed consent, embryo disposition, parentage of ART offspring, gestational agreements and quality assurance. A version of the Model Act is available at: http://apps.americanbar.org/dch/committee.cfm?com=FL142000. For an analysis of the ABA Model Act, *see* Charles P. Kindregan & Steven H. Snyder, *Clarifying the Law of ART: The New American Bar Association Model Act Governing Assisted Reproductive Technology*, 42 FAM. L. Q. 203 (2008).

ART regulatory review has also garnered presidential interest, expressed through a series of commissions established beginning in 1974. For a brief history of presidential bioethics commissions, *see* http://bioethics.gov/cms/history. The most recent executive level commission to comprehensively address the regulation of reproductive technologies was the President's Council on Bioethics (PCB), appointed by President George W. Bush in 2001. Its thorough ART report, issued in 2004, is titled, *Reproduction & Responsibility: The Regulation of New Biotechnologies*. The report is a "product of two years of research, reflection, and deliberation" according to the PCB's Chair, Leon Kass. An initial conclusion reached by the Council was that "[i]n the United States, existing institutions appear to be insufficient to handle the questions raised by the new biotechnologies." The President's Council on Bioethics, "Regulating the New Biotechnologies: Observations and Procedural Options for the Council," Staff Working Paper discussed at session 7 of the Council's meeting on October 18, 2002. The Council then heard invited presentations on various aspects of the subject, including testimony from federal agencies, ART professional organizations, and patient advocates. In addition, numerous groups and individuals responded to the Council's call for public comment, submitting voluminous written documentation for consideration.

The final report contains a detailed overview of existing regulatory structures, and it sets forth possible policy options for future examination and study. The Council makes interim recommendations for implementation by existing regulatory institutions, rather than suggesting any major changes or increased responsibility for these extant bodies. As you read the Council's recommendations, think about how federal and state lawmakers could translate the suggested reforms into clear, understandable, and workable legislation.

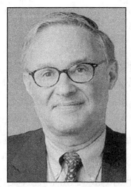

Dr. Leon Kass, Chair of the President's Council on Bioethics

President's Council on Bioethics
Reproduction & Responsibility: The Regulation of New Biotechnologies
205-218 (2004)

Recommendations

Over the past two years, the Council has devoted much time and energy to examining the current oversight and regulation of the uses of biotechnologies that touch the beginnings of human life — practices arising at the intersection of assisted reproduction, genetic screening, and human embryo research. The Council has heard from various experts and stakeholders, engaged in its own diagnostic review of current regulatory mechanisms and institutions, outlined the key findings emerging from that review, and surveyed various general and specific policy options . . .

In Sections I and II of this chapter, the Council proposes several measures it believes the federal government and the various relevant professional societies should adopt immediately . . . These include a call for comprehensive information gathering, data collection, monitoring, and reporting of the uses and effects of these technologies. They also address the needs for increased consumer protection, improved informed decision-making, and more conscientious enforcement of existing guidelines for practitioners of assisted reproductive technologies (ARTs) . . .

In offering these interim recommendations for improvements in data collection, monitoring, and professional self-regulation and in proposing limits and restraints on some potential applications of ARTs, the Council does not intend to challenge the current practices or impugn the ethical standards of most practitioners of assisted reproduction. The Council recognizes the efforts of professionals and patient groups working in this field to devise and implement appropriate ethical guidelines and standards of care. Yet we have identified areas of concern that have not been sufficiently studied or addressed. And there are at present no effective mechanisms for monitoring or regulating some of the more problematic practices or for preventing unwelcome innovations introduced by irresponsible practitioners. Indeed, it is our belief that responsible professional participants, patients, policymakers, and interested citizens should be able to recognize the merit of our proposals and work to see them implemented . . .

I. FEDERAL STUDIES, DATA COLLECTION, REPORTING, AND MONITORING REGARDING THE USES AND EFFECTS OF THESE TECHNOLOGIES

A. Undertake a Federally Funded Longitudinal Study of the Impact of ARTs on the Health and Development of Children Born with Their Aid

A most important unanswered question before the Council concerns the precise effects of ART and adjunct technologies on the health and normal development of children who are now being born or who will in the future be born with their aid. There have been a few studies, mostly undertaken abroad, reaching different and sometimes contradictory results . . . The Council strongly believes . . . that what is needed now is a *prospective* longitudinal study — national, comprehensive, and federally funded — that looks at both the short-term and the long-term effects of these technologies and practices on the health of children produced with their assistance, including any cognitive, developmental, or physical impairments. Such a study would require an adequate control sample, and a sufficiently large population of subjects to yield meaningful statistical results. Participation in such a study would, of course, be voluntary . . .

B. Undertake Federally Funded Studies on the Impact of ARTs on the Health and Well-Being of Women

Another area where better information is needed regards the health and well-being of women who use ARTs and of women who donate their eggs for the use of others. One or more studies, either in conjunction with or separate from the above-mentioned longitudinal study, should be conducted to discover the effects, if any, of the use of ARTs on women's health, including any short-term or long-term hormonal, physical, or psychological impairments. Participation in such a study would, of course, be voluntary.

C. Undertake Federally Funded Comprehensive Studies on the Uses of Reproductive Genetic Technologies, and on Their Effects on Children Born with Their Aid

. . . [A]ssisted reproduction and genomic knowledge are increasingly converging with one another. Practices such as preimplantation genetic diagnosis (PGD) and gamete sorting represent the first fusion of these disciplines. Before these practices become routine, it is desirable that policymakers and the public understand their present and projected uses and effects. To this end, there should be federally funded comprehensive studies, undertaken ideally with the full participation of ART practitioners and their professional associations, on how and to what extent such practices are currently and may soon be employed, and their effects on the health of children born with their aid . . .

D. Strengthen and Augment the Fertility Clinic Success Rate and Certification Act

As currently written, the Fertility Clinic Success Rate and Certification Act (FCSRCA) is aimed at providing consumers with key information about the pregnancy and live-birth success rates of assisted reproduction clinics in the United States. We believe that the Act should be augmented and strengthened, both to improve this original function of consumer protection and to allow for better public oversight (through the already existing ART surveillance program at the Centers for Disease Control [CDC]) of the development, uses, and effects of reproductive technologies and practices. Toward these ends, the Act, or the regulations propounded pursuant to it, or both, should be improved and strengthened in the following ways.

1. Enhance Reporting Requirements.

a. Efficacy. Provide more user-friendly reporting of data, including adding "patients" as an additional unit of measure.

Currently, data are reported only in terms of "cycles" of treatment (beginning when a woman starts ovarian stimulation or monitoring), rather than in terms of individual patients treated. Thus, it is impossible to know how many individuals undergo assisted reproduction procedures in a given year, how many patients achieve success in the first (or second or third) cycle, how many women fail to conceive, and the like. Presenting results in terms of "numbers of individuals" (in addition to "numbers of cycles") would be very helpful to prospective patients and would yield more precise information for policymakers. Also, this information should be presented with any qualifying language or additional information that would help to avoid confusion for prospective patients or the public.

b. Risks and side effects. Require the publication of all reported adverse health effects.

. . . At the present time, the CDC does collect data on complications and adverse outcomes of pregnancy, including low birthweight and birth defects for each live born and stillborn infant, but this information is not made public. Knowledge of such adverse effects is of paramount concern for prospective patients, policymakers, and the public at large. The CDC should publish its data on the incidence of adverse effects on women undergoing treatment, as well as on the health and development of children born with the aid of ART. In order not to confuse or unduly alarm prospective patients or the public, the CDC should include in its publication comparative data on the incidence of such effects in unassisted births . . .

*c. Costs to the patients. Require the reporting and publication
of the average prices of the procedures and the average cost (to patients)
of a successful assisted pregnancy.*

There is currently no comprehensive source of information regarding the costs borne by the patients seeking treatment involving assisted reproductive technologies. Not surprisingly, prospective patients are keenly interested in this information. Moreover, policymakers interested in questions regarding equality of access, insurance coverage, and related matters would greatly benefit from such information . . .

2. Enhance Patient Protections: Informed Decision-Making.

a. Provide model forms for decision-making.

The present Act would be greatly improved by providing for the promulgation of easy-to-read model consent forms that include information on the possible health risks to mother and child, the novelty of the various procedures used, the number of procedures performed to date, the outcomes, and the various safeguards in place to ensure that such procedures are safe and effective.

3. Improve Implementation.

a. Enforcement. Provide stronger penalties to enhance compliance with the Act's reporting requirements.

Under the Act as currently written the only penalty for noncompliance is the publication of the names of nonreporting clinics. This is insufficient, given the importance of clinic compliance to ART consumers and the greater public. The penalties should reflect the magnitude of harms to be avoided. We leave to legislators the question of what precisely these should be . . .

II. INCREASED OVERSIGHT BY PROFESSIONAL SOCIETIES AND PRACTITIONERS

Professional oversight has traditionally been the principal mechanism of regulation for the practice of medicine, and the practice of reproductive medicine is no exception. There is a well-developed body of professional guidelines and standards for the clinical practice of assisted reproduction, and as far as the Council can determine (in the absence of a more comprehensive investigation of physicians' actual conduct), the vast majority of practitioners abide by these guidelines and standards and are dedicated to the welfare of their patients. Yet the Council has identified the following substantive areas that it believes require attention and improvement:

A. Strengthen Informed Patient Decision-Making

Clinicians and their professional societies should make efforts to improve the current system of informed decision-making by patients to conform to the concerns and suggestions described above. ASRM and SART (the Society for Assisted Reproductive Technology) should pay attention not only to helping devise improved consent forms, but also to recommending procedures to their members for discussing the subject properly with patients and for securing their meaningful consent. For this purpose, they should consider making training sessions on this subject a requirement of membership.

B. Treat the Child Born with the Aid of Assisted Reproductive Procedures as a Patient

ART clinicians should take additional measures to ensure the health and safety of all participants in the ART process, *including the children who are born as a result*. Thus, in making decisions and undertaking clinical interventions, such practitioners should carefully consider how these actions will affect the health and well-being of these children . . . ART clinicians and their professional societies should consult with pediatricians (and their professional societies) to learn how their practices may be affecting the health and safety of the children born as a result. Clinicians and professional societies should also cooperate fully and vigorously with any efforts (such as the studies described in Section I of this chapter) to ascertain the effects of ART and related practices on the health and development of such children. In addition, the Council strongly endorses a specific substantive recommendation: clinicians and professional societies should take additional concrete steps to *reduce the incidence of multiple embryo transfers* and resulting multiple births, a known source of high risk and discernible harm to the resulting children.

C. Improve Enforcement of Existing Guidelines

There are today a host of reasonable guidelines in place for clinicians and practitioners engaged in ART, and, to repeat, they are apparently followed by most practitioners. However, the relevant professional societies need to take stronger steps to ensure that these guidelines are followed. For example, one such professional society "actively discourages" the use of PGD for sex selection for nonmedical purposes, yet several prominent members of that society openly advertise the practice. Professional societies must clarify the contours of appropriate conduct and adopt reasonable mechanisms of enforcement.

D. Improve Procedures for Movement of Experimental Procedures into Clinical Practice

Professional societies and clinicians should develop a more systematic mechanism for reviewing experimental procedures before they become part of standard clinical practice. Such a system might include requirements for animal studies, institutional review board (IRB) oversight, and formal discussion and ongoing (and prospective) monitoring of the significance and results of novel procedures.

E. Create and Enforce Minimum Uniform Standards for the Protection of Human Subjects Affected by Assisted Reproduction

At present there is no systematic, mandatory mechanism for protecting human subjects who are engaged in experimental ART protocols not affiliated with institutions receiving federal funds. This problem is compounded by the fact that in the practice of assisted reproduction (as in the practice of medicine more generally), there is not a clear distinction between research and innovative clinical practice. Investigational interventions that could affect the health and well-being of children born with the aid of ART should be subjected to at least as much ethical scrutiny and regulatory oversight as investigational interventions affecting other human subjects of research. Current research policies establish special protections for children and fetuses in research. For similar reasons, there is a need for special protections when research involves interventions in embryos that could later affect the health and welfare of the resulting live-born children. Clinicians and their professional societies should adopt measures (such as IRB-like oversight) to provide necessary safeguards.

F. Develop Additional Self-Imposed Ethical Boundaries

Clinicians and professional societies would be well-advised to establish for themselves additional clear boundaries defining what is and what is not ethically appropriate conduct, regarding both research and clinical practice. Without such guidance, irresponsible clinicians and scientists may engage in practices that will, fairly or unfairly, bring opprobrium on the discipline as a whole. Practices such as, among others, the fusion of male and female embryos, the use of gametes harvested from fetuses (or produced from stem cells) to create embryos, and the transfer of human embryos to nonhuman uteri for purposes of research fall squarely into this category. The relevant professional societies should preemptively take a firm stand against such practices and back that stand up with meaningful enforcement.

NOTES AND QUESTIONS

By admission, the Council's recommendations are modest, and envision greater study of the effect that ART has on women and children. The recommendations seem, for the most part, noncontroversial in substance, and may only raise an eyebrow or two when questions of funding are debated.

Following the above-excerpted recommendations for additional study of potential harms and greater professional self-regulation, the Council proposes a set of "targeted legislative measures." The measures suggest moratoria on "questionable practices" which the Council urges Congress to enact in short order to prevent "any individual from committing acts that could radically alter what the community regards as acceptable in human reproduction . . ." The council describes these practices as "some already in use, others likely to be tried in the foreseeable future," thus, emphasizing the urgency of action. The recommended bans are organized according to four principles, each pointing to one or two provisions that should be the subject of a legislative measure:

A. Preserving a Reasonable Boundary between the Human

and the Nonhuman (or, between the Human and the Animal) in Human Procreation

The question of the human-animal boundary in general can, in some respects, be quite complex and subtle, and the "mixing" of human and animal tissues and materials is not, in the Council's view, by itself objectionable. In the *context of therapy and preventive medicine*, we accept the transplantation of animal organs or their parts to replace defective human ones; and we welcome the use of vaccines and drugs produced from animals. Looking to the future, we do not see any overriding objection to the insertion of animal-derived genes or cells into a human body — or even into human fetuses — where the aim would be to treat or prevent a dread disease in the patient or the developing child (although issues would remain about indirect genetic modification of egg and sperm that could adversely affect future generations) . . . But in the *context of procreation* — of actually mixing human and nonhuman gametes or blastomeres at the very earliest stages of biological development — we believe that the ethical concerns raised by violating that boundary are especially acute, and at the same time that the prospects for drawing clear lines limiting permissible research are especially favorable. One bright line should be drawn at the creation of animal-human hybrid embryos, produced ex vivo by fertilization of human egg by animal (for example, chimpanzee) sperm (or the reverse): we do not wish to have to judge the humanity or moral worth of such an ambiguous hybrid entity (for example, a "humanzee," the analog of the mule); we do not want a possibly human being to have other than human progenitors. A second bright line would be at the insertion of ex vivo human embryos into the bodies of animals: an ex vivo human embryo entering a uterus belongs *only* in a *human* uterus. If these lines should be crossed, it should only be after clear public deliberation and assent, not by the private decision of some adventurous or renegade researchers. We therefore recommend that Congress should:

> **Prohibit the transfer, for any purpose, of any human embryo into the body of any member of a nonhuman species; and**

> **Prohibit the production of a hybrid human-animal embryo by fertilization of human egg by animal sperm or of animal egg by human sperm.**

B.   Respect for Women and Human Pregnancy, Preventing Certain Exploitative and Degrading Practices

Respect for women with regard to assisted reproduction encompasses many things, including respect for their health, autonomy, and privacy; these are by and large properly attended to in current assisted-reproduction practices. But in the face of some new technological possibilities, we recognize that respect for women also involves respecting their bodily integrity. A number of animal experiments using assisted reproductive technologies have shown the value of initiating pregnancies solely for the purpose of research on embryonic and fetal development or for the purpose of securing tissues or organs for transplantation. We generally do not object to such procedures being performed on other animals, but we do not believe they should, under any circumstances, be undertaken with humans, or that human pregnancy should be initiated using assisted reproductive technologies for any purpose other than to seek the birth of a child. A woman and her uterus should not be regarded or used as a piece of laboratory equipment, as an "incubator" for growing research materials, or as a "field" for growing and harvesting body parts. We therefore recommend that, in an effort to express our society's profound regard for human pregnancy and pregnant women, Congress should:

> **Prohibit the transfer of a human embryo (produced ex vivo) to a woman's uterus for any purpose other than to attempt to produce a live-born child.**

C. *Respect for Children Conceived with the Aid of Assisted Reproductive Technologies, Securing for Them the Same Rights and Human Attachments Naturally Available to Children Conceived In Vivo*

We believe that children conceived with the aid of ARTs deserve to be treated like all other children and to be afforded the same opportunities, benefits, and human attachments available to children conceived without such assistance . . . But . . . certain applications of embryo manipulation and assisted reproductive techniques could deny to children born with their aid a full and equal share in our common human origins, for instance by denying them the direct biological connection to *two* human genetic parents or by giving them a fetal or embryonic progenitor. We believe that such departures and inequities in human origins should not be inflicted on any child. We therefore recommend that, in an effort to secure for children who are born with the help of ARTs the same rights and human attachments naturally available to children conceived in vivo, Congress should:

> **Prohibit attempts to conceive a child by any means other than the union of egg and sperm.**

> **Prohibit attempts to conceive a child by using gametes obtained from a human fetus or derived from human embryonic stem cells.**

> **Prohibit attempts to conceive a child by fusing blastomeres from two or more embryos.**

D. *Setting Some Agreed-Upon Boundaries on How Embryos May Be Used and Treated*

What degree of respect is owed to early human embryos will almost certainly continue to arouse great controversy, as it does among members of this Council. But we all agree that human embryos deserve . . . (at least) special respect. Accordingly, we believe some measures setting upper age limits on the use of embryos in research and limits on commerce in human embryos may be agreeable to all parties to the ongoing dispute over the moral status of human embryos. Along these lines, we believe that Congress should:

> **Prohibit the use of human embryos in research beyond a designated stage in their development (between 10 and 14 days after fertilization); and**

> **Prohibit the buying and selling of human embryos.**

With these legislative proposals, the Council turns largely from the practiced to the prospective, aiming to "head off at the pass" anticipated conduct that it believes would be universally disfavored. Notice that many of the named practices involve the creation of a child by means other than those that are currently used (namely, in vivo and in vitro fertilization of a single egg by a single sperm). If British law had similarly banned IVF in the 1970s because it presented a novel method of conception, would society have been better off with this preservation of the status quo? Interestingly, at the time IVF was being developed, at least one commentator warned against further experimentation with in vitro fertilization, even suggesting a "voluntary moratorium on any attempts to create a child through IVF and embryo transfer until the safety of the procedures could be assessed." This commentator further argued that "[b]ecause the new procedures for in vitro fertilization and laboratory culture of human embryos probably carry a serious risk of damage to any child so generated, there appears to be no ethical way to proceed." This commentator was Leon Kass, the Chair of the President's Council of Bioethics, the person who stewarded the above suggested moratoria on novel methods of reproduction. *See* Leon R. Kass, *Babies By Means of In Vitro Fertilization: Unethical Experiments on the Unborn?*, 285 NEW ENG. J. MED. 1174 (1971). Do you agree with Dr. Kass that caution and respect for the human being as we are currently formed should translate into prohibition, or do you see a way to ethically and safely proceed to further investigate the wonders of human reproduction? The final two chapters of the book explore these outer edges of ART, investigating the scientifically and politically evolving topics of human stem cell research and human reproductive cloning.

Chapter 9

HUMAN EMBRYONIC STEM CELL RESEARCH

> Monitoring stem cell research can be a bit like watching Niagara Falls. Not only do scientific reports pour forth daily, . . . but a kind of mist rises up for the torrent of news flashes and editorials, making it difficult to separate knowledge from opinion and hope from hype. —

> *The President's Council on Bioethics*, in
> Monitoring Stem Cell Research
> (January 2004)

The last quarter of the twentieth century may be remembered as a period of great advancement in the field of reproductive medicine. Beginning with the debut IVF birth of Louise Brown in 1978, physicians and researchers succeeded in prodding many of nature's secrets surrounding the interworkings of human procreation, with discoveries ranging from embryo cryopreservation to intracytoplasmic sperm injection (ICSI) to preimplantation genetic diagnosis (PGD). Each of these advances allows ART practitioners to offer patients better and more successful treatments in their quest to conceive and give birth to healthy offspring. But as the twenty-first century dawned, a new era in reproductive medicine seemed to emerge. The ability to create embryos in the laboratory became of interest not just as a means to overcome infertility, but as a possible source of medical therapies and cures for all of humankind.

In the late 1990s, researchers discovered that cells taken from early embryos had two unique properties that distinguished them from other types of cells. First, these early or "stem" cells had the capacity to renew themselves for long periods of time through cell division, thus creating stem cell lines that could be available for study well into the future. In contrast, non-stem cells do not have the ability to proliferate indefinitely in a culture medium, making them less desirable as a source for cell research. Second, embryonic stem cells are undifferentiated, meaning they have not yet become a specific type of cell such as a blood or skin cell, but they could be coaxed into becoming specific cell types, including cardiac, nerve, liver, or muscle cells. This ability to induce embryonic stem cells to become working heart, pancreas, brain, or other cells of the human body posed the possibility of groundbreaking advancements in clinical medicine. If embryonic stem cells could be "manufactured" into other body cells, they could repair damage caused by innumerable diseases — diseases that have eluded therapy or cure since they first appeared in the human population.

As attractive as the idea of "repairing the body with the body" sounds, the fact remains that the source of these regenerating cells is the human embryo, which must be destroyed in order for its stem cells to be retrieved. Thus, the debate over human embryonic stem cell research emerges. The debate stirs up passion on all sides, from those who believe that society has a duty to yield the early embryo for the benefit of human health and well-being, to those who maintain the sanctity of life, even at its earliest stages, bars destruction of any form of human life. Controversy over the source of these potentially life-saving cells has also motivated scientists to try to derive renewable stem cell lines from material other than human embryos. In a little over a decade, the prospect of stem cell research has captured the attention of researchers, presidents, national commissions, lawmakers, and commentators, both in the United States and worldwide. A glimpse into the facts and fiction, hope and hype, follows.

SECTION I: THE SCIENCE OF EMBRYONIC STEM CELL RESEARCH

A. Introduction to the Terms

Jennifer L. Enmon
Stem Cell Research: Is the Law Preventing Progress?
2002 Utah Law Review 621, 622-628

A. Stem Cells: What Are They?

Stem cells are undifferentiated cells that have the ability to self replicate and differentiate into any cell type in the body.[1] Embryonic, fetal, and adult tissues are sources of stem cells. The resulting cells are referred to as embryonic stem (ES) cells, embryonic germ (EG) cells, and adult stem cells, respectively. ES and EG cells are the more controversial stem cells, because ES cell lines are derived from in vitro fertilized embryos and EG cells are derived from aborted fetal tissue. In contrast, adult stem cell lines are derived from a living donor who is unharmed by the process.

Stem cells that differentiate into all tissues in the body and can form an entire organism are referred to as totipotent stem cells. Those that can form most of the body's tissue are pluripotent stem cells, and those that can differentiate into only a few tissues are called multipotent stem cells. ES and EG cells are characterized as pluripotent stem cells. In contrast, adult stem cells are generally characterized as multipotent, meaning adult stem cells cannot differentiate into as many cell types as ES and EG cells. Moreover, adult stem cells "have not been isolated for all tissues of the body," further limiting their potential. Adult stem cells have also been difficult to isolate and purify. Because of the disadvantages associated with adult stem cells, they are limited as both a research tool and potential treatment tool. Hence, pluripotent cells derived from embryonic and fetal tissue currently hold the most promise in advancing the medical field.

---

[1] Much of the author's basic description of stem cells is based on publications by the National Institutes of Health, specifically its report entitled, "Stem Cells: Scientific Progress and Future Research Directions" (2001), available at http://www.nih.gov/news/stemcell/scireport.htm. -Ed.

1. Embryo Derived Pluripotent Stem Cells

ES cell lines are created from in vitro fertilized embryos. Approximately five days after a human egg is fertilized, the embryo (referred to as a blastocyst at this stage of development) begins to differentiate into two layers consisting of an inner cell mass (ICM) and an outer cell mass. The ICM gives rise to an ES cell line when removed from the outer cell mass and exposed to the proper conditions. Tests are performed on these cell lines to ensure that the isolated and cultured cells exhibit pluripotency and, therefore, that the isolated cells are actually ES cells.

ES cells as a research tool are useful only if the cell line can be maintained undifferentiated and, when desired, can be directed to form specific cell types. ES cell lines have been maintained without differentiating for several months, demonstrating the robustness of ES cell lines. In addition, ES cell lines can be cryopreserved for several months for use at a later time. Established ES cell lines have also been directed to differentiate into a variety of cell/tissue types by exposure to particular growth factors, an "initial step toward achieving fully directed cell differentiation." This initial step was greatly extended upon the report of directing ES cells to differentiate into blood cells. These results demonstrate that with time and appropriate funding, scientists will learn to direct ES cells to form other tissues, creating "the potential to treat a wide variety of diseases."

2. EG Derived Pluripotent Stem Cells

EG cells are derived from specific cells obtained from fetuses aborted five to nine weeks after fertilization. Researchers have been able to generate pluripotent cells from initial cultures of the fetal cells capable of long-term proliferation. However, it has not been shown that pluripotent cells derived from EG cells can be maintained undifferentiated for as long as ES cells can be maintained undifferentiated. Hence, pluripotent ES cells may prove to be more useful because ES cells can be maintained undifferentiated in culture longer than EG derived pluripotent stem cells.

B. How Can Pluripotent ES and EG Cells Treat Diseases?

Diseases, such as Parkinson's or Alzheimer's, are targets of pluripotent stem cell research, because these diseases are characterized by damaged cells and there are no cures for these diseases. However . . . basic research is routinely conducted on rodent models . . . [It] is hoped that success with rodent models is indicative of potential treatments of human disease.

There have been many promising results using rodent models. Type I Diabetes is caused when the body attacks its own insulin producing cells. Mouse ES cells have been differentiated into insulin producing cells; these cells, when transplanted into mice spleens, have resulted in the reversal of diabetes. Furthermore, insulin producing cells have been obtained from human ES cells.

Similarly, success has been achieved with neurological disorders such as Parkinson's and Lou Gehrig's diseases. Parkinson's disease is caused by decreasing dopamine neurons. Scientists hope that ES cells could be implanted in the brain and coaxed to differentiate into new neurons. Again, rodent models have shown promise, with mouse ES cells being used to treat Parkinson's-like symptoms in rats. Scientists have also made progress using pluripotent cells to treat degenerative motor neuron diseases such as amyotrophic lateral sclerosis, commonly known as Lou Gehrig's disease. Rats with Lou Gehrig's symptoms were injected with EG derived pluripotent cells and within three months many of the previously paralyzed rats were able to move their limbs. These are just a few examples of incurable diseases that debilitate people everyday that may, in the future, be treated with pluripotent stem cells, given appropriate funding and time.

C. Pluripotent ES Cells and Cloning

Pluripotent ES cell and cloning technology can be combined in what is referred to as "therapeutic cloning." Therapeutic cloning recently made headlines when Advanced Cell Technology, Inc., a Massachusetts based company, announced the cloning of a human embryo. However, the embryo was not created for reproductive purposes and was never intended to create a human. Instead, the blastocyst was created as a source of ES cells.

Using ES cells, researchers may eventually find treatments for numerous diseases. However, one potential problem is that treatments created with these cells may be rejected by a patient's immune system, similar to rejection experienced after an organ transplant. But, if the treatment could be derived from a patient's own cells, rejection or a lifetime of immunosuppressive therapy could be avoided. Therapeutic cloning represents such a treatment.

Therapeutic cloning involves the replacement of the DNA in a human egg or oocyte with a patient's own DNA. This new cell is activated and begins to divide, forming a blastocyst. However, as with ordinary ES cell line derivation, the blastocyst development is stopped by harvesting the ICM at approximately five days postfertilization. ES cells are then cultured and could be transplanted into the patient without immunosuppressive therapy or fear of rejection.

Given the great promises stem cells hold, especially pluripotent stem cells, carefully crafted legislation is required to ensure that medical advancement in this area is not overly inhibited.

NOTES AND QUESTIONS

1.   The current debate over embryonic stem cell research was launched in the fall of 1998 when two teams of researchers from American universities published independent reports that the groups had succeeded in isolating and culturing stem cells from human embryos and aborted fetuses. The first report described the work of John Gearhart and his colleagues at The Johns Hopkins University, who derived embryonic germ cells (EG cells) from the gonadal tissue of cadaveric fetal tissue.[2] Michael J. Shamblott et al., *Derivation of Pluripotent Stem Cells From Cultured*

---

[2] The gonadal tissue are cells that ultimately give rise to sperm cells or egg cells, depending on the sex of the fetus.

Human Primordial Germ Cells, 95 PROC. NAT'L ACAD. SCI. 13726 (1998). The second report issued from James Thomson and coworkers at the University of Wisconsin, who derived embryonic stem cells (ES cells) from the blastocyst of an early human embryo donated by a couple who had received fertility treatment.[3] James A. Thomson et al., *Embryonic Stem Cell Lines Derived From Human Blastocysts*, 282 SCIENCE 1145 (1998). These two reports of stem cell isolation and cultivation meant that scientists could move to the next step of inducing these undifferentiated cells to specialize into any cell of the human body, giving rise to cell-based therapies to treat disease. What had only been imagined was now coined the new field of regenerative medicine.

The import of these discoveries was immediately apparent, even to those outside the scientific community. On November 14, 1998, President Clinton wrote to the National Bioethics Advisory Commission (NBAC), a presidential commission established by Executive Order in October 1995, requesting the group "conduct a thorough review of the issues associated with . . . human stem cell research, balancing all medical and ethical issues." See Ethical Issues in Human Stem Cell Research, Vol. 1, Report and Recommendations of the National Bioethics Advisory Commission 1 (1999) (the NBAC Report). The stem cell debate, far from resolved at the turn of the century and the start of a new administration, prompted President Bush to turn to his bioethics advisors for counsel on the emerging science of regenerative medicine. In January 2004 the President's Council on Bioethics published its report, Monitoring Stem Cell Research, documenting the Council's two year study of the now highly public debate. We will take a closer look at both presidential reports throughout this Chapter.

---

[3] A blastocyst is an embryo at roughly five day post-fertilization, consisting of approximately 100-200 cells.

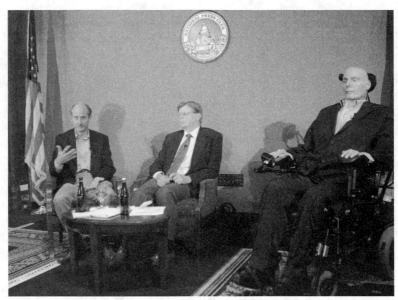

Actor and Stem Cell Research Advocate Christopher Reeve (right) confers with Dr. John Gearhart (center) and Dr. James Thomson (left) (October 2003)

2. *Sources of Embryonic Stem Cells.* The controversy over stem cell research rests primarily at the source — the source of the cells themselves. Embryonic stem cells, including ES and EG cells, can be derived from four different sources, each engendering its own set of ethical dilemmas. The four sources are:

1. *Embryos created by in vitro fertilization for infertility treatments that are donated by the progenitor couple.* In Chapters 6 and 7 we studied the common practice of couples undergoing fertility treatment using IVF to freeze excess embryos for use in later cycles. In some cases, couples succeed in their pursuit of parenthood, or abandon such quest, leaving embryos in frozen storage for long periods. A subset of progenitors who have no plans to implant the embryos donate them for research. These embryo donations serve as the source for embryonic stem cells. Once donated, the embryos are thawed and allowed to develop for two to three days, until they reach the blastocyst stage. Cells from the blastocyst's inner cell mass, which if implanted would become the fetus, are retrieved and placed in a culture medium that enables the undifferentiated cells to proliferate and maintain the potential to contribute to all adult cell types. Once the inner cell mass is disrupted in the blastocyst, it can no longer develop into a fetus and is thus discarded. See The NBAC Report, at 9.

2. *Embryos created by in vitro fertilization expressly for research purposes.* Researchers can create embryos using donated sperm and eggs, specifically and exclusively for the purpose of harvesting stem cells from those developing embryos. The difference between IVF embryos created for research and IVF embryos created for reproduction is the motivation of the creators at the time the embryos are formed. The original intent of an

infertile couple is to use the embryos for procreation, while the researchers intend to retrieve the stem cells and thereafter discard the embryo. There are two primary reasons offered for creating embryos strictly for research purposes. First, to provide a sufficient supply of embryos. If IVF couples are not willing to donate at the rate needed to keep pace with research, embryos could be created to satisfy scientific experimentation (assuming a sufficient supply of donated eggs and sperm). Second, specifically designed embryos may be more useful for research and medical purposes. If scientists can draw upon specific characteristics of the gametes, they may be able to create embryos that would be more useful either to a particular person in need of therapy, or for developing a particular line of therapy. At the current time, both of these rationales are more speculative than real, as there does not appear to be an insufficient supply of donated embryos, and a preference for research, rather than reproductive embryos, has not emerged. *See The NBAC Report*, at 55-56.

3. *Embryos created by somatic cell nuclear transfer or other cloning techniques.* Creating and using cloned embryos for stem cell research is referred to as "therapeutic cloning." A cloned embryo is an embryo created not by the union of a sperm and an egg, but by a technique known as somatic cell nuclear transfer (SCNT). SCNT begins when the nucleus is removed from an unfertilized human egg and replaced by the nucleus of a somatic cell (a non-sex cell, such as a skin cell) of the organism to be cloned. A chemical or an electric pulse is then applied to the egg to activate it, much the way a sperm activates an egg by penetrating its surface in the course of natural fertilization. Thereafter, the egg develops into an embryo and after five days, into a blastocyst.

The inner cell mass of a cloned embryo can be harvested just like the cells from an IVF embryo. The difference is that the stem cells are an exact match for an existing person, the one who supplied the non-sex cell for transfer into the enucleated egg. If these cells can be coaxed to become specific heart, nerve, liver, or other cells, they can be transplanted back into the person who contributed the cell, and will not face the tissue rejection that accompanies organ and tissue transplantation when one person donates body parts to another. Since the repairing cells are made from the donor's own cells, presumably the donor's body will not reject this "non-foreign" tissue. Therapeutic cloning offers the real possibility that the human body can heal itself, but the creation of an embryo using SCNT and its subsequent destruction continues to pose ethical concerns surrounding this source of embryonic stem cells.[4] See James A. Thomson, *Human*

---

[4] Cloning embryos for stem cell research is also referred to as "research cloning", with some arguing that this term is more accurate because the promise of any therapy resulting from cloned embryos is highly speculative. As one scholar remarked, "I think it amounts to a gross misrepresentation for those who favor research cloning to try to sell it to the public as "therapeutic cloning" and to suggest that a ban will prevent thousands — or millions — of patients with serious and even lethal diseases from obtaining rejection-proof transplants." Alexander Morgan Capron, *Placing a Moratorium on Research Cloning To Ensure Effective Control Over Reproductive Cloning*, 53 Hast. L. J. 1075 (2002).

Embryonic Stem Cells, in THE HUMAN EMBRYONIC STEM CELL DEBATE, 15-16 (Suzanne Holland et al., eds., 2001).[5]

4. *Embryonic germ cells derived from fetal tissue.* EG cells are derived from the primordial germ cells, which occur in a specific part of the fetus called the gonadal ridge, and which normally develop into mature gametes (eggs and sperm). The EG cells are collected from the bodies of five- to nine-week-old fetuses that have been donated after elective abortions. Once isolated and placed in culture, EG cells can give rise to undifferentiated cells capable of long-term proliferation, similar to the propensities of ES cells. Researchers caution that EG cells may not be as robust as ES cells in their capacity to proliferate long-term. According to the National Institutes of Health, EG cells can be maintained through approximately 70 doubling cycles while ES cells have been maintained for up to about 300 doubling cycles. Nevertheless, current scientific thinking remains optimistic that EG cells, like their ES counterparts, can be differentiated into a variety of cell types. *See* Nat'l Insts. Of Health, U.S. Dept. of Health & Human Servs., *Stem Cells: Scientific Progress and Future Research Directions* 14 (2001).

Do you believe stem cells should receive different legal treatment based solely on their source of origin? For example, do you think it would be appropriate to legalize embryonic stem cell research for ES cells derived from donated spare IVF embryos, but outlaw research using embryos created strictly for research purposes? Does the intent of the embryos' creator(s) at the time of creation forever determine the status of the embryo for research purposes? Suppose an embryo is created for research using donor gametes, but on day 3, when the embryo is eight cells in size and suitable for transfer back to the uterus, the egg donor changes her mind about the research and seeks to implant the embryo. Does the fact that the embryo was originally created for research bar its transformation to a reproductive embryo?

3. *Adult Stem Cells.* Adult stem cells refers to stem cells that are non-embryonic, and thus more differentiated. The primary roles of adult stem cells in the human body are to maintain and repair the tissue in which they are found. Adult stem cells can be retrieved from various places in the body, including bone marrow, skin, and portions of the small intestine. The term "adult stem cell" is a bit of a misnomer because these highly prolific cells are not just found in adults; they can be found in various tissues in children, as well as in the umbilical cord at the time of a baby's delivery. Like ES and EG cells, adult stem cells can give rise to cell lines that are more specialized than themselves, but because they have been partially differentiated, they are not thought to be as flexible as stem cells derived from embryos or fetal tissue. See, e.g., David Perlman, *Marrow Stem Cells Have Limited*

---

[5] Therapeutic cloning can be contrasted with reproductive cloning in which the embryo developed using SCNT is implanted in a woman's uterus with the hope that a child will be born. That cloned child would share the identical genome of the person whose cell was injected into the enucleated egg. Reproductive cloning is a type of asexual reproduction because the egg and sperm do not unite to form the embryo; the embryo is formed from a single egg that has been activated to divide into an embryo. Sperm is not a necessary element of reproductive cloning. We take up the topic of reproductive cloning in Chapter 10.

Use, Study Finds, S.F. CHRON., Oct. 16, 2003, at A6 (reporting on UCSF and Stanford study showing stem cells from adult bone marrow do not create a wide variety of cells the way embryonic stem cells do); compare *Tissue Regeneration: Unique Adult Stem Cell Identified*, HEART DISEASE WEEKLY, Feb. 27, 2005, at 215 (announcing researchers have identified adult stem cells that may have the capacity to repair and regenerate all tissue types in the body). Regenerative medicine research using adult stem cells is ongoing, with many hoping for great success using these bodily products that can be retrieved without the controversy that surrounds embryo research. See President's Council on Bioethics, *Monitoring Stem Cell Research* 10-11 (2004).

4. *Induced Pluripotent Stem Cells.* Perhaps the most exciting scientific advancement in stem cell research over the past several years has been the development of induced pluripotent stem cells (iPS cells). In 2007, scientists at Kyoto University in Japan and the University of Wisconsin announced they had reprogrammed human adult skin cells to regress back to their pluripotent state (as undifferentiated cell lines potentially capable of being transformed into any cell type in the body). The technique, in simplest terms, reverses the process of developing cell lines using embryonic stem cells. Instead of extracting cells from a 5-day-old embryo (and destroying the embryo in the process) and coaxing those undifferentiated cells to transform into specific cells of the body, iPS cells start with a specific cell, such as a skin cell, which is coaxed to revert back to its undifferentiated original form. This "coaxing" was at first achieved by injecting the skin cell with several genes that induced the cell to evolve backward to a state of pluripotency. Over a few years, refinements to this reprogramming method have been introduced, improving the production and quality of the iPS cell lines. *See* Nancy M.P. King, Christine Nero-Coughlin, Anthony Atala, *Pluripotent Stem Cells: The Search for the "Perfect" Source*, 12 MINN. J. L. SCI. & TECH. 715 (2011); Constance Holden & Gretchen Vogel, *A Seismic Shift for Stem Cell Research*, 319 SCIENCE 560 (2008).

The promise of undifferentiated cell lines derived from non-embryonic sources was greeted with much enthusiasm from across the scientific, ethical and political spectrum. If iPS cells were as robust and workable as human ES cells, then stem cell research could proceed unencumbered by the weighty and confounding dilemmas that surround the derivation of embryonic stem cells. To date, both ES and iPS cell lines continue to pose challenges to scientists working to develop usable pluripotent cells. Research using both types of cells reveals that both cells display higher genetic abnormalities than other cells. Since the goals of stem cell research is to produce therapies and cures for treating disease, the ingredients of those therapies must themselves be disease-free. The high level of genetic abnormality of ES and iPS cells may suggest that any product derived from these cells could cause a disease, such as cancer (which is associated with genetic abnormality), thus making the cell lines highly unsuitable for therapeutic application. *See* Eryn Brown, *Genetic Abnormalities Found in Stem Cell Lines*, L.A. TIMES, Jan. 6, 2011.

B. Human and Animal Stem Cell Studies

Initial reactions to the prospect of regenerative medicine as a means of curing human diseases — leaving aside for now the great debate over embryo destruction — were hopefulness, excitement and support for investment in the infrastructure and brainpower required to bring effective treatments to patients worldwide. In his excellent book, *Stem Cell Century*, Professor Russell Korobkin gathers some of the many predictions that "stem cell research will lead to the most important medical care advances in our lifetimes." He quotes the former National Institutes of Health director Harold Varmus telling Congress that "there is almost no realm of medicine that might not be touched by this innovation . . . It is not too unrealistic to say that this research has the potential to revolutionize the practice of medicine and improve the quality and length of life." Senator Orrin Hatch (R-Utah) called stem cell research "the most promising research in healthcare perhaps in [the] history of the world." *See* RUSSELL KOROBKIN (WITH STEPHEN R. MUNZER), STEM CELL CENTURY 2-3 (2007). With such high hopes and expectations, could any medical invention really deliver as hyped?

It is important to keep in mind that the initial reports of isolating and cultivating embryonic stem cells were only a first step in what was known at the time to be a complex, even elusive process. A decade and a half after the 1998 "proof of principle" reports, where does progress on human stem cell research stand? On the one hand, the so-called Holy Grail of stem cell research has not been realized. That is, to date, no human line of stem cells has been isolated, cultivated into specialized cells and transplanted into a patient who was cured of an ailment. On the other hand, some initial steps have been taken toward testing embryonic stem cell-derived therapies in human patients. As of 2012, the U.S. Food and Drug Administration has approved two clinical trials to test the safety of therapies derived from human embryonic stem cells. In 2010, Geron Corporation began the first such trial, injecting nervous system cells derived from embryonic cells into patients with severe spinal cord injuries. Promising animal studies had shown tremendous results, healing the severed spinal cords of mice injected with embryo-derived neuron cells. One year later in November 2011, Geron announced it was shutting down the study after enrolling only four patients, none of whom showed any improvement in condition. The company's chief executive reassured the public of his deep belief in the promise of stem cell therapy, but explained that the decision to exit the stem cell arena was based on economics. *See* Andrew Pollack, *Geron Is Shutting Down Its Stem Cell Clinical Trial*, N.Y. TIMES, Nov. 14, 2011 (reporting the small trial cost Geron $25 million).

The second clinical trial is being conducted by Massachusetts-based Advance Cell Technology on patients with an eye disease called macular degeneration. As of April 2012, three patients had enrolled in the study in which retinal cells derived from embryonic stem cells were injected into the eye. No results have yet been published. To follow the clinical trial's progress, check out the company website at www.advancecell.com.

To some, the lack of widespread and well-enrolled clinical trials is a sign that the initial excitement over stem cell therapy was a hype that led to dangerous exaggeration. Setting expectations at such a high level, argues Professor Rebecca

Dresser, "threatens scientific integrity." In making this particular claim, Professor Dresser reminds us of other early scientific breakthroughs that fell short of initial expectations such as the artificial heart, fetal tissue transplantation and gene therapy. *See* Rebecca Dresser, *Stem Cell Research as Innovation: Expanding the Ethical and Policy Conversation*, 38 J.L. MED. & ETHICS 332 (2010). To others, particularly scientists who are devoting their lives to unraveling the stem cell puzzle, the lack of significant progress in these early years is both expected and acceptable. One researcher who studies the application of stem cell therapies to Alzheimer's disease remarks on the "legitimate enthusiasm about stem cell therapies" but cautions that "we should not expect overnight success." He urges we "resist the temptation to delay starting important avenues of research because they might require hard work and an uncertain time-line." *See* Lawrence Goldstein, *Why Scientific Details Are Important When Novel Technologies Encounter Law, Politics and Ethics*, 38 J.L. MED. & ETHICS 204 (2010).

Today's aspirations for therapies are based largely on an array of animal studies in which damaged tissue in mice has seemingly been repaired, and, as noted above, on a smattering of studies involving human stem cells that appear to have differentiated into a few specific cell types. While large-scale studies on human subjects may be off in the future, a review of the current state of the science may be useful in informing and shaping your views on the moral and legal questions that surround stem cell research. Knowing where we are today may help you determine where we should head tomorrow.

What follows is a summary of clinical research and reporting on a variety of human ailments thought to be susceptible to stem cell-derived treatment or cure. To emphasize the progress, or lack thereof, over the past roughly 15 years since the introduction of the concept of regenerative medicine, each entry reflects the original description of the research contained in the first edition of this book (completed in 2005), followed by an update of activity over the past seven years.

1. Parkinson's Disease. Parkinson's is a chronic, progressive movement disorder in which brain cells — neurons — that produce the chemical dopamine begin to malfunction and eventually die. Dopamine is a neurotransmitter, or chemical messenger, that transports signals to the parts of the brain that control movement initiation and coordination. When Parkinson's disease occurs, for unexplained reasons, these neurons begin to die at a faster rate and the amount of dopamine produced in the brain decreases. The disease is characterized by tremors of the hands, arms, legs, jaw and face, and by impaired balance and coordination. See The Parkinson's Disease Foundation Website at www.pdf.org.

Stem cell research focusing on Parkinson's is aimed at prompting undifferentiated cells to become neurons that could replace the dopamine-producing brain cells that are lost to the disease. In 2003, scientists at New York's Memorial Sloan-Kettering Cancer Center reported initial success in treating a Parkinson's-like disease in mice. The team cloned mice embryonic stem cells and then coaxed the cells to become dopamine-producing cells. The stem cell-derived brain cells were then transplanted into the brains of mice which had been chemically damaged to produce Parkinson's-like symptoms. According to a published report, the treatment produced robust alleviation of the mice's symptoms, and autopsies of the mice's brains showed healthy colonies of transplanted cells. See Tiziano Barberi et al., *Neural Subtype Specification of Fertilization and Nuclear Transfer Embryonic Stem Cells and Application in Parkinsonian Mice*, 21 NATURE BIOTECHNOLOGY 1200-1207 (2003).

Update: Translation of successful animal experiments into human application has not yielded any significant results to date, at least measured by the opening of clinical trials for human subjects or the publication of scientific papers detailing promising results in human patients. In one review article surveying the state of stem cell research and neurologic disorders, including Parkinson's disease, the author laments, "There are still many obstacles to be overcome before clinical application of cell therapy in neurological disease patients is adopted . . . [I]t is still uncertain what kind of stem cells would be an ideal source for cellular grafts and . . . the mechanism by which transplantation of stem cells leads to an enhanced functional recovery has to be better understood." Seung U. Kim & Jean de Vellis, *Stem Cell-Based Cell Therapy in Neurological Diseases: A Review*, 87 J. NEURO-SCIENCE RESEARCH 2183 (2009). Other researchers report human nonembryonic cells have been reprogrammed into iPS cells that can be subsequently differentiated into the neurons needed to treat the disease. This means, in principle, a patient's own skin cells could be reprogrammed into healthy neurons for transplantation into the brain, but the researchers urge "caution is appropriate because of the risk of adverse events [as with other neurotransplantation trials]." *See* Bernard Lo & Lindsay Parham, *Resolving Ethical Issues in Stem Cell Clinical Trials: The Example of Parkinson Disease*, 38 J. L. MED. & ETHICS 257 (2010).

2. Amyotrophic Lateral Sclerosis (Lou Gehrig's Disease). ALS is a progressive neurodegenerative disease that affects nerve cells in the brain and the spinal cord. Motor neurons, cells that cause muscles to contract, reach from the brain to the spinal cord and from the spinal cord to the muscles throughout the body. The progressive degeneration of the motor neurons in ALS eventually leads to these cells' death. When the motor neurons die, the ability of the brain to initiate and control muscle movement is lost. With voluntary muscle action progressively affected, patients in the later stages of the disease may become totally paralyzed. See The ALS Association Website at *www.alsa.org.*

A January 2005 study at the University of Wisconsin showed, for the first time, that human stem cells could be made to become motor neurons, the cells of the nervous system destroyed by ALS. The UW team derived motor neurons from human embryonic stem cells, by exposing the stem cells to a specific acid early in development. The next step in the process is to test the stem cell-derived neurons in animals to see if they will replace the cells lost by ALS. See Xue-Jun Li, *Specification of Motoneurons from Human Embryonic Stem Cells.* 23 NATURE BIOTECHNOLOGY 215-221 (2005).

Update: Research continues at the University of Wisconsin where researchers developed neurons from human ES cells and implanted them into the brains of mice. Scans showed that the mice brains were able to send and receive electrical impulses in a normal way, creating hope that derived neurons can fully integrate into the brain. For more information, visit the University's Stem Cell and Regenerative Medicine Center website at www.stemcells.wisc.edu.

3. Diabetes. Diabetes is a chronic disorder in which the body is unable to regulate blood glucose, or blood sugar, levels. There are two major types of diabetes, Type 1 and Type 2. Type 1, also called juvenile or insulin-dependent diabetes, occurs when the body's immune system attacks and destroys beta cells in the pancreas. Beta cells produce insulin, a hormone that aids in moving glucose from the blood into cells throughout the body. Insulin enables the body to use glucose found in foods to produce energy for the body. When the beta cells are destroyed, insulin production is thwarted and glucose remains in the blood, a condition that can cause damage to all the body's organs. Because Type 1 diabetics produce no insulin, they must inject daily doses of the hormone to survive. Type 2, or adult onset diabetes, results when the body does not produce enough insulin and/or is unable to use insulin properly. This form of diabetes usually occurs in people who are over 40, overweight, and have a family history of diabetes, although today it is increasingly occurring in younger people, particularly adolescents. See The Joslin Diabetes Center website, www.joslin.org.

In 2003, a team of scientists at the John P. Robarts Research Institute in Canada reported that transplanted adult stem cells derived from bone marrow induced the recipient's pancreatic tissue to repair itself, restoring normal insulin production and reversing symptoms associated with diabetes in animal models of diabetes. In a 2002 study using animal models, researchers at Stanford University School of Medicine created insulin-producing cells from mouse embryonic stem cells. The insulin-producing cells formed pancreatic islet-like clusters, which when transplanted into diabetic mice, reduced blood sugar and increased lifespan. See www.jdrf.org.

Update: According to the Juvenile Diabetes Research Foundation, "In September 2008 researchers from the University of North Carolina at Chapel Hill were able to generate insulin-secreting cells from human skin cells. After turning the skin cells into induced pluripotent stem (iPS) cells, the researchers reprogrammed the cells to produce insulin. These reprogrammed cells not only secreted an insulin component but also produced insulin in response to glucose, raising the possibility that patient-specific stem cells derived from reprogramming could provide a treatment for type 1 diabetes." *See* JDRF Advocacy, Stem Cell Research, available at: http://advocacy.jdrf.org/index.cfm?page_id=109182.

4. Heart Failure. In a 2004 study of heart cells, researchers in Israel were able to prompt human embryonic cells to differentiate into beating heart cells. These heart cells were transplanted directly into a cluster of live rat heart cells in a lab dish. The cells from the two species beat at different rates at first, but within 24 hours the combined masses began pulsing at the same rate. To test whether the human heart cells derived from stem cells could function in a live organism, the researchers transplanted them into 13 pigs whose hearts had been damaged so they beat more slowly. The injury resembled a human heart rhythm disorder caused by disease or a small heart attack. Eleven of the 13 pigs receiving the cells returned to faster heart rates after the stem cell transplant. *See* Izhak Kehat et al., *Electromechanical Integration of Cardiomyocytes Derived from Human Embryonic Stem Cells*, 22 NATURE BIOTECHNOLOGY, 1282-1289 (2004).

Update: Scientists from the Institute of Bioengineering and Nanotechnology in Singapore have shown that human embryonic stem cells can be transformed into heart cells using a "decellularized" heart as a scaffold. For the study, the researchers stripped a mouse heart of its cells, leaving only the organ's scaffold, and replaced them with stem cells. After 14 days, the stem cells developed into two different types of cells found in the heart. The cell-laden scaffold was then implanted back into the mouse where it was observed to develop visible blood vessels, which are critical for the transport of nutrients and oxygen to the heart. *See* Institute of Bioengineering and Nanotechnology, Aug. 12, 2011, available at: http://stemcellaction.org/content/recent-advances-human-embryonic-stem-cell-research.

5. Blindness. In the fall of 2004, researchers at Advanced Cell Technology in Massachusetts described experiments in which retinal pigment epithelial cells (RPE cells) were grown from human embryonic stem cells. RPE cells are critical for vision because they provide nutrients and eliminate waste from the rods and cones — the light-sensitive cells in the retina. The deterioration of RPE cells in middle or old age produces age-related macular degeneration, the leading cause of vision loss in people 60 or older. In the study, human embryonic stem cells allowed to develop in a lab dish under specific conditions spontaneously turned into RPE cells. Researchers hope to test the cells in animals during the next year and, if they prove successful, get permission to conduct trials in humans with RPE-related vision loss. See Irina Klimanskaya et al., *Derivation and Comparative Assessment of Retinal Pigment Epithelial From Human Embryonic Stem Cells Using Transciptomics*, 6 CLONING AND STEM CELLS 217 (2004).

Update: As noted previously, in November 2010 the U.S. Food & Drug Administration approved a clinical trial (in which human patients are enrolled, treated and monitored) to assess the safety of an embryonic stem cell-based therapy for macular degeneration. Patients will receive injections of laboratory-derived retinal cells that have been differentiated from human embryonic stem cells. The treatment was shown to improve the vision in rats. To date, three patients have been enrolled in the study but no results have yet been published.

PROBLEM

Imagine one of your loved ones suffers a motor vehicle accident that damages his or her spinal cord. The treating physicians conclude after two weeks of treatment that the injury and resulting paralysis of the lower extremities is irreversible. At the same time, the doctors reassure you and your loved one that over time physical and psychological therapy can help the patient adjust to life as a paraplegiac. You learn of a clinical trial in an nearby city in which embryonic stem cell-derived spinal cord cells are being injected into the damaged spinal cords of recent accident victims. The research protocol is open to patients who have suffered spinal cord injuries with in the past month. Would you alert your loved one to this clinical trial? If so, would you encourage your loved one to enroll in this study? What are the pros and cons of pursuing stem cell therapy at this time?

C.   Framing the Debate Over Stem Cell Research

Public discourse over stem cell research, particularly research involving the destruction of human embryos, has been robust and steady since the isolation and cultivation of human embryonic stem cells in the late 1990s. Even today, hardly a day goes by without some mention of stem cell research in the news, whether a story about a recent scientific breakthrough, or news about a state legislature voting to endorse or ban research using embryonic cells, or coverage of the ongoing debate about the role of the federal government in funding stem cell research. A bare-bones assessment of all the dialogue surrounding stem cell research yields two basic questions: Should research using cells derived from embryos and aborted fetuses be legal, and if so, should it be funded by the federal government?

In 2004 the President's Council on Bioethics produced a report on the status of stem cell research, setting forth what it considered to be the essential ethical issues that shape the domestic debate. As you read the report, you will note that the questions of legality and funding break down into numerous components, each worthy of contemplation.

The President's Council on Bioethics
Monitoring Stem Cell Research 5-7
(January 2004)

While most of the public controversy has focused on the issue of embryo use and destruction, other ethical and policy issues have also attracted attention. Although entangled with the issue of embryos, the question of the significance and use of federal funds is itself a contested issue: Should moral considerations be used to decide what sort of research may or may not be funded? What is the symbolic and moral-political significance of providing national approval, in the form of active support, for practices that many Americans regard as abhorrent or objectionable? Conversely, what is the symbolic and moral-political significance of refusing to support potentially life-saving scientific investigations that many Americans regard as morally obligatory?

Even for those who favor embryo research, there are questions about its proper limits and the means of establishing and enforcing those limits through meaningful regulation. Under the present arrangement, with the federal government only recently in the picture, what is done with human embryos, especially in the private sector, is entirely unregulated (save in those states that have enacted special statutes dealing with embryo or stem cell research). Is this a desirable arrangement? Can some other system be devised, one that protects the human goods we care about but that does not do more harm than good? What are those human goods? What boundaries can and should we try to establish, and how?

Although well-established therapies based on transplantation of stem cell-derived tissues are still largely in the future, concern has already been expressed (as it has been about other aspects of health care in the United States) about access to any realized benefits and about research priorities: Will these benefits be equitably available, regardless of ability to pay? How should the emergence of the new field of stem cell research alter the allocation of our limited resources for biomedical research? How, in a morally and politically controverted area of research, should the balance be struck between public and private sources of support? As with any emerging discovery, how can we distinguish between genuine promise and "hype," and between the more urgent and the less urgent medical needs calling out for assistance?

There are also sensitive issues regarding premature claims of cures for diseases that are not scientifically substantiated and the potential exploitation of sick people and their families. Some advocates of stem cell research have made bold claims about the number of people who will be helped should the research go forward, hoping to generate sympathy for increased research funding among legislators and the public. A few advocates have gone so far as to blame (in advance) opponents of embryonic stem cell research for those who will die unless the research goes forward today. At the same time, other scientists have cautioned that the pace of progress will be very slow, and that no cures can be guaranteed in advance. Which of these claims and counterclaims is closer to the truth cannot be known ahead of time. Only once the proper scientific studies are conducted will we discover the potential therapeutic value of stem cells from any source. How, then, in the meantime should we discuss these matters, offering encouragement but without misleading or exploiting the fears and hopes of the desperately ill?

Finally, questions are raised by some about the social significance of accepting the use of nascent human life as a resource for scientific investigation and the search for cures. Such questions have been raised even by people who do not regard an early human embryo as fully "one of us," and who are concerned not so much about the fate of individual embryos as they are about the character and sensibilities of a society that comes to normalize such practices. What would our society be like if it came to treat as acceptable or normal the exploitation of what hitherto were regarded as the seeds of the next generation? Conversely, exactly analogous questions are raised by some about the social significance of refusing to use these 150-to-200-cell early human embryos as a resource for responsible scientific investigation and the search for cures. What would a society be like if it refused, for moral scruples about (merely) nascent life, to encourage every thoughtful and scientifically sound effort to heal disease and relieve the suffering of fully developed human beings among us?

SECTION II: THE LEGAL FRAMEWORK SURROUNDING STEM CELL RESEARCH

The freshness of advances in stem cell research has not made the science immune from the reach of existing and newly enacted laws. For example, statutes and regulations expressly governing research using human embryos and fetuses have been on the books for years, and their applicability to embryonic and fetal stem cell research seems straightforward. On the other hand, it can be argued that existing embryo and fetal research laws were drafted without reference to the promise of stem cell research, and thus their application to current scientific experimentation should be re-evaluated.

In addition to laws that pre-date the 1998 isolation of human embryonic stem cells, a handful of federal and state laws and policies have been enacted in the wake of the emerging science. The stem cell-specific laws vary greatly in scope, with some aimed at encouraging and facilitating research, and others explicitly banning, even criminalizing such research within the jurisdiction. In addition to laws regulating the actual conduct surrounding research (i.e., whether research can be conducted, which embryos can be used in research, how researchers must obtain embryos and fetuses for research, for example), legal structures have developed over the question of governmental funding for stem cell research. The federal government is the largest source of funding for medical research in the U.S., currently spending about $30 billion annually through grants from the National Institutes of Health (NIH). Many believe that the federal government's participation in funding stem cell research, or refusal to do so, will significantly shape the future of regenerative medicine.

In order to understand the current state of the law regarding experimentation and funding, we will review the history of federal and state laws surrounding fetal and embryonic research.

A. Laws Relating to Aborted Fetuses as Sources of Stem Cells

The law and policy governing research on fetal tissue evolved long before the 1998 discovery that stem cells could be derived from the tissue of aborted fetuses. In the main, the legal structures surrounding fetal tissue research track the national debate over abortion, with the first federal activity following on the heels of *Roe v. Wade*, the 1973 landmark decision legalizing pre-viability abortions. The materials that follow review the history of federal and state regulation and funding of fetal tissue research. As you become familiar with the laws, consider whether these pre-stem cell enactments should be applied to today's technologies.

1. Federal Law Relating to Aborted Fetuses as Sources of Stem Cells

National Bioethics Advisory Commission
***Ethical Issues in Human Stem Cell Research* 29-31**
(September 1999)

The Law Relating to Aborted Fetuses as Sources of EG Cells

Federal law permits funding of some research with cells and tissues from the products of elective as well as spontaneous abortions, and state law facilitates the donation and use of fetal tissue for research. Both state and federal law set forth several requirements for the process of retrieving and using material from this source, although amendments may be needed to federal law in order to make existing safeguards applicable to stem cell research.

Federal Law Regarding Research Using Cells and Tissues from Aborted Fetuses

Since as early as the 1930s, American biomedical research has utilized *ex utero* fetal tissue both as a medium and, increasingly, as an object for experimentation . . . "For many years, the production and testing of vaccines, the study of viral reagents, the propagation of human viruses, and the testing of biological products have been dependent on the unique growth properties of fetal tissue" . . . For example, the 1954 Nobel Prize for Medicine was awarded to American immunologists who used cell lines obtained from human fetal kidney cells to grow polio virus in cell cultures, a key advance in the development of polio vaccines . . .

In 1972, allegations (some of them quite shocking) about experiments with fetuses both *in* and *ex utero* created an air of controversy (fueled by the greater societal debate about elective abortion) over the use of fetal tissue in research. When Congress established the National Commission for the Protection of Human Subjects of Biomedical and Behavioral Research in 1974, it placed the topic of research using the human fetus at the top of the commission's agenda. Within four months of assuming office, the commissioners were mandated to report on the subject, with the proviso that the presentation of their report to the Secretary of the Department of Health, Education, and Welfare (DHEW) — now the Department of Health and Human Services (DHHS) — would lift the moratorium that Congress had imposed on federal funding of research using live fetuses On July 25, 1975, the National Commission submitted its conclusions and recommendations, which formed the basis for regulations that the Department issued later that year on research involving fetuses, pregnant women, and human IVF (1975).

General Regulation of Research with Human Beings Including Fetuses

The 1975 provisions remain as elements of the current federal regulations that aim to protect human subjects participating in research conducted with federal funds — rules that also are followed on a voluntary basis by many institutions in the case of research performed without federal support. The core regulations are set forth in the *Federal Policy for the Protection of Human Subjects*, known as the Common Rule, because the same regulatory provisions have been adopted by most federal agencies and departments that conduct or sponsor research in which human subjects are used. The DHHS regulations appear in Volume 45, Part 46 of the Code of Federal Regulations — 45 CFR 46. The Common Rule makes up Subpart A of the DHHS regulations, and additional protections for special populations of research subjects [including fetuses] appear in three further subparts of 45 CFR 46.

The special provisions applicable to fetal material appear in Subpart B, which covers research on "1) the fetus, 2) pregnant women, and 3) human *in vitro* fertilization" and applies to all DHHS "grants and contracts supporting research, development, and related activities" involving those subjects. The regulations primarily address research that could affect living fetuses adversely. They provide for stringent Institutional Review Board (IRB) consideration, which is based upon the results of preliminary studies on animals and . . . on assurances that living fetuses will be exposed only to minimal risk except when the research is intended to meet the health needs of the fetus or its mother . . .

The Conditions for Federal Support of Fetal Tissue Transplantation

In the 1980s, medical scientists began experimenting with implanting brain tissue from aborted fetuses into patients with Parkinson's disease as well as patients with other neurological disorders. NIH investigators were among those working in this field, and their protocol to use fetal tissue for transplantation was approved by an internal NIH review body. Although the research complied with Subpart B, then-NIH Director James B. Wyngaarden decided to seek approval from Assistant Secretary for Health Robert E. Windom before proceeding. In March 1988, Windom responded by declaring a temporary moratorium on federally funded transplantation research involving fetal tissue from induced abortions. He also asked NIH to establish an advisory body to consider whether such research should be conducted and under what conditions . . . The Human Fetal Tissue Transplantation Research Panel — composed of biomedical investigators, lawyers, ethicists, clergy, and politicians — deliberated until the fall of 1988. Panel members then voted 19-2 to recommend continued funding for fetal tissue transplantation research under guidelines designed to ensure the ethical integrity of any experimental procedures. In November 1989, after the transition had been made from the Reagan to the Bush administration, DHHS Secretary Louis Sullivan extended the moratorium indefinitely, based upon the position taken by the minority-voting panel members that fetal tissue transplantation research would increase the incidence of elective abortion . . . Attempts by Congress to override the Secretary's decision were not enacted or were vetoed by President [George H.W.] Bush.

On January 22, 1993, immediately after President Clinton took office, he instructed the incoming Secretary of DHHS to lift the ban on federal funding for human fetal tissue transplantation research. On February 5, 1993, DHHS Secretary Donna Shalala officially rescinded the moratorium, and, in March 1993, NIH published interim guidelines for research involving human fetal tissue transplantation (OPRR 1994). Provisions to legislate these safeguards were promptly proposed in Congress and included in the NIH Revitalization Act of 1993, which President Clinton signed into law on June 10, 1993.[6]

The 1993 act mirrors most prior statutory and regulatory provisions on research

---

[6] The 1993 law provides in relevant part:

(a) Establishment of program

(1) In general. The Secretary [of Health and Human Services] may conduct or support research on the transplantation of human fetal tissue for therapeutic purposes. (2) Source of tissue. Human fetal tissue may be used in research carried out under paragraph (1) regardless of whether the tissue is obtained pursuant to a spontaneous or induced abortion or pursuant to a stillbirth.

(b) Informed consent of donor (1) In general. In research carried out under subsection (a) of this section, human fetal tissue may be used only if the woman providing the tissue makes a statement, made in writing and signed by the woman, declaring that —

(A) the woman donates the fetal tissue for use in research described in subsection (a) of this section;

(B) the donation is made without any restriction regarding the identity of individuals who may be the recipients of transplantations of the tissue; and

(C) the woman has not been informed of the identity of any such individuals.

(2) Additional statement. In research carried out under subsection (a) of this section, human fetal tissue may be used only if the attending physician with respect to obtaining the tissue

involving tissue from dead fetuses. In general, the Revitalization Act states that any tissue from any type or category of abortion may be used for research on transplantation, but only for "therapeutic purposes." Most agree that this means that research on transplantation that has as its goal the treatment of disease is covered by the act, but that basic laboratory research — which only tangentially can be described as having a therapeutic purpose — would not be covered . . . [T]he attending physician must sign a statement affirming five . . . conditions of the abortion, aimed at insulating a woman's decision to abort from her decision to provide tissue for fetal research. Finally, the person principally responsible for the experiment must also affirm his or her own knowledge of the sources of tissue, that others involved in the research are aware of the tissue status, and that the researcher had no part in the abortion decision or its timing . . .

Research of the type conducted by Gearhart and his colleagues at The Johns Hopkins University, in which primordial germ cells were obtained from the gonadal ridge of human fetuses that had been aborted five to nine weeks after fertilization, arguably is not covered by the fetal tissue transplantation provisions of the 1993 NIH Revitalization Act, because these fetal cells are intended to be cultured and used in laboratory experiments, not transplanted . . . Someday, with the advancement of knowledge about cell differentiation and the like, EG cells derived from dead fetuses may be linked more directly or indirectly with transplantation, at which point the 1993 Act would arguably become applicable. In anticipation of that day, and in order to achieve simplicity in the meantime by applying the same rules to all federally supported research with fetal remains, whether or not for transplantation, it would appear desirable to amend the law to clarify that the safeguards of the 1993 Act apply to research in which EG cells are obtained from dead fetuses after a spontaneous or elective abortion.

NOTES AND QUESTIONS

1. The history of the federal government's regulation of fetal tissue research is complex, even ambiguous, as the authors of the NBAC report conclude, but at bottom, two certainties emerge. First, research using aborted human fetuses is not prohibited under federal law, and second, whether such research is federally funded is largely a matter of politics. One can trace the availability of federal funding for fetal tissue research mostly by noting the political party of the president in office at the time of inquiry. The first funding moratorium was enacted by Congress in 1974, and it was lifted during the Carter Administration from 1976 to 1980. When Ronald Reagan was elected in 1980, he banned the use of federal funds for research involving fetal tissue, a ban that remained in place during his two terms, and that of his Republican predecessor, George H. Bush.

Upon taking office in 1993, Democratic president Bill Clinton ordered the ban on

---

from the woman involved makes a statement, made in writing and signed by the physician, declaring that —

(A) in the case of tissue obtained pursuant to an induced abortion —

(i) the consent of the woman for the abortion was obtained prior to requesting or obtaining consent for a donation of the tissue for use in such research . . .

42 U.S.C. § 289g-1 (2005). - Ed.

federal funding of fetal tissue transplantation lifted. By the time George W. Bush took office in January 2001, the focus of federal funding had shifted from fetal tissue to embryonic stem cells, a topic he contemplated for nine months before announcing a new federal policy. But during the 2000 campaign, George Bush told the U.S. Conference of Catholic Bishops, "I oppose using federal funds to perform fetal tissue research from induced abortions." Jeremy Manier, *U.S. Quietly OKs Fetal Stem Cell Work; Bush Allows Funding Despite Federal Limits on Embryo Use*, CHI. TRIB., July 7, 2002, at 1. President Bush left undisturbed the Clinton-era policy of permitting, but highly regulating, the provision of federal funds for fetal tissue research because, according to White House officials, "Congress passed a law in 1993 that made it illegal for presidents to ban funding for such research."[7] *Id.* Under President Obama, research using fetal tissue remains lawful and funded. According to the FDA website listing active and completed clinical trials, at least a few research protocols using fetal tissue have been approved for funding by the federal government as of 2012. *See* U.S. National Institutes of Health, ClinicalTrials.gov, available at: http://clinicaltrials.gov/ct2/results?term=fetal+tissue (describing clinical trial to treat an eye disorder using product derived from fetal tissue). Should a president have the authority to ban federal funding of medical research?

2.   The restrictions surrounding the legalization of fetal tissue transplantation research contained in the 1993 NIH Revitalization Act were generated mainly in response to concerns that such research would encourage abortion. The thinking was that if a woman experienced an unwanted pregnancy, she could more easily justify or rationalize a decision to elect abortion on the grounds that the fetal remains could be used to promote medical research. Another feared scenario was that women would become pregnant for the sole purpose of aborting in order to aid an ailing relative with compatible fetal tissue for transplantation. Thus, the regulations prohibit directed donation (in which the tissue donor identifies the recipient of the donated tissue), and require that the woman consent to the abortion prior to being asked to donate the aborted fetal tissue.

Do you think a woman's decision to abort could be influenced by her knowledge about fetal tissue research? If so, do the regulations prohibiting directed donation and requiring prior consent to abort prevent a woman from electing abortion for the purpose of donating the fetal remains for research?

3.   At the end of the excerpted NBAC discussion above, the Commission argues that the derivation of EG cells is not covered by the 1993 federal law regulating fetal tissue transplantation because, under current technologies, the EG cells are merely cultured and used in laboratory experiments. Do you agree that both the letter and the spirit of the law does not govern EG cell research? If EG cells are prompted to transmute into say, heart cells, would injection of these new heart cells into a human subject be considered fetal tissue transplantation?

---

[7] Presumably the White House officials were referring to Section 113 of Pub. L. 103-43, Title I, Subtitle A, Part II, 107 Stat. 132 providing that: "no official of the executive branch may impose a policy that the Department of Health and Human Services is prohibited from conducting or supporting any research on the transplantation of human fetal tissue for therapeutic purposes." This provision was enacted on June 10, 1993.

2. State Laws Relating to Aborted Fetuses as Sources of Stem Cells

The 1993 federal law regulating the use of fetal tissue for research cedes to each state the ultimate authority to determine whether research may be conducted in any given state. "The Secretary may conduct research . . . only in accordance with applicable State and local law."42 U.S.C. § 289g-1(e)(2). If isolation, cultivation and transplantation of stem cells derived from fetal tissue is accomplished, state laws governing fetal tissue research will be an important, if not unitary, source of legal authority as to the propriety of such medical therapy. While states may amend their codes to directly address the issue of fetal stem cells research and therapy, the question of how and whether existing laws would treat such conduct looms large. The 1999 Presidential Commission considered the impact of current state regulation and provided the following interpretation.

National Bioethics Advisory Commission
Ethical Issues in Human Stem Cell Research 32-33
(September 1999)

State Law Regarding Using Aborted Fetuses as Sources of Stem Cells

As recognized by federal statutes and regulations, state law governs the manner in which cells and tissues from dead fetuses become available for research, principally by statutes, regulations, and case law on organ transplantation. The most basic legal provisions lie in the Uniform Anatomical Gift Act (UAGA), which was first proposed in 1968 and rapidly became the most widely adopted uniform statute. While the UAGA is largely consistent with relevant federal statutes and regulations and should facilitate researchers obtaining cadaveric fetal tissue, a number of states have adopted other statutes that limit or prohibit certain types of research with fetal remains.

Laws Facilitating Donation of Fetal Material for EG Cell Research: The UAGA

The UAGA is relevant not only because federal statutes and regulations explicitly condition funding for research with fetal tissue on compliance with state and local laws, but also because the act applies when EG cell research using fetal tissue does not receive federal funding. The original version of the UAGA was approved by all 50 states and the District of Columbia; a 1987 revision has been enacted by 22 states. The act establishes a system of voluntary donation of "anatomical gifts" for transplantation, education, and research. It was intended to make it easier for people to authorize gifts of their own body (or parts thereof) through a simple "donor card" executed before the occasion arose, as well as to allow donations to be made with the permission of the next-of-kin, following an order established by the statute. The revised UAGA includes "a stillborn infant or fetus" in the definition of "decedents," for whom parental consent is determinative . . .

However, federal law restricts the procedures authorized by the UAGA in one area. The UAGA permits donors to designate recipients — including individual patients — of anatomical gifts. The stricter provisions of the NIH Revitalization Act (which prohibits a donor from having knowledge of an individual transplant recipient) could override this state law in the case of federally supported fetal tissue transplantation, but the issue might not arise regarding stem cell research for two reasons. First, such research does not involve transplantation (and hence at this time is not relevant to the NIH Revitalization Act). Second, according to the Revitalization Act, the only recipient who may be designated by the parents of a dead fetus would be a stem cell researcher or research institution.

Laws Restricting Use of Donated Fetal Material for EG Cell Research

At present, 24 states do not have on their books any statutes "specifically addressing research on embryos or fetuses," and the restrictions in most of the remaining states principally involve embryos remaining after infertility treatments and limitations aimed at discouraging therapeutic abortions.[8] For example, in 12 states, the law applies only to research with fetuses prior or subsequent to an elective abortion.[9] Six states ban research that involves aborted fetuses or their organs, tissues, or remains,[10] which could cause difficulties for researchers using stem cell lines derived from aborted fetuses "if cell lines are considered 'tissue.' " Six other states permit fetal research when the fetus is deceased, but mandate that the donor must provide consent,[11] although none "specifically address[es] the type of information that must be provided to the progenitors before they are asked for consent." . . .

In order to diminish the impact that the potential use of a fetus in research might have on the decision to abort, states have enacted many restrictions on payment for fetal remains. The broadest prohibitions appear as part of state statutes regulating or prohibiting fetal research. Bans on sale vary in their terminology — an "aborted product of conception," an "aborted unborn child or the remains thereof," an "aborted fetus or any tissue or organ thereof," or an "unborn child" — and exist both in states that permit research on a dead fetus with the mother's consent and in those where it is illegal to conduct research upon any aborted product of conception . . .

The most widely adopted prohibitions on commercialization of fetal remains are

---

[8] A listing of state laws regulating research on embryos and fetuses can be found in Chapter 4, footnote 78. - Ed.

[9] [n.23] See Ariz. Rev. Stat. Ann. § 36-2302(A) (subsequent); Ark. Stat. Ann. § 20-17-802 (subsequent); Cal. Health and Safety Code § 123440 (subsequent); Fla. Stat. Ann. § 390.011(6) (prior or subsequent); Ind. Code Ann. § 16-34-2-6 (subsequent); Ky. Rev. Stat. § 436.026 (subsequent); Mo. Ann. Stat. § 188.037 (prior or subsequent); Neb. Rev. Stat. § 28-346 (subsequent); Ohio Rev. Code Ann. § 2919.14(A) (subsequent); Okla. Stat. Ann. Tit. 63, § 1-735(A) (prior or subsequent); Tenn. Code Ann. § 39-15-208 (subsequent); Wyo. Stat. Ann. § 35-6-115 (subsequent).

[10] [n.24] Ariz. Rev. Stat. Ann. § 36-2303, -2303; Ind. Code Ann. § 16.34-2-6; N.D. Cent. Code § 14-02.2-01 to -02; Ohio Rev. Code Ann. § 2919.14; Okla. Stat. Ann. Tit. 63, § 1-735; S.D. Codified Laws Ann. § 36-23A-17.

[11] [n.26] Ark. Stat. Ann. § 20-17-802(2); Mass. Ann. Laws ch. 112 § 12J(a)(II); Mich. Comp. Laws Ann. § 333.2687 (must also comply with state's version of the UAGA, Mich. Comp. Laws Ann. § 333.10101 et seq.): Pa. Cons. Stat. Ann. § 3216(b)(1) (mother's consent valid only after decision to abort has been made; no compensation allowed): R.I. Gen. Laws § 11-54-1(d); Tenn. Code Ann. § 39-15-208(a).

those in Sections 10(a) and (b) of the 1987 revision of the UAGA, which prohibit the sale or purchase of any human body parts for any consideration beyond that necessary to pay for expenses incurred in the removal, processing, and transportation of the tissue. On the federal level, what is in essence the same proscription is included both in the 1993 NIH Revitalization Act, which bars the acquisition or transfer of fetal tissue for "valuable consideration" with the same exceptions, and in the National Organ Transplant Act of 1984 (NOTA), which prohibits the sale of any human organ for "valuable consideration for use in human transplantation" if the sale involves interstate commerce. (In 1988, Congress amended NOTA to include fetal organs within the definition of "human organ," in order to foreclose the sale of fetal tissue as well.) Yet both federal statutes could be interpreted to apply only to sales for transplant or therapeutic purposes, not laboratory research. Moreover, the definition of reasonable processing fees in the federal law (and by extension, the UAGA) is arguably too vague, "leav[ing] . . . room for unscrupulous tissue processors to abuse the law". If special provisions are adopted to govern federal support of research with fetal material to create human EG cell lines, it would seem advisable to ensure that the provisions lay out more clearly what payments may be made to whom and on what basis for fetal cells and tissues . . .

MARGARET S. v. EDWARDS
United States Court of Appeals, Fifth Circuit
794 F.2d 994 (1986)

Before WILLIAMS, HIGGINBOTHAM, and DAVIS, Circuit Judges.

PATRICK E. HIGGINBOTHAM, CIRCUIT JUDGE:

We are asked to decide the constitutionality of two statutory provisions through which Louisiana has sought to regulate the practice of abortion. One provision requires that the attending physician inform his patient, within twenty-four hours after she undergoes an abortion, that she may exercise one of several options for the disposition of the fetal remains. The other forbids "experimentation" on the fetal remains of an abortion. We are persuaded that the first provision must be declared unconstitutional under *City of Akron v. Akron Center for Reproductive Health, Inc.*, 462 U.S. 416, 103 S.Ct. 2481, 2502, 76 L.Ed.2d 687 (1983), and that the second is unconstitutionally vague . . .

IV

La. Rev. Stat. Ann. § 40:1299.35.13 provides: "No person shall experiment on an unborn child or a child born as the result of an abortion, whether the unborn child or child is alive or dead, unless the experimentation is therapeutic to the unborn child or child." La. Rev. Stat. Ann. § 40:1299.35.18 imposes criminal penalties for violating this or any other section of the abortion statute.[12] The district court

---

[12] [n.11] The state's brief does not offer any explanation of the purpose of the prohibition of experiments on the fetus or child that emerges as a result of an abortion. We can hypothesize that

offered several alternative rationales for invalidating this provision. 597 F. Supp. at 673- 76. Although we agree that this statutory provision is unconstitutional, we neither approve nor disapprove any of the rationales put forth by the district court. Our holding is based solely on our conclusion that the use of the terms "experiment" and "experimentation" makes the statute impermissibly vague. A state's legislative enactment is void for vagueness under the due process clause of the fourteenth amendment if it "is inherently standardless, enforceable only on the exercise of an unlimited, and hence arbitrary, discretion vested in the state." *Ferguson v. Estelle*, 718 F.2d 730, 735 (5th Cir.1983). This test requires that the law be vague "not in the sense that it requires a person to conform his conduct to an imprecise but comprehensible normative standard, but rather in the sense that no standard of conduct is specified at all." *Coates v. City of Cincinnati*, 402 U.S. 611, 614, 91 S.Ct. 1686, 1688, 29 L.Ed.2d 214 (1971). The vagueness doctrine has been applied with considerable stringency to a law that required physicians to use professional diligence in caring for the life and health of a viable aborted fetus. *Colautti v. Franklin*, 439 U.S. 379, 99 S.Ct. 675, 58 L.Ed.2d 596 (1979).

The plaintiffs' expert witness offered unrebutted testimony, which we find quite plausible, that physicians do not and cannot distinguish clearly between medical experiments and medical tests. As the expert witness pointed out, every medical test that is now "standard" began as an "experiment" that became standard through a gradual process of observing the results, confirming the benefits, and often modifying the technique. Thus, as the witness concluded, "we have at one end things that are obviously standard tests and [at] the other end things that are complete experimentation. But in the center there is a very broad area where diagnostic procedures of testing types overlap with experimentation procedures. . . ." Indeed, as the challenged statute itself seems to acknowledge, even medical *treatment* can be reasonably described as both a test and an experiment . . . The whole distinction between experimentation and testing, or between research and practice, is therefore almost meaningless in the medical context. When one adds to this the fact that some innovative tests or treatments are done on fetal tissue in order to monitor the health of the mother, one can see that physicians who treat pregnant women are being threatened with an inherently standardless prohibition. We therefore think that this statute "simply has *no* core" that unquestionably applies to certain activities, *Smith v. Goguen*, 415 U.S. 566, 578, 94 S.Ct. 1242, 1249, 39 L.Ed.2d 605 (1974) (emphasis in original), and we hold that it is unconstitutionally vague.[13]

AFFIRMED.

Louisiana wanted to remove some of the incentives for research-minded physicians either to promote abortions or to manipulate the timing of abortions in an effort to acquire fetal remains of a desired maturity. The statute is therefore rationally related to an important state interest. *Cf. Maher v. Roe*, 432 U.S. 464, 473-74, 97 S.Ct. 2376, 2382-83, 53 L.Ed.2d 484 (1977).

[13] [n.13] This of course does not imply that the states are powerless to regulate medical experimentation. Because of the nature of the vagueness doctrine, any holding that a statute is unconstitutionally vague must necessarily be highly case-specific. A statute using more precise language than that used in R.S. 40:1299.35.13, whether it applied to fetal experimentation or other forms of medical research, would present a different case than the one we decided today.

JERRE S. WILLIAMS, CIRCUIT JUDGE, specially concurring:

I concur in the decision of the majority in affirming the district court's holding that the two provisions of the Louisiana Code at issue are unconstitutional. I write separately because the majority opinion does not address adequately the constitutional issues raised by these two statutory provisions. The majority's analysis strains unnecessarily to restrict the scope of this case, resulting in unrealistic and unconvincing justifications for the decision . . .

I. EXPERIMENTATION ON FETAL REMAINS

A. *Vagueness*

The majority opinion invalidates this provision on the ground that the terms "experiment" and "experimentation" are impermissibly vague, a ground not discussed by the district court nor raised by the parties on appeal. I cannot join in this conclusion.

In order to strike down a legislative enactment for vagueness, a court must determine that the enactment is impermissibly vague in all of its applications . . . An enactment is not vague merely because it is imprecise . . . A statute is unconstitutionally void for vagueness only when no standard of conduct is outlined at all; when no core of prohibited activity is defined. The result is an absence of objective standards by which to conform one's behavior. Invariably, enforcement must be subjective and erratic . . . This provision does not present such dangers.

The majority properly sets out that there are procedures that are undeniably medical "experiments" and procedures that are medical "tests." The majority finds a problem " 'in the center [where] there is a very broad area where diagnostic procedures of testing types overlap with experimentation procedures.' " This view, however, rests upon what I feel is a contrived definition of the term "experiment." It reasons that because medical "tests" are developed from medical "experiments," then many kinds of medical experiments may also be tests. This was the rationale offered by the witness upon whom the majority opinion relies, Dr. William Sternberg. He specifically emphasized that the ban "would inhibit further development in those areas of scientific endeavor." These are not words of vagueness, but words of scientific policy. It is my view that this attempted confusion between experimentation and tests is not in reality a vagueness claim. It is a claim that a ban on experimentation will inevitably preclude the development of tests that may prove beneficial in future medical and surgical treatment. This is in actuality a claim on the merits. Section 1299.35.13 prohibits general medical research on fetal remains that is not beneficial to the fetus. There is most certainly a "core" by which to apply this provision. Whatever other faults this ban on experimentation may harbor, vagueness is not one . . .

Although imprecisely drafted, § 1299.35.13 is not unconstitutionally vague. As against a claim of vagueness, it provides ample warning to those who undertake to act within its purview. A prospective researcher would be required only to inquire as to the source of the fetal tissue upon which he wishes to experiment.

B. *State Interest in Prohibiting Experimentation*

A state may exercise its police powers to ensure public health, safety and welfare . . . The regulation of medical experimentation is a proper exercise of this authority. A state's authority in this context is admittedly broad . . . The exercise of these police powers, however, must be rationally related to important state interests . . . Section 40:1299.35.13 fails to bear such a rational relationship to an important state interest.

Although Louisiana seeks to prohibit experimentation on tissue obtained from induced abortions it imposes no comparable restrictions on experimentation on human tissue. Indeed, Louisiana law specifically provides for the use of human corpses for the purposes of research. La.R.S.A. § 17:2353. The evidence presented at trial failed to establish that tissue derived from an induced abortion presents a greater threat to public health or other public concerns than the tissue of human corpses. Further, no rational justification is shown for prohibiting experimentation on fetal tissue from a lawful induced abortion as opposed to a spontaneous abortion . . . The record is lacking in showing valid state policy in any of these distinctions. I can only conclude that under the guise of police regulation the state has actually undertaken to discourage constitutionally privileged induced abortions. *Thornburgh v. American College of Obstetricians & Gynecologists*, 476 U.S. 747, ___, 106 S.Ct. 2169, 2178, 90 L.Ed.2d 779 (1986). I would affirm the judgment of the district court on this ground . . .

NOTES AND QUESTIONS

1.   Arizona law provides: "A person shall not knowingly use any human fetus or embryo, living or dead, or any parts, organs or fluids of any such fetus or embryo resulting from an induced abortion in any manner for any medical experimentation or scientific or medical investigation purposes except as is strictly necessary to diagnose a disease or condition in the mother of the fetus or embryo and only if the abortion was performed because of such disease or condition." Ariz. Rev. Stat. Ann. § 36-2302(A). Violation of this law is a felony. Is this Arizona law unconstitutionally vague? See *Forbes v. Napolitano*, 236 F. 3d 1009 (9th Cir. 2000).

Perhaps you see merit in Judge Williams' argument that a statute prohibiting experimentation on fetal remains is not vague, but may suffer a different infirmity — failure to demonstrate a rational relationship to important state interests. What state interests do you think Arizona lawmakers advanced in enacting the fetal experimentation law?

The Arizona statute was enacted in 1975, long before Dr. Gearhart isolated and cultivated fetal embryonic germ cells and noted their possible role in reparative medicine. If Dr. Gearhart's laboratory were located in Phoenix, rather than across the country in Baltimore, could the District Attorney successfully prosecute the researcher for a felony offense?

2.   *EG Stem Cell Research and Abortion.* One's view of the moral acceptability of fetal tissue research is inevitably and inextricably linked to one's view of elective abortion. As explained by the National Bioethics Advisory Commission:

Those who believe that elective abortions are morally acceptable are less likely to identify insurmountable ethical barriers to research that involves the derivation and use of EG cells derived from cadaveric fetal tissue . . . Those who view elective abortions as morally unjustified often — but not always — oppose the research use of tissue derived from aborted fetuses . . .

Opponents of the research . . . argue that those who obtain and use fetal material from elective abortion inevitably become associated, in ethically unacceptable ways, with the abortions that are the source of the material. They identify two major types of unacceptable association or cooperation with abortion: 1) casual responsibility for abortions and 2) symbolic association with abortions.

1. Casual Responsibility

. . . Those involved in research uses of EG cells derived from fetal tissue could be indirectly responsible for abortions if the perceived potential benefits of the research contributed to an increase in the number of abortions. Opponents of fetal tissue research argue that it is unrealistic to suppose that a woman's decision to abort can be kept separate from considerations of donating fetal tissue, as many women facing the abortion decision are likely to have gained knowledge about fetal tissue research through the media or other sources. The knowledge that having an elective abortion might have benefits for future patients through the donation of fetal tissue for research may tip the balance in favor of going through with an abortion for some women who are ambivalent about it. Some argue that the benefits achieved through the routine use of fetal tissue will further legitimize abortion and result in more permissive societal attitudes and policies concerning elective abortion . . .

2. Symbolic Association

People can become inappropriately associated with what they believe are wrongful acts for which they are not causally responsible. Particularly problematic for many is an association that appears to symbolize approval of the wrongdoing . . . [T]hose involved in research on fetal tissue enter a symbolic alliance with the practice of abortion in producing or deriving benefits from it.

National Bioethics Advisory Commission, *Ethical Issues in Human Stem Cell Research* 45-47 (September 1999).

A few questions. First, do you agree with the argument that the existence of EG stem cell research could "tip the balance" in favor of abortion for pregnant women who are "ambivalent" about the decision? Do you have any personal knowledge about a woman's decision to seek or shun an abortion? Was the woman ambivalent about her decision?

Is the prospect of aiding medical research an inducement or a justification? What is the difference, if any, between these two concepts?

Do you agree that a researcher who derives stem cells from fetal tissue symbolically condones the practice of abortion? Would a patient who accepts cells derived from EG cells also be an accomplice in approving abortion?

B. Laws Relating to Embryos as Sources of Stem Cells

1. Federal Law Relating to Embryos as Sources of Stem Cells

Kara L. Belew
Stem Cell Division: Abortion Law and Its Influence on the Adoption of Radically Different Embryonic Stem Cell Legislation in the United States, the United Kingdom, and Germany
39 Texas International Law Journal 479, 499-506 (2004)

The United States has taken a market-oriented approach to stem cell research allowing virtually unfettered research in the private sector. The federal government has not developed national stem cell legislation and there are no federal restrictions on private sector stem cell research. Regulation of reproductive technologies is left to the states, which have enacted inconsistent legislation . . . As a result of newly emerging IVF procedures, during the 1970s embryos became available for experimentation in the United States for the first time. Recognizing the impending moral implications of IVF research, Congress issued a moratorium banning human IVF experimentation until appropriate regulations could be adopted by the Department of Health and Human Services (DHHS). Within a year, the DHHS had adopted regulations to lift the moratorium. The regulations provided that "no application or proposal involving human in vitro fertilization may be funded by the Department or any component thereof until the application or proposal has been reviewed by the Ethical Advisory Board [EAB] and the Board has rendered advice as to its acceptability from an ethical standpoint."[14] As a result, no application involving IVF research could be funded without EAB approval. In 1978, the first EAB was appointed. That same year public interest in IVF increased after the birth of Louise Brown, the first so-called test tube baby, in England. In 1979, the EAB recommended the federal funding of IVF research after having been asked to consider the broader moral, legal, and ethical considerations of IVF research for an American IVF study. The EAB determined the research was acceptable from an ethical standpoint so long as it was not attainable by other means and the embryo would be maintained no longer than fourteen days. Despite obtaining EAB approval for IVF research, the DHHS did not fund any research involving IVF and allowed the EAB to expire. As a result, no human embryo experiments were ever financed following an EAB review. During the 1980s, the pro-life lobby pressured the Ronald Reagan and George Bush administrations against funding human embryo research. This helped to ensure that no federal funds were used in the research of human embryos, and an EAB was never re-appointed. The failure of these administrations to appoint an EAB resulted in a thirteen-year de facto moratorium on federally-

---

[14] [n.198] 45 C.F.R. 46.204(d) (1993). This provision was rescinded in 1994. Health and Human Services Policy for the Protection of Human Subjects Research, 59 Fed. Reg. 28,276 (June 1, 1994).

funded IVF research - since the EAB was the only lawful body that could recommend funding.

The election of Bill Clinton ushered in a different political approach towards embryo-related research. In January 1993, on Clinton's second day in office, he lifted the moratorium on federally-funded fetal tissue transplantation research. Thereafter, Clinton proposed and Congress passed sweeping new legislation, the National Institutes of Health Revitalization Act of 1993. Importantly, the Act eliminated the EAB approval requirement for research involving human embryos, resulting in embryo research going forward unless disapproved. Subsequently, the NIH began receiving applications for federal funding of human embryo research. The NIH responded by assembling an ethics board, the Human Embryo Research Panel, to "consider various areas of research involving the ex utero . . . human embryo and to provide advice as to those areas" that are and are not acceptable for federal funding . . . [I]n September 1994, the panel released a report recommending federal funding of human embryo research under certain conditions. Specifically, the panel identified the derivation of human embryos as ethically appropriate to receive federal funds, while discouraging the use of embryos after the fourteenth day of development . . . In an additional, highly controversial decision, the panel also recommended the funding of research on embryos created expressly for scientific purposes after concluding that fertilization studies were needed to answer crucial questions about reproductive medicine.

The panel report sparked a fierce ethical debate . . . In fact, before any official response on the report from the NIH, Clinton issued a directive barring the use of federal funds to create human embryos for scientific experimentation. Clinton stated explicitly that he deplored "the creation of human embryos for research purposes."

Although Clinton's directive had explicitly prohibited the NIH from allocating federal funds when such funding would support the creation of human embryos for research purposes, the directive did not forbid the funding of projects using "spare" embryos left over after infertility treatments. However, before any specific funding decisions by the NIH could be made, Republicans in Congress introduced an amendment to the DHHS appropriations bill. The "Dickey Amendment"[15] passed and effectively prohibited federal funding for any activity involving:

(1) the creation of a human embryo or embryos for research purposes; or

(2) research in which a human embryo or embryos are destroyed, discarded, or knowingly subjected to risk of injury or death greater than that allowed for research on fetuses in utero under 45 CFR 46.208(a)(2) and . . . [42 U.S.C. 289g(b)] . . .

For purposes of this section, the phrase "human embryo or embryos" shall include any organism, not protected as a human subject under 45 CFR 46 as of the date of enactment of this Act, that is derived by fertilization,

---

[15] [n.225] The amendment was called the "Dickey Amendment" because Rep. Jay Dickey (R-Ark.) co-authored the legislation.

parthenogenesis, cloning, or any other means from one or more human gametes.[16]

The ban was retained in each successive appropriations bill (appropriations bills are passed annually) through 2002.[17]

In 1998, following the University of Wisconsin's publication of scientific reports describing the successful isolation of human embryological stem cells in the private sector, debate arose over whether the NIH could provide federal funding for human ES cell research in a manner consistent with the Dickey Amendment. The breakthrough research of the Wisconsin scientists had not been eligible for federal funding.[18] The success in the private sector prompted Clinton to order the National Bioethics Advisory Commission (NBAC), a presidentially-appointed committee established to advise the federal government on bioethics issues and to perform a thorough review of the ethical issues associated with human stem cell research. The NBAC released its report in January 1999. The NBAC report recommended that "research involving the derivation and use of ES cells from embryos remaining after infertility treatments should be eligible for federal funding . . . under appropriate regulations that include public oversight and review." . . . Despite strong disagreement over the prohibition placed on the federal funding of research by the Dickey Amendment, in August 2000, the NIH adopted guidelines allowing for the funding of research using human pluripotent stem cells. Such funding did not extend to research for the derivation of pluripotent cells from human embryos, but did extend to research for the derivation of such cells from human fetal tissue. Immediately following the publication of the guidelines, the NIH began accepting grant applications for research projects utilizing human stem cells. Before any funding could be made available, however, the guidelines provided that all grant applications would have to be reviewed by the NIH Human Pluripotent Stem Cell Review Group (HPSCRG) for compliance with the guidelines . . . Before the HPSCRG could meet to review funding applications, the election of President George W. Bush ushered in a new national stem cell funding policy. During his campaign, Bush articulated the position that he was against federal funding of embryonic research that would "result in destruction of . . . a human embryo." . . . In order to prevent the NIH from funding stem cell research under the Clinton administration's policies . . . [in the spring 2001] the Bush administration froze federal funding of stem cell research and postponed the first scheduled meeting of the HPSCRG in anticipation of the announcement of his administration's own funding guidelines

On August 9, 2001, Bush announced in a televised address to the country his decision to allow federal funding of ES cell research, but funding would be limited to the roughly sixty "existing stem cell lines, where the life and death decision has already been made." According to Bush, his plan was designed to allow exploration into "the promise and potential of stem cell research without crossing a fundamental moral line, by providing taxpayer funding that would sanction or encourage

---

[16] [n226] Balanced Budget Downpayment Act, I, Pub. L. No. 104-99, 128, 110 Stat. 26, 34 (1996).

[17] As of 2012, the Dickey Amendment has been retained in each annual appropriation bill authorizing funding for the National Institutes of Health, which funds medical and scientific research in the U.S. - Ed.

[18] [n.230] The scientists' work was funded privately by Geron Corporation of Menlo Park, California.

further destruction of human embryos that have at least the potential for life." Bush's policy statement effectively replaced the NIH guidelines adopted by the Clinton administration.

The Bush plan allows for federal funding of research on an ES cell line if the line existed before his address on August 9, 2001, and the line was derived "(1) with the informed consent of the donors; (2) from excess embryos created solely for reproductive purposes; and (3) without any financial inducements to the donors." The plan also provides that "no federal funds will be used for: (1) the derivation or use of stem cell lines derived from newly destroyed embryos; (2) the creation of any human embryos for research purposes; or (3) the cloning of human embryos for any purpose." Bush also announced the establishment of a new Bioethics Council to monitor stem cell research, recommend guidelines and regulations, and consider the ethical ramifications of stem cell research.

NOTES AND QUESTIONS

1. Stay tuned for the next installment of presidential leadership on the matter of embryonic research and funding. The above article was written during the administration of President George W. Bush. The steps and policies undertaken by President Barack Obama are discussed in Section III(A)(2).

2. The history of federal law governing embryo research is a tale of funding, not prohibition. As succinctly phrased by the President's Council on Bioethics, the "Bioethics Council" referred to at the end of the above article, "At the federal level, research that involves the destruction of embryos is neither prohibited nor supported and encouraged." The President's Council on Bioethics, Monitoring Stem Cell Research 26 (January 2004). Why has Congress not (successfully) mobilized to ban all research on human embryos? If such a ban were enacted, would it be constitutional?[19]

3. Since 1996 Congress has successfully mobilized to ban federal funding of

---

[19] The lack of federal law pertaining to embryonic stem cell research is not for lack of interest on the part of Congress. Since the announcement of embryonic stem cell derivation in 1998, Congress has considered dozens of bills on the topic, and two of those bills passed the House but failed to pass the Senate. On July 31, 2001 and February 27, 2003, the House passed H.R. 2505, 107th Cong. And H.R. 534, 108th Cong., respectively. The bills prohibit both reproductive and therapeutic cloning, and would impose criminal penalties for up to 10 years in prison for any violations of the law. The bills failed to pass the Senate, largely because a majority of senators favor stem cell research, including research using cloned embryos, which would be prohibited under the House bills. In March 2005, a group of "influential conservatives," headed by Leon Kass, Chair of the President's Council on Bioethics, expressed their frustration over Congress' inability to pass legislation banning human cloning. In response, they drafted a bioethics agenda for President Bush's second term and began building a political coalition to support the policies contained therein. "We have today an administration and a Congress as friendly to human life and human dignity as we are likely to have for many years to come," reads the document, which was obtained by The Washington Post. "It would be tragic if we failed to take advantage of this rare opportunity to enact significant bans on some of the most egregious biotechnical practices." Dr. Kass maintains that his role in this group is independent of his role as Chair of the President's Council. See Rick Weiss, *Conservatives Draft a "Bioethics Agenda" for President*, Wash. Post, Mar. 8, 2005, at A6. The agenda, which calls for prohibitions on therapeutic cloning and the creation of embryos for research purposes, can be found at http://blog.bioethics.net/2005/03/kass-agenda-bioethics-for-second-term.html. For a discussion of the bioethics agenda, including its calls for prohibition on therapeutic cloning and the

human embryonic research with the annual passage of the Dickey Amendment (also known as the Dickey-Wicker Amendment for its two co-sponsors, Rep. Jay Wickey (R-Ohio) and Sen. Roger Wicker (R-Mississippi)), a provision attached to the appropriation bills funding the Department of Health and Human Services. The Amendment provides, "None of the funds made available in this Act may be used for (1) the creation of a human embryo or embryos for research purposes; or (2) research in which a human embryo or embryos are destroyed . . ." This clear ban on funding research in which embryos are destroyed would seem to quash any discussion about federal funding for embryonic stem cell research which, under current practices, requires that the embryo be destroyed in order for the stem cells to be retrieved. How is it that Presidents Clinton, Bush and Obama were and remain able to negotiate the stem cell funding issue, when federal law on the subject seems crystal clear?

The answer is attributable to a federal government attorney by the name of Harriet Raab. In 1999, Ms. Raab was General Counsel of the Department of Health and Human Services, when the Director of the National Institutes of Health sought her legal opinion as to whether embryonic research on existing stem cell lines, where the derivation process had already been completed, was permissible under the Dickey Amendment. Attorney Raab argued in a January 1999 memorandum to NIH Director Harold Varmus that the wording of the law would permit funding embryonic stem cell research because the amendment did not "apply to research utilizing human pluripotent stem cells because such cells are not a human embryo within the statutory definition." If stem cells were derived from embryos that had been developed using private funds, she reasoned, the subsequently developed cell lines might be considered eligible for public funding because the cells themselves were not embryos capable of becoming a fully formed human being.

Does Attorney Raab's interpretation of the federal law uphold the letter of the law? The spirit of the law? If federal funding did flow to support embryonic stem cell research based on the DHHS interpretation, who, if anyone, would have standing to challenge the federal government's decision to fund this form of medical research? Consider the following case.

DOE v. SHALALA
United State District Court, District of Maryland
862 F. Supp. 1421 (1994)

MESSITTE, District Judge.

Plaintiffs in this suit seek to enjoin the activity of the National Institutes of Health (NIH) Human Embryo Research Panel (Panel) on the grounds that . . . Section 101 of the NIH Revitalization Act of 1993 (Revitalization Act), 42 U.S.C. § 289a-1, violates the U.S. Constitution. More immediately, their objective is to prevent the Panel from holding any meetings or making any recommendations to NIH or the Secretary of Health and Human Services with regard to the issue of

---

creation of embryos for research, *see* Eric Cohen, *The Bioethics Agenda and the Bush Second Term,* 7 The New Atlantis 11 (Fall 2004/Winter 2005).

human fetal research. The matter comes before the Court in the form of a Motion for Preliminary Injunction, anticipating the imminent publication by the Panel of its report and recommendations.

The Court holds that Plaintiffs lack standing to litigate these claims . . . Accordingly, the Court finds no need to engage in the usual preliminary injunction analysis and will proceed directly to dismiss Plaintiffs' suit.

II.

Would-be Plaintiff Mary Doe is an unnamed baby girl who, according to the Amended Complaint, is "a pre-born child in being as a human embryo." She is allegedly one of more than 20,000 such embryos *ex utero* located in various in vitro laboratories within the United States. Plaintiff International Foundation for Genetic Research (The Michael Fund) is a non-profit organization whose primary purpose is to sponsor research involving the genetic disorder known as Down's Syndrome and similar inborn chromosomal disorders. Plaintiff Michael Policastro, after whom The Michael Fund was named, is 24 years of age and suffers from Down's Syndrome. Defendants, in addition to the Secretary of U.S. Department of Health and Human Services and NIH, are the Department of Health and Human Services, the Director of NIH individually, the NIH Human Embryo Research Panel and the individual members of the Panel. The Panel whose activities are challenged in this proceeding came into existence following the enactment of the NIH Revitalization Act of 1993, P.L. No. 103-43, codified at 42 U.S.C. § 281 et seq. Consideration of pertinent provisions of the Act will illuminate the nature of the litigation.

Under the Act, the Secretary of HHS may not withhold federal funds for clinical research "because of ethical considerations" unless she first convenes an ethics advisory board (EAB) which, in accordance with certain prescribed procedures, studies such considerations, and either (1) recommends, by majority vote, because of ethical considerations, that the Secretary withhold funds for their proposed research or (2) recommends, by majority vote, because of ethical considerations, that the Secretary *not* withhold funds for the proposed research, but the Secretary finds the recommendation to be arbitrary and capricious. See 42 U.S.C. § 289a-1(b). This law amended existing federal regulations governing research on human embryos, which required such research to be reviewed by an EAB before such research might proceed. See 45 C.F.R. § 46.204(d). Because prior presidential administrations apparently chose not to appoint an EAB, no funding for such research had in fact been approved. What the new law did was to reverse the conditions for in vitro fertilization research: it could go forward unless disapproved. Previously it could not go forward unless approved . . .

Not later than 180 days after an EAB is convened, it is required to submit to the Secretary and to the Committee on Energy and Commerce of the House of Representatives and the Committee on Labor and Human Resources of the United States Senate a report describing its findings regarding the proposed research project or projects and making recommendations as to whether the Secretary should or should not withhold funds for such project or projects on ethical grounds. 42 U.S.C. § 289a-1(b)(5)(B)(ii).

With the passage of the Revitalization Act, NIH in fact received a number of applications seeking financial support of research involving human embryos. During the fall of 1993, therefore, Secretary Shalala, acting pursuant to the law, decided to convene and appoint an EAB, to be known as the NIH Human Embryo Research Panel. The Panel was charged by the Secretary with addressing the moral and ethical issues raised by the use of human embryos in research and with developing "guidelines" as to which areas of research involving human embryos would be acceptable for funding, which would require additional review, and which would be unacceptable for federal support. The Committee has held five public meetings all of which were open to the public and is expected to render a report to the Advisory Committee to the Director of NIH in short order.

In the present suit Plaintiffs seek to block issuance of the report and any further activities of the Panel, contending in part that at least 10 of the 19 members of the Panel "are current or former NIH grantees who have firmly endorsed the principle and many of the protocols of extended and unfettered human embryo research." The Panel, say Plaintiffs, "is accordingly predisposed to and will most probably make recommendations in favor of the Secretary not withholding federal funding for at least some projects involving human embryo research."

If, Plaintiffs continue, the Panel makes recommendations in favor of the Secretary not withholding federal funding for proposed projects involving human research, Plaintiffs will be harmed in the following ways: would-be Plaintiff Mary Doe and the group of which she is a part will be deprived of "the right to life without due process of law"; Plaintiff The Michael Fund will have federal funding otherwise available to support research involving Down's Syndrome and related disorders diverted to projects involving human embryo research; and individual Plaintiff Michael Policastro will not only suffer the consequences of the Fund's reduced research support, but will, along with other mature persons affected with Down's Syndrome, be threatened with the loss of life by the activities of Defendants, "which will have the effect of making socially acceptable, and ultimately fully legal, the destruction of people affected with Down's Syndrome."

Plaintiffs challenge the existence and activities of the Panel in several counts. They contend:

— in Count I, that the lack of balance and conflicts of interest prevalent on the Panel violate the "fair balance" requirement of the Federal Advisory Committee Act, 5 U.S.C., App. 2, Section 5(b)(2);

— in Count II, that Section 101 of the Revitalization Act violates Article II, Section 2, Clause 2, the Appointments Clause of the U.S. Constitution, which requires Presidential appointments of certain government officers;

— in Count III, that Section 101 of the Act violates Article II, Section 3 of the Constitution in that it restricts the President's power to take care that the laws be faithfully executed;

— in Count IV, that Section 101 violates the doctrine of separation of powers; and

— in Count V, that the actions of Defendants violate the Fifth, Eighth, and Ninth Amendments to the Constitution, in that they will deprive would-be Plaintiff Mary Doe, others like her, and individual Plaintiff Michael Policastro, of life and liberty without due process of law, subject them to cruel and unusual punishment, and deprive them of their right to privacy.

Mindful of the imminent publication by the Panel of its report and recommendations to the Advisory Committee and the Secretary, Plaintiffs ask for a preliminary injunction to prevent the publication as well as a cessation of any further Panel activities pending trial.

In response, the United States argues primarily that the Panel is not an "advisory committee" subject to the Federal Advisory Committee Act, but only a group of consultants which will advise the Standing Advisory Committee of NIH, which in turn will advise the NIH Director. The Government also argues that Plaintiffs lack standing to pursue this suit and that certain issues are either non-justiciable or not ripe for decision. The Government opposes the issuance of a preliminary injunction.

The Court finds that considerations of standing and justiciability are dispositive of the case. The Court therefore considers the applicable legal concepts.

III.

The Court accepts that organizational Plaintiff The Michael Fund and individual Plaintiff Michael Policastro properly speak for themselves through designated counsel. The situation is considerably different, however, as to would-be Plaintiff Mary Doe, described as a "pre-born child in being as a human embryo." Putting aside for the moment the question of whether a human embryo has independent legal interests capable of protection, it is clear that any such interests would have to be protected through the person of a guardian ad litem. See Fed.R.Civ.P.17(c); Cf. *Hatch v. Riggs National Bank*, 361 F.2d 559 (D.C.Cir.1966) (proper to appoint guardian ad litem for unborn beneficiaries of trust). Indeed The Michael Fund has filed a motion that someone, presumably it, be appointed guardian ad litem of Mary Doe.

Ordinarily the inquiry with regard to appointment of a guardian ad litem would be limited to whether the guardian can adequately represent the interests of its ward . . . Here, however, the matter is complicated by the fact that Mary Doe seeks to represent not only herself, but "all others similarly situated," which the Court understands to be some 20,000 human embryos currently in storage in various facilities around the United States. In other words, although The Michael Fund does not pray or plead it as such, it seeks to have this action proceed as a class action pursuant to Fed.R.Civ.P. 23.

There are several reasons why the suit cannot proceed as to "Mary Doe." First, philosophical and religious considerations aside, the Supreme Court has made it clear that the word "person," as used in the Fourteenth Amendment, does not include the unborn. *Roe v. Wade*, 410 U.S. 113, 158, 93 S.Ct. 705, 729, 35 L.Ed.2d 147 (1973). It has thus been held that embryos are not persons with legally protectable interests within the meaning of Fed.R.Civ.P. 17(c) such that appointments of guardians ad litem are warranted or required. See *Roe v. Casey*, 464 F.Supp. 483 (E.D.Pa.1978), aff'd, 623 F.2d 829 (3d Cir.1980). The Court sees no distinction between fetuses *in utero* or *ex utero.*

Additionally, appointing a guardian ad litem for an unspecified embryo, much less for a class of some 20,000, would present the Court with an impossible task. While the Court in no sense questions the bona fides of The Michael Fund, it is asked to decide that The Michael Fund, which is apparently committed to the prevention of federal funding for fetal research, can fairly represent the interests of one unspecified fetus and 20,000 others . . .

Based on conventional considerations relating to the appointment of guardians ad litem and class representatives, the Court declines to designate the organizational Plaintiff as guardian ad litem for would-be Plaintiff Mary Doe. The suit will not be permitted to go forward and will be dismissed as to her. The Court proceeds with its review of the standing of Plaintiffs The Michael Fund and Michael Policastro to pursue the litigation.

IV.

Under Article III, Section 2, of the U.S. Constitution, the judicial power of the United States extends to cases and controversies. The two terms . . . refer to disputes which are "definite and concrete, touching the legal relations of parties having adverse legal interests. It must be a real and substantial controversy admitting of specific relief through a decree of a conclusive character, as distinguished from an opinion advising what the law would be upon a hypothetical state of affairs."

One component of the case or controversy requirement is the question of standing, which bears on the power of a court to entertain a party's claim . . . Standing involves determining whether a particular litigant is entitled to invoke the jurisdiction of a court to decide a particular issue . . .

Although there has been some uncertainty about the scope of the standing doctrine in the past, it is essentially settled that:

> at an irreducible minimum, Art. III requires the party who invokes the court's authority to "show that he personally has suffered some actual or threatened injury as a result of the putatively illegal conduct of the defendant," and that the injury "fairly can be traced to the challenged action" and "is likely to be redressed by a favorable decision." [Citations omitted]

The Court considers each of these elements.

With regard to the injury requirement, a party must have "such a personal stake in the outcome of the controversy as to assure that concrete adverseness which sharpens the presentation of issues upon which the court so largely depends for illumination of difficult constitutional questions." *Baker v. Carr*, 369 U.S. 186, 204, 82 S.Ct. 691, 702, 7 L.Ed.2d 663 (1962). The injury must be direct, distinct and palpable, not merely conjectural. *Allen v. Wright*, 468 U.S. 737, 751, 104 S.Ct. 3315, 3324-25, 82 L.Ed.2d 556 (1984). It must be an "injury-in-fact." *Association of Data*

Processing Serv. Orgs. v. Camp, 397 U.S. 150, 152 (1970) . . .

In . . . addition to injury-in-fact there must be causation-in-fact. The injury must be suffered "as a consequence of the alleged constitutional error," and must be "other than the psychological consequence presumably produced by observation of conduct with which one disagrees." *Valley Forge Christian College*, 454 U.S. at 482, 102 S.Ct. at 765 . . .

Against this legal background, the Court considers Plaintiffs' claims in the present case.

The Court turns first to the issue of constitutional standing and the questions of injury-in-fact, causation-in-fact, and the redressability of any injury by a favorable court decision.

Plaintiffs The Michael Fund and Michael Policastro allege that injury to them will result because "federal funds available for the support of research designed to discover a cure and treatment for persons afflicted with genetic disorders, such as Down's Syndrome, will be reduced in direct proportion to the extent that such funds are diverted to the support of human embryo research projects." Michael Policastro is said to be threatened with the loss of his life because the activities of Defendants "will have the effect of making socially acceptable, and ultimately fully legal, the destruction of people with Down's Syndrome."

These allegations of injury, sincerely felt though they may be, do not, in the Court's view, pass constitutional muster. Such injuries are remote and speculative, not immediate and palpable. Even if, following a report of the Panel, NIH were to elect to fund fetal research projects (and it is by no means certain to what extent it will), there is no basis for concluding that that decision would diminish funding for research projects involving Down's Syndrome or other genetic disorders. Nor is there any basis in the least for suggesting that Plaintiff Michael Policastro's life might be at risk if fetal research were to go forward.

Similarly, Plaintiffs cannot satisfy the second constitutional requirement for standing — that there be causation between the challenged action and the particularized injury sustained. There is, again, simply no basis for concluding that an ultimate decision by NIH to fund fetal research would concretely and demonstrably diminish the organizational Plaintiff's funding or put Michael Policastro's life in danger.

Finally, it is open to serious question whether a court decree in this case would actually redress the alleged harm. What Plaintiffs ask for is injunctive relief to prevent the Human Embryo Research Panel from reporting to the Advisory Committee and the Secretary about the ethics of pursuing human embryo research or, indeed, from carrying on any further activities. But preventing the Panel from issuing a report could well have no effect whatsoever on the ultimate decision of the Secretary to fund such research. The Revitalization Act allows that such research may go forward *unless* an EAB advises the Secretary that it should not and if she does not overrule the Panel. In sharp contrast to prior law, there is no requirement that an EAB be constituted at all before the research proceeds. In other words, it may be doubted — for constitutional purposes — whether blocking the Panel's report or its other activity would fairly redress the harms claimed here if the

Secretary of HHS decided to go forward with funding in the absence of a report from EAB and with the activities of the Board frozen by injunction . . . The Court concludes that Plaintiffs fail to meet the requisite constitutional requirements for standing to pursue this case . . .

ORDER

Upon consideration of Plaintiffs' Motion for Appointment of a Guardian Ad Litem for would-be Plaintiff Mary Doe and Defendants' Opposition thereto; and upon consideration of Plaintiffs' Motion for Preliminary Injunction and Defendants' Opposition thereto; and upon consideration of Defendants' Motion for Judgment on the Pleadings or, in the Alternative, for Summary Judgment and Plaintiffs' Opposition thereto; it is for the reasons set forth in the Court's Opinion of even date, this 26th day of September, 1994 ORDERED that Plaintiffs' Motion for Appointment of a Guardian Ad Litem is hereby DENIED; and it is further ORDERED that Plaintiffs' Motion for Preliminary Injunction is hereby DENIED; and it is further ORDERED that Defendants' Motion for Summary Judgment is hereby GRANTED and Plaintiffs' Complaint and Amended Complaint are hereby DISMISSED.

QUESTION

Michael J. Fox is an actor who suffers from Parkinson's Disease, an illness for which stem cell therapy has shown great promise in animal studies. Would he have standing to challenge the constitutionality of the Dickey Amendment by suing the Secretary of the Department of Health and Human Services for failing to authorize funding for embryonic stem cell research? Has he met the "injury-in-fact" and the "causation-in-fact" tests necessary to present a case or controversy under Article III, Section 2, of the U.S. Constitution?

2. State Laws Relating to Embryos as Sources of Stem Cells

National Bioethics Advisory Commission
Ethical Issues in Human Stem Cell Research 35-36
(September 1999)

State Law Regarding Research Using Cells and Tissues from Human Embryos

State legislatures have apparently been more concerned about regulating and restricting research using human fetuses or their remains instead of addressing research involving laboratory manipulation of human gametes and early stage embryos. Nonetheless, although the statutes usually ignore issues (other than commercialization) specific to IVF, some could be construed broadly enough to encompass a range of experimental activities involving IVF, including cryopreservation, pre- implantation screening, gene therapy, twinning, cell line development, and basic research. The latter two are of obvious relevance to creating stem cell cultures from embryonic sources.

States that regulate cell line development from human embryos either prohibit the practice entirely or restrict it substantially. "All ten states that prohibit embryological research have vaguely worded statutes which could encompass cell line development if the statutes were interpreted broadly . . . [although] some [activity] could be characterized as non-experimental, thus removing it from the scope of experimentation bans".[20] Issues inherent in cell line development will include the potential for restrictions on downstream commercialization and uncertainty over the extent to which gamete donors must be informed about the nature of and potential commercial uses of the biological materials they donate.

Basic research typically involves precommercial scientific activity designed to explore biological processes or to understand genetic and cellular control mechanisms. As noted previously, 24 states and the District of Columbia do not restrict research involving fetuses or embryos. Of the remaining 26 states that regulate embryo or fetal research in one form or another, basic embryological research is prohibited or restricted in 10.[21] Although the degree of regulation of experimental use of embryos under the New Hampshire statute is unlikely to impair ES cell research in that state, the remaining nine states have legislated more broadly, effectively banning all research involving *in vitro* embryos, with penalties mandated in some states, including civil fines and imprisonment. The subject of commercialization is a potentially important one, affecting both researchers who must acquire embryos from for-profit IVF clinics or other sources and downstream users who may develop derivative, commercial applications from basic embryological and stem cell research. Currently, five states prohibit payment for IVF embryos for research purposes. [Maine, Massachusetts, Michigan, North Dakota, and Rhode Island]. Eight additional states prohibit payment for human embryos for any purpose. [Florida, Georgia, Illinois, Louisiana, Minnesota, Pennsylvania, Texas, and Utah]. Five states apply ambiguous restrictions that may or may not prohibit sale of embryos, depending upon interpretation or, in some cases, action by state officials. More troubling, some statutes could be interpreted to prevent payment for ES cell lines derived from human embryos, although "it is possible that because a cell line is new tissue produced from the genetic material of, but not originally a part of, the embryo, laws proscribing the sale of embryonic tissue may not apply." In line with NOTA and the 1987 revisions of the UAGA, state statutes on organ transplantation now typically prohibit sale of human organs or parts, but none include language likely to impede research involving human embryos.

---

[20] Here NBAC cites June Coleman, *Playing God or Playing Scientists: A Constitutional analysis of State Laws Banning Embryological Procedures*, 27 Pac. L. J. 1331 (1996). -Ed.

[21] A report submitted to the President's Council on Bioethics pegs the number of states that ban research on embryos at 11 — 9 that ban research on IVF embryos altogether [Florida, Louisiana, Maine, Massachusetts, Michigan, Minnesota, North Dakota, Pennsylvania and Rhode Island], and 2 that ban "destructive" embryo research [Iowa and South Dakota]. See Lori B. Andrews, *Legislators as Lobbyists: Proposed State Regulation of Embryonic Stem Cell Research, Therapeutic Cloning and Reproductive Cloning*, at 203, Appendix E to Monitoring Stem Cell Research, a report of The President's Council on Bioethics (2004).

NOTES AND QUESTIONS

1. *Keeping Current on State Laws.* Several organizations keep track of state legislative activity surrounding embryo research. For a review of current law on fetal and embryonic research, visit the National Conference of State Legislatures' website, at www.ncsl.org.

2. State regulation of embryonic stem cell research creates a proverbial patchwork of laws, with about a fifth of all states banning any research activity, and another fifth or so placing restrictions on research that can lawfully take place within the state's borders. As noted in the excerpt above, it is not clear in every state whether existing law would prohibit the conduct associated with embryonic stem cell research. Would a researcher who derives stem cells from donated IVF embryos be in violation of the following laws?

Massachusetts General Laws Annotated
Chapter 12, Section 12J

§ 12J. Experimentation on human fetuses prohibited.

(a) I. No person shall use any live human fetus whether before or after expulsion from its mother's womb, for scientific, laboratory, research or other kind of experimentation . . .

A fetus is a live fetus for purposes of this section when, in the best medical judgment of a physician, it shows evidence of life as determined by the same medical standards as are used in determining evidence of life in a spontaneously aborted fetus at approximately the same stage of gestational development . . . (a) IV. No person shall knowingly sell, transfer, distribute or give away any fetus for a use which is in violation of the provisions of this section. For purposes of this section, the word "fetus" shall include also an embryo or neonate. (a) V. Except as hereafter provided, whoever violates the provisions of this section shall be punished by imprisonment in a jail or house of correction for not less than one year nor more than two and one-half years or by imprisonment in the state prison for not more than five years and by the imposition of a fine of up to ten thousand dollars.

Maine Revised Statutes Annotated
Title 22 Health and Welfare

§ 1593.   Sale and use of fetuses 1. Prohibition. A person may not use, transfer, distribute or give away a live human fetus, whether intrauterine or extrauterine, or any product of conception considered live born, for scientific experimentation or for any form of experimentation. 2. Consenting, aiding or assisting. A person may not consent to violating subsection 1 or aid or assist another in violating subsection 1.3. Penalty. A person who violates this section commits a Class C crime. Violation of this section is a strict liability crime as defined in Title 17-A, section 34, subsection 4-A.

§ 1595.   Live born and live birth, defined "Live born" and "live birth," as used in this chapter, shall mean a product of conception after complete expulsion or extraction from its mother; irrespective of the duration of pregnancy, which breathes or shows any other evidence of life such as beating of the heart, pulsation of the umbilical cord or definite movement of voluntary muscles, whether or not the umbilical cord has been cut or the placenta is attached. Each product of such a birth is considered live born and fully recognized as a human person under Maine law.

3. *Stem Cells Derived From Cloned Embryos.* Recall that embryonic stem cells can be derived from two types of embryos — embryos created through in vitro fertilization and embryos created through cloning (a process called somatic cell nuclear transfer). In theory, the benefit of using stem cells from cloned embryos is that they will be an exact tissue match for the person whose cell was used to create the embryo in the first place. Any tissue derived from the cloned embryo will not be rejected by the patient's body, because the tissue will be an exact match of existing organs and tissues. Harvesting and cultivating stem cells from cloned embryos is often referred to as therapeutic cloning. Therapeutic cloning is controversial for the same reasons that stem cell research in general is controversial — both involve the destruction of the embryo at the blastocyst stage. Therapeutic cloning faces additional challenges from those who oppose the creation of an embryo in a manner other than the fusion of an egg and a sperm.

A handful of states have enacted laws pertaining to stem cell research using cloned embryos. According to the Genetics & Public Policy Center based at Johns Hopkins University, seven states — Arkansas, Indiana, Iowa, Michigan, North Dakota, South Dakota and Virginia — ban therapeutic cloning, while five states — California, Connecticut, Missouri, New Jersey and Rhode Island. — explicitly legalize and support therapeutic cloning by enacted statute. Compare these two opposite state public policies. California Health & Safety Code, Section 125300 provides, "[t]hat research involving the derivation and use of human embryonic stem cells, human embryonic germ cells, and human adult stem cells from any source, including somatic cell nuclear transplantation, shall be permitted and that full consideration of the ethical and medical implications of this research be given." In contrast, Arkansas Code Section 20-16-1002 makes it unlawful "for any person or entity, public or private, to intentionally or knowingly: (1) Perform or attempt to perform human cloning; (2) Participate in an attempt to perform human cloning; (3) Ship, transfer, or receive for any purpose an embryo produced by human cloning; or (4) Ship, transfer, or receive, in whole or in part, any oocyte, embryo, fetus, or human somatic cell for the purpose of human cloning."

The states that ban therapeutic cloning also ban reproductive cloning, the creation of an embryo for purposes of producing a child who would have the same genome as an existing person. Reproductive cloning draws far more opponents than therapeutic cloning, with many people expressing revulsion at the prospect of birthing children whose conception was asexual, that is, not the result of fertilization. A few states have outlawed reproductive cloning, but specifically allowed therapeutic cloning. See, e.g., Cal. Health & Safety Code § 24185; R.I. Gen. Laws § 23-16.4-1; Va. Code Ann. § 32.1-162.22. The Rhode Island law provides:

The purpose of this legislation is to place a ban on the creation of a human being through division of a blastocyst, zygote, or embryo or somatic cell nuclear transfer, and to protect the citizens of the state from potential abuse deriving from cloning technologies. This ban is not intended to apply to the cloning of human cells, genes, tissues, or organs that would not result in the replication of an entire human being. Nor is this ban intended to apply to in vitro fertilization, the administration of fertility enhancing drugs, or other medical procedures used to assist a woman in becoming or remaining pregnant, so long as that procedure is not specifically intended to result in the gestation or birth of a child who is genetically identical to another conceptus, embryo, fetus, or human being, living or dead.

What is the public policy behind banning reproductive cloning but allowing therapeutic cloning? Should lawmakers be concerned that if embryo cloning is allowed for one purpose — developing stem cell therapies — that it will inevitably be used by occupationally curious scientists for another purpose — reproduction? If an embryo is cloned, is the temptation to implant it in a woman's womb too great such that all cloning should be banned? For such an argument, *see* Alexander Morgan Capron, *Placing a Moratorium on Research Cloning To Ensure Effective Control Over Reproductive Cloning*, 53 Hast. L. J. 1075 (2002). *See also* June Mary Zekan Makdisi, *The Slide From Human Embryonic Stem Cell Research to Reproductive Cloning: Ethical Decision-Making and the Ban on Federal Funding*, 34 Rutgers L. J. 463 (2003) (arguing federal funding of embryonic stem cell research will inevitably lead to government funding for reproductive cloning research).

SECTION III: GOVERNMENT FUNDING OF STEM CELL RESEARCH

The materials in Section 2 set out the current parameters surrounding the legality of embryonic stem cell research. Federal law does not explicitly prohibit such research, while laws in about a dozen states make the intentional destruction of a human embryo either a crime or a civilly prohibited act, thus banning such research in those state. The result is that embryonic stem cell research is legal in the majority of states. From this foundational reality, a question of public policy flows: Should the government make available public funds to support and advance the study of stem cells derived from human embryos? The national answer to this question is as divided as the electorate has been in recent presidential contests. For some, the idea of destroying an embryo to extract its stem cells is an immoral act of killing, and should not be in any way sanctioned by the federal government. For others, the potential cures hidden within the embryonic stem cells are so advantageous to humankind they impose a moral obligation on the federal government to aid in advancing those medical benefits.

The problem, perhaps, lies in the fact that the U.S. federal government has historically played a major role in supporting medical research. As reported by the President's Council of Bioethics, "The federal government makes significant public resources available to biomedical researchers each year — more than $20 billion in fiscal year 2003 alone — in the form of research grants offered largely through the National Institutes of Health (NIH). This level of public expenditure reflects the great esteem in which Americans hold the biomedical enterprise and the value we place on the development of treatments and cures for those who are suffering." In 2011, the NIH biomedical research budget reached approximately $30 billion. With this history as background, it seems natural for the government to be called upon to fund research in the emerging stem cell arena. But the source of those stem cells — the human embryo — create a controversy over whether taxpayer dollars should support an activity that some individuals find immorally objectionable and others consider morally obligatory.

The debate over funding occurs at the both federal and state levels, as researchers, patient advocates, private biomedical concerns, religious leaders and everyday citizens vie for support — financial, political, moral, and otherwise — for their respective positions.

A. Federal Funding of Stem Cell Research

1. The First Presidential Proclamation: August 9, 2001

The issue of federal funding for embryonic stem cell research became a subject for debate during the first presidential election to follow the discovery of derived embryonic stem cells in 1998. During the 2000 election, candidates Al Gore and George W. Bush staked out opposite positions on the question of federal funding, with Democratic Gore promising to release funding for research and Republican Bush vowing to block any federal involvement in the destruction of human embryos. After President Bush's inauguration, he no doubt gave great thought to the issue, reportedly consulting with numerous experts before arriving at a decision. That decision was announced to the nation by telecast on August 9, 2001, barely eight months into the president's first term in office. Recall that when President Bush took office in January 2001, the federal government had never funded any embryonic stem cell research, though it was poised to do so under the previous Clinton Administration guidelines that would have allowed funding for research on stem cell lines (though the support stopped short of funding the actual destruction of the embryos). Upon taking office, while President Bush wrestled with the question of federal funding, he froze any funding until the policies could be reviewed.

President Bush announced his stem cell funding policy in a nationally televised speech from his Crawford, Texas, Ranch beginning at 9:00 p.m. eastern standard time.

Remarks by the President on Stem Cell Research
The Bush Ranch, Crawford Texas
www.whitehouse.gov/news/releases/2001/08/20010809-2.html

Good evening. I appreciate you giving me a few minutes of your time tonight so I can discuss with you a complex and difficult issue, an issue that is one of the most profound of our time.

The issue of research involving stem cells derived from human embryos is increasingly the subject of a national debate and dinner table discussions. The issue is confronted every day in laboratories as scientists ponder the ethical ramifications of their work. It is agonized over by parents and many couples as they try to have children, or to save children already born.

The issue is debated within the church, with people of different faiths, even many of the same faith coming to different conclusions. Many people are finding that the more they know about stem cell research, the less certain they are about the right ethical and moral conclusions.

My administration must decide whether to allow federal funds, your tax dollars, to be used for scientific research on stem cells derived from human embryos. A large number of these embryos already exist. They are the product of a process called in vitro fertilization, which helps so many couples conceive children. When doctors match sperm and egg to create life outside the womb, they usually produce more embryos than are planted in the mother. Once a couple successfully has children, or if they are unsuccessful, the additional embryos remain frozen in laboratories . . .

Based on preliminary work that has been privately funded, scientists believe further research using stem cells offers great promise that could help improve the lives of those who suffer from many terrible diseases — from juvenile diabetes to Alzheimer's, from Parkinson's to spinal cord injuries. And while scientists admit they are not yet certain, they believe stem cells derived from embryos have unique potential . . .

Scientists further believe that rapid progress in this research will come only with federal funds. Federal dollars help attract the best and brightest scientists. They ensure new discoveries are widely shared at the largest number of research facilities and that the research is directed toward the greatest public good.

The United States has a long and proud record of leading the world toward advances in science and medicine that improve human life. And the United States has a long and proud record of upholding the highest standards of ethics as we expand the limits of science and knowledge. Research on embryonic stem cells raises profound ethical questions, because extracting the stem cell destroys the embryo, and thus destroys its potential for life . . .

As I thought through this issue, I kept returning to two fundamental questions: First, are these frozen embryos human life, and therefore, something precious to be protected? And second, if they're going to be destroyed anyway, shouldn't they be used for a greater good, for research that has the potential to save and improve other lives?

On the first issue, are these embryos human life — well, one researcher told me he believes this five-day-old cluster of cells is not an embryo, not yet an individual, but a pre-embryo. He argued that it has the potential for life, but it is not a life because it cannot develop on its own.

An ethicist dismissed that as a callous attempt at rationalization. Make no mistake, he told me, that cluster of cells is the same way you and I, and all the rest of us, started our lives. One goes with a heavy heart if we use these, he said, because we are dealing with the seeds of the next generation.

And to the other crucial question, if these are going to be destroyed anyway, why not use them for good purpose — I also found different answers. Many argue these embryos are byproducts of a process that helps create life, and we should allow couples to donate them to science so they can be used for good purpose instead of wasting their potential. Others will argue there's no such thing as excess life, and the fact that a living being is going to die does not justify experimenting on it or exploiting it as a natural resource.

At its core, this issue forces us to confront fundamental questions about the beginnings of life and the ends of science. It lies at a difficult moral intersection, juxtaposing the need to protect life in all its phases with the prospect of saving and improving life in all its stages . . .

My position on these issues is shaped by deeply held beliefs. I'm a strong supporter of science and technology, and believe they have the potential for incredible good — to improve lives, to save life, to conquer disease. Research offers hope that millions of our loved ones may be cured of a disease and rid of their suffering. I have friends whose children suffer from juvenile diabetes. Nancy Reagan has written me about President Reagan's struggle with Alzheimer's. My own family has confronted the tragedy of childhood leukemia. And, like all Americans, I have great hope for cures.

I also believe human life is a sacred gift from our Creator. I worry about a culture that devalues life, and believe as your President I have an important obligation to foster and encourage respect for life in America and throughout the world. And while we're all hopeful about the potential of this research, no one can be certain that the science will live up to the hope it has generated . . .

As a result of private research, more than 60 genetically diverse stem cell lines already exist. They were created from embryos that have already been destroyed, and they have the ability to regenerate themselves indefinitely, creating ongoing opportunities for research. I have concluded that we should allow federal funds to be used for research on these existing stem cell lines, where the life and death decision has already been made.

Leading scientists tell me research on these 60 lines has great promise that could lead to breakthrough therapies and cures. This allows us to explore the promise and potential of stem cell research without crossing a fundamental moral line, by providing taxpayer funding that would sanction or encourage further destruction of human embryos that have at least the potential for life.

I also believe that great scientific progress can be made through aggressive federal funding of research on umbilical cord placenta, adult and animal stem cells which do not involve the same moral dilemma. This year, your government will spend $250 million on this important research.

I will also name a President's council to monitor stem cell research, to recommend appropriate guidelines and regulations, and to consider all of the medical and ethical ramifications of biomedical innovation. This council will consist of leading scientists, doctors, ethicists, lawyers, theologians and others, and will be chaired by Dr. Leon Kass, a leading biomedical ethicist from the University of Chicago.

This council will keep us apprised of new developments and give our nation a forum to continue to discuss and evaluate these important issues. As we go forward, I hope we will always be guided by both intellect and heart, by both our capabilities and our conscience.

I have made this decision with great care, and I pray it is the right one.

Thank you for listening. Good night, and God bless America.

NOTES AND QUESTIONS

1. *A Solomonic Compromise?* Reaction to the President's stem cell funding policy was predictably diverse and wide-ranging, with opinions scattered from complete agreement with this "middle-of-the road" approach, to outrage that a single federal dollar would be spent to support research in which human life has been purposefully destroyed, to lament over the loss of essential resources in the fight against devastating diseases. The policy has been referred to as a "Solomonic compromise" because it permitted some federal funding of stem cell research without encouraging future embryo destruction.

The specific funding parameters of the Bush Administration policy were set out by the National Institutes of Health, the federal granting authority in charge of funding biomedical research. As you read the requirements and exclusions, consider in your own mind whether the policy meets the dual goals of assisting research and respecting nascent life.

Bush Administration NIH Guidelines for Embryonic Stem Cell Funding

Taken from the website of the National Institutes of Health on September 26, 2003

NOTICE OF CRITERIA FOR FEDERAL FUNDING OF RESEARCH ON EXISTING HUMAN EMBRYONIC STEM CELLS AND ESTABLISHMENT OF NIH HUMAN EMBRYONIC STEM CELL REGISTRY

Release Date: November 7, 2001

Office of the Director, NIH

On August 9, 2001, at 9:00 p.m. EDT, the President announced his decision to allow Federal funds to be used for research on existing human embryonic stem cell lines as long as prior to his announcement (1) the derivation process (which commences with the removal of the inner cell mass from the blastocyst) had already been initiated and (2) the embryo from which the stem cell line was derived no longer had the possibility of development as a human being.

In addition, the President established the following criteria that must be met:

The stem cells must have been derived from an embryo that was created for reproductive purposes;

The embryo was no longer needed for these purposes;

Informed consent must have been obtained for the donation of the embryo;

No financial inducements were provided for donation of the embryo.

In order to facilitate research using human embryonic stem cells, the NIH is creating a Human Embryonic Stem Cell Registry that will list the human embryonic stem cells that meet the eligibility criteria. Specifically, the laboratories or companies that provide the cells listed on the Registry will have submitted to the NIH a signed assurance. Each provider must retain for submission to the NIH, if necessary, written documentation to verify the statements in the signed assurance.

The Registry will be accessible to investigators on the NIH Home Page http://escr.nih.gov. Requests for Federal funding must cite a human embryonic stem cell line that is listed on the NIH Registry. Such requests will also need to meet existing scientific and technical merit criteria and be recommended for funding by the relevant National Advisory Council, as appropriate.

Imagine you are a biomedical scientist interested in conducting stem cell research. Using private funding in 2000 and early 2001, you derived five stem cell lines that continue to proliferate and remain undifferentiated, ideal clinical circumstances for investigating the limits of stem cells as medical therapy. If you apply for federal funds under the Bush policy, how can you prove that the embryos from which the five lines were derived were "no longer needed" for reproductive purposes? Could a childless infertile couple challenge this assertion by arguing that they would have been willing to adopt the embryos for their own reproductive needs? Are the embryos then needed for reproductive purposes?

2. *The Questions of Quantity and Quality.* When the Bush Administration's policy was first announced, some of the criticism focused on the quantity and quality of the existing stem cell lines that would be available for research funding. President Bush referred to "60 genetically diverse stem cell lines" that would be available for funding because they had been derived prior to the imposition of the new policy. Scientists wondered where the 60 lines were located, and whether they would be robust enough to sustain research well into the future.

As to the question of quantity, a 2004 unpublished NIH analysis revealed that only 15 cell lines were available for federally funded research. The numbers were arrived at as follows. After the August 2001 announcement of the Bush Administration policy, it was thought that 78 stem cell lines met the criteria set out in the newly-minted policy. However, follow-up interviews and searches found that 17 of those cell lines had been withdrawn or failed to grow, 31 lines belonged to foreign laboratories that were unwilling to ship them to U.S. researchers, seven lines were determined to be duplicates of other lines, and eight others were unavailable, but might become available at a later time. See Kaiser Daily Reproductive Health Report, *Fewer Embryonic Stem Cell Lines Than Expected Available for Federally Funded Research, NIH Analysis Says*, March 3, 2004, available at: kaisernetwork@cme.kff.org. *See also* Justin Gillis & Rick Weiss, *NIH: Few Stem Cell Colonies Likely Available for Research; Of Approved Lines, Many Are Failing*, Wash. Post, March 3, 2004, at A3 (quoting NIH administrator James Battey as describing the "best-case scenario" under the Bush administration policy as 23 cell colonies available in the U.S. for research).

Perhaps more crucial than the number of cell lines was the health and potential application of the existing lines to human therapeutics. Again, controversy swirled around this issue. According to the same unpublished NIH report noted above, some of the existing 15 cell lines had developed severe genetic abnormalities and were likely useless for creating therapies and impractical for research. In addition to concerns about genetic abnormalities in the cell lines, scientists questioned whether potential therapies derived from the original lines could be used in humans, as the federally sanctioned stem cell lines had been derived using feeder cells from mouse embryos, thus opening up the possibility that humans could be infected with mouse viruses contained in the cells.

In 2003 a scientific panel convened at Johns Hopkins University in Baltimore addressed the issue of mouse contamination in the stem cell lines available for federal dollars. The group of scientists, philosophers, ethicists and lawyers concluded that the cell lines eligible for federal funding were unethical to use for transplantation into human patients because of the risk of introducing mouse virus into the human population. *See* Julie Bell, *Scientist Panel Proposes Embryo Stem Cell "Bank"; Federally Approved Lines Inadequate, Pose Risk to Patients, Researchers Say*, Baltimore Sun, Nov. 11, 2003. The question of safety for human use was revisited in January 2005 by researchers at the University of California-San Diego. Reporting in the journal *Nature Medicine*, the group determined that all of the embryonic stem cell lines available for federal funding had molecules from mice attached to them that could be risky for use in medical therapies. *See* Andis Robeznieks, *Embryonic Stem Cell Line Found to be Contaminated*, AMERICAN MEDICAL NEWS, Feb. 14, 2005. Dr. James Battey, Chair of the NIH Stem Cell Task Force, appeared more sanguine about the presence of mouse molecules. He noted that humans routinely ingest animal products in meat and dairy products without experiencing immune responses, adding that the Food and Drug Administration has approved other health care products with animal molecules, and humans have been able to take those "with no evidence of rip-roaring immune rejection." Id.

If Dr. Battey was right and any therapies developed from the funding-eligible stem cell lines would be tolerated in humans, were there any other reasons to advocate for a change in the Bush Administration funding policy?

2. Defending and Questioning the Bush Administration Policy

O. Carter Snead
The Pedagogical Significance of the Bush Stem Cell Policy: A Window into Bioethical Regulation in the United States
5 Yale Journal of Health Policy & Ethics 491 (2005)

The enormous significance of the Bush stem cell funding policy has been evident since its inception. The announcement of the policy on August 9, 2001 marked the first time a U.S. president had ever taken up a matter of bioethical import as the sole subject of a major national policy address. Indeed, the August 9th speech was the President's first nationally televised policy address of any kind. Since then, the policy has been a constant focus of attention and discussion by political commentators, the print and broadcast media, advocacy organizations, scientists, elected officials, and candidates for all levels of office (including especially the 2004 Democratic nominee for President, Senator John Kerry, who made his opposition to the Bush policy a centerpiece of his domestic campaign, mentioning it explicitly in his acceptance speech at the Democratic National Convention). The biotechnology industry has taken a keen interest in stem cell research as a possible avenue for medical therapies; one study suggests that as of 2002 private sector companies had spent an aggregate of $208 million on research and development of stem cell technologies. In response to the policy, there has been a flurry of state legislation proposed and enacted, with some states affirming and others condemning the Administration's approach . . .

To date, the significance of the Bush stem cell policy has been framed and publicly debated in terms of its practical import: Does it impede the scientific and medical progress that the research seems to promise? Is it adequately protective and respectful of embryonic human life? Aside from its great practical significance, however, the Bush policy is arguably one of the most important recent legal developments for the field of bioethics for an additional reason: its deep pedagogical significance. The Bush policy provides an unparalleled window into the nature and substance of "bioethical regulation" within the unique framework of the American system of government. And it does so in dramatic fashion, against the backdrop of some of the most enduring and vexing questions in all of bioethics: What is owed to developing human life, and how does this obligation stand in relation to the aim of science to advance knowledge with the ultimate aspiration of alleviating human suffering? Reflecting on the nature and scope of the policy yields insights into a number of crucial matters that are central to the problem of whether and how to govern science and medicine according to bioethical principles . . .

I. The Bush Policy

[The author reviews the history of federal policy on embryo research funding, including enactment of the 1993 NIH Revitalization Act which effectively cleared the way for federal funding, followed by the 1996 Dickey Amendment which prohibited the use of federal funds for research in which a human embryo is destroyed, and the 1999 opinion by the Department of Health and Human Services' General Counsel that even under the Dickey Amendment it would be legally permissible to authorize federal funding for researchers who worked with stem cells acquired from embryos that had been destroyed using private funding.]

Against the backdrop of this twenty-five year history, President Bush was confronted with the question of whether and how to fund stem cell research. President Bush accepted the legal analysis of the former HHS General Counsel, but pursued a policy that sought to combine that analysis with the principle animating the Dickey Amendment, namely, that human life is worthy of profound respect at all of its developmental stages (from zygote to adult), and therefore, at the very least, the federal government should not provide financial incentives for its destruction, even for the sake of beneficial scientific research. President Bush thus formulated a stem cell funding policy that would, in his words, "aggressively promote stem cell research" without violating his aforementioned principle of respect for human embryonic life. In practice, the Bush policy authorizes federal funding for all forms of stem cell research that do not create incentives for the destruction of human embryos . . . So as not to encourage future destruction of human embryos, no federal funding is permitted for research on embryonic stem cell lines derived after August 9, 2001. For fiscal year 2003, the Bush Administration, through NIH, allocated $ 190.7 million for adult stem cell research, and $ 24.8 million for embryonic stem cell research . . . The Bush policy imposes no restrictions on privately funded embryonic stem cell research . . .

II. The Pedagogical Significance of the Bush Policy

What, then, is the pedagogical significance of the Bush policy? As noted above, a careful consideration of the policy's scope and substance yields . . . insights into the nature of bioethical regulation in the United States . . .

B. Principles of Federalism

The Bush policy further illustrates how matters of federalism — both horizontal and vertical — are implicated in the context of bioethical governance. Principles of horizontal federalism play an important role in the formulation and implementation of public policy that touches and concerns bioethics. In making such policy, each co-equal branch must act within the boundaries of its own enumerated powers, while respecting the prerogatives and domains of the others. This process is brought into sharp relief by a reflection on the Bush policy's origins and operation, described above. The Bush policy was written against the backdrop of the nearly thirty-year history of give and take between the executive and legislative branches over the question of federal funding for embryo research . . . [T]his inter-branch dialogue culminated in the enactment of the Dickey Amendment, whereby the legislative branch, acting pursuant to its constitutionally enumerated spending power, formally proscribed the use of federal funds for research in which human embryos are destroyed or discarded. In formulating a policy governing stem cell research and its funding, the Bush Administration (like the Clinton Administration before it) was required to work within the framework provided by Dickey out of respect for the federalist principle of separation of powers. The Bush policy accepted the Clinton Administration's refined interpretation of Dickey, but chose a policy that upheld a broad conception of the principle of respect for embryonic human life that provided the foundation for the original amendment. Thus, the Bush policy demonstrates both an acknowledgement of Congress's sole authority to appropriate federal funds and a robust exercise of the President's authority as head of the executive branch to allocate the appropriated funding according to the Administration's priorities.

In similar fashion, reflection on the Bush policy lends key insights into principles of vertical federalism in the context of bioethical governance. In enacting public policy, both state and federal governments are limited by their respective jurisdictional mechanisms. By virtue of the general police power to safeguard the health, welfare, and morals of citizens, states enjoy wide latitude to legislate according to bioethical principles. By contrast, the federal government is somewhat more limited in its options, consigned to act only pursuant to powers enumerated by the

Constitution. This division of responsibility allows in some cases for action and reaction between and among the federal and state governments.

Such is the case with the Bush policy. The Bush policy illustrates the use of the jurisdictional nexus of federal spending: The Administration is able to set ethical conditions on those practices to which it provides financial assistance, while remaining silent (and thus uninvolved) with respect to privately funded stem cell research. This leaves the state governments free to affirm or reject the policy within their own borders. Many states have taken this opportunity . . .

C. The Significance of Federal Funding

The Bush policy also offers noteworthy lessons regarding the nature and significance of federal funding. The U.S. government is a major provider of funds and resources for scientific and medical research. This is reflective of the esteem in which the American polity holds the scientific enterprise, as well as its great concern for the alleviation of human suffering. Federal funding has long played a significant role in the regulation of medicine and science according to bioethical principles. In the first instance, it is a jurisdictional nexus, allowing for the regulation of activities that might otherwise lie beyond the enumerated powers of the federal government by attaching certain conditions to the provision of funds. But perhaps more importantly for the present discussion, federal funding is a powerful device whereby the government expresses the polity's approval, disdain, or studied neutrality toward specified conduct. The government is under no obligation to provide federal funding for most activities — including those activities in which individuals may engage as a matter of constitutional right. Thus, the provision of federal funding can confer legitimacy on a given enterprise, signaling its worthiness for the allocation of otherwise scarce funds. The withholding of federal funds can signify a variety of sentiments: a lack of faith in the worthiness (moral or otherwise) of the enterprise, moral caution or affirmative disdain for the activity in question, or simply the judgment that there are more important priorities worthy of the expenditure of limited resources.

The Bush policy is instructive in this regard. It does, as mentioned above, utilize funding as a jurisdictional nexus. But it also conveys a message regarding the priorities of the Administration. First, it requires the federal government to adopt a posture of neutrality in the debate over the moral propriety of destructive embryo research. The Bush policy affirmatively and deliberately withholds the federal government's official approval for such practices, though it does allow these practices to proceed in the private sector. As such, no taxpayer is compelled to pay for and encourage an activity (i.e., embryo destruction) that a significant portion of the American public finds morally troublesome. At the same time, the Bush policy was designed in an effort to reflect the government's commitment "to fully exploring the promise and potential of stem cell research" without running afoul of the particular moral and ethical principles set forth and embraced by President Bush in announcing the policy.

D. Governance According to a "Bright Line" Moral Principle

The Bush policy provides a rich and complex example of one particular approach to "bioethical governance." It is not driven by a utilitarian weighing of commensurate values, but rather begins with a clear moral standard that may not be transgressed. In his August 9, 2001 speech . . . President Bush said: "There is at least one bright line: We do not end some lives for the medical benefit of others. For me, this is a matter of conviction: a belief that life, including early life, is biologically human, genetically distinct, and valuable." This is the moral and ethical foundation upon which the Bush policy is erected. The Administration's stated desire to better the human condition by eradicating dreaded diseases and debilitating injuries, and its attendant enthusiasm and support for scientific research aimed at these goals, are thus expressed and acted upon within the boundaries of this moral framework. Accordingly, the Bush policy is designed to endorse and actively promote all stem cell research (including embryonic) that does not encourage the future instrumentalization and destruction of human embryos . . .

E. Political Prudence and Respect for Pluralism

While the Bush policy provides insight into a particular species of moral governance, it also teaches one way in which the formulation of bioethical policies is influenced by considerations of political prudence and respect for pluralism. Although the moral foundation of the Bush policy is a view that human beings are worthy of maximal respect regardless of their developmental stage and that ending some human lives for the medical benefit of others is unethical, the Bush policy does not seek to ban destructive embryo research altogether. To the contrary, it steers a more moderate course, merely withholding the government's affirmative endorsement of the practice by way of federal funding . . .

[T]he restrained nature of the Bush policy might . . . serve to demonstrate how considerations of pluralism can affect the formulation of bioethical public policy. While the Bush approach begins with the moral judgment that human embryos should not be instrumentalized or destroyed for the sake of another's medical benefit, the ultimate legal expression of this policy implicitly acknowledges that there is great division among the American citizenry on this point by remaining neutral on the ultimate question of the legal permissibility of embryo research. The policy does not ban the destruction of human embryos to derive embryonic stem cells, but it does withhold the government's official approval and refuses to compel American taxpayers to subsidize an activity that is a source of great moral and ethical disquiet for a significant portion of the population. The Bush policy could thus be seen as an example of how the government can express its ethical approval (or disapproval) of a particular type of scientific activity while respecting the deep disagreements that persist in society . . .

James F. Childress
An Ethical Defense of Federal Funding for Human Embryonic Stem Cell Research
2 Yale J. Health Policy, Law & Ethics 157 (2001)

I. A Range of Ethically Acceptable Policies

Despite the thought and consideration that went into President Bush's announced policy on the use of federal funds in human embryonic stem cell research, I would argue that more flexible policies are ethically acceptable and even preferable. Three options merit consideration:

(1) Providing federal funds for research on cell lines derived (using non-federal funds) from embryos prior to August 9, 2001 within certain ethical guidelines (President Bush's announced policy).

(2) Providing federal funds for research on cell lines derived (using non-federal funds) from embryos, earlier or in the future, within certain ethical guidelines (the policy proposed earlier by the National Institutes of Health (NIH)).

(3) Providing federal funds for both the derivation of, and research on, cell lines derived from embryos within certain ethical guidelines (NBAC's recommendation).[22]

President Bush's announced policy (option 1) suggests that it is ethically acceptable to use federal funds for research on stem cell lines that were derived, using non-federal funds, prior to his announcement on August 9, if the derivation also met certain ethical requirements, including the informed consent of donors of embryos created solely for reproductive purposes and the absence of financial inducements. If policy option 1 is ethically acceptable — as I believe it is — then it should also be ethically acceptable to do the same thing prospectively (policy option 2). That is, it should be ethically acceptable to provide federal funds for research on stem cell lines derived in the future, after August 9 as well as before, with non-federal funds and within the same ethical guidelines. This prospective policy would offer greater — and needed — flexibility for the short-term and long-term future. And it would be ethically preferable because it would increase the possibilities for important research, without violating relevant ethical standards.

President Bush's statement noted that the first policy (option 1), which includes about sixty stem cell lines (about which there is considerable scientific uncertainty and controversy), "allows us to explore the promise and potential of stem cell

---

[22] NBAC refers to the National Bioethics Advisory Commission, established by Executive Order 12975, signed by President Clinton on October 3, 1995. NBAC was charged with providing advice and making recommendations to government entities, including the President, on bioethical issues arising from research on human biology and behavior. In 1999, NBAC issued a report on human stem cell research, favoring "federal sponsorship of research that involves the derivation and use of human embryonic stem (ES) cells" as long as funding was limited to "embryos remaining after infertility treatments." See Ethical Issues in Human Stem Cell Research, Vol. 1, Report and Recommendations of the National Bioethics Advisory Commission, Transmittal Letter (1999).

research without crossing a fundamental moral line by providing taxpayer funding that would sanction or encourage further destruction of human embryos that have at least the potential for life." However, I believe that ethically we can provide federal tax funds for research on stem cells derived after as well as before August 9, using non-federal funds, and that this can be accomplished without sanctioning or encouraging further destruction of human embryos. To do so, we must establish effective ethical safeguards. Those safeguards should ensure, to the greatest extent possible, the couple's voluntary and informed decision to destroy their embryos — rather than use them or donate them to another couple — and their voluntary and informed decision to donate them for research . . . [A]s matters stand in most jurisdictions, couples may determine how to dispose of their embryos.

It is possible to go further than either of these first two policies and recommend, as the NBAC did, a third option — the provision of federal funds for both the derivation of stem cells from embryos and research on those cell lines, again in accord with ethical requirements. One argument for this option is that a strict separation between derivation and use would adversely affect the development of scientific knowledge. For instance, the methods for deriving embryonic stem cells may affect their properties, and scientists may increase their understanding of the nature of such cells in the process of deriving them.

In short, I see no ethical reason for limiting federal funding to research with cell lines derived by some arbitrary date, as long as we can ensure that future derivation, with non-federal funds (option 2) or federal funds (option 3), also respects the same moral limits. Indeed, our collective moral duty to alleviate human suffering and reduce the number of premature deaths provides a strong ethical reason to support this research, within moral limits.

II. Respect for the Embryo

There is widespread agreement, as the NBAC observed, that "human embryos deserve respect as a form of human life," but at the same time, sharp disagreements exist "regarding both what form such respect should take and what level of protection is required at different stages of embryonic development." At the very least this "respect" implies that:

- Early embryos should not be used unless they are necessary for research;

- embryos remaining after in vitro fertilization (IVF), as well as cadaveric fetal tissue, should not be bought or sold; and

- alternative sources of stem cells should simultaneously be explored.

Indeed, given the promise of this research, and the uncertainty about which stem cells might be adequate and which might be superior for various purposes, research on stem cells derived from different sources should be eligible for federal funding. The goal of realizing the therapeutic promise of stem cell research is ethically significant. It is also ethically important to treat the different sources of stem cells with appropriate respect.

One interpretation of appropriate respect for early embryos would rule out their deliberate creation in order to use them in research. I supported the NBAC's recommendation that, at this time, federal agencies should not fund research involving the derivation or use of embryonic stem cells from embryos made solely for research purposes, whether they were made by IVF or by somatic cell nuclear transfer [cloning] into oocytes. However, in this area, it is ethically dangerous to say "never" . . . For now, it appears to be possible to develop enough cell lines without creating more embryos, and there appears to be no need for nuclear transfer unless and until therapy is possible. But if therapy becomes possible, matched tissue may be needed. And it may then be necessary to revisit the question about so-called "therapeutic cloning," which at the present is really experimental research rather than therapeutic . . .

Conclusion

If President Bush's announced policy is ethically acceptable, as I believe it is, there is no cogent ethical reason for stopping where his policy stops — with the use of stem cell lines that were derived from embryos by August 9, 2001. Indeed, that temporal restriction is difficult to defend from an ethical standpoint. It is possible to use non-federal funds (or even, I would argue, federal funds) to derive stem cell lines from embryos within certain ethical requirements, and to provide federal funds for research on those lines without sanctioning or encouraging the destruction of embryos or the creation of so-called "extra" or "surplus" embryos in clinical IVF. I would support these other policy options — derivation with non-federal funds or with federal funds — on the grounds that they will probably enable important research to proceed more rapidly, and will not breach crucial ethical boundaries . . .

Whichever policies are adopted to enable important and promising stem cell research to go forward, within ethical limits, we will need a strong public body to review protocols for deriving stem cells from embryos (and from fetal tissue) and to monitor this research. Perhaps the Council on Bioethics, which President Bush has announced, could fulfill these functions, but it is not yet clear what its mandate and structure will be . . .

It is safe to assume that no policy currently under discussion will be the final one. We will need to revisit this research again and again as the science develops and as its ethical implications become clearer, particularly through a public body's on-going review and oversight. Thus, no policy will end the national conversation about how to balance, over time, the relevant ethical considerations. Our public dialogue needs to continue with as much rigor and imagination as possible. As we continue to reflect on the important issues raised by human embryonic stem cell research, we need a policy with greater flexibility than the one President Bush announced, but also with close review and oversight . . .

NOTES AND QUESTIONS

1.   Compare the supportive, approving analysis by Professor Snead with the somewhat critical assessment provided by Professor Childress. It probably will not surprise you to learn that both men developed their views as members of the presidential commissions that studied and reported on the merits of government-sponsored stem cell research — but for different Presidents. O. Carter Snead was

the General Counsel for the President's Council on Bioethics, appointed by President Bush, and James Childress was a member of the Clinton-era National Bioethics Advisory Commission. What are the key differences between the positions the two men espouse? Do you see any common ground, areas in which both men would agree?

2. *Popular Opinion on Stem Cell Research.* On at least two occasions, Professor Snead supports his argument with an assertion that "a significant portion of the American public" finds the destruction of embryos for research purposes "morally troublesome." These statement, he asserts, are based on a variety of public opinion polls asking respondents their views on embryonic stem cell research. In citing to the polls, he appropriately warns the reader that "polling in this area has reached varied results, not surprisingly turning largely on how the question is framed and what information is provided to respondents." O. Carter Snead, *The Pedagogical Significance of the Bush Stem Cell Policy: A Window into Bioethical Regulation in the United States*, 5 YALE J. HEALTH POLICY & ETHICS 491, n. 37 (2005).

Another hazard of public opinion polls is the selectivity used to report results; if only one response is reported, rather than all responses, the reader may be left with the impression that the single result represents the majority view of the respondents. For example, Professor Snead cites to an April 9, 2002 poll conducted by the Pew Research Center for the People & the Press, titled, "Cloning Opposed, Stem Cell Research Narrowly Supported." He accurately reports that 35% of respondents oppose federal funding for stem cell research. But Professor Snead fails to include reference to the 50% of respondents who favor government funding for stem cell research. In that same poll, 47% of those surveyed said they felt conducting research toward medical cures was more important than not destroying human embryos, with 39% finding embryo preservation more important than medical research. Do you agree that 35% and 39% of Americans is a "significant portion" of the population? Does the author have a duty to disclose the percentage of Americans who hold opposite views? Are those who favor embryonic stem cell research a "significant portion" of Americans?

3.   What support does Professor Childress offer for his assertion that "it should be ethically acceptable to provide federal funds for research on stem cell lines derived in the future, after August 9"? He speaks of increasing the "possibilities for important research" but does he provide evidence that research will be stunted under the current policy? Do you believe Professor Childress has adequately addressed the concerns raised by Professor Snead and others that destroying early life cannot be justified by the prospect of medical therapies?

PROBLEM

You have just been elected Governor of your home state. Your state has no law directly addressing the legality of research on human embryos. During the campaign, you received campaign contributions, within the legal limits, from a variety of groups, including the National Right To Life Committee (RTL) and the American Juvenile Diabetes Foundation (JDF). You accepted these contributions without making any promises or assurances to these or any groups that supported your candidacy. Upon assuming the office, you are approached by both RTL and

JDF about the question of embryonic stem cell research. RTL asks you to introduce legislation that would ban all research on human embryos for any purpose, and JDF seeks your support for a bill that would legalize and fund embryonic stem cell research in the state. You decide that the best course of action is to appoint a statewide commission to study the legal and moral parameters of stem cell research and report back within one year.

Who should you appoint to the Stem Cell Commission? What research should your staff conduct before appointing each member? What guidelines should you provide to the Commission as they undertake their duties?

3.   President Obama and a New Era of Stem Cell Research Policy

The 2008 presidential campaign focused far less on stem cell research than had the previous two races in which Democratic candidates favored federal funding and the Republican candidates did not. The contest between Barack Obama (D) and John McCain (R) may have been contentious on matters of the economy and foreign policy, but both men agreed that the federal government should invest in stem cell research, including stem cell lines derived from human embryos. Senator McCain had long supported funding for embryonic stem cell research, breaking party lines and voting for several bills that would have permitted the federal government to fund embryonic stem cell research. In 2006, Senator McCain was one of 19 Republicans to vote for the Stem Cell Research Enhancement Act of 2006, a bill that President Bush vetoed.

Shortly after taking office in 2009, President Obama fulfilled a campaign promise and lifted the President Bush-era restrictions on federal funding of embryonic stem cell research. In March 2009, President Obama issued an Executive Order detailing the new policy and direction for this type of medical research.

THE WHITE HOUSE
Office of the Press Secretary
For Immediate Release March 9, 2009
EXECUTIVE ORDER

REMOVING BARRIERS TO RESPONSIBLE SCIENTIFIC RESEARCH INVOLVING HUMAN STEM CELLS

By the authority vested in me as President by the Constitution and the laws of the United States of America, it is hereby ordered as follows:

Section 1. Policy. Research involving human embryonic stem cells and human non-embryonic stem cells has the potential to lead to better understanding and treatment of many disabling diseases and conditions. Advances over the past decade in this promising scientific field have been encouraging, leading to broad agreement in the scientific community that the research should be supported by Federal funds.

For the past 8 years, the authority of the Department of Health and Human Services, including the National Institutes of Health (NIH), to fund and conduct human embryonic stem cell research has been limited by Presidential actions. The purpose of this order is to remove these limitations on scientific inquiry, to expand NIH support for the exploration of human stem cell research, and in so doing to enhance the contribution of America's scientists to important new discoveries and new therapies for the benefit of humankind.

Sec. 2. Research. The Secretary of Health and Human Services (Secretary), through the Director of NIH, may support and conduct responsible, scientifically worthy human stem cell research, including human embryonic stem cell research, to the extent permitted by law.

Sec. 3. Guidance. Within 120 days from the date of this order, the Secretary, through the Director of NIH, shall review existing NIH guidance and other widely recognized guidelines on human stem cell research, including provisions establishing appropriate safeguards, and issue new NIH guidance on such research that is consistent with this order. The Secretary, through NIH, shall review and update such guidance periodically, as appropriate . . .

Sec. 5. Revocations. (a) The Presidential statement of August 9, 2001, limiting Federal funding for research involving human embryonic stem cells, shall have no further effect as a statement of governmental policy . . .

NOTES AND QUESTIONS

1.   Section 3 of President Obama's Executive Order directs the Director of NIH to issue new guidance on the federal funding parameters surrounding human embryonic stem cell research. As directed, the NIH published guidelines on July 7, 2009. Reprinted in part below, notice that much of the focus in the guidelines is on the informed consent obtained from the embryo donors. As you read the excerpt, try to put yourself in the role of each party who might be affected by these guidelines, including the embryo donors, the stem cell researchers and the government funders.

National Institutes of Health Guidelines
for Research Using Human Stem Cells

<u>Scope of Guidelines</u>

These Guidelines apply to the expenditure of National Institutes of Health (NIH) funds for research using human embryonic stem cells (hESCs) . . .

These guidelines are based on the following principles:

Responsible research with hESCs has the potential to improve our understanding of human health and illness and discover new ways to prevent and/or treat illness.

Individuals donating embryos for research purposes should do so freely, with voluntary and informed consent . . .

<u>Eligibility of Human Embryonic Stem Cells for Research with NIH Funding</u>

For the purpose of these Guidelines, "human embryonic stem cells (hESCs)" are cells that are derived from the inner cell mass of blastocyst stage human embryos, are capable of dividing without differentiating for a prolonged period in culture, and are known to develop into cells and tissues of the three primary germ layers. Although hESCs are derived from embryos, such stem cells are not themselves human embryos. All of the processes and procedures for review of the eligibility of hESCs will be centralized at the NIH as follows:

A. Applicant institutions proposing research using hESCs . . . should have been derived from human embryos:

1. that were created using in vitro fertilization for reproductive purposes and were no longer needed for this purpose;

2. that were donated by individuals who sought reproductive treatment (hereafter referred to as "donor(s)") and who gave voluntary written consent for the human embryos to be used for research purposes; and

3. for which all of the following can be assured and documentation provided, such as consent forms, written policies, or other documentation, provided:

a. All options available in the health care facility where treatment was sought pertaining to the embryos no longer needed for reproductive purposes were explained to the individual(s) who sought reproductive treatment.

b. No payments, cash or in kind, were offered for the donated embryos.

c. Policies and/or procedures were in place at the health care facility where the embryos were donated that neither consenting nor refusing to donate embryos for research would affect the quality of care provided to potential donor(s).

d. There was a clear separation between the prospective donor(s)'s decision to create human embryos for reproductive purposes and the prospective donor(s)'s decision to donate human embryos for research purposes. Specifically:

i. Decisions related to the creation of human embryos for reproductive purposes should have been made free from the influence of researchers proposing to derive or utilize hESCs in research. The attending physician responsible for reproductive clinical care and the researcher deriving and/or proposing to utilize hESCs should not have been the same person unless separation was not practicable.

ii. At the time of donation, consent for that donation should have been obtained from the individual(s) who had sought reproductive treatment. That is, even if potential donor(s) had given prior indication of their intent to donate to research any embryos that remained after reproductive treatment, consent for the donation for research purposes should have been given at the time of the donation . . .

Other Research Not Eligible for NIH Funding

A. NIH funding of the derivation of stem cells from human embryos is prohibited by the annual appropriations ban on funding of human embryo research (Section 509, Omnibus Appropriations Act, 2009, Pub. L. 111-8, 3/11/09), otherwise known as the Dickey Amendment.

B. Research using hESCs derived from other sources, including somatic cell nuclear transfer, parthenogenesis, and/or IVF embryos created for research purposes, is not eligible for NIH funding.

A full version of the most recent NIH Guidelines is available at: www.stemcells. nih.gov.

2. *Availability of Stem Cell Lines.* Recall that President Bush's stem cell policy limited funding to lines developed before August 9, 2001 when he delivered his address to the nation on the topic. When President Obama took office in January 2009, estimates on the number of stem cell lines available for funding ranged from around 15 to 23, a number research enthusiasts believed was far too low. Have the new guidelines increased the number of available stem cell research lines since their issue in July 2009? According to the NIH Human Embryonic Stem Cell Registry, as of April 2012 there are 153 human embryonic stem cell eligible for funding under the new Obama policy. In terms of funding allocation under the Bush and Obama White House's - during the Bush Administration (2002-08) the NIH spent $294 million for human embryonic stem cell research; it is estimated that some $562 million will be expended during the years 2009-12 under President Obama. *See* The Witherspoon Council on Ethics and the Integrity of Science, *The Stem Cell Debates: Lessons for Science and Politics*, THE NEW ATLANTIS, No. 34 (Winter 2012).

3. *Legal Challenges to the Obama Policy.* The Obama NIH guidelines acknowledge that funding is not available for the derivation of human embryonic stem cells because such activity would violate the Dickey Amendment. Recall that the Dickey Amendment, first drafted in 1996, is a rider attached to each annual spending bill that prohibits NIH from funding "research in which a human embryo or embryos are destroyed, discarded, or knowingly subjected to risk of injury or death greater than that allowed for fetuses *in utero.*" Even though the Dickey Amendment was first drafted before scientists announced derivation of the first human embryonic stem cell line in 1998, those with concerns about this type of research have argued that this law prohibits funding altogether because embryos are necessarily destroyed in order for the research to be performed.

The application of the Dickey Amendment to federal funding of embryonic stem cell research had been formally addressed only once, in 1999 when Harriet Raab, General Counsel of DHHS issued a memorandum on the matter. She argued that the wording of the law would permit funding embryonic stem cell research because the amendment did not "apply to research utilizing human pluripotent stem cells because such cells are not a human embryo within the statutory definition." If stem cells were derived from embryos that had been developed using private funds, she reasoned, the subsequently developed cell lines might be considered eligible for public funding because the cells themselves were not embryos capable of becoming a fully formed human being. This interpretation remained in place under the Bush Administration.

Within a few weeks of issue of the new Obama NIH guidelines, several parties, including two researchers on adult stem cells, an adoption agency, and a Christian medical association filed a lawsuit seeking to block DHHS from implementing the new guidelines. The plaintiffs argued that the unambiguous language of the Dickey Amendment prohibits funding for both the derivation of and subsequent research on embryonic stem cells because such research depends upon the destruction of a human embryo. The suit was initially dismissed in October 2009 for lack of legal standing because the parties were not materially harmed by the new policy. *Shereley v. Sebelius*, 686 F. Supp. 2d 1 (Dist. D.C. 2009). On appeal the U.S. Court of Appeals for the D.C. Circuit overturned the trial judge's decision, holding that the two scientists had standing because the new Obama administration policy would divert federal funds away from their research on adult stem cells. *Sherley v. Sebelius*, 610 F.3d 69 (D.C. Cir. 2010). On remand, the D.C. trial judge sided with the plaintiffs and issued a preliminary injunction ordering DHHS to cease funding embryonic stem cell research. The Obama administration appealed this decision, and the D.C. Circuit, again, weighed in.

SHERLEY v. SEBELIUS
United States Court of Appeals. District of Columbia Circuit
644 F.3d 388 (2011)

GINSBURG, Circuit Judge:

Two scientists brought this suit to enjoin the National Institutes of Health from funding research using human embryonic stem cells (ESCs) pursuant to the NIH's 2009 Guidelines. The district court granted their motion for a preliminary injunction, concluding they were likely to succeed in showing the Guidelines violated the Dickey — Wicker Amendment, an appropriations rider that bars federal funding for research in which a human embryo is destroyed. We conclude the plaintiffs are unlikely to prevail because Dickey — Wicker is ambiguous and the NIH seems reasonably to have concluded that, although Dickey — Wicker bars funding for the destructive act of deriving an ESC from an embryo, it does not prohibit funding a research project in which an ESC will be used. We therefore vacate the preliminary injunction.

I. Background . . .

The plaintiffs in this case, Drs. James Sherley and Theresa Deisher, are scientists who use only adult stem cells in their research. They contend the NIH has, by funding research projects using ESCs, violated the Dickey — Wicker Amendment, which the Congress has included in the annual appropriation for the Department of Health and Human Services each year since 1996. Dickey — Wicker prohibits the NIH from funding:

> (1) the creation of a human embryo or embryos for research purposes; or
> (2) research in which a human embryo or embryos are destroyed, discarded, or knowingly subjected to risk of injury or death greater than that allowed for research on fetuses in utero under 45 C.F.R. 46.204(b) and section 498(b) of the Public Health Service Act (42 U.S.C. 289g(b)) . . .

In 1996, when the Congress first passed Dickey — Wicker, scientists had taken steps to isolate ESCs but had not yet been able to stabilize them for research in the laboratory. The historical record suggests the Congress passed the Amendment chiefly to preclude President Clinton from acting upon an NIH report recommending federal funding for research using embryos that had been created for the purpose of in vitro fertilization . . . Dickey — Wicker became directly relevant to ESCs only in 1998, when researchers at the University of Wisconsin succeeded in generating a stable line of ESCs, which they made available to investigators who might apply for NIH funding.

For that reason, on January 15, 1999, the General Counsel of the Department of Health and Human Services issued a memorandum addressing whether Dickey — Wicker permits federal funding of research using ESCs that had been derived before the funded project began; she concluded such funding is permissible because ESCs are not "embryos." . . .

Early in 2001, President Bush directed the NIH not to fund any project pursuant to President Clinton's policy; later that year he decided funding for ESC research would be limited to projects using the approximately 60 then-extant cell lines derived from "embryos that ha[d] already been destroyed." *See* 37 Weekly Comp. Pres. Doc.. 1149, 1151 (Aug. 9, 2001) . . . Meanwhile, the Congress continued to reenact Dickey — Wicker each year of the Bush Administration.

Upon assuming office in 2009, President Obama lifted the temporal restriction imposed by President Bush and permitted the NIH to "support and conduct responsible, scientifically worthy human stem cell research, including human embryonic stem cell research, to the extent permitted by law." Exec. Order 13,505, 74 Fed.Reg. 10,667, 10,667 (2009). The NIH, after notice-and-comment rulemaking, then issued the 2009 Guidelines, 74 Fed.Reg. 32,170(32,175 (July 7, 2009), which are currently in effect. [The court cites to the 1999 Raab interpretation that research involving ESCs that does not involve an embryo's destruction does not violate federal law.] . . .

II. Analysis . . .

We begin our review, of course, by looking to the text of Dickey — Wicker . . . The district court held, and the plaintiffs argue on appeal, this provision unambiguously bars funding for any project using an ESC. They reason that, because an embryo had to be destroyed in order to yield an ESC, any later research project that uses an ESC is necessarily "research" in which the embryo is destroyed. For its part, the Government argues the "text is in no way an unambiguous ban on research using embryonic stem cells" because Dickey — Wicker is written in the present tense, addressing research "in which" embryos "are" destroyed, not research "for which" embryos "were destroyed."

The use of the present tense in a statute strongly suggests it does not extend to past actions. The Dictionary Act provides "unless the context indicates otherwise . . . words used in the present tense include the future as well as the present. 1 U.S.C. § 1. As the Supreme Court has observed, that provision implies "the present tense generally does not include the past." . . .

The plaintiffs respond by reiterating their primary argument: Because "research" using an ESC includes derivation of the ESC, the derivation does not predate but is an integral part of the "research." The conclusion does not follow from the premise; at best it shows Dickey — Wicker is open to more than one possible reading. The plaintiffs also argue we must read the term "research" broadly because the Congress, had it intended a narrower reading, would have used a term identifying a particular action, as it did in subsection (1) of Dickey — Wicker, which specifically bars the "creation" of an embryo for "research purposes." We see no basis for that inference. The definition of research is flexible enough to describe either a discrete project or an extended process, but this flexibility only reinforces our conclusion that the text is ambiguous . . .

Broadening our focus slightly, however, we can see the words surrounding "research" in the statute support the NIH's reading. Because the Congress wrote with particularity and in the present tense — the statute says "in which" and "are" rather than "for which" and "were" — it is entirely reasonable for the NIH to understand Dickey — Wicker as permitting funding for research using cell lines derived without federal funding, even as it bars funding for the derivation of additional lines.

Further, adding the temporal dimension to our perspective, we see, as the NIH noted in promulgating the 2009 Guidelines, the Congress has reenacted Dickey — Wicker unchanged year after year "with full knowledge that HHS has been funding [ESC] research since 2001," when President Bush first permitted federal funding for ESC projects, provided they used previously derived ESC lines. As the plaintiffs conceded at oral argument, because this policy permitted the NIH to fund projects using ESCs, it would have been prohibited under their proposed reading of Dickey — Wicker. So, too, with the policy the Clinton Administration announced in 1999 and, of course, with the 2009 Guidelines promulgated by the Obama Administration. The plaintiffs have no snappy response to the agency's point that the Congress's having reenacted Dickey — Wicker each and every year provides "further evidence . . . [it] intended the Agency's interpretation, or at least understood the interpretation as statutorily permissible." . . .

III. Conclusion

Because the plaintiffs have not shown they are likely to succeed on the merits, we conclude they are not entitled to preliminary injunctive relief. We reach this conclusion under the sliding scale approach to the preliminary injunction factors; *a fortiori* we would reach the same conclusion if likelihood of success on the merits is an independent requirement. Therefore, the preliminary injunction entered by the district court must be and is

Vacated.

KAREN LeCRAFT HENDERSON, Circuit Judge, dissenting:

The majority opinion has taken a straightforward case of statutory construction and produced a result that would make Rube Goldberg tip his hat. Breaking the simple noun "research" into "temporal" bits, narrowing the verb phrase "are destroyed" to an unintended scope, dismissing the definition section of implementing regulations promulgated by the Department of Health and Human Services (HHS) (in case the plain meaning of "research" were not plain enough), my colleagues perform linguistic jujitsu. I must therefore respectfully dissent . . .

The district court correctly looked to the dictionary definition of "research" as "diligent and systematic inquiry or investigation into a subject in order to discover or revise facts, theories, applications, etc . . . Research, then, comprises a systematic inquiry or investigation. And "systematic" connotes sequenced action . . . The first sequence of hESC research is the derivation of stem cells from the human embryo. The derivation of stem cells destroys the embryo and therefore cannot be federally funded, as the Government concedes. I believe the succeeding sequences of hESC research are likewise banned by the Amendment because, under the plain meaning of "research," they continue the "systematic inquiry or investigation." . . .

In my view, the majority opinion strains mightily to find the ambiguity the Government presses. Treating "research" as composed of free-standing pieces, it concludes that the only piece that is banned is the derivation of the hESCs. The authority for this novel reading of "research" is not the dictionary but the Amendment's use of the phrase "in which a human embryo or embryos *are* destroyed" rather than "for which a human embryo or embryos *were* destroyed." The majority opinion correctly notes that the Dictionary Act, which provides that "unless the context indicates otherwise . . . words used in the present tense include the future as well as the present," . . . implies "that the present tense generally does not include the past." . . . There is no question that, here, context manifests that the present tense includes both the past as well as the future. As already discussed, the derivation of hESCs constitutes *at least* research development, which, in *context*, means that it is "research in which a human embryo or embryos are [at any point] destroyed." . . .

I believe the plaintiffs have made a strong showing of likelihood of success on the merits. Under the sliding scale approach that remains the law of our Circuit, "[i]f the movant makes an unusually strong showing on one of the factors, then it does not necessarily have to make as strong a showing on another factor." Having concluded the plaintiffs have indeed made "an unusually strong showing" on the first factor, I cannot say the district court abused its discretion in balancing all of the factors in favor of granting preliminary injunctive relief.

For the foregoing reasons, I respectfully dissent.

AFTERWARD

After the D.C. Circuit denied the plaintiffs' request for preliminary injunction to enjoin the NIH from funding human embryonic stem cell research, the case returned to the District Court where the plaintiffs then sought summary judgment on the merits. The motion was denied and thereafter the trial court judge dismissed the case against the government on July 27, 2011. In August 2012, the D.C. Circuit upheld the trial court's dismissal of the plaintiffs' challenge, leaving the Obama administration's embryonic stem cell funding policy in place.

B. State Funding of Stem Cell Research

The potential promise of stem cell research, coupled with the federal government's initial limitations on funding, prompted a handful of states to become active in promoting and funding such research within the state's borders. Perhaps the states saw a potential boon to the local economy, enticing high-tech, high-paying jobs to a locality friendly to this sophisticated, albeit controversial, form of medical research. Since 1998, when researchers first announced the cultivation of embryonic stem cells, a number of state laws have been enacted by lawmakers, approved by voters, and considered by legislative committees, all in the hope of capturing a piece of the stem cell pie. Whether that pie will amount to anything more than a hill of beans remains to be seen, but at the outset two coastal states served as anchors in the vast and uncertain stem cell sea, with a handful of states sailing into the fray thereafter. Having exhausted all metaphors, we proceed to explore the relevant state laws.

1. California

It is said that California prides itself on being a State of Firsts. In 1997, shortly after the birth of the world's first cloned mammal, Dolly the sheep, California became the first state to ban human reproductive cloning, placing a "five year moratorium on the cloning of an entire human being in order to evaluate the profound medical, legal, and social implications that such a possibility raises." Cal. Health & Safety Code § 24185 (the law was amended in 2002, making the ban on reproductive cloning permanent). In 2002, as interest and excitement over the prospect of stem cell cures mounted, California lawmakers enacted the first-ever law encouraging researchers to conduct stem cell experiments in the Golden State. The law provides:

> The policy of the State of California shall be as follows
>
> (a) That research involving the derivation and use of human embryonic stem cells, human embryonic germ cells, and human adult stem cells from any source, including somatic cell nuclear transplantation, shall be permitted and that full consideration of the ethical and medical implications of the research be given.

Cal. Health & Safety Code § 125300 (2005). Governor Gray Davis signed the bill into law, declaring "California is a leader in the field of biomedical and biotechnology research. It is important to the California biomedical research community to have access to stem cells for promising research. Stem cell research could realize great benefits for persons with incurable, debilitating or degenerative diseases including Parkinson's, Alzheimers, heart disease, diabetes and cancer . . . This bill does not affect California statute that prohibits cloning a human being or engaging in human reproductive cloning." Governor Davis Signing Message, Stats. 2003, c. 507 (S.B. 771) (Sept. 24, 2003).

The California law also required the Department of Health Services to establish an anonymous registry of embryos to provide researchers with access to embryos that are available for research purposes. The most likely source of those embryos are ART clinics in which patients agree to donate their unwanted embryos to research. Recall in Chapter 7 we reviewed the California law which requires fertility specialists to provide patients with written forms on which they can indicate their preference for the disposition of unwanted or disputed embryos. One option for patients is to donate the embryos to research. When the research option is elected, fertility doctors are required to inform the donor/patient about the potential use of her embryos, including a "statement that the early human embryos will be used to derive human pluripotent stem cells for research and that the cells may be used, at some future time, for human transplantation research." Cal. Health & Safety Code § 125315(c)(1) (reprinted in Chapter 7, Section 3(A)(1)).

The most notable addition to the California stem cell program became law in November 2004 when voters approved Proposition 71, an initiative that authorizes the issuance of $3 billion in state general obligation bonds to provide funding for stem cell research. Prop. 71, officially entitled the "California Stem Cell Research and Cures Act," establishes the California Institute for Regenerative Medicine which is "authorize[d] an average of $295 million per year in bonds over a 10-year period to fund stem cell research and dedicated facilities for scientists at California's universities and other advanced medical research facilities throughout the state." Constitution of the State of California, Art. XXXV, Sec. 3 (2004). By way of comparison, in fiscal year 2004, the NIH funded about $24 million in grants for human embryonic stem cell research, less than one-tenth of the ambitious California funding plan.

Prop. 71 establishes a constitutional right to conduct stem cell research in the state. This right includes "research involving adult stem cells, cord blood stem cells, pluripotent stem cells, and/or progenitor cells." The law gingerly defines the potential sources of pluripotent stem cells in this manner: "Pluripotent stem cells may be derived from somatic cell nuclear transfer or from surplus products of in vitro fertilization treatments when such products are donated under appropriate informed consent procedures." Constitution of the State of California, Art. XXXV, Sec. 5 (2004). The "surplus products of in vitro fertilization" clearly refer to leftover embryos, yet the word "embryo" appears nowhere in the law.

The administrative structure of the new California Institute for Regenerative Medicine is placed in the hands of the Independent Citizen's Oversight Committee (ICOC), a 29-member board comprised of representatives of specified University of California campuses, another public or private California university, nonprofit academic and medical research institutions, companies with expertise in developing medical therapies, and disease research advocacy groups. The Governor, Lieutenant Governor, Treasurer, Controller, Speaker of the Assembly, President pro Tempore of the Senate, and certain UC campus Chancellors were each authorized to make the appointments to the ICOC. The membership of the ICOC was established in early 2005, and the group began meeting to configure a scheme for evaluating and funding grants from stem cell researchers. For a current list of ICOC members, see www.cirm.ca.gov.

Though passed by more than 59% of California voters, Prop. 71 had, and continues to attract, detractors. During the campaign, even those in favor of advancing stem cell research argued against passage of the initiative, citing its behemoth fiscal impact and its flawed structure, which invited the appearance, if not the practice, of conflict-of-interest transactions. One UC professor warned:

> Contrary to what its name suggests, the ICOC is neither "independent" of interest-group politics nor does it include any "citizen" members. Hard-driving university scientists, disease group advocates and private industry executives who will make up the ICOC all have vested interests in how the money is to be used. Scientists want to cure disease, but they may be focused on building institutes and generating papers. Companies want to make money, and charge the public high prices for therapies. Advocates for research on particular diseases, although they deserve to be at the table, do not represent the collective public interest when they battle to make their diseases the highest priority for the public.

David Winickoff, *Prop. 71, A Risky Experiment In Squandering Public Monies*, SAN. FRAN. CHRONICLE, Oct. 17, 2004, at E3.

In February 2005, shortly after Prop. 71 took effect, several public-interest groups filed lawsuits seeking to invalidate the $3 billion stem cell research institution approved by voters the previous November. One suit, filed by the People's Advocate and the National Tax Limitation Foundation, alleges the California Institute for Regenerative Medicine violates state law because it is not governed exclusively by the state government, and the committee that controls the research money (the ICOC) is not publicly elected. A second suit filed by the newly created Californians for Public Accountability and Ethical Science alleges it is illegal to exempt members of the ICOC from some government conflict-of-interest laws, as Prop. 71 allows. Both lawsuits were filed with the California Supreme Court, in an effort to obtain quick relief from ongoing efforts to begin providing grants to stem cell researchers. *See* Suits Filed to Invalidate California's $3 Billion Stem Cell Institute, Health & Medicine Week, March 14, 2005, at 1476. Ultimately, after more than two years of back-and-forth litigation, the California Supreme Court upheld Prop 71 in May 2007 when it denied review of an appellate court decision upholding the measure as constitutional. *California Family Bioethics Council v. California Institute for Regenerative Medicine*, 147 Cal. App. 4th 1319, 55 Cal. Rptr. 3d 272 (*review denied* May 16, 2007).

To date, the California Institute for Regenerative Medicine has distributed about $1.3 billion of the $3 billion funds allocated by Prop 71. While the CIRM website lists hundreds of ongoing grants, a good part of the funding has gone to infrastructure such as buildings and equipment, and basic research. Some express frustration over the lack of progress toward cures and therapies, while others remain patient that the investment will pay off in the long run.

2. New Jersey

In early 2004 New Jersey Governor James McGreevey signed into law a measure that promotes stem cell research in the state, while banning human cloning for reproductive purposes. Like its west coast predecessor, the law requires fertility clinics to inform their patients of the right to donate unused embryos for stem cell research. At the law signing ceremony, Governor McGreavey was joined by actor and stem cell research activist Christopher Reeve, who was paralyzed in a 1995 horseback riding accident. Mr. Reeve called the occasion his "proudest day" because his home state of New Jersey had "the courage to protect the freedom of ethical and responsible scientific inquiry." See *State of Cloning*, NAT'L REVIEW, Jan. 5, 2004. The Roman Catholic Church and other groups, including the New Jersey Right To Life, opposed the bill because it permits the destruction of early embryos. Marie Tasy, public and legislative affairs director for New Jersey Right to Life remarked, "This law will allow human lives to be treated as a commodity, creating classes of lesser humans to be created and sacrificed for the good of humanity." She called "the unethical practices authorized" under the new law "the ultimate desecration of human life." Id.

The New Jersey law provides in relevant part:

§ 26:2Z-2. Public policy regarding derivation and use of certain human cellsa. It is the public policy of this State that research involving the derivation and use of human embryonic stem cells, human embryonic germ cells and human adult stem cells, including somatic cell nuclear transplantation, shall: (1) be permitted in this State; (2) be conducted with full consideration for the ethical and medical implications of this research; and

(3) be reviewed, in each case, by an institutional review board operating in accordance with applicable federal regulations.b. (1) A physician or other health care provider who is treating a patient for infertility shall provide the patient with timely, relevant and appropriate information sufficient to allow that person to make an informed and voluntary choice regarding the disposition of any human embryos remaining following the infertility treatment.(2) A person to whom information is provided pursuant to paragraph (1) of this subsection shall be presented with the option of storing any unused embryos, donating them to another person, donating the remaining embryos for research purposes, or other means of disposition.

(3) A person who elects to donate, for research purposes, any embryos remaining after receiving infertility treatment shall provide written consent to that donation.c. (1) A person shall not knowingly, for valuable consideration, purchase or sell, or otherwise transfer or obtain, or promote the sale or transfer of, embryonic or cadaveric fetal tissue for research purposes pursuant to this act; however, embryonic or cadaveric fetal tissue may be donated for research purposes in accordance with the provisions of subsection b. of this section or other applicable State or federal law. For the purposes of this subsection, "valuable consideration" means financial gain or advantage, but shall not include reasonable payment for the removal, processing, disposal, preservation, quality control, storage, transplantation, or implantation of embryonic or cadaveric fetal tissue. (2) A person or entity who violates the provisions of this subsection shall be guilty of a crime of the third degree and, notwithstanding the provisions of subsection b. of N.J.S.2C:43-3, shall be subject to a fine of up to $50,00 for each violation.

In May 2004 the Stem Cell Institute of New Jersey was created with an initial grant of $9.5 million in state funds, making the Garden State the first to fund embryonic stem cell research. Following the death of Christopher Reeve in October 2004, acting Governor Richard Codey took up the cause of funding stem cell research (James McGreavey resigned in the fall of 2004 amid a personal scandal that garnered generous coverage in the pages of the National Inquirer). In his State of the State address in January 2005, Gov. Codey called for the state to spend $380 million to fund stem cell research, a request later rebuffed by state lawmakers facing what one elected representative termed, "the worst budget year in recent memory." See Kaitlin Gurney, *Legislators Balk At Stem Cell Funding*, PHIL. INQUIRER, March 9, 2005. Instead, a more modest $23 million was allocated to stem cell research in 2005 and 2006, generating 17 grant awards to various New Jersey research institutions.

New Jersey, like California, allows voters to approve bond initiatives on statewide ballots, but the ballot measure requires legislative approval (as opposed to collected voter signatures in California) before it can be put before voters. In 2007, New Jersey voters rejected an initiative that would have directed $450 million in state bond sales to fund stem cell research. The New Jersey Commission on Science and Technology, which had been awarding grants to the state's Stem Cell Institute, closed its doors in July 2010.

3.   Other State Activities

In addition to California and New Jersey, other states have made legislative steps toward regulating funding for embryonic stem cell research. In Connecticut in 2005, Republican Governor Jodi Rell signed a law that provided $100 million in state funding over 10 years. The Connecticut Stem Cell Research Grant Project continues to operate, seeking research applications as recently as January 2012.

Illinois Governor-turned-federal inmate Rod Blagojevich signed an executive order in July 2005 establishing the Illinois Regenerative Medicine Institute and ordering $10 million to be transferred to the program. Two years later in 2007, the Illinois legislature validated the governor's action, enacting a law further regulating the stem cell institute. A 2012 visit to the Illinois Regenerative Medicine Institute Oversight Committee website shows that all positions on the Committee are vacant, suggesting it is not in operation.

In Maryland, lawmakers created the Maryland Stem Cell Research Fund to "promote scientific and medical stem cell research and cures through grants and loans to public and private entities in the state." 2006 Md. S.B. 144. In 2007, the State of Maryland allocated $15 million to the Fund for adult and embryonic stem cell research. The Fund's website remains active, advertising funding opportunities as recently as 2011.

In 2005, Massachusetts lawmakers overrode a veto by Republican Governor Mitt Romney to permit stem cell research to proceed in the Commonwealth. The law established institutes for research, which gained access to state funding after the 2006 election of Democratic Governor Deval Patrick, who signed a bill directing $1 billion in state funding to stem cell research over a 10-year period.

New York lawmakers established the Empire State Stem Cell Trust, earmarking approximately $600 million to be granted over a 10-year period beginning in 2008.

In at least one state, lawmakers fought to prevent state funds from being used to sponsor stem cell research involving therapeutic cloning. Arizona House Bill 2221 was introduced on January 11, 2005, and was passed and signed into law by Governor Janet Napolitano (and later Secretary of Homeland Security under President Obama) on April 22, 2005. The law provides:

35-196.04. Use of public monies for human cloning; prohibition; definition A. Notwithstanding any other law, tax monies of this state or any political subdivision of this state, federal monies passing through the state treasury . . . or any other public monies shall not be used by any person or entity, including any state funded institution or facility, for human somatic cell nuclear transfer, commonly known as human cloning . . .

C. For purposes of this section, "human somatic cell nuclear transfer" means human asexual reproduction that is accomplished by introducing the genetic material from one or more human somatic cells into a fertilized or unfertilized oocyte whose nuclear materials has been removed or inactivated so as to produce an organism, at any stage of development, that is genetically virtually identical to an existing or previously existing human organism.

The State of Missouri likewise prohibits public expenditure toward human cloning, as follows:

No state funds shall be used for research with respect to the cloning of a human person. For purposes of this section, the term "cloning" means the replication of a human person by taking a cell with genetic material and cultivating such cell through the egg, embryo, fetal and newborn stages of development into a new human person.

Mo. Stat. Ann. § 1-217 (2005).

PROBLEM

Assume you are counsel to an upstart biotechnology company, searching for a city to headquarter its new business enterprise. The company's main research is in medical therapies using human biologics, including human stem cells. Your client has received generous real estate packages from venture capitalists in St. Louis and Phoenix. In addition, you have explored possible locations in Northern California's "Silicon Valley," an area rich with high-tech businesses, but also much more expensive than the Missouri and Arizona options. What advice would you give your client about where to locate the headquarters? What factors weighed most heavily in your decision?

SECTION IV: INTERNATIONAL AND CROSS-CULTURAL PERSPECTIVES ON STEM CELL RESEARCH

A. International Perspectives

The hopes and fears over stem cell research do not just affect lawmakers in this country, they occupy governmental bodies worldwide. Ideally, any cures or therapies that emerge from stem cell research will benefit people according to their disease, not their geographical boundaries. Moreover, numerous countries across the globe are interested in securing whatever financial advantages stem cell research might procure. If public and private funds are being expended on developing stem cell processes and products, global competition for those resources is likely to be spirited.

The global regulatory landscape governing stem cell research, much like the picture within the U.S., is a checkerboard of countries adopting a variety of different approaches. This diversity is perhaps best displayed by the position taken in the United Nations General Assembly, which in 2001 established the Ad Hoc Committee on an International Convention Against the Reproductive Cloning of Human Beings. The Ad Hoc Committee met periodically over the next four years, but was never able to reach a consensus on an international convention against human cloning because some Member States believed that a ban on human cloning would also ban therapeutic cloning, a practice those countries thought should be strictly controlled but not prohibited.

In March 2005, the U.N General Assembly approved a nonbinding statement urging governments to ban all forms of human cloning, including cloning for embryonic stem cell research. In a press release, the U.N. stated, "The General Assembly this morning adopted the United Nations Declaration on Human Cloning, by which Member States were called on to adopt all measures necessary to prohibit all forms of human cloning inasmuch as they are incompatible with human dignity and the protection of human life." United Nations Press Release, GA/10333 (59th General Assembly, 82nd Meeting, March 8, 2005). The vote was 84-34 with 37 abstentions. Those voting in favor included the United States, Afghanistan, Austria, Germany, Iraq, Italy, Mexico, Poland, Saudi Arabia, Switzerland, and virtually all of Latin America. Those opposed included Belgium, Canada, China, North and South Korea, Netherlands, New Zealand, Singapore, Spain, and the United Kingdom.

In a statement released by the U.N., a representative of the U.K. explained he voted against the Declaration "because the reference to "human life" could be interpreted as a call for a total ban on all forms of human cloning." He worried that the language was "ambiguous . . . which might sow confusion about the acceptability of that important field of research." He further opined "The Declaration voted on today was a weak, non-binding political statement that did not reflect anything approaching consensus within the Assembly, and would not affect the United Kingdom's strong support of stem cell research." Id.

The White House released a statement by then President Bush in response to the U.N. vote:

> I applaud the strong vote of the United Nations General Assembly today urging countries to ban all forms of human cloning. I am also grateful for the strong statement against practices that exploit women. Human life must not be created for the purpose of destroying it. The United States and the international community have now spoken clearly that human cloning is an affront to human dignity and that we must work together to protect human life. I look forward to working with Members of Congress to enact legislation to ban all human cloning in the United States.

Statement by the President, Office of the Press Secretary, March 8, 2005, available at: http://www.whitehouse.gov/news/releases/2005/03/20050308-25.html.

The nonbinding UN Declaration on Human Cloning remains in place as of May 2012. In 2008, the UN's International Bioethics Committee began a four-year review of global cloning policies, ultimately urging more dialogue and education about the science and ethics of the technique. With respect to law, the IBC issued the following statement:

> [T]he IBC considers that the existing international legal frameworks and regulations are not sufficient to properly address the challenges posed by the most recent developments. They are non-binding and mutually inconsistent as a result of different views of Member States. A process should be initiated that could lead to the establishment of a more robust mechanism, such as an internationally effective and valuable convention or a moratorium, to prohibit reproductive cloning.

See United Nation Educational, Scientific and Cultural Organization, Human Cloning and International Governance, available at: http://www.unesco.org/new/en/social-and-human-sciences/themes/bioethics/international-bioethics-committee/ibc-sessions/eighteenth-session-baku-2011/human-cloning/.

When the prospect of embryonic stem cell research first appeared on the international scientific scene in the late 1990s, nations tended to line up as either in favor of allowing such research or opposed to sponsoring research in which human embryos were destroyed. A flurry of international activity surrounded stem cell research for several years, followed by a quieter period in the mid-2000s as discoveries lagged and a scandal in South Korea rocked the scientific community. What follows is a summary of stem cell law and/or policy of selected countries outside the U.S.

Australia

In December 2002 the Federal Parliament passed legislation banning cloning and regulating research involving human embryos. The Prohibition of Human Cloning Act 2002 prohibits all forms of human cloning, including cloning embryos for stem cell research. The Research Involving Human Embryos Act 2002 strictly regulates the use of embryos in research, establishing the Embryo Research Licensing Committee. The Committee is authorized to grant licenses for research involving "excess ART embryos" that were created before April 5, 2002. Research

Involving Human Embryos Act 2002, Sec. 24(3). Thus, like the 2001 Bush Administration policy in the U.S., Australian lawmakers struggled to balance their varying views on the destruction of the human embryo for research purposes, compromising on the population of embryos that could be used for research. But in contrast to the professed permanence of the Bush Administration policy, the law contains a sunset clause, repealing the restriction on pre-2002 embryos in April 2005. Research Involving Human Embryos Act 2002, Sec. 46.

In 2002 The National Stem Cell Centre was opened in Melbourne, funded in part by the State of Victoria and a private grant from a biotechnology consortium. See www.biomelbourne.org. Researchers expressed concern that state funding for stem cell research in general would decline in light of Australia's support for the nonbinding United Nations Declaration against all forms of cloning, passed in March 2005. The Australian vote was consistent with its law, which bans therapeutic cloning, but supporters of stem cell research using cloned embryos had hoped that its U.N. representative would vote against the Declaration, in part because Parliament was set to review the country's existing stem cell laws in 2005, a review supporters hoped would foster regulation rather than restriction of therapeutic cloning. See *Science Around the World*, THE SCIENTIST, Jan. 31, 2005, at 38. In fact, in 2006 Australian law was amended to allow for therapeutic cloning, while continuing to prohibit cloning for reproductive purposes. A review of national policy conducted in 2010-11 recommended no change from the permissive 2006 policy. Even though some research on cloned embryos was permitted, the Australian Stem Cell Centre closed in July 2011.

Canada

In March 2004 the Canadian Parliament passed the Assisted Human Reproduction Act, a law governing the use of embryos in research and assisted reproduction. The law prohibits the creation of human embryos explicitly for research purposes but allows research on unused human embryos created for fertility procedures. The law also bans human cloning for reproductive purposes, but allows limited embryonic stem cell research. Even though not explicitly stated, the new law would also ban therapeutic cloning because it limits embryo research to existing embryos created for fertility treatment.

The Canadian law authorizes the Assisted Human Reproduction Agency (AHRA) to implement and oversee the legislation and regulations. Researchers intending to use an in vitro embryo in their research must satisfy the AHRA that they have undertaken certain steps before being issued a licence to proceed. The Act allows for the in vitro embryo to be used only if the following conditions are met, including:

> it is demonstrated to the AHRA that the use of an in vitro embryo is necessary for the purposes of the research;

> the in vitro embryo is no longer needed for reproductive purposes, as an embryo cannot be specifically created for research purposes;

> fully informed and written consent was obtained from the individual(s) for whom the embryo was created;

> no one has purchased, sold or advertised to sell the in vitro embryo(s); and

the researcher has obtained a licence from the AHRA to undertake the research.

See Health Canada, *Research Involving the In Vitro Embryo* (March 2004), available at: http://www.hc-sc.gc.ca/english/media/releases/2004/2004_10bk3.htm. As discussed in Chapter 8, the comprehensive Canadian ART law was challenged as exceeding the legislative authority of the Canadian Parliament to rest regulation of ART in federal, rather than provincial (state-like) hands. After six years of litigation, in December 2010 the Supreme Court of Canada struck down several key features of the law, leaving much of the regulatory authority in the hands of provincial authorities. The above provisions governing human cloning and stem cell research were upheld as constitutionally within the jurisdiction of federal law. *See Patchwork Regulations Likely Outcome of Reproductive Technologies Ruling*, 183(4) Can. Med. Ass'n. J. E215 (2011).

China

In December 2003 the Chinese Ministry of Science and Technology and the Ministry of Health issued "Ethical Guiding Principles on Human Embryonic Stem Cell Research." The official translation of the policy provides as follows:

> The Ethical Guiding Principles for Research on Human Embryonic Stem Cell (hereinafter referred to as the Guiding Principle) are formulated for the purpose of bringing human embryonic stem cell research in biomedical domains conducted in the People's Republic of China to accord with bioethical norms, to ensure internationally recognized bioethical guidelines and domestic related regulations to be respected and complied with, and to promote a healthy development of human embryonic stem cell research.
>
> Human embryonic stem cells described in the Guiding Principles include stem cells derived from donated human embryos, those originated from germ cells and those obtained from somatic cell nuclear transfer technology.
>
> Any research activity related to human embryonic stem cells conducted in the territory of the People's Republic of China shall abide by the Guiding Principle.
>
> Any research aiming at human reproductive cloning shall be prohibited.
>
> Human embryonic stem cells used for research purpose can only be derived from the following means with voluntary agreement:
>
> > Spared gamete or embryos after in vitro fertilization (IVF);
> >
> > Fetal cells from accidental spontaneous or voluntarily selected abortions;
> >
> > Embryos obtained by somatic cell nuclear transfer technology or parthenogenetic split embryos; and
> >
> > Germ cells voluntarily donated.

All research activities related to human embryonic stem cells shall comply with the following norms:

Embryos obtained from IVF, human somatic cell nuclear transfer, parthenogenesis or genetic modification techniques, its in vitro culture period shall not exceed 14 days starting from the day when fertilization or nuclear transfer is performed.

It shall be prohibited to implant embryos created by means described above into the genital organ of human beings or any other species.

It shall be prohibited to hybridize human germ cells with germ cells of any other species.

It shall be prohibited to buy or sell human gametes, fertilized eggs, embryos and fetal tissues.

The principle of informed consent and informed choice shall be complied with, the form of informed consent shall be signed, and subject's privacy shall be protected in all research activities related to human embryonic stem cells.

The informed consent and informed choice mentioned above refer to that the researchers shall use accurate, clear and popular expressions to tell the subjects the expected aim of the experiment as well as the potential consequences and risks and to obtain their consent by signing on a form of informed consent.

Research institutions engaged in human embryonic stem cell shall establish an ethical committee, which consists of research and administrative expert in biology, medicine, law and sociology with the responsibilities for providing scientific and ethical review, consultation and supervision of the research activities related to human embryonic stem cells.

See China Regulations & Laws, available at: http://www.chinaphs.org/bioethics/regulations_&_laws.htm#EGPHECR.

The Chinese government's approval of all types of stem cell research, including therapeutic cloning, makes China, according to the newspaper China Daily, "one of the leading countries in stem cell research." See *Nation Needs Law To Prevent Cloning Misuse*, CHINA DAILY, Mar. 12, 2005. Some Chinese lawmakers worried that China's lack of restrictive legislation on reproductive cloning, coupled with its permissive approach to therapeutic cloning, would cause the line between the two practices to become blurred, with dire consequences. The lawmakers called for legislation to clarify China's opposition to reproductive cloning. *Id.* To date, no further legislation has been passed. China continues to permit researchers to conduct clinical trials in which terminally or chronically ill patients receive stem cell therapy.

Costa Rica

Costa Rica prohibits all forms of cloning as well as embryonic stem cell research. A February 2005 Decree provides:

Article 11: Any manipulation or alteration of an embryo's genetic code is prohibited, as is any kind of experimentation with embryos.

See Decree No. 24029-S: A Regulation on Assisted Reproduction, available at: http://www.netsalud.sa.cr/ms/decretos/dec5.htm (in Spanish).

France

The French Bioethics Law, amended in July 2004, specifically prohibits human cloning for reproductive and therapeutic purposes, germline gene therapy and the creation of embryos purely for research purposes. Research using imported surplus embryos, however, was permitted. Human reproductive cloning is considered a "crime against the human race" and has been criminalized with jail sentences of up to 20 years and the imposition of fines. Research or therapeutic cloning is punishable with up to seven years in prison and fines. See Bioethics Law (8 July 2004, amended Law No. 94-653 of July 29 1994, on Respect for the Human Body and Law No. 94-654 of July 29 1994, on the Donation and Use of Elements and Products of the Human Body, Medically Assisted Procreation, and Prenatal Diagnosis.)

French law was slightly revised in 2006 to encourage stem cell research. Under national guidelines, French scientists can now use domestic surplus embryos to develop cell lines. *See* The Pew Forum on Religion & Public Life, *Stem Cell Research Around the World* (July 2008), available at: http://www.pewforum.org/Science-and-Bioethics/Stem-Cell-Research-Around-the-World.aspx.

Germany

Germany has one of most restrictive policies of any nation on embryonic stem cell research, but the science is permitted under limited circumstances. To begin, Germany bans all use of embryos in research. The codification of this policy came in 1990 with the passage of the Embryo Protection Act. The Act placed a strict ban on the manipulation of human embryos for research, banning the creation of embryos that would not be transferred to the uterus. Thus, under the Act derivation of stem cells from human embryos is prohibited. See John A. Robertson, *Causative v. Beneficial Complicity in the Embryonic Stem Cell Debate*, 36 CONN. L. REV. 1099 (2004).

The impetus for Germany's position on the protection of human embryos stems from its experience of eugenic experimentation during the Nazi reign. In 1945, when the Federal Republic of Germany was reconstituting its government after the defeat of the Nazi Party, lawmakers enacted the Basic Law, which became the underlying regulations for the German Constitution. In an effort to demonstrate intolerance for Nazi era policies, the Basic Law included clauses aimed at protecting human dignity, bodily inviolability, and the right to life. The 1990 Embryo Protection Act is a reflection of the Basic Law, favoring human life and dignity and "founded on the principle that embryos in vitro are wholly worthy of protection." In essence, the German law assigns the embryo the same legal rights as fully developed human beings. *See* Kara L. Belew, *Stem Cell Division: Abortion Law and Its Influence on the Adoption of Radically Different Embryonic Stem Cell Legislation in the United States, the United Kingdom, and Germany*, 39 TEX. INT'L L. J. 479 (2004).

Scientists and others in Germany began to seek a change in the 1990 Act at the end of the twentieth century when stem cell research showed commercial and medical promise. A national debate over the issue of stem cell research erupted in 1999 after a scientist submitted a grant proposal requesting government funding for a stem cell research project using stem cells he proposed to import from outside of Germany. At the time, importation of embryonic stem cells was banned under the 1990 Act. An intense debate occupied many in Germany, from the Chancellor, to the Parliament, to ordinary citizens. On January 1, 2002, the German Parliament voted in favor of allowing scientists to import embryonic stem cells, so long as the cell lines were derived from surplus IVF embryos prior to January 1, 2002. A vote in 2008 moved up this cut-off date to May 2007.

The importation of stem cells remains controversial in Germany. In a news article appearing after the law was amended to allow importation, the opposite views were displayed quite clearly. "Supporters of imports warned that the German biotechnology industry risked losing important business if scientists went elsewhere to research on stem cells, . . . [b]ut others were concerned by the ethical implications of such research . . . Germany's president, Johannes Rau, . . . warned that the development of gene technology risked reviving memories of atrocities and human experiments committed by the Nazis." *Germany Authorises Stem Cell Imports*, BBC News, Jan. 30, 2002.

Italy

As a predominantly Roman Catholic country, Italy has prohibited experimentation that involves the ex vivo creation or intentional destruction of human embryos. In February 2004, the Italian Parliament passed a comprehensive law addressing assisted reproductive technologies. Article 13 of the Assisted Medical Procreation Law relates to embryonic stem cell research, and provides in relevant part:

1. Any experiment on a human embryo is prohibited.

2. Clinical and experimental research on each human embryo is only permitted on condition that it solely aims to reach therapeutic and diagnostic goals related to the health and development of the embryo itself, and if no other alternative procedure is available.

3. The following conditions are anyway banned:

1. the production of human embryos for research or experiment or anyhow for purposes different from those stated in this Law;

2. every form of eugenic selection of embryos and gametes, namely any procedure that, through selection techniques or manipulation or any artificial method, is directed at the alteration of the genetic inheritance of the embryo or gamete, or at the predetermination of its genetic characteristics, with the exception of the procedures performed for diagnostic and therapeutic purposes mentioned in clause 2 of this article;

3. procedures of cloning through nuclear transfer or early embryo splitting or of ectogenesis both for reproductive and research purposes;

See The European Society of Human Reproduction and Embryology website at:

http://www.eshre.eu/ESHRE/English/Guidelines-Legal/Legal-documentation/
Italy/page.aspx/167.

While Italian law does prohibit the creation of embryos and embryonic stem cell lines, it permits research on cell lines established in lawful ways outside the country. In 2009, several Italian stem cell researchers challenged the government's exclusion of embryonic stem cell research from federal funding of stem cell research in general. The scientists did not prevail, but vowed to continue to fight for what they believed were their constitutional rights and academic freedom. *See Italian Stem Cell Scientists Challenge Government — The Story Continues*, EuroStemCell, available at: http://www.eurostemcell.org/story/italian-stem-cell-scientists-challenge-government-story-continues.

Japan

Since the turn of the twenty-first century, the Japanese government has been actively involved in developing and enacting comprehensive law and policy pertaining to cloning and embryonic stem cell research. In November 2000, the Japanese Parliament, called the Diet, passed the "Law Concerning Regulation Relating to Human Cloning Techniques and Other Similar Techniques." The law permits cloning for research purposes only, prohibiting the implantation of cloned embryos into a woman's uterus, or transplantation of the embryo into a human or an animal. Specifically, Article 3 of the law provides, "No person shall transfer a somatic clone embryo, a human-animal amphimictic embryo, a human-animal hybrid embryo or a human-animal chimeric embryo into the uterus of a human or an animal." The law imposes criminal sanctions for the violation of its provisions. Presumably this law would ban therapeutic cloning, because it involves the transplantation of cloned stem cells back into the human body.

One commentator has noted the unusual language of the Japanese law, noting:

> One interesting, and somewhat shocking, aspect of the Japanese Human Cloning Regulation Act is the language regarding human-animal amphimictic embryos and human animal hybrid embryos. Scientists would be allowed to create animal-human embryos as long as the cells used to create the embryo are not from human embryos or fertilized eggs. It is forbidden to implant such an embryo into the uterus of a woman or animal. A Japanese scholar, Masahiro Morioka, expressed his concern that the law permits scientists to do just about anything with embryos as long as they are not implanted into the uterus. The scholar feels the Diet was more interested in catching up with the advances that biotechnology companies in the United States have made rather than considering the ethics of the broad legislation. Morioka points out that some of the issues that were part of the legislation, such as human-animals, were not discussed with scientists working in the field of cloning. Furthermore, he asserts that the public would not accept the law if they were made aware of its details.

Suzanne H. Rhodes, *The Difficulty of Regulating Reproductive and Therapeutic Cloning: Can the United States Learn Anything from the Laws of Other Countries?*, 21 PENN. STATE INT'L L. REV. 341, 353-54 (2003).

In 2001, one year after the Cloning Law was enacted, the Ministry of Education, Culture, Sports, Science and Technology tackled the legal issues surrounding embryonic stem cell research. The Ministry issued "Guidelines for the Derivation and Utilization of Human Embryonic Stem Cells," which authorized stem cell research on surplus IVF embryos, providing that the "derivation and utilization of ES cells shall be limited to basic research." *See* Rosario M. Isasi, Bartha M. Knoppers, Peter A. Singer, Abdallah S. Daar, *Legal and Ethical Approaches to Stem Cell and Cloning Research: A Comparative Analysis of Policies in Latin, America, Asia, and Africa*, 32 J. Law, Med. & Ethics 626 (2004). At that time a moratorium was placed on cloning embryos for research or therapeutic purposes so that it could be studied by the Council for Science and Technology Policy, the highest-ranking organization for setting the country's science and technology policy. The Council is chaired by the prime minister.

The question of stem cell research using cloned embryos remained a subject of debate until June 2004 when the Council approved a report issued by its Bioethics Committee that endorses the use of cloning technology to produce embryonic stem cells for research on basic regenerative medicine. The Council decided that only particular research institutes would be allowed to conduct the research and that the government would be responsible for potential embryonic production. *See* Gustav Ando, *Japan Gives Thumbs Up To Cloning*, World Markets Analysis (July 27, 2004). Initial stem cell research guidelines issued by the Council to Japan's Ministry of Health, Labour and Welfare, and the Ministry of Education, Culture, Sports, Science & Technology were considered restrictive and cumbersome, imposing administrative hurdles to research progress. In 2009, the guidelines were eased, though they continue to prohibit reproductive cloning but permit therapeutic or research cloning.

The Netherlands

The 2002 Embryos Act governs the use and creation of embryos for scientific research in the Netherlands. The Act bans the production of embryos purely for research purposes, as well as the cloning of human beings. Under the law, people who have successfully undergone IVF treatment may donate the gametes or embryos they no longer need to a third party to produce embryonic stem cells or for scientific research. Thus, stem cell research using spare IVF embryos is permitted, so long as the research is approved by the Central Committee on Research Involving Human Subjects, a division of the Ministry of Health. A 2007 review of Dutch law by the cabinet left existing law in place for the foreseeable future.

Norway

The law in Norway prohibits all embryos research, according to Law No. 100 on the use of biotechnology in human medicine (the Biotechnology Law), enacted in December 2003. Translated from Norwegian and appearing on a website maintained by the Global Lawyers and Physicians Working Together for Human Rights, the law provides:

3.1. *Prohibition of research on fertilized eggs, etc.*

Research on fertilized eggs, human embryos, and cell lines cultured from fertilized eggs or human embryos shall be prohibited.

3.2. *Prohibition of the production of human embryos by cloning, etc.*

It shall be prohibited: (a) to produce human embryos by cloning; (b) to carry out research on cell lines cultured from human embryos produced by cloning; and (c) to produce embryos by cloning through the introduction of heritable material from a human being into an egg cell of an animal. Cloning means techniques for producing heritable identical copies.

See http://www.glphr.org/genetic/europe2-7.htm.

Singapore

Singapore seemed to take an early lead in stem cell research, hosting what was then the world's largest conference on the emerging field in October 2003. At the time, Singapore was perceived to have some of the world's most liberal guidelines on stem cell research, where scientists were permitted to clone embryos and extract their stem cells for research. In September 2004, the Singapore Parliament tightened and clarified the country's law, enacting the Human Cloning and Other Prohibited Practices Law. The law bans human reproductive cloning, but permits cloning for research purposes and embryonic stem cell research. The relevant portions of the law provide as follows:

Sec. 5. No person shall place any human embryo clone in the body of a human or in the body of an animal.

Sec. 7. No person shall develop any human embryo, that is created by a process other than the fertilisation of a human egg by human sperm, for a period more than 14 days, excluding any period when the development of the embryo is suspended.

Sec. 8. No person shall develop any human embryo outside the body of a woman for a period of more than 14 days, excluding any period when the development of the embryo is suspended.

Do you see how the law permits stem cell research and therapeutic cloning while banning reproductive cloning?

South Korea

The story of embryonic stem cell research in South Korea is one of notoriety and malfeasance perpetrated by at least one ambitious researcher. In February 2004 a team of South Korean researchers reported in the journal *Science* that they had developed a cell line using stem cells derived from a human embryo that had been created using somatic cell nuclear transfer — cloning. *See* Woo Suk Hwang et al., *Evidence of a Pluripotent Human Embryonic Stem Cell Line Derived from a Cloned Blastocyst*, 303 Science 1669 (2004). This report was the world's first that it was possible to inject a somatic cell nucleus into an unfertilized egg, coax the egg to grow and divide, nurture the resulting embryo to the blastocyst stage and then remove the pluripotent stem cells from the five-day-old embryo. A further published paper reported that the same group of South Korean scientists had developed 11 patient-specific embryonic stem cell lines, meaning that the lines could be differentiated into any cell in the body for transplant back to the patient in the hope of providing compatible tissue for therapy or cure. *See* Woo Suk Hwang et al., *Patient-Specific Embryonic Stem Cells Derived from Human SCNT Blastocysts*, 308 SCIENCE 1777 (2005).

In early 2006, evidence of ethical lapses in Woo Suk Hwang's lab began to emerge. First, it was revealed that the researcher had pressured female members of his staff to "donate" eggs for the ongoing experiments, clearly in violation of national and international research ethics parameters. But further revelations were more devastating. Independent analysis of the reported data showed the research had been fabricated — that the cell lines had not been derived from cloning human embryos but by other already established techniques. Once hailed as a national hero, Woo Suk Hwang was quickly derided for his egregious conduct. In October 2009, following a three-year trial, Hwang was found guilty of embezzlement and bioethical violations, but cleared on charges of fraud. The judge expressed sympathy for Hwang's apparent dedication to Korean biotechnology. His two-year prison sentence was suspended for three years, thus paving the way for him to continue his research career. *See* Evan Y. Snyder & Jeanne F. Loring, *Beyond Fraud — Stem-Cell Research Continues*, 354 NEW ENG. J. MED. 321 (2006); David Cyranoski, *Woo Suk Hwang Convicted, but Not of Fraud*, 461 NATURE 1181 (2009).

As a result of the scandal, South Korea enacted the Bioethics and Safety Act in December 2008. The Act replaced a 2005 law which was criticized for failing to protect human embryos, as well as gamete and embryo donors. The 2008 law prohibits human reproductive cloning and the production of embryos for non-reproductive purposes. Nonetheless, sources of human embryonic stem cells permitted under the Act include somatic cell nuclear transfer, "for the purpose of conducting research aimed at curing rare or currently incurable diseases," and "spare" IVF embryos if they have exceeded a maximum storage period of five years or if researchers receive consent from their progenitors. Payment for gametes is prohibited as well, although oocyte donors may be reimbursed for costs associated with the procedure. *See* The Witherspoon Council on Ethics and the Integrity of Science, *Overview of International Human Embryonic Stem Cell Law, in* The Stem Cell Debates: Lessons for Science and Politics, 34 The New Atlantis 129 (Winter 2012), available at: http://www.thenewatlantis.com/publications/appendix-e-overview-of-international-human-embryonic-stem-cell-laws.

United Kingdom

It is fair to say that the U.K. has the most long-standing and comprehensive legal structure governing research on human embryos in the world. The Human Fertilisation and Embryology Act of 1990 authorized research on embryos up to 14 days post-fertilization, provided the research is licensed by the Human Fertilisation and Embryology Authority (HFEA), the British governmental body that licenses and monitors all human embryo research being conducted in the UK. Under the Act, research can be conducted on embryos donated from IVF clinics as well as embryos specifically created for research purposes.

In 2001 the U.K. became the first jurisdiction to pass a law allowing scientists to clone human embryos for embryonic stem cell research. The 2001 Human Embryology Act permits therapeutic cloning, but criminalizes reproductive cloning, imposing fines and a 10-year prison term on any violators. The HFEA, which reviews all license requests to perform therapeutic cloning, issued its first such license in August 2004 to researchers at the University of Newcastle upon Tyne. The Newcastle scientists hope to use stem cells to develop insulin-producing cells that could be transplanted into diabetic patients without risk of rejection. See David Adam, *Regulators Give Green Light to Stem Cell Clones*, THE GUARDIAN (London), Aug. 12, 2004, at 1. A second license was granted in February 2005 to a team at the Roslin Institute in Scotland, led by Ian Wilmut, famed for creating the cloned sheep known as "Dolly." The Roslin group proposed to study motor neurons, cells that degenerate in patients with Amyotrophic Lateral Sclerosis (Lou Gehrig's Disease). Like the license granted to the Newcastle scientists, the HFEA limited the teams to using only unfertilized eggs, eggs that failed to fertilize during infertility treatments — a compromise the government imposed to address ethical concerns about the use of healthy human eggs in experiments. See Rick Weiss, *British to Clone Human Embryos for Stem Cells*, WASH. POST, Feb. 9, 2005, at A2.

The HFEA publishes a list of granted and pending licenses for human embryonic stem cell research on its website, www.HFEA.gov.uk. As of 2009, the HFEA had approved 21 research protocols, and was considering one additional proposal.

For a deeper discussion of the regulatory framework in the U.K., *see* Eric Blyth, *The United Kingdom: Evolution of a Statutory Regulatory Approach*, in THIRD PARTY ASSISTED CONCEPTION ACROSS CULTURES, 226-245 (2004); ANDREA L. BONNICKSEN, CRAFTING A CLONING POLICY 152-160 (2002); Samantha Halliday, *A Comparative Approach to the Regulation of Human Embryonic Stem Cell Research in Europe*, 12 MEDICAL L. REV. 40 (2004); Denise Stevens, *Embryonic Stem Cell Research: Will President Bush's Limitation on Federal Funding Put the United States at a Disadvantage? A Comparison Between U.S. and International Law*, 25 HOUS. J. INT'L L. 623 (2003).

NOTES AND QUESTIONS

1.   The law, policy and science surrounding stem cell research is so fast moving no doubt some, if not most, of these country's stated positions will have changed by the time you review the materials in this chapter. Fear not — there are several sources that continually update the state of the international law in this emerging field. As of spring 2012, two of the most up to date websites detailing laws in the U.S. include one maintained by the National Conference of State Legislatures, available at: http://www.ncsl.org/issues-research/health/embryonic-and-fetal-research-laws. aspx, and another sponsored by the Kaiser Family Foundation called State Health Facts,   available   at   http://www.statehealthfacts.org/comparetable.jsp?ind= 111&cat=2. In early 2012, *The New Atlantis* published a comprehensive update on stem cell research in the U.S. and abroad, including a comprehensive appendix listing laws in dozens of countries. *See* The Witherspoon Council on Ethics and the Integrity of Science, *Overview of International Human Embryonic Stem Cell Law,* *in* The Stem Cell Debates: Lessons for Science and Politics, 34 THE NEW ATLANTIS

129 (Winter 2012), available at: http://www.thenewatlantis.com/publications/appendix-e-overview-of-international-human-embryonic-stem-cell-laws.

2. Does it matter that different countries have different laws on the question of stem cell research? If medical therapies are developed using stem cells derived from human embryos, will patients who live in countries which prohibit any experimentation on embryos be prohibited from accessing therapies that, if processed in that country would be considered the result of illegal activity?

3. On November 27, 2004, voters in Switzerland approved a national referendum that permits scientists to conduct stem cell research using embryos donated from IVF clinics (with the consent of the progenitor couple). Swiss law still prohibits the creation of embryos for research purposes, including forming embryos through the union of sperm and egg, or by cloning. The referendum, passed by a vote of 66 to 34%, was placed before voters after Parliament passed a similar law in 2003 that authorized stem cell research. Opponents of the 2003 Embryonic Research Act mobilized to place the issue before the Swiss voters, hoping to overturn the law. But voters approved the law by a 2-1 margin. *See* Fiona Fleck, *Swiss Voters Back Stem-Cell Research*, N.Y. TIMES, Nov. 28, 2004.

Is direct democracy (that is, popular voting on referenda or initiatives) the best way to create a nation's public policy? What relief is available to the third of Swiss voters who oppose embryonic stem cell research? What about people in, say, Costa Rica, who favor stem cell research in a country where all research involving human embryos is banned? Is a government's policy on stem cell research any different in its impact on the nation's citizens than other state-sponsored policies such as those on abortion, the death penalty or the provision of social services?

B.   Religious Perspectives on Embryonic Stem Cell Research

For many individuals, and for many countries, religious beliefs play a major role in guiding one's views about embryonic stem cell research. In 1999, when the U.S. National Bioethics Advisory Commission met at President Clinton's request to address the legal, medical and ethical issues surrounding the emerging science, the group recognized that learning and incorporating the views of the country's major religions was an essential component to a thorough and legitimate report. According to NBAC, "the Commission believed that testimony from scholars of religious ethics was crucial to its goal of informing itself about the range, content, and rationale of various ethical positions regarding research in this area." *See* Ethical Issues in Human Stem Cell Research, Vol. 1, Report and Recommendations of the National Bioethics Advisory Commission, 99 (1999). Thus, the Commission heard testimony from scholars who work within the Roman Catholic, Protestant, Eastern Orthodox, Jewish and Islamic faiths. NBAC's summary of those views is excerpted below.

National Bioethics Advisory Commission Summary of Presentations on Religious Perspectives Relating to Research Involving Human Stem Cells, May 7, 1999
Ethical Issues In Human Stem Cell Research 99-104
(September 1999)

Roman Catholic Perspectives

The restrictive, "official" position within Roman Catholicism opposes EG and ES cell research, primarily because obtaining stem cells from either aborted fetal tissue or embryos that remain following clinical in vitro fertilization (IVF) procedures involves the intentional destruction of a genetically unique, living member of the human species. According to this view, it is impermissible to obtain stem cells from in vitro fertilized blastocysts, because doing so results in the destruction of the blastocyst — a human life worthy of full moral protection from the moment of conception. No amount of benefit to others can justify the destruction of the blastocyst, an act that would be equivalent to murder.

Similarly, from this perspective, it is impermissible to obtain EG cells from the gonadal tissue of aborted fetuses, because although such harvesting is not directly responsible for the death of the fetus, it nevertheless involves complicity with the evil of abortion. Moreover, to make use of any therapy derived from research on either human embryonic or fetal tissue and to contribute to the development or application of such research through general taxation would involve complicity in the destruction of human life. Federal funding, which in a sense would make all citizens complicit in this research, thus would greatly impose upon the consciences of Catholics.

However, even the restrictive position of the Roman Catholic Church does not oppose stem cell research per se. The central moral impediment to such research concerns the sources from which stem cells are derived. The act of harvesting stem cells from other sources — miscarried fetuses, placental blood, or adult tissues — would not be intrinsically immoral. In fact, this perspective, recognizing the potential benefits to human health of stem cell research, encourages investigation into the feasibility of such alternative sources. In practice, however, stem cell research, even with alternative stem cell sources, would remain morally problematic for two reasons. First, some are concerned that any safeguards will be ineffective because, in the face of potentially promising and lucrative research, the temptation to transgress such safeguards might be irresistible. Second, many fear that the benefits of this research might not be distributed equitably and are concerned that stem cell research perhaps may not be the best use of national resources, given the preponderance of so many other unmet human needs.

Although all Roman Catholics share a variety of important basic convictions, individual Catholics often differ in how to interpret them in practice. According to a less restrictive Catholic perspective, this disagreement is due, at least in part, to a commitment to the theory of natural law — a commitment that, while a fundamental part of the Catholic tradition, also involves reliance upon an "imperfect science." A commitment to natural law involves belief in a moral order that can be "seen" by all human beings in the reality of creation itself. But because the act of "looking" entails "a complex process of discernment and deliberation, and a structuring of insights, a determination of meaning, from the fullest vantage point available, given a particular history — one that includes the illumination of Scripture and the accumulated wisdom of the tradition" — what any two human beings see will not always be the same.

With respect to stem cell research, the major areas of disagreement among Catholics are also those upon which the restrictive voice within Catholicism most strongly bases its opposition: the moral status of the embryo and the moral permissibility of using aborted fetuses as sources of stem cells. In contrast to this restrictive view of the embryo, another Catholic might, with the aid of science, look to the reality of the early human embryo and see that which is not yet an "individualized human entity with the settled inherent potential to become a human person." Because the early embryo, according to this less restrictive view, is not a person, it is sometimes permissible to use it in research, though as human life it must always be accorded some respect. Similarly, one might decide that adequate barriers — such as a prohibition against the directed donation of cadaveric fetal tissue, and the distinction between somatic cell nuclear transfer (SCNT) for research or therapy and SCNT for reproduction — can be erected between the use of aborted fetal tissue in research and the act of abortion itself so that engaging in the former does not amount to complicity in the latter. From this perspective, then, a Catholic may be able to support ES cell research without sacrificing a commitment to the fundamental principles that define Catholicism, including the duties to protect human life, honor the sacred, and promote distributive justice in health care. Finally, because of the diversity within and among ethical traditions, this perspective is congruent with the restrictive Catholic view that individuals who oppose this research should not be forced to contribute to it but, contrary to the restrictive view, favors an approach that would allow federal funding, but with accommodations made to permit conscientious objection.

To summarize the testimony of the Roman Catholic panel, all agree that in light of certain agreed-upon principles, major Catholic concerns with regard to both embryonic and nonembryonic stem cell research include the following issues: 1) the moral status of the early embryo, 2) complicity with abortion in using fetal tissue as a source of stem cells, 3) the need for safeguards, distributive justice, and just allocation of national resources, and 4) the difficulty in federally funding research to which many are opposed on moral and religious grounds. The major disagreements arise from conflicting interpretations of the broad principles, which in turn lead to different responses to these four major concerns.

Jewish Perspectives

The two main sources of Jewish ethics — theology and law — yield several principles relevant to a Jewish ethical analysis of stem cell research. First, human beings are merely the stewards of their bodies, which belong to God. Moreover, God has placed conditions on the use of the human body, including the command that health and life must be preserved. Second, human beings are God's partners in healing, and in order to fulfill God's command, they have a duty to use any means available to heal themselves, whether these means are natural or artificial. Third, because all human beings, regardless of ability, are created in the image of God, they are valuable. Fourth, human beings, unlike God, lack perfect knowledge of the consequences of their actions and in the process of trying to improve themselves or the world must, therefore, be careful to avoid causing harm to them.

Four potential moral impediments to EG and ES cell research arise from these Jewish principles: 1) the moral status of the fetus and of the act of abortion, 2) potential complicity with evil, 3) the commandments to respect the dead, and 4) the moral status of the embryo.

According to Conservative Judaism, the fetus until the 40th day after conception is "like water." Although the fetus becomes a potential and partial person after the 40th day, and is thus entitled to a certain amount of respect and protection, it remains primarily a part of the pregnant woman's body, and does not become an independent person with full moral rights until the greater part of its body emerges from the womb during birth. Because of the command to preserve human health and life, if either the health or the life of the woman is clearly threatened by the fetus, abortion is not only permissible but obligatory, as she is a full person while the fetus remains only a part of her and a potential person. When the woman's health is at some increased risk but is not clearly compromised by the pregnancy, abortion is permissible but not obligatory. More recently, some Jewish authorities also permit abortion in cases in which the fetus has a terminal disease or serious malformations.

According to Orthodox Judaism, on the other hand, after 40 days of gestation, the fetus becomes a person with full moral rights and may not be aborted except to protect the pregnant woman's health. Yet, even though abortion after 40 days is viewed by the Orthodox Jews as homicide, it does not follow from this perspective that life-saving use of stem cells procured from illegitimately aborted fetuses is impermissible (although the question of who can legitimately give consent to such procurement is problematic from this perspective). Although this perspective recognizes the possibility that therapeutic use of aborted fetuses may make abortion appear less heinous, the strength of the commandment to preserve life, for which all other laws must be suspended except those prohibiting murder, idolatry, and sexual transgressions, overrides this concern. Thus, despite the disagreement within Judaism regarding the moral status of the fetus and the permissibility of abortion after 40 days, all agree that neither source of stem cells is illegitimate. One caveat to this consensus is that some within Conservative Judaism who accept the permissibility of abortion to preserve the life or health of the woman nevertheless require that stem cells be procured only from fetuses that have been legitimately aborted; Orthodox Judaism, by contrast, appears to hold that although abortion after 40 days postconception is generally impermissible, there is no complicity involved in using these aborted fetuses as sources of stem cells.

Jewish thinkers agree that commandments to respect the dead, which require that corpses not be mutilated or left unburied longer than necessary, can be suspended in order to save lives. Because of the strong commandment to preserve life and health, for example, Jewish law permits both autopsies and organ procurement when they will benefit the living. Reasoning by analogy, if tissue procurement from the cadavers of full persons in order to benefit human health and life is permitted, then tissue procurement from dead fetuses — which according to some Jewish perspectives are less than full persons — must also be permitted for the same purpose provided that (for some interpreters) the abortion itself was permissible according to Jewish law.

There is also wide consensus within Judaism that no serious moral impediments exist to using IVF embryos as sources of stem cells because extra-corporeal embryos have no status under Jewish law. These entities lack status because all embryos prior to 40 days postconception are "like water" and because as extra-corporeal entities, they lack the status of potential and partial person that is accorded to fetuses, which develop from embryos implanted in a uterus. Although extra-corporeal embryos merit a certain respect as human life, they are closest in moral status to gametes and thus may be discarded, frozen, or used as life-saving sources of stem cells. In fact, so long as they are never implanted, there is no clear legal prohibition against creating embryos for research purposes, although extra-legal norms may raise ethical questions about this practice.

Because stem cells can be permissibly procured either from extra-corporeal embryos or from legitimately aborted fetuses, stem cell research is not considered intrinsically immoral. Rather, stem cell research becomes morally problematic when applied in a variety of contexts. First, Judaism views the provision of health care as a communal duty. Thus, a context in which the benefits of stem cell research are not accessible to all persons who are in need would be problematic. Similarly, it may be problematic to focus national resources in this area of research rather than in other areas of need. In addition, although obtaining consent to procure stem cells is necessary, it may be challenging. Finally, there is widespread agreement that stem cell research should not be used to enhance human beings, although some disagreement exists over whether it may be used to improve health or whether it must be reserved only for life-saving purposes.

Eastern Orthodox Perspectives

According to Eastern Orthodoxy, all human beings are created in the image of God and grow continuously toward the likeness of God. Although the embryo, fetus, and adult are each at different stages of this process, all share the same potential for attaining authentic personhood, and each, with God's grace, will attain such personhood. According to this belief, God has given us medicine in order to heal, and any misuse of this gift that results in the destruction of potentially authentic persons is considered illegitimate. Thus, although miscarried fetuses may be used as sources of EG cells, neither electively aborted fetuses nor blastocysts may be so used. However, despite the impermissibility of procuring ES cells from blastocysts, because cell lines from this source already exist and have the potential to save lives, it is considered wasteful to discard these lines, and it is in fact permissible to use them. No complicity is thought to arise from such use. On the other hand, it is not permissible to procure EG cells from aborted fetuses, as such procurement *would* involve complicity.

Even assuming that stem cells could be permissibly procured, Eastern Orthodoxy shares with other religious traditions a variety of concerns about the context in which stem cell research might be applied, including addressing the problems of equitable access to the benefits of the research and other problems that can occur when market forces control the research; using the research for eugenic or cosmetic purposes, rather than for healing; and obtaining the informed, voluntary consent of the woman or couple.

Islamic Perspectives

Islam consists of two major schools of thought — Sunni and Shi'I — both of which refer to the same historical sources. Although these two schools differ somewhat in their views of abortion, in general, Islam regards the life of the fetus as developing over several stages, and personhood is considered a process. Although from the moment of conception the embryo is a human life meriting some protection, it is not commonly thought to attain personhood until it is ensouled, some time around the fourth month of gestation. Thus, because of the enormous potential to improve human health through this type of research, the vast majority of followers of Islam would agree that it is permissible to use early human embryonic life for this purpose. Moreover, it is permissible to use the tissue from illegitimately aborted fetuses to save lives, just as it is permissible to use cadaveric organs to save lives, even when the cadaveric organ source has been wrongfully killed. Finally, with caution, it can be deduced that creating embryos for research purposes is also permissible from an Islamic perspective, as long as those embryos are not implanted.

Protestant Perspectives

Protestant positions range dramatically from the highly restrictive to the nonrestrictive in this area. For example, according to restrictive Protestant view, a person is not defined by his or her capacities; rather, a person is a human being with a personal history, regardless of whether he or she is aware of that history. From this perspective, embryos are simply the weakest and least advantaged people among us. Because procuring stem cells from embryos requires the destruction of the embryo, such procurement thus raises serious moral issues, despite the ease with which it might be used to attain undeniably positive consequences for others, and rather than accepting the use of illicit means to achieve a good end, we should search for alternative, permissible means. Similarly, using aborted fetuses as sources of EG cells amounts to complicity with evil, and procurement of EG cells even from permissibly aborted fetuses (however that category is defined) would involve using a human life twice for another's benefit — first, to benefit the woman who aborted and then to benefit society through EG cell research. Therefore, from this perspective, it is impermissible to derive stem cells from embryos, whether spare or created for this purpose, and from aborted fetuses, whether permissibly aborted or not. The use of alternative sources of stem cells — for example, from bone marrow or umbilical cord blood — would, however, be permissible.

For Protestants whose views are less restrictive on this issue, the moral status of the embryo is more ambiguous. Although even nascent human life — which retains the potential for full human life — deserves respect and protection from callous disregard, the early embryo and the late fetus are viewed in moral terms as significantly different. Because the potential benefits of ES and EG cell research are so substantial, the moral difference between the early embryo and the developed fetus becomes compelling in this case, and it is thus permissible to use human life at the blastocyst stage to benefit other lives. No embryos should be created solely for this purpose, however, unless no other sources are available, and attempts should be made to locate alternative sources of stem cells that do not involve the destruction of embryos. It is permissible to procure EG cells from aborted fetuses, as long as safeguards are erected to prevent the therapeutic use of aborted fetal tissue from either increasing the frequency of abortion or encouraging a callous view of early human life. Moreover, although less restrictive Protestant views permit the procurement of stem cells from both proposed sources, this procurement must occur within a context of respect for nascent human life, only when significant benefit can be derived from it, and only after broad public discussion and acceptance of such research. If the general public is excluded from a discussion of this research, then public support of this and future beneficial research may be compromised. Furthermore, the requirement that all members of society have the opportunity to participate in open, sustained dialogue about these decisions is critical from this perspective, and if federal funds are to be allocated toward this research, conscientious objectors should be accommodated. Finally, most Protestants share previously articulated contextual concerns regarding 1) ensuring global access to the benefits of this research, 2) avoiding the negative consequences that might come with market-controlled research, and 3) assessing the priority of these research efforts relative to other current and pending health-related research projects.

Summary of Broad Areas of Agreement and Disagreement

Not surprisingly, the panelists did not reach unanimity on all aspects of human ES and EG cell research. Although some differences exist among the various religious traditions, these mostly concern the appropriate sources and methods of religious-ethical reasoning. On substantive issues, less restrictive individuals across most religious traditions appear to have more in common with each other than with restrictive members of their own faiths. (The same is true for commonalities among restrictive members of all faiths.) The substantive issues relevant to stem cell research on which there is internal disagreement include the following:

1) *The moral status of the embryo.* The perceived status of the embryo ranges from full moral personhood with correlative inviolable rights to life to an early, extracorporeal biological entity lacking any significant moral status. Between these poles, although the embryo tends to be viewed as valuable because of its current status as a form of human life and its potential status as a person, it is ultimately, if tragically, subordinate to the health needs of actual persons.

2) *Whether the use of EG cells derived from aborted fetuses involves complicity with the perceived evil of abortion.* On one end of the spectrum is the view that many abortions are permissible. Thus, complicity with evil is either never or rarely a consideration. On the other end of the spectrum is the view that all deliberate abortions are immoral, and that any use of EG cells derived from aborted fetuses involves complicity. Those who take more moderate positions argue that even when

abortion is wrong, it is not wrong to use tissue that would otherwise be discarded, or that complicity can be avoided by erecting barriers between abortion and stem cell procurement, such as a prohibition of directed donation.

3) *Whether stem cell research should, ideally, be federally funded.* Some, based on their belief in the duty to heal, hold that stem cell research should proceed as quickly as possible (given certain conditions; see below), while others hold that any federal funding that enables immoral research is itself immoral and would involve conscientious citizens in complicity against their will. The moderate view holds that in the absence of agreement on such issues as the moral status of the embryo, conscientious objectors should be allowed to opt out of federal support for the research and that without any federal support, privatized human ES and EG cell research will make contextual goals such as distributive justice even more difficult to realize.

Despite these areas of disagreement, widespread consensus was reached both within and among the various religious traditions on several important issues in ES and EG cell research:

1) Stem cell research is not inherently immoral, and in fact has the potential to contribute important knowledge that can lead to therapies for certain diseases, provided that morally legitimate sources of cells are used (although this is defined differently), and provided that important contextual factors of justice and regulation are addressed. (See #3 below.)

2) If society chooses to embark upon federally funded ES and EG cell research, it must do so under conditions of respect for the humanity of the embryo. It would be preferable if there existed alternative sources of stem cells that did not involve the direct or indirect destruction of human life, and efforts should be made to identify such sources.

3) In order for the research to be morally permissible, several "background factors" must be in place, including:

- assurance of equitable access to the benefits of the research,

- appropriate prioritization of this research relative to other social needs,

- assurance that the research will be used to treat disease, not enhance humans,

- public education, discussion, and acceptance of human stem cell research, and

- public scrutiny, oversight, and regulation of the research.

4) Assuming that privately funded research will continue in this area, it is preferable that a public body — even one that is funded with tax dollars — be required by law to review all private sector research and to make this review part of the public record, despite the possibility that the connection between the government and ES and EG cell research may be perceived as legitimating research that some citizens will continue to consider immoral.

NOTES AND QUESTIONS

1. The full statements of each of the religious scholars who testified before the Commission are contained in the NBAC Report, *Ethical Issues In Human Stem Cell Research, Volume III, Religious Perspectives*, available at: http://bioethics. georgetown.edu/nbac/pubs.html. Another excellent summary of religious perspectives on stem cell research is contained in THE HUMAN EMBRYONIC STEM CELL DEBATE: SCIENCE, ETHICS, AND PUBLIC POLICY (Suzanne Holland, Karen Lebaqz, & Laurie Zoloth, eds., 2001).

2. *Religion and Public Policy.* What role, if any, should religion play in the formation of public policy? No doubt this is a question you have pondered in other law school classes, probably amid a variety of viewpoints from your fellow classmates. The National Bioethics Advisory Commission briefly considered this question, concluding, "Although it would be inappropriate for religious views to determine public policy in our country, such views are the products of long traditions of ethical reflection, and they often overlap with secular views." NBAC Report at 99. Based on this statement, do you believe NBAC considered the range of religious views on stem cell research in reaching its conclusions? Should NBAC have considered religion in forming its public policy recommendations?

3. *Feminist and Race Perspectives.* A person's perspective on the ethics of stem cell research may be influenced by factors either apart from or in addition to the individual's religious beliefs. Our gender or race may have a greater impact on shaping our world view than any other single influence in our lives. Suzanne Holland writes eloquently and persuasively about the role that gender and race will play in the ability of patients to access stem cell therapies in the future. She echoes the worries of many of the religious leaders cited above that the principle of distributive justice will not prevail in this niche area of health care, just as it has not prevailed in the overall provision of health care services in our country:

It is true that women, the poor, persons of color, and marginals could benefit from the regenerative medical therapies and drug therapies heralded by [embryonic stem] cell and [fetal] cell research, but it is not at all likely that they will be the ones who do benefit. Such therapies, when they are perfected, are likely to be cost-prohibited for all but the wealthy and the well-insured, assuming that insurance companies agree to such coverage, a big assumption in any case. The poor, who are largely female, and most persons of color will simply be marginalized from these therapies, even as is it possible that their eggs are commercialized downstream for profit.

Suzanne Holland, *Beyond the Embryo: A Feminist Appraisal of the Embryonic Stem Cell Debate*, in THE HUMAN EMBRYONIC STEM CELL DEBATE: SCIENCE, ETHICS, AND PUBLIC POLICY 83 (Suzanne Holland, Karen Lebaqz, & Laurie Zoloth, eds., 2001).

Professor Holland's final point about the commercialization of women's eggs is reminiscent of the debate over the propriety of a market in human gametes. (Recall our discussion of the benefits and burdens of a gamete market in Chapter 3, Section 3.) If the market for human eggs for reproductive purposes serves to commodify woman's attributes, measuring their value to society according to the physical characteristics rather than their inherent worth, will the expansion of the egg market for research purposes exacerbate or ameliorate the problem of commodification? Professor Holland observes that, at the very least, the market for women's eggs will be further stratified according to "preferred" physical characteristics. Caucasian Ivy League women will continue to garner higher sums for their eggs than their non-Caucasian, less well-educated counterparts when it comes to selling eggs to couples desiring to procreate using donor gametes. But a sub-market will also develop for research eggs, and this market is likely to pay less than the reproductive market because it will be less selective about the physical attributes of the egg donors. Again, poorer women and women of color who wish to participate in the research egg market will be paid less for their eggs than women who are selected for the reproductive market, further reinforcing the notion that a woman's value rests solely in her genes.

The concern about a secondary market in lower-priced eggs for research, as opposed to reproductive, purposes has not yet been realized because the market for research eggs barely exists. Many states explicitly ban payment to donors who provide gametes for research purposes. For example, in 2006 California lawmakers passed a law prohibiting payment to egg donors in excess of the amount of reimbursement of direct expenses incurred as a result of the procedure. The law further specifies that "[n]o human oocyte or embryo shall be acquired, sold, offered for sale, received, or otherwise transferred for valuable consideration for the purposes of medical research or development of medical therapies." Cal. Health & Safety Code § 125350. New York stands basically alone as a jurisdiction expressly permitting researchers to compensate egg donors on par with reproductive donors. In June 2009, the Empire State Stem Cell Board released a statement permitting compensation to women who donate oocytes for research purposes. The full report is available at: http://stemcell.ny.gov/news.html.

If compensation for donor research eggs does become a reality, a further area of concern is the "downstream commercialization" of human embryos, mentioned by Professor Holland above. If a woman agrees to donate an egg for research, and once fertilized that embryo produces a valuable and profitable cell line or medical therapy, the donor will receive no benefit from her donation other than the generalized benefit that every member of society may share as a healthier community. Should women who donate eggs and embryos be partnered, economically, with the biotechnology companies that develop biologic products from those donated human tissues? Certainly the biotech industry would answer in the negative. Would you? Is a modicum of profit-sharing an unreasonable demand for women to make? See *Moore v. Regents of the University of California*, 51 Cal. 3d 120, 271 Cal. Rptr. 146, 793 P.2d 479 (1990), *cert. denied*, 499 U.S. 936 (1991); *Greenberg v. Miami Children's Hospital Res. Inst.*, 264 F. Supp. 2d 1064 (S.D. Fla. 2003).

Chapter 10

HUMAN REPRODUCTIVE CLONING

The prospect of human cloning — creating an individual who has the identical genes as an existing person — soared from science fiction to reality with the birth of a single Scottish sheep. On February 23, 1997, it seemed that the world paused, if only for a moment, to reflect upon the future of the human species when Scottish scientists Ian Wilmut and Keith Campbell announced that they had orchestrated the birth of Dolly the sheep, the world's first cloned mammal. The manner of Dolly's conception ignited a worldwide debate about the glory and the tragedy of science, a debate that continues today. For many, Dolly was a shocking symbol of biotechnology raging out of control, warranting a swift and decisive halting of any further experimentation in the cloning arena before its inevitable spillover to the human race. For a smaller group, Dolly was a marvelous and long-awaited sign that a century-old inquiry into the possibility of asexual reproduction had yielded a tentative answer. For both groups, and for the myriad whose views land somewhere in between, the ensuing years since Dolly's birth have supplied sufficient fuel to ensure that the cloning fires will burn long into the future.[1]

We will view the cloning debate from three perspectives — the view from science, the view from politics, and the view from law. Though occasionally converging, these perspectives often operate independent of each other, provoking experts in each field to express concern about the rationale and motivation driving the other actors. Each perspective is worthy of review, and only a complete overview of the field will enable you to form your own view of human reproductive cloning.

SECTION I: THE SCIENCE OF HUMAN REPRODUCTIVE CLONING

The following statement is an essential starting point for any discussion about human reproductive cloning: As of the publication date of this book, there is no evidence that a human being has ever been born using cloning technology. Despite occasional claims that a cloned baby has been born, or that women have been successfully impregnated with cloned embryos, no proof of these claims has ever

---

[1] Drs. Wilmut and Campbell hail from the Roslin Institute in Edinburgh, Scotland, where they announced Dolly's unique birth to the public. Dolly, a Finn Dorset sheep, was born on July 5, 1996. The Scottish scientists revealed the technical aspects of their work in the peer-review journal Nature. See Ian Wilmut, et al., *Viable Offspring Derived from Fetal and Adult Mammalian Cells*, 385 Nature 810 (1997). The activity surrounding Dolly's birth, and premature death in 2003, are described in Judith F. Daar, *The Prospect of Human Cloning: Improving Nature or Dooming the Species?*, 33 Seton Hall L. Rev. 511 (2003).

been presented to the public.[2] That said, is it possible that someday a cloned human being will be born? Yes, it is possible, though scientists working in the area express profound skepticism that the technology to clone a human being will be perfected anytime soon. More on this in a moment. For now, let's learn the basic steps in the cloning process.

A. Three Types of Cloning

The word "clone" derives from the Greek word "klon," meaning twig, and refers to a twig that can give rise to an identical tree. Cloning is a scientific method in which the genome of an organism can be replicated. Though the technique is most often associated with reproduction — the creation of a human being who is genetically identical to an existing person — cloning is a broader concept not limited to use in reproduction. According to the American Society for Reproductive Medicine, the following three techniques are currently referred to as cloning: 1) reproductive cloning, 2) therapeutic cloning, and 3) embryonic cloning. *See* Michael R. Soules, *The President's Message: Cloning*, 35:1 ASRM News 3 (2001). The techniques associated with each are described below.

1. Reproductive Cloning

Reproductive cloning is a form of reproduction in which offspring result not from the union of egg and sperm (sexual reproduction) but from the replication of the genetic makeup of another single individual (asexual reproduction). See The President's Council on Bioethics, Human Cloning and Human Dignity, xxiv (2002), at www.bioethics.georgetown.edu. Reproductive cloning involves somatic cell nuclear transfer (SCNT). Using SCNT, the nucleus is removed from an unfertilized human egg. The nucleus is in the center of the egg cell and contains the genetic material (chromosomes) that direct the genetic characteristics of human beings. The egg is procured in the same way that eggs are retrieved from women undergoing IVF, or women agreeing to donate eggs to infertile couples — through surgical retrieval from the ovaries.

Once the nucleus is removed from the egg, it is replaced by a nucleus of a somatic (non-sex) cell of the human to be cloned. The somatic cell can be any cell in the body, such as a skin cell or a blood cell. The gametes (egg and sperm) cannot be used to create a cloned human being because they contain only 23 chromosomes, as opposed to the 46 chromosomes (organized into 23 pairs) that are necessary to form a human

---

[2] The most notorious cloning claimants are members of a group called Clonaid, a private company affiliated with the Raelian religious sect. Raelian doctrine teaches that space travelers created the human race by cloning. Among other things, Raelians believe cloning is the path to eternal life, transferring memories and consciousness from one copy to the next. Clonaid and the Raelians enjoyed their 15 minutes of fame in December 2002 when they announced the birth of the world's first human clone. The baby, nicknamed Eve, was alleged to have been born outside the U.S. to American parents. See Dana Canedy & Kenneth Chang, *Group Says Human Clone Was Born to an American*, N.Y. Times, Dec. 28, 2002, at A16. Even after failing to produce any proof of the baby's birth, Clonaid continues to announce the birth of clones, today boasting on its website, www.clonaid.com, "We are the world's leading provider of reproductive human cloning services . . . [W]e've been able to help a number of patients have their own children through our cloning technology very happy that we have been able to give birth successfully to five clone babies." No proof, not even a baby picture, supports these claims.

being. After the somatic cell nucleus is placed into the enucleated egg, a chemical or an electrical pulse is applied to the egg to activate it, much the way a sperm activates an egg by penetrating its surface in the course of natural fertilization. Thereafter, the egg develops into an embryo that can be implanted into the uterus of a woman who would carry the pregnancy to term.[3] Note that reproductive cloning differs from natural, or sexual, reproduction in that the offspring have the identical genetic make-up of the cell donor, rather than a mixture of two genomes from the male and female gamete providers. For more information on SCNT, *see* George E. Siedel, Jr., *Cloning Mammals: Methods, Applications, and Characteristics of Cloned Animals*, in HUMAN CLONING 28-31 (Barbara MacKinnon, ed., 2000).

Dolly the sheep was the first mammal to be born using SCNT, but her birth came 60 years after scientists first began to contemplate reproduction in this fashion. Experimentation in the field of reproductive cloning dates back to the 1930s when researchers attempted to clone a vertebrate. In the 1950s and 1960s, cloning efforts focused on amphibia, with some successes achieved using frog eggs. In 1975, scientists succeeded in cloning frogs, producing tadpoles after transferring cell nuclei from adult frogs. See *Significant Events in the History of Cloning*, 15:3 TRANSPLANT NEWS, Feb. 14, 2005. In the 1970s scientists began to experiment with mammals, but it would take until 1997 for the first cloned mammal to appear on the world scene.

2.   Therapeutic Cloning

Therapeutic cloning is discussed in Chapter 9 in connection with human embryonic stem cell research. The process begins with the same steps as reproductive cloning, but stops short of implanting the derived embryo into a woman's uterus for gestational purposes. Instead, the embryo is grown to the blastocyst state, at about five days post-fertilization. The blastocyst is composed of an inner cell mass and a trophectoderm, which is an outer layer of cells destined to become part of the placenta. The inner cell mass consists of embryonic stem cells, which researchers believe can be extracted, coaxed to differentiate into any number of cells in the human body, and then transplanted back into a human body where they can repair or replace diseased or missing cells. The potential medical benefit of therapeutic cloning rests in its ability to create tissue from stem cells which are genetically identical to the person/patient who donated the cell from which the nucleus was derived. It is speculated that tissues created by therapeutic cloning would not be rejected by a patient's immune system because they will be recognized as compatible with the donor's own tissue. See James A. Thomson, *Human*

---

[3] Once the cloned embryo implants in a woman's uterus, it will develop like any other embryo. One author cautions that this part of the cloning process is lost on many people, causing great misconceptions to arise. "Cloning has been described as 'more frightening than weapons of mass destruction.' However, cloning does not result in the immediate creation of a fully grown adult. A cloned being is formed by the same process as every other naturally occurring living thing. It starts as a cell which becomes an embryo, which grows into a fetus, and then is born as a baby. Cloning does not result in the mass production of genetically identical human beings who will become successively more flawed, as with a Xerox copy. Any embryos resulting from cloning must be implanted in a woman's uterus and carried to term one at a time." Yuriko Mary Shikai, *Don't Be Swept Away By The Mass Hysteria: The Benefits of Human Reproductive Cloning and Its Future*, 33 Southwestern U. L. Rev. 259, 273 (2004).

Embryonic Stem Cells, in THE HUMAN EMBRYONIC STEM CELL DEBATE, 15-16 (Suzanne Holland et al., eds., 2001).

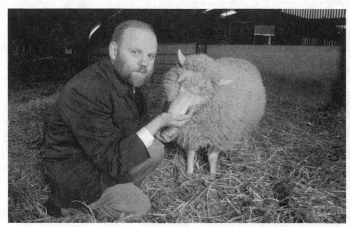

Dr. Ian Wilmut with Dolly, February 26, 1997

The inroads and controversies surrounding therapeutic cloning are discussed in Chapter 9, but it takes little piercing analysis to understand that foes of reproductive cloning may also oppose therapeutic cloning because it involves the creation of an "unnatural" embryo, and then requires destruction of that embryo in order for the stem cells to be harvested. *See* The President's Council on Bioethics, *Human Cloning and Human Dignity*, xxxv-xxxvi (2002) (summarizing the majority position of the Council recommending a ban on reproductive cloning and a four-year moratorium on therapeutic cloning). Conversely, some who oppose reproductive cloning are in favor of therapeutic cloning because the latter promotes medical cures and therapies without birthing a child who may be harmed by the cloning process. *See* National Bioethics Advisory Commission, Cloning Human Beings, iv (1997) (recommending legislation to prohibit reproductive cloning, so long as it does not interfere with biomedical advances such as stem cell research).

3. Embryo Cloning

Embryonic cloning, sometimes called embryo splitting, begins with an embryo formed the old-fashioned way, by a single sperm penetrating a single egg to form a human embryo. This embryo would have the same random mixing of genes from the male and female progenitor as any existing person. To clone the embryo, the cells or blastomeres of the early embryo are then separated and the nucleus from each of these blastomeres is removed and reinjected into an enucleated egg. Just as in SCNT, the new egg is prompted to develop into an embryo. Embryo cloning thus produces a finite number of genetically identical offspring, each having the same genome as the original embryo. Unlike reproductive or therapeutic cloning, embryonic cloning does not involve replicating an existing organism, but rather creates multiple offspring from the donors' combined DNA. Embryo cloning can be used, for example, if a couple has limited gametes and wants to maximize their chance for a successful pregnancy by creating multiple embryos. For more information on embryo cloning, *see* George E. Siedel, Jr., *Cloning Mammals:*

Methods, Applications, and Characteristics of Cloned Animals, in HUMAN CLONING 24-28 (Barbara MacKinnon ed., 2000).

The potential practice of embryo cloning raised a public stir in 1993 when researchers at George Washington University revealed at a meeting of the American Fertility Society that they had succeeding in splitting cells from 17 embryos and growing them into 48 new embryos, with the cloned embryos reaching between the 4- and 32-celled stage before they all died. The GWU researchers used abnormal embryos that would not have progressed to a fully formed child so as not to evoke concern that they had destroyed viable human life. But evoke they did. The university investigated the researchers when it was discovered they had failed to seek permission from the GWU institutional review board prior to conducting the research. Following the investigation, the researchers were disciplined and instructed to destroy their data. The university also voluntarily forwarded the records of the incident to the Office for Protection from Research Risks at the National Institutes of Health. The matter seemed to reach a frenzied end in 1994 when one of the researchers resigned his post at the university. *See* Ruth Macklin, *Cloning Without Prior Approval: A Response to Recent Disclosures of Noncompliance*, 5 KENNEDY INST. ETHICS J. 57 (1995).

B.   Advances in Animal Cloning

Successes and failures in animal cloning many serve as a precursor to the eventual introduction of human cloning, particularly if scientists are able to clone our closest neighbors in the animal kingdom. To date, the list of animals that have been successfully cloned using SCNT sits at around a dozen — the group of cloned animals includes sheep, rabbits, cattle, goats, mice, pigs, cats, horses, mules, deer, water buffalo and dogs. In addition, researchers at the Oregon Health & Sciences University in Portland have announced progress toward achieving a milestone in animal cloning, the cloning of a monkey. In November 2007, a team of OHSU scientists announced they succeeded in cloning monkey embryos, though none of the embryos were implanted for gestation. *See* Rick Weiss, *Monkey Embryos Cloned for Stem Cells*, WASH. POST, Nov. 15, 2007. Several years earlier, these same researchers announced using embryo splitting to form four genetically identical embryos by "splitting" a single eight-celled embryo (formed with sperm and egg, not by SCNT). A female monkey named Tetra was born of this advancement. *See* Sarah Ramsey, *Embryo Splitting Produces Primate "Clone,"* 355 THE LANCET 205 (2000).

Progress in the cloning of multiple animal species may seem a logical and necessary step in the march toward human cloning, but the results and reactions to animal cloning have stirred rather than quelled concerns over the prospect of human cloning. In the years since the announcement of Dolly's birth, reports on the safety and efficacy of animal cloning have ranged from "the health of clones is no different from that of non-clones" to "every clone is genetically and physically defective." Finding the reality amid these vastly diverging reports is a challenge, one complicated by the fact that the science continues to evolve daily.

1. Safety and Efficacy Concerns

If we are to be convinced that reproductive cloning will not wreak havoc on the human species, we might want proof that cloning in the animal world is both safe and effective. If cloning proves as good a method of animal reproduction as other forms of assisted conception, such as AID and IVF, then its introduction as an option for nonhuman procreation may invite less controversy than currently surrounds the technique. While studies on animal cloning are ongoing, we can look at a few of the myriad published reports to help us gauge the status of the emerging science.

In terms of cloning efficacy, it is fair to say that Dolly is not a model of reproductive efficiency. The facts surrounding Dolly's birth are now well-known. Dolly was the only sheep to survive the 277 attempts at SCNT, a ratio which far exceeds the number of live animal births using other forms of assisted conception. Dr. Wilmut reported that he and his colleagues made 277 attempts to fuse an adult sheep mammary gland nucleus with an enucleated oocyte and activate the egg to begin cell division. Of these attempts, 29 embryos reached the blastocyst stage (11 percent) and only 1 of 29 (3 percent) blastocysts transferred resulted in a live birth.

The statistics surrounding animal cloning are constantly in flux at this early stage. Some recent reports suggest that the success rates in cloning animals are between one and five percent, meaning that up to 99 percent of cloned animals do not survive birth. *See* Michele Grygotis, *Researchers Find Cloned Mice Prone to Obesity in Adulthood, Have Shortened Lifespans, Genetic Engineering Research,* 12 TRANSPLANT NEWS, Mar. 31, 2001. Other researchers report much higher overall survival rates. For example, animal researchers at the University of Georgia report that 14.3% of cloned bovine embryos developed into healthy, normal animals. See Rebecca McCarthy, *UGA Clones Calf From Dead Animal,* ATLANTA J. & CONSTIT., Apr. 26, 2002, at 1A. By comparison, it is estimated that about two-thirds of all human embryos that develop from the union of the sperm and the egg are in some way defective, meaning that the embryos never implant or perish very early in development. *See* Howard W. Jones & Lucinda Veeck, *What Is An Embryo?,* 77 FERTILITY & STERILITY 658 (2002) (reprinted in Chapter 1).

More worrisome than the ratio of cloning attempt to live birth are the health problems that seem to have plagued at least the first generations of cloned animals. Again, the data is somewhat conflicting. The most striking example of the poor health of cloned animals is Dolly herself. The newsmaking sheep died from lung disease on February 13, 2003 at the age of six and a half. A sheep's normal lifespan is about 12 years, thus Dolly's early death could have been related to the manner of her conception. Other signs of cloning-related health problems are discussed in several retrospective reports which list defects occurring regularly in cloned animals. Health related problems include gigantism (excessive size) in cloned sheep and cattle, placentas up to four times the normal size in mice, and heart defects in pigs. Researchers at the University of Cincinnati reported that cloned mice became obese after three weeks and grew to nearly three times larger than normal mice as they aged. See Grygotis, *supra.* Other experiments with cloned mice found damaged immune systems, spontaneous abortions, abnormal births, and premature deaths. *Id.*

Researchers who report these clinical findings on cloned animals are generally unsure why these defects occur. One theory holds that cloned animals have shortened telomeres, the bits of genetic material at the tips of chromosomes that wear down each time a cell divides. Shorter than normal telomeres essentially means that cells start out older and may die off sooner, possibly translating into a shorter lifespan for the cloned animal. Other researchers speculate that cloning problems are due to inadequate or inappropriate "reprogramming" of genes during the process of injecting DNA into an enucleated egg. Still others believe that the cloning process can turn any gene on or off at random with an unpredictable and potentially devastating impact on the health of the cloned animal. *See Health Dangers of the Human Clones*, DAILY MAIL, Apr. 29, 2002, at 33.

On the other end of the spectrum, reports that cloned animals are as healthy as their naturally conceived counterparts abound. To begin, the sheer number of successfully cloned species indicates the rapid progress of animal cloning research. But more persuasively, some cloning scientists have reported on the overall good health of cloned animals. In a study published in the prestigious journal *Science*, researchers compared cloned cows to cows conceived through artificial insemination and found no difference in their health status. *See* Robert Lanza, *Cloned Cattle Can Be Healthy and Normal*, 294 SCIENCE 1893 (2001). In addition, a 2002 survey of all cloned live-born animals concluded that the majority remained healthy. Moreover, the survey found that the health of the natural offspring of cloned animals is no different from non-cloned animal offspring. *See* Alan Coleman, *Comment & Analysis: Letters: Dolly, The Media Hog*, THE GUARDIAN, Apr. 24, 2002, at 17. A 2008 study by the U.S. Food & Drug Administration on animal cloning concluded, "cloning poses no unique risks to animal health, compared to the risks found with other reproduction methods, including natural mating." U.S. Food & Drug Administration, Animal Cloning and Food Safety (Jan. 2008), available at: www.fda.gov.

In terms of clones reproducing, Dolly herself became a mother in April 1998 when she gave birth to Bonnie, a lamb conceived "the old-fashioned way" with a mountain ram named David. In 1999, Dolly gave birth again, this time to triplets, and in 2000 she bore twins, with no complications reported for any of these offspring. In 2002, French researchers announced the birth of healthy rabbit clones. The rabbits had been born a year earlier, but researchers delayed announcing the births until the rabbits started to reproduce normally. In announcing the cloning achievement, researchers assured the public that "the animals were mature and their good health certain." See David Brown, *A Big Hop Forward: Rabbits Cloned; Research Promise Seen In Second Lab Animal to be Replicated*, WASH. POST, Mar. 30, 2002, at A1. And in a move that was literally suitable for the Guinness Book of World Records, a team of Japanese and American scientists succeeded in the feat of serial cloning a prized bull. Kamitakafuku, a 17-year-old Japanese bull that has been used to inseminate more than 350,000 cows, was cloned in 1998, an event celebrated by inclusion in the famous records book. Another record emerged in 2001 when one of Kamitakafuku's clones was himself cloned, producing a clone of a clone. By all accounts, all the bulls are healthy and enjoying their notoriety. See C. Kubota et al., *Serial Bull Cloning By Somatic Cell Nuclear Transfer*, NATURE BIOTECHNOLOGY, May 23, 2004.

2. Purposes of Animal Cloning

Whether the secrets of human cloning are bound up in the animal world remains to be seen, but even in the absence of such a link, the ability to replicate animals possesses its own independent merit. The purposes of animal cloning run the gamut from providing life-saving therapies for humans to reproducing a cherished pet. As you hear each stated purpose, consider whether the same regulations that prohibit human cloning for its potential menacing effect on society should apply likewise to cloning animals.

Cloned animals are used in medical and scientific research aimed at producing therapies and cures for human ailments. For example, researchers at the Roslin Institute in Scotland, the center that produced Dolly, use cloned sheep and other large animals to produce medicines in the milk of such animals. These researchers have succeeded in transferring human genes that produce useful proteins into sheep and cows, who in turn can produce substances such as a blood clotting agent to treat hemophilia and an agent used to treat cystic fibrosis and other lung conditions. Animal cloning has also been used to develop organs for possible transplantation into humans. Though still in the development stage, researchers hope to combine genetic techniques with cloning to someday produce solid organs that can be transplanted into humans whose organs are failing. This research, however, will not proceed at the Roslin Institute. In December 2011, the Scottish concern announced that it would not longer undertake research relating to the cloning of animals. One reason? Its lead researcher, Ian Wilmut, moved on to another institution — but not before being knighted by Queen Elizabeth II in 2008.

Animal cloning has also been used to protect, and even resurrect, endangered or extinct species. In March 2005, scientists in Chile announced a plan to clone the huemul, a native endangered species of the deer family. The stag is a national symbol which has become endangered due to excessive hunting. And in a move reminiscent of *Jurassic Park*, in 2002 Australian researchers announced plans to clone an extinct Tasmanian tiger. Declared extinct in 1936, the tiger's DNA had been successfully replicated using DNA from a preserved pup specimen. *See Researchers Announce Plans to Clone Extinct Tasmanian Tiger*, CHANNEL NEWS ASIA, May 28, 2002. Query the human benefit to such an attempt. The animal was hardly a beloved species — it was hunted as vermin for attacking sheep, garnering a bounty for every carcass produced. Alas, sheep worldwide baahed a sigh of relief when the tiger project was dropped in 2005 due to the poor quality of the DNA.

Human consumption of animal products has fed the market for animal cloning, while at the same time stirring debate about the ethical treatment of animals. Cattle ranchers are optimistic that cloning technology will give rise to large herds of cows capable of producing meat with heritable traits such as tenderness and marbling. But animal rights activists have rallied against animal cloning because of its potential to impose suffering on animals, by birthing offspring that are unhealthy or fail to survive the neonatal period. In the early 2000s, health activists expressed concern about animal cloning, asking the U.S. Food and Drug Administration to ban the sale of products derived from cloned animals. Despite evidence that meat and milk from cloned animals are essentially identical to that from naturally reproduced animals, in an abundance of caution the FDA asked the food industry to keep products from cloned animals out of the food chain while it studied their safety. *See Milk and Meat of Clones Seem Safe, Study Says,* N.Y. TIMES, April 12, 2005, at F2. In January 2008, the FDA issued its report confirming the safety of food products from cloned animals. Specifically, the federal agency found that "the composition of food products from cattle, swine, and goat clones, or the offspring of any animal clones, is no different from that of conventionally bred animals. Because of the preceding . . . there are no additional risks to people eating food from cattle, swine, and goat clones or the offspring of any animal clones traditionally consumed as food." Accordingly, the FDA concluded that food labels do not have to state if food is from animal clones or their offspring. *See* U.S. Food & Drug Administration, Animal Cloning and Food Safety (Jan. 2008), available at: www.fda.gov.

Perhaps the most hotly debated use of animal cloning is the revivification of a lost pet. Pet cloning was first contemplated in December 2001 when California-based Genetic Savings & Clone (GSC) teamed with researchers at Texas A&M University to clone a cat, appropriately named "cc" for "copycat." After "cc" was found to be healthy, even mugging it for the 2003 International Cat Show in Houston, GSC announced that it was open for business. For a mere $50,000, cat owners could be the first to own a clone of their beloved Whiskers or Friskey. In December 2004 the company delivered its first pet clone, proudly handing Little Nicky to a Texas woman who had mourned the death of her longtime feline companion Nicky. See *First Cloned-to-Order Cat Sold in U.S.,* BIRMINGHAM POST, Dec. 24, 2004, at 6. But in what became a sign of its economic woes, GSC reduced the price for a cat clone to $32,000 in 2005. Despite this bargain basement offer, there were few takers and GSC closed its doors at the end of 2006. Dog cloning, first described in 2007 by South Korean researchers, has also failed to attract a large market for the service. One reason could be the $100,000 price tag or the fact that cloned pets often do not look exactly like their "parent" owing to the influence of the gestational mother's uterine environment or the mitochondrial DNA contained in the enucleated egg used in the process. *See* Dan Harris, *Cloning Fido: South Korean's Dog Cloning Industry Raises Ethical Red Flags,* available at: http://abcnews.go.com/ Technology/south-koreas-dog-cloning-industry-raises-ethical-red/story?id= 15309415.

C.   Inroads Into Human Cloning

To reiterate what we learned at the outset of this chapter, there is no evidence that a human being has been born using cloning technology. Further, there is no evidence that a viable human embryo that could become a human being has ever been created using cloning technology. The field was much in the news and undoubtedly tarnished in 2006 when it was revealed that scientific reports of the world's first cloned human embryos were entirely fraudulent. As discussed in Chapter 9, in 2004 and 2005 South Korean researchers reported creating embryos and then deriving patient-specific stem cell lines using somatic cell nuclear transfer. The reports boasted that researchers had successfully transferred a living person's DNA into a hollowed-out egg and coaxed the egg to become an embryo that bore the identical genome to its DNA donor. If the embryo remained viable, it could have been implanted into a woman's uterus to produce the world's first human cloning. Once the reports were revealed as total fabrication, much suspicion hovered over the field. Today, the scientific literature suggests the closest we have come to human cloning is the ability to transfer the DNA-containing nucleus of a human cell into an enucleated egg and "reprogram" the egg to revert back to its embryonic state. These reprogrammed embryos seemed to display qualities similar to embryos formed when egg and sperm combine, but much work lies ahead before any clinical applications can be realized. *See* Young Chung et al., *Reprogramming of Human Somatic Cells Using Human and Animal Oocytes*, 11(2) CLONING AND STEM CELLS 213 (2009).

The prospect of human cloning generates strong public opinion, overwhelmingly on the negative side. Since the birth of Dolly, when we began to contemplate a world in which cloned human beings roamed the earth, editorial pages and scientific journals have brimmed with commentary about the evils of cloning, often conjuring up images of "hordes of Hitlers" or other dreaded historical figures returning to inflict even greater misery on human kind.[4] Public opinion polls consistently show that folks are strongly opposed to human cloning. In a November 2001 Gallup Poll, 88% of respondents said they oppose "cloning that is designed specifically to result in the birth of a human being," while only 9% approved such activity. *See* American Enterprise Institute for Public Policy Research, No. 2, vol. 13, at 60 (Mar. 1, 2002). A more recent poll shows little change. In 2010, 88% of American adults pegged human cloning as "morally wrong" while a mere 9% found it "morally acceptable." The survey is available at: http://www.gallup.com/poll/6028/cloning.aspx.

Why are humans so united in opposition to reproductive cloning? The next excerpts explore the potential benefits and harms that cloning could bring to cloned children, to their parents, and to society at large. As you read these proffered rationales for exploring or shunning scientific research into human cloning, keep in mind that any assessment of the practice's effect on society is entirely speculative. Since we do not yet know how a cloned child would look or act, our fears and our hopes are based on what we believe a cloning world would be like.

---

[4] "Scenarios of human cloning, propagated by fictional literature and popular culture, have engendered fear and loathing in the hearts of its surveyors. One particularly nefarious account is told in Ira Levin's The Boys From Brazil, in which Nazi escapees succeed in cloning multiple human versions of the twentieth century's most dreaded individual — Adolph Hitler. . . . The plot involved placement of ninety-four neonate Hitler clones into adoptive homes that roughly resembled the Fuhrer's own family situation. As each clone neared the age of fourteen, his father was to die, as did Hitler's own father at that time, so as to provide a near identical environment in which the clones could reach their diabolical potential. At one point in the novel, a biology professor explains the technique of human cloning to the protagonist Nazi hunter, remarking, "What planned society could resist the idea?" See Judith F. Daar, *The Future of Human Cloning: Prescient Lessons From Medical Ethics Past*, 8 So. Cal. Interdisciplinary L. J. 167 (1998) (citing several of the numerous commentaries predicting doom should a human being be conceived through cloning).

Judith F. Daar
The Prospect of Human Cloning: Improving Nature or Dooming the Species?
33 Seton Hall L. Rev. 511, 527-535 (2003)

Much has been written about the potential good and bad consequences that cloning portends, thus what follows is a brief overview of the anticipated consequences of human SCNT.

[a. Possible Benefits of Reproductive Cloning]

Identifying the possible benefits of cloning is the first step. If cloning proves a safe and effective method of reproduction, it could aid couples and individuals in several ways. Couples who are refractory to current infertility treatment would be able to have a genetically related child through cloning. For example, couples in which both the male and female lack gametes are unable to produce a child without the aid of gamete donors. Cloning would allow such a couple to experience the joys of parenting a child whose genes derive from one member of the pair. In this capacity, cloning would join a growing spectrum of assisted reproductive technologies that currently aids tens of thousands of individuals in realizing their dreams of parenthood. Because of its complexity and likely expense, it would serve as a last resort for most couples who desire to parent a genetically-related child, but nevertheless it would likely bring tremendous happiness to those couples who successfully avail themselves of the technique.

In addition to aiding infertile couples, cloning could also be used to avoid transmission of deleterious genetic traits to offspring. In light of our growing familiarity with genetically-based disease processes, we are increasingly aware that the key to maintaining our health lies more in the past than it does in the future. The Human Genome Project has revealed the genetic bases of many diseases and is now beginning to pinpoint the exact location of genes thought to be responsible for these ailments.[5] If a couple is aware that one member is a carrier for a genetically-linked disease, cloning may be a sure way to avoid passing that gene to the couple's offspring. As with infertility treatment, cloning may not necessarily be the first choice for a couple in this position, as current technologies offer numerous alternatives to prospective parents wishing to avoid deleterious gene transmission. In addition to the use of donor gametes, couples can use preimplantation genetic diagnosis (PGD) to learn about the health of their embryos before they are implanted into the uterus. Using PGD, the couple can select for implantation only the unaffected embryos in an effort to maximize the health of their child. Cloning, however, may be more attractive to couples wishing to avoid deleterious gene transmission because it does not involve the deliberate destruction of affected embryos. In the end, cloning could benefit those couples who wish to avoid passing on one partner's genome because of its health implications.

A third possible benefit of cloning would be to assist single individuals and same sex couples in their efforts to reproduce. These prospective parents may wish to

---

[5] The Human Genome Project is discussed in Chapter 4. -Ed.

procreate without the aid and potential entanglement of gamete donors. For single individuals and same sex couples wishing to parent a genetically-related child, cloning offers benefits that are unmatched by current reproductive technologies. For this group, the use of donor gametes may be particularly unattractive because of its potential to raise parentage issues. Lesbian couples that use artificial insemination by donor (AID) risk sperm donors' paternity claims once the child is born. In some cases, courts uphold these claims, warning that AID donors relinquish their parental rights only if the recipient woman follows a statutory protocol surrounding the insemination. Single and gay men also face claims by egg donors and genetic surrogates whose link to the child may also entitle them to parental rights. Cloning may alleviate some of these worries by eliminating gamete donors from the procreation equation.

Another beneficial use of cloning would be to aid parents who have suffered the loss of a child. This use would require that parents preserve some number of cells from their child, either before the child dies or even shortly after death.[6] Of course, the cloned child would not be the same human being as the deceased child, but his or her genetic similarity to the passed sibling may provide enormous solace to the parents. In fact, reproductive cloning to respond to the loss of a child has motivated couples to support underground cloning efforts in the United States. Clearly, these parents believe that cloning would be a benefit to them. Critics wonder, however, whether the cloned child, even if born healthy, would benefit from conception in this manner and under these circumstances. Would the parents harbor unrealistic expectations of the child that would negatively impact that child's life? . . .

In summary, at least four groups could reap benefits from reproductive cloning: infertile couples refractory to treatment with other assisted reproductive technologies; couples wishing to assure avoidance of a deleterious genetic trait; single and same sex couples who eschew the use of gamete donors, but who wish to have a child that is genetically related to them; and parents who wish to clone a deceased child. These individuals would argue that cloning is uniquely capable of providing them the parenting opportunities they seek. A ban on cloning would significantly harm these individuals because there are no alternatives that fulfill their specific desires. The overall utility of cloning, however, can only be evaluated by weighing both benefits and harms. The next section explores some of the counterbalancing perceived harms of reproductive cloning.

b. Possible Harms of Reproductive Cloning

. . . First, and perhaps most importantly, there are tremendous concerns over the safety and efficacy of human cloning. To date, despite claims to the contrary we have seen no evidence of any human being conceived through SCNT. As a result, we do not know what that process would yield in the human reproductive setting. Moreover, animal studies reveal that in some cases the cloned offspring suffer from

---

[6] [n.80] The idea of post-mortem reproductive cloning is no longer strictly a science fiction idea. In 2001, scientists announced that they had successfully cloned a calf from a cow that had been dead for 48 hours. Using a cooling method, the cow's cells were removed two days after death and then the nuclei were extracted and injected into enucleated egg cells. See Rebecca McCarthy, *UGA Clones Calf from Dead Animal*, Atlanta J. & Const., Apr. 26, 2002, at 1A.

health problems related to structural and functional abnormalities. While we do not yet know how the data collected on animals will translate to the human population, at the very least we know that the safety of human cloning is not assured. Of course, the safety of reproduction in any form is never certain, but at least with existing technologies we are familiar with the risk profiles associated with each technique.

A second harm often cited is the threat cloning poses to the individuality of the cloned child. The worry is that society would view the child as a mere replica of the cell donor and, therefore, undervalue the child's unique selfhood. Whatever talents or idiosyncrasies attached to the donor would be expected of the child, with no care paid to allowing the child to develop an individualized personality. Parents might expect the child to make the same life choices made by the cell donor and might mete out severe repercussions if the child fails to satisfy these expectations.[7] On a grander scale, cloning might threaten the individuality of the human race. If cloning becomes widespread, it would reduce the number of unique genomes born in our world, creating classification of persons according to the perceived worth of their genes. We would cease valuing individuality and instead fixate on the predetermined genetic destiny attached to the cloned person.

An oft-cited response to concerns about individuality is that a clone would be born as an infant in a different familial setting and in a different historical time frame. Unique circumstances and events would shape the child's life, as cloning certainly does not expose the child to the formative environment of the cell donor. The child's future would be as open as any naturally conceived child, both of whom may have parents who harbor great expectations for their children. A parent's expectations for his or her child would probably not change in a cloning scenario, as expectations are often based on the parent's own accomplishments and failures. Whether those accomplishments and failures derive from one genome or two would not likely alter parents' attitudes toward their children. Moreover, concerns that the same genetic diseases plaguing the cell donor will also affect the clone are not necessarily well-founded. Advances in genetic diagnosis and gene therapy have progressed at a rapid pace in the past ten years and are predicted to accelerate with each passing day. We have learned much about the genetic bases of certain diseases, such as coronary artery disease and hypertension, which are diseases that are highly responsive to newly developed therapies and studied lifestyle changes. Since many gene-linked diseases do not develop until adulthood, a cloned child could reasonably assume that a treatment for his or her particular disease would be available when needed.

A third harm expressed about cloning is the threat of commodification of children. If and when cloning becomes available for reproduction, it will likely enter

---

[7] [n.90] One author has labeled this phenomenon as depriving a child of "a right to an open future." See Joel Feinberg, *The Child's Right to An Open Future*, in Whose Child? Children's Rights, Parental Authority, and State Power 124 (W. Aiken & H. LaFollette eds., 1980); see also Dena S. Davis, *Genetic Dilemmas and the Child's Right to an Open Future*, 28 Rutgers L.J. 549 (1997). This argument rests on a notion of genetic determinism, that one's genome determines one's future. A child with a duplicated genome would lack the opportunity to determine his or her own future, or at the very least would be aware of the life choices and life struggles that afflicted the cell donor. This knowledge alone would limit the "open future" for cloned individuals who might be herded into the same life path followed by their predecessors.

the market at an extraordinarily high price. The expenses surrounding human cloning are already a topic of discussion, and these costs are out of reach for the vast majority of prospective parents.[8] For those few wealthy individuals who do avail themselves of the emerging technology, there is concern that they will treat their cloned children as commodities, rather than as individual human beings, because their births were orchestrated at an enormous financial cost. Parents, it is argued, will expect a return on their investment much in the way any investor seeks profit, and thus will be intolerant of any perceived imperfection in their "product."

It may be worth noting that similar concerns have been raised over other reproductive scenarios. These include surrogate parenting arrangements in which a woman is paid to gestate another couple's embryo, and the creation of embryos using donor gametes in which prospective parents pay for gametes that meet their specifications. Both of these arrangements involve the expenditure of significant funds, as does the use of assisted reproductive technologies in general. The average cost for a single treatment using in vitro fertilization and embryo transfer is between $8,000 and $10,500, as compared to the absence of expenses associated with natural conception. Yet nearly two decades of experience with collaborative and assisted reproduction, a process in which couples often spend their life savings in pursuit of parenthood, have not yielded a study showing that these parents regard their children as commodities. In fact, psychological profiles conducted on the children of assisted reproduction show they are no different from their naturally conceived counterparts.

A final harm worthy of inclusion is the prediction that cloning will advance eugenics in our society. Opponents postulate that through cloning it will be possible to develop both super- and sub-human individuals to meet society's needs, creating a class system beyond any naturally occurring division among the people of the world. The clear distinctions among individuals will lead us to revere and shun certain genotypes, perhaps ultimately leading to the enslavement or destruction of the lesser class.[9] What is so very sad about this Doomsday scenario is that history has proven that we do not need cloning to practice eugenics in our society. The examples abound, including the Holocaust in World War II Germany, ethnic cleansing in the former Yugoslavia in the late 1990s, and the implementation of forced sterilization statutes to weed out "mental defectives" from American society in the 1920s. Justice Holmes' words of seventy-five years ago still ring eerily from his opinion in *Buck v. Bell*, when the Court upheld a Virginia statute allowing involuntary sterilization of mental defectives because "three generations of imbeciles are enough."

Sadly, ordinary conception has already produced men capable of ferocious inhumanity unaided by any reproductive technology. Cloning will likely not provide

---

[8] [n.94] See James A. Haught & Tara Tuckwiller, *Cloning Effort Hidden in West Virginia Town; Father Wanted to Duplicate Dead Son*, Wash. Times, Aug. 14, 2001, at A1 (reporting payment of $500,000 by a Charleston lawyer to a cloning group to clone his dead son).

[9] [n.99] See George J. Annas et al., *Protecting the Endangered Human: Toward an International Treaty Prohibiting Cloning and Inheritable Alterations*, 28 Am. J.L. & Med. 151, 153 (2002) (describing human cloning as a crime against humanity "by taking human evolution into our own hands and directing it toward the development of a new species, sometimes termed the posthuman").

any greater opportunity for manipulating our offspring than we currently enjoy. Using preimplantation genetic diagnosis, we can screen embryos for genetic traits, either deleterious or benign, and select those traits we find most desirable. Moreover, the opportunities for collaborative reproduction allow parents to choose the phenotypes and genotypes that will combine to produce their child. Nothing in our current law prevents parents from selecting egg and sperm donors of a particular stature, intelligence, race, etc. in order to attempt to "engineer" their children.

To date, we have seen parents using the option of donor gametes in order to maximize the well-being of their children, with most families selecting donors who resemble them in appearance and family background. The children of assisted reproductive technology (ART), though they may have been engineered to some extent, are welcomed by their parents as any newborn is welcomed. There is no logical reason why a cloned child would not receive the same treatment. Children of cloned conception will be born into the world as any other child. Their parents' instincts for nurturing will or will not take hold, making these children no more or less likely than any other children to experience the joys and sorrows of life.

Lori B. Andrews
Is There a Right to Clone? Constitutional Challenges to Bans on Human Cloning
11 Harv. J. Law & Technology 643, 649-57 (1998)

B. The Potential Physical Risks in Cloning Humans

[Professor Andrews begins by suggesting we approach human cloning by first addressing the many safety concerns through animal research.]

Reactivating the genes of a cell is risky. An adult cell which has already been differentiated contains a complete complement of genes, but only a small proportion are activated in order to do the specialized task of that cell. Activating the slumbering genes may reveal hidden mutations . . .

Moreover, some differentiated cells rearrange a subset of their genes. For example, immune cells rearrange some of their genes to make surface molecules. Such rearrangement could cause problems for the resulting clone. Also, if all the genes in the adult DNA are not properly reactivated, there could be a problem for the clone at a later developmental stage. The high rate of laboratory deaths suggests that cloning may in fact damage the DNA of a cell . . .

Furthermore, because scientists do not fully understand the cellular aging process, they do not know what "age" or "genetic clock" Dolly inherited. On a cellular level . . . was she a normal seven month old lamb, or was she six years old (the age of the mammary donor cell)? There is speculation that Dolly's cells most likely are set to the genetic clock of the nucleus donor, and therefore are comparable to those of her six year old progenitor . . .

The gross deformities and early deaths among cloned animals raise concerns that initial trials in human nuclear transplantation will also meet with disastrous results. Dr. Wilmut [Dolly's creator] is specifically concerned with the ethical issues raised by any such defective births . . . [He] noted . . . that "[w]ith people, the possibility of 276 failures, many of which would involve miscarriages, sounds horrific and raises huge ethical barriers" to the possibility of human cloning in the near future. Roger Pederson, a physician at the University of California, San Francisco, stated that many scientific groups are voluntarily observing a moratorium on human cloning because "the chance of abhorrent offspring is high."

C. The Potential Psychological Impacts of Cloning

Concerns about the psychological impact of cloning focus on the parent/child relationship, the undermining of the clone's autonomy and free will, and the later-born twin's loss of ability to control private information.

The unique origins of a clone might create unreasonable expectations about her. When a clone is created from a dead child, the parents might expect the second child to be a replacement for the first. The similar physical appearance of the second child will bring to life the ghost of the first, perhaps underscoring expectations that the children will be identical in behavior and personality. But the clone will invariably be different. The parents will be older — even if just by a few years — than they were when rearing the first child. They will also have suffered an indelible grief, the death of their child, and thus may have a tendency to overprotect the clone. They may also narrow the experiences of the clone, exposing it only to the type of food, toys, or classes that the first child liked.

These two problems — the specter of difference, leading to disappointment, and the narrowing of experiences — are likely to haunt all cloning arrangements. Consider, for example, what might happen if a couple cloned a famous basketball player. If the clone breaks his knee at age ten, would his parents consider him a disappointment? Would he view himself as a failure? . . .

Family relationships could also be altered by the fact that a cloned child may seem more like an object than a person, since he or she is "designed and manufactured as a product, rather than welcomed as a gift." . . . [Cloning] might diminish the personhood of a clone if he were created to satisfy the vanity of the nucleic DNA donor or to meet the needs of a pre-existing individual, such as a child needing bone marrow. In attempting to cull out from the resulting child the favored traits of the loved one or celebrity who has been cloned, the social parents might limit the environmental stimuli to which the child is exposed. "Arguably a person cloned from a departed loved one . . . has less chance of being loved solely for his own intrinsic worth."

Some scientists argue that these concerns are unfounded, because a clone will be invariably different from the original. The NBAC [National Bioethics Advisory Commission] report observes that "the idea that one could make through somatic cell nuclear transfer a team of Michael Jordans, a physics department of Albert Einsteins, or an opera chorus of Pavarottis, is simply false."

However, we are in an era of genetic determinism. James Watson, co-discoverer of deoxyribonucleic acid ("DNA") and the first director of the Human Genome

Project, has stated, "[w]e used to think our fate was in our stars. Now we know, in large measure, our fate is in our genes."

Whether or not genetics actually play such a large role in human development, parents may raise a clone as if they do. After all, regardless of their belief in genetic determinism, the only reason people want to clone (as opposed to adopting or using an egg or sperm donor in the case of infertility) is to assure that a child has a certain genetic make-up. It seems absurd to think that they would forget about that genetic make-up once the clone was born. We already limit parents' genetic foreknowledge of their children because we believe it will improperly influence their rearing practices. Medical genetics groups often caution parents against having their children tested for late-onset genetic disorders, because a child who tested positive could "grow up in a world of limited horizons and may be psychologically harmed even if treatment is subsequently found for the disorder."

Cloning could undermine human dignity by threatening the replicant's sense of self and autonomy. A vast body of developmental psychology research has demonstrated children's need to have a sense of an independent self. This might be difficult for the clone of a parent or of a previous child who died. Even if the clone did not believe in genetic determinism, the original's life "would always haunt the later twin, standing as an undue influence on the latter's life, and shaping it in ways to which others lives are not vulnerable." . . .

Another problem is that a clone cannot control disclosure of intimate personal information. This may threaten her self-image. Studies of people's responses to genetic testing information show that learning genetic information about oneself (whether it is positive or negative information) can harm one's self image. Moreover, an individual might be stigmatized or discriminated against based on foreknowledge of her genotype. If an individual were cloned and later died young of an inheritable disease, the clone might suffer from insurance or employment discrimination.

D. The Potential Societal Impacts of Cloning Humans

The prospect of cloning humans raises several serious concerns about its overall effect on society. Cloning may interfere with evolution, because it promotes genetic uniformity, thus increasing the danger that a disease might arise in the future to which clones would have no resistance . . . Genetic adaptation has allowed the human species to survive; producing genetically identical humans may therefore be threatening to the species . . . Despite these overall risks, some commentators argue that if human cloning is restricted to very rare cases, then the evolution of the human species should not be stunted nor the human gene pool disturbed any more than the gene pool is currently affected by naturally occurring identical twins.

Cloning might also bring detrimental changes to the instituition [sic] of the family. Boston College theologian Lisa Sowhill Cahill is concerned that cloning may lead to the commodification of human beings and their genes and to the manipulation of human genetics to achieve more socially desirable children. Allen Verhey, a Protestant ethicist at Hope College in Holland, Michigan, warns that cloning would desensitize society into regarding children as "products." Other opponents envision a world where clones are "cannibalized for spare parts" — made solely for medical purposes and asked to donate their organs . . .

In addition to weakening an individual's sense of free will, cloning would "weaken the social constructs and political institutions that serve to foster the exercise of individual autonomy and to inhibit the coercive manipulation of individuals."

NOTES AND QUESTIONS

1. What was your view on reproductive cloning before you read the above materials? Has your view changed at all since learning more about the science, potential harms and possible benefits of human cloning?

2. The legal and scientific commentary on human cloning is massive. A few of the selective works, listed in alphabetical order by author last name, include: Erez Aloni, *Cloning and the LGBTI Family: Cautious Optimism*, 35 N.Y.U. REV. L. & SOC. CHANGE 1 (2011); George J. Annas, *Why We Should Ban Human Cloning*, 339 NEW ENG. J. MED. 122 (1998); Nigel M. De S. Cameron & Anna V. Henderson, *Brave new World at the General Assembly: The United Nations Declaration on Human Cloning*, 9 MINN. J. L. SCI. & TECH. 145 (2008); Ronald Chester, *To Be, Be, Be . . . Not Just to Be: Legal and Social Implications of Cloning for Human Reproduction*, 49 FLA. L. REV. 303 (1997); Daniel Mark Cohen, *Cloning and the Constitution, Cloning and the Constitution, Cloning and the Constitution, Cloning and . . .*, 26 NOVA L. REV. 511 (2002); Elizabeth Price Foley, *The Constitutional Implications of Human Cloning*, 42 ARIZ. L. REV. 647 (2000); Clarke D. Forsythe, *Human Cloning and the Constitution*, 32 VAL. U. L. REV. 469 (1998); Rudolf Jaenisch, *Human Cloning — The Science and Ethics of Nuclear Transplantation*, 351 NEW ENG. J. MED. 2787 (2004); Michael I. Kahn, *Clowning Around With Clones: The Moral and Legal Implications of Human Cloning*, 3 U.S.F. J.L. & SOC. CHALLENGES 161 (1999); Russell Korobkin, *Stem Cell Research and the Cloning Wars*, 18 STANFORD L. & POL'Y REV. 161 (2007); Anne Lawton, *The Frankenstein Controversy: The Constitutionality of a Federal Ban on Cloning*, 87 KY. L.J. 277 (1998); John A. Robertson, *Liberty, Identity, and Human Cloning*, 76 TEX. L. REV. 1371 (1998); Yuriko Mary Shikai, *Don't Be Swept Away By Mass Hysteria: The Benefits of Human Reproductive Cloning and Its Future*, 33 SW. U. L. REV. 259 (2004); Richard F. Storrow, *Equal Protection for Human Clones* (reviewing Kerry Macintosh, Human Clones and the Law), 40 FAM. L. Q. 529 (2006); Susan Tall, *Legal and Ethical Implications of Human Procreative Cloning*, 3 U.S.F. J.L. & SOC. CHALLENGES 25 (1999).

3. Aside from the substantial and understandable concerns about the safety of human cloning, most arguments against the technology focus on the social and psychological well-being of the cloned child, and to a lesser extent on the potential harms to society. Philosopher Bonnie Steinbock summarizes these harms in her work, *Cloning Human Beings: Sorting Through the Ethical Issues*, in HUMAN CLONING 68-84 (Barbara MacKinnon, ed., 2000). For ease of discussion, the harms are listed in no particular order:

1) Cloning undermines human individuality and dignity

2) Cloning encourages parents to treat their children as commodities rather than humans

3)   Cloning destroys the integrity of families

4)   Cloning tempts humans to "play God"

5)   Cloning deprives a child of a right to an open future

6)   Cloning encourages the manufacture of a sub-human species to serve non-clones

7)   Cloning promotes eugenics

8)   Cloning deprives a child of having two genetic parents

9)   Cloning disrupts family relations if donor is both parent and sibling.

Do you agree with each of these predicted harms? If so, are they collectively or even individually sufficient to justify a total ban on any attempt to create a human being? If not, how would you refute each claim? If you do not believe that cloning will cause these stated harms, can you justify continued research on human cloning by composing an equally long list of potential benefits?

PROBLEM

Imagine a world in which human reproductive cloning is proving safe and effective in preliminary clinical trials. A noted clonist, Dr. Anton, advertises his services in a local newspaper. His ad reads as follows: "Research scientist seeks volunteers to participate in a study on human cloning. Volunteers must be married and must be otherwise unable to have children naturally."

Adam and Eve Robinson see this ad and know immediately that they wish to apply to serve as volunteers in Dr. Anton's program. The Robinsons have a son, Kevin, who they adopted when he was a few days old, 12 years ago. Adam and Eve made the decision to not tell Kevin that he was adopted. The couple was unable to conceive on their own for reasons that doctors could not adequately explain, but after several years of failed fertility treatment, they decided to fulfill their dreams of parenthood through adoption. To the Robinsons, Kevin is the perfect child. They feel so blessed to parent him that they wish to clone Kevin to have the opportunity to parent another child. Their decision to have another child through cloning is based on their knowledge that they are unable to have a child naturally and their belief that they have a perfect child, one they would want to reproduce if they could. Though Eve could not herself conceive a child, she is capable of gestating an existing embryo, including an embryo developed through cloning.

The Robinsons apply for admission to Dr. Anton's protocol and are accepted. The next step will be to supply Dr. Anton with several of Eve's eggs and some of Kevin's DNA. The DNA can be obtained through any cell of the body, including cells that have been excised previously. The Robinsons wish to clone Kevin but they do not wish to tell him about this desire. Instead, they offer Dr. Anton DNA from Kevin's baby teeth which the Robinsons meticulously saved and labeled as each fell out. The teeth contain enough DNA from the enamel and blood residue to allow cloning to take place. But Dr. Anton is concerned about accepting DNA from a living person who has not given consent for the cloning process.

What advice would you give to Dr. Anton and to the Robinsons as to this proposed cloning scheme?

SECTION II: THE POLITICS OF HUMAN CLONING

A.   Initial Reaction from the Federal Government

The February 1997 announcement of Dolly's birth by cloning set off a firestorm of political activity unrivaled by any other scientific discovery in recent memory. In the days and months following the announcement, the federal government acted with uncharacteristic speed to assure the public that human cloning would not become a reality in the near future. On March 4, 1997, a mere 10 days after Dr. Wilmut made worldwide headlines, President Clinton issued an Executive Order banning the use of federal funding for human cloning research. At the same time, the President asked his previously assembled bioethics council, the National Bioethics Advisory Commission (NBAC), to review the legal and ethical issues associated with cloning and to report back to him in 90 days with recommendations on possible federal actions to prevent its abuse. In June 1997, right on schedule, NBAC responded to President Clinton's request and issued a report on human cloning.

The NBAC report recommended a temporary moratorium on all clinical and research efforts to clone a human being. The report was, by its own admission, a compromise position grounded in the issue of safety, the only area of common agreement among the diverse group of participants. As you read the report, think about whether the conclusions and assumptions drawn by NBAC are different today than they were a decade and a half or so ago.

National Bioethics Advisory Commission
Cloning Human Beings
Executive Summary, i-v (June 1997)

In its deliberations, NBAC reviewed the scientific developments which preceded the Roslin announcement, as well as those likely to follow in its path. It also considered the many moral concerns raised by the possibility that this technique could be used to clone human beings. Much of the initial reaction to this possibility was negative. Careful assessment of that response revealed fears about harms to the children who may be created in this manner, particularly psychological harms associated with a possibly diminished sense of individuality and personal autonomy. Others expressed concern about a degradation in the quality of parenting and family life.

In addition to concerns about specific harms to children, people have frequently expressed fears that the widespread practice of somatic cell nuclear transfer cloning would undermine important social values by opening the door to a form of eugenics or by tempting some to manipulate others as if they were objects instead of persons. Arrayed against these concerns are other important social values, such as protecting the widest possible sphere of personal choice, particularly in matters pertaining to procreation and child rearing, maintaining privacy and the freedom of scientific inquiry, and encouraging the possible development of new biomedical breakthroughs.

To arrive at its recommendations concerning the use of somatic cell nuclear transfer techniques to create children, NBAC also examined long-standing religious traditions that guide many citizens' responses to new technologies and found that religious positions on human cloning are pluralistic in their premises, modes of argument, and conclusions. Some religious thinkers argue that the use of somatic cell nuclear transfer cloning to create a child would be intrinsically immoral and thus could never be morally justified. Other religious thinkers contend that human cloning to create a child could be morally justified under some circumstances, but hold that it should be strictly regulated in order to prevent abuses.

The public policies recommended with respect to the creation of a child using somatic cell nuclear transfer reflect the Commission's best judgments about both the ethics of attempting such an experiment and its view of traditions regarding limitations on individual actions in the name of the common good. At present, the use of this technique to create a child would be a premature experiment that would expose the fetus and the developing child to unacceptable risks. This in itself might be sufficient to justify a prohibition on cloning human beings at this time, even if such efforts were to be characterized as the exercise of a fundamental right to attempt to procreate.

Beyond the issue of the safety of the procedure, however, NBAC found that concerns relating to the potential psychological harms to children and effects on the moral, religious, and cultural values of society merited further reflection and deliberation. Whether upon such further deliberation our nation will conclude that the use of cloning techniques to create children should be allowed or permanently banned is, for the moment, an open question. Time is an ally in this regard, allowing for the accrual of further data from animal experimentation, enabling an assessment of the prospective safety and efficacy of the procedure in humans, as well as granting a period of fuller national debate on ethical and social concerns. The Commission therefore concluded that there should be imposed a period of time in which no attempt is made to create a child using somatic cell nuclear transfer.

Within this overall framework the Commission came to the following conclusions and recommendations:

I. The Commission concludes that at this time it is morally unacceptable for anyone in the public or private sector, whether in a research or clinical setting, to attempt to create a child using somatic cell nuclear transfer cloning. The Commission reached a consensus on this point because current scientific information indicates that this technique is not safe to use in humans at this point. Indeed, the Commission believes it would violate important ethical obligations were clinicians or researchers to attempt to create a child using these particular technologies, which are likely to involve unacceptable risks to the fetus and/or potential child. Moreover, in addition to safety concerns, many other serious ethical concerns have been identified, which require much more widespread and careful public deliberation before this technology may be used.

The Commission, therefore, recommends the following for immediate action:

- A continuation of the current moratorium on the use of federal funding in support of any attempt to create a child by somatic cell nuclear transfer.

- An immediate request to all firms, clinicians, investigators, and professional societies in the private and non-federally funded sectors to comply voluntarily with the intent of the federal moratorium. Professional and scientific societies should make clear that any attempt to create a child by somatic cell nuclear transfer and implantation into a woman's body would at this time be an irresponsible, unethical, and unprofessional act.

II. The Commission further recommends that:

- Federal legislation should be enacted to prohibit anyone from attempting, whether in a research or clinical setting, to create a child through somatic cell nuclear transfer cloning. It is critical, however, that such legislation include a sunset clause to ensure that Congress will review the issue after a specified time period (three to five years) in order to decide whether the prohibition continues to be needed. If state legislation is enacted, it should also contain such a sunset provision. Any such legislation or associated regulation also ought to require that at some point prior to the expiration of the sunset period, an appropriate oversight body will evaluate and report on the current status of somatic cell nuclear transfer technology and on the ethical and social issues that its potential use to create human beings would raise in light of public understandings at that time.

III. The Commission also concludes that:

- Any regulatory or legislative actions undertaken to effect the foregoing prohibition on creating a child by somatic cell nuclear transfer should be carefully written so as not to interfere with other important areas of scientific research. In particular, no new regulations are required regarding the cloning of human DNA sequences and cell lines, since neither activity raises the scientific and ethical issues that arise from the attempt to create children through somatic cell nuclear transfer, and these fields of research have already provided important scientific and biomedical advances. Likewise, research on cloning animals by somatic cell nuclear transfer does not raise the issues implicated in attempting to use this technique for human cloning, and its continuation should only be subject to existing regulations regarding the humane use of animals and review by institution-based animal protection committees.

- If a legislative ban is not enacted, or if a legislative ban is ever lifted, clinical use of somatic cell nuclear transfer techniques to create a child should be preceded by research trials that are governed by the twin protections of independent review and informed consent, consistent with existing norms of human subjects protection.

- The United States Government should cooperate with other nations and international organizations to enforce any common aspects of their respective policies on the cloning of human beings.

IV. The Commission also concludes that different ethical and religious perspectives and traditions are divided on many of the important moral issues that surround any attempt to create a child using somatic cell nuclear transfer techniques. Therefore, the Commission recommends that:

- The federal government, and all interested and concerned parties, encourage widespread and continuing deliberation on these issues in order to further our understanding of the ethical and social implications of this technology and to enable society to produce appropriate long-term policies regarding this technology should the time come when present concerns about safety have been addressed.

V. Finally, because scientific knowledge is essential for all citizens to participate in a full and informed fashion in the governance of our complex society, the Commission recommends that:

- Federal departments and agencies concerned with science should cooperate in seeking out and supporting opportunities to provide information and education to the public in the area of genetics, and on other developments in the biomedical sciences, especially where these affect important cultural practices, values, and beliefs.

NOTES AND QUESTIONS

1. The NBAC Report recommends that Congress enact legislation prohibiting the creation of a child using cloning technology, but adds that any such law should include a "sunset provision," a clause that would render the law ineffective after a certain number of years unless action is taken to renew the measure. Are sunset provisions a good idea for all laws pertaining to emerging or developing technologies? Are there any problems that could arise, such as those related to legislative efficiency, when sunset provisions are used in prohibitory laws?

In this case, NBAC recommended a prohibition be evaluated in three to five years (the years 2000-2002). Using your 20/20 hindsight, if such a law were enacted in 1997, do you believe it would have been sunsetted at the dawn of the twenty-first century? In light of the lack of scientific progress toward human reproductive cloning, so you believe a federal prohibition is a good idea today?

2. *Cloning and Congress.* One might surmise that the near-universal condemnation of human reproductive cloning, including calls for its temporary prohibition by a Democratically appointed commission, would prompt Congress to act swiftly and decisively to ban all attempts at creating a cloned child. Politics being what they are, no such ban has passed ever both houses of Congress. As noted in Chapter 9, the fact that Congress has yet to pass a cloning ban is in no way an indication of its lack of interest in the field, or its support for research into reproductive cloning. The explanation seems to lie in the breadth and scope of the cloning bills that have been introduced into Congress by teams of legislators from both sides of the aisle. Since 1997, federal lawmakers have entertained dozens of bills pertaining to cloning, with most landing in one of two camps. Either the bills ban both reproductive and

therapeutic cloning, or they ban only reproductive cloning but allow therapeutic cloning.

Two bills that would have criminalized all forms of cloning passed the House, but failed to pass the Senate. See H.R. 2505, 107th Cong. (passed in 2001 by a vote of 265-162) and H.R. 534, 108th Cong. (passed in 2003 by a vote of 241-155). Political analysts explain the result by surmising that a majority of then-sitting senators favored stem cell research, including research using cloned embryos, and thus opposed a law which would have shut down research in this area. In March 2005, Senator Sam Brownback (R-Kan.) introduced another version of previous bills that criminalized all forms of human cloning, including therapeutic cloning designed to create immune-compatible medical products. Senate Bill 658, introduced on March 17, 2005, provided in relevant part:

SECTION 1. SHORT TITLE.

This Act may be cited as the 'Human Cloning Prohibition Act of 2005'.

SEC. 2. PROHIBITION ON HUMAN CLONING . . .

(a) Definitions- In this section:

(1) HUMAN CLONING - The term "human cloning" means human asexual reproduction, accomplished by introducing nuclear material from one or more human somatic cells into a fertilized or unfertilized oocyte whose nuclear material has been removed or inactivated so as to produce a living organism (at any stage of development) that is genetically virtually identical to an existing or previously existing human organism.

(2) ASEXUAL REPRODUCTION- The term "asexual reproduction" means reproduction not initiated by the union of oocyte and sperm.

(3) SOMATIC CELL- The term "somatic cell" means a diploid cell (having a complete set of chromosomes) obtained or derived from a living or deceased human body at any stage of development.

(b) Prohibition- It shall be unlawful for any person or entity, public or private, in or affecting interstate commerce, knowingly —

(1) to perform or attempt to perform human cloning;

(2) to participate in an attempt to perform human cloning; or

(3) to ship or receive for any purpose an embryo produced by human cloning or any product derived from such embryo.

(c) Importation- It shall be unlawful for any person or entity, public or private, knowingly to import for any purpose an embryo produced by human cloning.

(d) Penalties-

(1) CRIMINAL PENALTY- Any person or entity that violates this section shall be fined or imprisoned for not more than 10 years, or both.

(2) CIVIL PENALTY- Any person or entity that violates any provision of this section shall be subject to, in the case of a violation that involves the derivation of a pecuniary gain, a civil penalty of not less than $1,000,000 and not more than an amount equal to the amount of the gross gain multiplied by 2, if that amount is greater than $1,000,000.

(e) Scientific Research- Nothing in this section restricts areas of scientific research not specifically prohibited by this section, including research in the use of nuclear transfer or other cloning techniques to produce molecules, DNA, cells other than human embryos, tissues, organs, plants, or animals other than humans.

Bills similar to the above 2005 bill were introduced in both chambers of Congress in 2007 (110th Congress) and 2009 (111th Congress), but none made it out of the initial chamber. Each bore the same title, the Human Cloning Prohibition Act. No such bill was introduced in the 112th Congress in 2011, owing perhaps to lack of enthusiasm for pursuing a federal cloning ban at that time.

Do you support the aim of above bill? If so, do you believe it would have any impact on research in the field of cell-based regenerative medicine? If not, is it because you favor both reproductive and therapeutic cloning, or just the latter? If polls are accurate in their results that most Americans oppose reproductive cloning but favor therapeutic cloning, why would lawmakers tie the two techniques together in a single "all or nothing" bill?

Shortly after S. 658 was introduced, on April 21, 2005 another group of Senators introduced a counter measure in the form of Senate Bill 876, entitled the "Human Cloning Ban and Stem Cell Research Protection Act of 2005." The bill prohibits human reproductive cloning but also authorizes embryonic stem cell research. Relevant portions of the bill provided as follows:

———

SECTION 301. Prohibition on Human Cloning.

(a) Definitions - In this section:

(1) HUMAN CLONING - The term "Human cloning" means implanting or attempting to implant the product of nuclear transplantation into a uterus or the functional equivalent of a uterus.

(b) Prohibitions on Human Cloning - It shall be unlawful for any person or other legal entity, public or private —

(1) to conduct or attempt to conduct human cloning . . .

SECTION 499A. Ethical Requirements for Nuclear Transplantation Research

. . .

(c) Prohibition on Conducting Nuclear Transplantation on Fertilized Eggs — A somatic cell nucleus shall not be transplanted into a human oocyte that has undergone or will undergo fertilization.

Do you think S. 658 permits or prohibits therapeutic cloning?

3. *Professional and Scientific Organizations Weigh in on Reproductive Cloning.* Numerous blue-ribbon panels and professional organizations have reported on cloning in recent years; these reports illustrate general opposition to cloning, particularly reproductive cloning. Prominent among these panels is the prestigious National Academy of Sciences (NAS), which issued a tentative report in April 2002 addressing the scientific and medical aspects of human reproductive cloning. In its report, NAS recommends that "human reproductive cloning should not now be practiced [because] [i]t is dangerous and likely to fail." See Committee on Science, Engineering, and Public Policy, Policy and Global Affairs Division, Nat. Acad. of Sciences, Scientific and Medical Aspects of Human Reproductive Cloning, 6-6 (National Academy Press 2002). The report further recommends that there be a legally enforceable ban on the practice of human reproductive cloning. The NAS position is somewhat akin to that taken by President Clinton's National Bioethics Advisory Commission in suggesting that any ban be reconsidered within five years. Reconsideration, NAS argues, should be based on new scientific and medical evidence demonstrating that the cloning procedure is "likely to be safe and effective" and "a broad national dialogue on the societal, religious, and ethical issues suggests that a reconsideration of the ban is warranted."

Professional organizations have also responded hesitantly, but overwhelmingly negatively, to cloning. One professional organization that might be viewed as friendly to human cloning is the American Society for Reproductive Medicine (ASRM), a voluntary organization of fertility specialists founded in 1944. Recall that ASRM is a multidisciplinary organization whose members include physicians and other health care professionals practicing in the area of reproductive medicine. Because many of its members could benefit professionally and financially by offering cloning services, one might assume that ASRM would favor only minimal restrictions on the technique. Yet, in a November 2000 report from its Ethics Committee, ASRM joined the swell of anti-cloning sentiment. After discussing the possible ethical arguments for and against reproductive cloning, the ASRM Ethics Committee concluded that "[a]s long as the safety of reproductive SCNT is uncertain, ethical issues have been insufficiently explored, and infertile couples have alternatives for conception, the use of reproductive SCNT by medical professionals does not meet standards of ethical acceptability." See The Ethics Committee of the American Society for Reproductive Medicine, *Human Somatic Cell Nuclear Transfer (Cloning)*, 74 FERTILITY & STERILITY 873, 875 (2000). Thus, opposition to cloning continues to predominate even among physicians and researchers who are most knowledgeable about the science and potential benefits of this emerging reproductive technology.

B. Later Reactions from the Federal Government

When President George W. Bush took office in January 2001, mammalian cloning had been a reality for a scant four years, but its place in the public arena had been firmly established. As recounted in Chapter 9, the bioethics item that dominated President Bush's first months in office was the question of whether to allow federal funds to be used for human embryonic stem cell research. But the related concept of human reproductive cloning again jumped to center stage in November 2001 when the President appointed his newly constituted President's

Council on Bioethics. The very first topic selected by the Council to study and report on was the ethics of human cloning. In early 2002, the Council held hearings and gathered information on the topic, issuing its final report in July 2002.

Like its predecessor NBAC, the Bush executive-level bioethics panel was not of one mind on the topic of human cloning, especially when discussing the ethics of cloning for biomedical research. While the Council members did diverge on the question of therapeutic cloning (deemed "cloning-for-biomedical-research"), all the members were unanimous in their opposition to reproductive cloning ("cloning-to-produce-children"). An excerpt from the Council's Executive Summary sets forth the group's reasons and recommendations.

The President's Council on Bioethics
Human Cloning and Human Dignity
Executive Summary, xxvii–xxix (July 2002)

The Ethics of Cloning-to-Produce-Children

Two separate national-level reports on human cloning (NBAC, 1997; NAS, 2002) concluded that attempts to clone a human being would be unethical at this time due to safety concerns and the likelihood of harm to those involved. The Council concurs in this conclusion. But we have extended the work of these distinguished bodies by undertaking a broad ethical examination of the merits of, and difficulties with, cloning-to-produce-children.

Cloning-to-produce-children might serve several purposes. It might allow infertile couples or others to have genetically-related children; permit couples at risk of conceiving a child with a genetic disease to avoid having an afflicted child; allow the bearing of a child who could become an ideal transplant donor for a particular patient in need; enable a parent to keep a living connection with a dead or dying child or spouse; or enable individuals or society to try to "replicate" individuals of great talent or beauty. These purposes have been defended by appeals to the goods of freedom, existence (as opposed to nonexistence), and well-being — all vitally important ideals.

A major weakness in these arguments supporting cloning-to-produce-children is that they overemphasize the freedom, desires, and control of parents, and pay insufficient attention to the well-being of the cloned child-to-be. The Council holds that, once the child-to-be is carefully considered, these arguments are not sufficient to overcome the powerful case against engaging in cloning-to-produce-children.

First, cloning-to-produce-children would violate the principles of the ethics of human research. Given the high rates of morbidity and mortality in the cloning of other mammals, we believe that cloning-to-produce-children would be extremely unsafe, and that attempts to produce a cloned child would be highly unethical. Indeed, our moral analysis of this matter leads us to conclude that this is not, as is sometimes implied, a merely temporary objection, easily removed by the improvement of technique. We offer reasons for believing that the safety risks might be enduring, and offer arguments in support of a strong conclusion: that conducting experiments in an effort to make cloning-to-produce-children less dangerous would itself be an unacceptable violation of the norms of research ethics. There seems to be no ethical way to try to discover whether cloning-to-produce-children can become safe, now or in the future.

If carefully considered, the concerns about safety also begin to reveal the ethical principles that should guide a broader assessment of cloning-to-produce-children: the principles of freedom, equality, and human dignity. To appreciate the broader human significance of cloning-to-produce-children, one needs first to reflect on the meaning of having children; the meaning of asexual, as opposed to sexual, reproduction; the importance of origins and genetic endowment for identity and sense of self; the meaning of exercising greater human control over the processes and "products" of human reproduction; and the difference between begetting and making. Reflecting on these topics, the Council has identified five categories of concern regarding cloning-to-produce-children. (Different Council Members give varying moral weight to these different concerns.)

- *Problems of identity and individuality.* Cloned children may experience serious problems of identity both because each will be genetically virtually identical to a human being who has already lived and because the expectations for their lives may be shadowed by constant comparisons to the life of the "original."

- *Concerns regarding manufacture.* Cloned children would be the first human beings whose entire genetic makeup is selected in advance. They might come to be considered more like products of a designed manufacturing process than "gifts" whom their parents are prepared to accept as they are. Such an attitude toward children could also contribute to increased commercialization and industrialization of human procreation.

- *The prospect of a new eugenics.* Cloning, if successful, might serve the ends of privately pursued eugenic enhancement, either by avoiding the genetic defects that may arise when human reproduction is left to chance, or by preserving and perpetuating outstanding genetic traits, including the possibility, someday in the future, of using cloning to perpetuate genetically engineered enhancements.

- *Troubled family relations.* By confounding and transgressing the natural boundaries between generations, cloning could strain the social ties between them. Fathers could become "twin brothers" to their "sons"; mothers could give birth to their genetic twins; and grandparents would also be the "genetic parents" of their grandchildren. Genetic relation to only one parent might produce special difficulties for family life.

- *Effects on society.* Cloning-to-produce-children would affect not only the direct participants but also the entire society that allows or supports this activity. Even if practiced on a small scale, it could affect the way society looks at children and set a precedent for future nontherapeutic interventions into the human genetic endowment or novel forms of control by one generation over the next. In the absence of wisdom regarding these matters, prudence dictates caution and restraint.

Conclusion: For some or all of these reasons, the Council is in full agreement that cloning-to-produce-children is not only unsafe but also morally unacceptable, and ought not to be attempted.

NOTES AND QUESTIONS

1. The Council's stated reasons for opposing human reproductive cloning are fairly familiar to us at this point, having seen these same objections appear in the Daar and Andrews articles earlier in the chapter, as well as listed in Note 3 following those excerpted pieces. Let us spend a moment exploring the typical reasons given for opposing human reproductive cloning. The objections set forth by the PCB are reproduced below and examined with the hope that your own views on the subject will be informed and sharpened.

> 1) **Problems of Identity and Individuality.** Does the Council envision that cloning will be used to produce multiple children using the same genome, thus exacerbating the problem of identity? If so, could a regulation that limited the use of a particular genome, such as is sometimes done when sperm banks limit the use of a particular donor's sperm, solve the problem?

Is the problem of "constant comparisons" to another unique to cloning? Are naturally conceived children ever compared to, say, a sibling or a parent? Why would comparisons to a genetically identical human being be different/worse than comparisons that parents and society currently engage in?

> 2) **Concerns Regarding Manufacture.** Are cloned children more likely to be treated as manufactured than current children of ART whose parents expend a great deal of money in order to bring about their birth? Do parents already select the genetic make-up of their child through PGD, or by using gamete donors (or even more instinctively when they pick a mate)? If so, is selection based on a single genome more harmful than selection based on a mixed genome?

> 3) **The Prospect of New Eugenics.** If PGD already allows parents to avoid genetic defects in their children, how and why would cloning exacerbate this phenomenon? How and why is perpetuating outstanding genetic traits harmful to society?

> 4) **Troubled Family Relations.** Does the Council take into account the role that social rearing plays in developing parent-child relationships? Would a cloned child regard her mother as a sister if the woman who gave birth to the daughter consistently treated and regarded the child as her offspring rather than her sibling? Why would a parent who uses cloning for reproductive purposes want to treat the cloned child as a sibling?

Why is genetic relation to only one parent any more harmful to children than the current situation where gamete donors are used, or when a child's parent dies or abandons the child early in life possibly leaving the child to be reared by only one genetically related parent?

> 5) **Effects on Society.** Would cloning to produce children cause society to pay less regard to the cloned children as a future generation because of the circumstances of their conception? Did the introduction of IVF cause

society to treat these children as "other" or the subject of "control" in a manner that caused harm to these novel offspring? Why would cloning provoke a societal reaction different than that provoked by IVF?

2. *Dr. Kass, reprised.* The drafting of the Council's report is often largely attributed to its chair, Dr. Leon Kass, whose characteristic and erudite prose are recognizable to fans and foes alike. Perhaps as proof, consider the phraseology that appears at the end of the fourth paragraph in the excerpted summary. When speaking about whether reproductive cloning could ever be an acceptable practice, the Council concludes: "There seems to be no ethical way to try to discover whether cloning-to-produce-children can become safe, now or in the future."

Dr. Kass used this same phraseology in 1971 when warning against the newly-emerging technology of in vitro fertilization. Writing in the New England Journal of Medicine, he argued that "[b]ecause the new procedures for in vitro fertilization and laboratory culture of human embryos probably carry a serious risk of damage to any child so generated, *there appears to be no ethical way to proceed.*" See Leon R. Kass, *Babies By Means of In Vitro Fertilization: Unethical Experiments on the Unborn?*, 285 NEW ENG. J. MED. 1174 (1971) (italics added). Was Dr. Kass correct that there was no ethical way to proceed to discover whether IVF could be a safe method of assisted conception? Even if you believe he was not correct in that assessment, should his warning regarding cloning be given greater weight because the technology involves asexual, as opposed to sexual, reproduction?

3. *President Obama and Human Cloning.* The Obama Administration has not invested itself in studying and reporting on the prospect of human reproductive cloning as did the administrations of Presidents Bush and Clinton, perhaps because the science has seemingly failed to evolve in any perceptible way. Still, President Obama did mention his opposition to human reproductive cloning when he signed the Executive Order expanding federal funding for human embryonic stem cell research in March 2009 (as discussed in Chapter 9). In a White House ceremony, President Obama made clear, "we will ensure that our government never opens the door to the use of cloning for human reproduction. It is dangerous, profoundly wrong, and has no place in our society, or any society." President Obama's full remarks at the signing ceremony are available at: http://www.whitehouse.gov/the_press_office/Remarks-of-the-President-As-Prepared-for-Delivery-Signing-of-Stem-Cell-Executive-Order-and-Scientific-Integrity-Presidential-Memorandum/.

C. Reactions from the States

Reproductive cloning is at its heart a medical procedure, and thus would be subject to state regulation as a component of the practice of medicine. State lawmakers understood their jurisdiction to regulate cloning, and seemed to take up that mantle with enthusiasm. Since the announcement of Dolly's birth in 1997, a majority of U.S. states legislatures have considered bills that would ban human reproductive cloning in the jurisdiction.[10] According to the National Conference of

---

[10] According to report submitted to the President's Council on Bioethics, in 2002 and 2003, 27 states introduced bills that would ban reproductive cloning. See Lori B. Andrews, *Legislators as Lobbyists: Proposed State Regulation of Embryonic Stem Cell Research, Therapeutic Cloning and Reproductive*

State Legislatures, 13 states have enacted bans on reproductive cloning: Arkansas, California, Connecticut, Indiana, Iowa, Maryland, Massachusetts, Michigan, New Jersey, North Dakota, Rhode Island, South Dakota and Virginia.[11] The statutes range in scope from providing for civil penalties if cloning is achieved or attempted, to meting out criminal punishment for any attempts to clone a human being. Compare the civil penalty and criminal punishment approach in two states — Michigan and Arkansas.

Michigan Compiled Laws Annotated
Chapter 333. Health, Public Health Code

§ 333.16274. Prohibition of human cloning

(1) A licensee or registrant shall not engage in or attempt to engage in human cloning.

(2) Subsection (1) does not prohibit scientific research or cell-based therapies not specifically prohibited by that subsection.

(3) A licensee or registrant who violates subsection (1) is subject to the

---

Cloning, at 207, Appendix E to Monitoring Stem Cell Research, a report of The President's Council on Bioethics (2004). The anti-cloning bills pending as of late 2002 include: H.R. 218, 2002 Reg. Sess. (Ala. 2002); H.R. 2108, 45th Leg., 2nd Reg. Sess. (Ariz. 2002); Jt. Res. 38, 2001-01 Reg. Sess. (Cal. 2002); S. 1557, 2001-02 Reg. Sess. (Cal. 2002); S. 1230, 2001-02 Reg. Sess. (Cal. 2002); H.R. 1073, 63rd Gen. Assemb., 2nd Reg. Sess. (Colo. 2002); S. 344, 141st Gen. Assemb., 2nd Yr. (Del. 2002); S. 329, 141st Gen. Assemb., 2nd Yr. (Del. 2002); S. 1164, 104th Reg. Sess. (Fla. 2002); H.R. 805, 104th Reg. Sess. (Fla., 2002); H.R. Res. 1612, 146th Gen. Assemb., Reg. Sess. (Ga. 2002); S. Res. 864, 146th Gen. Assemb., Reg. Sess. (Ga. 2002); H.R. 3693, 92nd Gen. Assemb., 2001-02 Gen. Assemb. (Ill. 2001); S. 493, 92nd Gen. Assemb., 2001-02 Gen. Assemb. (Ill. 2002); S. 138, 112th Gen. Assemb., 2nd Reg. Sess. (Ind. 2001); S. 2118, 79th Gen. Assemb., 2nd Sess. (Iowa 2002); H.R. 2736, 79th Legis., 2002 Reg. Sess. (Kan. 2002); H.R. 138, 2002 Reg. Sess. (Ky. 2002); H.R. Res. 458, 2002 Reg. Sess. (Ky. 2001); S. 1809, 182nd Gen. Ct., 2001 Reg. Sess. (Mass. 2001); S. 1794, 182nd Gen. Ct., 2001 Reg. Sess. (Mass. 2001); S. 1673, 182nd Gen. Ct., 2001 Reg. Sess. (Mass. 2000); S. 192, 182nd Gen. Ct., 2001 Reg. Sess. (Mass. 2000); H.R. 354, 91st Legis., 2002 Reg. Sess. (Mich. 2002); H.R. 361, 2002 Reg. Sess. of Miss. Legis. (Miss. 2001); H.R. 1449, 91st Gen. Assemb., 2nd Reg. Sess. (Mo. 2002); H.R. 1028, 91st Gen. Assemb., 2nd Reg. Sess. (Mo. 2001); H.R. 947, 91st Gen. Assemb., 1st Reg. Sess. (Mo. 2001); H.R. 718, 91st Gen. Assemb., 1st Reg. Sess. (Mo. 2001); H.R. 1067, 97th Legis., 2nd Reg. Sess. (Neb. 2002); H.R. 1464, 2nd Year of the 157th Sess. of the Gen. Ct. (N.H. 2002); H.R. 2040, 210th Legis. (N.J. 2002); H.R. 1379, 209th Legis., 2nd Reg. Sess. (N.J. 2002); S. 542, 209th Legis., 2nd Reg. Sess. (N.J. 2002); H.R. 3978, 209th Legis., 2nd Reg. Sess. (N.J. 2001); S. 7638, 225th Annual Legis. Sess. (N.Y. 2002); H.R. 9292, 224th Annual Legis. Sess (N.Y. 2001); H.R. 2905, 224th Annual Legis. Sess. (N.Y. 2001); S. 1689, 224th Annual Legis. Sess. (N.Y. 2001); S. 1161, 224th Annual Legis. Sess. (N.Y. 2001); S. 670, 224th Annual Legis. Sess. (N.Y. 2001); S. 1552, 48th Legis. 2nd Sess. (Okla. 2002); H.R. 2036, 48th Legis, 2nd Sess. (Okla. 15, 2002); H.R. 2142, 48th Legis., 2nd Sess. (Okla. 2002); H.R. 2011, 48th Legis., 2nd Sess. (Okla. 2002); H.R. 3897, 71st Legis. Assemb. (Or. 2001); H.R. 7145, 2001-02 Legis. Sess. (R.I. 2002); S. 820, 114th Sess. of the S.C. Gen. Assemb. (S.C. 2001); H.R. 4408, 114th Sess. of the S.C. Gen. Assembly (S.C. 2001); S. Con. Res. 13, 77th Legis. Assembly (S.C. 2002); S. 1209, 77th Legis. (Tex. 2001); S. 102, 77th Legis. (Tex. 2000); H.R. 2463, 2001 Sess. (Va. 2001); S. 1305, 2001 Sess. (Va. 2001); S. 379, 95th Legis. Sess. (Wis. 2002); H.R. 699, 95th Legis. Sess. (Wis. 2002), as cited in Judith F. Daar, *The Prospect of Human Cloning: Improving Nature or Dooming the Species?*, 33 Seton Hall L. Rev. 511, 520, n. 41 (2003).

[11] The state of Louisiana enacted a cloning ban in 1999, but the measure contained a sunset clause which rendered the law null and void as of July 1, 2003. La. Rev. Stat. § 1299.36. As of this writing, no new law has been enacted. The state of Illinois enacted a human reproductive cloning ban, along with a law permitting therapeutic cloning, in 2008. *See* 410 Ill. Stat. Comp. 110/40 (2008).

administrative penalties prescribed in sections 16221 and 16226 and to the civil penalty prescribed in section 16275.

(4) This section does not give a person a private right of action.

(5) As used in this section:

(a) "Human cloning" means the use of human somatic cell nuclear transfer technology to produce a human embryo.

(b) "Human embryo" means a human egg cell with a full genetic composition capable of differentiating and maturing into a complete human being.

(c) "Human somatic cell" means a cell of a developing or fully developed human being that is not and will not become a sperm or egg cell.

(d) "Human somatic cell nuclear transfer" means transferring the nucleus of a human somatic cell into an egg cell from which the nucleus has been removed or rendered inert.

§ 333.16275. Penalties

(1) A licensee or registrant or other individual shall not engage in or attempt to engage in human cloning . . .

(3) A licensee or registrant or other individual who violates subsection (1) is subject to a civil penalty of $10,000,000.00. A fine collected under this subsection shall be distributed in the same manner as penal fines are distributed in this state.

Arkansas Code Annotated
Title 20. Public Health and Welfare, Chapter 16. Reproductive Health

§ 20-16-1001. Definitions

As used in this subchapter: . . .

(4) "Human cloning" means human asexual reproduction, accomplished by introducing the genetic material from one (1) or more human somatic cells into a fertilized or unfertilized oocyte whose nuclear material has been removed or inactivated so as to produce a living organism, at any stage of development, that is genetically virtually identical to an existing or previously existing human organism . . .

Massachusetts General Laws Annotated
Chapter 12, Section 12J

§ 20-16-1002. Prohibited acts — Penalties

(a) It is unlawful for any person or entity, public or private, to intentionally or knowingly:

(1) Perform or attempt to perform human cloning;

(2) Participate in an attempt to perform human cloning;

(3) Ship, transfer, or receive for any purpose an embryo produced by human cloning; or

(4) Ship, transfer, or receive, in whole or in part, any oocyte, embryo, fetus, or human somatic cell for the purpose of human cloning.

(b) A violation of subdivision (a)(1) or (2) of this section, or both, is a Class C felony.

(c) A violation of subdivision (a)(3) or (4) of this section, or both, is a Class A misdemeanor.

(d) (1) In addition to any criminal penalty that may be levied, any person or entity that violates any provision of this section shall be subject to a fine of not less than two hundred fifty thousand dollars ($250,000) or twice the amount of any pecuniary gain that is received by the person or entity, whichever is greater.

NOTES AND QUESTIONS

1. *Federal Preemption.* If Congress unifies to pass a cloning ban which criminalizes both reproductive and therapeutic cloning, will the state cloning measures have any legal force or effect? The answer rests in the Supremacy Clause of the U.S. Constitution, Article VI, which provides that the ". . . Laws of the United States . . . shall be the Supreme Law of the Land." Our Supreme Court has declared, "[U]nder the Supremacy Clause, from which our pre-emption doctrine is derived, 'any state law, however clearly within a State's acknowledged power, which interferes with or is contrary to federal law, must yield.' " *Gade v. National Solid Waste Management Association,* 505 U.S. 88, 108 (1992). As explained by constitutional law scholar Erwin Chemerinsky, "the Supreme Court has identified two major situations where preemption occurs. One is where a federal law expressly preempts state or local law. The other situation is where preemption is implied by a clear congressional intent to preempt state or local law." ERWIN CHEMERINSKY, CONSTITUTIONAL LAW: PRINCIPLES AND POLICIES 376 (2d. Ed. 2002).

Compare the Michigan and Arkansas laws with the proposed federal law, reprinted in Section 2(A), above. Does the proposed federal law contain a provision expressly preempting any state cloning laws? Does the federal bill imply a clear congressional intent to preempt state laws? Is there any conduct that would be permitted under the federal law but would be banned by either of the state laws?

2. *Commerce Clause Concerns.* An inverse conundrum to the federal preemption question is whether Congress has the authority to comprehensively regulate reproductive cloning under the Constitution's Commerce Clause. As Professor Russell Korobkin explains, "[u]nder our federal system, the national government lacks general regulatory authority: Congress's ability to enact legislation is limited to the powers granted to it by the Constitution." Those powers are, in part, contained in the Commerce Clause, which permits Congress "to regulate Commerce with foreign Nations, and among the several States." After reviewing the U.S. Supreme Court's interpretation of Congress's regulatory authority under the Commerce Clause, Professor Korobkin concludes that a federal cloning ban would likely survive attack on such grounds because recent case law has broadly defined

the kind of activity that falls within Congress's constitutional realm. Moreover, he opines, even if reproductive cloning is seen as a traditional state concern upon which federal legislation should not encroach, the recent expansive view of the Commerce Clause would likely permit formal congressional rejection of this form of reproduction. *See* Russell Korobkin, *Stem Cell Research and the Cloning Wars*, 18 STANFORD L. & POL'Y REV. 161, 176-80 (2007).

3. *Deterrence?* Do you think that cloning bans — either federal or state — will prevent people from attempting to create a cloned human being? To help answer this question, make a list of the following two groups: Who is most likely to be deterred from cloning research by the threat of criminal sanctions? Who is most unlikely to be deterred? Assuming for the sake of argument that experiments in human cloning will go forward despite laws to the contrary, which list of actors would you prefer to proceed with cloning research? Are these actors on your "likely" or "unlikely" to be deterred list?

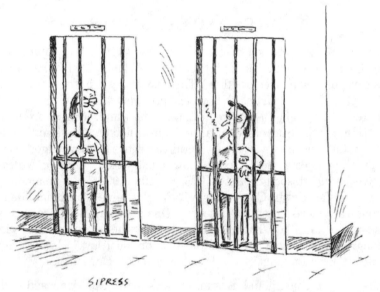

SIPRESS

"I cloned a guy in Reno. How 'bout yourself?"

4. *International Perspectives on Reproductive Cloning.* In Chapter 9 we discussed international perspectives on human therapeutic cloning. Section 4(A) of Chapter 9 lists a variety of countries and their laws on cloning. As you can see from the list, reproductive cloning is banned in Australia, Canada, China, Costa Rica, France, Germany, Italy, Japan, Holland, Norway, Singapore, South Korea and the United Kingdom. In addition, according to a 2012 survey, human reproductive cloning is banned in Austria, Argentina, Belgium, Brazil, Columbia, Denmark, Finland, Iceland, Israel, Latvia, Mexico, Panama, Peru, Romania, Russia, Slovakia, Slovenia, South Africa, Spain, Sweden, Switzerland and Turkey. *See* Countries with Bans on Human Cloning and/or Genetic Engineering, Public Agenda, available at: http://www.publicagenda.org/charts/countries-bans-human-cloning-andor-genetic-engineering.

SECTION III: CONSTITUTIONAL ASPECTS OF HUMAN CLONING

The groundswell of support for state, federal and international bans on human reproductive cloning proceed seemingly unencumbered by concerns about the legality of such measures. Lawmakers and other proponents of cloning bans speak little if at all about the legal or constitutional merits of forestalling scientific inquiry into the workings of human SCNT. The popularity of bans on reproductive cloning assumes the mantle of legality, perhaps based on a sense that widespread outrage would flow from contrary attempts to formally legalize, or even regulate, the practice. It may be the case that public support for cloning bans is so strong that any legal challenge to an enacted ban would be summarily dismissed, with no judge willing to be perceived as dooming the human species.

Despite their popular appeal, as thinkers in the law we should pause to consider whether state-sponsored prohibitions on a specific method of bearing children are constitutionally sound. In Chapter 2 we reviewed the vast jurisprudence surrounding procreation, often pondering whether the long-standing constitutionally protected right "to bear or beget a child"[12] includes the right to procreate using assisted conception. Reproductive cloning raises some of the same questions as other forms of noncoital reproduction such as IVF and artificial insemination — questions such as: Can the government regulate the practice to promote the health and well-being of children without unduly infringing on a couple's right to procreate?

But cloning can be distinguished from other forms of ART on at least two grounds. First, cloning is a form of asexual reproduction, which differs from every other currently known form of reproduction which involves sexual reproduction — the fusion of one egg and one sperm. Second, unlike any other reproductive method, cloning produces a child with a genetic make-up that is an exact copy of an existing person, rather than the random genome that every living person now sports. Whether these distinguishing characteristics are sufficient to toss cloning out of the parameters of constitutionally protected conduct surrounding procreation remains a topic of debate and exploration. The materials that follow explore the constitutionality of legislated bans on human reproductive cloning. The bans are considered in light of the two most likely challenges to be raised against them: cloning bans violate the Fourteenth Amendment guarantee of procreative liberty by depriving individuals of reproductive choice, and they violate the First Amendment right to medical and scientific inquiry.

A.   Cloning and Procreational Autonomy

The ability of any enacted cloning ban to withstand a constitutional attack based on procreational autonomy may rest upon the technique's perceived solidarity with natural reproduction. Briefly stated, we know that the Due Process Clause of the Fifth and Fourteenth Amendments prohibit, respectively, federal or state governments from depriving any individual of "life, liberty, or property without due

---

[12] Quoting Justice Brennan's opinion in *Eisenstadt v. Baird*, 405 U.S. 438, 453 (1972).

process of law." Through a series of Supreme Court decisions beginning with *Skinner v. Oklahoma*, 316 U.S. 535 (1942), this Due Process liberty interest has been interpreted to protect the right to have children. Today, the right to procreate has been established as a fundamental right, protecting an individual's right to have children against governmental interference unless the state can show a compelling reason for imposing restrictions.

The foundational inquiry here is: Would reproductive cloning be considered "procreation" and thus a fundamental right which can only be restricted for compelling state reasons? As you might expect, arguments flow on both sides.

Professor John Robertson argues that reproductive cloning is a form of procreation and thus should be considered to merit the same constitutional protections as other forms of reproduction:

> Is cloning sufficiently similar to current assisted-reproduction and genetic-selection practices to be treated similarly as a presumptively protected exercise of family or reproductive liberty? Couples who request cloning . . . are seeking to rear healthy children with whom they will have a genetic or biologic tie, just as couples who conceive their children sexually do. Whether described as "replication" or as "reproduction," the resort to cloning is similar enough in purpose and effects to other reproduction and genetic-selection practices that it should be treated similarly. Therefore, a couple should be free to choose cloning unless there are compelling reasons for thinking that this would create harm that the other procedures would not cause.

John A. Robertson, *Human Cloning and the Challenge of Regulation*, 339 NEW ENG. J. MED. 119 (1998).

Professor Lori Andrews disagrees, finding a significant distinction between natural and current forms of assisted conception on the one had, and cloning:

> [C]loning is too qualitatively different from normal reproduction and from the types of assisted reproduction [for] . . . the same Constitutional protections apply . . .

> Cloning is not a process of genetic mix, but of genetic duplication. In even the most high-tech reproductive technologies available, a mix of genes occurs to create an individual with a genotype that has never before existed on earth. Even in the case of twins, their futures are unknown and the distinction between the offspring and their parents is acknowledged. In the case of cloning, however, the genotype in question has already existed. Even though it is clear that a clone will develop into a person with different traits because of different social, environmental, and generational influences, there is strong speculation that the fact that he or she has a genotype that already existed will affect how the resulting clone is treated by himself, his family, and social institutions.

> . . . [E]ven if a fundamental constitutional right to clone were recognized, any legislation that would infringe unduly upon this right would be permissible if it were narrowly tailored to further a compelling state

interest . . . [T]he potential physical and psychological risks of cloning an entire individual are sufficiently compelling to justify banning the procedure. Further, the notion of replicating existing humans seems to fundamentally conflict with our legal system, which emphatically protects individuality and uniqueness.

Lori B. Andrews, *Is There a Right to Clone? Constitutional Challenges to Bans on Human Cloning*, 11 HARV. J. LAW & TECHNOLOGY 643, 666-67 (1998).

Elizabeth Price Foley
Human Cloning and the Right to Reproduce
65 Albany L. Rev. 625, 638-46 (2002)

III. Does the Right to Reproduce Extend to Asexual Reproduction?

Even assuming the Supreme Court would accept that the Constitution protects, at least to some extent, the right to reproduce by non-coital, sexual methods, such as artificial insemination or IVF, the question remains as to whether it would agree that the right of reproduction extends even further to include the use of non-coital, asexual methods.

As an initial matter, it is worth noting that, as recent research has indicated, asexual reproduction is not limited to cloning. Parthenogenesis, or "virgin birth," is a process whereby eggs spontaneously begin the process of cell division without the need for sperm. Parthenogenesis thus differs from nuclear transfer cloning because it does not require the re-nucleation of a donor egg using the differentiated cell of a donor. All it takes, in other words, is an egg and the right environment. In a situation not involving natural parthenogenesis, this likely means that the egg must be soaked in a combination of chemicals. If the mix of chemicals is right, the egg will begin spontaneously dividing as though fertilization had occurred.

Parthenogenesis occurs naturally in numerous animal species, including some mammals. And in late November 2001, the scientists at Advanced Cell Technology revealed that they had successfully induced parthenogenesis in human eggs stimulated by chemicals. Specifically, the study involved the use of twenty-two donor eggs from three volunteers that were incubated in certain substances, rinsed, and placed in a culture media. After twelve hours, twenty of the twenty-two eggs (ninety percent) had begun the process of cell division; after five days, six of the original twenty-two (thirty percent) had divided to the point of forming blastomeres.

Whether by parthenogenesis or cloning, some scholars adamantly insist that asexual reproduction is qualitatively different from reproduction by sexual means (including sexual ARTs such as IVF), and thus should be afforded little or no constitutional protection. The gist of this objection is that cloning, and presumably, parthenogenesis precisely because it is asexual, should be treated differently, even though the result is the same as with sexual reproduction — namely, the creation of a human being. Opponents of cloning thus assert that, although the ends are the same as that of sexual reproduction, the means are different, and the law should focus on the means, not the ends.

The difficulty with this objection is its vagueness. What is the difference between sexual and asexual reproduction? The only objectively apparent difference is that sexual reproduction requires the union of sperm and egg (whether in the bedroom or petri dish), whereas asexual reproduction does not. The other differences discussed thus far in the debate are merely speculative and based more on one's theological or ideological preferences than on any objective data. These include fears about the impact of asexual reproduction on the institutions of marriage and the family, personal autonomy and privacy, the sanctity of life, the health and safety of the developing human embryo, and genetic diversity.

Many of these fears were also vehemently voiced as the basis for opposing the use of sexual ARTs such as IVF and artificial insemination. Not surprisingly, these fears have significantly subsided as time has gone by, to the point where an overwhelming majority of Americans supports the use of sexual ARTs. Moreover, it seems axiomatic that fear should not provide a sufficient basis for legal prohibition of action. As Justice Brandeis eloquently put it in the context of the First Amendment, "[f]ear of serious injury cannot alone justify suppression. . . . [Because of fear] [m]en feared witches and burnt women."

Because these speculative fears about asexual reproduction are ineluctably rooted in one's subjective experience and beliefs (i.e., ethics and morality), many find it difficult, if not impossible, to move beyond them. I do not mean to suggest that there is no room for ethical considerations in the development of public policy and law — quite the contrary. I do mean to suggest however, that, absent objective evidence that damage to persons or valued institutions will occur, judges and lawmakers should resist the temptation to base public policy on such considerations. If majoritarian fears of harm — without evidence that such harms will indeed occur — can provide a valid basis for governmental prohibition of conduct, many of the liberties we now enjoy would undoubtedly be short-lived. If one puts aside, at least for the moment, these speculative fears about asexual reproduction, one is left with considering whether asexual reproduction — merely because it does not require union of sperm and egg — should be treated differently under the law.

As I have argued strenuously in the past the asexual nature of cloning (or, for that matter, parthenogenesis), standing alone, should not be sufficient to justify a ban on the practice. There is simply no evidence that the asexual nature of this particular means of reproduction will result in any harms not already presented by sexual reproduction. Moreover, the end result — the birth of a child — is undeniably the same, whether reproduction is accomplished by sexual or asexual means. If the affirmative right to reproduce means anything, should it not mean that we, as human beings, have the right to bear or beget biologically related offspring? If so, what difference should the means employed make? Why should the law care, in other words, how our children are conceived?

If the law does not care what sexual position we assume when we conceive our children and does not care whether our children are conceived in a petri dish, why should it care whether our children are conceived without the use of sperm? From a feminist perspective, a legal construct that allows reproduction by sexual intercourse or by the artificial sexual union of sperm and egg (e.g., IVF) but not by cloning or parthenogenesis smacks of sexism, or more precisely, spermism. How could the law justify allowing all means of reproduction except those requiring the use of sperm? Is there something magical about sperm that gives lawmakers comfort, other than the fact that most of them have it? Although the Founding Fathers certainly never envisioned the possibility of reproduction without the use of sperm, do we really believe they intended to deny the right to have a biologically related child simply because the means employed did not involve its use? Should the ability of an individual to fulfill the dream of raising and loving his or her own child hinge upon the presence or absence of this one substance? I think it clear that it is the ends that matter, not the means. So long as the object is to have a child of one's own, the means employed should be legally irrelevant.

Although my own conclusions with regard to this issue are rather clear, I am left wondering (as is any academic writing about an issue of first impression) whether a court would concur. In other words, what would be the likely reaction of a court to this question? If asked, would a court sanction the use of asexual reproduction as constitutionally protected activity? Answering these questions requires a different construct, for these questions are not normative ones (i.e., what should a court do?), but pragmatic ones (i.e., what will a court likely do?). This, in turn, requires something more than acknowledgment and assessment of legal doctrine. It requires acknowledgment and assessment of the inevitable human tendency towards outcome-orientation (i.e., what is the conclusion I wish to reach and how do I then justify it?).

With this in mind, we can now turn to the pragmatic question: What would a court likely do when asked whether the right to reproduce encompasses the use of asexual methods such as cloning? A court would undoubtedly start with the substantive due process analytical legal framework pronounced in *Washington v. Glucksberg* [521 U.S. 702 (1997)], a case in which terminally ill patients challenged the constitutionality of criminal assisted-suicide laws as applied to their requests for physician aid in dying]. Specifically, the Supreme Court has recognized two salient features that identify practices protected by substantive due process: (1) the practice is " 'deeply rooted in this Nation's history and tradition' " and " 'implicit in the concept of ordered liberty,' such that 'neither liberty nor justice would exist if they were sacrificed,' " and (2) there is a " 'careful description' " of the liberty interest being asserted.

The second feature — the careful description of the interest being asserted — is necessary, according to the *Glucksberg* Court, "because guideposts for responsible decisionmaking in this unchartered area are scarce and open-ended" and because "[b]y extending constitutional protection to an asserted right or liberty interest, we, to a great extent, place the matter outside the arena of public debate and legislative action," thus running the risk that "the liberty protected by the Due Process Clause be subtly transformed into the policy preferences of the Members of this Court." With a cognizance of the possibility of subjective Lochnerian judicial lawmaking thus firmly in mind, the *Glucksberg* Court went on to carefully describe the right asserted by the respondents as "a right to commit suicide which itself includes a right to assistance in doing so." The plaintiffs in Glucksberg had, not surprisingly, framed the issue quite differently. Specifically, they had argued that the right being asserted was a " 'right to die with dignity,' " to " 'choose a humane, dignified death' " or to "control[] the manner and timing of . . . death."

Once the *Glucksberg* Court had "carefully described" the right asserted as a "right to commit suicide," the outcome of the case was sealed. Applying the second feature of substantive due process analysis, the Court concluded that the Nation's history and traditions did not indicate that there was a "deeply rooted" right to commit suicide — quite the contrary, since hundreds of years of Anglo-American law have considered assistance with suicide a crime.

A similar fate could await those who may assert that there is a constitutional right to have access to or to use cloning, parthenogenesis, or other asexual reproductive technology. If the Court determined, as a normative matter, that asexual reproduction was undesirable, it could reject a substantive due process claim by "carefully describing" the right being asserted as a "right to engage in asexual reproduction." So described, there is little doubt that the second substantive due process inquiry — i.e., whether the asserted right is "deeply rooted" in our Nation's history and traditions — would be answered in the negative. Given the recent genesis of asexual means of human reproduction and the virtually uniform popular condemnation of such procedures, the use of asexual reproductive technology is not likely to be characterized by the court as "deeply rooted" in our nation's history and traditions.

Of course, the newness of a given action is not, ipso facto, the death knell for its constitutional protection. Even conservative justices such as Justice Scalia have recognized that activities that are not "old" enough to qualify as deeply rooted in our history and traditions may, nonetheless, be found to qualify for constitutional protection, so long as courts refer "to the most specific level at which a relevant tradition protecting, or denying protection to, the asserted right can be identified." In other words, in situations involving new phenomena, one must attempt to analogize as best as one can. Thus, the lawyer's job is to identify, as closely as possible, an analogous tradition that is either protected or not protected.

The constitutional protection afforded to asexual reproduction thus depends, once again, on how one frames the right being asserted. Specifically, proponents and opponents of human cloning must attempt to identify an analogous tradition and argue, respectively, that it historically has or has not been protected by law. Which analogy the courts ultimately embrace will thus seal the outcome of this substantive due process issue. But what are the possible analogies for which proponents and opponents of human cloning would argue?

Proponents of human cloning would, of course, argue for the use of a broad analogue. Specifically, they would argue that the most closely analogous tradition that can be identified is reproduction. If a court agreed with this characterization, it would necessarily conclude that asexual reproduction (such as cloning) is but a subset of the larger category of reproduction; hence, because reproduction historically has been protected, so should asexual reproduction. This approach, however, probably would not satisfy conservative jurists, such as Justice Scalia, who presumably would emphasize that the Court's task, in assessing the constitutional protection of a new activity under substantive due process analysis, is to identify the most specific — i.e., most narrowly drawn — analogue possible in order to avoid Lochnerian pitfalls.

Proponents of asexual reproduction could, however, also argue for a more narrow analogue — specifically, the use of sexual ARTs such as IVF and artificial insemination. A court wishing to adopt such a middle ground approach would be required to decide whether and to what extent sexual ARTs are constitutionally protected. The constitutional protection afforded to human cloning (and parthenogenesis) would thus be coextensive with that of other ARTs. Since other ARTs appear to enjoy a high degree of constitutional protection, asexual reproductive methods would be similarly protected.

A court could also conclude that there is no apt analogy to be drawn between asexual reproduction and sexual reproduction — that these are, in other words, sui generis, "apples and oranges. In order to conclude, however, that asexual and sexual reproduction are apples and oranges, the court would need to catalog the differences between the two types of reproduction. Given the strong similarities between cloning and existing sexual ARTs such as IVF, this would be a difficult task.

The differences between reproduction via sexual intercourse and reproduction via ARTs (sexual or asexual), on the other hand, are rather apparent. The former requires a physical intimacy between a man and woman, the latter does not, at least not in the traditional sense. Indeed, once one moves away from old-fashioned intercourse (and perhaps artificial insemination), reproduction is accomplished in essentially the same way: an ovum is somehow stimulated to begin the process of cell division. With IVF, the stimulation is achieved by the addition of sperm. With parthenogenesis, the stimulation is achieved by chemicals. With cloning, the stimulation is achieved by a combination of a mild jolt of electricity followed by cell starvation. Traditional physical intimacy between man and woman is neither implicated nor threatened.

Given the rather stark difference between sexual intercourse and all forms of assisted reproduction, and the equally stark similarities among the various types of artificial reproduction, a court wishing to say that sexual and asexual reproduction are "apples and oranges" would thus have a difficult time. A more apt characterization would be that sexual intercourse is the "apple" and all other artificial reproductive technologies are the "oranges." The difficulty with this conclusion, of course, is that it leaves all of the oranges (ARTs) constitutionally unprotected and hence, vulnerable to complete prohibition. IVF, GIFT, ZIFT, and other ARTs could be as easily banned as cloning — a result that is, pragmatically speaking, unacceptable.

An outcome-oriented court preferring not to leave all types of ARTs vulnerable to legislative attack could, as an alternative, conclude that all forms of reproduction are constitutionally protected but vary the degree of constitutional protection according to the means employed. A court could thus acknowledge a hierarchy of constitutional protection, similar to the hierarchy recognized in equal protection jurisprudence. Under this approach, presumably, reproduction via sexual intercourse would receive the highest degree of constitutional protection, given its inherent privacy implications and undoubted characterization as a right which is deeply rooted in our nation's history and traditions. Laws attempting to infringe upon an individual's ability to engage in reproduction via sexual intercourse would thus be subjected to the strictest judicial scrutiny. Just below this category of judicial protection would fall laws regulating reproduction by assisted (i.e., noncoital) means. A court opting for this approach would likely reason that although many ARTs have achieved a broad level of acceptance and use, they do not enjoy the same historical and traditional reverence as reproduction via sexual intercourse. Moreover, while there are certain intimacy and privacy interests implicated by reproduction via ARTs, these interests are somewhat diminished. When an egg is stimulated to begin division in a petri dish, whether by sperm, chemicals, or a jolt of electricity, the specter of "bedroom police" is not as apparent or threatening. For this reason, under a hierarchical approach, a court could uphold a law regulating the personnel and facilities employed in IVF cloning or other ARTs — regulations that would not be tolerated for reproduction via sexual intercourse. Thus, while the government would be able to restrict the use of ARTs to certain places (e.g., licensed facilities) and prohibit the application of ARTs except by certain personnel (e.g., physicians), it certainly would not be able to impose the same kinds of restrictions on sexual intercourse.

George J. Annas, Lori B. Andrews and Rosario M. Isasi
Protecting the Endangered Human: Toward an International Treaty Prohibiting Cloning and Inheritable Alterations
28 Am. J.L. & Med. 151, 157-162 (2002)

[At the outset of the article, the authors suggest language for a proposed international "Convention of the Preservation of the Human Species" that would outlaw all efforts to initiate a pregnancy by using either intentionally modified genetic material or human replication cloning, such as through somatic cell nuclear transfer. The excerpt that follows presents the legal and policy justifications for such an international ban.]

III. An International Convention: Why Now?

Five years after the announcement of the cloning of Dolly the sheep it is time to ask not if cloning and inheritable alterations should be regulated, but how. Had a five-year moratorium for further thought and discussion been placed on cloning humans, as the National Bioethics Advisory Commission (NBAC) recommended in 1997, for example, the time would now have expired. What new have we learned in the last five years?

First, virtually every scientist in the world with an opinion believes it is unsafe to attempt a human pregnancy with a cloned embryo. This is, for example, the unanimous conclusion of a 2002 report from the U.S. National Academy of Sciences, which recommended that human "reproductive" cloning be outlawed in the United States following a study that included the viewpoints of the only two scientists in the world who publicly advocate human cloning today. Although scientists seldom like to predict the future without overwhelming data to support them, many believe that human cloning or inheritable genetic alternations at the embryo level will never be safe because they will always be inherently unpredictable in their effects on the children and their offspring. As Stewart Newman has noted, for example, it is unlikely that a human created from the union of "two damaged cells" (an enucleated egg and a nucleus removed from a somatic cell) could ever be healthy . . . It is worth underlining that the dangers are not just physical, but also psychological.

Whether cloned children could ever overcome the psychological problems associated with their origins is unknown and perhaps unknowable. In short, the safety issues, which inherently make attempts to clone or genetically alter a human being unethical human experiments, provide sufficient scientific justification for the treaty alone.

If and when safety can be assured, assuming this will ever be possible, two primary arguments have been set forth in favor of proceeding with cloning (and its first cousin, inheritable genetic alterations). First, cloning is a type of human reproduction that can help infertile couples have genetically-related children. Second, cloning is a part of human "progress" that could lead to a new type of genetic immortality, therefore, to prevent it is to be anti-scientific.

The infertility argument is made by physiologist Panos Zavos and his former Italian colleague, infertility specialist Severino Antinori. They argue that the inability of a sterile male to have a genetically-related child is such a human tragedy that it justifies human cloning. This view not only ignores the rights and interests of women and children (even if only males are to be cloned, eggs must be procured from a woman, the embryos must be gestated by a woman and the child is the subject of the experiment), but also contains a highly-contested assertion: that asexual genetic replication or duplication should be seen as "human reproduction." In fact, humans are a sexually reproducing species and have never reproduced or replicated themselves asexually.

Asexual replication may or may not be categorized by future courts as a form of human reproduction, but there are strong arguments against it. First, asexual reproduction changes a fundamental characteristic of what it means to be human (i.e., a sexually reproducing species) by making sexual reproduction involving the genetic mixture of male and female gametes optional. Second, the "child" of an asexual replication is also the twin brother of the male "parent," a relationship that has never existed before in human society. The first clone, for example, will be the first human being with a single genetic "parent" (unless the biological grandparents are taken to be the actual "parents" of the clone). Third, the genetic replica of a genetically sterile man would be sterile himself and could only "reproduce" by cloning. This means either that infertility is not a major problem (because if it were, it would be unethical for a physician to intentionally create a child with this problem), or that the desire of existing adults should take precedent over the welfare of children. We find neither conclusion persuasive, and this is probably why, although some ethicists believe that cloning could be considered a form of human reproduction, infertility specialists have not joined Antinori's call for human cloning as a treatment for infertile males. In fact the organization that represents infertility specialists in the United States, and is generally opposed to the regulation of the infertility industry, the American Society of Reproductive Medicine, has nonetheless consistently opposed human cloning.

There are, nonetheless, legal commentators who believe that human cloning should be classified as a form of human reproduction, and protected as such, at least if it is the only way for an individual to have a "genetically-related child." . . . Suffice it to say here that it is very unclear that human reproduction or procreation of a kind protected by principles of autonomy and self-fulfillment can be found in a "right to have a genetically-related child." It cannot be just the genetic tie that is important in human reproduction, because if it were, this could be accomplished by having one's twin brother have a child with one's wife — the genetic tie would be identical, yet few, if any, would argue that this method of reproduction should satisfy the twin's right to have a "genetically-related child." Genes are important, but there is more to human reproduction, as protected by the U.S. Constitution, than simple genetic replication.

The second major argument in favor of human cloning is that it can lead to a form of immortality. This is the premise of the Raelian cult that has chartered its own corporation, Clonaid, to engage in human cloning. The leader of the cult, who calls himself Rael (formerly Claude Vorilhon, the editor of a French motor sport magazine), believes that all humans were created in the laboratories of the planet Elohim and that the Elohims have instructed Rael and his followers to develop cloning on Earth to provide earthlings with a form of immortality. The Raelians, of course, can believe whatever they want to; but just as human sacrifice is illegal, experiments that pose a significant danger to women and children can also be outlawed, and the religious beliefs of this cult do not provide a sufficient justification to refrain from outlawing cloning.

Just as two primary arguments in favor of cloning and inheritable genetic alterations have emerged over the past five years, so have two basic arguments about the future regulation of these technologies. The first, exemplified by Lee Silver, is that these technologies, while not necessarily desirable, are unstoppable because the market combined with parental desire will drive scientists and physicians to offer these services to demanding couples. Similar to the way parents now seek early educational enrichment for their children, he believes that parents of the future will seek early genetic enhancement to give them a competitive advantage in life. Silver thinks this will ultimately lead to the creation of two separate species or subspecies, the GenRich and "the naturals."

A related "do nothing" argument is that regulation may not be needed because the technologies will not be widely used. The thought is that humans may muddle through, either because the science of human genetic alterations may never prove possible, or because it will be used by only a handful of humans because most will instinctively reject it. Colin Tudge, a proponent of this argument, also accepts Silver's argument that the market is powerful and often determinative, but nonetheless believes that the three fundamental principles of all religions — personal humility, respect for fellow humans and reverence for the universe as a whole — could lead the vast majority of humans to reject cloning and genetic alterations. In his words:

> The new technologies, taken to extremes, threaten the idea of humanity. We now need to ask as a matter of urgency who we really are and what we really value about ourselves. It could all be changed after all — we ourselves could be changed — perhaps simply by commercial forces that we have allowed to drift beyond our control. If that is not serious, it is hard to see what is.

We agree with Tudge that the issues are serious. We think that they are too serious to be left to religions or human instinct, or even to individual national legislation, to address.

In this regard, we find a second approach, that of a democratically-formed regulatory scheme more reasonable. Indeed, in our view the widespread condemnation of human replicative cloning by governments around the world means that cloning provides a unique opportunity for the world to begin to work together to take some control over the biotechnology that threatens our very existence.

The primary arguments against cloning and inheritable genetic alterations, which we believe make an international treaty the appropriate action, have been summarized in detail elsewhere. In general, the arguments are that these interventions would require massive dangerous and unethical human experimentation, that cloning would inevitably be bad for the resulting children by restricting their right to an "open future," that cloning would lead to a new eugenics movement for "designer children" (because if an individual could select the entire genome of their future child, it would seem impossible to prohibit individuals from choosing one or more specific genetic characteristics of their future children), and that it would likely lead to the creation of a new species or subspecies of humans, sometimes called the "posthuman." In the context of the species, the last argument has gotten the least attention, and so it is worth exploring.

Specifically, the argument is that cloning will inevitably lead to attempts to modify the somatic cell nucleus not to create genetic duplicates of existing people, but "better" children. If this attempt fails, that is the end of it. If it succeeds, however, something like the scenario envisioned by Silver and others such as Nancy Kress, will unfold: a new species or subspecies of humans will emerge. The new species, or "posthuman," will likely view the old "normal" humans as inferior, even savages, and fit for slavery or slaughter. The normals, on the other hand, may see the posthumans as a threat and if they can, may engage in a preemptive strike by killing the posthumans before they themselves are killed or enslaved by them. It is ultimately this predictable potential for genocide that makes species-altering experiments potential weapons of mass destruction, and makes the unaccountable genetic engineer a potential bioterrorist. It is also why cloning and genetic modification is of species-wide concern and why an international treaty to address it is appropriate. Such a treaty is necessary because existing laws on cloning and inheritable genetic alterations, although often well-intentioned, have serious limitations.

NOTES AND QUESTIONS

1.   Compare the views of Professor Foley and Professors Annas, Andrews and Isasi on human cloning as a method of reproduction. Do you see any areas of agreement among the authors? What are the major areas of disagreement? If you were asked to mediate a resolution between the two sides on the question — should human cloning be banned? — can you envision a solution that would be acceptable to both sides?

2.   Note the colorful use of language both sides of the cloning debate invoke. Do you agree with Professor Foley that opposition to asexual reproduction using

cloning is a form of "spermism?" What is spermism? On the other hand, do you agree that reproductive cloning is a potential "weapon of mass destruction" and that professionals that aid in the birth of a cloned child should be considered "bioter-rorists?" Does use of emotional language advance or detract from a productive national (or international) dialogue on the issue of cloning?

3.   The question of whether the Constitution would protect the right to clone is only partially answered by a determination of whether cloning is akin to procreation and thus a fundamental right. As explained by Professor Cass Sunstein, "For purposes of substantive due process, the first question is whether the right to clone counts as a fundamental one, with which the government can interfere only to protect a 'compelling' interest. If there is no fundamental right, the government is required merely to show a 'rational basis' for its action, a much easier burden to meet." Cass R. Sunstein, *Is There a Constitutional Right to Clone?*, 53 Hast. L. J. 987, 989 (2002). Professor Sunstein concludes that reproductive cloning is not a fundamental right and thus could be the subject of government interference, and perhaps total prohibition, with the state required to show only a rational basis for taking such legislative action. What would be a state actor's rational basis be for enacting a ban on reproductive cloning? Do any of these reasons rise to the level of a compelling state interest sufficient to satisfy strict scrutiny in the event cloning were found to be akin to a fundamental right to procreate?

If reproductive cloning were banned, even criminalized, in the U.S., who would be harmed by such a law? Certainly our first thoughts probably turn to the prospective parents who would be denied the right to have children in this manner. Are there any other identifiable groups who would be harmed by a cloning ban? Consider the materials that follow.

B.   Cloning and the Right to Scientific Inquiry

John Charles Kunich
The Naked Clone
91 Kentucky L. J. 1, 48-55 (2002)

When the facts diverge from the naked clone situation[13], somewhat different legal issues become relevant. For example, some of the more sweeping bans include prohibitions on the cloning of humans for any purposes, including scientific or medical research. Some researchers may want to use cloned humans, presumably limited to early stages of embryonic development, to explore stem cell options and other issues. Such experiments would in no event lead to the birth of a living infant

---

[13] Earlier in his article, Professor Kunich explains that, "The term 'naked clone' is used to highlight one particularly propitious concatenation of circumstances, in which well-meaning, loving, child-focused people are barred from cloning despite being motivated by some of the best, most altruistic, and most basic human impulses. The parents, perhaps already devastated by the terminal illness of their child, would be bereft a second time, having lost the chance to give life another chance through cloning. The child of cloning would be naked in the sense of being devoid of protection, stripped of legal rights, and without any refuge from the government that forbids him or her even to exist. The privacy rights of the parents and child would be subordinated to the state interests, leaving the child of cloning naked and exposed to the dictates of the government." 91 Ky L. J. at 31-32. -Ed.

and, as such, would fall within a different category from the several variants of the naked clone scenario. Presumably there would be no implantation in any woman's uterus and no implication of a woman's privacy rights. There would be no issues of parental rights, nor of reproductive liberty.

However, these cases would implicate important rights too. It can be argued that scientific or medical research constitutes a form of expression within the meaning of the First Amendment. The research process involves a quest for truth, a hunt for more information, which is at the heart of the First Amendment, as an indispensable prerequisite to the more familiar dissemination of information. Also, perhaps the performance of research itself could be viewed as a type of expressive conduct or symbolic speech, making the statement that such research is valuable and the furtherance of knowledge concerning a hypothesis is a worthy aim.

If one accepts either of these premises, a total ban on one particular form of research, i.e., that involving the cloning of humans, should be considered a content-based restriction on expression, invoking strict scrutiny by the courts. The ban would be explicitly aimed at one specific type of research, not neutrally applicable to scientific research in general, and it would be deliberately and precisely targeted against human clonal experimentation. The gathering and dissemination of scientific data specific to the cloning of humans would be the entire focal point, tantamount to an explicit ban on expressive conduct that proclaims the worthiness of pursuing human clonal research. This is content-based regulation of expression, and it calls for strict scrutiny. A compelling state interest is required in order to survive strict scrutiny and, as we have discussed, it could be difficult to cobble together such an interest in banning cloning, given its similarities to other forms of reproduction and the implausibility of the worst-case arguments. Moreover, it is a bedrock pillar of the First Amendment that government may not ban or punish speech, including expressive conduct, based on its content merely because that content is deemed repugnant, unpopular, or inadvisable.

The right or liberty to conduct scientific research — to search for knowledge and truth — has some support in Supreme Court precedent. In several cases, the Court has stated that the First Amendment safeguards a "marketplace of ideas," and, as with any marketplace, it must be continually stocked with new supplies, whether obtained by the press or by scientific researchers. The actions of those who produce information and ideas for the marketplace of ideas are deserving of First Amendment protection, at least as much as the actions of those who disseminate information and ideas. Before ideas and information can be expressed, they necessarily must first be created or discovered by someone. The Court has recognized, in dicta, a Fourteenth Amendment liberty interest in conducting research or inquiry as well, although some lower federal courts have held that there is no fundamental right to conduct research on human fetuses. Substantive and procedural due process requirements have also been postulated as sources of constitutional protection for scientific inquiry.

Modern events seldom recall the official condemnation and persecution suffered by the renowned seventeenth-century scientist Galileo Galilei, but the bans on research and exploration into cloning have done just that. The Inquisition forced Galileo publicly to deny, under threat of torture, what he had learned through scientific study — that the earth revolved around the sun, i.e., the Copernican theory — in order to escape execution for the crime of heresy. Found guilty and sentenced to life imprisonment, he spent the last ten years of his life under house arrest. This infamous travesty was made possible by a society in which the line between Church and State was blatantly breached and a person could be criminally punished for activities that discomforted the religious sensibilities of the dominant elite. When those in power use that authority in a preemptive strike to seal off entire categories of learning and inquiry, the loss is unfathomable. No one can ever know what might have been known had the freedom to discover not been denied. Second and third generations of valuable breakthroughs into tangentially related areas might have been gained but for the prior restraint on research, and again, we can never know what we might have learned. This is a loss without limits.

When the law places Galileo in chains, the entire society of humankind is likewise shackled. We are forced, like Galileo, to kneel before the power of the state and abjure the reality we have found through so many years of work and sacrifice, pretending instead that modern discoveries were never made. We artificially and arbitrarily close the collective mind of the people to the facts, because myths are safer and more familiar to those in command of the coercive force of government. It would require a compelling state interest indeed to justify such a breathtaking curtailment of the freedom of inquiry.

Attempts to find this elusive state interest have led some to liken cloning research to the vilest, most extreme, pseudo-scientific examples available in the bottom of the dustbin of history, such as the notorious experiments by Josef Mengele on living prisoners in Nazi concentration camps. There are such vast differences between the two situations that one scarcely knows where to begin. Legitimate experiments and laboratory procedures involving very early stage human cells are legally and morally indistinguishable from other contemporary activities that are free from governmental censorship. This is not a case of compelling already-born, sentient human beings to diabolical, excruciating, and ultimately fatal surgical procedures to satisfy the perverse curiosity of an evil doctor. There is no legal basis for placing modern cloning research either into an unprotected class by itself, or into a locked room with Mengele as the only cellmate.

Some would nonetheless assert that there is a compelling state interest in preventing the creation and use of living human embryos for the explicit purpose of serving as the raw materials for laboratory experiments. In this view, such cloned embryos might be deemed human beings, and the clinical exploitation and commodification of them an evil well within the power of government to ban. Notwithstanding the potential benefits that might be reaped from these experiments, the sacredness of human life would stand as an insurmountable obstacle to using cloned human embryos for medical or scientific research.

A related point deals with the large numbers of failures likely to be endured en route to every successful cloning. This concern applies not only to laboratory research but also to the naked clone scenario in which parents seek to create a live baby. Recall the dismal success rate experienced during the process that resulted in Dolly. Until and unless massive progress is made toward improving the lopsided ratio of failures to successes, it is possible that every live child of cloning would be outnumbered many times over by embryos that never make it to a live birth, never survive the earliest stages of infancy, or are deformed. If cloning produces dozens or even hundreds of doomed, damaged, or discarded embryos and infants for every healthy baby, this could spark intense opposition on the grounds that this is an appalling waste of nascent human life. Again, it appears to reduce people to commodities and to accept many dead embryos and deformed babies as just another of the costs of doing business for the production of every viable, normal child of cloning.

There is a certain visceral power to these objections. If the cloning dilemma had developed prior to *Roe v. Wade*, there is little doubt that the opponents of cloning would have prevailed in the courts, including the Supreme Court. There was a long history of legal recognition and protection of unborn human life under the common law. Modern criminal law and tort law also accommodated the interests of the state in the protection of pre-birth humans. But the lens through which the judiciary views inchoate human life has been radically altered since *Roe*. The courts have accepted, and indeed ensured, the legality of millions of abortions annually, with myriad embryos and fetuses intentionally eliminated at all stages of gestation, under all circumstances, and for any and all reasons. The process of in vitro fertilization is also now well-established and is afforded the full complement of legal protections, notwithstanding the significant numbers of unsuccessful attempts to bring about a healthy baby and the frequency with which embryos are discarded.

There has not been a surfeit of restrictive legislation or regulation pertaining to in vitro fertilization, despite some moral and religious objections. No state has banned it, and the legal measures that are in effect generally require only data collection, certification of practitioners and facilities, and the provision for informed consent. The parallels with cloning are both obvious and significant. Some critics initially predicted that in vitro fertilization would result in the mass-production of infants. Public outrage at the dawn of in vitro fertilization was extreme, at least in some quarters, and dire consequences were prophesied. In the early years, legal commentators decried the technology and urged restrictions. Yet, as the reality juggernaut inexorably encroached on speculation, the law has actually moved to protect and foster the use of in vitro fertilization, primarily because it has been demonstrably successful and a boon to infertile couples and individuals.

Realistically, it is highly unlikely that the cloning of humans would be attempted by most medical professionals, nor would people want to try it as a form of assisted reproduction, until the technology has moved beyond the stage of high failure rates and abnormal births, with or without legislation restricting the practice. It would be prohibitively expensive and ethically dubious to persist in efforts to clone people unless additional experiments involving animals, especially higher primates, dramatically improved the probability of a normal, live birth. On the pragmatic level, cloning would need to attain something approaching the success rate of in vitro fertilization before it becomes a real option, both for would-be parents and for the medical and technological professionals involved. The process would be self-regulating to a significant degree. If legislation were narrowly tailored to regulate human reproductive cloning and/or research, perhaps with a very short-term temporary ban until the requisite progress is achieved through non-human research, there could be a legitimate judicial imprimatur as well.

Potentially, courts might draw a distinction between "casualties" unavoidably incurred in the process of cloning a human being under the naked clone situation and cloned embryos intentionally created and "harvested" for the express purpose of scientific/medical research. The naked clone position is buttressed by powerful additional constitutional rights not available in the research setting, and this might justify greater judicial deference to the former than the latter. Restrictions and regulations, although probably not an outright permanent ban, could be tolerated in the research setting, while cloning for reproduction would be much more fully protected. However, in light of the analogous collateral loss of human embryos during in vitro fertilization experiments and actual in vitro fertilization attempts to reproduce and the many millions of pre-natal fetuses and embryos deliberately destroyed through various forms of abortion, it is possible that courts would not find an outcome-determinative distinction between the two. We have blazed a path that may lead to even large-scale, intentional sacrifice of research-only cloned human embryos, and a fortiori the unintentional loss of embryos associated with the presumed low success rate of live-birth directed cloning efforts.

NOTES AND QUESTIONS

1. Do you agree with Professor Kunich that a ban on human cloning unduly interferes with a right of scientific inquiry? If such a right does exist as a fundamental right protected either by the Fourteenth Amendment right to personal liberty, or the First Amendment right to free speech, could a ban be justified as fulfilling a compelling state interest? Are the government's reasons for banning scientific inquiry surrounding cloning the same as those for banning individuals and physicians from attempting to create a child through cloning?

If you are interested in learning more about cloning and the Constitution, Professor Kunich has expanded his arguments into a full-length book titled, *The Naked Clone: How Cloning Bans Threaten Our Personal Rights* (2003).

2. Professor Lori Andrews has given thought to the question of whether a cloning ban would infringe upon a constitutional right of scientific inquiry, concluding:

> Cloning is sufficiently analogous to embryo research that restrictions on it should not be considered protected by a right of scientific inquiry. In holding that the right to conduct medical research is not fundamental under the Constitution, a federal court [*Margaret S. v. Edwards*, 448 F. Supp. 181 (E.D. La. 1980] held that a state could regulate experimentation involving the unborn so long as the regulation was rational. The court explained, in words that are particularly applicable to cloning, "[g]iven the dangers of abuse inherent in any rapidly developing field, it is rational for a State to act to protect the health and safety of its citizens."

> Even if cloning research on humans were protected by the Constitution, certain restrictions would be permissible. The freedom to pursue knowledge is distinguishable from the right to choose the method for achieving that knowledge, which may permissibly be regulated to some extent. Although the government may not prohibit research in an attempt to

prevent the development of new knowledge, it may restrict or prohibit the means used by researchers that threaten interests in which the state has a legitimate concern. Research may be restricted, for example, to protect the subject's right to autonomy and welfare by requiring informed, free and competent consent.

Therefore, federal and state government may regulate the researcher's methods in order to protect the rights of research subjects and community safety.

Lori B. Andrews, *Is There a Right to Clone? Constitutional Challenges to Bans on Human Cloning*, 11 HARV. J. LAW & TECHNOLOGY 643, 663 (1998). If research on human reproductive cloning is not considered a protected right within the ambit of scientific research, and thus subject to total prohibition, would there be any legal way to experiment in the cloning field? Is banning scientific inquiry in the field of human cloning a benefit or harm to humankind?

If research on IVF had likewise been prohibited in the 1970s, which parts of this book would be available for you to read today? Perhaps you are of the mind that less is more, especially if you have read from cover to cover, but it is apparent the world that IVF has spawned is vast and growing. Whether cloning will take its place at the far end of the ART spectrum, stirring initial controversy but gradually settling in as another technology in the array of reproductive choices, remains a question for editions to come.

GLOSSARY

AID Artificial Insemination by Donor. Assisted insemination in which semen is obtained from a donor who does not intend to act as the resulting child's father, as opposed to the woman's husband or partner.

AIH Artificial Insemination Heterologous. Assisted insemination in which semen is obtained from a woman's husband or partner, as opposed to a donor who does not intend to act as the resulting child's father.

ART Assisted reproductive technologies. A variety of medical procedures in which pregnancy is accomplished by means other than sexual intercourse. ART includes all fertility treatments in which the egg, the sperm, or both, are handled outside the body. The two most common ART procedures are: 1) artificial insemination, in which sperm is introduced into the female reproductive tract using an injection device, and 2) in vitro fertilization (IVF), which involves surgically removing eggs from a woman's ovaries, combining them with sperm in a laboratory, and returning the product of that union to the woman's uterus.

Artificial Insemination See Assisted Insemination.

Assisted Insemination A medical procedure used to treat male factor infertility (for example, low sperm count or poor motility) or to assist women with no male partner achieve pregnancy. Assisted insemination requires that semen be obtained from the male, and then placed in the woman's reproductive tract using an injection device.

Blastocyst The developing embryo at approximately five days after fertilization. The blastocyst is composed of an inner cell mass and a trophectoderm, which is an outer layer of cells destined to become part of the placenta. The cells from the inner cell mass have the potential to form any cell type of the body and are commonly referred to as embryonic stem cells.

Egg The female sexual cell or gamete from inception until fertilization. Medical literature favors the term "oocyte".

Embryo The developing human organism from approximately 14 days after fertilization of the egg by the sperm until the period when organs and organ systems begin to develop, at approximately the end of the second month.

Embryonic Stem Cells In humans, these cells are contained in a five-day-old embryo (blastocyst) and are pluripotent, meaning they are undifferentiated and have the capacity to form of all of the cells of the human body. The study of regenerative medicine involves the isolation, cultivation and transformation of embryonic stem cells into different body cell types, such as nerve cells, heart cells and insulin-producing cells, which can be transplanted into patients who suffer from diseases that damage these cell types in their bodies. Embryonic stem cells are taken from the blastocyst, which is then no longer able to develop into a fully formed human being.

Fertilization   The union of male and female gametes leading to formation of a unique one-cell entity known as a zygote. Fertilization begins with the penetration of the oocyte by the sperm and is completed with the fusion of the male and female pronuclei (nuclear material containing chromosomes). When the pronuclei merge in human fertilization, the zygote contains the number of chromosomes characteristic of the species.

Fetus   The developing human organism after the embryonic stage until birth. The fetus is described as the product of conception from approximately the end of the eighth week (or second month) until the moment of birth.

Gamete   The oocyte (egg) or the spermatozoon (sperm); a mature reproductive cell that, upon union with another gametic cell, results in the development of a new individual.

GIFT   Gamete intrafallopian transfer. A medical procedure in which a woman's eggs are retrieved following ovarian stimulation, mixed in the laboratory with sperm, and reintroduced into the fallopian tube using a fiber-optic instrument called a laparoscope which is inserted through small incisions in the woman's abdomen. GIFT assists the gametes (eggs and sperm) in reaching the fallopian tube, the location where natural fertilization takes place. In order to use GIFT, a woman must have at least one healthy fallopian tube.

ICSI   Intracytoplasmic sperm injection. A medical procedure in which a single sperm is injected directly into the egg in order to achieve fertilization. ICSI involves placing sperm in a solution to slow their movement; a single sperm is selected from the solution and immobilized. Using a slim injection pipette, the sperm is inserted into the cytoplasm of the egg (the material surrounding the egg cell nucleus). ICSI is performed in the laboratory using eggs that have been retrieved from a woman's ovaries. Once the injection has taken place, the eggs are later studied to see if fertilization has occurred. The resulting embryos are then placed into the woman's uterus.

iPS Cells   Induced Pluripotent Stem Cells. These cells were first created in 2006 by scientists interested in creating undifferentiated cell lines that could be transformed into any cell type in the body. Ideally, these newly transformed cells could be used to treat diseases in which healthy cells replace damaged cells associated with a variety of illnesses. iPS cells begin as adult cells, such as skin cells, that are reprogrammed to regress back to their pluripotent state. Pluripotent cells are capable of forming into any adult cell type. iPS cells are being developed as part of the study of regenerative medicine in which blank or undifferentiated cells are coaxed (by chemicals, genetic processes or other methods) to become specific cell types such as nerve cells, heart cells or insulin-producing cells that can be transplanted into patients as therapies or cures for diseases that cause damage to these cells.

IVF   In vitro fertilization. A medical procedure in which a woman's eggs are extracted from her ovaries, mixed with sperm in the laboratory, the resulting embryos are grown for three to five days, then transferred back to the woman's uterus through the cervix. An IVF cycle has four phases: **Phase 1: Ovarian Stimulation and Monitoring**. A woman is treated with a sequence of drugs, generally administered through injection, to induce multiple follicles to mature so that several eggs can be retrieved. Drug treatment usually begins midway through a woman's menstrual cycle and continues until the eggs are retrieved. **Phase 2: Egg Collection**. Egg retrieval is done in a surgical procedure in which either general anesthesia, or a combination of sedation and pain medications are administered to the woman. Physicians insert an ultrasound-guided needle through the vaginal wall and into a developed ovarian follicle. Using suction, the fluid inside the follicle is withdrawn, along with the egg it contains. This removal technique is repeated for each follicle that has developed. **Phase 3: Fertilization and Embryo Culture**. Each normal appearing egg is placed in a separate petri dish containing culture medium. Semen is obtained from the male partner and is processed to obtain a high concentration of motile sperm. The sperm is then introduced into the dish. The contents of the dish are examined under a microscope after one day to determine if the egg is fertilized. **Phase 4: Embryo Transfer**. Embryos are generally transferred to the woman's uterus two or three days after egg retrieval, when they are comprised of four to eight cells. Under certain circumstances the embryo will be transferred after five days when it has become a blastocyst. The transfer is accomplished using a sterile tube with a syringe on one end. Droplets of fluid containing one embryo are drawn into the tube which is inserted through the cervix and then injected into the uterus. Embryo transfer generally requires no anesthesia or sedation. Following embryo transfer, a woman will wait approximately 10 to 14 days before undergoing a blood test to determine if she is pregnant.

Morula The developing human organism from the 16-cell preembryo stage until blastocyst formation; the stage commonly observed between 72 and 96 hours after fertilization.

PGD Preimplantation genetic diagnosis. PGD is a technique in which one cell of three-day-old eight-celled embryo is removed and studied for its genetic composition. The cell is removed through an opening made in the covering of the embryo. The extracted cell is analyzed using different techniques, including fluorescence in-situ hybridization or FISH. This technique uses probes — small pieces of DNA — that are a match for the chromosomes present in the cell. Each probe is labeled with a different fluorescent dye. These fluorescent probes are applied to the extracted cell and they attach to the chromosomes. Under a fluorescent microscope, scientists can visualize the dye-colored chromosomes that are in that cell. This visualization allows scientists to count if the cell has the correct number of chromosomes and also to determine the gender of the embryo because the sex chromosomes can be dyed and seen under the microscope.

Posthumous Reproduction The birth of a child after the death of one or both of the gamete providers. Posthumous reproduction refers to a child who is conceived and in utero during the lifetime of a gametic parent but born after that parent's death.

Postmortem Conception The conception or gestation and birth of a child after the death of one or both of the gamete providers. Posthumous conception can be accomplished by freezing sperm, eggs or embryos during the lifetime of the gamete provider(s), and then thawing and implanting any resulting embryo after death. Sperm and eggs may also be retrieved from the gamete provider shortly after the person's death, and any resulting child born of that process would be considered a postmortem conception child.

Preembryo   The developing human organism during early cleaving stages, which immediately follow fertilization, until development of the embryo. The preembryonic period immediately follows the zygote stage and ends at approximately 14 days after fertilization with the development of the primitive streak.

Reproductive Cloning   A form of reproduction in which offspring result not from the union of egg and sperm (sexual reproduction) but from the replication of the genetic makeup of another single individual (asexual reproduction). Reproductive cloning involves somatic cell nuclear transfer (SCNT), a technique in which the nucleus is removed from an unfertilized human egg and is replaced by the nucleus of a somatic, or non-sex, cell of the person to be cloned. A chemical or an electric pulse is then applied to the egg to activate it to begin dividing and forming an embryo. Once the embryo reaches the eight-celled stage, it can be transferred to a woman's uterus for implantation, gestation and birth. To date, no child has ever been born using reproductive cloning.

Somatic Cell Nuclear Transfer (SCNT)   SCNT begins when the nucleus is removed from an unfertilized human egg and replaced by the nucleus of a somatic (non-sex) cell of the organism to be cloned. A chemical or an electric pulse is then applied to the egg to activate it, in much the same way a sperm activates an egg by penetrating its surface in the course of natural fertilization. Thereafter, the egg develops into an embryo and after five days, into a blastocyst.

Sperm   The male sexual cell or gamete, which serves to fertilize the female oocyte (egg). It consists of a head, neck, midpiece and tail. Medical literature uses the term "spermatozoon."

Therapeutic Cloning   Also known as "Research Cloning." A technique in which embryos are created using somatic cell nuclear transfer and grown to the blastocyst stage, approximately five days after the embryo first begins to divide. The blastocyst contains an inner cell mass of approximately 100-200 stem cells which are retrieved and prompted to differentiate into specific cell types. The goal of therapeutic cloning is to develop compatible cells or tissues that can be transplanted back into the cell donor to replace lost or damaged cells, without immunosuppressive therapy or fear of rejection.

ZIFT   Zygote intrafallopian transfer. A medical procedure in which a woman's eggs are retrieved following ovarian stimulation, mixed in the laboratory with sperm, and allowed to develop into early embryos (also called zygotes, usually seen approximately one day after fertilization). The zygotes are transferred into a woman's fallopian tubes using a laparoscope, placed through the woman's abdomen, to guide placement of the early embryos. ZIFT combines some of the laboratory elements of IVF and the tubal transfer of GIFT.

Zygote   The one-cell stage of the developing human organism before the first cleavage, usually seen 18-24 hours after the sperm penetrates the egg.

TABLE OF CASES

[References are to pages]

A

A.H.W. v. G.H.B. 427
A.L.S. v. E.A.G. 414
A.Z. v. B.Z. 607; 612; 630, 631
Abbott v. Bragdon. 19, 20
Adoption of (see name of party) . . . .
Adoptions of B.L.V.B. and E.L.V.B. 487
Akron v. Akron Center for Reproductive Health.153;
726
Alexander v. Alexander 563
Alexandra S. v. Pacific Fertility Medical Center,.481
Allen v. Wright. 739
American Academy of Pediatrics v. Lungren. . .202
Anderson v. Liberty Lobby, Inc.. 272
Anna J. v. Mark C 424
Association of Data Processing Serv. Orgs. v.
Camp 739
Astrue v. Capato 559

B

Baby Girl, L.J., Matter of Adoption of 405
Baby M, In re 394; 397; 427, 428; 442; 457
Baird v. Eisenstadt. 106
Baird; Commonwealth v.. 106
Baker v. Carr. 739
Bartels; State v. 82
Becker v. Schwartz. 367, 368
Beeler v. Astrue 559
Bellotti v. Baird 160
Belsito v. Clark. 424; 443
Blessing v. Freestone 20
Block v. Rutherford 167
Board of Trustees of University of Alabama v.
Garrett 94
Bolger v. Youngs Drug Products Corp. 109
Bolling v. Sharpe. 110
Bowers v. Hardwick. 90
Bragdon v. Abbott 18; 252; 271; 276
Buck v. Bell. 88, 89; 92; 159
Building a Better Baby Business 667
Buzzanca, In re Marriage of . . . 464; 494; 504; 620
Byrn v. New York City Health & Hosps. Corp. . 595

C

C.M. v. C.C.. 479
C.O. v. W.S.. 478

California Family Bioethics Council v. California
Institute for Regenerative Medicine 770
Capato v. Comm'r of Soc. Sec. 559
Capitol Square Review and Advisory Bd. v.
Pinette 20
Carey v. Population Services International . 109; 152;
159
Castellano v. City of New York 275
City and County of (see name of city and county). .
City of (see name of city) . . . .
Cleveland Board of Education v. LaFleur. .160; 617
Coates v. City of Cincinnati. 727
Colautti v. Franklin. 727
Commonwealth v. (see name of defendant). . . . . .
County of (see name of county). . . . .
Crandall v. Woodard 650
Cruzan v. Director, Missouri Department of
Health. 90
Culliton v. Beth Israel Deaconess Medical
Center 426; 441; 556

D

D'Ambra v. United States 576
Dahl, In the Marriage of 598
Daniels v. Williams 124
Davis v. Berry 88; 155
Davis v. Carlson 167
Davis v. Davis . . . 60; 66; 154; 158; 577; 585; 594,
595; 607
Del Zio v. Columbia Presbyterian Hospital. . . .584
Doe v. Bolton. 112
Doe v. Doe 414; 617
Doe v. Kelley. 404
Doe v. Shalala 735
Doolan v. IVF America, Inc.. . . . . .675; 680
Doornbos v. Doornbos. 34

E

EEOC v. Staten Island Savings Bank 278
Egert v. Connecticut General Life Insurance
Company 25; 267
Eisenstadt v. Baird. . .106; 113, 114; 152; 159; 348;
456; 629; 831
Elisa B. v. Superior Court 493
Ex rel. (see name of relator). . . . .

[References are to pages]

F

Feilen; State v.. 88
Ferguson v. Estelle. 727
Ferguson v. McKiernan 384
Finley v. Astrue 557
Florida Dept. Children & Families v. Adoption of
     X.X.G. .488
Forbes v. Napolitano. 729
Ford v. Schering-Plough Corp. 278
Frisina v. Women & Infants Hosp. of R.I. 575

G

Gade   v.   National   Solid   Waste   Management
     Association 829
Gaines v. Canada 89
Gerber v. Hickman. 165; 171
Geroge, In re. 505
Gillett-Netting v. Barnhart. 559
Gonzales v. Carhart. 130
Goodridge v. Dep't Public Health. 476; 484
Goodwin v. Turner. 167, 168
Greenberg   v.   Miami   Children's   Hospital   Res.
     Inst.. 795
Griswold v. Connecticut . . 100; 113; 152; 155; 159,
                   160; 170; 354; 629
Griswold; State v.. 100
Gursky v. Gursky. 29; 372; 375

H

Hall v. Fertility Inst.. 525
Harper v. Wausau Ins. Co.. 200
Harris v. McRae 121
Hatch v. Riggs National Bank. 738
Hawkins v. Scituate Oil 578
Health and Human Services Policy for the Protection
     of Human Subjects Research. 731
Hecht v. Superior Court 69; 529; 552
Hernandez v. Coughlin. 167, 168
Hill v. National Collegiate Athletic Assn.. 202
Hodas v. Morin. 427
Huddleston v. Infertility Center of America. . . .423
Hudson v. McMillian. 168
Hudson v. Palmer 166

I

In re Adoption of (see name of party). . . . .
In re Estate of (see name of party) . . . .
In re Marriage of (see name of party). . . . .

In re (see name of party) . . . .
In the Interest of (see name of party). . . . .
In the Matter of (see name of party) . . . .
International Shoe Co. v. Washington. 157

J

J.B. v. M.B.. . . . . .607; 625; 630
J.F. v. D.B.. . . . . 425; 443; 472
J.R. v. Utah. 444; 453
Jacob v. Shultz-Jacob 482
Jacobson v. Massachusetts 93
Jane L. v. Bangerter 355
Janicki v. Hospital of St. Raphael 69
Janis, In re Estate of. 563
Jeter v. Mayo Clinic Arizona 583
Jhordan C. v. Mary K.. . . . . .379; 481
Johnson v. Calvert. . .415; 428; 440; 464; 466; 489;
               492; 495; 504; 508; 512; 636
Johnson v. Superior Court 196; 204

K

K.M. v. E.G.. 489
K.M.H. and K.C.H., In the Interest of 393
Karin T. v. Michael T.. 482
Karlin v. IVF Am., Inc.. 669
Kass v. Kass. 69; 591; 594; 607; 615; 631; 670
Kentucky Dep't of Corrs. v. Thompson. 167
Kerrigan v. Comm'r of Pub. Health. 476
Kesler v. Weniger 387
Khabbaz v. Commissioner. 557
Kievernagal, In re Estate of. 529
Kinzie   v.   Physician's   Liability   Insurance
     Company 25; 268
Kolacy, In re Estate of 546; 552
Krauel v. Iowa Methodist Medical Center . . 20; 271
Kristine H. v. Lisa R.. 496

L

L.A.L. v. D.A.L.. 480
The L Teaching Hospitals NHS v. Mr. A 516
Lamaritata v. Lucas 479
Laporta v. Wal-Mart Stores, Inc.. 280
Lawrence v. Texas. 90; 129
Lawton v. Steele. 83
Leonard F. v. Israel Discount Bank of New York.279
Lifchez v. Hartigan. 151
Litowitz v. Litowitz. 69; 164; 229; 604
Lockyer v. City and County of San Francisco . . 487

[References are to pages]

Lofton v. Secretary of Department of Children and
 Family Services, ... 488
Loving v. Virginia 114

M

Maher v. Roe 120, 121; 726
Mansfield v. Hyde 201
Marchetti v. Parsons 578
Margaret S. v. Edwards 355; 726; 846
Margaret S. v. Treen 727
Marriage Cases, In re 476; 487
Marriage of (see name of party) . . . .
Marsh v. Reserve Life Insurance Co. 267
Martin B, In re 557
Matter of Estate of (see name of party) . . . .
Matthew B.M., In re Adoption of 414
McDonald v. McDonald 471; 636
McDonald v. State Farm Fire & Cas. Co. 610
McFall v. Shimp 505
McGraw v. Sears Roebuck & Co. 277
McIntyre v. Crouch 479
McNulty v. McDowell. 682
Metropolitan Creditors Service v. Sadri 200
Meyer v. Nebraska 81; 101; 115; 155; 159
Meyer v. State 82
Miccolis v. Amica Mutual Insurance Co. 577
Michael H. v. Gerald D. 90
Mickle v. Henrichs 88
Miller v. Am. Infertility Group of Ill. 580
Miller v. Elliott 32
Monterey Plaza Hotel, Ltd. v. Local 483 166
Moore v. East Cleveland. 617
Moore   v.   Regents   of   the   University   of
 California 232; 795
Morgan v. Christman 675
Morris v. Hamilton. 650
Morrissey v. Brewer 167
Mugler v. Kansas. 124

N

NAACP v. Alabama 101
Nebraska District of Evangelical Lutheran Synod, etc.
 v. McKelvie et al. (Neb.) 83
New York, etc., Comr. of Public Welfare of City of v.
 Koehler. .30
North Coast Women's Care Medical Group, Inc. v.
 Superior Court. 256; 691
North Dakota, State of v. Coliton. 31

O

O. G. M., In the Interest of 634
Olmstead v. United States. 159
Oswego Laborers' Local 214 Pension Fund v. Marine
 Midland Bank, N. A. 672

P

Parentage of J.M.K. and D.R.K., In the Matter
 of 393
Paretta   v.   Med.   Offices   for   Human
 Reproduction 366; 683
Patsone v. Pennsylvania. 89
Payton v. Abbott Labs 681
Pell v. Procunier. 166
People v. (see name of defendant). . . . .
Perry-Rogers v. Fasano 510
Phillips v. United States. 681
Pierce v. Society of Sisters 101; 114; 160
Planned   Parenthood   of   Central   Missouri   v.
 Danforth. . . .128; 152; 155, 156; 160; 586; 620
Planned Parenthood of Southeastern Pennsylvania v.
 Casey. 90; 120; 123; 129; 354; 620
Poe v. Ullman 101
Poelker v. Doe 126
Pohl v. State. 82
Pope v. Moore 513
Prato-Morrison v. Doe 500; 508
Prince v. Massachusetts 114; 160
Principal Mutual Life Ins. Co. v. Vars, Pave, McCord
 & Freedman. 202

R

R.C., In the Interest of 479; 636
R.R. v. M.H. 409; 441; 617
Raftopol v. Ramey 415; 440
Rains v. Belsh 202
Re C.K.G, C.L.G & C.L.G. 376; 471
Reber v. Reiss 625
Reed v. Reed. 107
Regents of the University of California v. Bakke . 94
Reilly v. Blue Cross & Blue Shield United. . . .269
Reilly v. United States. 578
Reproductive Health Serv. v. Webster. 121
Reuss v. Time Insurance Co. 267
Robert B. v. Susan B. 506; 676
Roberto D. B., In re 425
Roberts v. United States Jaycees 167

[References are to pages]

Roe v. Casey. 739
Roe v. Wade. .66; 94; 112; 115; 120; 123; 125; 127; 152; 153; 155; 160; 354; 595; 738
Roman v. Roman. 598
Royster Guano Co. v. Virginia. 107

S

Saks v. Franklin Covey Co. 271; 280
Schafer v. Astrue. 559
Sharon S. v. Superior Court. 497
Sherley v. Sebelius. 764
Shin v. Kong. 384
Skinner v. Oklahoma. .87; 114; 159; 168; 354; 402; 455; 629; 832
Skinner v. State. 88
Smith v. Brown. 428
Smith v. Goguen 355; 727
Smith v. Organization of Foster Families for Equality and Reform. 455
Soos v. Superior Court in and for County of Maricopa. 439; 461
Sorensen; People v.. . . . . .373; 464
Stanley v. Illinois. 155; 455
State v. (see name of defendant). . . . .
State of (see name of state) . . . .
Stenberg v. Carhart. 130
Stephen K. v. Roni L. 468; 620
Stone v. Regents of University of California. . . .501
Stowe v. Davis. 594
Strnad v. Strnad 31; 33; 371; 372; 375
Surrogate Parenting Assocs. v. Commonwealth ex. rel. Armstrong. 405
Sutton v. United Air Lines. 25; 276
Syrkowski v. Appleyard 404; 405

T

T.M.H. v. D.M.T.. 497
Tammy, Adoption of. 483

Thornburgh v. American College of Obstetricians and Gynecologists. 63; 66; 122; 729
Toussaint v. McCarthy. 167
Turner v. Safley. 166–168; 170
Twigg v. Mays. 513

U

Union Pacific R. Co. v. Botsford 114
Valley Forge Christian College, v. 740

V

Varnum v. Brien 476, 477
Vernoff v. Astrue. 534
Viccaro v. Milunsky. 681

W

Walker v. Rinck 682
Washington v. Glucksberg. 90; 129; 835
Webster v. Reproductive Health Services . . .66, 67; 120; 126; 160
West v. Superior Court. 508
Williams v. Smith. 88
Winn v. Aleda Construction Co.. 651
Wisconsin v. Yoder. 160
Witcraft v. Sundstrand Health and Disability Group Benefit Plan. 267
Witten, Re Marriage of 633
Woodward v. Comm'r of Soc. Sec. 551

Y

Yick Wo v. Hopkins. 89
York v. Jones. 67; 154; 648

Z

Zablocki v. Redhail 94

INDEX

[References are to sections.]

A

ABORTION
Generally . . . 2[I][B][2]; 2[I][B][2][c]
Roe progeny . . . 2[I][B][2][b]
Roe v. Wade . . . 2[I][B][2][a]

ANIMAL CLONING (See CLONING, HUMAN REPRODUCTIVE, subhead: Animal cloning, advances in)

ART (See ASSISTED REPRODUCTIVE TECHNOLOGIES (ART))

ASSISTED CONCEPTION
Generally . . . 1[III]
ART (See ASSISTED REPRODUCTIVE TECHNOLOGIES (ART))
Conception in laboratory
    Advances in IVF . . . 1[III][B][2]
    Body, investigating possibility of conception outside . . . 1[III][B][1]
    Future of ART . . . 1[III][B][3]
    Glossary of ART terms . . . 1[III][B][3]
    Investigating possibility of conception outside body . . . 1[III][B][1]
Infertility (See HUMAN REPRODUCTION, subhead: Infertility)
In vitro fertilization (See subhead: Conception in laboratory)

ASSISTED REPRODUCTIVE TECHNOLOGIES (ART)
Business of (See BUSINESS OF ART)
Divorce and (See DIVORCE, ART AND)
Effectiveness of ART . . . 1[III][C][1]
Failures in ART medicine (See subhead: Successes and failures in ART medicine)
Family law issues in (See FAMILY LAW ISSUES IN ART)
Fundamental right, as
    Arguments against . . . 2[II][B]
    Arguments for . . . 2[II][A]
    Judicial perspectives on
        Generally . . . 2[II][C]
        Distinguishing natural conception and ART . . . 2[II][C][1]
        Equating natural conception and ART . . . 2[II][C][2]
Future of . . . 1[III][B][2]
Gender selection in (See CHILDREN'S TRAITS, CHOOSING)
Genetic selection in (See CHILDREN'S TRAITS, CHOOSING)
Glossary of ART terms . . . 1[III][B][3]
History of
    Generally . . . 1[III][A][1]
    Human artificial insemination . . . 1[III][A][2]
Human artificial insemination . . . 1[III][A][2]

ASSISTED REPRODUCTIVE TECHNOLOGIES (ART)—Cont.
Regulations (See REGULATING REPRODUCTIVE TECHNOLOGIES)
Safety in
    Adult . . . 1[III][C][2]; 1[III][C][2][b]
    Children . . . 1[III][C][2]; 1[III][C][2][a]
Successes and failures in ART medicine
    Adult, safety for . . . 1[III][C][2]; 1[III][C][2][b]
    Children, safety for . . . 1[III][C][2]; 1[III][C][2][a]
    Effectiveness of ART . . . 1[III][C][1]

B

BUSINESS OF ART
Benefits and burdens of
    Generally . . . 3[III]
    ART market, concept of open
        Age, exclusions based on . . . 3[III][B][1]
        Health status, exclusions based on . . . 3[III][B][2]
        Marital status, exclusions based on . . . 3[III][B][3]
        Sexual orientation, exclusions based on . . . 3[III][B][3]
    Sale of gametes, market ban for
        Gamete market, arguments in support of . . . 3[III][A][2]
        Market inalienability, arguments for . . . 3[III][A][1]
Burdens of, benefits and (See subhead: Benefits and burdens of)
Egg donations
    Generally . . . 3[II]; 3[II][B]
    Business of . . . 3[II][B][1]
    Ethics of . . . 3[II][B][2]
    Informed consent and
        Benefits . . . 3[II][B][3][a]
        Gamete placement, informing donors about . . . 3[II][B][3][b]
        Risks . . . 3[II][B][3][a]
Insuring (See INSURANCE OF ART SERVICES)
Reproductive technologies, understanding market for
    Fertility clinics as providers of ART services
        Patient's perspective . . . 3[I][A][1]
        Physician's perspective . . . 3[I][A][2]
    Profiles of ART clients . . . 3[I][B]
Sperm donations
    Generally . . . 3[II]; 3[II][A]
    Child's perspective . . . 3[II][A][1]
    Donor disclosure . . . 3[II][A][1]
    Pitfalls of sperm donation . . . 3[II][A][2]

[References are to sections.]

C

CHILDREN'S TRAITS, CHOOSING
Generally . . . Ch 4
Gender, choosing child's
    Generally . . . 4[I][A]
    Constitutional analysis surrounding gender selection . . . 4[III][A]
    Ethical debate surrounding gender selection . . . 4[III][B]
    Legal debate surrounding gender selection . . . 4[III][A]
    Postconception gender selection . . . 4[I][A][2]
    Preconception gender selection . . . 4[I][A][1]
Genetic make-up, choosing child's
    Generally . . . 4[I][B]
    Ethical dilemmas surrounding genetic selection . . . 4[IV][A]
    Legal dilemmas surrounding genetic selection . . . 4[IV][B]
    Preimplantation genetic diagnosis (See PREIMPLANTATION GENETIC DIAGNOSIS (PGD))
Law, current state of . . . 4[II]
Technology, current state of . . . 4[I]

CLONING, HUMAN REPRODUCTIVE
Generally . . . Ch 10
Animal cloning, advances in
    Generally . . . 10[I][B]
    Efficacy concerns . . . 10[I][B][1]
    Purposes of . . . 10[I][B][2]
    Safety concerns . . . 10[I][B][1]
Constitutional aspects of
    Generally . . . 10[III]
    Procreational autonomy, cloning and . . . 10[III][A]
    Right to scientific inquiry, cloning and . . . 10[III][B]
Embryo cloning . . . 10[I][A][3]
Politics of
    Federal government
        Initial reaction . . . 10[II][A]
        Later reaction . . . 10[II][B]
    Reactions from States . . . 10[II][C]
Procreational autonomy, cloning and . . . 10[III][A]
Reproductive cloning . . . 10[I][A][1]
Right to scientific inquiry, cloning and . . . 10[III][B]
Science of
    Generally . . . 10[I]
    Animal cloning (See subhead: Animal cloning, advances in)
    Inroads into human cloning . . . 10[I][C]
    Types of cloning (See subhead: Types of cloning)
Therapeutic cloning . . . 10[I][A][2]
Types of cloning
    Generally . . . 10[I][A]
    Embryo cloning . . . 10[I][A][3]
    Reproductive cloning . . . 10[I][A][1]
    Therapeutic cloning . . . 10[I][A][2]

CONCEPTION
Assisted (See ASSISTED CONCEPTION)
Methods of, natural and assisted (See HUMAN REPRODUCTION)
PGD to achieve . . . 4[I][B][3]

CONTRACEPTION, HUMAN
Emerging advances in . . . 2[I][B][1]

D

DIVORCE, ART AND
Generally . . . Ch 7
Abandoned embryos, problem of . . . 7[III]; 7[III][B]
Donation of embryos
    Another couple, to . . . 7[III][A][4]
    Research
        Prohibitions on research, state law . . . 7[III][A][1][b]
        Types . . . 7[III][A][1][a]
Embryo cryopreservation, popularity and frailty of . . . 7[I]
Excess embryos, problem of
    Generally . . . 7[III]
    Discarding embryos after designated time frame . . . 7[III][A][2]
    Donations (See subhead: Donation of embryos)
    Maintaining embryos in frozen storage . . . 7[III][A][3]
    Patient choice, excess embryos and . . . 7[III][A]
Legal landscape surrounding frozen embryo disputes
    Contract approach . . . 7[II][B]
    Davis v. Davis . . . 7[II][A]
    Parental rights, question of . . . 7[II][D]
    Public policy approach . . . 7[II][C]

DONATIONS
Egg (See BUSINESS OF ART, subhead: Egg donations)
Embryos (See DIVORCE, ART AND, subhead: Donation of embryos)
Sperm (See BUSINESS OF ART, subhead: Sperm donations)

E

EGGS
Donations (See BUSINESS OF ART, subhead: Egg donations)
Freezing . . . 6[I][B]

EMBRYO, HUMAN
Cloning . . . 10[I][A][3]
Freezing
    Generally . . . 6[I][C]
    Disputes over frozen embryos (See DIVORCE, ART AND)
Status and nature of (See HUMAN REPRODUCTION, subhead: Status of human embryo)

[References are to sections.]

F

FAMILY LAW ISSUES IN ART
Dilemmas in family law
    Changes in law . . . 5[I][B]
    Donors, problem of known . . . 5[I][C]
    Paternity in AID families, determining
      . . . 5[I][A]
    Problem of known donors . . . 5[I][C]
Donor gametes, building families through
    Generally . . . 5[III][A]
    State of law in donor gametes
        Judicial perspectives . . . 5[III][B][1]
        Statutory perspectives . . . 5[III][B][2]
Gamete mix-ups (See subhead: Laboratory, mishaps
  in)
Laboratory, mishaps in
    Generally . . . 5[V][A]
    Judicial perspectives on gamete mix-ups
        Malfeasance, case of physician
          . . . 5[V][B][1]
        Negligence, case of physician
          . . . 5[V][B][2]
    Legislative perspectives on gamete mix-ups
      . . . 5[V][C]
Same-sex relationships, building families in
    Generally . . . 5[IV]
    Paternity for same-sex parents, determining
      . . . 5[IV][B][1]
    Prevalence of same-sex parents . . . 5[IV][A]
Surrogate parenting agreements, building families
  through
    Distinguishing traditional and gestational sur-
      rogacy
        Generally . . . 5[II][B]
        Gestational surrogacy . . . 5[II][B][2]
        Traditional surrogacy . . . 5[II][B][1]
    In The Matter of Baby M . . . 5[II][A]
    Profiles in
        Generally . . . 5[II][B][3]
        Gestational surrogate mother
          . . . 5[II][B][3][b]
        Intended mother . . . 5[II][B][3][c]
        Traditional surrogate mother
          . . . 5[II][B][3][a]
    Statutory responses to
        Constitutionality of surrogacy laws
          . . . 5[II][C][2]
        Laws regulating surrogacy
          . . . 5[II][C][1]
        State laws regulating surrogacy
          . . . 5[II][C][1][a]
        Uniform laws regulating surrogacy
          . . . 5[II][C][1][b]

**FERTILITY CLINICS AS PROVIDERS OF ART
  SERVICES**
Patient's perspective . . . 3[I][A][1]
Physician's perspective . . . 3[I][A][2]

G

GAMETES
Donor, building families through (See FAMILY
  LAW ISSUES IN ART, subhead: Donor gametes,
  building families through)
Market ban for sale
    Arguments in support of . . . 3[III][A][2]
    Inalienability, arguments for market
      . . . 3[III][A][1]
Mix-ups (See FAMILY LAW ISSUES IN ART, sub-
  head: Laboratory, mishaps in)

GENDER SELECTION (See CHILDREN'S
  TRAITS, CHOOSING)

GENETIC SELECTION (See CHILDREN'S
  TRAITS, CHOOSING)

H

HUMAN ARTIFICIAL INSEMINATION
Generally . . . 1[III][A][2]

HUMAN EMBRYO (See HUMAN REPRODUC-
  TION, subhead: Status of human embryo)

**HUMAN EMBRYONIC STEM CELL RE-
  SEARCH**
Generally . . . Ch 9
Government funding of
    Generally . . . 9[III]
    Federal funding of stem cell research
        Bush administration policy, defending
          and questioning . . . 9[III][A][2]
        First Presidential Proclamation (August 9,
          2001) . . . 9[III][A][1]
        President Obama and new era of stem
          cell research policy . . . 9[III][A][3]
    State funding of stem cell research
        Generally . . . 9[III][B]; 9[III][B][3]
        California . . . 9[III][B][1]
        New Jersey . . . 9[III][B][2]
International and cross-cultural perspectives on stem
  cell research
    International perspectives . . . 9[IV][A]
    Religious perspectives . . . 9[IV][B]
Legal framework surrounding
    Generally . . . 9[II]
    Aborted fetuses as sources of stem cells, laws
      relating to
        Generally . . . 9[II][A]
        Federal law . . . 9[II][A][1]
        State laws . . . 9[II][A][2]
    Embryos as sources of stem cells, laws relating
      to
        Federal law . . . 9[II][B][1]
        State law . . . 9[II][B][2]
Science of
    Generally . . . 9[I][A]
    Animal stem cell studies, human and
      . . . 9[I][B]
    Debate over stem cell research . . . 9[I][C]

[References are to sections.]

HUMAN EMBRYONIC STEM CELL RESEARCH—Cont.
Science of—Cont.
    Human and animal stem cell studies . . . 9[I][B]

HUMAN REPRODUCTION
Assisted conception (See ASSISTED CONCEPTION)
Bragdon v. Abbott . . . 1[II][A]
Infertility
    Generally . . . 1[I][B]
    Causes of . . . 1[I][B][1]
    Incidence of . . . 1[I][B][2]
Judicial perspectives on modern role of reproduction . . . 1[II]
Natural conception
    Generally . . . 1[I][A]
    Distinguishing natural conception and ART . . . 2[II][C][1]
    Equating natural conception and ART . . . 2[II][C][2]
    Occurrence where natural conception does not happen (See subhead: Infertility)
Nature of human embryo (See subhead: Status of human embryo)
Status of human embryo . . . 1[IV]
    Biological status of human embryo . . . 1[IV][A]
    Legal status of human embryo
        Generally . . . 1[IV][B][1]
        Legal responses to . . . 1[IV][B][2]
    Moral status of human embryo . . . 1[IV][C]
Wonders of
    Generally . . . 1[I]
    Infertility (See subhead: Infertility)
    Natural conception (See subhead: Natural conception)

I

INSURANCE OF ART SERVICES
Effect on clinical outcomes . . . 3[IV][B]
Market landscape
    Infertility insurance coverage, status of
        Case law . . . 3[IV][A][1][b]
        Statutory law . . . 3[IV][A][1][a]
    Politics of ART insurance coverage . . . 3[IV][A][2]

IN VITRO FERTILIZATION (See Assisted Conception, subhead: Conception in laboratory)

L

LABORATORY
Conception (See ASSISTED CONCEPTION, subhead: Conception in laboratory)
Mishaps in (See FAMILY LAW ISSUES IN ART, subhead: Laboratory, mishaps in)

N

NATURAL CONCEPTION (See HUMAN REPRODUCTION, subhead: Natural conception)

P

PATERNITY
AID families, determination . . . 5[I][A]
Same-sex parents, determination . . . 5[IV][B][1]

PGD (See PREIMPLANTATION GENETIC DIAGNOSIS (PGD))

POSTMORTEM REPRODUCTION
Generally . . . Ch 6
Eggs, freezing . . . 6[I][B]
Embryos, freezing
    Generally . . . 6[I][C]
    Disputes over frozen embryos (See DIVORCE, ART AND)
Legal dilemmas in postmortem reproduction
    Death benefits, awarding . . . 6[II][B]
    Family law questions . . . 6[II][A]
    Inheritance rights, awarding . . . 6[II][B]
    Probate law . . . 6[II][B]
Possibilities for . . . 6[I]
Rights of postmortem conception children
    Generally . . . 6[III]
    Laws governing rights of posthumous children . . . 6[III][B]
    Model laws
        ABA Model Act . . . 6[III][C][1]
        New York state task force on life and law . . . 6[III][C][2]
    Task force reports
        ABA Model Act . . . 6[III][C][1]
        New York state task force on life and law . . . 6[III][C][2]
    Uniform laws governing postmortem reproduction
        Uniform Parentage Act . . . 6[III][A][1]
        Uniform Probate Code . . . 6[III][A][2]
Sperm, freezing
    Generally . . . 6[I][A][1][a]
    Legal disputes over frozen sperm . . . 6[I][A][1][b]
    Retrieval, sperm
        Death, after . . . 6[I][A][2]
        Life, during . . . 6[I][A][1]

PREGNANCY
Assisted (See ASSISTED CONCEPTION)
PGD to achieve . . . 4[I][B][3]

PREIMPLANTATION GENETIC DIAGNOSIS (PGD)
Avoid illness, to
    Generally . . . 4[I][B][2]
    Adult-onset diseases, PGD and . . . 4[I][B][2][b]
    Disability, PGD and meaning of . . . 4[I][B][2][a]
Cure illness, to . . . 4[I][B][1]

PREIMPLANTATION GENETIC DIAGNOSIS (PGD)—Cont.
Pregnancy, to achieve . . . 4[I][B][3]

PROCREATIONAL LIBERTY
Generally . . . Ch 2
Assisted reproduction as fundamental right (See AS-
   SISTED REPRODUCTIVE TECHNOLOGIES
   (ART))
Avoid procreation, right to
   Abortion (See ABORTION)
   Contraception, emerging advances in human
     . . . 2[I][B][1]
Constitution (See subhead: Traditional reproduction
   and constitution)
Reproduction as fundamental right, establishing
   Early cases . . . 2[I][A][1]
   State support for mandatory sterilization
     . . . 2[I][A][2]
   Sterilization, State support for mandatory
     . . . 2[I][A][2]
Traditional reproduction and Constitution
   Avoid procreation, right to
     Abortion (See ABORTION)
     Contraception, emerging advances in hu-
       man . . . 2[I][B][1]
   Reproduction as fundamental right establishing
     (See subhead: Reproduction as fundamental
     right, establishing)

R

**REGULATING REPRODUCTIVE TECHNOLO-
GIES**
Generally . . . Ch 8
Increased ART regulation, need for
   Generally . . . 8[II]
   Offspring, protecting ART . . . 8[II][B]
   Patients, protecting ART
     Generally . . . 8[II][A]
     Deceptive statements . . . 8[II][A][1]
     False advertising . . . 8[II][A][1]
     Fraud . . . 8[II][A][3]
     Lack of informed consent
       . . . 8[II][A][2]
     Luring patients . . . 8[II][A][1]
     Negligence . . . 8[II][A][3]
     Theft . . . 8[II][A][3]

**REGULATING REPRODUCTIVE
TECHNOLOGIES**—Cont.
Increased ART regulation, need for—Cont.
   Patients, protecting ART—Cont.
     Treatment errors . . . 8[II][A][3]
   Physicians, protecting ART
     Generally . . . 8[II][C]
     Public confidence, enhancing
       . . . 8[II][C][1]
     Treatment denials, authorizing
       . . . 8[II][C][2]
Legal landscape for ART
   Current state of regulation
     Generally . . . 8[I][B]
     Direct regulation . . . 8[I][B][1];
       8[I][B][3]
     Indirect regulation . . . 8[I][B][2];
       8[I][B][4]
     Self-regulation by fertility industry
       . . . 8[I][B][5]
   Goals of regulation . . . 8[I][A]
Proposed regulatory schemes . . . 8[III]

REPRODUCTION
Fundamental right of (See PROCREATIONAL LIB-
   ERTY)
Human reproductive cloning (See CLONING, HU-
   MAN REPRODUCTIVE)
Judicial perspectives on modern role of . . . 1[II]
Postmortem (See POSTMORTEM REPRODUC-
   TION)

S

SPERM
Donations (See BUSINESS OF ART, subhead:
   Sperm donations)
Freezing (See POSTMORTEM REPRODUCTION,
   subhead: Sperm, freezing)

**STEM CELL RESEARCH, HUMAN EMBRY-
ONIC** (See HUMAN EMBRYONIC STEM
CELL RESEARCH)

SURROGATE PARENTING AGREEMENTS
(See FAMILY LAW ISSUES IN ART, subhead:
   Surrogate parenting agreements, building families
   through)